Management of Severe Traumatic Brain Injury

AF694010

Terje Sundstrøm • Per-Olof Grände
Teemu Luoto • Christina Rosenlund
Johan Undén • Knut Gustav Wester
Editors

Management of Severe Traumatic Brain Injury

Evidence, Tricks, and Pitfalls

Second Edition

Springer

Editors
Terje Sundstrøm
Department of Neurosurgery
Haukeland University Hospital
Bergen
Norway

Department of Clinical Medicine
University of Bergen
Bergen
Norway

Teemu Luoto
Department of Neurosurgery
Tampere University Hospital
Tampere
Finland

Johan Undén
Department of Operation
and Intensive Care
Halmstad Hospital
Halmstad
Sweden

Per-Olof Grände
Department of Anaesthesia
and Intensive Care
Lund University Hospital
Lund
Sweden

Christina Rosenlund
Department of Neurosurgery
Odense University Hospital
Odense
Denmark

Knut Gustav Wester
Department of Clinical Medicine K1
University of Bergen
Bergen
Norway

ISBN 978-3-030-39385-4 ISBN 978-3-030-39383-0 (eBook)
https://doi.org/10.1007/978-3-030-39383-0

© Springer Nature Switzerland AG 2020
This work is subject to copyright. All rights are reserved by the Publisher, whether the whole or part of the material is concerned, specifically the rights of translation, reprinting, reuse of illustrations, recitation, broadcasting, reproduction on microfilms or in any other physical way, and transmission or information storage and retrieval, electronic adaptation, computer software, or by similar or dissimilar methodology now known or hereafter developed.
The use of general descriptive names, registered names, trademarks, service marks, etc. in this publication does not imply, even in the absence of a specific statement, that such names are exempt from the relevant protective laws and regulations and therefore free for general use.
The publisher, the authors, and the editors are safe to assume that the advice and information in this book are believed to be true and accurate at the date of publication. Neither the publisher nor the authors or the editors give a warranty, expressed or implied, with respect to the material contained herein or for any errors or omissions that may have been made. The publisher remains neutral with regard to jurisdictional claims in published maps and institutional affiliations.

This Springer imprint is published by the registered company Springer Nature Switzerland AG
The registered company address is: Gewerbestrasse 11, 6330 Cham, Switzerland

Foreword I

Traumatic brain injury (TBI) constitutes a vast global health problem, impacting over 50 million people worldwide each year and costing the global economy $400 million USD. TBI has been described as "the most complex disease in our most complex organ." We now recognize that it is a process, not an event. A disproportionate burden of death and disability exists in low- and middle-income countries (LMICs). Concerted efforts are required to address this global pandemic. Concerted efforts in the sense of both international collaborations and of interactions between basic neuroscience and clinical research.

This second edition of the textbook *Management of Severe Traumatic Brain Injury: Evidence, tricks, and pitfalls* constitutes an amazing concerted effort, bringing together contributions from world-leading experts, linking basic neuroscience to clinical research and practice, and presenting this in a very clear and educational format. The Scandinavian Neurotrauma Committee (SNC) deserves a huge compliment for this achievement. Importantly, this textbook also bridges the neurotrauma gap between high-income countries (HICs) and LMICs, true to the long-standing interest of Scandinavian neurosurgery in promoting educational activities in Africa. Over 90% of neurotrauma occur in LMICs, whilst over 90% of TBI publications originate from HICs. LMICs are severely underrepresented in TBI research. Surgery for neurotrauma represents more than 40% of neurosurgical procedures performed all over the world and more than 60% in developing areas of the world. Acquiring detailed knowledge of TBI, its pathophysiology and management, should thus be a priority for all neurosurgeons and neurosurgical trainees. This knowledge needs to extend far beyond a narrow focus on surgical management.

As past and current presidents of the Neurotrauma Committee of the World Federation of Neurosurgical Societies, we greatly welcome this new edition for its pragmatic approach, which will serve clinicians and researchers across the world. This book is relevant to basic scientists who wish to understand more about clinical dilemmas, to neurosurgical trainees across the world, and also to seasoned experts like ourselves who are sure to find something new!

The book should belong on the shelf of every neurosurgical department.

Edegem, Belgium Andrew I. R. Maas
Peshawar, Pakistan Tariq Khan

Foreword II

The book is the result of a carefully concerted venture from the most dedicated neurosurgeons, neurointensivists, neuroanaesthesiologists, trauma surgeons, neuroradiologists, rehabilitation physicians, and psychologist throughout Scandinavia working on traumatic brain injury (TBI). Together, and through the Scandinavian Neurotrauma Committee (SNC), they have described the current knowledge—and sometimes the lack thereof—in a structured and easily readable form. The book covers all topics from the epidemiology and organizational considerations of trauma management, via evidence-based treatment strategies and monitoring, to long-term follow-up and rehabilitation.

The first edition of this book was published in 2012. Although brain injury research is clearly under-financed, the field is making rapid progress. The SNC has published treatment guidelines for the management of minimal, mild, and moderate head injuries, paediatric injuries, and the prehospital management of severe TBI. This work has structured the treatment of these patients throughout, and beyond, Scandinavia. Importantly, it has also fostered a range of studies on implementation and follow-up of such guidelines, giving rise to further improvements—as well as this second edition *Management of severe traumatic brain injury: Evidence, tricks, and pitfalls*. Overall, the SNC is a great example on how a regional multinational effort can make an impact. The epidemiology of TBI is vastly different throughout the globe, but the underlying challenges on organization, clinical decision-making, prevention of secondary damage, and rehabilitation remain very similar.

This book covers the topic of severe head trauma in a well-written and pedagogical way. It is a "must read" for all residents in neuro- or trauma surgery, anaesthesiology, and intensive care medicine. It should also be an important resource to all seasoned clinicians for updated information. The layout of the book makes it a good everyday reference. This book should be found in any and all units dealing with trauma patients.

I am very proud of the work performed by the SNC, and I am sure that you will enjoy reading this book as much as I did.

Einar Osland Vik-Mo
The Scandinavian Neurosurgical
Society, Oslo, Norway

In Memoriam Bertil Romner

Bertil Romner was one of the founders and a leading member of the Scandinavian Neurotrauma Committee (SNC). He died of cancer when he was 59 years old in August 2013. He was trained as a neurosurgeon at the Department of Neurosurgery, Lund University Hospital, Sweden. He defended his Ph.D. thesis in 1991, became associate professor in 1994 and led the neurointensive care unit in Lund from 1996 to 2006. In 2006, he became professor of neurosurgery at the University Hospital of Copenhagen, Denmark. In 2010, he became professor of neurosurgery at the Lund University, Sweden. From 1999 to his death, he held a second professorship at the Arctic University of Norway in Tromsø, Norway.

Bertil will be remembered as an active scientist, supervisor, and inspirator. He was a popular speaker with tremendous scenic talent and had a huge network of collaborators and friends all over the world. He spent countless afternoons together with members of his "research family," and through his leadership he raised the bar for scientific and clinical excellence. He was internationally acclaimed for his contributions to neurosurgery and neurointensive care and published more than 150 articles. His main research field was transcranial Doppler measurement of blood flow and, in more recent years, noninvasive Doppler measurement of intracranial pressure. He also made seminal contributions on treatment of subarachnoid hemorrhage, low-pressure hydrocephalus, and clinical use of and research on brain biomarkers, such as S100B. Over the last years, his research was focused on management of head injuries. Notably, he spear-headed the development of Scandinavian guidelines for minimal, mild, and moderate head injuries published in 2013, including for the first time a biomarker as an alternative to CT in the diagnostic workup of head injuries. He was also the main organizer of several congresses in Lund on clinical and research applications for biomarkers.

"I'm on my way," Bertil often replied on the phone when he was late to a meeting. He was always on the move. He constantly initiated new projects and always participated with infectious enthusiasm. When matters became difficult, he always said: "It'll be solved" ("*Det löser sig*"). He was almost always right.

Bertil truly enjoyed life. He had a great sense of humor and a strong social competence. His warm personality and genuine consideration for others were clearly reflected with patients, relatives, colleagues, and neighbors. In spite of his disease, he refused to give up and kept on working full time as a professor, both in clinic and research. Before he died, he said "I have so much undone."

Through Bertil's death, we have lost a dear friend and a dedicated clinician and scientist. He has left a great void that is impossible to fill. We all really miss him and honor his memory.

On behalf of the SNC.

Lund, Sweden	Per-Olof Grände
Copenhagen, Denmark	Vagn Eskesen
Tromsø, Norway	Tor Ingebrigtsen

Scandinavian Neurotrauma Committee

The Scandinavian Neurotrauma Committee (SNC; www.neurotrauma.nu) was founded in 1998 after an initiative from the Scandinavian Neurosurgical Society. The committee comprises dedicated neurosurgeons, neurologists, intensivists, anaesthesiologists, radiologists, and paediatricians from Denmark, Finland, Norway, and Sweden (population 27 million, 22 neurosurgical centers). The SNC is independent of industry funding and members are supported by their respective institutions. The biannual Nordic Neurotrauma Conference is hosted by the SNC.

The major objective of the SNC is to improve the management of neurotrauma patients in the Nordic countries.

Members of the Scandinavian Neurotrauma Committee

Knut Gustav Wester (president)
Neurosurgeon
Bergen, Norway

Terje Sundstrøm
Neurosurgeon
Bergen, Norway

Mads Aarhus
Neurosurgeon
Oslo, Norway

Tor Brommeland
Neurosurgeon
Oslo, Norway

Anders Christian Feyling
Anaesthesiologist
Oslo, Norway

Kent Gøran Moen
Radiologist
Trondheim, Norway

Carsten Kock-Jensen
Neurosurgeon
Aarhus, Denmark

Bent Lob Dahl
Anaesthesiologist
Aarhus, Denmark

Stig Dyrskog
Anaesthesiologist
Aarhus, Denmark

Ramona Åstrand
Neurosurgeon
Copenhagen, Denmark

Christina Rosenlund
Neurosurgeon
Odense, Denmark

Olli Tenovuo
Neurologist
Turku, Finland

Teemu Luoto
Neurosurgeon
Tampere, Finland

Rahul Raj
Neurosurgeon
Helsinki, Finland

Bo-Michael Bellander
Neurosurgeon/Anaesthesiologist
Stockholm, Sweden

David Nelson
Anaesthesiologist
Stockholm, Sweden

Peter Reinstrup
Anaesthesiologist
Lund, Sweden

Johan Undén
Anaesthesiologist
Halmstad, Sweden

Per-Olof Grände
Anaesthesiologist
Lund, Sweden

Niklas Marklund
Neurosurgeon
Lund, Sweden

Zandra Olivecrona
Neurosurgeon
Örebro, Sweden

Johan Ljungqvist
Neurosurgeon
Gothenburg, Sweden

Olga Calcagnile
Paediatrician
Gothenburg, Sweden

Introduction

Traumatic brain injury (TBI) is an important public health problem. In Europe, TBI has been estimated to annually account for 82,000 deaths and 2.1 million hospital discharges (Majdan et al. 2016). Many survivors suffer long-term disabilities incurring significant personal and societal costs.

TBI incidence rates are increasing in elderly people, especially in high-income countries (HICs) (Roozenbeek et al. 2013). The situation in low- and middle-income countries (LMICs) is particularly concerning, with a significant increase in the number of TBIs coupled with substantial resource limitations, poorly developed trauma management systems, and lack of qualified medical personnel (Rubiano et al. 2015).

Many different TBI guidelines have been developed, all aiming to improve the quality of care in and between prehospital services, primary hospitals, neurosurgical departments, neurointensive care units, and rehabilitation facilities. The Brain Trauma Foundation (BTF; www.braintrauma.org) has been instrumental in this work. Their first evidence-based guidelines were published in 1995 and have been updated several times, most recently in 2017.

The Scandinavian Neurotrauma Committee (SNC) published their first guidelines for the management of minimal, mild, and moderate head injuries in adults in 2000 (Ingebrigtsen et al. 2000a, b; Romner et al. 2000a, b). These guidelines were extensively updated in 2013 (Undén et al. 2013), and separate paediatric guidelines were published in 2016 (Åstrand et al. 2016). In collaboration with the BTF, the SNC published guidelines for the prehospital management of severe traumatic head injury in 2008 (Bellander et al. 2008; Juul et al. 2008; Sollid et al. 2008).

The groundwork for the first edition of this book was started in 2007. The major goal was to create a comprehensive, yet practical, manual for severe TBI management throughout the entire chain of care. In this perspective, it was of significant importance to recruit recognized professionals from most centers in the Nordic countries, and from most of the involved specialties in neurotrauma care. The first edition—*Management of Severe Traumatic Brain Injury: Evidence, Tricks, and Pitfalls*—was published in 2012. It was a welcome addition to the TBI literature and has been actively used in many clinics to improve TBI management. Two years ago, in conjunction with the first Nordic Neurotrauma Conference, the SNC therefore decided to embark on the second edition.

The second edition is a major update on severe TBI. Most of the previous chapters have undergone substantial revisions and 24 new chapters have been added, reflecting both advances and key challenges within the field. The first edition included 59 authors from 36 departments at 19 hospitals or universities in 5 countries. Notably, almost all of the authors from the first edition have also contributed to this second edition, and more than 40 new authors have participated.

The authors performed literature searches, not only with reference to the BTF guidelines from 1995 and later revisions, but also within other areas of the medical field, which is reflected in the index of this book. Based upon the literature, clinical recommendations were made (influenced by grading systems such as the United States Preventive Services Task Force, the National Health Services (UK) Centre for Reviews and Dissemination, the Cochrane Collaboration and the GRADE guidelines (Guyatt et al. 2011)). In order to achieve a high degree of clinical practicality, the classifications were refined through an independent review process and consensus discussion in the SNC group.

Levels of recommendation:

- Level I recommendation: Based upon properly designed (prospective) randomized controlled trials (the gold standard of clinical practice).
- Level II recommendation: Prospectively collected data or retrospective analyses concerning relevant studies and based on clearly reliable data in well-defined populations. This includes prospective trials that did not meet the strict criteria for Level I recommendations, as well as non-randomized studies, observational studies, case-control studies, and cohort studies.
- Level III recommendation: Descriptive studies, consensus reports, and expert opinions.

Most of the provided recommendations are Level II or III. As a whole, the scientific foundation for management of severe TBI is extensive, but rarely grounded on high-quality evidence. These recommendation levels allow the reader to appreciate the scientific background behind the recommendation whilst also providing a practical and clinically useful message (in particular in the absence of high-quality evidence).

Each chapter has been given a standardized setup, with the exception of a few chapters where this approach was not practical. The reader is given initial *Recommendations*. An *Overview* gives a short summary of the relevant literature with emphasis on more recent studies, also including older, but important, research. A section with *Tips, Tricks, and Pitfalls* provides practical advice and expert views. The relevant literature is reviewed in the *Background* section. When applicable, a final section entitled *Specific Paediatric Concerns* is provided.

The SNC hope that this updated book will prove useful for those faced with the clinical and scientific problems of severely brain-injured patients.

The aim is to help establish a systematic and sustainable healthcare system, including all aspects of TBI, from injury to long-term recovery.

This book would not have been possible without the initiative and support from the SNC. We are grateful to all the authors for their enthusiasm and hard work. We would like to thank all the section editors for their consistency and imperative scientific input. We are also deeply indebted to all of the above affiliated institutions for financial support and facilitation. Finally, we would like to extend our sincerest appreciation to Springer International Publishing AG for their invaluable editorial assistance.

Terje Sundstrøm
Per-Olof Grände
Teemu Luoto
Christina Rosenlund
Johan Undén
Knut Gustav Wester

References

Åstrand R, Rosenlund C, Undén J. Scandinavian Neurotrauma Committee (SNC). Scandinavian guidelines for initial management of minor and moderate head trauma in children. BMC Med. 2016;14:33.

Bellander BM, Sollid S, Kock-Jensen C, Juul N, Eskesen V, Sundstrøm T, Wester K, Romner B. Prehospital management of patients with severe head injuries. Scandinavian guidelines according to Brain Trauma Foundation. Lakartidningen. 2008;105:1834–38.

Guyatt GH, Oxman AD, Schünemann HJ, Tugwell P, Knottnerus A. GRADE guidelines: a new series of articles in the Journal of Clinical Epidemiology. J Clin Epidemiol. 2011;64:380–2.

Ingebrigtsen T, Rise IR, Wester K, Romner B, Kock-Jensen C. Scandinavian guidelines for management of minimal, mild and moderate head injuries. Tidsskr Nor Laegeforen. 2000a;120:1985–90.

Ingebrigtsen T, Romner B, Kock-Jensen C. Scandinavian guidelines for initial management of minimal, mild, and moderate head injuries. J Trauma. 2000b;48:760–6.

Juul N, Sollid S, Sundstrøm T, Kock-Jensen C, Eskesen V, Bellander BM, Wester K, Romner B. Scandinavian guidelines on the pre-hospital management of traumatic brain injury. Ugeskr Laeger. 2008;170:2337–41.

Majdan M, Plancikova D, Brazinova A, Rusnak M, Nieboer D, Feigin V, Maas A. Epidemiology of traumatic brain injuries in Europe: a cross-sectional analysis. Lancet Public Health. 2016;1:e76–83.

Romner B, Ingebrigtsen T, Kock-Jensen C. Scandinavian guidelines for management of head injuries. Evidence-based management of minimal, mild and moderate head injuries. Ugeskr Laeger. 2000a;162:3839–45.

Romner B, Ingebrigtsen T, Kock-Jensen C. Scandinavian guidelines for management of head injuries. Evidence-based management of minimal, mild and moderate head injuries. Lakartidningen. 2000b;97:3186–92.

Roozenbeek B, Maas AI, Menon DK. Changing patterns in the epidemiology of traumatic brain injury. Nat Rev Neurol. 2013;9:231–6.

Rubiano AM, Carney N, Chesnut R, Puyana JC. Global neurotrauma research challenges and opportunities. Nature. 2015;527:S193–7.

Sollid S, Sundstrøm T, Kock-Jensen C, Juul N, Eskesen V, Bellander BM, Wester K, Romner B. Scandinavian guidelines for prehospital management of severe traumatic brain injury. Tidsskr Nor Laegeforen. 2008;128:1524–7.

Undén J, Ingebrigtsen T, Romner B, Scandinavian Neurotrauma Committee (SNC). Scandinavian guidelines for initial management of minimal, mild and moderate head injuries in adults: an evidence and consensus-based update. BMC Med. 2013;11:50.

Contents

Part IV Admission, Diagnostics and Planning

Part V Acute Surgical Treatment

Part X Outcome and Prognosis

Part XI Research in Severe TBI

Contributors

Catherine Aaro Jonsson Child and Youth Rehabilitation, Östersunds Hospital, Östersund, Sweden

Nada Andelic Department of Physical Medicine and Rehabilitation, Oslo University Hospital Ullevål, Oslo, Norway

Research Centre for Habilitation and Rehabilitation Models and Services, Faculty of Medicine, Institute of Health and Society, University of Oslo, Oslo, Norway

Ramona Åstrand Department of Neurosurgery, Rigshospitalet, Copenhagen University Hospital, Copenhagen, Denmark

Aniko Bartfai Division of Rehabilitation Medicine, Department of Clinical Sciences, Danderyd Hospital, Karolinska Institute, Stockholm, Sweden

Bo-Michael Bellander Department of Clinical Neuroscience, Karolinska Institutet, Stockholm, Sweden

Department of Neurosurgery, Karolinska University Hospital, Stockholm, Sweden

Jan-Erik Berdal Infectious Diseases Department, Akershus University Hospital, Nordbyhagen, Norway

Eric L. Bloomfield Department of Anesthesiology, Mayo Clinic, Rochester, MN, USA

Tor Brommeland Department of Neurosurgery, Oslo University Hospital Rikshospitalet, Oslo, Norway

Department of Neurosurgery, Oslo University Hospital Ullevål, Oslo, Norway

Olga Calcagnile Department of Paediatric Medicine, Halland Regional Hospital, Halmstad, Sweden

Aqeel Chaudhry Department of Neurosurgery, Haukeland Trauma Center, Haukeland University Hospital, Bergen, Norway

Bent Lob Dahl Department of Anesthesia and Intensive Care, Silkeborg Regional Hospital, Silkeborg, Denmark

Geir Olav Dahle Department of Anaesthesia and Intensive Care, Haukeland University Hospital, Bergen, Norway

Bram Johan de Hoog Department of Anaesthesia and Intensive Care, Haukeland University Hospital, Bergen, Norway

Erik Edström Department of Clinical Neuroscience, Karolinska Institute, Stockholm, Sweden

Department of Neurosurgery, Karolinska University Hospital, Stockholm, Sweden

Per Enblad Section of Neurosurgery, Department of Neuroscience/ Neurosurgery, Uppsala University Hospital, Uppsala University, Uppsala, Sweden

Martin Engström Department of Health Care, Region Halland, Halmstad, Sweden

Vagn Eskesen University Clinic of Neurosurgery, Copenhagen University Hospital, Copenhagen, Denmark

Ulla Feldt-Rasmussen Department of Medical Endocrinology, Copenhagen University Hospital, Copenhagen, Denmark

Vibeke Fink-Jensen Department of Neuroradiology, Aarhus University Hospital, Aarhus, Denmark

Alexander Fletcher-Sandersjöö Department of Neurosurgery, Karolinska University Hospital, Solna, Sweden

Jon Axel Forsse Department of Neurosurgery, Odense University Hospital, Odense, Denmark

Jan Frennström Department of Neurosurgery, Skåne University Hospital, Lund, Sweden

Kristian Dahl Friesgaard Department of Anesthesiology and Intensive Care, Aarhus University Hospital, Aarhus, Denmark

Christine Gaarder Department of Traumatology, Oslo University Hospital Ullevål, Oslo, Norway

Faculty of Medicine, University of Oslo, Oslo, Norway

Thomas Geisner Department of Vascular Surgery, Haukeland Trauma Center, Haukeland University Hospital, Bergen, Norway

Mads Gilbert The Clinic of Emergency Medicine, University Hospital of North Norway, Tromsø, Norway

The Anaesthesia and Critical Care Research Group, Institute of Clinical Medicine, The Arctic University of Norway, Tromsø, Norway

Alison K. Godbolt University Department of Rehabilitation Medicine, and Department of Clinical Sciences, Karolinska Institute, Danderyd Hospital, Stockholm, Sweden

Per-Olof Grände Department of Anaesthesia and Intensive Care, Lund University and Lund University Hospital, Lund, Sweden

Anne Berit Guttormsen Department of Anaesthesia and Intensive Care, Haukeland University Hospital, Bergen, Norway

Department of Clinical Medicine, University of Bergen, Bergen, Norway

Nikolaj Preus Hatting Department of Neuroanesthesiology and Neurointensive Care, Odense University Hospital, Odense, Denmark

Christian A. Helland Department of Neurosurgery, Haukeland University Hospital, Bergen, Norway

Department of Clinical Medicine, University of Bergen, Bergen, Norway

Eirik Helseth Institute of Clinical Medicine, University of Oslo, Oslo, Norway

Department of Neurosurgery, Oslo University Hospital, Oslo, Norway

Ann Hermansson ENT Department, University Hospital, Lund, Sweden

Department of Otorhinolaryngology, Lund University Hospital, Lund, Sweden

Jennie Witte Hernæs Eating Disorders Unit, Skaraborgs Hospital, Skövde, Sweden

Lars Hillered Department of Neuroscience, Neurosurgery, Uppsala University, Uppsala, Sweden

Tim Howells Department of Neuroscience, Neurosurgery, Uppsala University, Uppsala, Sweden

Tor Ingebrigtsen Department of Clinical Medicine, Faculty of Health Sciences, UiT the Arctic University of Norway, Tromsø, Norway

Department of Neurosurgery, Ophthalmology and ENT, University Hospital of North Norway, Tromsø, Norway

Daniel Isacson Department of Plastic and Maxillofacial Surgery, Uppsala University Hospital, Uppsala, Sweden

Birger Johnsen Department of Clinical Neurophysiology, Aarhus University Hospital, Aarhus, Denmark

Niels Juul Department of Anaesthesia, Aarhus University Hospital, Aarhus, Denmark

Tariq Khan Department of Neurosurgery, Northwest School of Medicine, Peshawar, Pakistan

Svein Kleiven Division of Neuronic Engineering, KTH Royal Institute of Technology, Huddinge, Sweden

Marianne Klose Department of Medical Endocrinology, Copenhagen University Hospital, Copenhagen, Denmark

Jens Aage Kølsen-Petersen Department of Anaesthesia, Aarhus University Hospital, Aarhus, Denmark

Salla Koponen Department of Psychiatry, Hospital District of Helsinki and Uusimaa, Helsinki, Finland

Lars-Owe D. Koskinen Department of Clinical Science-Neurosciences/ Neurosurgery, Umeå University and Umeå University Hospital, Umeå, Sweden

Ingela Kristiansen Department of Women's and Children's Health, Uppsala University and Uppsala University Childrens' Hospital, Uppsala, Sweden

Tsegazeab Laeke Department of Clinical Medicine, University of Bergen, Bergen, Norway

Department of Neurosurgery, Addis Ababa University, Addis Ababa, Ethiopia

Christian Sigvald Langfrits Department of Anesthesia and Intensive Care, Aalborg University Hospital, Aalborg, Denmark

Hege Linnerud Department of Neurosurgery, Oslo University Hospital Ullevål, Oslo, Norway

Johan Ljungqvist Department of Neurosurgery, Sahlgrenska University Hospital, Gothenburg, Sweden

Institute of Neuroscience and Physiology, Sahlgrenska Academy University of Gothenburg, Gothenburg, Sweden

Pia Löwhagen Hendén Department of Anesthesiology and Intensive Care, Sahlgrenska University Hospital, Gothenburg, Sweden

Morten Lund-Johansen Department of Clinical Medicine, University of Bergen, Bergen, Norway

Department of Neurosurgery, Haukeland University Hospital, Bergen, Norway

Teemu Luoto Department of Neurosurgery, Tampere University Hospital and Tampere University, Tampere, Finland

Andrew I. R. Maas Department of Neurosurgery, Antwerp University Hospital and University of Antwerp, Edegem, Belgium

Marek Majdan Department of Public Health, Faculty of Health Sciences and Social Work, Trnava University, Trnava, Slovak Republic

Niklas Marklund Department of Clinical Sciences Lund, Neurosurgery, Lund University, Skåne University Hospital, Lund, Sweden

David K. Menon Division of Anaesthesia, University of Cambridge, Cambridge, UK

Neurosciences Critical Care Unit, Addenbrooke's Hospital, Cambridge, UK

Ronni Mikkelsen Department of Neuroradiology, Aarhus University Hospital, Aarhus, Denmark

Department of Biomedicine, Aarhus University, Aarhus, Denmark

Kent Gøran Moen Faculty of Medicine and Health Sciences, Department of Neuromedicine and Movement Science, Norwegian University of Science and Technology (NTNU), Trondheim, Norway

Department of Radiology, Nord-Trøndelag Hospital Trust, Levanger Hospital, Levanger, Norway

Jens Kjølseth Møller Department of Clinical Microbiology, Vejle Hospital, Vejle, Denmark

Kirsten Møller Department of Neuroanaesthesiology, The Neuroscience Centre, Rigshospitalet, University of Copenhagen, Copenhagen, Denmark

Department of Clinical Medicine, University of Copenhagen, Copenhagen, Denmark

Pål Aksel Næss Department of Traumatology, Oslo University Hospital Ullevål, Oslo, Norway

Faculty of Medicine, University of Oslo, Oslo, Norway

David W. Nelson Department of Physiology and Pharmacology, Section of Perioperative Medicine and Intensive Care, Karolinska Institutet, Stockholm, Sweden

Rasmus Philip Nielsen Department of Anaesthesiology, Regional Hospital West Jutland, Herning, Denmark

Troels Halfeld Nielsen Department of Neurosurgery, Odense University Hospital, Odense, Denmark

Carl-Henrik Nordström Department of Neurosurgery, Odense University Hospital, Odense, Denmark

Daniel Nowinski Department of Plastic and Maxillofacial Surgery, Uppsala University Hospital, Uppsala, Sweden

Department of Surgical Sciences, Plastic Surgery, Uppsala University, Uppsala, Sweden

Magnus Olivecrona Department of Medical Sciences, Faculty of Medicine, Örebro University, Örebro, Sweden

Section for Neurosurgery, Department of Anaesthesia and Intensive Care, University Hospital, Örebro, Sweden

Zandra Olivecrona Department of Medical Sciences, Faculty of Medicine, Örebro University, Örebro, Sweden

Section for Neurosurgery, Department of Anaesthesia and Intensive Care, University Hospital, Örebro, Sweden

Jussi P. Posti Clinical Neurosciences, Department of Neurosurgery and Turku Brain Injury Centre, Turku University Hospital and University of Turku, Turku, Finland

Christian Rahbek Department of Neuroradiology, Aarhus University Hospital, Aarhus, Denmark

Mads Rasmussen Department of Anaesthesia and Intensive Care, Section of Neuroanaesthesia, Aarhus University Hospital, Aarhus, Denmark

Peter Reinstrup Department of Intensive and Perioperative Care, Skånes University Hospital, Lund, Sweden

Department of Anaesthesia and Intensive Care, Lund University and Lund University Hospital, Lund, Sweden

Jens Jakob Riis Department of Neurosurgery, Aalborg University Hospital, Aalborg, Denmark

Elisabeth Ronne-Engström Department of Neuroscience, Neurosurgery, Uppsala University, Uppsala, Sweden

Pål A. Rønning Department of Neurosurgery, Oslo University Hospital, Oslo, Norway

Christina Rosenlund Department of Neurosurgery, Odense University Hospital, Odense, Denmark

Elham Rostami Department of Neurosurgery, Uppsala University Hospital, Uppsala, Sweden

Department of Neuroscience, Karolinska Institutet, Stockholm, Sweden

Thoralph Ruge Department of Emergency and Internal Medicine, Skåne University Hospital, Lund, Sweden

Department of Internal Medicine, Skåne University Hospital, Lund, Sweden

Department of Clinical Sciences, Lund University, Malmö, Sweden

Malin Rundgren Neurointensive Care Unit, Department of Intensive and Preoperative Care, Skåne University Hospital, Lund, Sweden

Department of Clinical Sciences, Anesthesiology and Intensive Care Medicine, Skåne University Hospital, Lund University, Lund, Sweden

Ulrika Sandvik Department of Clinical Neuroscience, Karolinska Institute, Stockholm, Sweden

Department of Neurosurgery, Karolinska University Hospital, Stockholm, Sweden

Ulf Schott Department of Anaesthesia and Intensive Care, Institution of Clinical Sciences, Lund University, Lund, Sweden

Rico Frederik Schou Department of Neuroanesthesia and Neurocritical Care, Odense University Hospital, Odense, Denmark

Section of Neuroanesthesia and Neurointensive Care, Department of Anesthesia and Intensive Care Medicine, Odense University Hospital, Odense, Denmark

Solrun Sigurdardottir Department of Research, Sunnaas Rehabilitation Hospital, Bjørnemyr, Norway

Toril Skandsen Faculty of Medicine and Health Sciences, Department of Neuromedicine and Movement Science, Norwegian University of Science and Technology (NTNU), Trondheim, Norway

Department of Physical Medicine and Rehabilitation, St. Olav's Hospital, Trondheim University Hospital, Trondheim, Norway

Steinar Skrede Department of Medicine, Section of Infectious Diseases, Haukeland University Hospital, Bergen, Bergen, Norway

Leif Hovgaard Sørensen Department of Neuroradiology, Aarhus University Hospital, Aarhus, Denmark

Jacob Bertram Springborg Department of Neurosurgery, University Clinic of Neurosurgery, Copenhagen University Hospital, Copenhagen, Denmark

Morten Zebitz Steiness Spine Section, Department of Neurosurgery, Aalborg University Hospital, Aalborg, Denmark

Terje Sundstrøm Department of Neurosurgery, Haukeland University Hospital, Bergen, Norway

Department of Clinical Medicine, University of Bergen, Bergen, Norway

Riikka Takala Perioperative Services, Intensive Care Medicine and Pain Management, Turku University Hospital, Turku, Finland

Olli Tenovuo Turku Brain Injury Centre, Turku University Hospital, Turku, Finland

Department of Clinical Medicine, University of Turku, Turku, Finland

Department of Clinical Medicine, Turku Brain Injury Centre, Turku University Hospital, University of Turku, Turku, Finland

Eric Peter Thelin Department of Clinical Neuroscience, Karolinska Institutet, Stockholm, Sweden

Division of Neurosurgery, Department of Clinical Neurosciences, University of Cambridge, Cambridge, UK

Johan Undén Department of Anaesthesia and Intensive Care, Hallands Hospital, Halmstad, Sweden

Department of Operation and Intensive Care, Hallands Hospital, Halmstad, Sweden

Lund University, Lund, Sweden

Arne Einar Vaaler Department of Mental Health, Norwegian University of Science and Technology (NTNU), Trondheim, Norway

Eirik Vikane Department of Physical Medicine and Rehabilitation, Haukeland University Hospital, Bergen, Norway

Anne Vik Department of Neuromedicine and Movement Science, Norwegian University of Science and Technology (NTNU), Trondheim, Norway

Department of Neurosurgery, St. Olav's Hospital, Trondheim University Hospital, Trondheim, Norway

Einar Osland Vik-Mo Department of Neurosurgery, Oslo University Hospital Rikshospitalet, Oslo, Norway

Karen-Lise Kobberø Welling Neurointensive Care Unit, Section 6021, Department of Neuroanaesthesiology, The Neuroscience Centre, Rigshospitalet, University of Copenhagen, Copenhagen, Denmark

Knut Gustav Wester Department of Clinical Medicine K1, University of Bergen, Bergen, Norway

Part I

Traumatic Brain Injury as a Public Health Problem

Olli Tenovuo

1 Epidemiological Aspects

Marek Majdan, Tor Ingebrigtsen, and Olli Tenovuo

1.1 Introduction

Injuries are a significant cause of disability and death. Based on the estimations of the Global Burden of Diseases study (GBD), in 2013 globally 973 million people sustained an injury requiring medical attention and about 4.8 million died from an injury (Haagsma et al. 2016). TBIs are among the most severe injuries. In the European Union (EU), estimated 2.5 million people sustain a TBI annually (Maas et al. 2017), of which about 1.5 million people are admitted to hospital, and 57,000 people die (Majdan et al. 2016).

M. Majdan (✉)
Department of Public Health, Faculty of Health Sciences and Social Work, Trnava University, Trnava, Slovak Republic
e-mail: mmajdan@truni.sk

T. Ingebrigtsen
Department of Clinical Medicine, Faculty of Health Sciences, UiT the Arctic University of Norway, Tromsø, Norway

Department of Neurosurgery, Ophthalmology and ENT, University Hospital of North Norway, Tromsø, Norway
e-mail: tor.ingebrigtsen@unn.no

O. Tenovuo
Turku Brain Injury Centre, Turku University Hospital, Turku, Finland

Department of Clinical Medicine, University of Turku, Turku, Finland

Epidemiological data are key for influencing the occurrence and outcome of any disease. They provide data on how often diseases occur, what their causes are, which populations are at highest risk, and the impacts on the level of individuals and populations.

Valid epidemiological data on TBI are not yet sufficient, but both the quality and quantity of available information have improved over the past decades. Three systematic reviews have summarized epidemiological data on TBI for Europe (Brazinova et al. 2018; Peeters et al. 2015; Tagliaferri et al. 2006). The most recent study (Brazinova et al. 2018) identified 84 methodologically valid studies presenting data on regional or national level.

It should be noted that systematic reviews synthesize data from epidemiological studies with substantial differences in study population, case ascertainment procedures, study period, and other aspects. This potentially causes bias and complicates pooled estimates. Some of these limitations can be overcome by using uniform case ascertainment procedures and a common study period, and by overseeing or validating the data collection. Examples of such practices are surveillance systems, such as the one implemented in the US (Taylor et al. 2017), trauma registries, or studies using uniform data for their analyses (Majdan et al. 2016, 2017).

Incidence, prevalence, mortality, and case fatality rates are all traditional epidemiological

© Springer Nature Switzerland AG 2020
T. Sundstrøm et al. (eds.), *Management of Severe Traumatic Brain Injury*,
https://doi.org/10.1007/978-3-030-39383-0_1

indicators used to describe the occurrence and outcome of diseases and injuries. They provide excellent data on the number of occurring and existing cases, but are not able to fully capture the impact of a disease in its full width, especially in case of heterogenic conditions as TBI. Therefore, modern indicators providing more detailed information about the true burden to individuals and populations are increasingly used. Among these are years of lost life (YLL), years lived with disability (YLD), disability adjusted life years (DALY), and healthy life expectancy (HALE). These indicators were introduced and used for example in the GBD study (GBD 2017 DALYs and HALE Collaborators 2018). Table 1.1 provides an overview of all these indicators and their use.

When estimating epidemiological patterns of TBI, case ascertainment is of key importance. While studies on hospital cohorts of patients with TBI have their limitations in terms of generalizability, they usually provide a good opportunity to define and characterize TBI in detail. On the other hand, studies relying on administratively collected data using ICD definitions (such as databases of causes of deaths or hospital discharges) provide a convenient way to compare epidemiological characteristics over time, or between populations of different countries. The disadvantage is that investigators do not have the possibility to validate the given diagnosis and therefore have to rely on the coding provided. This may cause biased results. A number of studies using administratively collected data use the ICD definition of head injuries to describe TBI epidemiology (Majdan et al. 2016, 2017; Brazinova et al. 2018; Mauritz et al. 2014). Although some of the minor head injuries do not include a TBI, the similarities in the incidence of TBI-related hospital discharges estimated using data from hospital cohorts (Brazinova et al. 2018; Peeters et al. 2015; Tagliaferri et al. 2006) and administrative sources (Majdan et al. 2016) suggest that ICD-10 head injury codes provide a reasonable estimate of hospital discharges due to TBI. In fact, in multiple investigations, ICD

Table 1.1 Indicators of occurrence, outcome, and burden used to describe the epidemiological patterns and impact of TBI in populations

Measure	How to calculate	What it expresses
Incidence rate	The number of new cases in a given time period divided by the total population from which they are drawn	A measure of the risk of developing some new condition within a specific period of time
Prevalence rate	The total number of persons with the observed condition (old and new cases) divided by the total population from which they are drawn	A measure of how common a condition is within a population at a certain time
Mortality rate	The number of persons dying from the condition per unit time (e.g. year) divided by the total population from which they are drawn	A measure of the number of deaths in a population, scaled to the size of the population within a specific period of time
Case fatality rate	The number of persons dying from the condition per unit time (e.g. year) divided by the total number of persons in the population with the same condition	A measure of the ratio of deaths within a designated population of people with a particular condition over a certain period of time
Years of life lost (YLL)	Reference age (life expectancy in the population) minus age of death = years of life lost	A measure of potential years of life lost. The reference age corresponds to the life expectancy of the population, commonly set at age 75
Years lived with disability (YLD)	Reference age minus age of onset of condition/disease = YLD	A measure of the years lived with the impact of disability
Disability-adjusted life year (DALY)	YLL + YLD = DALY	A measure of overall disease burden, expressed as the number of years lost due to ill health, disability or early death

Adopted from Management of Severe Traumatic Brain Injury—Evidence, Tricks and Pitfalls (Sundstrom et al. 2012*)*

codes have been shown to underestimate the incidence of TBI (Barker-Collo et al. 2016; Deb 1999; Shore et al. 2005).

1.2 Causes

In general, road traffic accidents (RTAs) and falls are the two major external causes of injury leading to TBI (Maas et al. 2017; Majdan et al. 2016; Brazinova et al. 2018; Peeters et al. 2015; Tagliaferri et al. 2006). Previously, RTAs were the most important cause. In recent years, a decline in the number of road traffic accidents and ageing of the population has caused a transition in the relative proportions of RTAs and falls as causes for TBI in high-income countries (Roozenbeek et al. 2013). The Nordic countries have a zero-vision for traffic deaths, and this goal has been approached for several months in a row in some regions (https://www.ssb.no/en/transport-og-reiseliv/statistikker/vtu). Falls are indeed nowadays the dominant cause in many countries (Maas et al. 2017). Based on data extracted from death certificates, falls were the predominant cause of fatal TBI in Europe in 2012, followed by RTAs, suicides, and violence (Majdan et al. 2016; Brazinova et al. 2018; Peeters et al. 2015). The causes of non-fatal TBI can be estimated from hospital cohorts, registry-based studies, or surveillance data, and they display a similar pattern: falls are predominant, followed by RTAs (Brazinova et al. 2018; Peeters et al. 2015; Tagliaferri et al. 2006).

1.3 Incidence

The reported incidence of TBI varies widely in published studies. In Europe, it ranges from 47 to 694 new cases per 100,000 people per year (Brazinova et al. 2018). Much of this variation is probably caused by differences in study designs or case ascertainment. Two summary estimates of TBI incidence for Europe were recently published (Majdan et al. 2016; Brazinova et al. 2018), and they are close to each other; 262 and 287.2 per 100,000 people per year, respectively. The former estimate is based on a meta-analysis of incidences from published studies (including hospital cohorts and studies using administrative data and the broader definition of head injuries) (Peeters et al. 2015) and the latter on hospital records from a single year from 25 European countries (using the broader definition of head injuries based on ICD-10) (Majdan et al. 2016). An estimate of the relative proportion of the head vs. brain injuries suggested that about 56% of all head injuries treated as inpatient were also intracranial injuries (Majdan et al. 2016). Capturing TBI in the whole range of its severity can lead to incidences, which are substantially higher; for example, a community-based study in New Zealand about TBIs of all severities resulted in 790 cases of TBI per 100,000 person years (Feigin et al. 2013).

1.4 Mortality and Case Fatality

Deaths as a consequence of TBI are usually reported using two different indicators: case fatality rates indicate the proportion of fatal cases of all TBI cases per unit of space and time, and mortality indicates the number of cases relative to the overall population.

Most studies of hospital cohorts report case fatalities, and these vary widely based on the characteristics of the cohort: in a systematic review, they ranged from 1 to 60%, with recent studies on TBI of all severities reporting 16–25% and those based on cohorts of severe TBI reporting about 50% (Brazinova et al. 2018). With increasing age, case fatality rates increase: a meta-analysis of TBI cases in those over 60 years of age showed a rate of 57% (McIntyre et al. 2013).

The close correlation with age is apparent in mortality rates as well. Based on data from death certificates, the proportion of persons 65 years or older among deaths due to TBI was 55%, and in females as high as 68% (Majdan et al. 2016). Mortality also varies from study to study and between countries, although not to a degree observed in case of incidences: in a systematic review, mortality ranged from 6 to 12 per 100,000 population (Brazinova et al. 2018), and in an analysis of death certificate data from 25 European countries, between 2.8 and 20.3 per 100,000 (Majdan et al. 2016). The pooled mortality rate in Europe has been estimated to 11.7 cases per 100,000 people, and TBIs caused 37% of injury deaths in Europe (Majdan et al. 2016). An important aspect of mortality after a TBI is the time after injury at which the death occurs. Usually, deaths in the ICU, before hospital discharge and by 6 months post injury are reported in the literature. The time of survival after the injury in general has implications for the burden and cost of TBI to society. This is dealt with in other parts of this book in greater detail.

1.5 The Burden of TBI and Global Aspects

The epidemiology of TBI is increasingly being studied using modern indicators of the burden of disease. A recent study from New Zealand estimated that 20,300 DALYs can be attributed to TBI in New Zealand (Te Ao et al. 2015), while a study from the Netherlands estimated 171,200 TBI-related DALYs (Scholten et al. 2014). A study based on detailed data on causes of death from 16 European countries estimated that about 17,000 TBI-related deaths resulted in about 375,000 YLLs, which translates to about 259 TBI-related YLLs per 100,000 people, or to about 24.3 years of lost life per TBI death (Majdan et al. 2017). For the year 2016, the burden of TBI is estimated on a global scale within the GBD study, but due to limitations of causes of death data, it is restricted to YLDs, resulting in 8.1 million YLDs (GBD 2016 Traumatic Brain Injury and Spinal Cord Injury Collaborators 2019).

Greatly contributing to the global occurrence of TBI are developing countries with growing economies, where road traffic is increasing rapidly while authorities are not able to keep up with preventive and control measures. It is estimated that one TBI death occurs in India every 3 min, and annually about one million people become disabled due to TBI, of which 60–70% are caused by RTAs (Maas et al. 2017). Similarly in China, RTAs are the main cause of TBI, accounting for about 54% of cases (Maas et al. 2017). The age-adjusted TBI mortality rate increased from 13 in 2003 to 17 per 100,000 population in 2008 (Cheng et al. 2017). In the USA, each year about 2.5 million are admitted to EDs, hospitalized, or die due to TBI, as estimated in 2010 by the CDC (Taylor et al. 2017). There is a massive lack of information from low- and middle-income countries where the incidence, mortality, and general burden is presumably much higher than in Europe and the USA.

Disease prevalence is the most appropriate indicator for assessing the need for care and continuous health services. In case of TBI, the information on prevalence (e.g. the number of people alive with a sequelae after TBI at a point in time) is very limited. Those few estimates that are available are mostly based on self-report surveys and may thus be biased. A systematic review summarized the available findings and reported lifetime history of TBI in about 12% of the interviewed persons, 17% in males and 9% in females (Frost et al. 2013). A more precise estimation was derived from a Swedish birth cohort where 9.1% of the cohort members sustained a TBI before the age of 25 years, but the percentage of those with permanent symptoms was not studied (Sariaslan et al. 2016). Another approach of estimating the prevalence is mathematical modelling. With this approach, the prevalence in the general population of New Zealand was calculated at 13% (11.4% in females and 14.8% in males) (Te Ao et al. 2015). On the global scale, the prevalence has been modelled in the GBD study, where the global prevalence of TBI was estimated at 55.5 million cases (GBD 2016 Traumatic Brain Injury and Spinal Cord Injury Collaborators 2019).

References

Barker-Collo S, Theadom A, Jones K, Feigin VL, Kahan M. Accuracy of an international classification of diseases code surveillance system in the identification of traumatic brain injury. Neuroepidemiology. 2016;47(1):46–52.

Brazinova A, Rehorcikova V, Taylor MS, Buckova V, Majdan M, Psota M, et al. Epidemiology of traumatic brain injury in Europe: a living systematic review. J Neurotrauma. 2018. [Epub ahead of print].

Cheng P, Yin P, Ning P, Wang L, Cheng X, Liu Y, et al. Trends in traumatic brain injury mortality in China, 2006-2013: a population-based longitudinal study. PLoS Med. 2017;14(7):e1002332.

Deb S. ICD-10 codes detect only a proportion of all head injury admissions. Brain Inj. 1999;13(5):369–73.

Feigin VL, Theadom A, Barker-Collo S, Starkey NJ, McPherson K, Kahan M, et al. Incidence of traumatic brain injury in New Zealand: a population-based study. Lancet Neurol. 2013;12(1):53–64.

Frost RB, Farrer TJ, Primosch M, Hedges DW. Prevalence of traumatic brain injury in the general adult population: a meta-analysis. Neuroepidemiology. 2013;40(3):154–9.

GBD 2016 Traumatic Brain Injury and Spinal Cord Injury Collaborators. Global, regional, and national burden of traumatic brain injury and spinal cord injury, 1990-2016: a systematic analysis for the Global Burden of Disease Study 2016. Lancet Neurol. 2019;18(1):56–87.

GBD 2017 DALYs and HALE Collaborators. Global, regional, and national disability-adjusted life-years (DALYs) for 359 diseases and injuries and healthy life expectancy (HALE) for 195 countries and territories, 1990-2017: a systematic analysis for the Global Burden of Disease Study 2017. Lancet. 2018;392(10159):1859–922.

Haagsma JA, Graetz N, Bolliger I, Naghavi M, Higashi H, Mullany EC, et al. The global burden of injury: incidence, mortality, disability-adjusted life years and time trends from the global burden of disease study 2013. Inj Prev. 2016;22(1):3–18.

Maas AIR, Menon DK, Adelson PD, Andelic N, Bell MJ, Belli A, et al. Traumatic brain injury: integrated approaches to improve prevention, clinical care, and research. Lancet Neurol. 2017;16(12):987–1048.

Majdan M, Plancikova D, Brazinova A, Rusnak M, Nieboer D, Feigin V, et al. Epidemiology of traumatic brain injuries in Europe: a cross-sectional analysis. Lancet Public Health. 2016;1(2):e76–83.

Majdan M, Plancikova D, Maas A, Polinder S, Feigin V, Theadom A, et al. Years of life lost due to traumatic brain injury in Europe: a cross-sectional analysis of 16 countries. PLoS Med. 2017;14(7):e1002331.

Mauritz W, Brazinova A, Majdan M, Leitgeb J. Epidemiology of traumatic brain injury in Austria. Wien Klin Wochenschr. 2014;126(1–2):42–52.

McIntyre A, Mehta S, Aubut J, Dijkers M, Teasell RW. Mortality among older adults after a traumatic brain injury: a meta-analysis. Brain Inj. 2013;27(1):31–40.

Peeters W, van den Brande R, Polinder S, Brazinova A, Steyerberg EW, Lingsma HF, et al. Epidemiology of traumatic brain injury in Europe. Acta Neurochir. 2015;157(10):1683–96.

Roozenbeek B, Maas AI, Menon DK. Changing patterns in the epidemiology of traumatic brain injury. Nat Rev Neurol. 2013;9(4):231–6.

Sariaslan A, Sharp DJ, D'Onofrio BM, Larsson H, Fazel S. Long-term outcomes associated with traumatic brain injury in childhood and adolescence: a Nationwide Swedish cohort study of a wide range of medical and social outcomes. PLoS Med. 2016;13(8):e1002103.

Scholten AC, Haagsma JA, Panneman MJ, van Beeck EF, Polinder S. Traumatic brain injury in the Netherlands: incidence, costs and disability-adjusted life years. PLoS One. 2014;9(10):e110905.

Shore AD, McCarthy ML, Serpi T, Gertner M. Validity of administrative data for characterizing traumatic brain injury-related hospitalizations. Brain Inj. 2005;19(8):613–21.

Sundstrom T, Grände P-O, Juul N, Kock-Jensen C, Romner B, Wester KG. Management of severe traumatic brain injury—evidence, tricks, and pitfalls. Berlin: Springer; 2012.

Tagliaferri F, Compagnone C, Korsic M, Servadei F, Kraus J. A systematic review of brain injury epidemiology in Europe. Acta Neurochir. 2006;148(3):255–68; discussion 68.

Taylor CA, Bell JM, Breiding MJ, Xu L. Traumatic brain injury-related emergency department visits, hospitalizations, and deaths—United States, 2007 and 2013. MMWR Surveill Summ. 2017;66(9):1–16.

Te Ao B, Tobias M, Ameratunga S, McPherson K, Theadom A, Dowell A, et al. Burden of traumatic brain injury in New Zealand: incidence, prevalence and disability-adjusted life years. Neuroepidemiology. 2015;44(4):255–61.

Challenges in Low- and Middle-Income Countries

2

Tsegazeab Laeke, Knut Gustav Wester, Morten Lund-Johansen, and Terje Sundstrøm

2.1 Overview

According to data from the World Health Organization (WHO), trauma causes more deaths than tuberculosis, HIV and malaria combined (World Health Organization 2014). It accounts for 15% of the burden of death and disability worldwide, and this is expected to rise to 20% by the year 2020 (WHO 1996). Trauma has now been recognized as a significant public health burden in LMICs (Nordberg 2000). In a recent global survey, trauma accounted for 12% of all deaths in LMICs, compared to 6% in HICs (Norton and Kobusingye 2013), and nearly 90% of all trauma-related deaths in the world occur in LMICs (Hofman et al. 2005). Poor safety measures within road traffic as well as within professional and domestic life lead to a manifold increase in the frequency of injuries compared to HICs.

The leading causes of injuries worldwide include road traffic accidents (RTAs), falls and violence. Injury mechanisms differ geographically. RTAs contributed to 30–86% of all trauma admissions in LMICs (Odero et al. 1997) and are projected to be the fifth leading cause of death worldwide (WHO 2008). Interpersonal violence is also found to be one of the commonest injury mechanisms in some LMICs (Seedat et al. 2009). Fall from heights in young construction workers is a common mechanism encountered in LMICs, where occupational safety is poorly implemented.

Neurotrauma is the most common cause of permanent disability, causing the highest loss of disability-adjusted life years (DALYs) (Rubiano et al. 2015). TBI causes half of all trauma-related deaths, and the number of victims is increasing at an alarming rate. The WHO has therefore predicted TBI to be the third leading cause of death in the world in 2030 (WHO 2015; Mathers and Loncar 2006). TBI, along with stroke, constitutes nearly 60% of the causes of death related to brain disorders (Dewan et al. 2018). Sixty percent of all head injuries are due to RTAs in LMICs, and mortality and disability from TBIs are higher in LMICs. Cost of care and treatment for patients with severe TBI are big challenges for families and caretakers in resource-limited settings, given

T. Laeke (✉)
Department of Clinical Medicine, University of Bergen, Bergen, Norway

Department of Neurosurgery, Addis Ababa University, Addis Ababa, Ethiopia

K. G. Wester
Department of Clinical Medicine, University of Bergen, Bergen, Norway
e-mail: Knut.Wester@uib.no

M. Lund-Johansen · T. Sundstrøm
Department of Clinical Medicine, University of Bergen, Bergen, Norway

Department of Neurosurgery, Haukeland University Hospital, Bergen, Norway
e-mail: mljo@helse-bergen.no; tjsu@helse-bergen.no

© Springer Nature Switzerland AG 2020
T. Sundstrøm et al. (eds.), *Management of Severe Traumatic Brain Injury*,
https://doi.org/10.1007/978-3-030-39383-0_2

the high expenses incurred and prolonged recovery time for the patients.

Despite alarming figures drawn from available data, there is no centralized database to exactly quantify trauma deaths in LMICs. This shortage poses a challenge when quantifying the problem, and hence, it becomes difficult to propose preventive and tailored treatment guidelines (Dewan et al. 2018). It is believed that this absence of structured neurotrauma registries leads to an underestimation of the true burden of TBIs (Rubiano et al. 2015).

Treatment of severe TBI in LMICs is characterized by significant resource limitations, poorly developed trauma management systems and lack of qualified medical personnel.

2.2 Prehospital Care

Prehospital care is at its early stage in most LMICs (Meskere et al. 2015). Incidental witnesses to the accident or patient relatives often bring trauma victims to the hospital. According to a study from Ethiopia, only 10% of hospital-admitted TBI patients were transported by ambulance from the accident site (Laeke et al. 2019). Ambulances are rarely staffed with medically trained personnel, and they lack appropriate life support equipment. Inadequate care at the accident scene and during transport may lead to impaired outcome due to secondary brain injuries, and hospitals giving trauma care are usually far away. Patients therefore have to be transported for a long time with inadequate care before arriving at the hospital. This leads to poor survival rates. In conclusion, suboptimal prehospital care and long transportation time both play a significant role for poor patient outcomes.

2.3 In-hospital Care

The Lancet Commission report documents a significant lack of surgical care worldwide. Reports show that about 74% of all surgeries globally were performed in HICs, which comprise only one third of the world's population. Neurosurgical care is particularly needed in many parts of the world (Servadei et al. 2018), and dedicated trauma centres fully equipped to treat severely injured patients are lacking. Most centres in LMICs lack clinical protocols for TBI and organized trauma teams (Newgard et al. 2015).

Most patients with TBI have no access to basic neurosurgical care, mainly due to lack of infrastructure and treatment costs (Park et al. 2016). Very few hospitals, if any, are adequately equipped to treat these patients in most of the resource-limited setups, and they are often inaccessible in a timely manner because of very long distances and poor transportation facilities. Hence, patients get neurosurgical care late and at an advanced stage of their condition; this makes the management and treatment challenging (Punchak et al. 2018).

Surgical infrastructure to give emergency care is severely compromised. Reports show that as many as 65% of 231 district hospitals in 12 Sub-Saharan countries lack continuous supply of electricity, and oxygen supplies are only available in 40% of surgical hospitals in East Africa (8 MDG 2015). These limitations can have detrimental consequences for patients with severe TBI.

CT scanners are not necessarily easily available, and there is a paucity of intensive care unit (ICU) beds. Facilities such as mechanical ventilators and equipment for arterial blood gas analysis are scarce, if at all present. Thus, in-hospital limitations force physicians to improvise and to do hard prioritizations based on salvageability.

2.4 Clinical Protocols and Guidelines

Most treatment guidelines on the management of severe TBI are based on evidence generated from HICs with affluent resources (Rubiano et al. 2015). They do not take into account the challenges with regard to both infrastructure and human resources that are faced in LMICs. This has made it difficult to directly transfer advanced treatment guidelines into resource-limited settings (Gosselin 2009). Moreover, there are very few studies on TBI management and outcome from LMICs (Sitsapesan et al. 2013). Notably, only 4.3% of all surgical research papers come from LMICs. This poses a challenge when trying to tailor the surgical management based on locally generated evidence.

2.5 Lack of Specialty Care

Neurotrauma care in LMICs is also characterized by a large deficiency of human resources. The ratio of neurosurgeons in the population is 1 per 6.4 million in Sub-Saharan Africa as compared to 1 per 62,500 in the United States (El Khamlichi 2014). In a recent study, Dewan et al. estimated the global deficit in neurosurgical care to be 5.2 million cases per year, of which Southeast Asia and Africa take the lion's share with 2.5 and 1.8 million unaddressed neurosurgical cases, respectively (Dewan et al. 2018). The huge manpower deficiency has made optimal neurosurgical care very difficult.

Patients succumb before getting the appropriate neurosurgical expertise. Neurotrauma care is often provided by non-neurosurgeons in an attempt to salvage life before patients are referred to hospitals where neurosurgical care can be given. Trained ICU doctors and nurses are also scarce.

2.6 Lack of Rehabilitation Care

Rehabilitation care is less developed in LMICs. Patients with severe TBI will usually be sent home directly after treatment of acute neurotrauma. Rehabilitation mainly relies on family members who are trained a few days in the hospital while visiting patients. Follow-up of patients is challenging due to a general lack of infrastructure in the community; lack of postal addresses and changing mobile telephone numbers are only a few of the factors that may hamper follow-up and consequently result in poor patient outcomes (Sitsapesan et al. 2013).

2.7 Interventions to Strengthen and Improve Care

2.7.1 Education and Training

Locally tailored training programs in neurosurgery have been developed in several LMICs. The Ethiopian neurosurgical training program has shown that this strategy has a significant impact by increasing the number of neurosurgeons in the country (Lund-Johansen et al. 2017). The quality of care is significantly increased with more timely and efficient treatment, especially as neurosurgical services are developed at district hospitals. Improved patient follow-up is a key element. Only 20–30% of patients are currently followed after treatment (Araki et al. 2017). Efforts are ongoing to train healthcare providers at district hospitals in monitoring patients for complications, diagnosing conditions that need further neurosurgical care, referring patients and registering data in centralized registry systems.

2.7.2 Research

Studies on the management of neurotrauma from LMICs are unfortunately underrepresented in the international literature relative to the scale of the problem. This is important, as different regions have their own needs and obstacles; neurotrauma research and management need to be contextualized. It is not possible to directly transfer cost demanding, evidence-based guidelines from Western counties to LMICs, which lack the necessary finances, equipment and human resources (Rubiano et al. 2015; Laeke et al. 2019; Lund-Johansen et al. 2017). Thus, there is a great need for more and better data on epidemiological aspects, in-hospital care and patient follow-up to facilitate development of locally tailored guidelines, to improve the quality of care provided and to identify region-specific focus areas for preventive efforts. A key issue for further development of neurosurgical training programs is to stimulate more research and formal research training (e.g. PhD), particularly within the most prevalent disease conditions.

2.8 Specific Paediatric Aspects

TBI affects more than three million children worldwide every year (WHO 2008; CDC 2015). In comparison, two million children are diagnosed with HIV and 500,000 with meningitis. The frequency of trauma deaths in children in LMICs is more than twice that of HICs (Dewan et al. 2016). In a Nigerian 12-year retrospective analysis of paediatric trauma deaths, TBI was the most common injury (Newgard et al. 2015).

Falls and RTAs are the most common causes of paediatric TBI in LMICs (Dewan et al. 2016). Children injured in RTAs are more likely to be pedestrians in LMICs as compared to vehicle occupants in HICs (Dewan et al. 2016). Many children in LMICs work from a very young age without proper safety precautions, and children are often unattended, predisposing them to unintentional injuries.

Children and adults with TBI in LMICs face many of the same challenges when it comes to prehospital care, hospital treatment and rehabilitation (Dewan et al. 2016; Fink et al. 2018). Very few centres are actually capable of treating severe paediatric TBI patients. Management of children with TBI remains basic and focused on initial care at healthcare facilities when comprehensive care is needed. Inter-hospital transport is relatively frequent and associated with a significant treatment delay and a negative impact on outcome (Newgard et al. 2015; Fink et al. 2018).

Educational and research efforts are needed to support the development of tailored diagnostic and treatment protocols for children with TBI in LMICs (Fink et al. 2018).

References

8 MDG. MDG Gap Task Force Report 2015. Taking stock of the global partnership for development. 2015.

Araki T, Yokota H, Morita A. Pediatric traumatic brain injury: characteristic features, diagnosis, and management. Neurol Med Chir. 2017;57(2):82–93.

CDC—Overview. GHAa. 2015. www.cdc.govglobalaids/resources.

Dewan MC, Mummareddy N, Wellons JC 3rd, Bonfield CM. Epidemiology of global pediatric traumatic brain injury: qualitative review. World Neurosurg. 2016;91:497–509.e1.

Dewan MC, Rattani A, Fieggen G, Arraez MA, Servadei F, Boop FA, et al. Global neurosurgery: the current capacity and deficit in the provision of essential neurosurgical care. Executive summary of the global neurosurgery initiative at the program in global surgery and social change. J Neurosurg. 2018:1–10.

El Khamlichi A. The World Federation of Neurosurgical Societies Rabat Reference Center for training African neurosurgeons: an experience worthy of duplication. World Neurosurg. 2014;81(2):234–9.

Fink EL, von Saint Andre-von Arnim A, Kumar R, Wilson PT, Bacha T, Tirsit A, Laeke T. Traumatic brain injury and infectious encephalopathy in children from four resource-limited settings in Africa. Pediatr Crit Care Med. 2018;19(7):649–57.

Gosselin R. The increasing burden of injuries in developing countries. Direct and indirect consequences. Tech Orthop. 2009;24:230–2.

Hofman K, Primack A, Keusch G, Hrynkow S. Addressing the growing burden of trauma and injury in low- and middle-income countries. Am J Public Health. 2005;95(1):13–7.

Laeke T, Tirsit A, Debebe F, Girma B, Gere D, Park KB, et al. Profile of head injuries: pre hospital care, diagnosis and severity in an Ethiopian tertiary hospital. World Neurosurg. 2019;127:e186–92.

Lund-Johansen M, Laeke T, Tirsit A, Munie T, Abebe M, Sahlu A, et al. An Ethiopian training program in neurosurgery with Norwegian support. World Neurosurg. 2017;99:403–8.

Mathers CD, Loncar D. Projections of global mortality and burden of disease from 2002 to 2030. PLoS Med. 2006;3:e442.

Meskere Y, Dinberu MT, Azazh A. Patterns and determinants of pre-hospital care among trauma patients treated in Tikur Anbessa Specialized Hospital, Emergency Department. Ethiop Med J. 2015;53(3):141–9.

Newgard CD, Meier EN, Bulger EM, Buick J, Sheehan K, Lin S, et al. Revisiting the "golden hour": an evaluation of out-of-hospital time in shock and traumatic brain injury. Ann Emerg Med. 2015;66(1):30–41, 41.e1–3.

Nordberg E. Injuries as a public health problem in sub-Saharan Africa: epidemiology and prospects for control. East Afr Med J. 2000;77(12 Suppl):S1–43.

Norton R, Kobusingye O. Injuries. N Engl J Med. 2013;368(18):1723–30.

Odero W, Garner P, Zwi A. Road traffic injuries in developing countries: a comprehensive review of epidemiological studies. Trop Med Int Health. 1997;2(5):445–60.

Park KB, Johnson WD, Dempsey RJ. Global neurosurgery: the unmet need. World Neurosurg. 2016;88:32–5.

Punchak M, Mukhopadhyay S, Sachdev S, Hung YC, Peeters S, Rattani A, et al. Neurosurgical care: availability and access in low-income and middle-income countries. World Neurosurg. 2018;112:e240–e54.

Rubiano AM, Carney N, Chesnut R, Puyana JC. Global neurotrauma research challenges and opportunities. Nature. 2015;527(7578):S193–7.

Seedat M, Van Niekerk A, Jewkes R, Suffla S, Ratele K. Violence and injuries in South Africa: prioritising an agenda for prevention. Lancet. 2009;374(9694):1011–22.

Servadei F, Rossini Z, Nicolosi F, Morselli C, Park KB. The role of neurosurgery in countries with limited facilities: facts and challenges. World Neurosurg. 2018;112:315–21.

Sitsapesan HA, Lawrence TP, Sweasey C, Wester K. Neurotrauma outside the high-income setting: a review of audit and data-collection strategies. World Neurosurg. 2013;79(3–4):568–75.

WHO. The global burden of disease. In: World Health Organization Bulletin; 1996.

WHO. The global burden of disease: 2004 update. 2008.

WHO. Global status report on road safety 2015. 2015.

World Health Organization. Injuries and violence: the facts. Geneva: WHO; 2014. https://www.who.int/healthinfo/global_burden_disease/en/.

3 Challenges in the Elderly

Teemu Luoto and Thoralph Ruge

Tips, Tricks and Pitfalls

- The most common cause of TBI in elderly are ground-level falls and not high energy impacts such as motor vehicle accidents as in younger patients.
- Early suspicion of an underlying TBI event may be essential for a favorable outcome in elderly patients.
- The clinical signs of acute TBI in elderly patients may initially be masked, mimicked or magnified due to age-related issues such as brain atrophy and general functional impairment.
- Pre-injury health problems worsen the prognosis of TBI in elderly patients, however prior health issues do not disqualify for further treatment.
- Chronological age and TBI severity alone are insufficient to predict outcome, instead management should be based on biological age, pre-injury health and functional capacity.
- Evidence-based treatment guidelines of geriatric TBI are lacking.

3.1 Overview

The number of elderly TBI patients is growing rapidly, especially in high-income countries (Gardner et al. 2018; Harvey and Close 2012). Elderly patients with TBI experience both a higher mortality and pre- and post-injury morbidity compared to younger patients (Brazinova et al. 2015; Kumar et al. 2018). In contrast to younger patients, elderly patients also have a different injury mechanism profile. The majority of elderly TBIs are sustained in low-energy impacts, especially ground-level falls (Brazinova et al. 2018). Younger patients are more prone to high-energy injuries, with motor vehicle accidents being the major cause of severe TBI. Women are more affected in higher ages than men (Gardner et al. 2018).

In relation to geriatric TBI, there is a clear lack of evidence-based guidelines. Major barriers

T. Luoto (✉)
Department of Neurosurgery, Tampere University Hospital and Tampere University, Tampere, Finland
e-mail: teemu.luoto@pshp.fi

T. Ruge
Department of Emergency and Internal Medicine, Skåne University Hospital, Lund, Sweden

Department of Internal Medicine, Skåne University Hospital, Lund, Sweden

Department of Clinical Sciences, Lund University, Malmö, Sweden
e-mail: thoralph.ruge@med.lu.se

© Springer Nature Switzerland AG 2020
T. Sundstrøm et al. (eds.), *Management of Severe Traumatic Brain Injury*,
https://doi.org/10.1007/978-3-030-39383-0_3

in the management of geriatric TBI include under-representation of older adults in TBI research, lack of systematic measurement of pre-injury health and lack of geriatric-specific TBI common data elements (Gardner et al. 2018). In elderly patients, pre-injury health may be a better predictor of outcome and response to treatment than age and TBI severity. Without proper guidelines and evidence-based guidance, the management of severe geriatric TBI is challenging. Clinicians are frequently faced with difficult ethical decisions on how to treat this growing and challenging patient population. Neurointensive (Dang et al. 2015) and neurosurgical care (De Bonis et al. 2011) and also rehabilitation require complex medical judgement. Pursuing active treatment can be futile and inhumane. On the other hand, decision-making on treatment withholding and withdrawing can be excruciating while proper guidelines and prognostic models are missing, and pessimistic prognosis becomes easily a self-fulfilling prophecy (Robertsen et al. 2017; McCredie et al. 2016).

3.2 Pre-injury Health

Pre-injury health problems are extremely common among patients with geriatric TBI and become more abundant with ageing. Cardiovascular, respiratory, metabolic, neurological and psychiatric conditions are all common comorbidities. Additionally, a substantial number of elderly patients have a history of earlier TBI (Hamill et al. 2015). Chronic medical conditions are usually accompanied by multiple medications (Catapano et al. 2017). Along with diseases and polypharmacy, many older adults suffer from frailty. Frail individuals have impaired adaptability to stressors such as acute illness or trauma. This increased vulnerability contributes to higher risk for diverse adverse outcomes (Joseph et al. 2017; Chen et al. 2014). Pre-injury comorbidity, polypharmacy, frailty and functional dependence are associated with worse outcome post-trauma (Evans et al. 2012; Joseph et al. 2014) and are also risk factors for sustaining a TBI (Dams-O'Connor et al. 2013).

3.3 Management

Acute management of geriatric TBI is challenged by pre-injury conditions, medication side effects and lack of proper information on prior functioning. Moreover, medication history can be unreliably attainable. Clinical assessment may inadequately capture the true burden of acute TBI. For example, age-related brain atrophy can allow an extra-axial hematoma to expand substantially before resulting in clinical signs or symptoms of TBI. Elderly patients have a higher incidence of CT-detectable traumatic lesion compared to younger patients; subdural hematomas being the most frequent TBI lesions among elderly. Hypothetically, this increased risk is multifactorial: age-related changes in vasculature and white matter, which render vessels more vulnerable to rupture and white matter tracts more susceptible to shear injury; weakened musculature in the neck and trunk; pre-existing conditions and medications such as antithrombotics (Gardner et al. 2018). Furthermore, acute evaluation of TBI-related mental, physical and cognitive alterations can be mimicked or masked by pre-injury illnesses or deficits.

There is a huge lack of evidence on neurosurgical and neurocritical management of geriatric TBI (Gardner et al. 2018). A few recent observational, largely retrospective studies have assessed the value of various acute neurosurgical interventions, including intracranial pressure (ICP) monitoring (Dang et al. 2015; You et al. 2016), craniotomy (Kinoshita et al. 2016) and decompressive craniectomy (De Bonis et al. 2011; Kinoshita et al. 2016) in older adults with moderate to severe TBI. However, these studies may be limited/confounded by indication and other potential sources of bias, such as the physician's opinion of a patient's prognosis, which may impact treatment decisions (Gardner et al. 2018). No generalizable evidence is available to guide clinicians in relation to neurosurgical and neurocritical management of geriatric TBI.

It is generally thought that older patients have less potential for rehabilitation than younger individuals due to prior functional deficits, limited cognitive capability and physiological receptiveness.

However, there is substantial evidence that intensive inpatient rehabilitation greatly benefits also older adults with TBI (Uomoto 2008). Geriatric severe TBI is less studied in the context of long-term rehabilitation. Patients with geriatric TBI with different injury severities have shown to gain functional independence after rehabilitation (Yap and Chua 2008; Graham et al. 2010). Limited rehabilitation resources often force to prioritize long-term treatment to younger individuals. Nevertheless, age should not be used as a main denominator for rehabilitation suitability. On the contrary, overall evaluation that takes into account a wide range of pre-injury factors (e.g., health, frailty, functional impairment, realistic rehabilitation goals) should be applied.

Prognostication in TBI is difficult, and the existing prediction models can explain only approximately 35% of the variance in outcome in populations with severe and moderate TBI (Maas et al. 2015). Withholding and withdrawing decision on life-sustaining therapies are mainly based on a poor prognosis (Delaney and Downar 2016; Souter et al. 2015). As evidence-based decision tools and prognostic models for elderly with TBI are lacking, alignments on conservative versus aggressive management should be made cautiously, avoiding age discrimination (Gardner et al. 2018). Management should rather be based on biological than chronological age and account for the patient's pre-injury health and functional capability, as well as considering patient's wishes about life-saving and aggressive treatments.

3.4 Outcome

Chronological age and TBI severity alone are insufficient to accurately predict the outcome. A subset of older adults, even those with severe TBI, may achieve outcomes similar to younger patients (Lilley et al. 2016; De Bonis et al. 2010; Taussky et al. 2012; Mak et al. 2012). Nevertheless, the generally reported in-hospital mortality of elderly with severe TBI is high, up to 70–80% (Mitra et al. 2008; Brazinova et al. 2010). Among older adults who survive the initial hospitalization and rehabilitation period post-TBI, the observed higher mortality among older versus younger individuals may predominantly be accounted for by expected age-related mortality observed in the general ageing population (Gardner et al. 2018).

Cognitive symptoms and impairment are common after elderly TBI, and the prevalence of these sequels correlate with the severity of the injury (Graham et al. 2010). Older patients tend to recover slower cognitively than younger patients with TBI (Cifu et al. 1996; Green et al. 2008). Apart from cognitive problems post-TBI, elderly patients with TBI are at increased risk for post-traumatic epilepsy (Gardner et al. 2018) compared to younger patients. Geriatric TBI is also associated with a higher incidence of dementia (Fann et al. 2018), Parkinson's disease (Ascherio and Schwarzschild 2016; Perry et al. 2016), stroke (Albrecht et al. 2015; Kowalski et al. 2017), and depression (Menzel 2008).

References

Albrecht JS, Liu X, Smith GS, Baumgarten M, Rattinger GB, Gambert SR, Langenberg P, Zuckerman IH. Stroke incidence following traumatic brain injury in older adults. J Head Trauma Rehabil. 2015;30(2):E62–7.

Ascherio A, Schwarzschild MA. The epidemiology of Parkinson's disease: risk factors and prevention. Lancet Neurol. 2016;15(12):1257–72.

Brazinova A, Mauritz W, Leitgeb J, Wilbacher I, Majdan M, Janciak I, Rusnak M. Outcomes of patients with severe traumatic brain injury who have Glasgow coma scale scores of 3 or 4 and are over 65 years old. J Neurotrauma. 2010;27(9):1549–55.

Brazinova A, Mauritz W, Majdan M, Rehorcikova V, Leitgeb J. Fatal traumatic brain injury in older adults in Austria 1980-2012: an analysis of 33 years. Age Ageing. 2015;44(3):502–6.

Brazinova A, Rehorcikova V, Taylor MS, Buckova V, Majdan M, Psota M, Peeters W, Feigin V, Theadom A, Holkovic L, Synnot A. Epidemiology of traumatic brain injury in Europe: a living systematic review. J Neurotrauma. 2018. [Epub ahead of print]. https://doi.org/10.1089/neu.2015.4126.

Catapano JS, Chapman AJ, Horner LP, Lu M, Fraser DR, Fildes JJ. Pre-injury polypharmacy predicts mortality in isolated severe traumatic brain injury patients. Am J Surg. 2017;213(6):1104–8.

Chen X, Mao G, Leng SX. Frailty syndrome: an overview. Clin Interv Aging. 2014;9:433–41.

Cifu DX, Kreutzer JS, Marwitz JH, Rosenthal M, Englander J, High W. Functional outcomes of older adults with traumatic brain injury: a prospective, multicenter analysis. Arch Phys Med Rehabil. 1996;77(9):883–8.

Dams-O'Connor K, Gibbons LE, Bowen JD, McCurry SM, Larson EB, Crane PK. Risk for late-life re-injury, dementia and death among individuals with traumatic brain injury: a population-based study. J Neurol Neurosurg Psychiatry. 2013;84(2):177–82.

Dang Q, Simon J, Catino J, Puente I, Habib F, Zucker L, Bukur M. More fateful than fruitful? Intracranial pressure monitoring in elderly patients with traumatic brain injury is associated with worse outcomes. J Surg Res. 2015;198(2):482–8.

De Bonis P, Pompucci A, Mangiola A, D'Alessandris QG, Rigante L, Anile C. Decompressive craniectomy for the treatment of traumatic brain injury: does an age limit exist? J Neurosurg. 2010;112(5):1150–3.

De Bonis P, Pompucci A, Mangiola A, Paternoster G, Festa R, Nucci CG, Maviglia R, Antonelli M, Anile C. Decompressive craniectomy for elderly patients with traumatic brain injury: it's probably not worth the while. J Neurotrauma. 2011;28(10):2043–8.

Delaney JW, Downar J. How is life support withdrawn in intensive care units: a narrative review. J Crit Care. 2016;35:12–8.

Evans DC, Cook CH, Christy JM, Murphy CV, Gerlach AT, Eiferman D, Lindsey DE, Whitmill ML, Papadimos TJ, Beery PR 2nd, Steinberg SM, Stawicki SP. Comorbidity-polypharmacy scoring facilitates outcome prediction in older trauma patients. J Am Geriatr Soc. 2012;60(8):1465–70.

Fann JR, Ribe AR, Pedersen HS, Fenger-Grøn M, Christensen J, Benros ME, Vestergaard M. Long-term risk of dementia among people with traumatic brain injury in Denmark: a population-based observational cohort study. Lancet Psychiatry. 2018;5(5):424–31.

Gardner RC, Dams-O'Connor K, Morrissey MR, Manley GT. Geriatric traumatic brain injury: epidemiology, outcomes, knowledge gaps, and future directions. J Neurotrauma. 2018;35:889. https://doi.org/10.1089/neu.2017.5371. [Epub ahead of print].

Graham JE, Radice-Neumann DM, Reistetter TA, Hammond FM, Dijkers M, Granger CV. Influence of sex and age on inpatient rehabilitation outcomes among older adults with traumatic brain injury. Arch Phys Med Rehabil. 2010;91(1):43–50.

Green RE, Colella B, Christensen B, Johns K, Frasca D, Bayley M, Monette G. Examining moderators of cognitive recovery trajectories after moderate to severe traumatic brain injury. Arch Phys Med Rehabil. 2008;89(12 Suppl):S16–24.

Hamill V, Barry SJ, McConnachie A, McMillan TM, Teasdale GM. Mortality from head injury over four decades in Scotland. J Neurotrauma. 2015;32(10):689–703.

Harvey LA, Close JC. Traumatic brain injury in older adults: characteristics, causes and consequences. Injury. 2012;43(11):1821–6.

Joseph B, Pandit V, Zangbar B, Kulvatunyou N, Hashmi A, Green DJ, O'Keeffe T, Tang A, Vercruysse G, Fain MJ, Friese RS, Rhee P. Superiority of frailty over age in predicting outcomes among geriatric trauma patients: a prospective analysis. JAMA Surg. 2014;149(8):766–72.

Joseph B, Orouji Jokar T, Hassan A, Azim A, Mohler MJ, Kulvatunyou N, Siddiqi S, Phelan H, Fain M, Rhee P. Redefining the association between old age and poor outcomes after trauma: the impact of frailty syndrome. J Trauma Acute Care Surg. 2017;82(3):575–81.

Kinoshita T, Yoshiya K, Fujimoto Y, Kajikawa R, Kiguchi T, Hara M, Wakayama A, Yoshimine T. Decompressive craniectomy in conjunction with evacuation of intracranial hemorrhagic lesions is associated with worse outcomes in elderly patients with traumatic brain injury: a propensity score analysis. World Neurosurg. 2016;89:187–92.

Kowalski RG, Haarbauer-Krupa JK, Bell JM, Corrigan JD, Hammond FM, Torbey MT, Hofmann MC, Dams-O'Connor K, Miller AC, Whiteneck GG. Acute ischemic stroke after moderate to severe traumatic brain injury: incidence and impact on outcome. Stroke. 2017;48(7):1802–9.

Kumar RG, Juengst SB, Wang Z, Dams-O'Connor K, Dikmen SS, O'Neil-Pirozzi TM, Dahdah MN, Hammond FM, Felix ER, Arenth PM, Wagner AK. Epidemiology of comorbid conditions among adults 50 years and older with traumatic brain injury. J Head Trauma Rehabil. 2018;33(1):15–24.

Lilley EJ, Williams KJ, Schneider EB, Hammouda K, Salim A, Haider AH, Cooper Z. Intensity of treatment, end-of-life care, and mortality for older patients with severe traumatic brain injury. J Trauma Acute Care Surg. 2016;80(6):998–1004.

Maas AI, Lingsma HF, Roozenbeek B. Predicting outcome after traumatic brain injury. Handb Clin Neurol. 2015;128:455–74.

Mak CH, Wong SK, Wong GK, Ng S, Wang KK, Lam PK, Poon WS. Traumatic brain injury in the elderly: is it as bad as we think? Curr Transl Geriatr Exp Gerontol Rep. 2012;1:171–8.

McCredie VA, Alali AS, Xiong W, Rubenfeld GD, Cuthbertson BH, Scales DC, Nathens AB. Timing of withdrawal of life-sustaining therapies in severe traumatic brain injury: impact on overall mortality. J Trauma Acute Care Surg. 2016;80(3):484–91.

Menzel JC. Depression in the elderly after traumatic brain injury: a systematic review. Brain Inj. 2008;22(5):375–80.

Mitra B, Cameron PA, Gabbe BJ, Rosenfeld JV, Kavar B. Management and hospital outcome of the severely head injured elderly patient. ANZ J Surg. 2008;78(7):588–92.

Perry DC, Sturm VE, Peterson MJ, Pieper CF, Bullock T, Boeve BF, Miller BL, Guskiewicz KM, Berger MS, Kramer JH, Welsh-Bohmer KA. Association of traumatic brain injury with subsequent neurological and psychiatric disease: a meta-analysis. J Neurosurg. 2016;124(2):511–26.

Robertsen A, Førde R, Skaga NO, Helseth E. Treatment-limiting decisions in patients with severe traumatic brain injury in a Norwegian Regional Trauma Center. Scand J Trauma Resusc Emerg Med. 2017;25(1):44.

Souter MJ, Blissitt PA, Blosser S, Bonomo J, Greer D, Jichici D, Mahanes D, Marcolini EG, Miller C, Sangha K, Yeager S. Recommendations for the critical care management of devastating brain injury: prognostication, psychosocial, and ethical management: a position statement for healthcare professionals from the Neurocritical Care Society. Neurocrit Care. 2015;23(1):4–13.

Taussky P, Hidalgo ET, Landolt H, Fandino J. Age and salvageability: analysis of outcome of patients older than 65 years undergoing craniotomy for acute traumatic subdural hematoma. World Neurosurg. 2012;78(3–4):306–11.

Uomoto JM. Older adults and neuropsychological rehabilitation following acquired brain injury. NeuroRehabilitation. 2008;23(5):415–24.

Yap SG, Chua KS. Rehabilitation outcomes in elderly patients with traumatic brain injury in Singapore. J Head Trauma Rehabil. 2008;23(3):158–63.

You W, Feng J, Tang Q, Cao J, Wang L, Lei J, Mao Q, Gao G, Jiang J. Intraventricular intracranial pressure monitoring improves the outcome of older adults with severe traumatic brain injury: an observational, prospective study. BMC Anesthesiol. 2016;16(1):35.

4 Challenges in Children

Olga Calcagnile, Ulrika Sandvik, and Erik Edström

4.1 Incidence and Global Perspectives

Severe TBI in children and adolescents is a complex disorder, with large heterogeneity in both pathology and mechanisms. The impact of severe TBI is enormous as it is the leading cause of death and life-long disability in children and causes significant societal costs and consequences (Murphy and Duhaime 2012; Maas et al. 2017; Hawley et al. 2002).

The real incidence of paediatric TBI injury is difficult to assess due to the lack of definitive classification and lack of reliable data. The incidence numbers also seem to vary between publications, reflecting the difficulty in extracting data out of different hospital systems and regional differences in data collection. Usually the annual incidence rates in the paediatric population for European countries are in the range of 180–300 per 100,000 population. These rates include all severities. The majority (80–90%) of these are mild and approximately 10% is believed to be moderate to severe TBI (Astrand et al. 2016). In developing countries, the incidence of TBI is increasing, probably due to increasing use of motor vehicles. According to the WHO, TBI is expected to surpass many other diseases as a major cause of disability and death by 2020 (Murphy and Duhaime 2012). Boys are generally at a higher risk for TBI. Among children younger than 3 years, the gender distribution is split evenly, but with increasing age, boys have nearly twice the injury rate of girls (Faul and Coronado 2015). Data on the impact of ethnicity and socioeconomic status is generally lacking (Dewan et al. 2016).

4.2 Age Distribution and Mechanisms

Activities and thus vulnerabilities vary greatly within the paediatric population, which is reflected in the mechanisms of injury. Incidences vary with age and societal factors. The majority of TBIs among infants and young children are due to falls, while adolescents are mostly injured during sports, recreational activities, and motor

O. Calcagnile (✉)
Department of Paediatric Medicine, Halland Regional Hospital, Halmstad, Sweden

U. Sandvik · E. Edström
Department of Clinical Neuroscience, Karolinska Institute, Stockholm, Sweden

Department of Neurosurgery, Karolinska University Hospital, Stockholm, Sweden
e-mail: ulrika.sandvik@sll.se; erik.edstrom@sll.se

© Springer Nature Switzerland AG 2020
T. Sundstrøm et al. (eds.), *Management of Severe Traumatic Brain Injury*,
https://doi.org/10.1007/978-3-030-39383-0_4

vehicle accidents (MVAs). In the age group between these two (5–14 years), falls are as common as collisions (Maas et al. 2017; Trefan et al. 2016). The highest incidence of TBI registered in the paediatric population is among infants and young children (0–4 years old). The second peak of incidence is reported among adolescents.

Most paediatric TBI injuries are due to MVAs (6–80%) and falls (5–87%). Abuse and other forms of non-accidental trauma represent 2–12%, and sports-related injury <1–29%. As can be seen from the wide ranges, regional and cultural differences are great. Among sports, soccer, cycling, and horseback riding are most commonly associated with paediatric TBI in Europe. In Africa, Asia, and India more than half of the MVAs in the paediatric population involved pedestrians, while in China 43% of MVAs involved a bicycle. In Australia, Europe, and the United States, however, the MVAs typically involve vehicle occupants. Falls seem to be a more frequent cause of paediatric TBI in Asian populations than in western countries. Sports-related paediatric TBI was more common in Australia and the United States (2–29%) than in Asian countries (0.7–2%) (Dewan et al. 2016; Davies et al. 2015).

4.3 Child Abuse

The incidence of child abuse or non-accidental trauma (NAT) is difficult to determine. Reported data varies widely between countries. Published data indicate an incidence of 2–12% of TBI in children, and NAT is the most common cause of severe paediatric TBI in infants and small children (Dewan et al. 2016; Davies et al. 2015). A newly published Scandinavian study on the epidemiology of subdural haemorrhage (SDH) during infancy shows an incidence of 2.3 per 100,000 infants for abusive SDH in the Swedish population (Högberg et al. 2018). NAT is often very difficult to distinguish from accidental injuries. The clinical presentation may range from normal neurological findings to unstable vital signs and coma. Often no external signs of injury are present. As the victims typically are either too young or too injured to report the assault, the clinical challenge is profound.

The term “shaken baby syndrome” was introduced in the 1970s, indicating the triad of encephalopathy (irritability, vomiting, altered level of consciousness), SDHs, and retinal bleedings. It has been considered to indicate a mechanism of violent shaking of the infant. However, some reports have shown that the presence of this triad is not exclusively associated with abusive head injury (Swedish Agency for Health Technology Assessment and Assessment of Social Services (SBU) 2016). The outcome of abusive head injuries has the worst prognosis among all forms of paediatric TBI. Mortality rates range from 13 to 23%. Approximately 55% suffer from neurological deficits, among which visual impairments are common (Keenan et al. 2004).

4.4 Prevention

At best modern trauma care prevents secondary injuries, but preventive measures are absolutely needed to diminish the burden of TBI. Many causes of paediatric TBI are preventable and have obvious remedies, which need to be implemented effectively. For instance, the introduction of a road safety program in Brazil, China, Kenya, Mexico, Turkey, and Vietnam is estimated to have a profound effect, resulting in 109,000 lives saved during 2014–2023. The program includes legislation on drunk driving, motorcycle helmets, safety belt use, and use of fines to improve adherence to traffic regulations. Albeit with a great variability between countries, reduced drunk driving was the single most important factor (84%) in reducing lives lost (Miller et al. 2018). While it is obvious that reduced numbers of MVAs will result in reduced numbers of severe TBI (Chen et al. 2018), data also suggests that helmet use during biking in children reduces the risk of hospital stay and head and neck injuries (McAdams et al. 2018) and that this translates into reductions in severe TBI and trauma deaths (Socialstyrelsen 2017). This holds true also for sports-related TBI, where helmet use in biking and horseback riding translates into reduced frequencies of trauma-induced amnesia, unconsciousness, and epidural hematomas (Bandte et al. 2018).

4.5 Features of Paediatric TBI

The peripheral and central nervous system in children differs from adults both in its anatomy and physiology; as a direct consequence, TBI in paediatric population shows some specific features and challenges. Anatomically the proportions between head and body differ between children and adults and vary during childhood. In newborns and infants, the head is large and heavy in respect to the rest of the body, and it will take several years to reach adult proportions. The brain of a newborn is around 25% of the size of an adult brain, while the total body weight is only 5% on average of that of an adult (Figaji 2017). Moreover, the heavy head is supported by weak neck muscles and stretchy ligaments that make it easier for both head and spine to get injured after a fall or other traumatic events (Hickman et al. 2015).

The skull and the cervical region reach different maturity stages at different ages. The posterior fontanel is the first to close around 2 months after birth while the anterior fontanel may stay open until 18 months of age. Even sutures close at different times, and this, together with fontanel, allows some adaptive margins when the intracranial volume increases. However, the level of volume increase is limited and does not adapt in case of quickly expanding volumes. Moreover, children have a lower intracranial pressure (ICP) than adults and tolerate only limited changes in ICP (Figaji 2017). (More details on ICP physiology, monitoring and treatment will be discussed elsewhere in this book.)

The skull in young children is thinner and more easily bendable than in adults. The skull may be easily deformed affecting the underlying parenchyma, even without any visible fractures. Typical fractures in infants and young children are for instance "ping-pong" fractures that will often remodel spontaneously; linear fractures may develop into "growing fractures", where the underlying dural tear will result in herniation of the brain. On the other hand, if the dura is intact, small skull fractures will heal completely thanks to the high osteogenic capacity of children's bones (Singh et al. 2016).

Special considerations should be taken for the vulnerability of the parenchyma of the developing brain. At birth the axons lack their protective myelin sheet, and it will take several years before the myelinisation process will be completed. It has been shown that unmyelinated axons are more vulnerable to injury leaving the young child brain more easily subjected to diffuse injury patterns (Babikian et al. 2015).

In this chapter, we have presented only some aspects that characterize and differ paediatric TBI from TBI in adults. The anatomical and physiological differences are clear; however, we are still lacking paediatric-specific data and guidelines. There are only few studies available, and at the moment, there is not enough evidence to support clinical recommendations. More paediatric-specific studies are needed.

References

Astrand R, Rosenlund C, Undén J, et al. Scandianavian guidelines for initial management of minor and moderate head trauma in children. BMC Med. 2016;14:33.

Babikian T, Merkley T, Savage RC, Giza CC, Levin H. Chronic aspects of Pediatric traumatic brain injury: review of the literature. J Neurotrauma. 2015;32:1849–60.

Bandte A, Fritzsche FS, Emami P, Kammler G, Püschel K, Krajewski K. Sport-related traumatic brain injury with and without helmets in children. World Neurosurg. 2018;111:e434–9.

Chen C, Peng J, Sribnick EA, Zhu M, Xiang H. Trend of age-adjusted rates of pediatric traumatic brain injury in U.S. emergency departments from 2006 to 2013. Int J Environ Res Public Health. 2018;15.

Davies FC, Coats TJ, Fisher R, Lawrence T, Lecky FE. A profile of suspected child abuse as a subgroup of major trauma patients. Emerg Med J. 2015;32:921–5.

Dewan MC, Mummareddy N, Wellons JC 3rd, Bonfield CM. Epidemiology of global pediatric traumatic brain injury: qualitative review. World Neurosurg. 2016;91:497–509.

Faul M, Coronado V. Epidemiology of traumatic brain injury. Handb Clin Neurol. 2015;127:3–13.

Figaji AA. Anatomical and physiological differences between children and adults relevant to traumatic brain injury and the implications for clinical assessment and care. Front Neurol. 2017;8:685.

Hawley CA, Ward AB, Magnay AR, Long J. Children's brain injury: a postal follow-up of 525 children from one health region in the UK. Brain Inj. 2002;16:969–85.

Hickman ZL, McDowell M, Anderson RCE. Principles of pediatric spinal column trauma. In: Albright AL, Pollack IF, Adelson PD, editors. Principles and practice of pediatric neurosurgery. 3rd ed; 2015. p. 789–805.

Högberg U, Andersson J, Squier W, Högberg G, Fellman V, Thiblin I, Wester K. Epidemiology of subdural haemorrhage during infancy: a population-based register study. PLoS One. 2018;13:e0206340.

Keenan HT, Runyan DK, Marshall SW, Nocera MA, Merten DF. A population-based comparison of clinical and outcome characteristics of young children with serious inflicted and noninflicted traumatic brain injury. Pediatrics. 2004;114:633–9.

Maas AIR, Menon DK, Adelson PD, et al. Traumatic brain injury: integrated approaches to improve prevention, clinical care, and research. Lancet Neurol. 2017;16:987–1048.

McAdams RJ, Swidarski K, Clark RM, Roberts KJ, Yang J, Mckenzie LB. Bicycle-related injuries among children treated in US emergency departments, 2006-2015. Accid Anal Prev. 2018;118:11–7.

Miller TR, Levy DT, Swedler DI. Lives saved by laws and regulations that resulted from the Bloomberg road safety program. Accid Anal Prev. 2018;113:131–6.

Murphy S, Duhaime A. Update in pediatric neurotrauma. Curr Trauma Rep. 2012;2:222–31.

Singh I, Rohilla S, Siddiqui SA, Kumar P. Growing skull fractures: guidelines for early diagnosis and surgical management. Childs Nerv Syst. 2016; 32:1117–22.

Socialstyrelsen. The Swedish National Board for Health and Welfare. Statistical database. 2017. http://www.socialstyrelsen.se/statistics/statisticaldatabase.

Swedish Agency for Health Technology Assessment and Assessment of Social Services (SBU). Traumatic shaking: the role of the triad in medical investigations of suspected traumatic shaking. Report 255E/2016.

Trefan L, Houston R, Pearson G, Edwards R, Hyde P, Maconochie I, Parslow RC, Kemp A. Epidemiology of children with head injury: a national overview. Arch Dis Child. 2016;101:527–32.

5 Biomechanics and Prevention

Svein Kleiven

5.1 Biomechanics of Traumatic Head Injuries

The interior and exterior surfaces of a car are designed to protect the occupants from injury at accidents through the use of energy-absorbing materials and clever structural solutions. The primary verification tool in the design process is the head injury criterion (HIC) applied in a free motion head-form experimental set-up, where a rigid dummy head is launched towards specific locations (National Highway Traffic Safety Administration (NHTSA), U.S. Department of Transportation (DoT) 1995). Linear accelerations in three perpendicular directions are measured in the head-form during the impact, and the performance is evaluated according to the HIC. The test procedure is established internationally and thus used by automotive manufacturers all over the world. Sports and automotive helmets are also only tested for pure radial impacts to the helmet, except for the Bbs 6658 and eEn 22.05 oblique impact tests for motorcycle helmets. These tests are, however, only used to assess external projections and surface friction by measuring the tangential force. A pure radial impact will cause primarily linear acceleration of the head, while a pure tangential impact around the head's centre of gravity will cause both rotational and linear acceleration of the head. In reality, pure radial impacts are very rare and would mainly cause skull fractures and injuries secondary to those fractures. Bicycle, motorcycle and equestrian accident statistics from Germany, Canada, Belgium and Finland have, on the other hand, found the most common accident situation to be an oblique impact, with an average angle to the ground of 30–40° (Harrison et al. 1996; Otte et al. 1999; Richter et al. 2001; Verschueren 2009). Thus, the highest likelihood for oblique impacts is causing both linear and rotational head kinematics (Fig. 5.1).

The human brain is sensitive to rotational motion (Holbourn 1943; Gennarelli et al. 1987; Kleiven 2013). In a pioneering work, Holbourn (1943) observed shear strain patterns in 2D gel models and claimed that translation is not injurious, while rotation could explain the majority of TBIs due to the nearly incompressible properties of brain tissue. The bulk modulus of brain tissue is roughly five to six orders of magnitude larger than the shear modulus (McElhaney et al. 1976), so that for a given impact, it tends to deform primarily in shear. Therefore, distortional strain has

Parts of the text has previously been published in "Kleiven S. Why most traumatic brain injuries are not caused by linear acceleration but skull fractures are. Front Bioeng Biotechnol. 2013;1:15."

S. Kleiven (✉)
Division of Neuronic Engineering, KTH Royal Institute of Technology, Huddinge, Sweden
e-mail: sveink@kth.se

© Springer Nature Switzerland AG 2020

T. Sundstrøm et al. (eds.), *Management of Severe Traumatic Brain Injury*,
https://doi.org/10.1007/978-3-030-39383-0_5

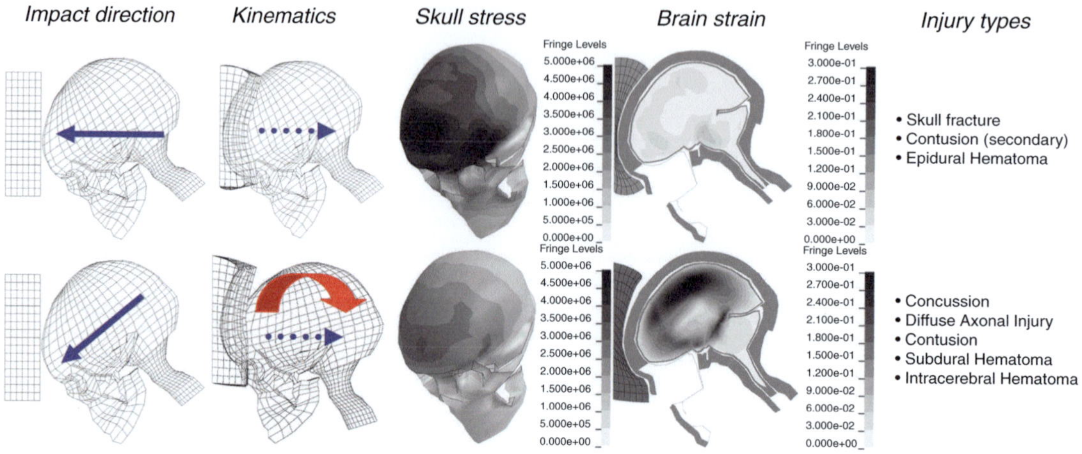

Fig. 5.1 Illustration of the biomechanics of an oblique impact (lower), compared to a corresponding perpendicular one (upper), when impacted against the same padding using an identical initial velocity of 6.7 m/s. Maximum principal strain (Green-Lagrange) at maximum for the brain are illustrated together with the maximum von Mises stress for the skull bone. (Modified from Kleiven 2013)

been used as an indicator for the risk of TBI in the current chapter. The maximal principal Green Lagrange strain was chosen as a predictor of CNS injuries, since it has been shown to correlate with diffuse axonal injuries (Gennarelli et al. 1989; Galbraith et al. 1993; Bain and Meaney 2000; Morrison et al. 2003), as well as with mechanical injury to the blood–brain barrier (Shreiber et al. 1997). This gives a large sensitivity of the strain in the brain to rotational loading and a small sensitivity to linear kinematics (Kleiven 2006). Therefore, rotational kinematics should be a better indicator of TBI risk than linear. It has also been shown that the most common severe injuries, such as subdural haemorrhage and diffuse axonal injury, are more easily caused by rotational head motion (Gennarelli et al. 1972, 1987). Gurdjian and Gurdjian (1975) suggested that a combination of skull deformation, pressures and inertial brain lag could present a clearer picture of head injury. Gennarelli et al. (1982) stated that all types of brain injury could be produced by angular acceleration. According to Ommaya (1985), rotation can produce both focal and diffuse brain injuries, while translation is limited to focal effects.

The aim of this chapter is to point out future directions when it comes to the prediction of head injuries, based on the predominant mechanisms behind each type of injury. To illustrate the difference between radial and oblique impacts, perpendicular impacts through the centre of gravity of the head and 45° oblique impacts have been simulated (Kleiven 2013). It is obvious that substantially higher strain levels in the brain are obtained for an oblique impact, compared to a corresponding perpendicular one, when impacted towards the same padding of expanded polypropylene using an identical initial velocity of 6.7 m/s. It is also clearly illustrated that the radial impact causes substantially higher stresses in the skull, with an associated higher risk of skull fractures (Fig. 5.1, upper).

5.2 Brain Injuries Primarily Induced by Rotational Kinematics

5.2.1 Concussion

The classical cerebral concussion involves immediate loss of consciousness following impact loading (Melvin et al. 1993). This is the most commonly occurring type of TBI injury, accounting for around 70% of the total, where more than 99% of the patients have left the hospital within 14 days (Kleiven et al. 2003). Gennarelli et al. (1972) subjected squirrel monkeys to controlled sagittal plane head motions. It was found that in animals subjected to pure translation of the head, cerebral concussion was not observed. In contrast, the animals that were subjected to head rotations were all concussed. Visible brain lesions were noted in both translated and rotated groups, but with a greater frequency and severity after rotation. Patton et al. (2012) suggested rotational kinematics above 4500 rad/s^2 and 33 rad/s for peak resultant angular acceleration and maximum change in resultant angular velocity, respectively, to predict concussions involving loss of consciousness lasting longer than 1 min in rugby and Australian football impacts. Recently, Rowson et al. (2012) recorded 57 concussions and a large number of sub-concussive impacts during the 2007–2009 collegiate American football seasons and proposed 6383 rad/s^2 in rotational acceleration associated with 28.3 rad/s in rotational velocity to represent a 50% risk of concussion. Studies on giant squid axons (Thibault 1993) suggested a maximal principal strain of around 0.10 to cause reversible injury to the axons, which could be used as an approximate axonal strain threshold for concussion. During simulations of concussions in the National Football League (NFL), the strain magnitude in the brain was found to be sensitive to only the rotational kinematics and not the translational motion (Kleiven 2007a).

5.2.2 Diffuse Axonal Injury (DAI)

DAI is associated with mechanical disruption of many axons in the cerebral hemispheres and subcortical white matter, illustrated as shear strain in Fig. 5.2. Severe memory and motor deficits may be present, and posttraumatic amnesia may last for weeks (Melvin et al. 1993). DAI is the prevailing mechanism also in mild TBI—it is only a matter of extent and severity. High-resolution imaging may show small haemorrhages and axonal swelling. The maximum strain needed to cause damage to the axons has been discussed above in previous publications. Studies have been performed with giant squid axons (Ueno and Melvin 1995), and a strain of 0.3 was suggested as threshold for DAI. Bain and Meaney (Bain and Meaney 2000) proposed a threshold of 0.2 in maximal principal strain in the brain tissue for the onset of the malfunction of the neurons in the brain, which could be seen as a first stage of DAI. Maximum principal Green Lagrange strain of 0.2 has also been shown to correlate with cell death and neuronal dysfunction associated with DAI (Morrison et al. 2003). Ueno and Melvin (Löwenhielm 1975) found, when applying kinematics to a 2D head model, that the rotational acceleration has a dominant effect on shear deformation, while linear acceleration is related to pressure.

5.2.3 Contusions

Cerebral contusion is one of the most frequently found lesions following head injury. It consists of heterogeneous areas of necrosis, pulping, infarction, haemorrhage and oedema (Melvin et al. 1993). Contusions generally occur at the site of impact (coup contusions) and at the opposite remote sites from the impact (contrecoup contusions) (Fig. 5.2). In the absence of skull fracture, contusions are likely induced by shearing and scratching of the brain tissue against edges and sharper ridges in the dura/skull and therefore caused by excessive head rotational loading (Gennarelli 1981). Moreover, Shreiber et al. (1997) derived a threshold of 0.19 in principal logarithmic strain in the cortex for a 50% risk of cerebral contusions induced by vacuum. As previously mentioned, this strain is sensitive only to only the rotational kinematics and not to the translational motion (Kleiven 2007a; Löwenhielm 1975).

5.2.4 Subdural Hematoma (SDH)

Acute SDH together with DAI injury account for more head injury deaths than all other lesions combined (Gennarelli and Thibault 1982). SDH is the most common of the severe TBIs, accounting for around 50% of the total of this category in Sweden (Kleiven et al. 2003). The most common mechanism of SDH is tearing of veins that bridge the subdural space as they go from the brain surface to the various dural sinuses (Fig. 5.2) (Gennarelli and

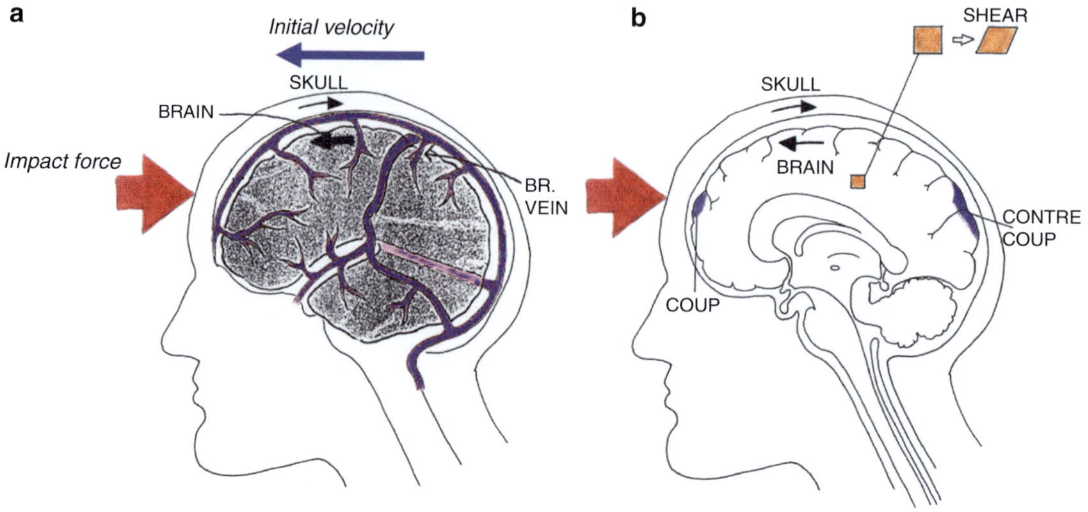

Fig. 5.2 (**a**) Schematic description of the biomechanics of subdural hematoma caused by tearing of blood vessels such as the bridging veins induced by relative motion between the skull and brain during impact. (**b**) Illustration of the biomechanics of concussions, contusions, intracerebral hematomas and diffuse axonal injuries caused by brain tissue deformation when impacted against a surface as illustrated in Fig. 5.1. (Modified from Kleiven 2013)

Thibault 1982). Based on previous primate experiments, Gennarelli (1983) suggested that SDH was produced by short duration and high amplitude of angular accelerations. Lee and Haut (1989) studied the effects of strain rate on tensile failure properties of human bridging veins and determined the ultimate strain to be about $\varepsilon_f = 0.5$, which was found to be independent of the strain rate ($\varepsilon = 0.1$–$250\ s^{-1}$). Earlier research done by Löwenhielm (1974) showed that the failure strain was markedly reduced from about 0.8 to 0.2 as the rate was increased. Lee et al. (1987) used a 2D sagittal model and Huang et al. (1999) used a 3D model (previously presented in Shugar 1977) to study the mechanisms of SDH. They found that the contribution of angular acceleration to tearing of bridging veins (measured as observed change in distance between a node in the interior of the skull and a node in the brain) was greater than the translational acceleration. Substantially larger relative motions between the skull and the brain as well as higher strain in the bridging veins have been found, when switching from a translational to a rotational mode of motion using a detailed 3D head model, including 11 pairs of the largest bridging veins (Kleiven 2003).

5.2.5 Intracerebral Hematoma (ICH)

ICHs are well-defined homogeneous collections of blood within the cerebral parenchyma. It was possible, through the reconstruction of a motocross accident, to re-create the injury pattern in the brain of the injured rider using maximal principal strains (Kleiven 2007a). The strain levels at maximum for two locations of intra-cerebral hematomas were around 0.4–0.5, which is close to the known thresholds for rupture of cerebral veins and arteries (Lee and Haut 1989; Lövenhielm 1974; Monson et al. 2003), indicating that the risk of intra-cerebral hematomas can be predicted by the pattern and magnitude of maximum principal strain.

5.3 Head Injuries Primarily Induced by Linear Kinematics

5.3.1 Skull Fracture

It is obvious that a purely radial impact produces higher contact forces and larger linear accelerations increasing the stresses in the skull bone, which predicts the risk of skull fractures (Fig. 5.1). Consistent mean fracture force levels in the range of 4.8–5.8 kN for the frontal bone and 3.5–3.6 kN for the temporoparietal area of the skull have been reported (Nahum et al. 1968; Allsop et al. 1988; Schneider and Nahum 1972). The reported fracture forces do, however, vary depending on the impact surface area (Hodgson and Thomas 1971, 1973). These force values can be related to the linear acceleration of the head through Newton's second law. A study by Mertz et al. (1997) estimated a 5% risk of skull fractures for a peak acceleration of 180 gravities (g) and a 40% risk of fractures for 250 g.

5.3.2 Epidural Hematoma (EDH)

EDH is a relatively infrequently occurring sequel to head trauma (0.2–6%) (Kleiven et al. 2003; Cooper 1982). It occurs as a result of trauma to the skull and the underlying meningeal vessels and is not due to brain injury (Melvin et al. 1993).

5.3.3 Contusions (Secondary to Skull Fracture)

Cerebral contusion at the site of impact in the presence of skull fracture is likely induced by the direct impression of the skull against the underlying brain tissue and therefore, as for skull fracture, caused by the contact force and well predicted by the linear acceleration.

5.4 Prevention of Traumatic Brain Injuries

The results presented and discussed in this chapter deal with TBIs induced by inertia or due to impacts and exclude penetrating injuries due to projectiles, fluid percussion injury systems or blast-induced TBIs, where the mechanisms are not yet well understood. Nevertheless, it can be concluded that minimizing the magnitudes of rotational kinematics would probably best prevent the following impact- or inertia-induced TBIs:

- Concussion
- Diffuse axonal injury
- Contusion (in absence of skull fracture)
- Subdural hematoma
- Intracerebral hematoma

This can be accomplished by built-in rotational protection systems in helmets such as MIPS (Multi-directional Impact Protections System) (Halldin et al. 2003). In a helmet with MIPS, a low friction layer separates the shell and the liner. When subjected to an angled impact, the low friction layer allows the helmet to slide relative to the head (Fig. 5.3). This reduces rotational motion when implemented in a helmet by absorbing and redirecting rotational energies and forces transferred to the brain.

On the other hand, minimizing the magnitudes of linear acceleration or the impact force would probably best prevent the following TBIs by minimizing the magnitudes of linear acceleration or the impact force:

- Skull fracture
- Epidural hematoma
- Contusions (secondary to skull fracture)

This can be achieved by introducing an energy absorbing liner, usually polymer foams such as expanded polystyrene or expanded polypropylene, which absorbs energy when compressed (Fig. 5.4a), and thereby reducing the linear acceleration and radial impact forces endured by the head (Fig. 5.4b). The density and strength of the helmet liner has to be chosen so that as much energy is absorbed in compression as possible, while keeping the linear accelerations and radial impact forces into a minimum. It is obvious from Fig. 5.4a that most energy is absorbed for the medium density foam (area under the curve of a force–deformation or stress–strain curve) for a compressive stress level of 0.3 MPa. Choosing a too stiff and strong, high-density liner will produce a large

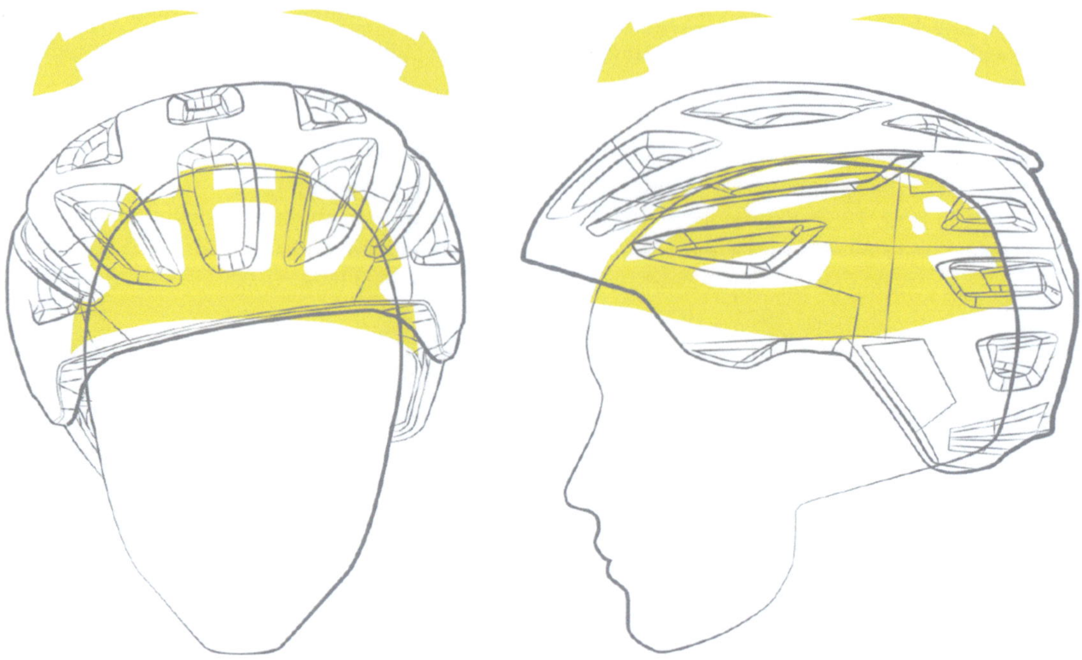

Fig. 5.3 MIPS (Multi-directional Impact Protection System) where the shell and the liner are separated by a low friction layer (Halldin et al. 2003), reducing the rotational motion by absorbing and redirecting rotational energies and forces transferred to the brain. (Modified from http://mipsprotection.com/technology/)

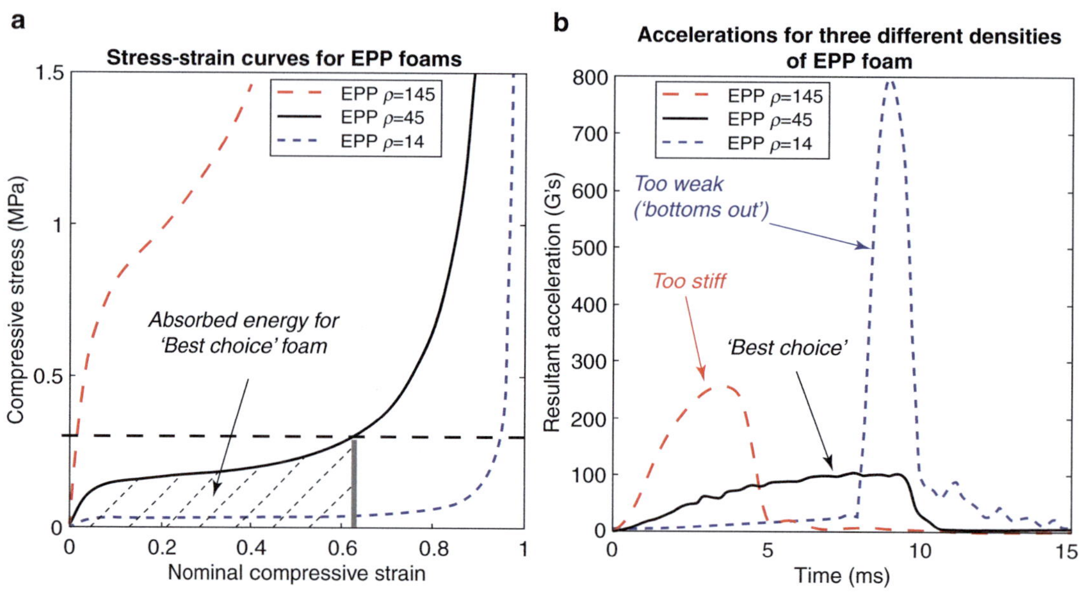

Fig. 5.4 (**a**) Three different energy-absorbing liners of expanded polypropylene, which absorbs energy when compressed. (**b**) The resulting linear acceleration magnitude for the three different liners illustrating a too soft, too stiff and best choice liner material for a 6.7 m/s radial impact. (Modified from Kleiven 2007b)

magnitude of linear acceleration with little liner deformation, while a too soft liner will bottom-out creating a large acceleration spike, where a large part of the load is transferred to the scalp, skull, dura, CSF and brain, when the foam is crushed to almost 100% deformation in compression (Fig. 5.4b).

References

Allsop D, Warner C, Wille M, Schneider D, Nahum, A. Facial impact response—a comparison of the hybrid III dummy and human cadaver. In: Proceedings of the 32nd Stapp Car Crash Conference, Society of Automotive Engineers, Warrendale, PA; 1988.

Bain BC, Meaney DF. Tissue-level thresholds for axonal damage in an experimental model of central nervous system white matter injury. J Biomech Eng. 2000;16:615–22.

Cooper PR. Post-traumatic intracranial mass lesions. In: Cooper PR, editor. Head injury. Baltimore: Williams and Wilkins; 1982. p. 185–232.

Galbraith JA, Thibault LE, Matteson DR. Mechanical and electrical responses of the squid giant axon to simple elongation. J Biomech Eng. 1993;115:13–22.

Gennarelli TA. Mechanistic approach to head injuries: clinical and experimental studies of the important types of injury. In: Ommaya AK, editor. Head and neck injury criteria: a consensus workshop. US Department of Transportation, National Highway Traffic Safety Administration, Washington DC; 1981. pp. 20–25.

Gennarelli TA. Head injuries in man and experimental animals: clinical aspects. Acta Neurochir Suppl. 1983;32:1–13.

Gennarelli TA, Thibault LE. Biomechanics of acute subdural hematoma. J Trauma. 1982;22:680–6.

Gennarelli T, Thibault L, Ommaya A. Pathophysiological responses to rotational and translational accelerations of the head. In: Proceedings of the 16th Stapp Car Crash Conference, Society of Automotive Engineers, Warrendale, PA; 1972.

Gennarelli TA, Thibault LE, Adams JH, Graham DI, Thompson CJ, Marcincin RP. Diffuse axonal injury and traumatic coma in the primate. Ann Neurol. 1982;12:564–74.

Gennarelli TA, Thibault LE, Tomei G, Wiser R, Graham DI, Adams J. Directional dependence of axonal brain injury due to centroidal and non-centroidal acceleration. In: Proceedings of the 31st Stapp Car Crash Conference, Society of Automotive Engineers, Warrendale, PA; 1987.

Gennarelli TA, Thibault LE, Tipperman R, et al. Axonal injury in the optic nerve: a model of diffuse axonal injury in the brain. J Neurosurg. 1989;71:244–53.

Gurdjian E, Gurdjian E. Re-evaluation of the biomechanics of blunt impact of the head. Surg Gynecol Obstet. 1975;140:845–50.

Halldin P, Aare M, Kleiven S, Von Holst H. Reduced risk for Dai by use of a new safety helmet. In: Proceedings of the international conference on closed head trauma, US Army Medical Research and Material Command, and US Department of Transportation, San Juan, Puerto Rico; 2003.

Harrison T, Mills N, Turner M. Jockeys head injuries and skull cap performance. In: Proceedings of the Ircobi Conference September 11–13, 1996; Dublin.

Hodgson V, Thomas L. Breaking strength of the human skull vs. impact surface curvature. Wayne State University School of Medicine, Department of Neurosurgery, Final Report, Contract No. Fh-11-7609; 1971.

Hodgson V, Thomas L. Breaking strength of the human skull vs. impact surface curvature. Wayne State University School of Medicine. NHTSA Dot-H-S-801-002. Pb 233041; 1973.

Holbourn A. Mechanics of head injury. Lancet. 1943;2:438–41.

Huang HM, et al. Three-dimensional finite element analysis of subdural hematoma. J Trauma. 1999;47:538–44.

Kleiven S. Influence of impact direction to the human head in prediction of subdural hematoma. J Neurotrauma. 2003;20:365–79.

Kleiven S. Evaluation of head injury criteria using a Fe model validated against experiments on localized brain motion, intra-cerebral acceleration, and intra-cranial pressure. Int J Crashworthiness. 2006;11:65–79.

Kleiven S. Predictors for traumatic brain injuries evaluated through accident reconstructions. In: 51st Stapp Car Crash Journal. 2007a. pp. 81–114.

Kleiven S. A parametric study of energy absorbing materials for head injury prevention (Paper No. 07- 0385-O). In: Proceedings of the 20th enhanced safety of vehicles conference, Lyon, France; 2007b.

Kleiven S. Why most traumatic brain injuries are not caused by linear acceleration but skull fractures are. Front Bioeng Biotechnol. 2013;1:15.

Kleiven S, Peloso PM, Von Holst H. The epidemiology of head injuries in Sweden from 1987 to 2000. J Inj Control Saf Promot. 2003;10:173–80.

Lee MC, Haut RC. Insensitivity of tensile failure properties of human bridging veins to strain rate: implications in biomechanics of subdural hematoma. J Biomech. 1989;22:537–42.

Lee MC, Melvin JW, Ueno K. Finite element analysis of traumatic subdural hematoma. In: Proceedings of the 31st Stapp Car Crash Conference, Sae Paper No. 872201, Society of Automotive Engineers, Warrendale, PA; 1987.

Lövenhielm P. Strain tolerance of the Vv. Cerebri Sup. (bridging veins) calculated from head-on collision tests with cadavers. Z Rechtsmedizin. 1974;75:131–44.

Löwenhielm P. Mathematical simulations of gliding contusions. J Biomech. 1975;8:351–6.

McElhaney J, Roberts V, Hilyard J. Properties of human tissues and components: nervous tissues. In: Handbook of human tolerance. Tokyo: Automobile Research Institute Inc; 1976. p. 143.

Melvin JW, Lighthall JW, Ueno K. Brain injury biomechanics. In: Nahum A, Melvin J, editors. Accidental injury. New York: Springer; 1993. p. 269–90.

Mertz H, Prasad P, Irwin A. Injury risk curves for children and adults in frontal and rear collisions. In: Proceedings of the 41st Stapp Car Crash Conference, Society of Automotive Engineers, Warrendale, PA; 1997.

Monson KL, Goldsmith W, Barbaro NM, Manley GT. Axial mechanical properties of fresh human cerebral blood vessels. J Biomech Eng. 2003;125:288–94.

Morrison BC, Cater HL, Wang CC-B, Thomas FC, Hung CT, Ateshian GA, Sundström LE. A tissue level tolerance criterion for living brain developed with an in vitro model of traumatic mechanical loading. In: 47th Stapp Car Crash Journal. 2003. pp. 93–105.

Nahum AM, Gatts JD, Gadd CW, Danforth JP. Impact tolerance of the skull and face. In: Proceedings of the 12th Stapp Car Crash Conference, Society of Automotive Engineers, Warrendale, PA; 1968.

National Highway Traffic Safety Administration (NHTSA), U.S. Department Of Transportation (DoT). Laboratory test procedures for Fmvss 201, Tp-201uu-00, Safety Assurance, Ovsc, Washington, DC; 1995.

Ommaya AK. Biomechanics of head injury: experimental aspects. In: Nahum A, Melvin J, editors. Biomechanics of trauma. Appleton & Lange: Norwalk; 1985. p. 245–69.

Otte D, Chinn B, Doyle D, et al. Contribution to final report of cost 327 project: University of Hannover, Hannover, Germany. 1999.

Patton D, Mcintosh A, Kleiven S, Frechede B. Injury data from unhelmeted football head impacts evaluated against critical strain tolerance curves. J Sports Eng Technol. 2012;226:177–84.

Richter M, Otte D, Lehmann U, et al. Head injury mechanisms in helmet protected motorcyclists: prospective multicenter study. J Trauma. 2001;51:949–58.

Rowson S, Duma S, Beckwith J, Chu J, Greenwald R, Crisco M, Brolinson P, Duhaime A, McAllister T, Maerlender A. Rotational head kinematics in football impacts: an injury risk function for concussion. Ann Biomed Eng. 2012;40:1–13.

Schneider D, Nahum A. Impact studies of the facial bones and skull. In: Proceedings of the 16th Stapp Car Crash Conference, Society of Automotive Engineers, Warrendale, PA; 1972.

Shreiber DI, Bain AC, Meaney DF. In vivo thresholds for mechanical injury to the blood-brain barrier. In: 41st Stapp Car Crash Conference, Society of Automotive Engineers, Warrendale, PA; 1997.

Shugar T. A finite element head injury model, final report, vol 1 Contract DoT Hs 289-3-550-Ia, NHTSA, Washington, DC; 1977.

Thibault LE. Brain injury from the macro to the micro level and back again: what have we learned to date? In: Proceedings of the international conference on impact trauma, Eindhoven, The Netherlands; 1993:3–25.

Ueno K, Melvin JW. Finite element model study of head impact based on hybrid III head acceleration: the effects of rotational and translational acceleration. J Biomech Eng. 1995;117:319–28.

Verschueren P. Biomechanical analysis of head injuries related to bicycle accidents and a new bicycle helmet concept. Doctoral thesis, Katholieke Universiteit Leuven, Belgium; 2009.

Part II

Classification and Assessment

Johan Undén

6 Pathophysiology of Severe Traumatic Brain Injury

Niklas Marklund and Olli Tenovuo

Recommendations

Level I

There are no Level I recommendations for this topic.

Level II

There are no current Level II recommendations for this topic.

Level III

There are numerous observational and mechanistic studies evaluating the pathophysiology of TBI, where available data shows that a) TBI is a disease process rather than a single incident, b) there is a vast heterogeneity of TBI at both clinical and molecular levels, and c) improvement of TBI care needs to better address inter-individual differences (including age, gender, genetic/epigenetic/metabolic factors, co-morbidities) by developing targeted personalized medicine therapies.

N. Marklund (✉)
Department of Clinical Sciences Lund, Neurosurgery, Lund University, Skåne University Hospital, Lund, Sweden
e-mail: niklas.marklund@med.lu.se

O. Tenovuo
Turku Brain Injury Centre, Turku University Hospital, Turku, Finland

Department of Clinical Medicine, University of Turku, Turku, Finland

6.1 Summary

TBI should be regarded as a disease process initiated at time of injury, complicated and markedly exacerbated by a complex set of secondary injury factors. The vulnerability of the injured brain partly explains the progressive deterioration that contributes to increased cell death, white matter atrophy, and brain network dysfunction over a period ranging from hours, days, or even years post-injury (Masel and DeWitt 2010). The damage sustained at primary impact is caused by mechanical deformation of brain tissue, resulting in neuronal and glial cell death, axonal shearing, and injury to cerebral vessels with ensuing blood–brain barrier (BBB) disruption and disturbed regulation of the cerebral blood flow (CBF) (Marklund and Hillered 2011). Key pathophysiological events are summarized in Fig. 6.1. The damage caused by the initial impact cannot be treated, only prevented. At present, rapid surgical treatment and modern neurocritical care may be lifesaving and attenuate the TBI-induced secondary injuries. However, no pharmacological treatments with proven clinical benefit are available for severe TBI, although increased understanding of the secondary injury and late

© Springer Nature Switzerland AG 2020
T. Sundstrøm et al. (eds.), *Management of Severe Traumatic Brain Injury*,
https://doi.org/10.1007/978-3-030-39383-0_6

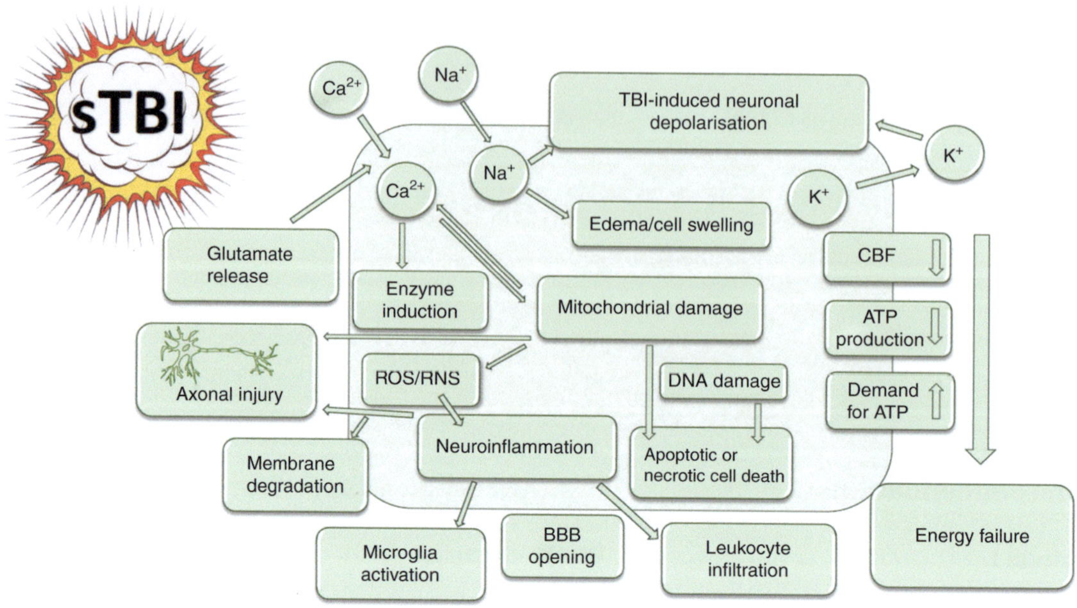

Fig. 6.1 Schematic overview of the pathophysiology of TBI. *ROS* reactive oxygen species, *RNS* reactive nitrogen species, *Ca* calcium, *Na* Sodium, *K* potassium, *CBF* cerebral blood flow, *BBB* blood–brain barrier, *ATP* adenosine triphosphate, *sTBI* severe TBI

processes raise hope for the development of novel treatments targeting both the short- and long-term factors contributing to the progressive injury. Such therapies need to target the vast heterogeneity of TBI and consider patient-specific factors, moving towards more individualized therapies (Saatman et al. 2008). Plausibly, such approaches are needed to further decrease morbidity and mortality, which remain high without marked improvements during the last decades (Stein et al. 2010).

Some of the secondary injury processes may be monitored clinically, although the detailed molecular events worsening the injury are incompletely known. Examples of the systemic factors monitored clinically in neurocritical care are covered elsewhere in this volume and include hypotension, hypoxia, hyperthermia, infectious complications, electrolyte disturbances, and hypo/hyperglycemia. Intracranial factors detected clinically using neurocritical care monitoring, clinical evaluation, and/or neuroimaging include enlargement of TBI-induced hemorrhages, cerebral edema, raised ICP/decreased CPP, seizures, and CBF impairments leading to ischemia (Kinoshita 2016). Furthermore, neuroinflammatory and neurodegenerative cascades initiated early may be prolonged and continue for years following TBI (Johnson et al. 2012, 2013a; Smith et al. 2013a; Ding et al. 2008). In the following paragraphs, the pathophysiology of severe TBI from a clinical and molecular perspective is outlined.

6.2 Pathophysiology of Severe TBI: Clinical Perspectives

6.2.1 Primary and Secondary Injuries

TBI can be classified in several ways. One of the clinically most important is the classification into primary and secondary injuries. Primary injuries include those pathophysiological events and brain lesions, which are caused by the primary trauma energy affecting the brain. These energies may be caused by a direct impact (such as when the head hits the ground in a fall), acceleration/deceleration, or from a penetrating object. Blast-induced TBIs belong to primary injuries and comprise complex multiple mechanisms, but are rare outside war zones. Different types of primary injury mechanisms are not mutually exclusive, and it is very common that both direct impact and deceleration occur in the same incident.

Primary injuries may be either extra-parenchymal or intra-parenchymal (Table 6.1). Extra-parenchymal injuries include epidural hematomas (EDHs), subdural hematomas (SDHs), and traumatic subarachnoid hemorrhages (tSAH). Intra-parenchymal lesions are traumatic intracerebral hemorrhages, contusions, or traumatic axonal injuries. Traumatic axonal injury is usually widespread and diffuse, known clinically as diffuse axonal injury (DAI). Regularly, many of these may co-occur in the same injury, e.g. a combination of SDH, tSAH, contusions, and axonal injury is common in cases of severe TBI. The presence of a certain type of primary injury is not directly linked to TBI severity, and all types may be seen in both mild and severe cases.

Secondary injuries are various pathophysiological events that are either triggered by the primary injury or consequences of other injuries or complications, with a detrimental effect on the injured brain. Traditionally, secondary injuries have been classified into systemic and intracranial. Systemic secondary injuries include events that may exacerbate the consequences of the primary injury, often by impairing oxygen supply or cellular homeostasis. The most important and common systemic secondary injuries are hypotension and hypoxia. Intracranial secondary injuries are often consequences of the primary brain injury but not unrelated to systemic secondary injuries. Among the most important and common intracranial secondary injuries are increased intracranial pressure, brain edema, and cerebral ischemia. Table 6.2 lists the most important systemic and intracranial secondary injuries, most of which have been discussed in detail elsewhere in this book.

The devastating consequences of the secondary injuries may be exemplified by the axonal injury process. Primary axonal injury from shearing forces may occur from the initial, primary impact although it is a rare event in TBI survivors. Instead, worsening axonal injury is a slow pathological process reaching full extent weeks or months after the trauma event (Ljungqvist et al. 2017), if ever in some cases (Cole et al. 2015), as discussed later in this chapter. Similarly, brain contusions (Figs. 6.2

Table 6.1 Classification of primary brain injuries

Extra-parenchymal	Intra-parenchymal
Epidural hematoma	Contusions
Subdural hematoma	Intracerebral hematoma
Traumatic subarachnoid bleeding	Diffuse axonal injury
	Diffuse vascular injury

Table 6.2 The most important systemic and intracranial secondary injuries

Systemic	Intracranial
Hypoxia	Increased ICP
Hypotension	Brain edema
Hypo-/hyperglycemia	Convulsions/seizures
Hypertermia	Brain ischemia (focal or global)
Electrolyte imbalance	Delayed intracranial bleedings
Coagulation disturbance	
Infections	

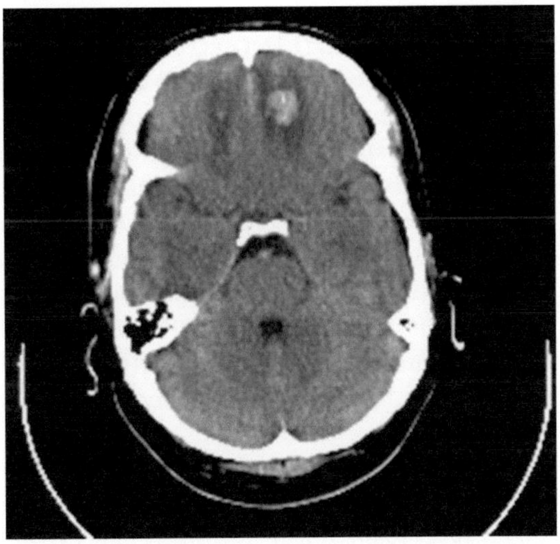

Fig. 6.2 A typical bilateral frontal contusion after hitting the occiput on the ground

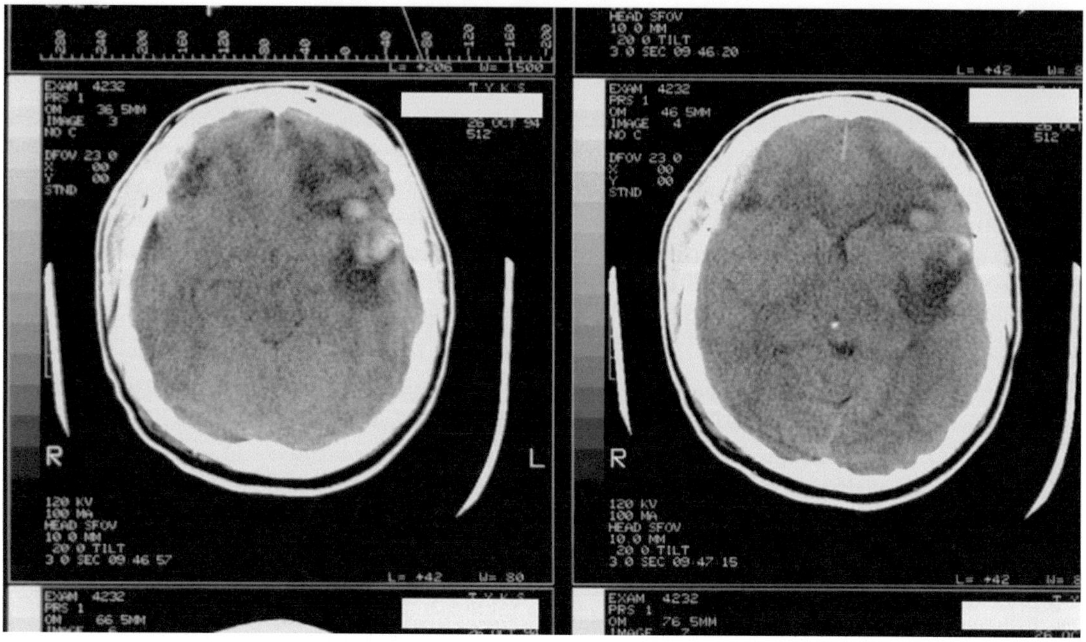

Fig. 6.3 Edema rings surrounding hemorrhagic contusions

and 6.3) may progress markedly within the first post-injury days leading to clinical deterioration. Thus, TBI is a highly dynamic disease where both rapid deterioration and a gradual, progressive decline can be observed.

6.2.2 Epidural Hematomas (EDH)

Epidural hematoma (EDH) is, according to its name, located between the skull and dura. It usually originates from a rupture of a meningeal artery, caused by a skull fracture. The middle meningeal artery injury is the most common source of the bleeding. EDH may be caused also from a venous injury, most often from a ruptured sinus in the posterior fossa, or from venous channels in the skull bone. In both cases, the amount of bleeding is often significant; hence, these usually require rapid neurosurgery.

EDH is typically the cause of the classical 'talk and die' or 'walk and die' course, when after a head trauma there is a lucid interval and the patient is in good clinical condition. The patient may not have lost consciousness at all, and the skull fracture easily escapes clinical examination if it is not depressed. As the blood collects between the skull and dura, it may rapidly lead to a deteriorating clinical situation, manifesting itself as lowering consciousness, hemiparesis, and clinical signs of brain herniation. EDH is often the reason for deaths in jail and is a main reason why patients with head trauma need frequent observation and monitoring of vital signs in the emergency department (ED). Once treated in time, the prognosis of EDH is very good if not accompanied by intracerebral lesions. Small EDHs may not require neurosurgery but need careful observation until the risk for progression is over.

EDH is more frequent in young people, because with age the dura adheres more tightly to the skull, leaving no room for an EDH. EDH is usually easy to separate from SDH on CT-imaging, by its lens-like structure, and frequent association with a skull fracture at the site of hematoma. However, a skull fracture is not a prerequisite for an EDH. In addition, EDHs do not cross epidural compartments, which are defined by the skull sutures, whereas SDHs often cover the whole hemisphere.

6.2.3 Subdural Hematomas (SDH)

Acute SDH has the worst prognosis and highest mortality of traumatic intracranial lesions (Ryan et al. 2012). SDH is usually of venous origin and located according to its name between the dura and the brain. SDH may also be caused by an arterial bleeding, but rupture of the bridging veins on brain surface is the typical cause of SDH.

SDH has much worse prognosis than EDH for many reasons, even if treated in time. First, contusions and DAI frequently accompany it. Second, SDH has a higher risk of rebleeding. Third, SDH frequently causes ischemia and metabolic disturbance in the underlying brain tissue. Fourth, brain edema frequently develops after SDH, causing elevated ICP and brain ischemia. As in the case with EDHs, small SDHs may be observed without neurosurgery, and they may spontaneously resolve within a few days or more. On the other hand, it is also common that an acute SDH leads to subacute and chronic forms of SDH, where the subdural blood has partly or wholly turned into subdural fluid collection.

The neurological symptoms from SDH are usually caused because of its influence on the underlying brain tissue, either from pure compression or ischemia and metabolic dysfunction. Because of its tendency to cause ischemia, SDH may also mimic stroke or transient ischemic attacks. Compressive effects are often easily visible on brain CT, but the neurological symptoms do not always correlate with the degree of compression because of these other potential mechanisms. If sufficiently large, the compressive effect and edema may lead to brain herniation.

SDH is usually fairly easy to recognize in brain imaging, especially when presenting as a large subdural collection of blood covering most of the hemispheric surface. SDHs may also be quite small, when distinction from an EDH is not always easy. Small SDHs located on the inferior surface of the brain may escape detection by CT imaging and be better visible on MR imaging.

6.2.4 Traumatic Subarachnoid Hemorrhage (tSAH)

Similar to other intracranial bleedings, tSAH may appear as the sole injury, or be accompanied with other types of injuries. It is usually easily separable from spontaneous aneurysmal SAH because of different localization of the blood and presentation after a trauma, as well as from SAH caused by an arteriovenous malformation. However, in some cases, this differential diagnosis is not straightforward, and it may be difficult to tell if the SAH caused the fall/injury or if the fall/injury caused a tSAH. If clinical doubt of the origin of SAH exists, imaging of brain vasculature is needed.

The severity of tSAH is very variable, ranging from small amount of blood in one cortical sulcus to large amounts of blood in the subarachnoid space, including the ventricles. If not confounded by other concomitant lesions, the amount of blood correlates strongly with the severity of clinical symptoms. Similarly as in non-traumatic SAH, subarachnoid blood disposes to vasospasms in cerebral arteries and to impaired CSF flow and hydrocephalus.

In many studies, the presence of tSAH has been a poor prognostic sign and is included in some of the CT scores with predictive value in TBI (Thelin et al. 2017). Yet, there are studies with opposite results (Nassiri et al. 2017), showing nicely the complexity of TBIs, where no single variable is able to give reliable prognostic predictions. In case of tSAH, the amount of blood, other concomitant intracranial lesions, and level of consciousness together largely determine the prognosis and not the lack/presence of tSAH itself. Indeed, small amount of tSAH without other signs of severe TBI usually has a fairly benign course (Thelin et al. 2017; Nassiri et al. 2017).

6.2.5 Contusions and Traumatic Intracerebral Bleedings

Contusion is the most common type of intracranial visible traumatic lesions. It is a typical impact lesion, although it may be caused also from pure acceleration/deceleration, when the moving brain bruises either against the bony ridges of the skull base or inner skull surface. The vast majority of contusions are located either frontally or temporally and often bilaterally. These predilection sites are caused either by the aforementioned skull base anatomy, with bony ridges causing bruises in the overlaying frontal and/or temporal lobes in a sudden movement, or by a contra-coup injury where the side opposite to the skull impact shows the greatest brain movement against the skull. This coup/contra-coup mechanism is typical for contusions, where there may be a small contusion at the site of impact and a larger contusion on the opposite side of the brain (Fig. 6.2). In a typical ground-level fall, the posterior part of the head strikes the ground, resulting in bilateral contusions in the frontal lobes and often to a lesser extent bilaterally in the temporal lobes. Consequently, injuries of several brain lobes simultaneously are fairly common. When a person falls frontwards, usually the outstretched arms absorb most of the impact energy; hence, occipital contusions are less common. The tentorium also protects the occipital parts of the brain from contusions.

Although many contusions are visible on admission, they may also develop with delay, often becoming visible not before the second or third day from the injury. Often neurological deterioration is caused by delayed contusion progression with surrounding edema. Some of the contusions are resolving while others are expanding, with expanding ones often surrounded with a "ring" of edema and ischemia (Newcombe et al. 2013) (Fig. 6.3), resembling the classical penumbra surrounding a brain infarction or hemorrhage. Most contusions contain a hemorrhagic core and surrounding edema, with variable relationships. The terms "intracerebral traumatic hemorrhage" and "traumatic intracranial bleeding" are often used interchangeably with contusion, especially if bleeding predominates instead of local edema. Most contusions do not require surgical measures, but large superficial bleedings may require evacuation if they cause marked compression, elevated ICP, and neurological deterioration.

6.2.6 Diffuse Axonal Injury (DAI)

In the original report by Strich in 1956, widespread axonal injury was observed at autopsy 5–15 months following severe TBI. Extensive experimental and clinical results later characterized the clinical entity of DAI (Adams et al. 1982) and showed that axons and other components of the white matter were vulnerable to rotational acceleration–deceleration forces causing shear injuries. It was suggested that axonal injury was the mechanism explaining unconsciousness and prolonged coma post-TBI in the absence of focal injuries (Gennarelli et al. 1982). At autopsy, DAI was found to be characterized by β-amyloid precursor protein (βAPP) accumulations observed as either a classical axonal bulb, caused by a single large axonal swelling, or axonal varicosities with several localized swellings in a single axon (Johnson et al. 2013b). The βAPP accumulation is caused by impaired axonal transport by injury and is described in more detail in the following paragraphs.

Diffuse injuries can be classified using the Marshall CT classification, or other CT classification scores. None of these are specific for DAI. The commonly used classification proposed by Adams in 1989 is based on histopathology obtained at autopsy (Adams et al. 1989), where Grade 1 is axonal injury in the cerebral hemispheres, in particular the grey–white interface, Grade 2 axonal injury in the corpus callosum, and Grade 3 axonal injury in the brainstem. Increasing use of MRI enabled adoption of this grading scale to modern neuroimaging. In patients with severe TBI, MRI commonly reveals Grade 3 DAI, although it must be noted that also high-resolution MRI is unable to depict the full extent of axonal injury (Abu Hamdeh et al. 2017; Skandsen et al. 2010). Several recent studies have attempted to improve the prognostic use of the Adams classification by using a detailed evaluation of brain stem pathology post-TBI (Moe et al. 2018). It should be emphasized that e.g. microhemorrhages observed on CT and/or MRI is not diagnostic of DAI—it merely suggests the presence of axonal injury. Furthermore, the link between vascular injury and DAI cannot be confirmed on regular MRI imaging. It is now established that axonal injury is not only observed in patients with a severely depressed level of consciousness, but isolated DAI in the absence of any focal mass lesions is yet a rather infrequent finding acutely in patients with severe TBI (Skandsen et al. 2010). Instead, in up to 50% of those with focal lesions, widespread axonal pathology is also present at autopsy, and some degree of axonal injury is plausibly present in a majority of severe TBI patients (Tsitsopoulos et al. 2017).

Axonal injury commonly has a profoundly negative impact on outcome (Adams et al. 2011; Kampfl et al. 1998; Graham et al. 2005). In severe TBI, patients with "pure" DAI presenting with deep unconsciousness have a poor prognosis reflected by the extent of brain stem and/or thalamic injury. Axonal injury also induces brain network disconnections with consequences such as impairment of cognition, executive functions and attention, visualized by newer MRI methodologies such as resting state MRI and diffusion tensor imaging studies. Disruptions in important white matter tracts such as the thalamo-frontal network, corpus callosum, limbic fibers, and interconnecting pathways related to the hippocampus and the diencephalon have been revealed and are linked to cognitive deficits (Kinnunen et al. 2011; Hayes et al. 2016; Fagerholm et al. 2015).

6.3 Pathophysiology of Severe TBI: Molecular Perspectives

6.3.1 Excitotoxicity, Mitochondrial Disturbance, and Cell Death

A pivotal initiating event in TBI is the massive release of the excitatory neurotransmitter glutamate, which may act on different types of glutamate receptors. These receptors may be divided into ionotropic (α-amino-3-hydroxy-5-methyl-4-isoxazolepropionic acid (AMPA/kainate) and *N*-methyl-D-aspartate (NMDA)) and metabotropic (mGluR1-5) receptor subtypes. In TBI, increased extracellular levels of glutamate lead to excitotoxicity due to excess activation of these receptors and the ensuing cascades that lead to detrimental intracellular effects. When high concentrations of glutamate in the synaptic cleft act on post-synaptic NMDA receptors, cation channels for calcium and sodium are opened in an uncontrolled fashion. This leads to the failure of Na+/K+ ATPase ion pump and excessive intracellular calcium levels. Furthermore, the increased intracellular calcium, which is another crucial pathophysiological event in TBI, leads to mitochondrial swelling. This, in turn, has numerous negative consequences for cell function, including impaired generation of ATP, which would be needed to restore membrane pump dysfunction. The depletion of high-energy phosphates (ATP) may be a rapid event and is associated with the increase of lactic acid and local acidosis (See Fig. 6.1).

Additionally, impaired mitochondrial function leads to increased generation of reactive oxygen species, impaired radical scavenging and release of cell death promoting molecules such as B-cell lymphoma 2 (BCl-2), apoptosis-inducing factor (AIF), and cytochrome-C. Furthermore, elevated levels of peroxynitrite contribute to the oxidation of cellular components in a process named lipid peroxidation, resulting in cell membrane dysfunction and impairment of cell function. The increased calcium levels also lead to increased activation of enzymes with destructive properties (lipases, proteases, nucleases) including caspases and calpains, dysfunction of the Golgi apparatus, and disaggregation of polyribosomes leading to impairment or dysfunction of protein synthesis.

TBI may also disrupt the delicate balance between neurons, astroglia, and the cerebral vasculature, further making the neurons vulnerable. It must be stated that although neurons have received most attention in TBI, other cell types such as glial and endothelial cells may be highly vulnerable to TBI as well. The key role of glutamate has been repeatedly ascertained, and blockade of glutamate receptors protects neurons from excitotoxicity and attenuates experimental neuronal damage in vivo. To date, attenuation of excitotoxicity has not translated into clinical treatment options, probably due to the difficulty of achieving sufficiently high concentrations of a pharmacological compound at the immediate post-injury time point (Cheng et al. 2012; Lamade et al. 2019).

Neurons are highly complex, are not replaced following injury to a significant degree during adulthood, and may live over 100 years. A constant protection against endogenous and exogenous toxins, replacement and repair of intracellular constituents, and a continuous production of energy is needed. For cellular function, an intact cell structure and maintenance of intra–extracellular osmotic and ionic gradients is crucial. The ability to maintain membrane integrity—cellular compartmentalization—is of paramount importance and when disrupted by the previously mentioned cascades, cell death ensues. Although cell death may be considered a continuum across a spectrum of cell death mechanisms, some key mechanisms may be identified.

- **Necrosis** is considered an uncontrolled, passive, and non-programmed form of cell death, without the intricate regulatory mechanisms as observed in apoptosis. It induces inflammation of surrounding tissues due to release of intracellular contents. It is also characterized by variable morphology, loss of cell membrane integrity, and lysosomal involvement, leading to autophagic and nonlysosomal disintegration.
- **Apoptosis** is a "programmed" and active form of cell death with complex regulatory mechanisms, which require energy. In the cell nucleus, chromatin condensation and nuclear fragmentation are observed. Membranes and organelles including mitochondria are preserved during early apoptotic cell death, including the formation of apoptotic bodies densely packed with cellular organelles and nuclear fragments. These cellular constituents are phagocytized by surrounding cells, and compared to necrosis, apoptosis is "cleaner" and does not induce an inflammatory response. Apoptosis is also observed during normal development.
- **Autophagocytosis** is mainly a morphologic definition and is considered a type of cell death associated with autophagosomes and autolysosomes. There is some controversy whether this is a specific mechanism of cell death.

Under normal conditions, proteolysis of regulatory, oxidized, and misfolded proteins, as well as aggregated proteins and even organelles takes place in the proteasome. Misfolded proteins may avoid detection by the ubiquitine system, and thus escape degradation in the proteasome system. This may allow certain proteins (tau, beta-amyloid, α-synuclein, etc.) to aggregate and accumulate in the injured brain, ultimately leading to cell dysfunction and/or cell death.

Thus, a mix of cell death patterns is anticipated in TBI. Importantly, severe TBI results in a progressive atrophy of the injured brain—to the same extent to that observed in Alzheimer's disease (Cole et al. 2015). Both neuronal cell death and, most importantly, white matter atrophy contribute to the ongoing loss of brain tissue. Importantly, oligodendrocyte death has been observed in severe TBI (Flygt et al. 2016), which may contribute to the observed white matter pathology.

6.3.2 Alterations of Cerebral Blood Flow (CBF)

The delivery of sufficient blood flow is imperative after severe TBI. Under normal conditions, the brain receives about 15% of the total blood volume, uses 20% of all oxygen, and consumes 25% of all glucose, despite constituting only ~2% of total body weight. In uninjured conditions, the brain receives a CBF of 50–54 mL/100 g brain tissue/min. Critical level is considered 18–20 mL/100 g brain tissue/min, and imminent cell death occurs at a CBF <10 mL/100 g brain tissue/min. Physiologically, the energy need at rest is, to a vast majority, fully met by aerobic oxidative phosphorylation.

After TBI, the energy requirement of the brain increases tremendously for the reasons described in the previous paragraphs. Furthermore, a CBF/energy metabolism mismatch is common

(Fig. 6.1). Although the CBF levels following TBI are markedly heterogeneous and may depend on a variety of individual factors, some characteristic CBF changes may be identified. First, in severe TBI patients who have died from their injury, 90% show widespread ischemic changes at autopsy (Graham et al. 1989). However, although there is a clear reduction of CBF during the first 12 post-injury hours in about 1/3 of patients, PET studies indicate that the metabolic needs are usually met and that frank ischemia has not developed (Kawai et al. 2008; Rostami et al. 2014). During the first few days, a reduced CBF down to about 50% of normal values may be observed. Thereafter for up to 4–5 days, either a normal or increased ("luxury perfusion") CBF emerges, again followed by a second phase of reduced CBF lasting up to 2 weeks post-injury (Rostami et al. 2014). In severe TBI, the tight coupling between CBF and neuronal metabolism is typically lost. Impaired energy metabolism in TBI is not only related to CBF, but it is also related to the increased energy requirements of the brain and on the availability and use of energy substrates. Both PET and microdialysis data suggest that a metabolic depression due to mitochondrial dysfunction is common. Furthermore, early hyperglycolysis, defined as increased cerebral glucose utilization relative to cerebral energy demand, is a common feature of TBI (Glenn et al. 2003). Finally, in severe TBI frank ischemia may occur, and if so it is strongly correlated with clinical outcome, as observed in fatal TBI cases. Thus, in severe TBI cases, ischemia should be avoided at all costs, although it may be less common than previously thought.

6.4 Cerebral Edema Post-TBI

Normal ICP is commonly stated to be in the range of 7–15 mmHg. However, due to the invasive methods used to measure ICP, the assessment of a completely normal ICP has been difficult. Recently, using implanted ICP sensors following unruptured aneurysm surgery or following removal of small brain tumors, the normal ICP was estimated to be ~0.5 ± 4.0 mmHg in the supine position (Andresen and Juhler 2014). Following severe TBI, there is an inevitable increase in ICP due to e.g. hemorrhages and the accumulation of cerebral edema. The accumulation of edema may lead to increased mass effect, increased ICP, and potentially herniation. When tissue pressure increases due to swelling, there may be a capillary lumen collapse leading to cerebral ischemia, thus exacerbating the edema. In fact, cerebral edema and brain swelling after traumatic brain injury were estimated to account for up to 50% of patient mortality (Donkin and Vink 2010).

Cerebral edema can be defined as a pathological increase in the water mass contained by the brain interstitial space. The current concept of edema formation post-TBI includes a sequence of events from an initial cytotoxic edema that is rapidly followed by ionic edema and then vasogenic edema, elegantly reviewed in Stokum et al. (2016).

Cytotoxic edema occurs in the immediate post-injury minutes after TBI and is caused by influx of mainly Na+, Cl− and water from the interstitial spaces. It occurs in all cell types in the brain, although predominately in astrocytes. An important difference to the transvascular types of edema (ionic and vasogenic edema) is that cytotoxic edema does not generate tissue swelling, since it merely rearranges water in the brain. Ionic edema arises following the cytotoxic edema, occurs extracellularly, and is characterized by an intact blood–brain barrier (BBB). It is caused by the Na+ gradient generated by cytotoxic edema and is the result of extravasation of Na+ and water, with Na+ accumulating in brain parenchyma. The vasogenic edema also arises extracellularly hours after the injury and in contrast to ionic edema it includes extravasation of plasma proteins and breakdown of the BBB, allowing IgG and albumin to enter the brain interstitial space, although not erythrocytes. Surrounding TBI-induced hematomas, a perihematomal edema arises triggered by the marked toxicity of blood to brain tissue. The hematoma, and its degradation products, leads to the formation of ionic edema, vasogenic edema, and delayed vasogenic edema. Thrombin, one of the key components in a cerebral hemorrhage, is a major contributor to the formation of perihematomal vasogenic edema by inducing an inflammatory response with the release of cytokines and infiltration of leucocytes from the circulation. The delayed vasogenic edema is mainly formed in response to hemoglobin degradation products such as methemoglobin, its heme moiety, and free iron which reaches peak tissue levels in ~3 days post-injury. Free iron is then known to lead to ROS production and BBB breakdown. BBB breakdown, known to persist up to a year or more in a significant proportion of TBI survivors (Hay et al. 2015), is another key component of edema formation in TBI. Numerous factors contribute to the maintenance of an intact BBB such as the interaction of the endothelium with e.g. neurons and glial cells that constitute the neurovascular unit (Nag et al. 2011). The BBB is crucial for maintaining cerebral homeostasis and TBI matrix metalloproteinases, as well as angiogenic factors and growth factors may be future treatment targets post-injury. Cerebral edema is a crucial injury mechanism in TBI that can partly (and briefly) be attenuated by hyperosmolar solutions such as hypertonic saline and mannitol, although much more research is needed to better refine pharmacological treatment options.

6.5 Inflammation and Immunity

Traditionally, TBI has been considered as an acute mechanical injury, and only recently, the possible major role of immunological aspects has been recognized. The disruptive energy forces of TBI predispose the brain for immunological cascades at least by two different mechanisms: cell death and necrosis liberating pro-inflammatory substances from cells; and disruption of the BBB allowing circulating immune cells to enter the brain. In addition, some aspects of the immune reactions triggered by a TBI can be classified as beneficial, aiming at limiting the injury and destroying harmful constituents released by the injury, whereas others are detrimental, considered to exaggerate and prolong immune responses resulting in chronic inflammation and progressive damage. Furthermore, the immunological responses and cascades can be classified as local, affecting the brain and injured brain regions; or systemic, affecting the whole body.

The immunological reactions triggered by a TBI involve a variety of immunological cells and mediators: neutrophils, macrophages, microglia, T-cells, and a large number of cytokines and other immunological mediators (McKee and Lukens 2016). The rapid immunological events occurring after TBI are purposeful protective reactions, aiming at neutralizing harmful mediators, cell constituents, and other potentially toxic substances. This complex acute immunological reaction subsides, and slower, reactive inflammatory processes will be activated. These aim at stabilizing the pathophysiological cascades, and initiating scarring and other healing measures. It appears that these physiological mechanisms may be considered a double-edged sword, turning into prolonged and exaggerated inflammatory reaction escaping proper control, and leading to chronic neuroinflammation and secondary brain damage (Simon et al. 2017).

Although still quite poorly known, the immune system may have a major role as a predictive factor in patients with TBI. Elevated cytokine levels are strongly associated with poor outcome (Di Battista et al. 2016). This is logical: the more severe TBI, the stronger is the immunological response. More interesting is the role of the immune and inflammatory systems in long-term processes and outcome. For reasons still poorly known, about 20% of patients with TBI do not show expected recovery after the acute phase, but rather show a slow constant and chronic decline (Wilson et al. 2017). Although the explanations for these poor outcomes are apparently multifactorial, there is increasing evidence from both experimental and human studies that chronic neuroinflammation may be a cause of this unfavorable outcome (Faden and Loane 2015). This has also raised hope that this course could be inhibited or reversed by anti-inflammatory therapies and that the time window for these interventions may be very long. Thus far, clinically useful interventions have not been found, but research in this field is active. Why only some patients with TBI have this adverse clinical course is not known, but it seems likely that genetic properties might play a role.

Not only does the immune system affect the injured brain, since experimental studies suggest that a severe TBI has a permanent effect on the immune system, leading to accelerated immune aging and chronic deficits in the immune system (Ritzel et al. 2018). This might be one explanation for TBI as chronic disease, which not only has an additive effect with aging phenomena but also is disease-causative (Masel and DeWitt 2010).

6.5.1 Pathophysiology of Axonal Injury

The principal mechanism resulting in axonal injury is rotational acceleration–deceleration forces resulting in deformation of the brain tissue, surpassing the resilience to mechanical stretch of the uninjured brain. Due to the variable densities of gray and white matter, rotational forces result in tension at the gray/white matter interface (Andriessen et al. 2010), and a rapid stretch of the axon will result in injury to the axonal membrane, then leading to injury of the axonal cytoskeleton. Primary axotomy has been observed in very severe TBI in patients dying at or shortly after the injury, but it seems to be rare in those who survive longer times after a TBI. Instead, a cascade of events will trigger axonal pathology leading to delayed axotomy (Smith et al. 2013b; Hill et al. 2016). The TBI-induced axonal stretch initiates opening of sodium channels, with ensuing calcium influx. The rapid increase of intracellular calcium then leads to the activation of calpains and caspases, which then causes disruption of microtubuli and neurofilaments. The injury to the cytoskeleton leads to impaired axonal transport, both antero- and retrogradely. This disturbs neuronal functions and leads to intra-axonal accumulation of numerous proteins and axonal swelling, which in turn may cause delayed axonal transection. In severe axonal injury, rapid opening of the axolemma with loss of control of membrane permeability—axonal mechanoporation—leads to further exacerbation of calcium influx, distal axonal fragmentation and axonal disconnection. Furthermore, the rapid calcium influx results in local mitochondrial damage with subsequent increase in the release of reactive oxygen species (ROS) and an impaired energy metabolism. In the event of axonal transection, the distal axonal segment will undergo a process of disintegration—the Wallerian degeneration.

These events are initiated early post-injury and then progress over the course of days to weeks or even longer. As noted in the previous section, βAPP is the hallmark histopathological finding of axonal injury and is detected in injured and swollen axons. βAPP is the precursor of β-amyloid (Aβ) species, found aggregated in the brains of Alzheimer's disease (AD) victims. βAPP-degrading enzymes such as presenilin-1 and beta-site APP-cleaving enzyme (BACE-1) also aggregate within injured axons, leading to the accumulation of Aβ peptides (Chen et al. 2004). In addition, immunohistochemistry and PET studies have shown prolonged accumulations of Aβ years after the injury (see Chap. 86). The small, monomeric Aβ peptides may also assemble as large soluble oligomers, forming protofibrils. Plausibly, the Aβ oligomers and protofibrils may be important factors resulting in neurotoxicity following TBI (Abu Hamdeh et al. 2018). The soluble protofibrils may subsequently form the insoluble fibrils typical of Aβ plaques observed in TBI and in AD. Intriguing data show that Aβ plaques, developing over many years in AD, are deposited in the brains of about a third of TBI victims within the first post-injury days. The aggregation of Aβ seems to be linked to the genetic presence of the ε4 allele for the lipid transporter protein apolipoprotein E (APOE ε4), a well-known risk factor for both AD and worse outcome following TBI (see Chap. 86).

In AD, the hallmark histopathological finding is not only the Aβ plaque but also neurofibrillary tangles (NFTs) consisting of hyperphosphorylated tau (P-tau) protein. Tau is microtubule-associated, and its physiological activity is regulated by the degree of phosphorylation. Hyperphosphorylation may cause aggregation of tau into NFTs, and increased tau release is associated with axonal injury and a worse clinical outcome (Magnoni et al. 2012, 2015). In long-time survivors of TBI, increased numbers of NFTs were observed at autopsy, similar to Aβ deposits (Johnson et al. 2012), suggesting a persistent pathophysiological process causing NFT aggregation that may be linked to axonal injury. Severe TBI is a known environmental risk factor for AD (see Chap. 82). The mechanisms outlined here may be contributing to the link between TBI and various neurodegenerative disorders, although the exact role of axonal injury in these processes remains to be established.

Although axonal injury has received and deserved most scientific attention, there are other components of the white matter that may contribute to the pathophysiology of TBI. Importantly, white matter degradation has been shown to persist for years following TBI, linked and associated with a persistent inflammation (Johnson et al. 2013a). Myelin injury has also been observed in both the experimental and clinical TBI setting. Recently, death of the myelin-producing oligodendrocytes (OLs) was observed in human TBI, associated with an increased number of the resident oligodendrocyte progenitor cells (OPCs). Obviously, loss of mature OLs may lead to impaired neuronal signaling and to increased axonal vulnerability. Whether the increased number of OPCs may replace the lost OLs and/or lead to remyelination of demyelinated axons remains to be established. Also, even though myelinated axons have been more extensively studied, unmyelinated axons may have a higher vulnerability to injury, which needs further studies.

Unfortunately, central nervous system (CNS) axons do not spontaneously regenerate after injury. Important contributors to the restriction of CNS plasticity are the myelin-associated inhibitors (MAI (Johnson et al. 2012), Fig. 6.4), including the molecules Nogo-A, myelin-associated glycoprotein (MAG), and oligodendrocyte-associated glycoprotein (OMgp), all sharing the NgR1 receptor. After injury, the expression of Nogo-A increases, which may lead to the activation of numerous down-stream cascades, ultimately leading to a failure of axonal regeneration. Furthermore, neuronal-intrinsic factors specific to the CNS may be additional contributing factors to the inability of CNS axon regeneration (Armstrong et al. 2016; Geoffroy and Zheng 2014).

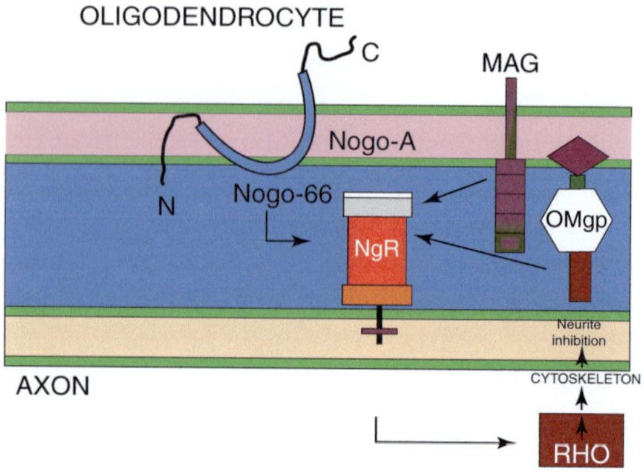

Fig. 6.4 Heavily simplified overview of the factors contributing to the absence of outgrowth possibilities following axonal injury in the adult CNS. *NgR* Nogo-66 receptor 1, *MAG* myelin-associated glycoprotein, *OMgp* oligodendrocyte-myelin glycoprotein

6.5.2 Temporal Aspects

TBI and especially severe TBI is a very dynamic injury. Both rapid recovery and sudden deterioration are common and well-known clinically. At the molecular and cellular level, all the various pathophysiological cascades have different temporal courses, both what comes to the initiation and duration of the injury process. During the first hours and days, edema formation, neutrophil activation, necrosis, excitotoxicity, and calcium influx are the prevailing events. After a few days post-injury, apoptosis and microglial activation emerge, while e.g. necrotic cell death has subsided. Later, demyelination, neuronal disconnection, neuroinflammation, and Wallerian degeneration become important, and epileptogenesis may start developing. Although all these different pathophysiological processes have their typical courses and time windows, individual differences may be marked due to several reasons, both injury- and treatment-related, as well as genetic.

One of the main reasons for lack of major progress and lack of targeted therapies for TBI has been insufficient knowledge of the pathophysiological cascades, and especially lack of tools to detect and monitor them. Targeted interventions cannot be developed, if ways to measure the presence and severity of the target pathophysiology are not available. This temporal variability and complexity are big challenges both for the clinical conventional diagnostics and for new diagnostic tools. For example, the optimal time for using different MRI sequences to detect TBI-related pathology is not known. Continuous monitoring of the gross cerebral physiology at the ICU tries partly to overcome these challenges and helps to prevent and treat some secondary injuries. However, the cellular mechanisms behind most events remain unknown, and thus the treatments are often made on a "best guess" basis. Microdialysis (see Chap. 42) may aid in solving these problems, and it helps to determine if deterioration is caused by ischemia or mitochondrial failure, guiding treatment decisions.

The active research on brain-injury biomarkers has also suffered from simplistic views, as if one sample (and one biomarker) at admission could give sufficient information. It has become evident that the complex and dynamic events of TBI have to be measured and monitored by serial samples of a panel of biomarkers, thus enabling to determine which processes are emerging and which ones are subsiding. This kind of approach is especially important in severe TBI, where multiple mechanisms may be operating at different time points.

6.6 Recovery Mechanisms and Plasticity

As discussed in more detail elsewhere in this book, the unpredictable outcome remains a major challenge for the clinicians. This is true for both short- and long-term predictions. During the acute stage, the clinical course of a severe TBI may take sudden turns, not only towards worse outcome but often also unexpectedly towards recovery. While these may often have obvious treatment-related causes, such as drug-related effects, there are also biological processes, which may manifest unpredictably.

During the acute phase, recovery mechanisms are only beginning to emerge, but fairly rapid improvement of the clinical stage may be observed due to resolving edema, cessation of cortical spreading depression or epileptiform activity, or reversal of subtle brain ischemia. During the first days and weeks, true recovery mechanism will become active (Mannino et al. 2018) and start by both limiting the injury and its consequences, as well as promoting regeneration and plasticity.

During the subacute period following severe TBI, it is clinically difficult to separate the contribution of resolving pathology from active recovery as a driver for clinical recovery. Biological mechanisms favoring recovery during this period include at least partly remyelination, immunological neutralization of toxic substances and constituents, and metabolic adjustment including increased CBF and glucose and energy metabolism. However, at least on an individual level, it is difficult or impossible to determine when these phenomena are signs of active recovery and when caused by chronic damage. All these alterations have been reported also at the chronic stage (McGuire et al. 2019) obviously reflecting the increased needs of the injured brain.

Long-term follow-up studies show that at least 50% of patients with TBI gradually improve over time, in some cases substantially. The mechanisms for recovery are intriguing in view of the lack of axonal regeneration and that lost neuronal cells are not replaced to a significant degree within the injured brain. Instead, a key mechanism for recovery is endogenous plasticity, which is in turn affected by both environmental and genetic factors. The molecular mechanisms leading to brain plasticity after TBI remain poorly understood, although sprouting of both local and long-range axonal projections, synaptic plasticity with altered neurotransmission, and re-shaping of the neuronal networks (Bose et al. 2015) may all be involved. Several neurotrophic substances and neurotransmitters have been shown or suggested to regulate and/or promote plasticity. Most experimental studies have focused on cortical mechanisms (Wolpaw 2007; Pruitt et al. 2017; Axelson et al. 2013; Combs et al. 2016), although recent data suggest that plasticity may occur in the entire CNS, including the spinal cord, and be related to behavioral recovery (Wolpaw 2007; Sist et al. 2014; Tennant 2014). Rehabilitative efforts such as enriched environment as used in the experimental setting and/or physical activity may stimulate endogenous neuroplasticity pathways (see e.g. Petzinger et al. 2013) and factors known to reduce brain plasticity may lead to a worse long-term outcome (Yue et al. 2017) implying an important role for plasticity in the CNS. It must be noted that CNS plasticity may be both beneficial and maladaptive (Tennant 2014), where examples of maladaptive post-injury plasticity include the development of spasticity and epilepsy. Still, promotion of plasticity is likely a key future treatment option for severe TBI. As such treatments are yet to come, the only clinical options are to promote plasticity with rehabilitation and to avoid factors that may interfere with these mechanisms. There is experimental evidence that some commonly used CNS-active drugs such as phenytoin, classical antipsychotics, and benzodiazepines may be detrimental and should possibly be avoided (Goldstein 1995). The timing of these agents may be crucial in this respect, and acute use does not possibly interfere with plasticity, which is a later process. This seems to be supported by clinical experience.

6.7 Conclusion

Severe TBI is among the most complex diseases known, and the vast individuality in injury mechanisms, genetic properties, and brain health makes the treatment of severe TBI extremely challenging. Although the macroscopic injury mechanisms are fairly well known, our knowledge of the cellular and molecular mechanisms is still insufficient. Research efforts should address ways to detect and assess these mechanisms, which would then enable developing of targeted therapies for various pathophysiological cascades. Past failures in bringing promising pharmacological agents from experimental studies to clinics are mainly due to lack of tools to control the vast heterogeneity of human severe TBI.

References

Abu Hamdeh S, Marklund N, Lannsjo M, Howells T, Raininko R, Wikstrom J, et al. Extended anatomical grading in diffuse axonal injury using MRI: hemorrhagic lesions in the Substantia Nigra and Mesencephalic Tegmentum indicate poor long-term outcome. J Neurotrauma. 2017;34(2):341–52.

Abu Hamdeh S, Waara ER, Moller C, Soderberg L, Basun H, Alafuzoff I, et al. Rapid amyloid-beta oligomer and protofibril accumulation in traumatic brain injury. Brain Pathol. 2018;28(4):451–62.

Adams JH, Graham DI, Murray LS, Scott G. Diffuse axonal injury due to nonmissile head injury in humans: an analysis of 45 cases. Ann Neurol. 1982;12(6):557–63.

Adams JH, Doyle D, Ford I, Gennarelli TA, Graham DI, McLellan DR. Diffuse axonal injury in head injury: definition, diagnosis and grading. Histopathology. 1989;15(1):49–59.

Adams JH, Jennett B, Murray LS, Teasdale GM, Gennarelli TA, Graham DI. Neuropathological findings in disabled survivors of a head injury. J Neurotrauma. 2011;28(5):701–9.

Andresen M, Juhler M. Intracranial pressure following complete removal of a small demarcated brain tumor: a model for normal intracranial pressure in humans. J Neurosurg. 2014;121(4):797–801.

Andriessen TM, Jacobs B, Vos PE. Clinical characteristics and pathophysiological mechanisms of focal and diffuse traumatic brain injury. J Cell Mol Med. 2010;14(10):2381–92.

Armstrong RC, Mierzwa AJ, Marion CM, Sullivan GM. White matter involvement after TBI: clues to axon and myelin repair capacity. Exp Neurol. 2016;275(Pt 3):328–33.

Axelson HW, Winkler T, Flygt J, Djupsjo A, Hanell A, Marklund N. Plasticity of the contralateral motor cortex following focal traumatic brain injury in the rat. Restor Neurol Neurosci. 2013;31(1):73–85.

Bose P, Hou J, Thompson FJ. Traumatic brain injury (TBI)-induced spasticity: neurobiology, treatment, and rehabilitation. In: Kobeissy FH, editor. Brain neurotrauma: molecular, neuropsychological, and rehabilitation aspects, Frontiers in neuroengineering. Boca Raton: CRC Press; 2015.

Chen XH, Siman R, Iwata A, Meaney DF, Trojanowski JQ, Smith DH. Long-term accumulation of amyloid-beta, beta-secretase, presenilin-1, and caspase-3 in damaged axons following brain trauma. Am J Pathol. 2004;165(2):357–71.

Cheng G, Kong RH, Zhang LM, Zhang JN. Mitochondria in traumatic brain injury and mitochondrial-targeted multipotential therapeutic strategies. Br J Pharmacol. 2012;167(4):699–719.

Cole JH, Leech R, Sharp DJ, Alzheimer's Disease Neuroimaging Initiative. Prediction of brain age suggests accelerated atrophy after traumatic brain injury. Ann Neurol. 2015;77(4):571–81.

Combs HL, Jones TA, Kozlowski DA, Adkins DL. Combinatorial motor training results in functional reorganization of remaining motor cortex after controlled cortical impact in rats. J Neurotrauma. 2016;33(8):741–7.

Di Battista AP, Rhind SG, Hutchison MG, Hassan S, Shiu MY, Inaba K, et al. Inflammatory cytokine and chemokine profiles are associated with patient outcome and the hyperadrenergic state following acute brain injury. J Neuroinflammation. 2016;13:40.

Ding K, Marquez de la Plata C, Wang JY, Mumphrey M, Moore C, Harper C, et al. Cerebral atrophy after traumatic white matter injury: correlation with acute neuroimaging and outcome. J Neurotrauma. 2008;25(12):1433–40.

Donkin JJ, Vink R. Mechanisms of cerebral edema in traumatic brain injury: therapeutic developments. Curr Opin Neurol. 2010;23(3):293–9.

Faden AI, Loane DJ. Chronic neurodegeneration after traumatic brain injury: Alzheimer disease, chronic traumatic encephalopathy, or persistent neuroinflammation? Neurotherapeutics. 2015;12(1):143–50.

Fagerholm ED, Hellyer PJ, Scott G, Leech R, Sharp DJ. Disconnection of network hubs and cognitive impairment after traumatic brain injury. Brain. 2015;138(Pt 6):1696–709.

Flygt J, Gumucio A, Ingelsson M, Skoglund K, Holm J, Alafuzoff I, et al. Human traumatic brain injury results in oligodendrocyte death and increases the number of oligodendrocyte progenitor cells. J Neuropathol Exp Neurol. 2016;75(6):503–15.

Gennarelli TA, Thibault LE, Adams JH, Graham DI, Thompson CJ, Marcincin RP. Diffuse axonal injury and traumatic coma in the primate. Ann Neurol. 1982;12(6):564–74.

Geoffroy CG, Zheng B. Myelin-associated inhibitors in axonal growth after CNS injury. Curr Opin Neurobiol. 2014;27:31–8.

Glenn TC, Kelly DF, Boscardin WJ, McArthur DL, Vespa P, Oertel M, et al. Energy dysfunction as a predictor of outcome after moderate or severe head injury: indices of oxygen, glucose, and lactate metabolism. J Cereb Blood Flow Metab. 2003;23(10):1239–50.

Goldstein LB. Prescribing of potentially harmful drugs to patients admitted to hospital after head injury. J Neurol Neurosurg Psychiatry. 1995;58(6):753–5.

Graham DI, Ford I, Adams JH, Doyle D, Teasdale GM, Lawrence AE, et al. Ischaemic brain damage is still common in fatal non-missile head injury. J Neurol Neurosurg Psychiatry. 1989;52(3):346–50.

Graham DI, Adams JH, Murray LS, Jennett B. Neuropathology of the vegetative state after head injury. Neuropsychol Rehabil. 2005;15(3–4):198–213.

Hay JR, Johnson VE, Young AM, Smith DH, Stewart W. Blood-brain barrier disruption is an early event that may persist for many years after traumatic brain injury in humans. J Neuropathol Exp Neurol. 2015;74(12):1147–57.

Hayes JP, Bigler ED, Verfaellie M. Traumatic brain injury as a disorder of brain connectivity. J Int Neuropsychol Soc. 2016;22(2):120–37.

Hill CS, Coleman MP, Menon DK. Traumatic axonal injury: mechanisms and translational opportunities. Trends Neurosci. 2016;39(5):311–24.

Johnson VE, Stewart W, Smith DH. Widespread tau and amyloid-beta pathology many years after a single traumatic brain injury in humans. Brain Pathol. 2012;22(2):142–9.

Johnson VE, Stewart JE, Begbie FD, Trojanowski JQ, Smith DH, Stewart W. Inflammation and white matter degeneration persist for years after a single traumatic brain injury. Brain J Neurol. 2013a;136(Pt 1):28–42.

Johnson VE, Stewart W, Smith DH. Axonal pathology in traumatic brain injury. Exp Neurol. 2013b;246:35–43.

Kampfl A, Franz G, Aichner F, Pfausler B, Haring HP, Felber S, et al. The persistent vegetative state after closed head injury: clinical and magnetic resonance imaging findings in 42 patients. J Neurosurg. 1998;88(5):809–16.

Kawai N, Nakamura T, Tamiya T, Nagao S. Metabolic disturbance without brain ischemia in traumatic brain injury: a positron emission tomography study. Acta Neurochir Suppl. 2008;102:241–5.

Kinnunen KM, Greenwood R, Powell JH, Leech R, Hawkins PC, Bonnelle V, et al. White matter damage and cognitive impairment after traumatic brain injury. Brain. 2011;134(Pt 2):449–63.

Kinoshita K. Traumatic brain injury: pathophysiology for neurocritical care. J Intensive Care. 2016;4:29.

Lamade AM, Kenny EM, Anthonymuthu TS, Soysal E, Clark RSB, Kagan VE, et al. Aiming for the target: mitochondrial drug delivery in traumatic brain injury. Neuropharmacology. 2019;145(Pt B):209–19.

Ljungqvist J, Nilsson D, Ljungberg M, Esbjornsson E, Eriksson-Ritzen C, Skoglund T. Longitudinal changes in diffusion tensor imaging parameters of the corpus callosum between 6 and 12 months after diffuse axonal injury. Brain Inj. 2017;31(3):344–50.

Magnoni S, Esparza TJ, Conte V, Carbonara M, Carrabba G, Holtzman DM, et al. Tau elevations in the brain extracellular space correlate with reduced amyloid-beta levels and predict adverse clinical outcomes after severe traumatic brain injury. Brain. 2012;135(Pt 4):1268–80.

Magnoni S, Mac Donald CL, Esparza TJ, Conte V, Sorrell J, Macri M, et al. Quantitative assessments of traumatic axonal injury in human brain: concordance of microdialysis and advanced MRI. Brain. 2015;138(Pt 8):2263–77.

Mannino C, Glenn TC, Hovda DA, Vespa PM, McArthur DL, Van Horn JD, et al. Acute glucose and lactate metabolism are associated with cognitive recovery following traumatic brain injury. J Neurosci Res. 2018;96(4):696–701.

Marklund N, Hillered L. Animal modelling of traumatic brain injury in preclinical drug development: where do we go from here? Br J Pharmacol. 2011;164(4):1207–29.

Masel BE, DeWitt DS. Traumatic brain injury: a disease process, not an event. J Neurotrauma. 2010;27(8):1529–40.

McGuire JL, DePasquale EAK, Watanabe M, Anwar F, Ngwenya LB, Atluri G, et al. Chronic dysregulation of cortical and subcortical metabolism after experimental traumatic brain injury. Mol Neurobiol. 2019;56(4):2908–21.

McKee CA, Lukens JR. Emerging roles for the immune system in traumatic brain injury. Front Immunol. 2016;7:556.

Moe HK, Moen KG, Skandsen T, Kvistad KA, Laureys S, Haberg A, et al. The influence of traumatic axonal injury in thalamus and brainstem on level of consciousness at scene or admission: a clinical magnetic resonance imaging study. J Neurotrauma. 2018;35:975.

Nag S, Kapadia A, Stewart DJ. Review: molecular pathogenesis of blood-brain barrier breakdown in acute brain injury. Neuropathol Appl Neurobiol. 2011;37(1):3–23.

Nassiri F, Badhiwala JH, Witiw CD, Mansouri A, Davidson B, Almenawer SA, et al. The clinical significance of isolated traumatic subarachnoid hemorrhage in mild traumatic brain injury: a meta-analysis. J Trauma Acute Care Surg. 2017;83(4):725–31.

Newcombe VF, Williams GB, Outtrim JG, Chatfield D, Gulia Abate M, Geeraerts T, et al. Microstructural basis of contusion expansion in traumatic brain injury: insights from diffusion tensor imaging. J Cereb Blood Flow Metab. 2013;33(6):855–62.

Petzinger GM, Fisher BE, McEwen S, Beeler JA, Walsh JP, Jakowec MW. Exercise-enhanced neuroplasticity targeting motor and cognitive circuitry in Parkinson's disease. Lancet Neurol. 2013;12(7):716–26.

Pruitt DT, Danaphongse TT, Schmid AN, Morrison RA, Kilgard MP, Rennaker RL 2nd, et al. Traumatic brain injury occludes training-dependent cortical reorganization in the contralesional hemisphere. J Neurotrauma. 2017;34(17):2495–503.

Ritzel RM, Doran SJ, Barrett JP, Henry RJ, Ma EL, Faden AI, et al. Chronic alterations in systemic immune function after traumatic brain injury. J Neurotrauma. 2018;35(13):1419–36.

Rostami E, Engquist H, Enblad P. Imaging of cerebral blood flow in patients with severe traumatic brain injury in the neurointensive care. Front Neurol. 2014;5:114.

Ryan CG, Thompson RE, Temkin NR, Crane PK, Ellenbogen RG, Elmore JG. Acute traumatic subdural hematoma: current mortality and functional outcomes in adult patients at a level I trauma center. J Trauma Acute Care Surg. 2012;73(5):1348–54.

Saatman KE, Duhaime AC, Bullock R, Maas AI, Valadka A, Manley GT, et al. Classification of traumatic brain injury for targeted therapies. J Neurotrauma. 2008;25(7):719–38.

Simon DW, McGeachy MJ, Bayir H, Clark RSB, Loane DJ, Kochanek PM. The far-reaching scope of neuroinflammation after traumatic brain injury. Nat Rev Neurol. 2017;13(9):572.

Sist B, Fouad K, Winship IR. Plasticity beyond peri-infarct cortex: spinal up regulation of structural plasticity, neurotrophins, and inflammatory cytokines during recovery from cortical stroke. Exp Neurol. 2014;252:47–56.

Skandsen T, Kvistad KA, Solheim O, Strand IH, Folvik M, Vik A. Prevalence and impact of diffuse axonal injury in patients with moderate and severe head injury: a cohort study of early magnetic resonance imaging findings and 1-year outcome. J Neurosurg. 2010;113(3):556–63.

Smith DH, Johnson VE, Stewart W. Chronic neuropathologies of single and repetitive TBI: substrates of dementia? Nat Rev Neurol. 2013a;9(4):211–21.

Smith DH, Hicks R, Povlishock JT. Therapy development for diffuse axonal injury. J Neurotrauma. 2013b;30(5):307–23.

Stein SC, Georgoff P, Meghan S, Mizra K, Sonnad SS. 150 years of treating severe traumatic brain injury: a systematic review of progress in mortality. J Neurotrauma. 2010;27(7):1343–53.

Stokum JA, Gerzanich V, Simard JM. Molecular pathophysiology of cerebral edema. J Cereb Blood Flow Metab. 2016;36(3):513–38.

Tennant KA. Thinking outside the brain: structural plasticity in the spinal cord promotes recovery from cortical stroke. Exp Neurol. 2014;254:195–9.

Thelin EP, Nelson DW, Vehvilainen J, Nystrom H, Kivisaari R, Siironen J, et al. Evaluation of novel computerized tomography scoring systems in human traumatic brain injury: an observational, multicenter study. PLoS Med. 2017;14(8):e1002368.

Tsitsopoulos PP, Abu Hamdeh S, Marklund N. Current opportunities for clinical monitoring of axonal pathology in traumatic brain injury. Front Neurol. 2017;8:599.

Wilson L, Stewart W, Dams-O'Connor K, Diaz-Arrastia R, Horton L, Menon DK, et al. The chronic and evolving neurological consequences of traumatic brain injury. Lancet Neurol. 2017;16(10):813–25.

Wolpaw JR. Spinal cord plasticity in acquisition and maintenance of motor skills. Acta Physiol. 2007;189(2):155–69.

Yue GH, Clark BC, Li S, Vaillancourt DE. Understanding neuromuscular system plasticity to improve motor function in health, disease, and injury. Neural Plast. 2017;2017:2425180.

Further Reading

Shetty AK, Mishra V, Kodali M, Hattiangady B. Blood brain barrier dysfunction and delayed neurological deficits in mild traumatic brain injury induced by blast shock waves. Front Cell Neurosci. 2014;8:232. https://doi.org/10.3389/fncel.2014.00232. eCollection 2014.

Classification of Head Injury

7

Ramona Åstrand and Johan Undén

Recommendations

Level I

There is insufficient data to support Level I recommendation for this topic.

Level II

The Glasgow Coma Scale score (GCS) is a reliable and widespread indicator of the severity of TBI.

Level III

Guidelines, such as the ones from the Scandinavian Neurotrauma Committee (SNC) for adults and children, respectively, often stratify patients into severity. The SNC stratification has been validated in external cohorts for both adults and children.

R. Åstrand (✉)
Department of Neurosurgery, Rigshospitalet, Copenhagen University Hospital, Copenhagen, Denmark

J. Undén
Department of Operation and Intensive Care, Hallands Hospital, Halmstad, Sweden

Lund University, Lund, Sweden

7.1 Overview

Head injuries can be categorised in several ways: by mechanism of injury (closed or penetrating injury), morphology (fractures, focal intracranial injury and diffuse intracranial injury) or severity of injury (minimal to severe).

Immediate triage and assessment of the severity and probable survival of the traumatised patient should be made whenever possible already at the scene of injury. Of useful help are the various trauma scores that have been developed to triage patients for care and to evaluate the severity of injury. The scores are based on physiological and/or anatomical features, as well as patient responses. Physiological scores are exemplified by Glasgow Coma Score (GCS) scale (Teasdale and Jennett 1974), the Revised Trauma Score (RTS) (Champion et al. 1989) and the Paediatric Trauma Score (PTS) (Tepas et al. 1987). The Injury Severity Score (ISS) is an anatomical score based on the Abbreviated Injury Scale (AIS) that provides an overall score of the patient (Baker et al. 1974).

The GCS scale has been the most valuable and frequently used scoring system for assessing the level of consciousness and thereby the severity of head trauma. It has, however, some limitations, especially with regard to the verbal component, which is difficult to use in intubated and comatose patients and in patients with aphasia. The Swedish Reaction Level Scale 85 (RLS) is a somewhat simpler scale than the GCS, though

© Springer Nature Switzerland AG 2020
T. Sundstrøm et al. (eds.), *Management of Severe Traumatic Brain Injury*,
https://doi.org/10.1007/978-3-030-39383-0_7

seldom used outside of Sweden (Starmark et al. 1988a, b).

The Full Outline of UnResponsiveness (FOUR) score is a relatively new coma score with four components: eye response, motor response, brainstem reflex and respiration. It does not include assessment of verbal response and has therefore an advantage in assessing critically ill patients in the intensive care setting (Wijdicks et al. 2005).

To estimate severity of brain injury after head trauma, various classification systems of head injury have been proposed and modified throughout the years. Most of them are based on the patients' level of consciousness according to the GCS, as e.g. the Head Injury Severity Scale (HISS) and the Mayo Classification System (Malec et al. 2007; Stein and Spettell 1995).

Tips, Tricks and Pitfalls

- Severe head injury is defined as a patient with conscious level of GCS 3–8 (RLS 4–8) after head injury.
- Traumatic brain injury is defined as primary or secondary injury to the brain after trauma.
- The definition of a paediatric patient varies in Scandinavian hospitals, with an upper age limit either below 16 or 18 years.
- Neurologic assessment, including GCS and pupil response, should be assessed as soon as possible either pre-hospital or at admission, before sedation and intubation for a more correct classification of the severity.
- Intoxicated patients are challenging to classify and should be treated with higher awareness. The GCS score may be decreased by 2–3 points due to heavy alcohol intoxication or drug use; a problematic confounding factor when assessing the level of consciousness in a head-injured patient.

7.2 Background

In the 1960s, there was a common belief amongst neurosurgeons that, aside from evacuating occasional hematomas or elevating depressed fractures, little could be done to influence outcome after head injury. However, with improvement of intensive care and resuscitation, the challenge for neurosurgeons was to assist in reducing mortality and morbidity for these severely head-injured patients. Studies in Glasgow showed that by avoiding potentially preventable secondary brain damage, one could limit the degree of disabilities in survivors (Reilly et al. 1975).

Complications, such as the development of intracranial haematomas or increased intracranial pressure, were difficult to recognise and treatment could be delayed. These concerns lead to the development of the GCS by Jennett and Teasdale in 1974 (Teasdale and Jennett 1974). The scale was initially designed as a research tool for the assessment of the comatose patient, but is now one of the most frequently used scales in triage of head injuries and in daily assessment of severe head injury. The drawback of using the GCS is the confounding effect of alcohol or other drugs, especially during the first few hours after injury. Heavy alcohol intoxication has been associated with a reduction of 2–3 points in GCS in assaulted patients (Brickley and Shepherd 1995).

7.2.1 Classification Systems

In 1981, Rimel and colleagues defined minor head injury as a head trauma with a GCS score of 13–15 at admission, loss of consciousness (LOC) less than 20 min and a duration of hospital admission less than 48 h (Rimel et al. 1981). Approximately a decade later, Stein and Spettell introduced a modified classification system, the Head Injury Severity Scale, a five-interval severity scale (minimal through critical) based primarily on initial GCS score. The HISS scale also includes the aspects of retrograde amnesia, loss of consciousness and focal neurological deficits for each severity interval (Stein and Spettell 1995). Other definitions of mild and moderate head injury vary in the literature, especially with regard to the importance of a GCS score of 13 and the duration of loss of consciousness.

In 2000, the Scandinavian Neurotrauma Committee (SNC) presented management guidelines for head injury (Ingebrigtsen et al. 2000), using a modified version of the HISS classification, dividing head injuries into minimal, mild, moderate and severe (Table 7.1). In the revised Scandinavian head injury guidelines from 2013

Table 7.1 Classification of head injuries according to SNC in 2000 (Ingebrigtsen et al. 2000)

HISS category	Clinical characteristics
Minimal	GCS = 15, no loss of consciousness
Mild	GCS = 14 or 15, brief (<5 min) loss of consciousness or amnesia, or impaired alertness or memory
Moderate	GCS = 9–13, or loss of consciousness ≥5 min, or focal neurologic deficit
Severe	GCS = 3–8

(Fig. 7.1), the classification system has been even further modified (Unden et al. 2013):

- Severe head injury includes all patients with an initial GCS score of 8 or below, hence, unconscious patients.
- Moderate head injury defines a patient with an initial GCS of 9–13.
- Mild head injury is split into three categories: the high-risk, the medium risk and the low-risk, each with defined risk factors for the development of an intracranial complication after head trauma. Mild, high-risk head injury includes patients with GCS of 14–15 and at least one of the following risk factors: post-traumatic seizures, focal neurological deficits, depressed skull fracture or basal skull fracture, shunt-treated hydrocephalus or therapeutic anticoagulation or coagulation disorder. Mild, medium-risk injury includes patients with GCS of 14–15 and being older or equal to

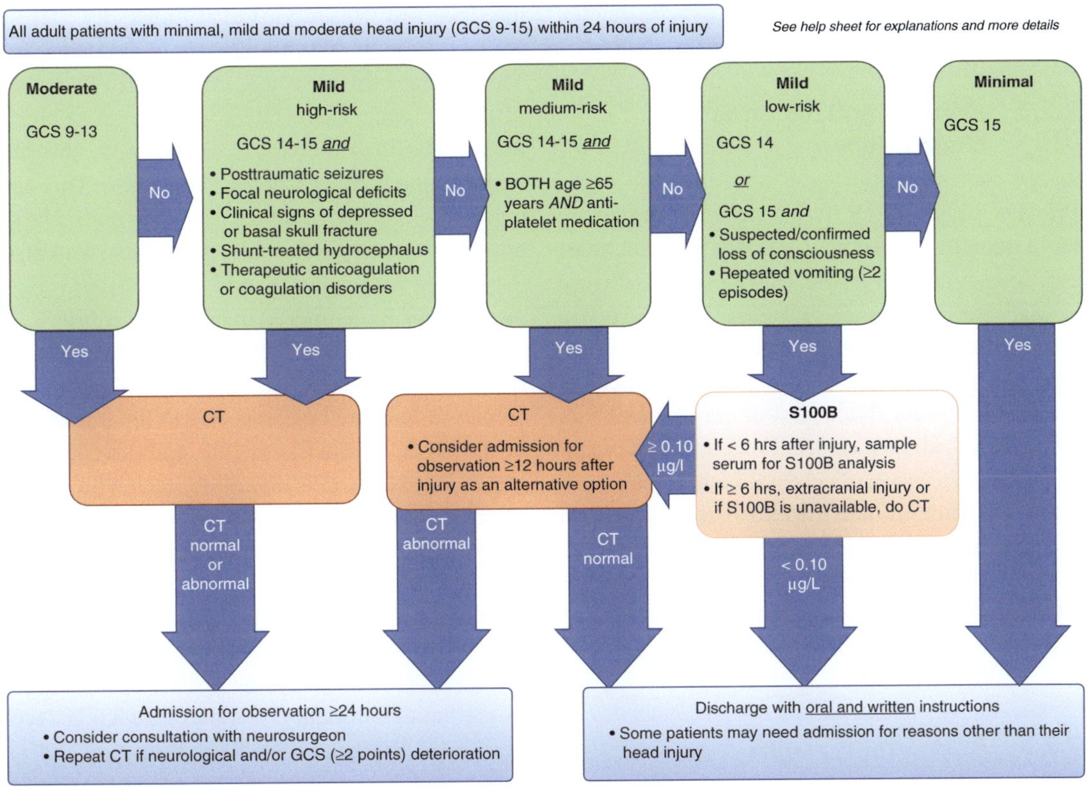

Fig. 7.1 Flowchart and classification of severity according to Scandinavian head trauma guidelines for adults (Unden et al. 2013)

65 years of age and on anti-platelet medication. Mild, low-risk head injury are patients with a GCS of 14 or GCS of 15 and suspected loss of consciousness or repeated vomiting after head trauma.

- Minimal head injury is presented by a patient with GCS 15 at admission and with none of the other risk factors from the previous categories.

The above risk stratification has been externally validated (Ananthaharan et al. 2018; Unden et al. 2015). "Commotio cerebri", or concussion, is a post hoc clinical definition of an awake patient with posttraumatic amnesia, possibly due to brief LOC after head trauma, but without any apparent brain injury. This is a diagnosis used after discharge when complications to the head injury have been ruled out, hence, not useful in the acute setting. Amnesia is most often retrograde, but in some cases even antegrade amnesia is present, i.e. the inability to recall new memories after the head injury event.

7.2.2 Primary and Secondary Brain Injury

Primary brain injury refers to the immediate brain damage caused upon impact. This includes cerebral contusions, shearing lesions (diffuse axonal injuries—DAI) and lacerations from a foreign body. Secondary brain injury refers to progressive brain damage due to development of the primary brain injury and/or extracranial factors. This includes cerebral oedema, hypoxia/ischemia, expansion of cerebral hematomas (subdural and epidural) and the expansion of cerebral contusions and the surrounding focal oedema, all which causes an increase in intracranial pressure (ICP) within the confined skull and can lead to cerebral herniation and death.

7.2.3 Assessment Scales

The Glasgow Coma Scale has been the most valuable and frequently used scoring system for assessing severity of neurologic injury after head trauma. The scale is divided into three parts: eye response, verbal response and motor response, adding to a total score of 3–15 points.

The GCS scale has, however, been considered difficult to apply on especially preverbal children (Yager et al. 1990), since their ability to express themselves verbally or non-verbally in a consistent manner is limited. The response from an infant is also clearly different from an adult. Reilly et al. were the first to design the paediatric version of the GCS, where verbal responses were reported as appropriate words, social smiles, cries, irritability and agitation (Reilly et al. 1988; Simpson and Reilly 1982). Later, some modifications of the scale have also been made to suite even the youngest children and infants (Table 7.2). The paediatric GCS scale has proved to be accurate in evaluating preverbal children with head trauma with regard to the need for acute intervention (Holmes et al. 2005).

In Sweden, the most frequently used scale for the assessment of the level of consciousness is the Swedish Reaction Level Scale 85 (RLS) (Johnstone et al. 1993; Starmark et al. 1988a, b). This scale evaluates the consciousness in an inverted manner to the GCS, with a scoring range from 1 (best) to 8 (worst), and without specific focus on the verbal response (Table 7.3). This has made the score more practical to use, particularly on neurologically traumatised patients (who also may suffer from aphasia) and children, as well as more easily remembered in acute situations.

The Full Outline of UnResponsiveness (FOUR) score was developed to improve assessment of comatose intubated patients due to the limitations of the GCS. It consists of four components: eye, motor, brainstem and respiration, each with a maximum score of 4 (Table 7.4). It is considered to be superior to the GCS due to it being more neurologically detailed and can also recognise a locked-in syndrome and different stages of herniation. The FOUR scale has been validated in the neuro-ICU and medical ICU showing some advantages in predicting mortality compared to GCS (Iyer et al. 2009; Wijdicks et al. 2005; Wolf et al. 2007). A few studies have assessed the use of the FOUR score in adult and paediatric patients in an emergency setting after head trauma. None of the studies showed an advantage of the FOUR score in

Table 7.2 The Glasgow Coma Scale

	Standard	Paediatric version	
		1–4 years	<1 year
Eye opening			
4	Spontaneous	Open	
3	To speech	To voice	
2	To pain	To pain	
1	None	No response	
Verbal response			
5	Orientated	Oriented, speaks, interacts	Coos, babbles
4	Confused conversation	Confused speech, consolable	Irritable cry, consolable
3	Words (inappropriate)	Inappropriate words, inconsolable	Persistent cry, inconsolable
2	Sounds (incomprehensible)	Incomprehensible, agitated	Moans to pain
1	None	No response	No response
Best motor response			
6	Obey commands	Normal spontaneous movement	
5	Localises pain	Localises pain	
4	Flexion, withdraws to pain	Withdraws to pain	
3	Flexion, abnormal to pain	Decorticate flexion	
2	Extension (to pain)	Decerebrate extension	
1	No response	No response	
3–15	Total score		

Table 7.3 The Swedish Reaction Level Scale

Reaction Level Scale (RLS 85)	Score
Fully awake, oriented	1
Lethargic, confused, contact after mild stimuli	2
Stupor, confused, contact after rough stimuli or pain	3
Unconscious, localises to pain	4
Unconscious, withdraws to pain	5
Unconscious, abnormal flexion to pain	6
Unconscious, abnormal extension to pain	7
No response to painful central stimuli	8

predicting morbidity and mortality compared to the GCS (Buyukcam et al. 2012; Eken et al. 2009).

The Revised Trauma Score (RTS) is a numeric grading system for estimating the severity of injury. It is composed of the GCS, systolic blood pressure and respiratory rate, each giving rise to a coded value score between 0 and 4 (Table 7.5). The severity of injury is estimated by the total sum of the three physiological parameters (GCS score, systolic blodd pressure and respiratory rate), ranging from a total RTS of 0 (no sign of life) to 12 (normal vital signs). The trauma scale was revised in 1989 into the RTS (Champion et al. 1989) and is primarily used in the prehospital setting to triage trauma patients to the most appropriate emergency care. A total RTS score < 11 indicates a more severe trauma and need for immediate treatment.

The Injury Severity Score (ISS) is an anatomical score that provides an overall score of the patient with multiple injuries after severe trauma (Table 7.6). It is based on the AIS score, which determines six body regions (head, face, chest, abdomen, extremities and pelvis, and external). The three most severely injured regions are squared and added to produce the ISS. The ISS correlates to mortality, morbidity, hospital stay and other measures of severity but is not considered a good tool for triage (Baker and O'Neill 1976; Baker et al. 1974).

7.3 Specific Paediatric Concerns

In some hospitals, the level of consciousness is more properly evaluated with the use of the paediatric GCS score (Reilly et al. 1988). The Paediatric Trauma Score (PTS) has been developed as an assessment score for trauma severity in children (Table 7.7), but its use in Scandinavia has so far been limited.

Table 7.4 The FOUR score

Scores	Eye response	Motor response	Brainstem	Respiration
4	Eyelids open or opened, tracking or blinking to command	Thumbs-up, fist or peace sign	Pupil and corneal reflexes present	Not intubated, regular breathing pattern
3	Eyelids open but not tracking	Localising to pain	One pupil wide and fixed	Not intubated, Cheyne-Stokes breathing pattern
2	Eyelids closed but open to loud voice	Flexion response to pain	Pupil or corneal reflexes absent	Not intubated, irregular breathing
1	Eyelids closed but open to pain	Extension response to pain	Pupil and corneal reflexes absent	Breathes above ventilatory rate
0	Eyelids remain closed with pain	No response to pain or generalised myoclonus status	Absent pupil, corneal and cough reflex	Breathes at ventilator rate or apnoea

Table 7.5 The Revised Trauma Score (RTS) scale

GCS score	Systolic blood pressure (mmHg)	Respiratory rate (breaths/min)	Coded value
13–15	>89	10–29	**4**
9–12	76–89	>29	**3**
6–8	50–75	6–9	**2**
4–5	1–49	1–5	**1**
3	0	0	**0**

Table 7.6 The Injury Severity Scale (ISS)

Region	Injury description (examples)	AIS	Square top three
Head and neck	No injury	0	
Face	Minor injury	1	
Thorax	Moderate injury	2	
Abdomen and viscera	Serious injury	3	[a]
Bony pelvis and extremities	Severe injury	4	[a]
External structures	Critical injury	5	[a]
Injury Severity Score = sum			0–75

Lethal injury (incompatible with life) = AIS 6 = ISS 75

[a]The three most severe injuries are squared and added, to produce the final ISS score

The head injury classification systems mainly apply to adults, although in clinical practice the previous Scandinavian head injury classification has also been used for children and adolescents. Definitions of mild to moderate head injury in children vary even more extensively in the literature than for adults, especially with regard to the duration of LOC (Committee on Quality Improvement, American Academy of Pediatrics and Commission on Clinical Policies and Research, American Academy of Family Physicians 1999; Schutzman et al. 2001). Other clinical factors such as scalp haematoma, low age (<2 years), history of excessive vomiting and suspected skull fracture and posttraumatic seizures have in former studies and proposed guidelines been considered as risk factors for developing an intracranial complication (Dunning et al. 2006; Holmes et al. 2004; Schutzman et al. 2001), requiring hospitalisation or further radiological investigation.

The Scandinavian head trauma guideline for children was published using similar, but not identical, definitions for the different severity levels as for the adult population (Astrand et al. 2016). The head trauma guideline is applicable to children younger than 18 years of age and with minimal to moderate head trauma within the last 24 h. Head trauma is classified into five categories based on the different risk factors present (Fig. 7.2):

- Moderate head trauma is defined as the child having a GCS of 9–13 on admission.
- Mild head trauma is classified into high risk, medium risk and low risk, depending on different risk factors for development of intracranial complications. The mild, high-risk category includes children with an admission GCS of 14–15 and with at least one of the

Table 7.7 The Paediatric Trauma Score (PTS)

	Category		
Component	+2	+1	−1
Size	≥20 kg	10–20 kg	<10 kg
Airway	Normal	Maintainable	Unmaintainable
Systolic blood pressure	≤90 mmHg	90–50 mmHg	<50 mmHg
CNS	Awake	Obtunded/LOC	Coma/decerebrate
Open wound	None	Minor	Major/penetrating
Skeletal	None	Closed fracture	Open/multiple fractures

Sum total points: −6 to +12. Scores <9 = potentially significant trauma

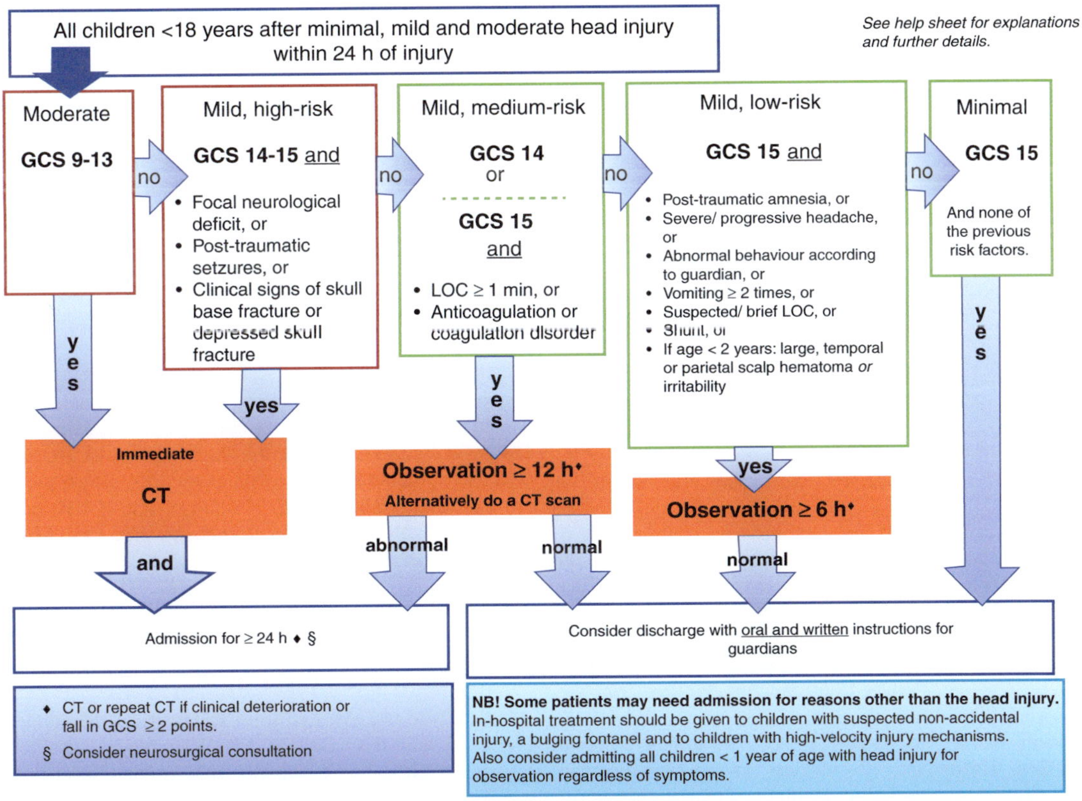

Fig. 7.2 Flowchart and classification of severity according to the Scandinavian guidelines for initial management of head trauma in children (Astrand et al. 2016)

following symptoms present: focal neurological deficit, posttraumatic seizure or clinical signs of skull base fracture or depressed skull fracture. The mild, medium risk includes children with admission GCS of 14 (and none of the high risk symptoms) or GCS 15 *and* loss of consciousness for more than 1 min, or in treatment with anticoagulation medicine or having a known coagulation disorder. Mild, low risk is the largest category and includes children with initial GCS of 15 and at least one of the following: posttraumatic amnesia, severe/progressive headache, abnormal behaviour according to guardian, repeated vomiting, suspected or brief LOC, or intracranial shunt system. If the child is younger than 2 years of age, have an initial GCCS of 15 and have a large temporal/parietal scalp hematoma or if the child is irritable, this is also classed as mild, low risk.

- Minimal head injury includes children who are fully awake on admission and do not have any of the previously mentioned symptoms.

The paediatric guidelines have been externally validated in a large independent cohort with encouraging results (Unden et al. 2018). Also, as for the adult guidelines, the risk stratification seems justified (Unden et al. 2015). The Scandinavian paediatric head trauma guidelines are currently being validated in a Nordic multicentre study.

The definition of severe head injury in children still include all children with GCS 3–8 after head trauma (Adelson et al. 2003).

7.4 Note

The flowcharts of the Scandinavian head injury guidelines for adults (Unden et al. 2013) and for children (Astrand et al. 2016) are presented in Figs. 7.1 and 7.2, respectively.

References

Adelson PD, Bratton SL, Carney NA, Chesnut RM, du Coudray HE, Goldstein B, Kochanek PM, Miller HC, Partington MD, Selden NR, Warden CR, Wright DW. Guidelines for the acute medical management of severe traumatic brain injury in infants, children, and adolescents. Chapter 1: introduction. Pediatr Crit Care Med. 2003;4:S2–4.

Ananthaharan A, Kravdal G, Straume-Naesheim TM. Utility and effectiveness of the Scandinavian guidelines to exclude computerized tomography scanning in mild traumatic brain injury—a prospective cohort study. BMC Emerg Med. 2018;18:44.

Astrand R, Rosenlund C, Unden J. Scandinavian guidelines for initial management of minor and moderate head trauma in children. BMC Med. 2016;14:33.

Baker SP, O'Neill B. The injury severity score: an update. J Trauma. 1976;16:882–5.

Baker SP, O'Neill B, Haddon W Jr, Long WB. The injury severity score: a method for describing patients with multiple injuries and evaluating emergency care. J Trauma. 1974;14:187–96.

Brickley MR, Shepherd JP. The relationship between alcohol intoxication, injury severity and Glasgow Coma Score in assault patients. Injury. 1995;26:311–4.

Buyukcam F, Kaya U, Karakilic ME, Cavus UY, Turan Sonmez F, Odabas O. Predicting the outcome in children with head trauma: comparison of FOUR score and Glasgow Coma Scale. Ulus Travma Acil Cerrahi Derg. 2012;18:469–73.

Champion HR, Sacco WJ, Copes WS, Gann DS, Gennarelli TA, Flanagan ME. A revision of the trauma score. J Trauma. 1989;29:623–9.

Committee on Quality Improvement, American Academy of Pediatrics and Commission on Clinical Policies and Research, American Academy of Family Physicians. The management of minor closed head injury in children. Pediatrics. 1999;104:1407–15.

Dunning J, Daly JP, Lomas JP, Lecky F, Batchelor J, Mackway-Jones K. Derivation of the children's head injury algorithm for the prediction of important clinical events decision rule for head injury in children. Arch Dis Child. 2006;91:885–91.

Eken C, Kartal M, Bacanli A, Eray O. Comparison of the full outline of unresponsiveness score Coma Scale and the Glasgow Coma Scale in an emergency setting population. Eur J Emerg Med. 2009;16:29–36.

Holmes JF, Palchak MJ, Conklin MJ, Kuppermann N. Do children require hospitalization after immediate post-traumatic seizures? Ann Emerg Med. 2004;43:706–10.

Holmes JF, Palchak MJ, MacFarlane T, Kuppermann N. Performance of the pediatric Glasgow Coma Scale in children with blunt head trauma. Acad Emerg Med. 2005;12:814–9.

Ingebrigtsen T, Romner B, Kock-Jensen C. Scandinavian guidelines for initial management of minimal, mild, and moderate head injuries. The Scandinavian Neurotrauma Committee. J Trauma. 2000;48:760–6.

Iyer VN, Mandrekar JN, Danielson RD, Zubkov AY, Elmer JL, Wijdicks EF. Validity of the FOUR score coma scale in the medical intensive care unit. Mayo Clin Proc. 2009;84:694–701.

Johnstone AJ, Lohlun JC, Miller JD, McIntosh CA, Gregori A, Brown R, Jones PA, Anderson SI, Tocher JL. A comparison of the Glasgow Coma Scale and the Swedish Reaction Level Scale. Brain Inj. 1993;7:501–6.

Malec JF, Brown AW, Leibson CL, Flaada JT, Mandrekar JN, Diehl NN, Perkins PK. The mayo classification system for traumatic brain injury severity. J Neurotrauma. 2007;24:1417–24.

Reilly PL, Graham DI, Adams JH, Jennett B. Patients with head injury who talk and die. Lancet. 1975;2:375–7.

Reilly PL, Simpson DA, Sprod R, Thomas L. Assessing the conscious level in infants and young children: a paediatric version of the Glasgow Coma Scale. Childs Nerv Syst. 1988;4:30–3.

Rimel RW, Giordani B, Barth JT, Boll TJ, Jane JA. Disability caused by minor head injury. Neurosurgery. 1981;9:221–8.

Schutzman SA, Barnes P, Duhaime AC, Greenes D, Homer C, Jaffe D, Lewis RJ, Luerssen TG, Schunk J. Evaluation and management of children younger than two years old with apparently minor head trauma: proposed guidelines. Pediatrics. 2001;107:983–93.

Simpson D, Reilly P. Pediatric coma scale. Lancet. 1982;2:450.

Starmark JE, Stalhammar D, Holmgren E. The Reaction Level Scale (RLS85). Manual and guidelines. Acta Neurochir. 1988a;91:12–20.

Starmark JE, Stalhammar D, Holmgren E, Rosander B. A comparison of the Glasgow Coma Scale and the Reaction Level Scale (RLS85). J Neurosurg. 1988b;69:699–706.

Stein SC, Spettell C. The Head Injury Severity Scale (HISS): a practical classification of closed-head injury. Brain Inj. 1995;9:437–44.

Teasdale G, Jennett B. Assessment of coma and impaired consciousness. A practical scale. Lancet. 1974;2:81–4.

Tepas JJ 3rd, Mollitt DL, Talbert JL, Bryant M. The pediatric trauma score as a predictor of injury severity in the injured child. J Pediatr Surg. 1987;22:14–8.

Unden J, Ingebrigtsen T, Romner B, Snc SN. Scandinavian guidelines for initial management of minimal, mild and moderate head injuries in adults: an evidence and consensus-based update. BMC Med. 2013;11:50.

Unden L, Calcagnile O, Unden J, Reinstrup P, Bazarian J. Validation of the Scandinavian guidelines for initial management of minimal, mild and moderate traumatic brain injury in adults. BMC Med. 2015;13:292.

Unden J, Dalziel SR, Borland ML, Phillips N, Kochar A, Lyttle MD, Bressan S, Cheek JA, Neutze J, Donath S, Hearps S, Oakley E, Dalton S, Gilhotra Y, Babl FE. External validation of the Scandinavian guidelines for management of minimal, mild and moderate head injuries in children. BMC Med. 2018;16:176.

Wijdicks EF, Bamlet WR, Maramattom BV, Manno EM, McClelland RL. Validation of a new coma scale: the FOUR score. Ann Neurol. 2005;58:585–93.

Wolf CA, Wijdicks EF, Bamlet WR, McClelland RL. Further validation of the FOUR score coma scale by intensive care nurses. Mayo Clin Proc. 2007;82:435–8.

Yager JY, Johnston B, Seshia SS. Coma scales in pediatric practice. Am J Dis Child. 1990;144:1088–91.

Primary Clinical Assessment

8

Jacob Bertram Springborg

Recommendations

Level I

Data are insufficient to support Level I recommendations for this subject.

Level II

The Glasgow Coma Scale score (GCS) is a reliable indicator of the severity of TBI; the Injury Severity Score (ISS) can be used to predict severity in patients with multitrauma.

Level III

When pupil fixation or dilation is observed, cerebral herniation should be suspected and appropriate interventions initiated. However, like other patients, patients with TBI may demonstrate iridoplegia, which is not due to cerebral herniation.

Tips, Tricks, and Pitfalls

- Do not use simultaneous verbal and tactile stimuli when evaluating the GCS. Start with verbal commands and proceed only to painful stimuli if the patient does not follow commands. Also, remember to start with a near midline painful stimulus to appreciate if the patient localises.
- Remember that not all 'fixed and blown' pupils are caused by ipsilateral cerebral herniation. Most neurosurgeons know of patients who have been operated on the wrong side because of a false localising sign and because a CT scan was not done for time reasons.
- Pupillary abnormalities in a patient who is conscious are almost never a sign of cerebral herniation.

8.1 Background

8.1.1 Measures of Consciousness

In 1974, Teasdale and Jennett introduced the GCS as an objective measure of the level of consciousness 6 h after TBI (Teasdale and Jennett 1974), and in 1976 the scale was adjusted to its current form (Teasdale and Jennett 1976) (Table 8.1). It has since become the most widely

J. B. Springborg (✉)
Department of Neurosurgery, University Clinic of Neurosurgery, Copenhagen University Hospital, Copenhagen, Denmark
e-mail: jacob.bertram.springborg@regionh.dk

© Springer Nature Switzerland AG 2020
T. Sundstrøm et al. (eds.), *Management of Severe Traumatic Brain Injury*,
https://doi.org/10.1007/978-3-030-39383-0_8

Table 8.1 Glasgow Coma Scale (GCS)

Adult GCS		Paediatric GCS	
Eye opening		*Eye opening*	
Spontaneous	4	Spontaneous	4
To speech	3	To speech	3
To pain	2	To pain	2
None	1	None	1
Verbal response		*Verbal response*	
Oriented	5	Coos, babbles	5
Confused	4	Irritable cries	4
Inappropriate words	3	Cries to pain	3
Sounds	2	Moans to pain	2
None	1	None	1
Motor response		*Motor response*	
Obey commands	6	Normal spontaneous movements	6
Localises to pain	5	Withdraws to touch	5
Withdraws to pain	4	Withdraws to pain	4
Abnormal flexion	3	Abnormal flexion	3
Abnormal extension	2	Abnormal extension	2
None	1	None	1

Table 8.2 Full Outline of UnResponsiveness (FOUR) Score

FOUR score	
Eye response	
Eyelids open or opened, tracking or blinking to command	4
Eyelids open but not tracking	3
Eyelids closed but open to loud voice	2
Eyelids closed but open to pain	1
Eyelids remain closed with pain	0
Motor response	
Thumbs-up, fist or peace sign	4
Localising to pain	3
Flexion response to pain	2
Extension response to pain	1
No response to pain or generalised myoclonus status	0
Brainstem reflexes	
Pupil and corneal reflexes present	4
One pupil wide and fixed	3
Pupil or corneal reflexes absent	2
Pupil and corneal reflexes absent	1
Absent pupil, corneal and cough reflex	0
Respiration	
Not intubated, regular breathing pattern	4
Not intubated, Cheyne–Stokes breathing pattern	3
Not intubated, irregular breathing	2
Breathes above ventilator rate	1
Breathes at ventilator rate or apnoea	0

used early clinical measure of the severity of TBI. The GCS allows repetitive and relatively reliably recordings of the level of consciousness and a standardised method of reporting the findings (Braakman et al. 1977; Menegazzi et al. 1993; Matis and Birbilis 2008). The GCS evaluates three independent responses to stimuli: eye opening, verbal response, and best motor response. In patients unable to follow commands, a painful blunt stimulus is applied, first near the midline, e.g. to the supraorbital nerve, to see if the patient localises, and if not so, peripherally, e.g. to the nail bed, to see if the patient withdraws. The motor score is based on the extremity with the best response and the eye opening score on the eye with the best response.

Other scales have been designed to evaluate the level of consciousness and predict outcome. Examples are the Swedish Reaction Level Scale (Starmark et al. 1988), which has eight values and resembles an enhanced GCS motor score, the Full Outline of UnResponsiveness (FOUR) score (Table 8.2), which besides eye and motor function, includes brain stem and respiratory function (Wijdicks et al. 2005) and the GCS-Pupils score, which is a simple arithmetic score (1–15) deducting the number of non-reacting pupils (0–2) from the GCS score (Brennan et al. 2018). Most of these scales are reliable and valid, but none have gained the same general acceptance and use as the GCS, which should therefore be considered gold standard. However, one should keep in mind that the use of the GCS scale has expanded beyond the original intension, and the limitations of the scale should be acknowledged (Matis and Birbilis 2008).

In intubated patients or in patients with lesions causing aphasia or cervical medullary dysfunction, the use of the GCS is problematic as the verbal or motor scores of these patients may be difficult to interpret. Likewise, patients may have additional injuries to the extremities complicating the assessment of the best motor score. Furthermore, the GCS score can be affected by a number of pre- and posttraumatic systemic factors that may impair the neurological response, e.g. alcohol, drugs, hypoglycaemia, hypotension, hypoxia or sedation. Intoxication is a common phenomenon in the trauma population. Therefore, these conditions should be corrected prior to the evaluation of the GCS, or if not possible, the GCS should be recorded as a modified GCS. Finally, ocular or facial trauma can hinder the evaluation of the eye or verbal response, and pre-existing factors such as hearing impairment, dementia, or psychiatric diseases may affect the evaluation of especially the verbal response. To overcome the problem with the evaluation of the verbal score of intubated patients, different models have been proposed to predict the verbal score from the eye and motor score (Rutledge et al. 1996; Meredith et al. 1998). However, the applicability of these attempts has been questioned (Chesnut 1997).

Several studies have confirmed the predictive value of the GCS in estimating outcome after TBI (Narayan et al. 1981; Rocca et al. 1989; Fearnside et al. 1993; Alvarez et al. 1998). However, as the CGS is a combined score of 120 different possible eye–verbal–motor score combinations summing up to just 13 different scores (3–15), it is not surprising that different patients with the same initial GCS score may have different outcomes, which has in fact been demonstrated in the general trauma population (Healey et al. 2003). In addition, these authors have demonstrated that most of the predictive power of the GCS resides in the motor score and that a mathematical transformation of the motor score gives an almost perfectly calibrated line between predicted and actual mortality (Healey et al. 2003). However, the design of that study leaves some unanswered questions about the reliability of the collected GCS values and the external validity of the study, which as mentioned included general trauma patients (National Trauma Data Bank). Nevertheless, others have confirmed that in patients with TBI, the motor score is the single most precise predictor of mortality (Kung et al. 2010). However, the National Trauma Data Bank end point 'survival to discharge' and mortality are poor indices of outcome for the head injury population, completely neglecting the quality of life in survivors.

8.1.2 Clinical Examination of the Pupils

This is an important aspect of neurological assessment and is not included in the GCS score. Pupil assessment is defined as each pupil's size and response to light stimulation. Pupil asymmetry is defined as more than 1 mm difference between the two pupils, and an absent light response ('fixed pupil') is defined as less than 1 mm constriction on bright light. The light reflex depends on a normally functioning lens, retina, optic nerve, brain stem, and oculomotor nerve. The parasympathetic pupillary constrictory nerve fibres run from the Edinger-Westphal nucleus in the high midbrain with the oculomotor nerve to the ciliary ganglion and from that with the short ciliary nerves to the pupillary constrictory muscles. The direct light response assesses the ipsilateral optic and oculomotor nerve, and the consensual light response assesses the ipsilateral optic and contralateral oculomotor nerve. The examination is generally easy and quick.

Increased intracranial pressure causing cerebral uncal herniation may compress the oculomotor nerve resulting in a reduction of parasympathetic tone in the pupillary constrictory muscles and thereby ipsilateral pupil dilation and an absent light reflex. Bilateral fixed and dilated pupils are consistent with direct brain stem injury or marked elevation of ICP with central herniation. Metabolic or circulatory disturbances including hypoxia, hypotension or hypothermia may, however, also be associated with pupil asymmetry or abnormal light reactivity (Meyer et al. 1993). Therefore, resuscitation and stabilisation should be initiated before evaluation of the pupils. Direct trauma to the eye or oculomotor nerve, e.g. from skull fracture through the sphenoid bone, may cause pupil dilation and thereby mimic severe intracranial injury or herniation. Moreover, traumatic carotid dissection may cause Horner's syndrome with ipsilateral pupil constriction from decreased sympathetic tone making the contralateral pupil appear dilated (Fujisawa et al. 2001). However, in Horner's syndrome, there is ptosis associated with the miotic eye, and the contralateral pupil appearing dilated will have a normal reaction to light. This assessment may be tricky in the acute setting. Finally, in patients with severe swelling of the orbital regions, the evaluation of the pupils can be impossible.

In summary, pupillary function may be an indicator of brain injury after trauma, but is not a specific indicator of severity or involved anatomy. Nonetheless, studies support the assessment of pupils after severe TBI as both a guide to decision-making and for prognostic reasons (Braakman et al. 1977; Chesnut et al. 1994; Halley et al. 2004).

8.1.3 Systems Designed to Grade Patients with Multiple Injuries

The most commonly used is the ISS (Baker et al. 1974), which is based on the Abbreviated Injury Scale (AIS). The AIS is an anatomical scoring system first introduced in 1969 (MacKenzie et al. 1985). The system describes single injuries, and injury severity is ranked on an ordinal scale of 1–6 with 1 being minor, 3 serious, 5 severe, and 6 an unsurvivable injury. The ISS provides an overall score for patients with multiple injuries. Each injury is assigned an AIS score and is allocated to one of six body regions (head, face, chest, abdomen, extremities including pelvis, and external). Only the highest AIS score in each body region is used. The three most severely injured body regions have their scores squared and added to produce the ISS score. The ISS score takes values from 0 to 75. If an injury is assigned an AIS score of 6 (unsurvivable injury), the ISS score is automatically assigned to 75. The ISS score correlates linearly with mortality, morbidity, hospital stay, and other measures of severity. Its weaknesses are that any error in AIS scoring increases the ISS error, many different injury patterns can give the same ISS score and injuries to different body regions are not weighted. Also, as a full description of patient injuries is not known prior to a full clinical investigation and potential surgery, the ISS, along with other anatomical scoring systems, is not useful as a triage tool. As multiple injuries within the same body region are only assigned a single score, a modification of the ISS, the "New Injury Severity Score" (NISS), has been proposed (Osler et al. 1997). This is calculated as the sum of the squares of the top three AIS scores regardless of body region. The NISS has been found to statistically outperform the traditional ISS score and is possibly a more accurate predictor of mortality in TBI (Lavoie et al. 2004).

8.2 Specific Paediatric Concerns

Standard GCS scoring of non-verbal children is inapplicable. The responses of children change with development, so the GCS requires modification for paediatric use (Table 8.1) (Matis and Birbilis 2008). In children with severe TBI, the GCS is an independent predictor of mortality, as in adults (White et al. 2001; Holmes et al. 2005; Tude Melo et al. 2010). However, in children, pupil examination seems to be of less value (Halley et al. 2004; Chan et al. 2005).

References

Alvarez M, Nava JM, Rué M, Quintana S. Mortality prediction in head trauma patients: performance of Glasgow Coma Score and general severity systems. Crit Care Med. 1998;26:142–8.

Baker SP, O'Neill B, Haddon W, Long WB. The injury severity score: a method for describing patients with multiple injuries and evaluating emergency care. J Trauma. 1974;14:187–96.

Braakman R, Avezaat CJ, Maas AI, Roel M, Schouten HJ. Inter observer agreement in the assessment of the motor response of the Glasgow "Coma" Scale. Clin Neurol Neurosurg. 1977;80:100–6.

Brennan PM, Murray GD, Teasdale GM. Simplifying the use of prognostic information in traumatic brain injury. Part 1: the GCS-pupils score: an extended index of clinical severity. J Neurosurg. 2018;128:1612–20.

Chan HC, Adnan WAW, Jaalam K, Abdullah MR, Abdullah J. Which mild head injured patients should have follow-up after discharge from an accident and emergency ward? A study in a University Hospital setting in Kelantan, Malaysia Southeast. Asian J Trop Med Public Health. 2005;36:982–93.

Chesnut RM. Appropriate use of the Glasgow Coma Scale in intubated patients: a linear regression prediction of the Glasgow verbal score from the Glasgow eye and motor scores. J Trauma. 1997;42:345.

Chesnut RM, Gautille T, Blunt BA, Klauber MR, Marshall LE. The localizing value of asymmetry in pupillary size in severe head injury: relation to lesion type and location. Neurosurgery. 1994;34:840–5.

Fearnside MR, Cook RJ, McDougall P, McNeil RJ. The Westmead Head Injury Project outcome in severe head injury. A comparative analysis of pre-hospital, clinical and CT variables. Br J Neurosurg. 1993;7:267–79.

Fujisawa H, Marukawa K, Kida S, Hasegawa M, Yamashita J, Matsui O. Abducens nerve palsy and ipsilateral Horner syndrome: a predicting sign of intracranial carotid injury in a head trauma patient. J Trauma. 2001;50:554–6.

Halley MK, Silva PD, Foley J, Rodarte A. Loss of consciousness: when to perform computed tomography? Pediatr Crit Care Med. 2004;5:230–3.

Healey C, Osler TM, Rogers FB, Healey MA, Glance LG, Kilgo PD, Shackford SR, Meredith JW. Improving the Glasgow Coma Scale score: motor score alone is a better predictor. J Trauma. 2003;54:671–8.

Holmes JF, Palchak MJ, MacFarlane T, Kuppermann N. Performance of the pediatric Glasgow coma scale in children with blunt head trauma. Acad Emerg Med. 2005;12:814–9.

Kung W-M, Tsai S-H, Chiu W-T, Hung K-S, Wang S-P, Lin J-W, Lin M-S. Correlation between Glasgow Coma Score components and survival in patients with traumatic brain injury. Injury. 2010;49:940–4.

Lavoie A, Moore L, LeSage N, Liberman M, Sampalis JS. The new injury severity score: a more accurate predictor of in-hospital mortality than the injury severity score. J Trauma. 2004;56:1312–20.

MacKenzie EJ, Shapiro S, Eastham JN. The abbreviated injury scale and injury severity score. Levels of inter- and intrarater reliability. Med Care. 1985;23:823–35.

Matis G, Birbilis T. The Glasgow Coma Scale—a brief review. Past, present, future. Acta Neurol Belg. 2008;108:75–89.

Menegazzi JJ, Davis EA, Sucov AN, Paris PM. Reliability of the Glasgow Coma Scale when used by emergency physicians and paramedics. J Trauma. 1993;34:46–8.

Meredith W, Rutledge R, Fakhry SM, Emery S, Kromhout-Schiro S. The conundrum of the Glasgow Coma Scale in intubated patients: a linear regression prediction of the Glasgow verbal score from the Glasgow eye and motor scores. J Trauma. 1998;44:839–44.

Meyer S, Gibb T, Jurkovich GJ. Evaluation and significance of the pupillary light reflex in trauma patients. Ann Emerg Med. 1993;22:1052–7.

Narayan RK, Greenberg RP, Miller JD, Enas GG, Choi SC, Kishore PR, Selhorst JB, Lutz HA, Becker DP. Improved confidence of outcome prediction in severe head injury. A comparative analysis of the clinical examination, multimodality evoked potentials, CT scanning, and intracranial pressure. J Neurosurg. 1981;54:751–62.

Osler T, Baker SP, Long W. A modification of the injury severity score that both improves accuracy and simplifies scoring. J Trauma. 1997;43:922–5.

Rocca B, Martin C, Viviand X, Bidet PF, Saint-Gilles HL, Chevalier A. Comparison of four severity scores in patients with head trauma. J Trauma. 1989;29:299–305.

Rutledge R, Lentz CW, Fakhry S, Hunt J. Appropriate use of the Glasgow Coma Scale in intubated patients: a linear regression prediction of the Glasgow verbal score from the Glasgow eye and motor scores. J Trauma. 1996;41:514–22.

Starmark JE, Stålhammar D, Holmgren E. The Reaction Level Scale (RLS85). Manual and guide- lines. Acta Neurochir. 1988;91:12–20.

Teasdale G, Jennett B. Assessment of coma and impaired consciousness. A practical scale. Lancet. 1974;2:81–4.

Teasdale G, Jennett B. Assessment and prognosis of coma after head injury. Acta Neurochir. 1976;34:45–55.

Tude Melo JR, Di Rocco F, Blanot S, Oliveira-Filho J, Roujeau T, Sainte-Rose C, Duracher C, Vecchione A, Meyer P, Zerah M. Mortality in children with severe head trauma: predictive factors and proposal for a new predictive scale. Neurosurgery. 2010;67:1542–7.

White JR, Farukhi Z, Bull C, Christensen J, Gordon T, Paidas C, Nichols DG. Predictors of outcome in severely head-injured children. Crit Care Med. 2001;29:534–40.

Wijdicks EFM, Bamlet WR, Maramattom BV, Manno EM, McClelland RL. Validation of a new coma scale: the FOUR score. Ann Neurol. 2005;58:585–93.

Part III

Prehospital Management

Johan Undén

9 Prehospital Guidelines

Riikka Takala

Recommendations

Level I

There are insufficient data to support a Level I recommendation for this topic.

Level II

Hypoxemia and hypotension increase morbidity and mortality after TBI.

Level III

Securing the airway, maintaining adequate blood pressure, oxygenation and ventilation are all key factors in the prevention of secondary brain injury. After stabilization, rapid transport of patients with severe TBI to a neurosurgical centre is crucial.

9.1 Overview

Traumatic brain injury (TBI) is a worldwide health problem with an incidence rate of 262 per 100,000/year. Most TBIs are mild, approximately 70–80%, with the rest being classified as moderate or severe TBIs. Severe TBI is associated with a high mortality, 30–40% (Maas et al. 2017).

TBI is a dynamic process where the primary injury occurs at the time of insult. Secondary injuries start to develop immediately after the insult and may continue to progress even days or weeks after the insult. The aim of treatment and care is to prevent and decrease secondary injuries. Quick and correct emergency treatment is therefore a corner stone of TBI care. Severe TBI patients should be transferred to a hospital with neurosurgical facilities as quickly as possible.

Tips, Tricks and Pitfalls

- Secondary injuries start to develop within minutes of the insult.
- Hypotension and hypoxia increase morbidity and mortality.
- Hyper- and hypoventilation increase mortality.
- Repeat neurological assessment often: GCS and pupils.
- Continuous monitoring: ECG, SpO_2, blood pressure.
- GCS < 9 patients need to be intubated.

R. Takala (✉)
Perioperative Services, Intensive Care Medicine and Pain Management, Turku University Hospital, Turku, Finland

© Springer Nature Switzerland AG 2020
T. Sundstrøm et al. (eds.), *Management of Severe Traumatic Brain Injury*,
https://doi.org/10.1007/978-3-030-39383-0_9

9.2 Summary of Prehospital Treatment

Hypoxemia (SpO_2 < 90%) and hypotension (RRsys < 120 mmHg) increase morbidity and mortality. They must be avoided and promptly treated. The rule of ABC (ensure protected airway and provide adequate oxygenation and ventilation (breathing) and circulation) applies to the emergency care of TBI.

Patients who have impaired consciousness (Glasgow Coma Scale ≤ 8) are unable to maintain their airway, may have impaired respiratory drive and are at risk of aspiration. Endotracheal intubation and controlled ventilation are therefore needed. Intubation is also needed if the patient has better consciousness than GCS of 9, but has concomitant multitrauma and supplemental oxygen does not correct hypoxemia. One must always assume that head-injured patients also have an injured neck, until otherwise proven. Normoventilation is recommended ($etCO_2$ 35–40 mmHg, 4.5–5.5 kPa) as both hyper- and hypoventilation increase mortality. However, if there are signs of cerebral herniation (i.e. pupil dilatation, Cushing's triad), short lasting hyperventilation may be considered. Hypertonic saline or mannitol may be used to decrease increased intracranial pressure (ICP) and in situations with cerebral herniation.

Hypotension is treated with isotonic or hypertonic crystalloids and vasopressors such as noradrenaline or phenylephrine.

9.3 Background

9.3.1 Prehospital Assessments

9.3.1.1 Oxygenation and Blood Pressure

Hypoxemia, defined as peripheral oxygen saturation (SpO_2) < 90%, and hypotension (previously defined as systolic blood pressure (SBP) < 90 mmHg) are both associated with high mortality and morbidity. A recent study including 13,151 patients observed that 20.7% and 28.1% patients died if they had only hypotension or hypoxemia, respectively, and mortality was 43.9% if both conditions existed (Spaite et al. 2017a).

Of those patients who did not have hypotension or hypoxemia, only 5.6% died. Updated Brain Trauma Foundation (BTF, www.braintrauma.org) guidelines from 2017 recommends systolic blood pressure values higher than 90 mmHg. They recommend that SBP should be kept at ≥100 mmHg for patients 50–69 years and at ≥110 mmHg or higher for patients 15–49 or >70 years old. In a TBI patient material consisting of over 3800 patients, aged 10 years or older, there was a linear association between systolic blood pressure, ranging from 40 to 119 mmHg, and death. An increase of systolic blood pressure of 10 mmHg was associated with an 18.8% decreased adjusted odds of death (Spaite et al. 2017b). A bimodal distribution of death has been observed in TBI patients, optimal SBP being between 120 and 140 mmHg (Zafar et al. 2011).

Cerebral perfusion pressure (CPP) is calculated as: mean arterial pressure (MAP) − intracranial pressure (ICP). BTF recommends that CPP should be kept between 60 and 70 mmHg.

Blood pressure should be monitored frequently if it is measured noninvasively. If possible, an arterial cannulation and continuous blood pressure measurement would be preferable as it is less prone to disturbances during the transportation and allows simple sampling for blood gas analysis. Electrocardiography and SpO_2 must also be monitored continuously.

9.3.1.2 Glasgow Coma Scale

The most common tool for assessing level of consciousness is the Glasgow Coma Scale (GCS) (Table 9.1). Chapter 3 discusses this topic further, and www.glasgowcomascale.org demonstrates in detail how it should be performed. GCS is a clinically important tool, and it should be performed immediately after the ABC evaluation. When evaluating GCS, hypoxaemia, hypoventilation, hypotension and hypoglycaemia must be corrected, otherwise GCS is not reliable. There are also confounding factors that may decrease the summed GCS score, such as alcohol and narcotic drugs, spinal cord injury, orbital swelling and dysphasia. Repeated and documented GCS are valuable means for monitoring the trend of con-

Table 9.1 GCS

GCS	
Eye opening	
Spontaneous	4
Speech	3
Pain	2
None	1
Verbal response	
Oriented	5
Confused	4
Inappropriate	3
Incomprehensible	2
None	1
Motor response	
Obey command	6
Localize pain	5
Flexor withdrawal (normal flexion)	4
Abnormal flexion	3
Extension	2
None	1

sciousness and for identifying possible worsening in neurological status. GCS is known to correlate with the severity of TBI. However, GCS at the scene is not such a reliable outcome predictor as GCS obtained upon admission, and motor score has the best predictive power (Marmarou et al. 2007; Lesko et al. 2013). GCS is performed by evaluating the patient's eye opening (1–4 points), verbal response (1–5 points) and best motor response (1–6 points) to speech or painful stimulus. When testing eye opening to pain, a peripheral stimulus should be used as the grimace associated with central pain may cause eye closure. If patients do not obey commands and motor response to painful stimulus is used, then central stimulus should be used. This is done by pressing the supraorbital notch. However, in cases of facial fractures adjacent to supraorbital notch, a peripheral stimulus is safer and is performed by applying slowly increasing pressure to nail tip. The points of each area are recorded separately, and the summed GCS score must be documented.

9.3.1.3 Pupils and Their Reactivity

Chapter 3 elaborates on this topic in detail. Evaluating and documenting the size of the pupils (in mm) and their reactivity to light are also essential as any changes in them give valuable information. Normal pupils may have a 1 mm diameter difference. A bright flashlight is used to assess the light reactivity. In a normal situation, the pupil constricts to a light and so does the contralateral pupil (direct and consensual reaction). Both the right and left pupil findings must be documented.

Before pupil evaluation, hypoxemia, hypoventilation and hypotension must be treated.

An important sign of uncal herniation is a unilaterally dilated and unreactive (fixed) pupil. In this situation, the ipsilateral anterior temporal lobe is pushed through the tentorium and the uncus of the temporal lobe compresses the oculomotor nerve (III cranial nerve). Damage to the medulla results in bilaterally dilated and fixed pupils. Acute pupil dilation is considered a neurological emergency.

Orbital trauma or a direct trauma to the eye may injure short ciliary nerve and pupillary sphincter muscle, respectively, also resulting in a dilated pupil. Documentation of traumas to the aforementioned areas is therefore important.

9.4 Prehospital Treatment

9.4.1 Airway, Ventilation and Oxygenation

A TBI patient with GCS ≤ 8 must be intubated as they are not able to maintain their airway and may have low respiratory drive, and they are at risk of aspiration. Short-acting anaesthetic agents should be used for intubation and maintaining sedation during the transport as the neurological status is often reassessed when the patient arrives to the emergency department. Short-acting opioids, propofol and short-acting benzodiazepines are suitable for intubation. Ketamine has become popular in the emergency medicine due to its stable haemodynamical properties, but there are currently not enough data regarding its safety in TBI patients, used as a sole anaesthetic agent. Some data shows that, when it is used in conjunction with other anaesthetics such as midazolam or propofol and patients are already mechanically ventilated, it does not increase ICP (Chang et al. 2013). In addition, hallucinations associated with ketamine administration may impair reliable neurological assessment upon admission to the hospital. However, in haemodynamically unstable patients with multiple trauma, ketamine is probably a safe choice as propofol is known to decrease blood pressure.

Prehospital intubation of TBI patients has resulted in conflicting results regarding their survival and neurological outcome. These contradictory results seem to arise from the experience and skills of the personnel. Data supports that unexperienced and untrained personnel should not intubate TBI patients (Bossers et al. 2015). The correct endotracheal tube placement must be ensured by pulmonary auscultation and end-tidal CO_2 ($etCO_2$) measurement. Endotracheal tubes should be secured with drapes, and the head of the bed should be elevated 15–30° and neck and head positioned in neutral position to ensure cerebral venous return. Of note, semi-rigid collars may also obstruct cerebral venous return.

Normoventilation ($etCO_2$ 35–40 mmHg, 4.5–5.5 kPa) is recommended as both hypoventilation and hyperventilation result in increased mortality (Davis et al. 2010). Hypoxaemia is corrected by administering supplemental oxygen. SpO_2 is aimed to be maintained at >90%. Hyperoxia may be harmful in critically ill patients and normoxia is suggested in TBI patients, although high-quality studies on the topic are still lacking.

9.4.2 Fluid Resuscitation

Isolated head trauma does not lead to hypovolaemia but may cause hypotension (Mahoney et al. 2003). However, if the patient has concomitant high cervical injury, this may cause neurogenic shock with hypotension and bradycardia. In addition, TBI with concomitant multitrauma with haemorrhage may result in hypovolaemia and hypotension. Both result in reduced cerebral perfusion pressure and oxygen delivery, predisposing the already injured and vulnerable brain to secondary injuries. Fluid resuscitation aims to restore oxygen delivery and adequate cerebral perfusion pressure and cerebral blood flow. Isotonic or hypertonic crystalloids (Gantner et al. 2014) are suitable for fluid resuscitation in the TBI patients. Hypertonic crystalloids can also be used as they decrease the ICP, but they do not improve the outcome of the patients (Cooper et al. 2004). The use of colloids and albumin are not recommended (Myburgh et al. 2007; Reinhart et al. 2012; Cooper et al. 2013; Oddo et al. 2018) as they may increase the mortality in TBI patients. Glucose containing fluids should be avoided, unless the patient has hypoglycaemia (B-gluck <5 mmol/L). If fluid therapy does not increase the blood pressure, vasoactive agents should be used. Noradrenaline and phenylephrine are recommended as continuous infusion.

9.4.3 Cerebral Herniation

Frequent neurological assessment is important as the patient's clinical status can worsen rapidly due to ongoing processes such as mass lesions, cerebral oedema or hydrocephalus. Clinical signs of increased ICP and cerebral herniation are loss of consciousness or progressive neurologic deterioration (at least 2 points decrease in GCS), one or both pupils dilated and unreactive to light, Cushing's triad (hypertension and bradycardia) and extension or no reaction to painful stimulus.

Sedation and analgesia must be sufficiently provided, preferably with a continuous infusion.

Hyperosmolar therapy with either mannitol or hypertonic saline is recommended. They both increase osmotic gradient, which induces water to move from cerebral tissue to the extracellular space, thus reducing cerebral oedema. Mannitol may cause electrolyte disturbances and hypovolemia due to excessive diuresis (Torre-Healy et al. 2012). Hypertonic saline increases cardiac output, blood pressure and cerebral blood flow (Torre-Healy et al. 2012; Tyagi et al. 2007). Hypertonic saline may be more effective and have longer lasting property to reduce ICP than mannitol (Kamel et al. 2011; Mortazavi et al. 2012).

Hyperventilation constricts cerebral arterial vessels and reduces cerebral flow (CBF) and ICP. CBF is often reduced in the acute phase of TBI and further decrease in CBF may lead to cerebral ischemia. In a small study of TBI patients, hyperventilation decreased ICP and improved CPP but increased hypoperfused brain volume (Coles et al. 2002). Hyperventilation worsens the neurological outcome in TBI patients (Stocchetti and Maas 2014). However, short-term hyperventilation can be useful in cases of imminent herniation and may outweigh its harmful effects. In such a case, hyperventilation should be titrated to $etCO_2$ of 30–35 mmHg, 3.9–4.6 kPa.

In patients with concomitant multitrauma, increased ICP can also result from increased venous pressure due to pneumothorax or abdominal injury. Pneumothorax must be treated promptly at the scene with chest drain or with thoracosentesis if drainage is not possible.

9.4.4 Seizure Treatment

TBI patients are at risk of epileptic seizures, which may cause and worsen secondary injuries. They must be promptly treated. Intravenous propofol or benzodiazepines such as lorazepam or midazolam are first-line choices. Of antiepileptic drugs, phosphenytoine and levetiracetam are currently the most widely used. They both seem to prevent early seizures in TBI, but in long-term use, phosphenytoine may worsen neurological outcome (Szaflarski et al. 2010; Bhullar et al. 2014).

9.4.5 Hypothermia

Hypothermia has been considered as neuroprotective, and several studies have assessed its role in the outcome of TBI patients. The recent POLAR study demonstrated that early prophylactic hypothermia in TBI patients does not improve neurological outcome or reduce mortality (Cooper et al. 2018), and its use is not recommended.

9.5 Transport

TBI patients should be transported to Level I or Level II trauma centres with 24 h coverage of neurosurgery, anaesthesiology, radiology (CT), traumatology and intensive care. There are no prospective randomized studies comparing "scoop and run" with "stay and play" on the outcome of TBI patients, and both the approaches are used in Nordic countries (Cnossen et al. 2018).

Severe TBI patients seem to benefit from a rapid transfer directly to a neurotrauma centre, and during transport all efforts must be done to prevent secondary injuries.

9.6 Paediatric TBI

Paediatric patients are not small adults, and the aetiology and pathology of paediatric TBI differ from that of adults. However, like in adults, hypotension and hypoxia increase mortality in paediatric TBI patients. Accordingly, assessment, treatment approaches and principals, such as avoiding hypoxemia and hypotension, are applied in the same way as in adults.

Paediatric patients should be transferred to Level I or II trauma centres familiar with paediatric TBI patients or to trauma centres familiar with paediatric TBI patients.

9.6.1 Oxygenation and Blood Pressure

Paediatric SpO_2 target is also >90%, whereas blood pressure targets are age dependent. In the paediatric population, hypotension is defined according to American College of Surgeons as follows:

Age 0–28 days, SBP < 60 mmHg, 1–12 months, SBP < 70 mmHg, 1–10 years, SBP < 70 + 2× age in years, >10 years, SBP < 90 mmHg. Current paediatric TBI guidelines from 2019 state that in children minimal CPP is 40 mmHg and threshold 40–50 mmHg should be considered, with infants at the lower end and adolescents at the upper end (Kochanek et al. 2019).

However, it may be that these hypotension and CPP thresholds in paediatric TBI patients are too low (Suttipongkaset et al. 2018), and they should

Table 9.2 Paediatric GCS

PGCS	
Eye opening	
Spontaneous	4
Speech	3
Pain	2
None	1
Verbal response	
Coos, babbles	5
Irritable cries	4
Cries to pain	3
Moans to pain	2
None	1
Motor response	
Normal spontaneous movement	6
Withdraws to touch	5
Withdraws to pain	4
Abnormal flexion	3
Extension	2
None	1

be more age specific (Allen et al. 2014), but data is currently too limited.

9.6.2 Paediatric GCS

Just like in adults, in paediatric patients GCS is assessed after stabilization. In children over 2 years old, adult GCS can be employed, whereas the paediatric GCS is used in pre-verbal children (Table 9.2).

References

Allen BB, Chiu Y-L, Gerber LM, Ghajar J, Greenfield JP. Age-specific cerebral perfusion pressure thresholds and survival in children and adolescents with severe traumatic brain injury. Pediatr Crit Care Med. 2014;15:62–70.

Bhullar IS, Johnson D, Paul JP, Kerwin AJ, Tepas JJ III, Frykberg ER. More harm than good. Antiseizure prophylaxis after traumatic brain injury does not decrease seizure rates but may inhibit functional recovery. J Trauma Acute Care Surg. 2014;76:54–61.

Bossers SM, Schwarte LA, Loer SA, Twisk JWR, Boer C, Schober P. Experience in prehospital endotracheal intubation significantly influences mortality of patients with severe traumatic brain injury: a systematic review and meta-analysis. PLoS One. 2015;10:e0141034–26.

Chang LC, Raty SR, Ortiz J, Bailard NS, Mathew SJ. The emerging use of ketamine for anesthesia and sedation in traumatic brain injuries. CNS Neurosci Ther. 2013;19:390–5.

Cnossen MC, van der Brande R, Lingsma HF, Polinder S, Lecky F, Maas AIR. Prehospital trauma care among 68 European neurotrauma centers: results of the CENTER-TBI provider profiling questionnaires. J Neurotrauma. 2018. https://doi.org/10.1089/neu.2018.5712.

Coles JP, Minhas PS, Fryer TD, Smielewski P, Aigbirihio F, Donovan T, et al. Effect of hyperventilation on cerebral blood flow in traumatic head injury: clinical relevance and monitoring correlates. Crit Care Med. 2002;30:1950–9.

Cooper DJ, Myles PS, McDermott FT, Murray LJ, Laidlaw J, Cooper G, et al. Prehospital hypertonic saline resuscitation of patients with hypotension and severe traumatic brain injury—a randomized controlled trial. JAMA. 2004;291:1350–7.

Cooper DJ, Myburgh J, Heritier S, Finfer S, Bellomo R, Billot L, et al. Albumin resuscitation for traumatic brain injury: is intracranial hypertension the cause of increased mortality? J Neurotrauma. 2013;30(7):512–8.

Cooper DJ, Nichol AD, Bailey M, Bernard S, Cameron PA, Pili-Floury S, et al. Effect of early sustained prophylactic hypothermia on neurologic outcomes among patients with severe traumatic brain injury. JAMA. 2018;320:2211–20.

Davis DP, Peay J, Sise MJ, Kennedy F, Simon F, Tominaga G, et al. Prehospital airway and ventilation management: a trauma score and injury severity score-based analysis. J Trauma. 2010;69:294–301.

Gantner D, Moore EM, Cooper DJ. Intravenous fluids in traumatic brain injury. Curr Opin Crit Care. 2014;20:385–9.

Kamel H, Navi BB, Nakagawa K, Hemphill JC III, Ko NU. Hypertonic saline versus mannitol for the treatment of elevated intracranial pressure: a meta-analysis of randomized clinical trials. Crit Care Med. 2011;39:554–9.

Kochanek PM, Tasker RC, Carney N, Totten AM, Adelson PD, Selden NR, et al. Guidelines for the management of pediatric severe traumatic brain injury, third edition. Pediatr Crit Care Med. 2019;20:S1–S82.

Lesko MM, Jenks T, O'Brien SJ, Childs C, Bouamra O, Woodford M, Lecky F. Comparing model performance for survival prediction using total Glasgow Coma Scale and its components in traumatic brain injury. J Neurotrauma. 2013;30:17–22.

Maas AIR, Menon DK, Adelson PD, Andelic N, Bell MJ, Belli A, et al. The lancet neurology commission traumatic brain injury: integrated approaches to improve prevention, clinical care, and research. Lancet Neurol. 2017;16:1–62.

Mahoney EJ, Biffl WL, Harrington DT, Cioffi WG. Isolated brain injury as a cause of hypotension in the blunt trauma patient. J Trauma. 2003;55(6):1065–9.

Marmarou A, Lu J, Butcher I, McHugh GS, Murray GD, Steyerberg EW, et al. Prognostic value of the Glasgow Coma Scale and pupil reactivity in traumatic brain injury assessed pre-hospital and on

enrollment: an IMPACT analysis. J Neurotrauma. 2007;24:270–80.
Mortazavi MM, Romeo AK, Deep A, Griessenauer CJ, Shoja MM, Tubbs RS, Fisher W. Hypertonic saline for treating raised intracranial pressure: literature review with meta-analysis. J Neurosurg. 2012;116:210–21.
Myburgh J, Cooper DJ, Finfer S, Bellomo R, Norton R, Bishop N, et al. Saline or albumin for fluid resuscitation in patients with traumatic brain injury. N Engl J Med. 2007;357:874–84.
Oddo M, Poole D, Helbok R, Meyfroidt G, Stocchetti N, Bouzat P, et al. Fluid therapy in neurointensive care patients: ESICM consensus and clinical practice recommendations. Intensive Care Med. 2018;44:449–63.
Reinhart K, Perner A, Sprung CL, Jaeschke R, Schortgen F, Johan Groeneveld AB, et al. Consensus statement of the ESICM task force on colloid volume therapy in critically ill patients. Intensive Care Med. 2012;38:368–83.
Spaite DW, Hu C, Bobrow BJ, Chikani V, Barnhart B, Gaither JB, et al. The effect of combined out-of-hospital hypotension and hypoxia on mortality in major traumatic brain injury. Ann Emerg Med. 2017a;69:62–72.
Spaite DW, Hu C, Bobrow BJ, Chikani V, Sherrill D, Barnhart B, et al. Mortality and prehospital blood pressure in patients with major traumatic brain injury. JAMA Surg. 2017b;152:360–9.
Stocchetti N, Maas AIR. Traumatic intracranial hypertension. N Engl J Med. 2014;370:2121–30.
Suttipongkaset P, Chaikittisilpa N, Vavilala MS, Lele AV, Watanitanon A, Chandee T, Krishnamoorthy V. Blood pressure thresholds and mortality in pediatric traumatic brain injury. Pediatrics. 2018;142:e20180594–9. https://doi.org/10.1542/peds.2018-0594.
Szaflarski JP, Sangha KS, Lindsell CJ, Shutter LA. Prospective, randomized, single-blinded comparative trial of intravenous levetiracetam versus phenytoin for seizure prophylaxis. Neurocrit Care. 2010;12:165–72.
Torre-Healy A, Marko NF, Weil RJ. Hyperosmolar therapy for intracranial hypertension. Neurocrit Care. 2012;17:117–30.
Tyagi R, Donaldson K, Loftus CM, Jallo J. Hypertonic saline: a clinical review. Neurosurg Rev. 2007;30:277–90.
Zafar SN, Millham FH, Chang Y, Fikry K, Alam HB, King DR, et al. Presenting blood pressure in traumatic brain injury: a bimodal distribution of death. J Trauma. 2011;71:1179–84.

10 What the Neurosurgeon and the Trauma Team Want to Know: What, Who, When, and Where?

Mads Gilbert and Knut Gustav Wester

10.1 Overview

Poor communication causes fragmented care. Important information is often missing during interhospital transfers. Improved, standardised communication during interhospital transfers can close the information gap and improve patient safety and time-critical clinical decisions.

The responsible MD in the neurosurgical unit in the receiving hospital must be given updated, correct, and sufficient information by the Emergency Medical Services (EMS) staff during the clinical handover. This information must build on information gathered by those who had the first contact with the neurotrauma patient or from the local hospital's emergency department (ED) or both. The transfer needs effective communication with concise, rational, clear, and time-efficient exchange of information. The exact and quality-assured patient history and clinical and logistical information should be transferred to the responsible neurosurgeon of the neurosurgical unit during the first contact with the referring hospital or the ambulance medical staff.

The information must be documented using a paper form, preferably a standard hand-written checklist type of form or digital format (see the end of this chapter). Updated information should be given by the referring partner or asked for by the receiving neurosurgical unit. This sheet may be copied and used in the neurosurgical unit.

In many emergency medical systems, patient and logistical information is best conveyed via the emergency medical dispatch centre by medically trained dispatchers during a multi-party telephone or radio/telephone conference.

Telemedicine is also an efficient tool in many emergency medical scenarios and will become more relevant also in neurosurgical patient care. Telemedicine solutions are more efficient when combined with web-based 'live' transmission of dynamic numeric and waveform data from a patient-connected multimonitor. More and systematic use of digital medical tools can facilitate timely and precise patient clinical information and safeguard earlier diagnosis and emergency management. Smartphone-based social media clients such as WhatsApp may be the future for even faster and reliable communication of clinical as well as radiological data during on-call neurosurgical referrals. The 'SBAR' (Situation—Background—Assessment—Recommendation) has also been launched as a structured way of communicating information that requires a

M. Gilbert (✉)
The Clinic of Emergency Medicine, University Hospital of North Norway, Tromsø, Norway

The Anaesthesia and Critical Care Research Group, Institute of Clinical Medicine, The Arctic University of Norway, Tromsø, Norway

K. G. Wester
Department of Clinical Medicine K1, University of Bergen, Bergen, Norway
e-mail: Knut.Wester@uib.no

© Springer Nature Switzerland AG 2020
T. Sundstrøm et al. (eds.), *Management of Severe Traumatic Brain Injury*,
https://doi.org/10.1007/978-3-030-39383-0_10

response from the receiver: http://www.ihi.org/resources/Pages/Tools/SBARToolkit.aspx.

10.2 What?

Vital Functions: ABC

- Any A, B, or C problem?
- Open airways?
  - Airway adjuncts needed?
  - Suction needed?
- Adequate ventilation?
- Respiratory rate?
- Oxygen saturation?
- $EtCO_2$?
- Updated blood gases?
- Adequate blood pressure (BP)?
  - BP over last 20–30 minutes?
- External or internal blood losses?
- Ongoing bleeding, not controlled?
- Hypothermia?
- Indications of fractures (extremities, pelvic, spine)?

Current Level of Consciousness and Neurological Status

- GCS score (total and each function score)
  - Current score?
  - Trended scores?
- Signs of herniation
  - Pupillary dilatation (uni- or bilateral)?
  - Extension spasms?
  - Cushing reflex (irregular breathing, bradycardia, hypertension)?
- Any other crude neurological deficit (hemi-, para-, or tetraparesis)?

Other Signs and Symptoms Following Injury

- Vomiting?
- Amnesia (duration)?
- Loss of consciousness following impact (duration)?
- Any focal neurological deficit since the injury?
- Any suspicion of a skull fracture or penetrating head injury?
- Any seizure since the injury?

Injury Mechanism

- High velocity (yes/no)?
- Road traffic accident (RTA)?
  - Car collision?
    - Driver?
    - Passenger?
    - Speed?
    - Roll-over?
    - Ejection from the vehicle?
  - Motorcycle?
    - Speed?
    - Helmet used?
    - More vehicles involved?
  - Bicycle?
    - Other vehicles involved?
    - Helmet used?
  - Pedestrian?
    - Hit by what?
    - Speed?
- Fall?
  - From which height?
- Violence?
  - Blunt blow? By what?
  - Penetrating injuries?
  - Gunshot injury?
- Multitrauma (yes/no)?
  - Any A, B, or C problem?
  - Adequate ventilation?
  - Adequate blood pressure?
  - Hypothermia?
  - External/internal blood loss?
  - Indications of fractures (extremities, pelvic, spine)?
- Hypothermia prevention started?
- Current core temperature?
- Any indication of a neck injury?
  - Para- or tetraparalyses?
  - Localised neck pain?
  - Is the neck stabilised before the transport?
- Is the patient otherwise stable for transport?
  - If not, what needs to be done and where?

Radiological Examinations

- Radiological examinations performed and findings?
- Can emergency CT or MRI-images be transferred via telemedical systems?

10.3 Who?

Name
Age
Gender

Previous medical conditions? Intoxication?

- Any history of bleeding or clotting disorders?
- Anticoagulant medication now (yes/no)?
  - Type of anticoagulation medication? Antidote available?
  - If warfarin, last INR value?
- Hydrocephalus with CSF shunt (yes/no)?
- Actual alcohol or drug intoxication?
- Other?

10.4 When?

- Approximate time of accident?
- Time of contact with the neurosurgical unit?
- Estimated exact time of arrival at the neurosurgical unit?
- Potential delays (weather, capacity, other potential delays)?

10.5 Where?

- Site of accident?
- Weather (hypothermia)?

10.6 Logistics?

Present Location, Transport, and Professional Companion to the Neurosurgical Unit?

- Is the patient in a hospital or in an ambulance?
- Professional capacity of ambulance unit?
  - Emergency physician present?
  - Paramedic?
  - Airway management expertise?
    Endotracheal intubation?
    Supraglottic airway?
- Established treatment and monitoring?
  - IV line(s)?
  - Intraosseous line(s)?
  - Pulse oximetry with $SatO_2$?
  - Repeated non-invasive blood pressure measurement (NIBP)? Intra-arterial line with intra-arterial blood pressure (IABP)?
  - ECG?
  - Capnography with end-tidal CO_2 (Et CO_2)?
  - Body temperature?
  - Anti-oedema treatment given (mannitol, hyperventilation)?
  - Blood transfusions given?
  - Damage control surgery performed at local hospital?
- Telemetry and telemedicine possibilities?
  - Live transfer of ongoing patient monitoring?
  - Digital transfer of diagnostic imaging (CT, MRI)?
  - Videoconferencing from local hospital?

Appendix

Neurotrauma emergency sheet	
Name:	Gender: M/F
Date of birth:	Date and time of first contact:
What?	
Vital functions—ABC:	
• Any A, B, or C problem:	Yes_/ No_/
• Open airways:	Yes_/ No_/
• Adequate ventilation:	Yes_/ No_/
• Adequate blood pressure:	Yes_/ No_/
• External or internal blood losses:	Yes_/ No_/
• Fractures (extremities, pelvic, spine):	Yes_/ No_/

(continued)

Neurotrauma emergency sheet	
Current level of consciousness and neurological status:	
GCS score (total and each category):	Total: E: M: V:
Herniation:	
• Unilateral pupillary dilatation:	Yes_/ No_/
• Bilateral pupillary dilatation:	Yes_/ No_/
• Extension spasms:	Yes_/ No_/
Any other coarse neurological deficit: • If yes, what?	Yes_/ No_/
Injury mechanism:	
• High velocity:	Yes_/ No_/
• Multitrauma:	Yes_/ No_/
• Road traffic accident (RTA):	Yes_/ No_/
• Car collision:	Yes_/ No_/
• Motorcycle:	Yes_/ No_/
• Bicycle:	Yes_/ No_/
• Pedestrian:	Yes_/ No_/
• Fall:	Yes_/ No_/
• From which height: • Other injury mechanisms—what? • Neck stabilised before the transport? • Patient otherwise stable for transport? • If not, what needs to be done and where?	
Radiological examinations: • Radiological examinations performed and findings: • Can emergency radiology be transferred via telemedical systems?	
When?	
• Approximate time of accident: • Time of contact with the neurosurgical unit: • Estimated time of arrival at the neurosurgical unit:	
Where? • Site of accident:	
Logistics: Present location, transport, and professional companion to the neurosurgical unit: • Patient in hospital or ambulance: • Professional capacity of ambulance unit: • Emergency physician present: • Paramedic: • Anti-oedema treatment given (mannitol, hyperventilation):	

Suggested Reading

Harl FN, Saucke MC, Greenberg CC, et al. Assessing written communication during interhospital transfers of emergency general surgery patients. J Surg Res. 2017;214:86–92.

Mason S, Kuczawski M, Teare MDell J, et al. AHEAD study: an observational study of the management of anticoagulated patients who suffer head injury. BMJ Open. 2017;7(1):e014324.

Aktüre E, Goodwin A, Tranmer B. Rescue strategies to facilitate emergency neurosurgery in patients on antiplatelet or anticoagulant agents. In: Loftus CM, editor. Anticoagulation and hemostasis in neurosurgery. Basel: Springer; 2016. p. 243–56.

Surveillance report 2017—Head injury: assessment and early management. NICE guideline CG176. 2014. https://www.nice.org.uk/guidance/cg176/resources/surveillance-report-2017-head-injury-assessment-and-early-management-2014-nice-guideline-cg176-4476227152/chapter/How-we-made-the-decision?tab=evidence.

Fahim Yegane SA, et al. Clinical information transfer between EMS staff and emergency medicine assistants during handover of trauma patients. Prehosp Disaster Med. 2017;32(5):541–7.

Kim DK, Yoo SK, Kim SH. Instant wireless transmission of radiological images using a personal digital assistant phone for emergency teleconsultation. J Telemed Telecare. 2005;11(2_suppl):58–61.

Nanah A, Bayoumi AB. The pros and cons of digital health communication tools in neurosurgery: a systematic review of literature. Neurosurg Rev. 2018:1–12.

Joshi SS, Murali-Krishnan S, Patankar P, et al. Neurosurgical referral service using smartphone client WhatsApp: preliminary study at a tertiary referral neurosurgical unit. Br J Neurosurg. 2018;32(5):553–7.

Transportation

11

Magnus Olivecrona and Zandra Olivecrona

Recommendations

Level I

There are no data to support a Level I recommendation on this topic.

Level II

There are no data to support a Level II recommendation on this topic.

Level III

The recommendations given are based on physiological knowledge and clinical experience and expertise.

There are some observational and retrospective studies to support the recommendations.

Tips, Tricks and Pitfalls

An uneventful transport is a good transport.

The fundamental requirement is that every doctor, nurse and paramedic likely to be involved in the transfer of seriously brain-injured patients has had formal training in the theoretical and practical aspects of the subject. This will include the following:

- The principles of managing a patient with an acute brain injury.
- The principles and practice of ATLS.
- Better one too many intubations than too few.
- Always perform a neurological examination before an intubation—there is time.
- The adverse physiological changes associated with moving the patient.
- Practical aspects of working in an ambulance or aircraft.
- Knowledge of the equipment and drugs used in transfer.
- Communications.

The sending physician is responsible for securing a smooth and medically safe transportation.

M. Olivecrona (✉) · Z. Olivecrona
Department of Medical Sciences, Faculty of Medicine, Örebro University, Örebro, Sweden

Section for Neurosurgery, Department of Anaesthesia and Intensive Care, University Hospital, Örebro, Sweden
e-mail: zandra.olivecrona@regionorebrolan.se

© Springer Nature Switzerland AG 2020
T. Sundstrøm et al. (eds.), *Management of Severe Traumatic Brain Injury*,
https://doi.org/10.1007/978-3-030-39383-0_11

11.1 Overview

Patients with severe traumatic brain injuries are often primarily treated or triaged at a local hospital without direct access to neurosurgery. Thus, many patients with serious brain injuries have to be transferred between hospitals. Other patients with suspected significant head injury may be transported directly to a facility with comprehensive trauma care and neurosurgery. Consequently, a large number of patients with severe head injury will experience two transportations within a short time, i.e. from the accident to the primary receiving hospital and from this hospital to a hospital with comprehensive neurotrauma care.

Transfer of patients with brain injury is potentially unsafe, and patients may suffer from secondary insults and brain injury due to a poorly performed transport. This can unfavourably affect the outcome and can be avoided if basic principles are applied. The main causes of secondary brain injury are raised intracranial pressure (ICP), hypoxia, hypotension, hypercarbia, hypocarbia, hyperpyrexia and cardiovascular instability. The principles guiding the safe transfer of a head-injured patient are common to all seriously injured persons, but there are some specific considerations that have to be made in the case of head injury. These principles apply equally to transfer of patients both between and within hospitals.

11.2 Principles of the Preparation Before Transportation

11.2.1 Basic Preparations and Considerations Before Transportation of the Head-Injured Patient

An uneventful, boring transport is a good transport.

All preparations before a transport should have the aim of anticipating possible adverse events and making interventions and preparations in order to prevent those. As an example, endotracheal intubation *during transportation* should be avoided, as it is both challenging and dangerous.

The principles of ATLS are valid on the scene of the accident, as well as in the hospital. This includes securing a patent airway, good breathing and an acceptable blood pressure.

The securing of the airway has the highest priority. As a basic principle, all unconscious patients (i.e. GCS ≤ 8) should be intubated. Other reasons for placing an endotracheal tube is a drop in GCS of two (2) or more points or a restless, agitated patient. It is better to have intubated one too many patients rather than too few. Intubation requires adequate sedation and muscle relaxation to avoid an increase in ICP.

The person doing the intubation should use the drugs she or he is familiar with. Ketamine and S-ketamine seem to be safe in persons with head injuries (Cornelius et al. 2018; Kramer et al. 2018; Zeiler et al. 2014). Preferably, short-acting drugs and/or drugs that can easily be reversed should be used in order to allow for clinical neurological examination on arrival to the destination.

In the evaluation of a potentially head-injured patient, it is important that the neurological condition is evaluated before the patient is sedated and intubated. A neurological evaluation consists of examination of the level of consciousness (GCS), pupillary reaction, corneal reflex and, if the patients is unconscious, an evaluation of the reactions to central and peripheral pain stimulation. This is easily done in less than 1 min and so there is *always* time for this essential evaluation. The information attained is very important for the receiving neurosurgeon.

A patient that is still hypotensive despite resuscitation at the local hospital must not be transported until all possible causes of the hypotension have been identified and the patient stabilized. In this situation, the correction of major haemorrhage is superior to transfer. It is important that these measures are not overlooked in an attempt to speed the transfer of the patient, as resulting complications may be impossible to deal with once the transfer has begun. Persistent hypotension will adversely affect neurological outcome. When other causes of hypotension are excluded, consider the use of inotropes/vasopressors to offset the hypotensive effects of sedative agents.

Almost all patients with head injury will have been given a neck collar. A neck collar can restrict the venous flow on the neck, with an increase in ICP as result, and should therefore be so loose as possible. In the intubated, ventilated, sedated and muscle-relaxed patient, one might consider loosening it or even to remove the collar during transportation.

11.2.2 Special Treatment Goals in the Transportation of the Severely Head-Injured Patient

The main goal during transportation of a head-injured patient is to avoid secondary brain injury. This is achieved by avoiding hypoxia, hypercapnia, hypocapnia, hypotension, cardiovascular instability, hyperpyrexia and seizures. The aims of ventilation and blood pressure differ from that of a non-head-injured patient, in order to avoid secondary brain injury during transportation.

The following treatment goals during transportation are set with the injured brain in mind:

1. **A**irway
   (a) Secure a patent airway.
      - Consider endotracheal airway, and be generous.
2. **B**reathing
   (a) $S_aO_2 > 95\%$
   (b) $P_aO_2 > 12$ kPa by $F_iO_2 < 0.5$
      - By a $F_iO_2 > 0.5$, $P_aO_2 > 10$ kPa
   (c) P_aCO_2 4.5–5.5 kPa
3. **C**irculation
   (a) Systolic blood pressure > 100 (110) mmHg
   (b) MAP >70 mmHg

Patients ventilated by hand are in danger of being hyperventilated. Hyperventilation to a $P_aCO_2 < 3.5$ kPa can cause ischaemic brain damage due to vasoconstriction (Curley et al. 2010).

Other measures to prevent secondary brain damage:

1. Tranexamic acid—give 1 g intravenously (New evidence points in the direction that tranexamic acid may prevent progression of intracranial bleeding. A large study is underway) (Chakroun-Walha et al. 2019; Fakharian et al. 2018; Perel et al. 2012; Yutthakasemsunt et al. 2013).
2. Fluid substitution—aim at normovolaemia.
   (a) Try to avoid crystalline fluids.
   (b) Give blood.
   (c) Give plasma.
   (d) If crystalloids are used, use isotonic solutions such as saline.
3. If the patient is treated with anticoagulants, actively reverse the drug using specific antidotes as soon as possible, irrespective of the indication for the anticoagulation.
   (a) If not antidote is available, discuss other options with a coagulation expert.
4. If necessary, use noradrenalin or phenylephrine to maintain an acceptable blood pressure.
5. Seizures should be treated immediately.
   (a) Diazepam or midazolam
   (b) Loading dose of levetiracetam
   (c) Propofol (risk for hypotension)

The sending physician is responsible for the transportation and should be aware of the special considerations before and during the transportation of a head-injured patient. She or he should, regardless of the competence of the transportation crew, communicate these to the person(s) directly responsible for the transportation. In most cases, a physician should accompany a person with severe head injury during the transportation, especially in a potentially unstable patient where transport interventions may be necessary.

11.2.3 Monitoring During Transportation

During transportation, the following parameters are recommended for monitoring:

- Oxygen saturation
- Capnography

- Blood pressure—preferably invasive
- ECG
- Urinary output
- Pupillary size
- Pupillary reaction to light

If the patient is not intubated, repeated examinations of the level of consciousness (according to the GCS) should be performed more often, not fewer times, than upon departure and upon arrival.

11.3 Signs of Herniation and Rising Intracranial Pressure During Transport

During transportation, the patient may deteriorate and show signs of herniation due to rising ICP. Signs of a threatening rise of the ICP and herniation are anisocoria, bilateral dilatation of the pupils, loss of corneal reflex, increasing blood pressure and decreasing heart rate (Cushing's response).

If this occurs during transportation:

1. Increase ventilation, i.e. lower the P_aCO_2.
2. Give mannitol 15 mg/mL, 250–500 mL rapidly.
3. Give hypertonic saline.
4. Increase sedation, and consider using thiopental.

11.4 Special Consideration Concerning Mode of Transport

The transfer can be made by land or by air. If the transfer is made by air, it can be made by helicopter or by fixed-wing aircraft. The latter involves a combination of land and air transport, i.e. transportation to and from airfields and the air transport. All kind of transports can be noisy and rough. This calls for special considerations concerning the need of treatment for motion sickness and the level of sedation. Motion sickness and noise can elevate the ICP, and thus a deeper sedation may be needed than in patients who do not have head injuries. There can be an indication for antiemetics. Hearing protection should be considered.

11.4.1 Air Transport

Specific considerations have to be taken for head-injured patients during air transport. The gravitational forces during take-off and landing, cabin pressure, temperature and the humidity can all affect the ICP.

11.4.1.1 Fixed-Wing Transportation

1. Gravitational forces

   The positioning of the patient in relation to the movement direction of the aircraft is important. The aim is to give the gravitational forces as little influence as possible on the patient. Ideally, this can be achieved if the patient is positioned across the aircraft. In most aircrafts, this is not possible. If the patient is positioned with the head forward and the feet aft, then due to the gravitational force the ICP will be lowered during take-off and raised during landing. The latter can then be counteracted by tilting the head upwards to a sitting position. The opposite is true if the patient is positioned with feet forward and head aft, and then the gravitational forces at the take-off can cause a rise in ICP, which can be counteracted by head elevation.
2. Cabin pressure

   At cruising altitude, most airplanes have at cruising altitude a cabin pressure, which is significantly lower than the pressure at sea level. The cabin pressure usually corresponds to the air pressure at 2400 m (8000 ft). This means that the partial pressure of oxygen is almost 30% lower than at sea level. This implies the need for supplementary oxygen for the head-injured patient in order to keep the goals stated above.

   The lower pressure in the cabin also means, in accordance with the general gas equation, that the volume of gas enclosed in the skull, e.g. after a skull base fracture or after an operation, increases in volume with the decreasing pressure in the cabin. From this, it follows that with the increasing volume of the gas, the ICP may rise. This can especially be true if the volume of the gas exceeds approximately 10 mL (Brandstrom et al. 2017). If there is a suspicion or knowledge of intracranial air especially over the volume of 10 mL, or if the patient has undergone an emergency craniotomy, the physician sending the patient should consider asking for ground pressure in the cabin, in order to avoid the risk of increasing ICP.

3. Humidity

   The air in an airplane has very low humidity, often below 5%. This means an increased loss of water for the patient and thus an increase in the need for volume substitution. This is especially important during longer transfers.

11.4.1.2 Helicopter Transportation

1. Gravitational forces

   The position of a helicopter accelerating or flying is not horizontal but tilted downwards ahead. This means that a patient lying on the gurney in the helicopter with the head forward and with no head elevation de facto is in a Trendelenburg position, i.e. with the head lower than the heart. Because of this, the ICP may rise due to reduced venous outflow and/or increased pressure in the jugular veins. The recommendation would be to elevate the headrest on the gurney during flight to counteract the venous outflow resistance (Maissan et al. 2018).

11.4.2 Land Transport

1. Gravitational forces

   The same principles of acceleration and deceleration apply to ground transport, e.g. in an ambulance. Depending on the positioning of the patient, there can be an influence on the ICP during acceleration and deceleration. It is important to drive as smoothly as possible.

11.5 Organising Transportation

There should be local instructions for how to organise a transport of a head-injured patient. There should also be agreements in place between the referring hospital and the trauma service/hospital to which the person is referred. This means that every physician that can be involved in taking care of a head-injured person in a hospital without neurosurgical competence has to familiarise herself/himself with the treatment protocols and transport organisation in the specific hospital and in the specific healthcare organisation.

11.6 Specific Paediatric Concerns

The transfer of paediatric patients will require size-specific equipment and, if possible, staff experienced in the transfer of critically ill children.

References

Brandstrom H, Sundelin A, Hoseason D, Sundstrom N, Birgander R, Johansson G, et al. Risk for intracranial pressure increase related to enclosed air in post-craniotomy patients during air ambulance transport: a retrospective cohort study with simulation. Scand J Trauma Resusc Emerg Med. 2017;25(1):50. https://doi.org/10.1186/s13049-017-0394-9.

Chakroun-Walha O, Samet A, Jerbi M, Nasri A, Talbi A, Kanoun H, et al. Benefits of the tranexamic acid in head trauma with no extracranial bleeding: a prospective follow-up of 180 patients. Eur J Trauma Emerg Surg. 2019;45(4):719–26. https://doi.org/10.1007/s00068-018-0974-z.

Cornelius BG, Webb E, Cornelius A, Smith KWG, Ristic S, Jain J, et al. Effect of sedative agent selection on morbidity, mortality and length of stay in patients with increase in intracranial pressure. World J Emerg Med. 2018;9(4):256–61. https://doi.org/10.5847/wjem.j.1920-8642.2018.04.003.

Curley G, Kavanagh BP, Laffey JG. Hypocapnia and the injured brain: more harm than benefit. Crit Care Med. 2010;38(5):1348–59. https://doi.org/10.1097/CCM.0b013e3181d8cf2b.

Fakharian E, Abedzadeh-Kalahroudi M, Atoof F. Effect of tranexamic acid on prevention of hemorrhagic mass growth in patients with traumatic brain injury. World Neurosurg. 2018;109:e748–e53. https://doi.org/10.1016/j.wneu.2017.10.075.

Kramer N, Lebowitz D, Walsh M, Ganti L. Rapid sequence intubation in traumatic brain-injured adults. Cureus. 2018;10(4):e2530. https://doi.org/10.7759/cureus.2530.

Maissan IM, Verbaan LA, van den Berg M, Houmes RJ, Stolker RJ, den Hartog D. Helicopter transportation increases intracranial pressure: a proof-of-principle study. Air Med J. 2018;37(4):249–52. https://doi.org/10.1016/j.amj.2018.02.010.

Perel P, Al-Shahi Salman R, Kawahara T, Morris Z, Prieto-Merino D, Roberts I, et al. CRASH-2 (Clinical Randomisation of an Antifibrinolytic in Significant Haemorrhage) intracranial bleeding study: the effect of tranexamic acid in traumatic brain injury—a nested randomised, placebo-controlled trial. Health Technol Assess. 2012;16(13):iii-xii, 1–54. https://doi.org/10.3310/hta16130.

Yutthakasemsunt S, Kittiwatanagul W, Piyavechvirat P, Thinkamrop B, Phuenpathom N, Lumbiganon P. Tranexamic acid for patients with traumatic brain injury: a randomized, double-blinded, placebo-controlled trial. BMC Emerg Med. 2013;13:20. https://doi.org/10.1186/1471-227X-13-20.

Zeiler FA, Teitelbaum J, West M, Gillman LM. The ketamine effect on ICP in traumatic brain injury. Neurocrit Care. 2014;21(1):163–73. https://doi.org/10.1007/s12028-013-9950-y.

Some Guidelines

Accident Compensation Corporation, New Zealand. 2011. https://www.acc.co.nz/assets/research/tbi-review-transfer.pdf.

Intensive Care Society Guidelines for the transport of the critically ill adult. 2011. http://www.ics.ac.uk/ICS/Guidelines___Standards/ICS/guidelines-and-standards.aspx?hkey=4ed20a1c-1ff8-46e0-b48e-732f1f4a90e2.

The Association of Anaesthetists of Great Britain and Ireland. Recommendations for the safe transfer of patients with brain injury. 2006. https://www.aagbi.org/sites/default/files/braininjury.pdf.

Part IV

Admission, Diagnostics and Planning

Christina Rosenlund

12 The Trauma Team Concept

Christina Rosenlund and Rico Frederik Schou

Recommendations

Level I

There are insufficient data to support a Level I recommendation.

Level II

Patient outcome is directly related to the time elapsed between trauma and properly delivered definite care.

Trauma outcome is improved if critically injured patients are cared for in trauma centers.

Implementation of standardized trauma evaluation, trauma centers, and better prehospital care has shortened the time from the trauma scene to definite care.

Level III

Level and timing of communication between the prehospital system and the primary receiving hospital influences timeliness in patient treatment and transfer to definite care.

Implementation of trauma teams has reduced the time spent on primary trauma care and the frequency of overseen injuries.

12.1 Overview

Receiving and treating severely injured patients involve many different groups of personnel and medical specialties which constitute the trauma team. The trauma team is formed by a team leader (often a surgeon or anesthesiologist in Scandinavia, an emergency medicine physician in other European countries), a dedicated anesthesiologist and nurse—emergency department nurses and a radiologist. Other specialties will be called forth as necessary, e.g., thoracic or general surgeon.

It is important that the trauma team and the trauma team settings are well organized and of high quality since the acute diagnostics and treatment can be very challenging. The foundation for optimal patient care is knowing your way around the trauma bay area, keeping the equipment most necessary for patient treatment close at hand, and

C. Rosenlund (✉)
Department of Neurosurgery, Odense University Hospital, Odense, Denmark
e-mail: christina.rosenlund2@rsyd.dk

R. F. Schou
Department of Neuroanesthesia and Neurocritical Care, Odense University Hospital, Odense, Denmark

Section of Neuroanesthesia and Neurointensive Care, Department of Anesthesia and Intensive Care Medicine, Odense University Hospital, Odense, Denmark
e-mail: rico.frederik.schou@rsyd.dk

© Springer Nature Switzerland AG 2020
T. Sundstrøm et al. (eds.), *Management of Severe Traumatic Brain Injury*,
https://doi.org/10.1007/978-3-030-39383-0_12

preparing two steps ahead whenever possible. Make sure all equipment is tested regularly and fully functioning.

Systematic and strict procedures should be outlined in a trauma manual. The trauma team leader is ultimately responsible for coordinating the process, gathering information, and making the final decisions for further treatment.

Optimally, the trauma patient is delivered to definite care in a trauma center with specialties capable of treating the injuries in question. A well-organized prehospital triage system will preferably prevent secondary transfers from other hospitals, should the trauma patient initially have been delivered to closest treating facility without the necessary specialties or competences available.

Before a secondary transfer is effectuated:

1. Ensure that the patient's ABCDEs are appropriately managed (see other chapter).
2. Do not wait for test results other than those necessary to ensure hemodynamic and respiratory stability.
3. Ensure that the level of care does not deteriorate, including the care delivered during transport to definite care.
4. Ensure that the proper written information is following the patient or available electronically/online.
5. Contact the trauma team leader when transfer is initiated.

Information provided directly to the trauma team leader at the receiving hospital should include:

1. Patient identification
2. Brief history of the incident, including pertinent prehospital data
3. Initial findings in the primary hospital
4. Patient's response to the therapy administered

Tips, Tricks, and Pitfalls

- The team leader should not participate in the practical management of the patient but should concentrate on keeping track of the process.
- Communicate in closed loops whenever you take an assignment. Teamwork is essential.
- Step away from the scene whenever you are without an assignment.

12.2 Background

Death due to injury occurs in one of three periods, first described in 1982. The primary injury during trauma is inevitable and occurs within seconds to minutes after the injury. The second period is within minutes to several hours following injury and trauma, and the timing and prioritizing of treatment in this period is of crucial importance to the patient outcome. It is the responsibility of the prehospital personnel and their medical director to ensure that appropriate patients arrive at appropriate hospitals and to alert the receiving hospital as early as possible.

The third peak occurs within hours to days or weeks following trauma and is due to sepsis or multiple organ failure, MOF.

The development of standardized trauma training, better prehospital care, trauma centers, and protocols for intensive care of injured patients has improved the prognosis and altered the picture (Sarkar et al. 2011). The golden hour of care after injury is characterized by rapid assessment and resuscitation, which are the fundamental principles of Advanced Trauma Life Support—the ATLS program. Many countries worldwide are now providing this program to doctors. Studies have shown significant effect on morbidity and mortality following implementation (Ali et al.

1993; Anderson et al. 1997; van Olden et al. 2004; Williams et al. 1997; Magnone et al. 2016). The principles are founded on the fact that the injuries causing the deaths within the second period are intracranial hematomas (epi- and subdural); thoracic injuries causing problems with the airways, breathing or circulation; and abdominal or extremity injuries causing massive bleeding; for the ABCDE principle, see other chapter.

It is essential that doctors assess their own capabilities and limitations, as well as those of their institution, to allow for early recognition of patients who may be safely cared for in the local hospital and those who require transfer for definite care. Once the need for transfer is recognized, arrangements should be expedited and not be delayed for diagnostic procedures that do not change the immediate plan of care. Transfer agreements must be established as early as possible to provide for the consistent and efficient movement of patients between institutions. The patient must be as respiratory and circulatory stabile as possible and should be transferred with personnel capable of monitoring and giving treatment to the trauma patient. The information accompanying the patient should include a written record of the problem, clinical findings, treatment given, and patient's status at the time of transfer in addition to demographic and historical information pertinent to the patient's injury (Mullins et al. 1994; Schoettker et al. 2003; Sharar et al. 1988).

12.3 Specific Pediatric Concerns

The recommendation regarding pediatric trauma patients follows the adult protocol. Pediatric patients with TBI should be treated in a pediatric trauma center, if possible (Orliaquet et al. 2008).

References

Ali J, et al. Trauma outcome improves following the advanced trauma life support program in a developing country. J Trauma. 1993;34:890–9.

Anderson ID, et al. Advanced trauma life support in the UK: 8 years on. Br J Hosp Med. 1997;57:272–3.

Magnone S, et al. Impact of ATLS guidelines, trauma team introduction, and 24-hour mortality due to severe trauma in a busy, metropolitan Italian hospital: a case control study. Ulus Travma Acil Cerrahi Derg. 2016;22(3):242–6.

Mullins PJ, et al. Outcome of hospitalized injured patients after institution of a trauma system in an urban area. JAMA. 1994;271:1919–24.

Orliaquet, et al. Management of critically ill children with traumatic brain injury. Paediatr Anaesth. 2008;18(6):455–61.

Sarkar B, et al. American College of Surgeons' Committee on Trauma Performance Improvement and Patient Safety program: maximal impact in a mature trauma center. J Trauma. 2011;71(5):1447–53. discussion 1453–4.

Schoettker P, et al. Reduction of time to definite care in trauma patients: effectiveness of a new checklist system. Injury. 2003;34:187–90.

Sharar SR, et al. Air transport following surgical stabilization: an extension of regionalized trauma care. J Trauma. 1988;28:794–8.

van Olden GDJ, et al. Clinical impact of advanced trauma life support. Am J Emerg Med. 2004;22:522–5.

Williams MJ, et al. Improved trauma management with advanced trauma life support (ATLS) training. J Accid Emerg Med. 1997;14:81–3.

Trauma Protocol (ABCDE)

13

Christina Rosenlund and Rico Frederik Schou

Recommendations

Level I

There are insufficient data to support a Level I recommendation.

Level II

There are insufficient data to support a Level II recommendation.

Level III

Implementation of systematic trauma protocols has shortened the time interval to definitive care and reduces the frequency of overseen injuries. A lateral (or mini-) thoracostomy is recommended to relieve tension pneumothorax. Rapid four-step procedure is the preferred method for emergency cricothyroidotomy.

13.1 Overview

Systematic evaluation and re-evaluation of the patient following the ABCDE principles will diminish the risk of overlooking injuries in the trauma patient. Primary focus in the first 5 min is to discover the most critical injuries and treat those first. The secondary survey is more thorough and will reveal the injuries causing problems later.

Tips, Tricks and Pitfalls

- (**A**irway) Nasopharyngeal airway is *not* an option in patients with skull base fractures.
- (**A**) The presence of gastric contents (vomiting) in the oropharynx represents a significant risk of aspiration. Suction and rotation (log roll) are indicated.
- (**A**) Abusive and belligerent patients may in fact have hypoxia and should not be presumed intoxicated.
- (**A**) Performing a needle cricothyroidotomy with jet insufflation can provide the time necessary to establish a definite airway when all other options have

C. Rosenlund (✉)
Department of Neurosurgery, Odense University Hospital, Odense, Denmark
e-mail: christina.rosenlund2@rsyd.dk

R. F. Schou
Department of Neuroanesthesia and Neurocritical Care, Odense University Hospital, Odense, Denmark

Section of Neuroanesthesia and Neurointensive Care, Department of Anesthesia and Intensive Care Medicine, Odense University Hospital, Odense, Denmark
e-mail: rico.frederik.schou@rsyd.dk

© Springer Nature Switzerland AG 2020
T. Sundstrøm et al. (eds.), *Management of Severe Traumatic Brain Injury*,
https://doi.org/10.1007/978-3-030-39383-0_13

failed, and hypoxia and patient deterioration are a threat. The rapid four-step tracheotomy procedure is recommended over standard technique for emergency tracheotomy.

- (**B**reathing) Patients with a penetrating thoracic trauma are presumed to have a pneumothorax until proven otherwise.
- (**B**) Both tension pneumothorax and massive haemothorax are associated with decreased breath sounds. Hyperresonance in percussion confirms a pneumothorax and dullness a haemothorax. Definite diagnosis, however, is made by lung ultrasound, LUS or X-ray (noise in the trauma settings can make the differentiation impossible!)
- (**B/C**irculation) Pressure pneumothorax and cardiac tamponade can cause shock. Pneumothorax is much more frequent than tamponade.
- (**C**) Until proven otherwise, bleeding is the reason for shock in a trauma patient! Replace the volume loss.
- (**D**isability) Intracranial haemorrhage is almost never the reason for shock—at least not because of bleeding! Important exception: infants!
- (**ABCDE**) Initial monitoring and tests:
  - Pulse oximetry
  - Capnography (intubated patients)
  - Invasive blood pressure
  - Continuous ECG
  - Temperature
  - Urinary catheter
  - Plain X-ray (thorax, pelvis)
  - FAST (abdomen)

13.2 Background

The initial 5 min is the primary survey and should include a rapid and prioritized attention to life-threatening injuries (Enderson et al. 2001; Esposito et al. 2005; American College Committee on Trauma 2012). The patient is quickly assessed and the injuries are managed, as they reveal themselves according to the ABCDE mnemonic. The greatest threat to life is treated first.

13.2.1 Airway

- Assess airway patency simultaneously with securing the cervical spine. Bleeding, facial fractures, direct trauma against head/neck or unconsciousness can cause problems handling the airway.
- GCS < 9 indicates intubation.
- Endotracheal intubation includes sedation, especially in the presence of TBI.
- See (alertness, colour, breathing movements, lesions/obstructions).
- Listen (breathing sounds/noise, speech).
- Feel (trachea in midline).

Endotracheal intubation for secure/definitive airway is a multiple-person procedure: one person fixating the head and cervical spine, a person giving medication and providing suction and tube whenever necessary and an intubator to do the laryngoscopy and insert the tube. There is no longer general consensus to the use of cricoid pressure application during rapid sequence induction. It may be detrimental and worsen the conditions for laryngoscopy (Algie et al. 2015; Salem et al. 2017; Caruana et al. 2017; Bohman et al. 2018).

If a definite airway is not obtainable through endotracheal intubation, a surgical airway is necessary. This is done through the cricothyroid membrane either as a needle or surgical cricothyroidotomy, in which the latter is to consider as a definite airway with insertion of a small endotracheal or a tracheostomy tube through the membrane. The rapid four-step technique is the recommended procedure of choice (Holmes et al. 1999; Schober et al. 2009).

Temporary options to a definite airway includes chin lift, jaw thrust, oro- and nasopharyngeal airways (see Tips, Tricks and Pitfalls), laryngeal mask airway, multilumen oesophageal airway, laryngeal tube airway and of course oxygen provided either directly through the established airway, through a nasal catheter or through a mask (American College Committee on Trauma 2012).

13.2.2 Breathing

- See (movement of the thorax, lesions).
- Listen (percussion, stethoscope).
- Feel (fractures of the ribs/sternum, subcutaneous emphysema).
- Measure respiratory frequency, pulse oximetry and end-tidal CO_2.
- Check for signs of tension pneumothorax, haemothorax, unstable thorax (at least two fractured adjacent ribs, flail chest) and cardiac tamponade.

Open pneumothorax can be immediately handled by placing a closed bandage on the lesion, fastening it to the skin on three sides and with the fourth open as a one-way valve. This turns it into a closed and simple pneumothorax.

A tension pneumothorax can potentially be managed by placing a large-calibre needle into the second intercostal space in the midclavicular line of the affected hemithorax. However, these needles tend to bend and loose effectiveness—or they are simply too short and quickly end up with the tip outside the pleural cavity—the latter being very probable and should be anticipated especially in adipose or very muscular patients. A failure rate of up to 80% is described with needle thoracocentesis (Kaserer et al. 2017).

An alternative in managing a tension pneumothorax in the emergency setting is a lateral/mini-thoracostomy or tube thoracostomy in case of coexisting massive haemothorax (Drinhaus et al. 2016).

More than one chest tube may be needed. Treatment of an unstable thorax is primarily intubation and ventilation.

Cardiac tamponade is diagnosed using ultrasound/focused assessment with sonography in trauma (FAST) and treated initially by pericardiocentesis under ECG monitoring (American College Committee on Trauma 2012). Definite treatment is surgery.

13.2.3 Circulation

Shock is defined as insufficient perfusion of the organs and is presented by a clinical picture with symptoms and objective findings from all the organ-related systems. It is imperative to recognise the presence of shock in order to treat it accordingly.

- Stop apparent bleeding by compression.
- Introduce two large-calibre intravenous catheters. Other peripheral lines and intraosseous and central venous lines or cutdowns should be used when necessary in accordance with the shock level of the patient and the skill level of the doctor.
- Draw blood samples for blood type, cross-match, haemoglobin, electrolytes, arterial blood gases, toxicology studies, and, if indicated, pregnancy test.
- Administer warmed crystalloids (lactated Ringer's or normal isotonic saline) and initial bolus of 20 mL/kg, which can be repeated.
- If continued need for volume arises, transfusions with blood products (SAG-M, plasma, platelets) are warranted. Use of colloids is controversial. They have been associated with a worsened outcome if administered in the patient with burns, multitrauma, renal insufficiency or severe coagulopathy (Rehm et al. 2017; Mullier et al. 2016). Other studies don't find a significant difference in mortality or morbidity (Orbegozo et al. 2014), and yet newer literature suggest a favourable outcome if designed colloids, such as polygelenes, are used (Singh et al. 2017).
- It is recommended with goal-directed therapy including viscoelastic haemostatic assays for early and management of trauma-induced coagulopathy (Stensballe et al. 2017).
- Evaluate response. Circulatory parameters have to normalise, not just stabilise!
- The goal of resuscitation is a systolic blood pressure >90–100 mmHg. Permissive hypotension where lower targets are accepted has been suggested for patients awaiting definitive haemostasis. This is by delaying aggressive fluid resuscitation until haemostasis is

achieved (American College Committee on Trauma 2012). Head trauma patients, though, should have a systolic blood pressure >110–120 mmHg to ensure sufficient cerebral blood flow.

- Seek the source of bleeding! Damage control surgery, DCS, may be necessary in the emergency setting (Rodrigues et al. 2016).
- Reasons for shock are the following: bleeding, tension pneumothorax and neurogenic (medullary compression) and cardiac tamponade (American College Committee on Trauma 2012).

13.2.4 Disability

A rapid neurological exam is performed.

- Glasgow Coma Scale score.
- Pupil reaction, size and form.
- Movement of the extremities, lateralizing signs?
- Indication for intubation at GCS < 9.
- Rule out hypoglycaemia.

13.2.5 Exposure

Hypothermia is of great concern in the trauma patient. A cascade of hypothermia, acidosis and coagulopathy (resuscitative haemodilution) is nick-named the "Trauma Triad of Death" or "The Lethal Triad" (Gerecht 2014; Michail 1999; Martini 2016). Coagulopathy alone is a prognostic factor for increased mortality and a challenge if the patient is being resuscitated and in need of DCS (Samuels et al. 2017).

- Undress the patient in order to make a complete and thorough examination/inspection including the back. At the same time avoid hypothermia.
- Use warmed fluids.
- Use blankets to cover the patient.
- High room temperature should be maintained in the resuscitation area.

Continuously reassess ABCDE throughout the initial treatment period. Make sure that the intervention actually provides the response expected (American College Committee on Trauma 2012).

13.3 Specific Paediatric Concerns

The recommendations regarding paediatric patients follow the adult protocol, apart from the different reference values in children and the alertness regarding the shorter interval between seemingly normal values during monitoring and the sudden deterioration leading to a shorter period for resuscitation, if alertness is not appropriate.

NB! Intracranial bleeding may on rare occasions cause hypovolaemic shock before neurological deterioration in small infants!

References

Algie CM, et al. Effectiveness and risks of cricoid pressure during rapid sequence induction for endotracheal intubation. Cochrane Database Syst Rev. 2015;18(11):CD011656.

American College Committee on Trauma. Advanced trauma life support. 9th ed. Chicago: American College of Surgeons; 2012. p. 1–366.

Bohman JK, et al. A pilot randomized clinical trial assessing the effect of cricoid pressure on risk of aspiration. Clin Respir J. 2018;12(1):175–82.

Caruana E, et al. Effect of cricoid pressure on laryngeal view during prehospital tracheal intubation: a propensity-based analysis. Emerg Med J. 2017;34(3):132–7.

Drinhaus H, et al. Chest decompression in emergency medicine and intensive care. Anaesthesist. 2016;65(10):768–75.

Enderson BL, et al. The tertiary trauma survey: a prospective study on missed injury. J Trauma. 2001;50:367–83.

Esposito TJ, et al. General surgeons and the advanced trauma life support course: is it time to refocus? J Trauma. 2005;59(6):1314–9.

Gerecht R. The lethal triad. Hypothermia, acidosis & coagulopathy create a deadly cycle for trauma patients. JEMS. 2014;39(4):56–60.

Holmes JF, et al. Comparison of 2 cricothyrotomy techniques: standard method versus rapid 4-step technique. Ann Emerg Med. 1999;32(4):442–6.

Kaserer A, et al. Failure rate of prehospital chest decompression after severe thoracic trauma. Am J Emerg Med. 2017;35(3):469–74.

Martini WZ. Coagulation complications following trauma. Mil Med Res. 2016;22(3):35. eCollection 2016.

Michail J. The trauma triad of death: hypothermia, acidosis, and coagulopathy. AACN Clin Issues. 1999;10(1):85–94.

Mullier F, et al. Facing coagulation disorders after acute trauma. B-ENT. 2016;Suppl 26(1):67–85.

Orbegozo CD, et al. Colloids for fluid resuscitation: what is their role in patients with shock? Minerva Anestesiol. 2014;80(8):963–9.

Rehm M, et al. State of the art in fluid and volume therapy: a user-friendly staged concept. Anaesthesist. 2017;66(3):153–67.

Rodrigues RR, et al. Bleeding and damage control surgery. Curr Opin Anaesthesiol. 2016;29(2):229–33.

Salem MR, et al. Cricoid pressure controversies: narrative review. Anesthesiology. 2017;126(4):738–52.

Samuels JM, et al. Damage control resuscitation. Chirurgia (Bucur). 2017;112(5):514–23.

Schober P, et al. Emergency cricothyrotomy-a comparative study of different techniques in human cadavers. Resuscitation. 2009;80(2):204–9.

Singh A, et al. Effectiveness and safety of polygeline in patients with hypovolemia due to trauma. J Emerg Trauma Shock. 2017;10(3):116–20.

Stensballe J, et al. Early haemorrhage control and management of trauma-induced coagulopathy: the importance of goal-directed therapy. Curr Opin Crit Care. 2017;23(6):503–10.

14 Hospital Response to Mass Casualty Incidents

Pål Aksel Næss and Christine Gaarder

Recommendations

Level I

There are insufficient data to support a Level I recommendation.

Level II

There are insufficient data to support a Level II recommendation.

Level III

In most multiple casualty incidents, the number of severely injured patients is modest. Still, these incidents pose a huge challenge to the involved hospitals.

Abstract

In an MCI, the strategy of medical care must be switched from optimal treatment of the individual patient to do the greatest good for the greatest number of patients.

P. A. Næss (✉) · C. Gaarder
Department of Traumatology, Oslo University Hospital Ullevål, Oslo, Norway

Faculty of Medicine, University of Oslo, Oslo, Norway
e-mail: paanae@ous-hf.no; tingaa@ous-hf.no

14.1 Overview

Mass casualty incidents (MCIs) are events incurring casualties large enough to overcome the capacity of even large trauma centres in certain situations. In an MCI, the strategy of medical care must be switched from optimal treatment of the individual patient to do the greatest good for the greatest number of patients. The MCI hospital response should clearly reflect such a strategy and must be based on an updated disaster plan. Trauma-competent staff is a limited resource in most hospitals. Key personnel must be regularly trained.

Tips, Tricks and Pitfalls

- Retriage patients at the entrance of the ED.
- Keep walking wounded away from areas designated to the treatment of severely injured.
- Trauma-competent surgical personnel is a limited resource.
- Split surgical command, triage and supervision.
- Start planning for the following days immediately.

© Springer Nature Switzerland AG 2020

T. Sundstrøm et al. (eds.), *Management of Severe Traumatic Brain Injury*,
https://doi.org/10.1007/978-3-030-39383-0_14

14.2 Background

While the spectrum of MCIs is unlimited, they share similar medical and public health concerns. Most MCIs affect a limited area, and although the number of severely injured is often moderate, the medical capacity of the receiving hospital is challenged. A consistent predefined reaction to MCIs is the accepted practice worldwide (Roth et al. 2013). This MCI response is aiming to provide the greatest good for the greatest number of people based on optimal use of available resources.

All hospitals must have an institution-specific disaster management plan. The plan should be updated regularly and cover all aspects relevant to various scenarios anticipated during an MCI. The plan should include relevant protocols and standing orders. All designated personnel should undergo educational programs, and key roles must be trained regularly.

In an MCI, prehospital triage is challenging and overtriage is more common. Moreover, less severely injured patients, i.e. the walking wounded, tend to migrate to the nearest hospital. To avoid resuscitation areas in the emergency department (ED) being overwhelmed by less severely injured casualties, all patients should enter the hospital through a single entrance and be triaged by a trauma-competent team to predefined admitting areas. These areas must be designated to different patient categories based on severity of injuries and staffed accordingly with trained personnel. To make these areas ready for incoming patients from the MCI, evacuation of regular patients from the ED must take place immediately.

In most institutions worldwide, the surgical trauma competence is a limited resource (Gaarder et al. 2012). Moreover, the entire treatment chain cannot be supervised from the ED entrance. On that background, the dual command concept as a universal principle to conserve resources and provide optimal patient care during an MCI was put forward (Hirshberg et al. 2001). The idea was that one physician should be responsible for the overall medical and administrative operation in the ED during an MCI, including patient flow and personnel deployment. A second physician should supervise the delivery of trauma care by the trauma teams and assign priorities for surgery. The use of the dual command concept has been reported to make supervision of trauma teams possible and allow effective use of trauma-experienced personnel (Gaarder et al. 2012).

Triage errors will inevitably occur in most MCIs especially in the initial phase of patient influx. The importance of trauma-trained staff in core control positions for retriage and optimisation of resources after the patients have left the ED has been underlined in several reports (Aylwin et al. 2005; Cushman et al. 2003; Gaarder et al. 2012).

The ideal situation during an MCI is to maintain adequate capacity at all treatment locations (Aylwin et al. 2005; Hirshberg et al. 2001). In the ED, this can be achieved by maximum mobilisation of personnel. Additionally, the standard of care must be set at a different level compared to the normal situation, termed minimal acceptable care (or institutional damage control). As part of this approach, time spent in the ED should be kept to a minimum. The use of imaging tests should be restricted to diagnosing life-threatening conditions (Roth et al. 2013). Ultrasound (i.e. focused assessment with sonography for trauma, FAST) has been recommended to be used liberally for detection of free fluid in the abdomen or the pericardial sac (Roth et al. 2013). However, if a positive FAST is followed by mandatory laparotomy in all patients during an MCI, a high rate of negative operations must be expected (Aylwin et al. 2005; de Ceballos et al. 2005; Gaarder et al. 2012). If available in the ED, computed tomography scan should be restricted to patients with suspected severe head injuries (Young et al. 2017). Radiological capacity elsewhere in the hospital should be increased as part of the MCI response and should be offered patients after transfer to an intensive care unit (ICU) or wards.

In the initial phase of an MCI, the operating room (OR) resource use should be minimised by applying damage control surgical principles or delaying operations when possible. Planned elective activity should be postponed and ongoing procedures completed as quickly as possible (Roth et al. 2013). When patient influx is under control and available OR capacity is deemed sufficient, the transition to a more definitive treatment approach should be initiated.

ICU bed is another limited resource in most hospitals, and once the MCI alert is activated, the staff in the ICU should start planning for patient arrival. Extra ventilator beds should be staffed with competent personnel.

Some patients with complex injuries will require multiple operations and long-time stay in the ICU. Such patients should be discussed in multidisciplinary meetings on a daily basis. Planning for "tomorrow" to provide continuity and optimal timing of treatment should be an integrated part of the MCI response from day 1.

14.3 Specific Paediatric Concerns

The recommendations regarding paediatric patients follow the adult protocols in principle.

References

Aylwin CJ, et al. Reduction in critical mortality in urban mass casualty incidents: analysis of triage, surge and resource use after the London bombings on July 7, 2005. Lancet. 2005;368:2219–25.

Cushman JG, et al. Two New York Hospitals' surgical response to the September 11, 2001 terrorist attack in New York City. J Trauma. 2003;54:147–55.

de Ceballos JP, et al. 11 March, 2004: the terrorist bomb explosions in Madrid, Spain—an analysis of the logistics, injuries sustained and clinical management of casualties treated at the closest hospital. Crit Care. 2005;9:104–11.

Gaarder C, et al. The twin terrorist attacks in Norway on July 22, 2011: the trauma center response. J Trauma Acute Care Surg. 2012;73:269–75.

Hirshberg A, et al. Hospital trauma care in multiple-casualty incidents: a critical view. Ann Emerg Med. 2001;37:647–52.

Roth RN, et al. Chapter 18: disaster, mass casualty incidents. In: The trauma manual: trauma and acute care surgery. Philadelphia: Lippincott Williams & Wilkins; 2013.

Young VS, et al. Radiology response in the emergency department during a mass casualty incident: a retrospective study of the two terrorist attacks on 22 July 2011 in Norway. Eur Radiol. 2017;27:2828–34.

15 Cervical Spine Injury

Tor Brommeland and Hege Linnerud

Recommendations

Level I

There is no clinically significant effect using high-dose steroid infusion in patients with spinal cord injury (SCI), and the complication risk is increased. Patients with concomitant traumatic brain injury (TBI) may have increased mortality rates using steroid infusion (Edwards et al. 2005).

In trauma patients that are awake, sober, without neck or distracting pain, neurologically intact, and able to complete a functional range of motion (ROM) examination, spinal stabilization and radiographic assessment of the cervical spine are not recommended (Theodore et al. 2013).

Level II

The American Spinal Injury Association (ASIA) score is recommended as the preferred neurological examination tool in the assessment of acute SCI patients (Hadley et al. 2013).

Level III

One can attempt to prevent secondary neurologic injury following spinal trauma by applying a spine board, a collar, and/or manual in-line stabilization of the cervical spine (Kornhall et al. 2017). Patients with SCI seem to benefit from early decompression and stabilization (<24 h) as well as maintaining a middle arterial pressure (MAP) above 85 mmHg for 5–7 days (Saadeh et al. 2017).

15.1 Overview

Attend to life-threatening injuries first, minimizing the movement of the patient until spinal trauma has been excluded. Obtain as much information as possible from the patient history and physical examination in order to establish a baseline in the patient's neurological status. Physical examination of the spine includes palpation of the vertebral column (log-rolling the patient), neurologic evaluation (motor and sensory deficits including reflexes), and rectal exploration. An alert, awake, sober, pain-free, and neurologically intact patient with normal ROM does not need stabilization or radiological investigations of the spine (Theodore et al. 2013). All other patients should have a radiological examination. CT imaging of the cervical spine is the method of choice. X-ray (AP, lateral, and odontoid view) should only be used as an initial evaluation if CT is not available. Based on CT findings and/or neurological status of the patient, MRI of the cervical spine may be necessary to complete the

T. Brommeland (✉) · H. Linnerud
Department of Neurosurgery, Oslo University Hospital Ullevål, Oslo, Norway
e-mail: uxegfr@ous-hf.no

© Springer Nature Switzerland AG 2020
T. Sundstrøm et al. (eds.), *Management of Severe Traumatic Brain Injury*,
https://doi.org/10.1007/978-3-030-39383-0_15

radiological investigation. MRI is superior in order to reveal injuries to ligamentous structures, the spinal cord, and intervertebral discs as well as displaying hematomas within the spinal canal. All patients with neurologic symptoms such as paresis, sensory disturbances, or radiating pain should have MRI of the cervical spine, even if the primary CT investigation is considered normal.

In the obtunded trauma patient not eligible for clinical examination and with a normal CT of the cervical spine, the available evidence is not sufficient to support a uniform strategy. However, there is increasing support in favor of cervical collar removal after a negative high-quality cervical spine CT scan alone (Ryken et al. 2013, Patel et al. 2015).

15.2 Background

The distribution of spinal injury shows the thoracolumbar region (Th12/L1) to be the most commonly affected followed by the cervical region (Leucht et al. 2009). Approximately 20% of patients admitted to a trauma center with a cervical fracture also have a SCI. The prevalence of a concomitant cervical spinal injury of any kind in patients with TBI is ca. 6.5% (Pandrich et al. 2018).

15.2.1 Classification of Cervical Spine Injuries

Based on the radiological and clinical investigations, the aim is to classify the injuries of the cervical spine as stable or unstable. We recommend using either the Subaxial Cervical Spine Injury Classification System (SLICS) or the latest AO classification for this purpose.

15.2.2 Treatment of Cervical Spine Injuries

Based on stability assessment and degree of compression of neurological structures, we sort cervical spine injuries into three treatment groups: (1) open surgery, (2) external immobilization, and (3) no stabilizing treatment needed. Surgical treatment consists of internal fixation, with or without additional reduction and/or decompression. This can be done by either an anterior or posterior approach. In cases with severe instability, such as subluxation injuries, a combined anterior and posterior procedure is required. Patients with SCI seem to benefit from early surgical intervention with decompression of the spinal cord as this may improve the final neurological outcome, as well as decreasing systemic complications. Some studies indicate that this should be done within 24 h after the trauma and that very early decompression (<8 h), if possible, may even further add benefits to the neurological result (Fehlings et al. 2012; Lee et al. 2018). In addition to decompression and stabilization of the injury, these patients should maintain middle arterial pressure (MAP) above 85 mmHg for 5–7 days (Saadeh et al. 2017). External stabilization is usually performed using a rigid collar for 6–12 weeks, less frequently a cranio-thoracic orthosis. A minor group of injuries (isolated spinous or transverse process fractures) do not need any stabilizing treatment.

15.3 Specific Pediatric Concerns

In pediatric trauma patients >3 years of age that are alert, not intoxicated, not having midline neck or distracting pain, neurologically intact, and not having unexplained hypotension, radiographic assessment of the cervical spine is not recommended.

For pediatric patients <3 years of age, the same criteria for cervical spine clearance apply, but additionally a high-energy trauma mechanism (motorized vehicle accidents, falls from more than 3 m, and non-accidental trauma) should be ruled out to clear the cervical spine without radiographic assessment (Rozzelle et al. 2013).

The incidence of cervical spine fractures in pediatric patients is less than in adults, and the type of injuries shows a higher share of pure ligamentous disruption like atlanto-occipital injuries, C1-C2 subluxations, and SCIWORA. There is no literature supporting elevated MAP in pediatric patients with SCI, but adult guidelines are usually adapted.

Tips, Tricks, and Pitfalls

- Immobilization on the spine board should be of as short duration as possible (less than 2 h) in order to prevent decubitus ulcers.
- CT scanning is the radiological examination of choice, but you should be aware that disc and ligament lesions are difficult and in some cases impossible to see on CT imaging.
- Spinal shock is a reversible condition and defined by the flaccidity and loss of reflexes seen after spinal cord injury, whereas neurogenic shock refers to impairment of the sympathetic pathways in the cervical or upper thoracic spinal cord. Both conditions, however, indicate spinal cord injury.
- Neurogenic shock includes loss of vasomotor tone and sympathetic innervations to the heart, causing vasodilatation, hypotension, and bradycardia.
- The ASIA (American Spinal Injury Association) score can be used to classify the spinal cord injury.
- Injuries located at C6 or higher can result in partial or total loss of respiratory function.

References

Edwards, et al. Final results of MRC CRASH, a randomized placebo-controlled trial of intravenous corticosteroids in adults with head injury—outcomes at 6 months. Lancet. 2005;365:1957–9.

Fehlings, et al. Early versus delayed decompression for traumatic cervical spinal cord injury: results of the surgical timing in acute spinal cord injury study. PLoS One. 2012;7:e32037.

Hadley, et al. Clinical assessment following acute cervical spinal cord injury. Neurosurgery. 2013;72(Suppl 2):40–53.

Kornhall, et al. The Norwegian guidelines for the prehospital management of adult trauma patients with potential spinal injury. Scand J Trauma Resusc Emerg Med. 2017;25:2.

Lee, et al. Early surgical decompression within 8 hours for traumatic spinal cord injury: is it beneficial? A meta-analysis. Acta Orthop Traumatol Turc. 2018;52:101–8.

Leucht, et al. Epidemiology of traumatic spine fractures. Injury. 2009;40:166–72.

Pandrich, et al. Prevalence of concomitant traumatic cranio-spinal injury: a systematic review and meta-analysis. Neurosurg Rev. 2018:1–9. https://doi.org/10.1007/s10143-018-0988-3.

Patel, et al. Cervical spine collar clearance in the obtunded adult blunt trauma patient: a systematic review and practice management guideline from the Eastern Association for the Surgery of Trauma. J Trauma Acute Care Surg. 2015;78(2):430–41.

Rozzelle, et al. Management of pediatric spine and spinal cord injuries. Neurosurgery. 2013;72(2):205–26.

Ryken, et al. Guidelines for the management of acute cervical spine and spinal cord injury: 2013 update. Neurosurgery. 2013;60:81–92.

Saadeh, et al. The impact of blood pressure management after spinal cord injury: a systematic review of the literature. Neurosurg Focus. 2017;43:E20.

Theodore, et al. Prehospital cervical spinal immobilization after trauma. Neurosurgery. 2013;72(Suppl 2):22–34.

16 Blast-Induced Brain Injury

Niklas Marklund

Recommendations

Level I

There is no Level I evidence for a treatment with proven clinical benefit for severe blast traumatic brain injury (bTBI).

Level II

There are no current Level II recommendations for this topic.

Level III

Numerous observational studies at a Level III evidence exist. These studies imply that blast traumatic brain injury represents a unique subtype of TBI. Although there are features of severe bTBI with similarities to other head impact or penetrating TBIs, the pressure wave-induced brain injuries are unique to bTBI.

N. Marklund (✉)
Department of Clinical Sciences Lund, Neurosurgery, Lund University, Skåne University Hospital, Lund, Sweden
e-mail: niklas.marklund@med.lu.se

16.1 Overview

During warfare, individuals may be exposed to explosives caused by e.g., bombs, artillery shells, land mines, grenades, and roadside/antipersonnel improvised explosive devices (IEDs). These explosives lead to injuries referred to as blast injuries. A bomb blast may lead to a traumatic brain injury (TBI) of all injury severities from a mild concussion-like disorder to a severe, life-threatening TBI (Rosenfeld et al. 2013). Blasts are the primary cause of TBI in war zones, at least among military staff. Blast-induced TBI (bTBI) was recognized as the hallmark brain injury among American soldiers during the Operation Enduring Freedom in Afghanistan in 2001 and Operation Iraqi Freedom in 2003 (Miller et al. 2018; Terrio et al. 2009; Warden 2006). Up to 70% of blast injuries are caused by IEDs (Warden 2006; Clark et al. 2007). The severity of the bTBI depends on the energy released by the blast and the distance from the individual to the epicenter of the blast. The bTBI induced by the explosion may be divided into four (or five) different injury mechanisms (Masel et al. 2012). The *primary blast injury* is caused by the explosion itself resulting in a sudden rise in atmospheric pressure, and as part of the blast wave the primary blast injury is induced. This also represents the mechanism unique to bTBI. The *secondary blast injury* results from fragments, released by the explosion, which may

© Springer Nature Switzerland AG 2020

T. Sundstrøm et al. (eds.), *Management of Severe Traumatic Brain Injury*,
https://doi.org/10.1007/978-3-030-39383-0_16

cause a penetrating TBI. The pathology of this secondary blast injury is similar to that observed in "regular" ballistic penetrating TBI discussed elsewhere in this volume. The *tertiary blast injury* occurs when an individual is thrown against or into a solid object by the blast forces and may be similar to other high-energy TBIs such as those observed in high-speed motor vehicle accidents. The *quaternary blast injury* may result from e.g. significant blood loss from associated injuries or from exposure to burns, chemicals, or radiation (DePalma et al. 2005). A fifth (the *quinary blast injury*) more controversial mechanism has also been proposed, resulting in markedly delayed injuries due to the chemical, biological, or radiological substances, released at time of explosion.

Thus, although both blunt and penetrating TBI may be caused by the blast, the distinct pathophysiology of bTBI results from the primary blast wave. When the primary blast waves traverse across a human head, widespread brain tissue injury may ensue leading to either mild, moderate, or severe bTBI (Wang et al. 2014). A new classification for bTBI was proposed, in which a blast-induced mild bTBI is characterized by loss of consciousness (LOC) <1 h and post-traumatic amnesia (PTA) for <24 h post-injury, moderate bTBI characterized by LOC for 1–24 h and PTA for 1–7 days, and severe bTBI characterized by LOC > 24 h and PTA > 7 days (Ling et al. 2009).

Of all bTBIs, more than 80% are mild. The severity of injury is determined also by the presence of obstacles, entrapment, and protective clothing, as well as if the explosion occurs in a closed or open space (Masel et al. 2012). Severe bTBI may result from any of these causative factors and is characterized by cerebral edema, intracranial hemorrhage, delayed vasospasm, and pseudoaneurysm formation (Rosenfeld et al. 2013). The treatment of these severe bTBIs follows principles outlined for the treatment of severe TBI. Examples found efficacious for the massive brain swelling and increased intracranial pressure include early decompressive craniectomy (Armonda et al. 2006), which may also render the patient sufficiently stable to be transported by air to the nearest experienced trauma center (Bell et al. 2010a; Ragel et al. 2010). Other surgical measures include wound debridement and/or dural repair, removal of accessible foreign bodies, hematoma evacuation, removal of superficial foreign bodies, and insertion of an intraventricular drainage (Rosenfeld et al. 2013).

Tips, Tricks, and Pitfalls

- Blast traumatic brain injury (bTBI) results from explosive devices, most commonly the antipersonnel improvised explosive devices (IEDs), resulting in rapid formation of a blast wave.
- The distinct pathophysiology of bTBI is caused by the primary blast wave, and evidence point to predominant roles for axonal injury and blood-brain barrier disturbance.
- The vast majority of bTBIs are mild and accompanied with a high degree of symptoms (headaches, memory problems, irritability, sleep problems)—even in those not obviously wounded by the explosion.
- Biomarkers in serum for diagnosis and prognosis as well as neuroimaging are rapidly advancing areas of research and might help to further categorize these injuries.
- Although helmets protect against regular blunt *impact* or missiles/penetrating TBI, and should be recommended for that reason, they may in fact impair the blast wave-induced brain injury.
- The use of rapid decompressive craniectomy, wound debridement with watertight dural closure, as well as repair of cranial vault and/or skull base defects following severe bTBI may result in outcomes at least similar to those observed in other forms of severe TBI.

16.2 Background

The use of explosives to inflict injury to others is not a novel invention. For instance, the first recorded terrorist bombing occurred in Belgium in 1585, where a bridge was destroyed resulting in the death of 800 soldiers. Explosions resulting in brain injuries may occur also in civilians, caused by industrial accidents, fireworks, and others, although they are much more common in warfare/terrorism. In modern warfare, explosion-induced TBI, commonly referred to as blast-induced traumatic brain injury (bTBI), is frequently observed. Blast injuries were increasingly acknowledged since the early 1970s, initially as a cause for lung injury which led to the development of improved body armors. The cause of these explosions is mainly antipersonnel improvised explosive devices (AP-IED), or simply IEDs, commonly in the form of roadside bombs using high-order explosives such as nitroglycerine, dynamite, TNT, C4, ammonium nitrate fuel oil, and others. Other IEDs use low-order explosives in pipe bombs, Molotov cocktails, and so forth, although no shock waves are created from those. When a chemical explosive detonates, enormous amounts of energy are rapidly released in a very short time, expanding quickly and compressing the surrounding air (Chandra and Sundaramurthy 2015). Thus, it has been estimated that at time of detonation, the explosive material is converted to combustion gases at extreme pressure (up to 400,000 atmospheres) and temperature (>2500 °C) in the course of a few microseconds (Masel et al. 2012). Then, a shock wave, a sphere, is formed which travels at supersonic speed. This rapid positive pressure wave is then followed by a negative pressure wave, named a Friedlander wave. The size of the IED determines the blast wave velocity and the duration of the pressure increases (Chandra and Sundaramurthy 2015). It is estimated that a peak pressure of 1 pound per square inch (PSI) is sufficient to knock over a soldier, 5 PSI ruptures the tympanic membrane, 7–8 PSI overturns a railway car, and at a PSI of >80, mortality exceeds 90%. For obvious reasons, explosions are worse in confined spaces than in open air (Elder and Cristian 2009). If the explosive compounds harbor metallic fragments, these may be converted into projectiles by the released energy (Chandra and Sundaramurthy 2015).

The blast mechanism may be divided into four, or five, phases. The *primary blast injury* is caused by the explosion and the resulting increased atmospheric pressure striking the affected individual. The blast wave is influenced by the surrounding environment and is markedly increased in a closed environment causing reflections of the pressure wave from, e.g., walls, floor, and ceiling. Many roadside explosives including the IEDs are filled with metal fragments, and the *secondary blast injury* results from fragments released with high energy which may cause penetrating injury to the brain or other parts of the body. The *tertiary blast injury* is the result of the individual being thrown by the blast into a solid object and may cause brain injuries similar to those observed in civilian high-energy motor vehicle accidents. These types of injuries are associated with acceleration/deceleration forces and blunt force trauma to the brain similar to that observed in blunt TBI by the acceleration/deceleration type of injury observed in high-speed motor vehicle accidents. The *quaternary blast injury* is a secondary injury resulting from e.g. blood loss from traumatic amputations or even from inhalation of toxic gases resulting from the explosion, heat, chemicals, or radiation. A quinary blast injury mechanism has also been proposed and results from markedly delayed injury due to chemical, biological, or radioactive substances released by the explosion.

In particular, air-fluid interfaces such as those at the ear, lung, heart, and gastrointestinal tract are vulnerable to the extreme pressure differences caused by the blast (Mayorga 1997). In the lung, the alveoli-capillary interface may be disrupted, and a high percentage of blast-induced mortality is due to lung injury. Furthermore, the pressure increases within the thorax may cause vagal nerve-induced hypotension typically resolving in 1–2 h (Eskridge et al. 2012).

To date, improvements in the personnel protection have led to increased survival of soldiers since penetrating injuries are reduced and the effects of the blast wave on the heart and lungs were attenuated. Unfortunately, although body armors saves many lives, they also make individuals more susceptible to sustain brain injuries. Commonly, a majority of blast victims is wearing a helmet at time of injury (Clark et al. 2007). However, although helmets work well against ballistic impact, they may actually aggravate bTBI (Chandra and Sundaramurthy 2015). The two most important mechanisms of bTBI are (1) direct transmission of pressure into the skull cavity leading to an increase in intracranial pressure (ICP) and (2) indirect transmission through the skull flexure (Chandra and Sundaramurthy 2015). The short pressure pulse and a potential propagation of the pressure wave via the blood vessels produce brain injuries unique to bTBI (Rosenfeld et al. 2013). In addition to the increased ICP, the blast pressure wave may impair cerebral blood flow and brain oxygenation. Many details of the pathophysiology of bTBI have not been established although much experimental and clinical work suggest an important role for axonal injury, due to shear stress induced by the pressure wave, that may evolve during the first post-injury year or more (Davenport et al. 2015).

Furthermore, bTBI may be accompanied by a blood-brain barrier disruption (Shetty et al. 2014), correlating with blast intensity with IgG accumulating in cells located in the cerebral cortex and the hippocampus. Improvements in neuroimaging and biomarkers, both rapidly advancing fields, are needed to further outline the mechanisms of bTBI see (Chandra and Sundaramurthy 2015; Agoston and Kamnaksh 2015).

To manage warfare severe bTBI, management systems and protocol including, e.g., early injury management, rapid transport to a military hospital experienced in trauma care, early damage control and resuscitation, and neurointensive care, have resulted in improved outcome for these critically injured individuals (Rosenfeld et al. 2013): As previously noted, severe bTBI is characterized by dynamic changes in ICP due to the presence of cerebral edema and intracranial hemorrhage, as well as vascular complications such as delayed vasospasm and pseudoaneurysm formation (Ling et al. 2009). A key management strategy is the use of early decompressive craniectomy for the treatment of brain swelling and increased ICP which also enables air transport (Bell et al. 2010a; Ragel et al. 2010). Furthermore, wound debridement and removal of easily accessible foreign material, evacuation of mass lesions, and placement of an external ventricular drainage are all part of the management strategies. Of utmost importance is the closure of all associated dural defects. Liberal use of the angiography and transcranial Doppler enables the detection of pseudoaneurysms and vasospasm, respectively (Bell et al. 2010b).

As expected, the initial Glasgow Coma Scale score is associated with clinical outcome (Weisbrod et al. 2012; Ecker et al. 2011). However, the outcome of severe bTBI is surprisingly favorable and compares well to that of a matched civilian severe TBI population. As examples, at 2 years following severe bTBI, 32% of patients with initial GCS scores of 3–5, and 63% of those with a GCS score of 6–8, had achieved functional independence (Weisbrod et al. 2012).

References

Agoston DV, Kamnaksh A. Modeling the neurobehavioral consequences of blast-induced traumatic brain injury spectrum disorder and identifying related biomarkers. In: Kobeissy FH, editor. Brain neurotrauma: molecular, neuropsychological, and rehabilitation aspects. Frontiers in neuroengineering. Boca Raton: CRC Press/Taylor & Francis; 2015.

Armonda RA, Bell RS, Vo AH, Ling G, DeGraba TJ, Crandall B, et al. Wartime traumatic cerebral vasospasm: recent review of combat casualties. Neurosurgery. 2006;59(6):1215–25. discussion 25.

Bell RS, Mossop CM, Dirks MS, Stephens FL, Mulligan L, Ecker R, et al. Early decompressive craniectomy for severe penetrating and closed head injury during wartime. Neurosurg Focus. 2010a;28(5):E1.

Bell RS, Vo AH, Roberts R, Wanebo J, Armonda RA. Wartime traumatic aneurysms: acute presentation, diagnosis, and multimodal treatment of 64 craniocervical arterial injuries. Neurosurgery. 2010b;66(1):66–79. discussion.

Chandra N, Sundaramurthy A. Acute pathophysiology of blast injury-from biomechanics to experiments and computations: implications on head and polytrauma. In: Kobeissy FH, editor. Brain neurotrauma: molecular, neuropsychological, and rehabilitation aspects.

Frontiers in neuroengineering. Boca Raton: CRC Press/Taylor & Francis; 2015.

Clark ME, Bair MJ, Buckenmaier CC 3rd, Gironda RJ, Walker RL. Pain and combat injuries in soldiers returning from operations enduring freedom and Iraqi freedom: implications for research and practice. J Rehabil Res Dev. 2007;44(2):179–94.

Davenport ND, Lim KO, Sponheim SR. White matter abnormalities associated with military PTSD in the context of blast TBI. Hum Brain Mapp. 2015;36(3):1053–64.

DePalma RG, Burris DG, Champion HR, Hodgson MJ. Blast injuries. N Engl J Med. 2005;352(13):1335–42.

Ecker RD, Mulligan LP, Dirks M, Bell RS, Severson MA, Howard RS, et al. Outcomes of 33 patients from the wars in Iraq and Afghanistan undergoing bilateral or bicompartmental craniectomy. J Neurosurg. 2011;115(1):124–9.

Elder GA, Cristian A. Blast-related mild traumatic brain injury: mechanisms of injury and impact on clinical care. Mt Sinai J Med. 2009;76(2):111–8.

Eskridge SL, Macera CA, Galarneau MR, Holbrook TL, Woodruff SI, MacGregor AJ, et al. Injuries from combat explosions in Iraq: injury type, location, and severity. Injury. 2012;43(10):1678–82.

Ling G, Bandak F, Armonda R, Grant G, Ecklund J. Explosive blast neurotrauma. J Neurotrauma. 2009;26(6):815–25.

Masel BE, Bell RS, Brossart S, Grill RJ, Hayes RL, Levin HS, et al. Galveston brain injury conference 2010: clinical and experimental aspects of blast injury. J Neurotrauma. 2012;29(12):2143–71.

Mayorga MA. The pathology of primary blast overpressure injury. Toxicology. 1997;121(1):17–28.

Miller L, Pacheco GJ, J CJ, Grimm RC, Dierschke NA, Baker J, et al. Causes of death in military working dogs during operation Iraqi freedom and operation enduring freedom, 2001–2013. Mil Med. 2018;183(9–10):e467–74.

Ragel BT, Klimo P Jr, Martin JE, Teff RJ, Bakken HE, Armonda RA. Wartime decompressive craniectomy: technique and lessons learned. Neurosurg Focus. 2010;28(5):E2.

Rosenfeld JV, McFarlane AC, Bragge P, Armonda RA, Grimes JB, Ling GS. Blast-related traumatic brain injury. Lancet Neurol. 2013;12(9):882–93.

Shetty AK, Mishra V, Kodali M, Hattiangady B. Blood brain barrier dysfunction and delayed neurological deficits in mild traumatic brain injury induced by blast shock waves. Front Cell Neurosci. 2014;8:232.

Terrio H, Brenner LA, Ivins BJ, Cho JM, Helmick K, Schwab K, et al. Traumatic brain injury screening: preliminary findings in a US Army Brigade Combat Team. J Head Trauma Rehabil. 2009;24(1):14–23.

Wang C, Pahk JB, Balaban CD, Miller MC, Wood AR, Vipperman JS. Computational study of human head response to primary blast waves of five levels from three directions. PLoS One. 2014;9(11):e113264.

Warden D. Military TBI during the Iraq and Afghanistan wars. J Head Trauma Rehabil. 2006;21(5):398–402.

Weisbrod AB, Rodriguez C, Bell R, Neal C, Armonda R, Dorlac W, et al. Long-term outcomes of combat casualties sustaining penetrating traumatic brain injury. J Trauma Acute Care Surg. 2012;73(6):1525–30.

17 Radiological Evaluation of Head Trauma

Christian Rahbek, Ronni Mikkelsen, and Vibeke Fink-Jensen

Recommendations

Level I

Data are insufficient to support Level I recommendations for this subject.

Level II

Data are insufficient to support Level II recommendations for this subject.

(Please note that there are no cohort or randomized studies in part due to the fact that head CT is the gold standard for evaluation of head trauma, and therefore it would be unethical to make randomized studies.)

Level III

A CT scan of the head is recommended as first-line examinations for a patient with head injury.

Evaluation of vascular injuries requires specific angiography series with contrast (CT, MRI, DSA) (Shetty et al. 2016).

MRI within the first days after trauma should be reserved for patients where the CT does not sufficiently explain the clinical state of the patient (Shetty et al. 2016).

17.1 Overview

CT imaging is the examination of choice in the acute setting because it is readily available and fast, offers full-body investigation with detailed imaging including imaging of bones with reconstruction in all planes and allows close observation of the patient.

In unstable patients, the teamwork between the radiologist, anaesthesiologist and trauma surgeon becomes vital to select the correct examination, to monitor the patient and to avoid motion artefacts. In these cases, immediate radiological assessment should be carried out to ensure the quality of images and the need for supplementary examination (i.e. angio).

The time of examination has significantly decreased with recent advances in technology, allowing for full-body imaging in a few minutes.

CT of the head is in most places performed with helical technique, as multidetector CT scanners are readily available in most trauma centres. This will allow reconstruction in all planes and

C. Rahbek (✉) · V. Fink-Jensen
Department of Neuroradiology, Aarhus University Hospital, Aarhus, Denmark
e-mail: chrirahb@rm.dk; vibfin@rm.dk

R. Mikkelsen
Department of Neuroradiology, Aarhus University Hospital, Aarhus, Denmark

Department of Biomedicine, Aarhus University, Aarhus, Denmark
e-mail: ronni.mikkelsen@clin.au.dk, ronni.mikkelsen@rm.dk

© Springer Nature Switzerland AG 2020
T. Sundstrøm et al. (eds.), *Management of Severe Traumatic Brain Injury*,
https://doi.org/10.1007/978-3-030-39383-0_17

evaluation of both soft tissues and bones from one scan series. It is recommended to include the facial skeleton from the hard palate in cranial direction including the mandible if there is clinical evidence of that region being involved. Some centres perform one scan series that cover the cervical spine, facial skeleton, brain and skull in one. Some neurosurgical centres use neuronavigation for emergency procedures such a placement of an external ventricular drain, and in such setting it is beneficial to ensure that the primary trauma protocol is compatible with their navigation software.

Haematomas will appear white (hyperdense) in the right window setting, whereas ongoing bleeding will appear darker (hypodense), and older haematomas will be similar to grey matter (isodense).

Contusions of the brain parenchyma appear as focally darker areas around punctate haemorrhages, often more apparent on later scans.

Diffuse cerebral oedema is seen as a diminished differentiation of grey-white matter boundaries, sulcal obliteration and narrowing of the basal cisterns and often also the ventricular system.

Also the falx and tentorium will appear whiter than normal against the brain parenchyma. Focal oedema is seen darker against the surrounding more normal parenchyma, but also with the above-mentioned signs.

Diffuse axonal injury (DAI) is often underestimated or not seen on CT. MRI is the examination of choice for DAI, where lesions will appear as small black spots on T2-weighted gradient echo series, but MRI is not as readily available as CT and is far more complex to perform with traumatized patients. MRI should therefore be reserved for those patients where CT within the first days after trauma does not sufficiently explain the clinical state of the patient.

One should always evaluate:

- Scalp lesions—lacerations, foreign bodies, oedema and/or subgaleal haematomas.
- Skull fractures—including the facial bones.
- Extra-axial lesions—epidural haemorrhage, subdural haemorrhage, subarachnoid haemorrhage and/or intraventricular haemorrhage.
- Intra-axial lesions—intraparenchymal haematomas, contusions, oedema with or without herniation and/or DAI.

The possibility of vascular injuries should also be considered. Cranial CT is usually performed as a non-contrast study, and more specific angiography series (CT, MRI or angiography) with contrast may be necessary.

Tips, Tricks and Pitfalls: CT Imaging of the Head

To avoid overlooking critical injuries in the immediate setting, perform a systematic evaluation using three different window settings:

- Brain parenchyma window (Level 30–40 Hounsfield Units (HU); window: 65–120 HU).
  - Is the ventricular system of normal size, and symmetrical around the midline?
  - Is there any extra- or intra-axial blood?
  - Is the grey-white matter differentiation normal? Are there any focal lesions?
  - Are the cortical sulci discernible and symmetrical, or are they narrowed or even obliterated?
  - Are the basal cisterns of normal size and symmetrical?
  - Are there any scalp lesions?
- Subdural window (L: 70–100 HU; W: 150–300 HU):
  - To avoid overlooking smaller subdural haematomas due to the density of bone and artefacts at the interface between the bone and soft intracranial tissue, use a subdural window. This will allow you to detect a thin layer of sub- or epidural blood.
- Bone window (L: 500 HU; W: 2000–4000 HU):
  - Are there any fractures involving the skull base or the calvarium? If so, are there dislocations and/or fragments?

- Is the optical canal intact?
- Is the carotid canal intact?
- Are there any indirect signs of fracture, i.e. opacification of the nasal sinuses and/or mastoid cells or intracranial air bubbles?
- Are there fractures of the facial bones?
- Are there any foreign bodies extra- or intracranially?

Especially regarding fractures, make good use of the possibility of three-dimensional reconstructing.

17.2 Background

Intracranial lesions can be subdivided into extra- and intra-axial lesions.

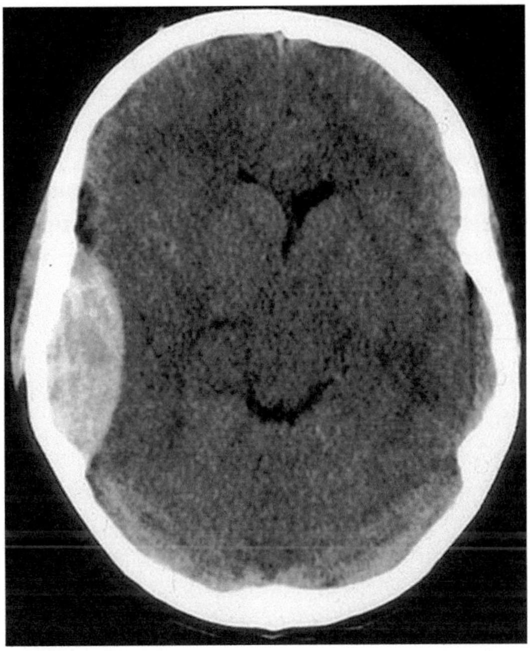

Fig. 17.1 Epidural haematoma

17.2.1 Extra-axial Lesions

Epidural haematomas (Fig. 17.1)

- Located between tabula interna and dura.
- Ninety per cent of cases occur in association with skull fractures involving the middle meningeal artery or less common one of the venous sinuses.
- Rarely crosses sutures but can cross the midline.
- Usually a biconvex appearance.

Subdural haematomas (Fig. 17.2)

- Located between the dura and arachnoid.
- Venous bleeding from superficial bridging cortical veins.
- Cross sutures but not midline.
- Often located along the falx cerebri or tentorium cerebelli.

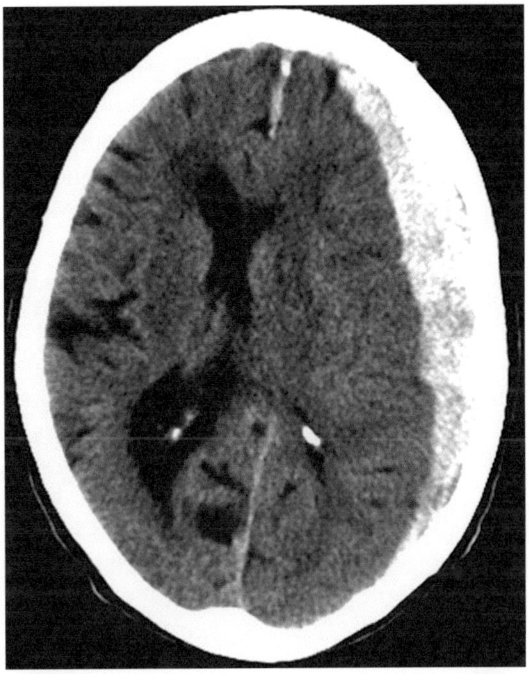

Fig. 17.2 Acute subdural haematoma

- Concave appearance towards brain surface.
- Chronic subdural haematomas appear dark; fresh bleeding in a chronic subdural haematoma will appear as white areas, often in compartments.
- After 2 days to 2 weeks, subdural haematomas can become isodense and very difficult to discern from the brain. Look for shift of midline or difference of right and left hemisphere sulci.

Traumatic subarachnoid haemorrhage (Fig. 17.3)

- Fresh blood found focally in most cases in a few sulci over the convexities or in the basal cisterns often the interpeduncular.
- It may look as though the sulci are effaced, when in fact it is blood replacing the CSF.
- If there is abundant and diffuse spread of SAH, one should always consider rupture of an aneurysm. Perhaps that was the cause for the traumatic incident to happen.

Intraventricular haemorrhage

- Seen as fresh blood (white on CT) in the ventricular system.
- Can be caused from direct trauma with tearing of subependymal veins, breakthrough from parenchymal hematoma or reflux from SAH.

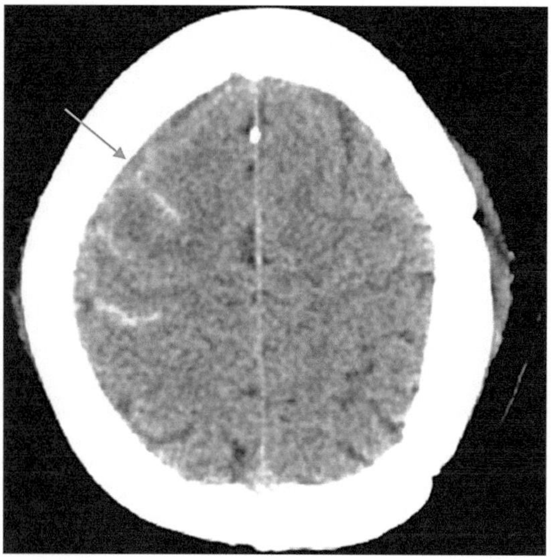

Fig. 17.3 Acute traumatic subarachnoid haemorrhage

- Often, the intraventricular bleeding is seen as blood in the posterior part of the occipital horns with a blood-CSF level. Even very small amounts of blood can be detected here (Parizel et al. 2005).

17.2.2 Intra-axial Lesions

Cerebral contusions (Fig. 17.4)

- The most common injury of the parenchyma.
- Are seen as punctate haemorrhages that after a few days are surrounded by oedema, often multiple, located near the brain surface supratentorially.
- Are caused as the brain hits the skull base or the falx/tentorium and are therefore often located inferiorly and anteriorly in the frontal and temporal lobes.

Intracerebral haematomas

- Larger than contusions.
- Located deeper within the brain parenchyma.

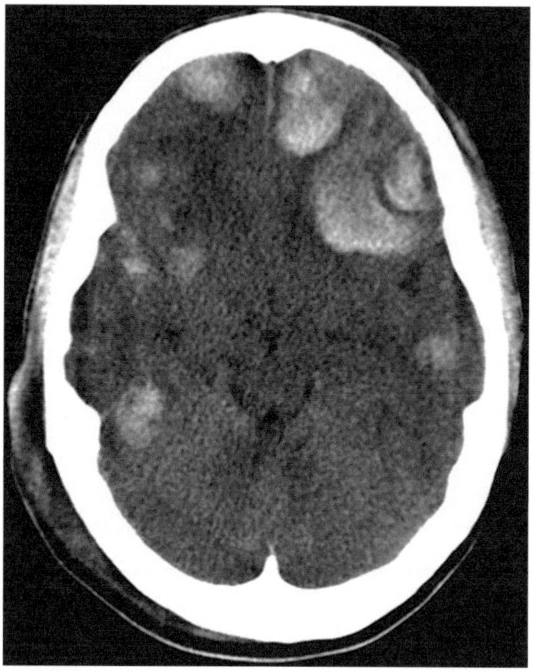

Fig. 17.4 Multiple brain contusions

- Frequently progress during the first few post-traumatic days, especially if a surgical decompression of epi- or subdural haematomas has been performed.
- A few days after the trauma, an oedema around the haematoma will occur.

Diffuse axonal injury (Fig. 17.5)

- Caused by shearing of the axons in rotational acceleration/deceleration closed head injuries.
- Most often not seen on the initial CT or only as very small haemorrhages at the grey-white matter boundaries.
- Can appear during the next few days, but as over 50% are non-haemorrhagic, they will not appear on CT with certainty.

MRI is much more reliable for showing DAI. The patient's clinical condition will often be worse than expected from the first CT. The use of advanced MRI techniques such as diffusion tensor images/tractographies, MR spectroscopies and functional MRI have shown promise in experimental settings, but is not yet standard in the clinical setting.

Cerebral oedema (Fig. 17.6)

- Can be diffuse.
- Associated with DAI or hypoxia, but can also develop without concomitant traumatic lesions.
- Develops during the first 24–48 h.
- Focal oedema can be associated with intra- or extra-axial haemorrhage.
- Can cause compression of blood vessels and eventually evolve into ischaemic areas of the brain.

Cerebral herniations

- Occur secondary to intra- or extra-axial expansive lesions and/or oedema.
- Subfalcine herniation is radiologically the most common type. It involves displacement of the cingulate gyrus under the inferior margin of the falx, compression of the ipsilateral

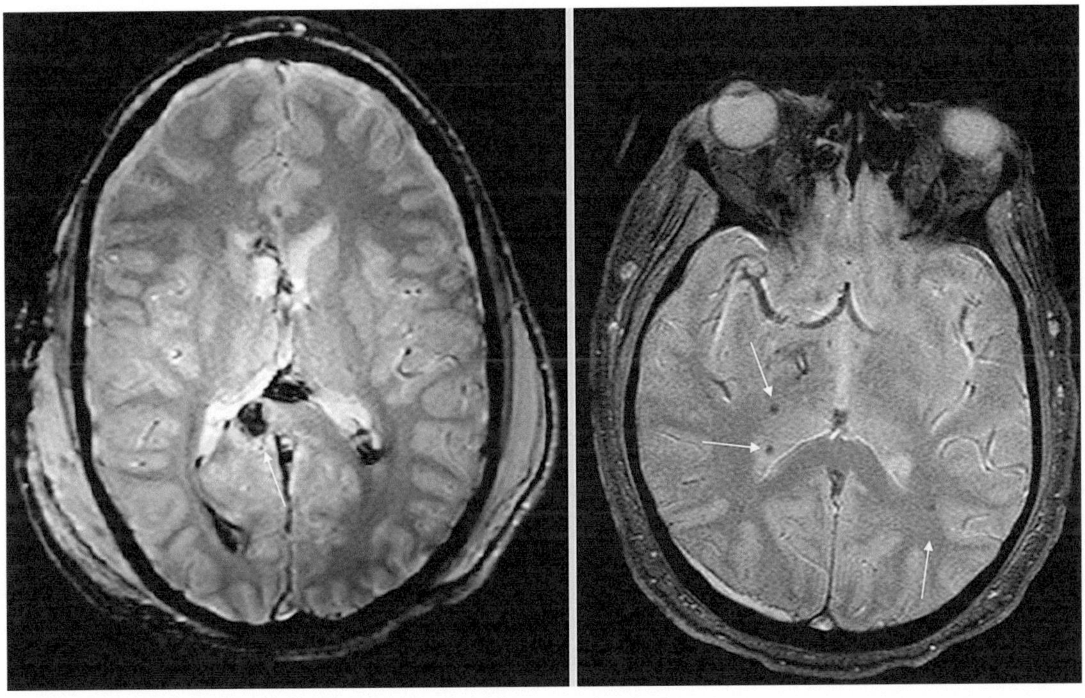

Fig. 17.5 Diffuse axonal injury, DAI and intraventricular haemorrhage

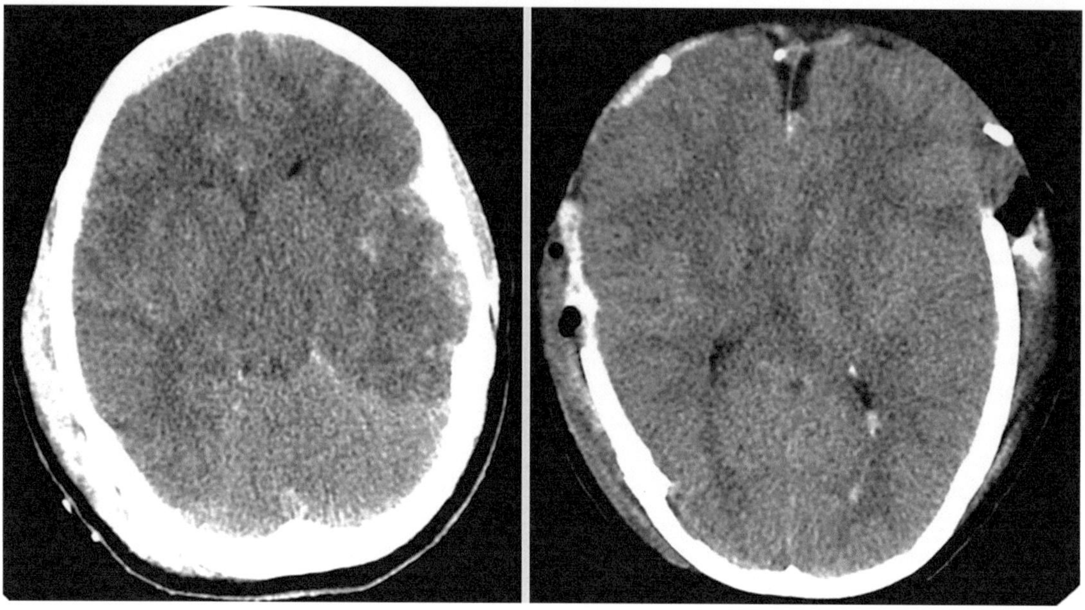

Fig. 17.6 Cerebral oedema. Day 1 and day 2 with bilateral craniectomy

lateral ventricle, blocking of the foramen of Monro and dilatation of the opposite lateral ventricle and midline shift.

- The anterior cerebral artery can be compressed until occlusion with infarction following.
- Transtentorial herniation is most often descending, where the medial part of the temporal lobe is pressed downwards, narrowing the ipsilateral basal cisterns and compressing the oculomotor nerve and eventually the posterior cerebral artery with infarction following.
- Can also be ascending with the vermis dislocated upwards, obliteration of the fourth ventricle and subsequent hydrocephalus.
- If the intracranial pressure increases, eventually herniation and incarceration at the foramen magnum will occur (Parizel et al. 2005).

17.2.3 Vascular Injuries

- Compression of vessels due to raised ICP can cause hypoperfusion and eventually infarction.
- Trauma can cause dissection or laceration of vessels either intra- or extra-cranially and hypoperfusion or thrombus (Fig. 17.7).

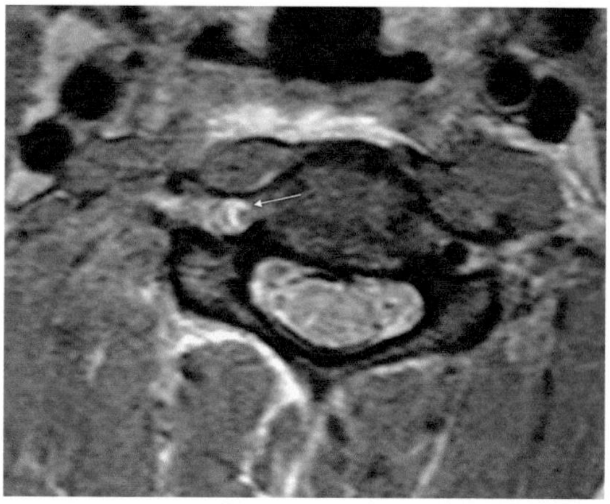

Fig. 17.7 Dissection of the right vertebral artery

- Subarachnoid haemorrhage can cause vasospasm and subsequent infarction, although the clinical course is often milder than in aneurysmal haemorrhage (Kramer 2013).

17.2.4 Skull Fractures

Skull fractures will not be presented in detail. Facial fractures, however, represent the risk of respiratory problems and should be assessed on the first CT scan. One should pay particular attention to the orbits, especially the optic canal, the central skull base, especially the carotid canal, and the temporal bone as fractures here may require immediate surgical intervention. Intracranial air bubbles imply fractures involving the nasal sinuses or temporal bone.

17.2.5 Specific Intracranial and Cervical Vascular Concerns

Suspected vascular injury and in particular vascular dissection require MRI or CT angiography. A conventional angiography may be necessary.

Lack of cerebral circulation confirms brain death. In these cases, filling of the intracerebral vessels during conventional angiography is absent due to extremely increased intracranial pressure. Angiography is considered to be a confirmatory test in doubtful situations, where brain death has to be stated before possible organ donation (Yousem and Nadgir 2017).

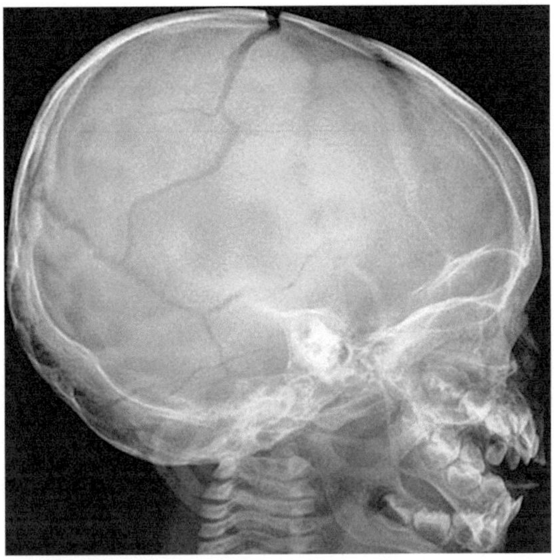

Fig. 17.8 Complex skull fracture in a child

17.3 Specific Paediatric Concerns

In children with trauma, unilateral infarction is seen in association with acute subdural haematoma. Also, cerebral oedema is more common in children than in adults.

17.3.1 Non-accidental Injury (NAI) or 'Battered Child Syndrome'

Always consider NAI in young children with head trauma, particularly in those without appropriate trauma history. Most NAI head injuries occur under the age of 2 years. The neurological presentation is often non-specific. CT is the most appropriate acute imaging procedure (Lonergan et al. 2003). For additional information on possible "Child abuse", see also Chap. 4.3.

Typical imaging findings in NAI are:

- Skull fractures (Fig. 17.8)
- Subdural haematomas, often of different age (Fig. 17.9)
- Cerebral oedema
- Hypoxic ischaemic encephalopathy (Figs. 17.9 and 17.10)
- Rarely intraventricular, intracerebral or epidural haematomas

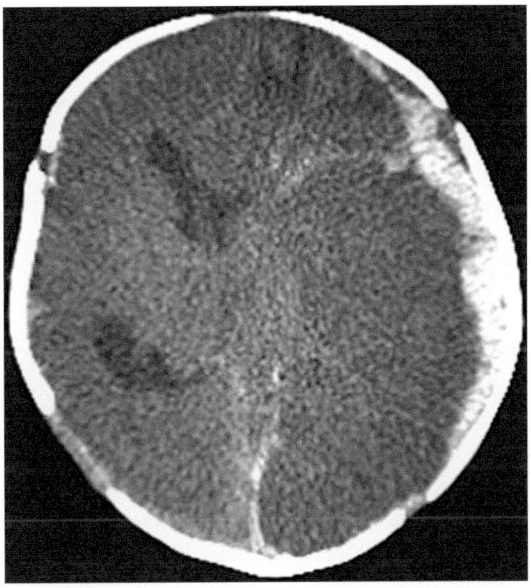

Fig. 17.9 Subdural haematoma, hypoxic ischaemic encephalopathy and subfalcine herniation

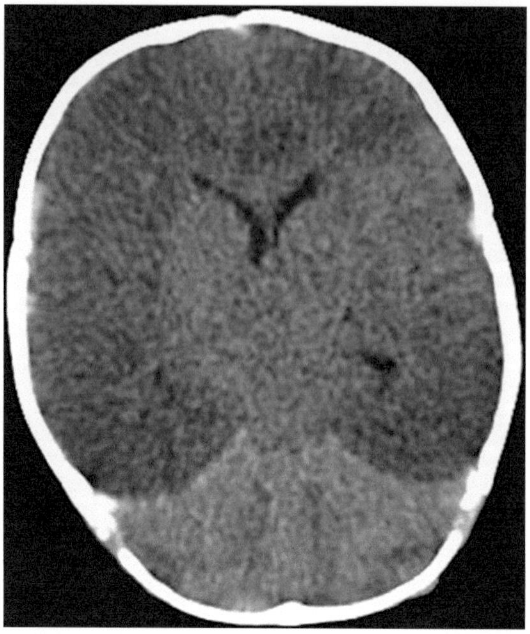

Fig. 17.10 Acute reversal sign ('white cerebellum') due to diffuse hypoxic brain injury

> **Tips, Tricks and Pitfalls: Paediatric Head Traumas**
>
> - Accidental skull fractures are usually linear and unilateral, affect the parietal bones and do not cross sutures.
> - Non-accidental fractures are often more complex.
> - Linear skull fractures can be missed on axial CT scans!
> - Accidental subdural haematomas are more often unilateral, non-accidental more often bilateral.
> - Non-accidental subdural haematomas extend more often into the interhemispheric fissure.
> - Acute reversal sign ('white cerebellum') + loss of grey-white matter differentiation + interhemispheric subdural haematoma is suggestive of NAI.
> - Subdural haematomas become isodense after about a week (depends on size), but dating of subdural collections is very imprecise.
> - MRI gives greater detail of subdural haematomas, may help to date the injury and is helpful to assess the extent of the parenchymal injury.
> - Remember: None of the aforementioned features are pathognomonic!
> - Remember also that children with temporal arachnoid cysts may get subdural and/or intra-cystic haematomas even after mild head traumas!
>
> A child suspected for NAI should not be sent home! Contact the paediatrician on call! Refer to a complete skeletal survey if NAI is suspected in infants and young children. Occult injury is rare in children over 3 years of age.

References

Daniel R. Kramer, Jesse L. Winer, B. A. Matthew Pease, Arun P. Amar, William J. Mack, (2013) Cerebral Vasospasm in Traumatic Brain Injury. Neurology Research International 2013:1–7.

Lonergan GJ, et al. From the archives of the AFIP. Child abuse: radiologic-pathologic correlation. Radiographics. 2003;23(4):811–45.

Parizel PM, et al. New developments in the neuroradiological diagnosis of craniocerebral trauma. Eur Radiol. 2005;15:569–81.

Shetty, et al. ACR appropriateness criteria head trauma. J Am Call Radiol. 2016;13:668–79.

Yousem DM, Nadgir R. Neuroradiology: the requisites. Philadelphia: Mosby/Elsevier; 2017. p. 150–73. Chapter 4.

18 Radiological Evaluation of Cervical Spine Trauma

Christian Rahbek, Ronni Mikkelsen, and Vibeke Fink-Jensen

Recommendations

Level I

Data are insufficient to support Level I recommendations for this subject.

Level II

A 3D CT of the cervical spine is far superior to plain X-ray (Holmes and Akkinepalli 2005).

Level III

MRI scan reveals damage to soft tissue that often isn't visible on a CT scan.

C. Rahbek (✉) · V. Fink-Jensen
Department of Neuroradiology, Aarhus University Hospital, Aarhus, Denmark
e-mail: chrirahb@rm.dk; vibfin@rm.dk

R. Mikkelsen
Department of Neuroradiology, Aarhus University Hospital, Aarhus, Denmark

Department of Biomedicine, Aarhus University, Aarhus, Denmark
e-mail: ronni.mikkelsen@rm.dk

18.1 Overview

CT should be the examination of choice, as it has a very high sensitivity and specificity for detecting injuries. Supplemental MRI for ligamentous or disc injuries should be reserved to cases with persisting neurological disability.

Particularly, multiplanar reconstruction and 3D reconstructions are valuable to visualize fractures and bone fragments.

Fractures of the cervical spine can be divided based on the mechanism of injury into *flexion*, *extension* or *compression* fractures or according to stability into *stable* or *unstable* fractures, using the three-column model (Fig. 18.1). There are multiple classification and scoring systems for spine injuries, some based on their anatomical location and others based on the osseous and ligamentous injuries.

Description/classification of injuries should be systematic and reflect a consensus between radiologist and treating physicians in regard to the classification systems used.

Tips, Tricks and Pitfalls: Cervical Spine Traumas

- Always do reconstructions and evaluate sagittal and coronal images.
- Be systematic when evaluating cervical images; look for:

© Springer Nature Switzerland AG 2020
T. Sundstrøm et al. (eds.), *Management of Severe Traumatic Brain Injury*,
https://doi.org/10.1007/978-3-030-39383-0_18

- Maintained height of the vertebral bodies.
- Alignment.
- Normal distances and parallel surfaces between endplates in disc spaces, facet joints and spinous processes.
- Continuous cortical margins.
- Paraspinal haematomas and disruption of the architecture of the muscles of the posterior neck.

• Alignment is evaluated along the lines of the anterior and posterior longitudinal ligament, the posterior margin of the spinal canal and along the posterior margin of the spinous processes.

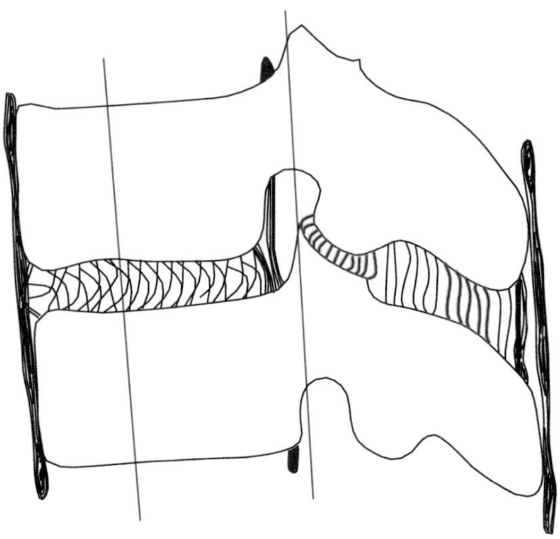

Fig. 18.1 The three-column model. Instability occurs when two of the three columns (anterior, middle or posterior) are injured

18.2 Background

18.2.1 Atlanto-occipital Dislocation

Atlanto-occipital dislocation in anterior-posterior or longitudinal direction results in increased distance between the basion and the odontoid. This injury can be associated with odontoid or condylar fractures and results often in severe soft tissue damage and brainstem injury.

18.2.2 Atlanto-axial Distraction

Atlanto-axial distraction causes widening of the distance between C1 and C2 with concomitant prevertebral soft tissue swelling and ligamentous tears. Dislocation in the transverse plane with rupture of the transverse ligament and associated fractures results in increased distance between the anterior surface of the odontoid and the posterior surface of C1.

18.2.3 Jefferson's Fracture

Jefferson's fracture is a compression "burst" fracture of C1 and involves disruptions of the anterior and posterior arches of the atlas. Tears of the transverse ligament are associated. More often, a hyperextension injury is seen with compression of the posterior arch of C1, resulting in a stable posterior arch fracture (Fig. 18.2).

18.2.4 Hangman's Fractures

Hangman's fractures are fracture dislocations of C2 caused by hyperextension injuries. If there are bilateral neural arch fractures, anterior displacement of C2 on C3 occurs. The posterior ring is usually fixed by the inferior articular process, unless there is accompanying facet disloca-

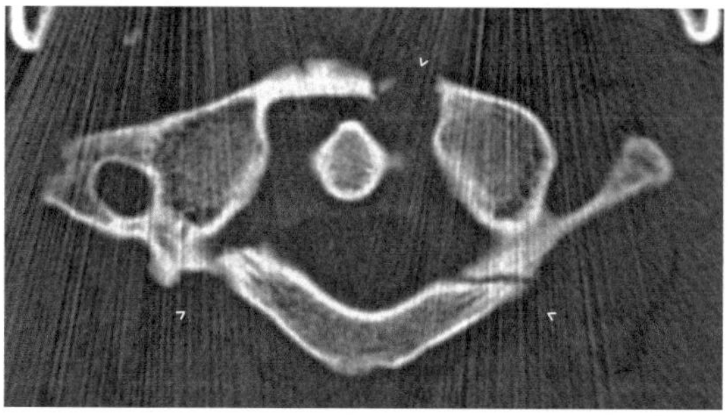

Fig. 18.2 Jefferson's fracture. *Arrow heads* indicate fractures disrupting anterior and posterior arches of C1

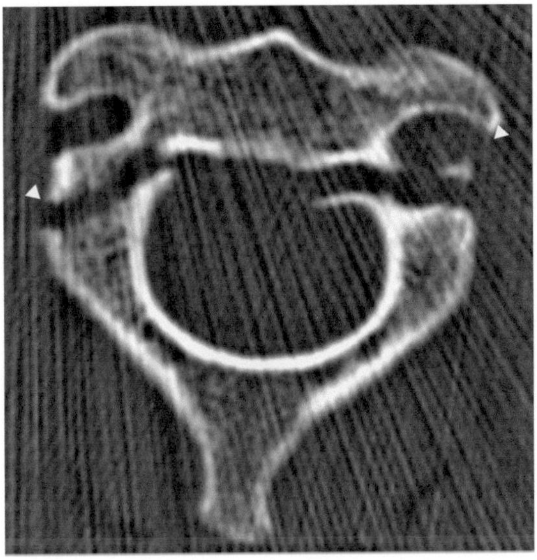

Fig. 18.3 Hangman's fracture: *Arrow heads* mark bilateral fracture through the posterior arch of C2

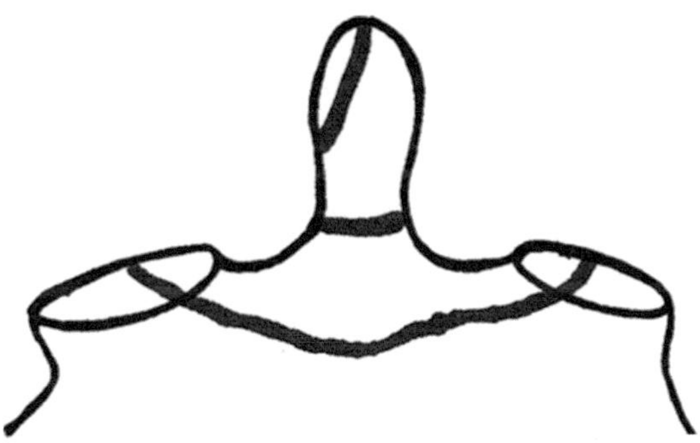

Fig. 18.4 Odontoid fractures. Type I: upper portion of the dens. Type II: junction of the dens with the body. Type III: through the body of the axis

tion. However, most Hangman's fractures result only in minimal translation and angulation (Fig. 18.3).

18.2.5 Odontoid ("Dens") Fractures

Odontoid ("dens") fractures are divided into three types according to Anderson and D'Alonzo with type II being unstable and type III relatively stable unless significantly displaced (Figs. 18.4 and 18.5).

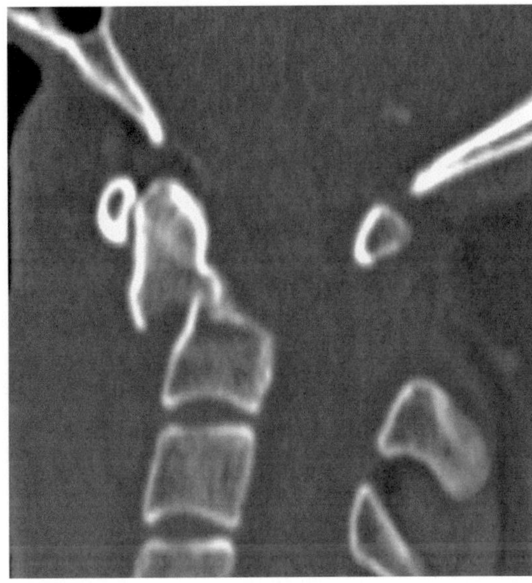

Fig. 18.5 Odontoid fracture, type II

18.2.6 Associated Vascular Injury

Due to the anatomy of the vertebral artery, high cervical injuries (predominantly C1 and 2) can be associated with vascular injury (including both dissection and transection). In cases with significant dislocation or high injury, a supplemental CT-angio should be considered.

18.2.7 Compression Fractures

Compression fractures of a vertebral body can involve one or both endplates. Most are wedge-shaped without involving the posterior cortex. Burst fractures also affect the posterior cortex of the vertebral body, and fragments can be displaced into the spinal canal.

18.2.8 Teardrop Fractures

Teardrop fractures can be caused by hyperflexion or hyperextension injuries (Fig. 18.6).

In hyperflexion injuries, a triangular fragment can be found at the anterior-inferior border of the vertebral body with reduction of the anterior body height and soft tissue swelling. Disruption

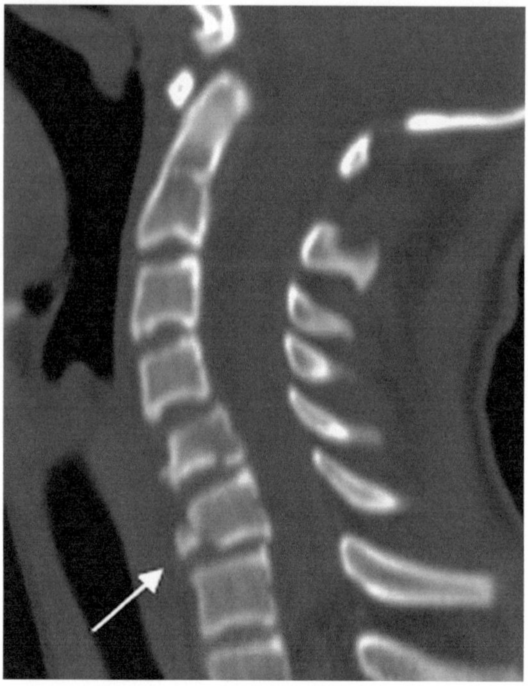

Fig. 18.6 Teardrop fracture C6 (*arrow*)

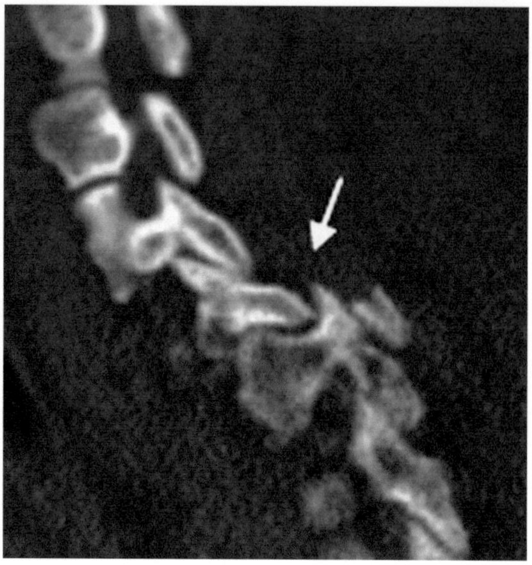

Fig. 18.7 Locked facets. Anterior displacement of inferior articular process is marked by the (*arrow*). Note the concomitant fracture of the articular process

of the anterior part of the disc and the posterior ligament complex results in posterior displacement of the fractured vertebra and diastasis of the interfacetal joints. These fractures are unstable.

Hyperextension injuries may also result in an avulsion of the anterior-inferior corner of the vertebral body, but leave the posterior columns intact and are stable.

18.2.9 Locked Facets

Locked facets are the result of anterior displacement with interfacetal dislocation and the articular mass of the vertebra above lying anterior to the articular mass of the vertebra below.

This occurs uni- or bilaterally. The facet capsule is the strongest part of the cervical ligamentous complex, and so dislocation of the facet joint is often associated with severe ligamentous injuries with disruption of the interosseous ligaments and discs (Fig. 18.7).

18.3 Imaging of Intraspinal Injuries

MRI is the modality of choice to visualize spinal soft tissue lesions such as spinal cord haemorrhage and oedema, transections, ligamentous tears, epidural haematomas, disc herniations, nerve root avulsion and cord compression and also visualizes subluxations and fractures. Be aware that most of these lesions may occur without fractures or dislocations. Spinal cord oedema and ligamentous or disc lesions will appear bright on T2-weighted images (Fig. 18.8). Bright signal on T1-weighted images is related to acute haemorrhage. Medullary haemorrhage is associated with poor prognostic outcome.

18.4 Specific Paediatric Concerns

In children under the age of 8 years, distraction and subluxation injuries (such as atlanto-occipital dislocation and rotatory subluxation of the atlas upon the axis) are more common than fractures

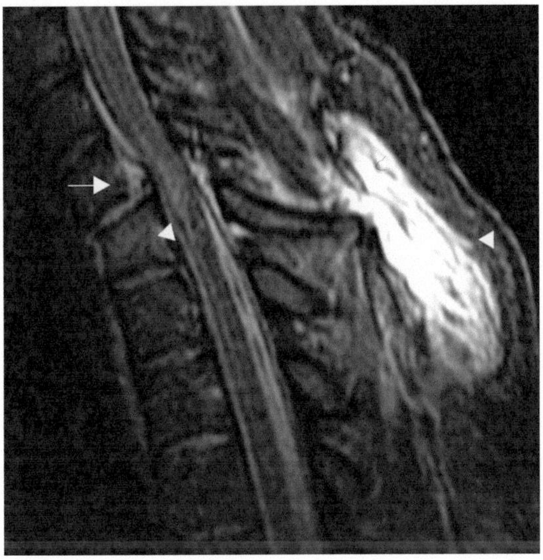

Fig. 18.8 T2-weighted STIR image. Cervical fracture and dislocation with oedema of the spinal cord and posterior soft tissue laceration (*bright areas posterior*)

and often involve the occipito-atlanto-axial segment. Keep the congenital variants in mind including the absence of the posterior arch of C1 and the os odontoideum arising from the secondary ossification centre of the odontoid.

Suggested Reading

Grainger RD, Allison DJ, et al. Diagnostic radiology: a textbook of medical imaging. London: Churchill Livingstone; 2001. p. 1815–33.

Holmes JF, Akkinepalli R. Computed tomography versus plain radiography to screen for cervical spine injury: a meta-analysis. J Trauma. 2005;58:902–5.

Lockwood M, et al. Screening via CT angiogram after traumatic cervical spine fractures: narrowing imaging to improve cost effectiveness. Experience of a Level I trauma center. J Neurosurg Spine. 2016;24(3):490–5.

Panczykowski D, et al. Comparative effectiveness of using computed tomography alone to exclude cervical spine injuries in obtunded or intubated patients: meta-analysis of 14,327 patients with blunt trauma. J Neurosurg. 2011;115(3):541–9.

Parizel PM, et al. New developments in the neuroradiological diagnosis of craniocerebral trauma. Eur Radiol. 2005;15:569–81.

Shah L, Ross J. Imaging of spine trauma. Neurosurgery. 2016;79(5):626–42.

Yousem DM, Nadgir R. Neuroradiology: the requisites. Philadelphia: Mosby/Elsevier; 2017. p. 393–604. Chapter 14.

19 Blood Samples

Bo-Michael Bellander and Rasmus Philip Nielsen

Recommendations

Level I

Data are insufficient data to support Level I recommendations for this subject.

Level II

Data are insufficient data to support Level II recommendations for this subject.

Level III

Recommendations from other topics implicate the use of certain blood samples. There is Level III evidence for avoiding hypoxia and hypo−/hyperglycemia. For this reason, measuring PaO2 and blood glucose is evident.

B.-M. Bellander (✉)
Department of Clinical Neuroscience, Karolinska Institutet, Stockholm, Sweden

Department of Neurosurgery, Karolinska University Hospital, Stockholm, Sweden
e-mail: bo-michael.bellander@sll.se

R. P. Nielsen
Department of Anaesthesiology, Regional Hospital West Jutland, Herning, Denmark
e-mail: rpn@dadlnet.dk

Tips, Tricks, and Pitfalls

- In the acute setting, have a predefined list of routine blood samples to be taken.
- Consider saving a blood sample in the freezer for later analysis.
- Take additional blood samples later, when the patient is stable and the patient's history is known.
- Evaluate the need for "routine" blood samples every day.
- Hyponatremia may occur rapidly and is dangerous due to the development of brain edema.
- Unconsciousness may be due to other issues than the traumatic brain injury.

19.1 Overview

Blood tests on patients suffering from traumatic brain injury should help the physician to identify potential conditions that may cause secondary brain damage that is avoidable if adequate intervention is instituted. Avoidable secondary insults that can lead to ischemia have been well described (Jones et al. 1994) of which some are detectable using adequate blood samples. A specific blood test is also indicated to make a proper diagnosis. Other explanations for impaired consciousness, such as substrate deficiency or electrolyte disturbances,

© Springer Nature Switzerland AG 2020
T. Sundstrøm et al. (eds.), *Management of Severe Traumatic Brain Injury*,
https://doi.org/10.1007/978-3-030-39383-0_19

must be ruled out. An episode with severe hypoglycemia increases mortality significantly (Krinsley and Grover 2007). Hyponatremia is a well-known explanation for brain edema formation. Circulatory impairment with a subsequent metabolic acidosis needs to be rapidly corrected. In addition, there are conditions leading to progressive bleeding due to platelet dysfunction caused by the trauma itself (Nekludov et al. 2007; Zhang et al. 2018) but also other bleeding disorders caused by ongoing anticoagulant (Wiegele et al. 2019) or platelet inhibiting therapy (Tollefsen et al. 2018) that need to be managed. Furthermore, blood samples, e.g. biomarkers, may also help in grading the severity of injury and predict outcome (Thelin et al. 2019).

When the unconscious TBI patient arrives to the trauma center or emergency room, an arterial blood gas (ABG) is mandatory to analyze pH, PaO_2, $PaCO_2$, base excess (BE) and/or bicarbonate. Venous samples may as well be obtained via the arterial line and should at least include sodium, potassium, creatinine, hemoglobin, leucocytes, C-reactive protein (CRP), platelets, INR/PP, glucose, ethanol and methanol, ABO blood type, activated partial thromboplastin time (APTT), fibrinogen and myoglobin.

Depending on the patient's premorbid condition, known illnesses and other extra-cranial injuries, additional blood sampling may be necessary, such as liver enzymes and amylase. Signs of extensive hemorrhage indicate blood cross-matching in case of a subsequent need for blood transfusion. A more extensive toxic screening may be indicated, and it is always wise to keep an additional blood sample in the freezer for later analysis.

Normal values for adults (over 18 years) may differ between laboratories and equipment, why it is important to know the specific normal values at the actual site.

19.2 Background

19.2.1 Arterial Blood Sample

Two very prominent and frequently found secondary insults with serious impact on outcome following traumatic brain injury are hypoxia and hypotension (Chesnut et al. 1993; Stocchetti et al. 1996; McHugh et al. 2007). An arterial blood gas (ABG) at admission will reveal hypoxia by presenting a low pO_2 and hypotension by presenting a negative base excess. Furthermore, pCO_2 in the ABG will also disclose an ongoing hyperventilation due to stress, pain and anxiety or due to excessive artificial ventilation negatively affecting the cerebral blood flow. A high pCO_2 indicates a ventilatory insufficiency that needs immediate correction.

19.2.2 Hematology

Oxygenation is dependent on the hemoglobin level; that is why it is important to detect anemia. Low hemoglobin is an independent predictor of poor outcome (Murray et al. 2007), but blood transfusion does not appear to significantly improve outcome in anemic patients with TBI (Salim et al. 2008). A recent review by East and co-workers stated that "there is insufficient evidence to make strong recommendations regarding which hemoglobin threshold to use as a transfusion trigger in critically-ill patients with TBI" (East et al. 2018).

When deciding on transfusion, it is important to differ between a patient with pre-shock anemia and circulatory instability due to an ongoing hemorrhage and an anemic circulatory stable patient with no signs of ongoing secondary brain damage. Laboratory values are to be assessed in relation to other clinical factors.

19.2.3 Electrolytes

S-Osmolality and *s-Sodium* are important in the development of brain edema. A rapid decline in osmolality due to hyponatremia may be deleterious to the patient and must be restituted acutely unlike chronic hyponatremia that may be corrected over days, as a rapid restitution bears the risk of inducing osmotic demyelination (George et al. 2018).

Magnesium Hypomagnesemia following traumatic brain injury is associated with neurological dysfunction, and restitution in the experimental setting attenuates these neurological changes. Unfortunately, substitution in the clinic has not been proven effective (Temkin et al. 2007).

Phosphate acts as a substrate for adenosine triphosphate (ATP) and plays a crucial role in energy metabolism. Hypophosphatemia is a serious condition that may lead to a decrease in cardiac and respiratory muscle contractility with a subsequent acute cardiac and respiratory failure, cardiac arrhythmia and cardiac arrest.

Osmotherapy to lower ICP will increase urinary output and affect the levels of electrolytes. Accurate balancing of fluid in- and output is essential, including control of the serum concentrations of electrolytes.

19.2.4 Coagulation

Acute traumatic coagulopathy has 19 different definitions in 22 studies (Epstein et al. 2015), but an INR of >1.3 appears to be a stable indicator despite that it only measures the extrinsic pathway of the coagulation cascade. The tissue injury and hypoperfusion are important factors for coagulopathy, but the brain trauma also appears to create a platelet dysfunction. Furthermore, the elderly group of TBI patients often are treated with anticoagulants or platelet inhibitors adding more hemorrhagic issues to the emergency room (Uccella et al. 2018). Basic coagulation parameters are necessary to determine, especially INR, APT-time and fibrinogen. The number of thrombocytes does not add any information on platelet function; that is why thrombelastography (TEG) or rotation thromboelastometry (ROTEM) may be used to assess clot formation and the subsequent fibrinolysis. Furthermore, by analyzing the receptors located on the platelets using multiple platelet function analyzer, e.g. Multiplate®, further information concerning ongoing antiplatelet treatments or trauma-induced platelet dysfunction may be gathered (Ganter and Hofer 2008).

19.2.5 Glucose

Glucose is the main substrate for the glycolytic pathway, and hypoglycemia may lead to energy failure and increased mortality (Krinsley and Grover 2007). On the other hand, severely head-injured patients frequently develop hyperglycemia (Lam et al. 1991) that also has been shown to be an independent predictor of poor outcome (Nelson et al. 2012). Tight glycemic control has been suggested (Van den Berghe et al. 2005), but contradictory findings (Oddo et al. 2008; Vespa et al. 2012) have led to the finding that the majority of European intensive care units today prefer conventional glucose management over tight glycemic control (Huijben et al. 2018).

19.2.6 Myoglobin

Patients suffering from general trauma often show a release of myoglobin from injured tissue with a subsequent risk for acute renal insufficiency (Polderman 2004).

19.3 Pre-existing or Concomitant Disease and Differential Diagnosis

At our hospital, the basic blood samples obtained at admission to the intensive care unit include a simple screening shown in Table 19.1. Furthermore, unconsciousness may be due to other issues than the traumatic brain injury. Encephalitis, uremia, epileptic seizures, Korsakoff syndrome and Wernicke encephalopathy, meningitis, septicemia, intoxication, hypo- or hyperglycemia and respiratory insufficiency are medical conditions that should be considered and might need additional blood samples.

19.4 Specific Pediatric Concerns

Blood samples should be obtained with micro techniques due to the reduced volume of circulating blood in children. The use of routine blood

Table 19.1 Specific sampling (adults) at NCCU Karolinska

1. Blood
(a) Erythrocytes, EVF, hemoglobin, MCH, MCV
2. Acid-base status
(a) Arterial blood gas including b-glucose
3. Electrolytes
(a) P-Sodium
(b) S-Osmolality
(c) P-Phosphate
(d) P-Potassium
(e) P-Magnesium
4. Coagulation
(a) Thrombocytes
(b) P-fibrin soluble
(c) P-fibrinogen
(d) P-PK(INR)
(e) ROTEM and/or Multiplate in certain cases
5. Infection
(a) Leukocytes
(b) p-CRP
(c) s-Procalcitonin
6. Glucose
(a) b-HbA1c (IFCC)
7. Renal
(a) p-Creatinine
8. Liver and pancreas:
(a) p-ASAT
(b) p-Urea
(c) p-Bilirubin
(d) p-GT
(e) p-Pancreas-amylase
9. Muscle injuries
(a) p-Myoglobin
10. Biomarkers
(a) s-S100B
11. Heart
(a) p-Troponin T

samples should be avoided due to the risk of anemia in small children. Some reference values will differ from the adult values.

References

Chesnut RM, Marshall LF, Klauber MR, Blunt BA, Baldwin N, Eisenberg HM, Jane JA, Marmarou A, Foulkes MA. The role of secondary brain injury in determining outcome from severe head injury. J Trauma. 1993;34:216–22.

East JM, Viau-Lapointe J, McCredie VA. Transfusion practices in traumatic brain injury. Curr Opin Anaesthesiol. 2018;31:219–26.

Epstein DS, Mitra B, Cameron PA, Fitzgerald M, Rosenfeld JV. Acute traumatic coagulopathy in the setting of isolated traumatic brain injury: definition, incidence and outcomes. Br J Neurosurg. 2015;29:118–22.

Ganter MT, Hofer CK. Coagulation monitoring: current techniques and clinical use of viscoelastic point-of-care coagulation devices. Anesth Analg. 2008;106:1366–75.

George JC, Zafar W, Bucaloiu ID, Chang AR. Risk factors and outcomes of rapid correction of severe hyponatremia. Clin J Am Soc Nephrol. 2018;13:984–92.

Huijben JA, Volovici V, Cnossen MC, Haitsma IK, Stocchetti N, Maas AIR, Menon DK, Ercole A, Citerio G, Nelson D, Polinder S, Steyerberg EW, Lingsma HF, van der Jagt M, C.-T. investigators, and participants. Variation in general supportive and preventive intensive care management of traumatic brain injury: a survey in 66 neurotrauma centers participating in the Collaborative European NeuroTrauma Effectiveness Research in Traumatic Brain Injury (CENTER-TBI) study. Crit Care. 2018;22:90.

Jones PA, Andrews PJD, Midgley S, Anderson SI, Piper IR, Tocher JL, Housley AM, Corrie JA, Slattery J, Dearden NM, Miller JD. Measuring the burden of secondary insults in head-injured patients during intensive care. J Neurosurg Anesthesiol. 1994;6:4–14.

Krinsley JS, Grover A. Severe hypoglycemia in critically ill patients: risk factors and outcomes. Crit Care Med. 2007;35:2262–7.

Lam AM, Winn HR, Cullen BF, Sundling N. Hyperglycemia and neurological outcome in patients with head injury. J Neurosurg. 1991;75:545–51.

McHugh GS, Engel DC, Butcher I, Steyerberg EW, Lu J, Mushkudiani N, Hernández AV, Marmarou A, Maas AI, Murray GD. Prognostic value of secondary insults in traumatic brain injury: results from the IMPACT study. J Neurotrauma. 2007;24:287–93.

Murray GD, Butcher I, McHugh GS, Lu J, Mushkudiani NA, Maas AI, Marmarou A, Steyerberg EW. Multivariable prognostic analysis in traumatic brain injury: results from the IMPACT study. J Neurotrauma. 2007;24:329–37.

Nekludov M, Bellander BM, Blombäck M, Wallen HN. Platelet dysfunction in patients with severe traumatic brain injury. J Neurotrauma. 2007;11:1699–706.

Nelson DW, Rudehill A, MacCallum RM, Holst A, Wanecek M, Weitzberg E, Bellander BM. Multivariate outcome prediction in traumatic brain injury with focus on laboratory values. J Neurotrauma. 2012;29:2613–24.

Oddo M, Schmidt JM, Carrera E, Badjatia N, Connolly ES, Presciutti M, Ostapkovich ND, Levine JM, Le Roux P, SA M. Impact of tight glycemic control on cerebral glucose metabolism after severe brain injury: a microdialysis study. Crit Care Med. 2008;36:3233–8.

Polderman KH. Acute renal failure and rhabdomyolysis. Int J Artif Organs. 2004;27:1030–3.

Salim A, Hadjizacharia P, DuBose J, Brown C, Inaba K, Chan L, Margulies DR. Role of anemia in traumatic brain injury. J Am Coll Surg. 2008;207:398–406.

Stocchetti N, Furlan A, Volta F. Hypoxemia and arterial hypotension at the accident scene in head injury. J Trauma. 1996;40:764–7.

Temkin NR, Anderson GD, Winn HR, Ellenbogen RG, Britz GW, Schuster J, Lucas T, Newell DW, Mansfield PN, Machamer JE, Barber J, SS D. Magnesium sulfate for neuroprotection after traumatic brain injury: a randomised controlled trial. Lancet Neurol. 2007;6:29–38.

Thelin E, Al Nimer F, Frostell A, Zetterberg H, Blennow K, Nyström H, Svensson M, Bellander BM, Piehl F, Nelson DW. A serum protein biomarker panel improves outcome prediction in human traumatic brain injury. J Neurotrauma 2019;36:1–13.

Tollefsen MH, Vik A, Skandsen T, Sandrod O, Deane SF, Rao V, Moen KG. Patients with moderate and severe traumatic brain injury: impact of preinjury platelet inhibitor or warfarin treatment. World Neurosurg. 2018;114:e209–17.

Uccella L, Zoia C, Bongetta D, Gaetani P, Martig F, Candrian C, Rosso R. Are antiplatelet and anticoagulants drugs a risk factor for bleeding in mild traumatic brain injury? World Neurosurg. 2018;110:e339–45.

Van den Berghe G, Schoonheydt K, Becx P, Bruyninckx F, Wouters PJ. Insulin therapy protects the central and peripheral nervous system of intensive care patients. Neurology. 2005;64:1348–53.

Vespa P, McArthur DL, Stein N, Huang SC, Shao W, Filippou M, Etchepare M, Glenn T, Hovda DA. Tight glycemic control increases metabolic distress in traumatic brain injury: a randomized controlled within-subjects trial. Crit Care Med. 2012;40:1923–9.

Wiegele M, Schochl H, Haushofer A, Ortler M, Leitgeb J, Kwasny O, Beer R, Ay C, Schaden E. Diagnostic and therapeutic approach in adult patients with traumatic brain injury receiving oral anticoagulant therapy: an Austrian interdisciplinary consensus statement. Crit Care. 2019;23:62.

Zhang J, Zhang F, Dong JF. Coagulopathy induced by traumatic brain injury: systemic manifestation of a localized injury. Blood. 2018;131:2001–6.

20 To Treat or Not to Treat in the Acute Setting (Withholding) and Withdrawal of Treatment

Magnus Olivecrona

Recommendations

Level I

There are no data supporting an individual prognosis at this level.

Level II

There are no data supporting an individual prognosis at this level.

There is prognostic value in age, GCS, GCS motor score, pupillary reaction, hypotension, hypoxia, CT findings, blood chemistry, ethnic origin, and social background.

Level III

There are some data supporting individual prognosis using prognostic models and calculators at this level.

There seems to be some prognostic value in ICP, CPP and PR_x.

There is insufficient evidence for the prognostic value of biomarkers.

There is insufficient evidence to base treatment decisions solely on prognostic calculators and instruments.

Tips, Tricks and Pitfalls

- Be aware that the presentation of poor prognostic factors such as bilateral dilated and fixed pupils does not necessarily mean that the patient will not survive or even have a favourable outcome.
- Be aware of not letting poor prognostic factors become self-fulfilling prophecies.
- There is, at present, no prognostic instrument or tool which allows for prognostication in an individual case, and thus no sole instrument or tool can be used to make treatment decisions in an individual case.

M. Olivecrona (✉)
Department of Medical Sciences, Faculty of Medicine, Örebro University, Örebro, Sweden

Section for Neurosurgery, Department of Anaesthesia and Intensive Care, University Hospital, Örebro, Sweden

20.1 Overview

Prognosis is derived from the Greek πρόγνωση which means literally “fore-knowing” and “foreseeing”.

© Springer Nature Switzerland AG 2020
T. Sundstrøm et al. (eds.), *Management of Severe Traumatic Brain Injury*, https://doi.org/10.1007/978-3-030-39383-0_20

The prognosis of a condition can be used to discuss the seriousness or likely outcome. It can as such be used as an aid in the information process to the patient and/or her/his relatives. It also gives information to the treating physician about what she/he could expect.

The accuracy of prognosis on group or population level can be very precise. At the individual level, the prognosis is most often considerably less accurate.

There are several factors that prognosticate poor outcome in severe traumatic brain injury. Among these are age, GCS, pupillary dilatation with loss of light reflex, hypoxia, hypotension, intradural mass lesions on the CT scan and presence of subarachnoidal or intraventricular blood on CT scan.

The ultimate use of the prognostication would be that the prognosis was so precise, on an individual level, that it allowed for treatment decisions and thus to individualisation of the treatment and care.

The treating physician has to be aware of the limitations of the prognosis and thus show caution in using the estimated prognosis for making treatment decisions for the individual patient.

There is a risk that a single negative prognostic factor, e.g. bilaterally dilated and fixed pupils, which is, on the group level, a strong negative prognostic factor, will be used as foundation for a treatment decision in an individual patient and thus becomes a self-fulfilling prognostic factor.

20.2 Background

Prognosis of the outcome in head trauma has always interested man. In the ancient literature, references to the prognosis of head trauma are found, e.g. in the Edgar Smith papyrus (n.d.) and in the writings of Hippocrates (1999).

Today, the prognosis of outcome of severe traumatic brain injury is mostly defined in relation to the outcome, measured as GOS or GOSE (Jennett and Bond 1975; Wilson et al. 1998). This can be in relation to every single level of the scales or to different dichotomisations, such as dead/alive or favourable/unfavourable. More recent attempts to prognosticate in relation to more refined outcomes such as quality of life have been attempted (Haller 2017; Norup et al. 2017).

The influence of different prognostic factors on the outcome can be analysed using statistical methods. The influence of a single factor on outcome can be analysed using univariate analysis. This result is of limited value. To adjust for confounders, and/or the influence of other prognostic factors, more advanced statistical methods have to be used, e.g. logistic regression or multivariate analysis. Further statistical modelling can result in prognostic models, which even can have the intension of prognosis at individual level.

Factors analysed for prognostic value can be of different kinds: patient characteristics (e.g. age, sex), admission data (e.g. GCS, blood pressure), or data from the clinical course (e.g. ICP, CPP, seizures). These factors are then analysed against different outcome measures such as GOS, GOSE, or quality of life.

Several attempts have been made to create complex prognostic models using several of the prognostic factors. An interesting observation is that in most of these attempts to create a prognostic model for severe traumatic brain injury, the treatment protocols used are not taken into account.

20.3 Prognostic Factors

20.3.1 Patient Characteristics

Sex: In severe traumatic brain injury, the majority of the patients are men. There is no difference between the sexes in regard to prognosis (Ellenberg et al. 1996; Husson et al. 2010; MRC CRASH Trial Collaborators et al. 2008; Butcher et al. 2007).

Age: Increasing age is a strong predictor for poorer outcome (MRC CRASH Trial Collaborators et al. 2008; Combes et al. 1996; Hukkelhoven et al. 2003; Mushkudiani et al. 2007). Some studies show a breaking point around 30–40 years (Hukkelhoven et al. 2003; Mushkudiani et al. 2007). The most head injury trials have an upper age limit of 60–70 years; so not so much is known of the prognosis in the elderly (Ostermann et al. 2018; Patel et al. 2010; Wan et al. 2017).

The relation between age and outcome in the paediatric population is not very well studied.

Ethnic origin: There are some studies that indicate that the prognosis in black patients is found to be poorer as compared with Caucasians (Mushkudiani et al. 2007; Perrin et al. 2014; Shafi et al. 2007; Sorani et al. 2009).

Minority status and poorer socio-economic status: There are some publications indicating poorer outcome after moderate and severe traumatic brain injury in people of minority status or in poorer socio-economic status (Arango-Lasprilla et al. 2007a, b).

20.3.2 Injury Severity, Clinical Characteristics

Glasgow Coma Score, Glasgow Motor Score: Both are strong predictors for outcome irrespective of time point for assessment (Husson et al. 2010; MRC CRASH Trial Collaborators et al. 2008; Marmarou et al. 2007a). The assessment of GCS is time dependent in the course of severe traumatic brain injury (Arbabi et al. 2004; Stocchetti et al. 2004). The time point has to be taken into consideration, if the assessment is done in the site of trauma, in the emergency room, after stabilisation, or even after intubation.

In unconscious patients, the motor score has been claimed to be more reliable than the total GCS score (Healey et al. 2003).

The modern care of severe traumatic brain injury includes early intubation and sedation, which has to be taken into consideration (Stocchetti et al. 2004; Balestreri et al. 2005).

We have to bear in mind that a GCS of 3 is an exclusion criterion in many studies; however, papers reporting good outcome (GOS 4–5) in patients with an initial GCS of 3 have been published (Chamoun et al. 2009; Mauritz et al. 2009; Olivecrona et al. 2009a).

Pupillary reaction: The absence of pupillary reaction in one or both eyes is a strong, negative prognostic factor (MRC CRASH Trial Collaborators et al. 2008; Marmarou et al. 2007a). This factor is claimed to be less sensitive for changes over time. In many studies of severe traumatic brain injury, dilated fixed pupil or pupils are an exclusion criterion. There are papers that report good outcome (GOS 4–5) in patients with dilated and fixed pupils (Mauritz et al. 2009; Olivecrona et al. 2009a; Clusmann et al. 2001).

Also loss of pupillary reaction unilaterally is a bad prognostic sign, though not as bad as the loss of pupillary reactivity bilaterally. For poorer outcome, an odds ratio of around 7 for bilateral loss of pupil reactivity has been reported, as compared with an odds ratio of 3 for unilateral loss of pupil reactivity (Marmarou et al. 2007a).

Hypotension: Hypotension, defined as a systolic blood pressure <90 mmHg, is a strong prognostic factor (Butcher et al. 2007; Chesnut et al. 1993a; Miller et al. 1978; Murray et al. 2007; Walia and Sutcliffe 2002). A bell-shaped curve for the impact of blood pressure on outcome has been reported. This curve shows a better prognosis for systolic blood pressures between 120 and 150 mmHg, corresponding to mean arterial blood pressure of 85–100 mmHg (Butcher et al. 2007).

Hypoxia: Hypoxia is a factor for poor outcome (Chesnut et al. 1993a; Miller et al. 1978; Hukkelhoven et al. 2005; McHugh et al. 2007). The definition of hypoxia varies between studies ($S_aO_2 < 90/92\%$ or $P_aO_2 < 8$ kPa).

Abbreviated Injury Scale (AIS), Injury Severity Score (ISSS): These scores are commonly used to describe extracranial injury (Rating the severity of tissue damage 1971; Baker et al. 1974). Whether extracranial injuries affect the prognosis or not has been discussed, and findings in both directions have been reported. It seems that the extent of the extracranial injury has a larger influence in persons with milder brain injury than in persons with severe brain injury. It also seems that the extent of extracranial injury mostly affects the early mortality (van Leeuwen et al. 2012).

20.3.3 Laboratory Parameters

Initial blood glucose: A high blood glucose level correlates positively with poor outcome (Helmy et al. 2010; Van Beek et al. 2007).

Initial sodium levels: Low and high sodium levels are associated with poor outcome (Van Beek et al. 2007).

Haemoglobin: Low haemoglobin is a factor in poor prognosis (Helmy et al. 2010; Van Beek et al. 2007).

Biomarkers: Biomarkers such as S-100B, neuron-specific enolase, and ApoE (ε) have attracted much attention for their possible prognostic value. The findings have been confounding. Some authors find prognostic value in the biomarkers (Nylen et al. 2008; Rainey et al. 2009; Rothoerl et al. 2000; Teasdale et al. 1997; Vos et al. 2010) and some authors do not (Alexander et al. 2007; Olivecrona et al. 2009b; Teasdale et al. 2005).

No biomarker has yet been proven to have a strong predictive value.

20.3.4 Structural Imaging

Computerised tomography: In 1991, Marshall and collaborators introduced a system to classify CT scans. This system was initially designed as a descriptive method (Marshall et al. 1991). The Marshall classification, which focuses on mass lesions, has been correlated to prognosis (Servadei et al. 2000). The importance of the CT scan features for the prognosis was well established in the treatment guidelines published in 2000 (The Brain Trauma Foundation 2000). A combination of different CT features, such as shift of the midline structures, the presence of subarachnoid blood and epidural haematoma, or compression of basal cisterns, increases the prognostic value (Maas et al. 2005, 2007). The presence of subarachnoid blood seems to be one of the strongest predictors of poor outcome (Maas et al. 2005). The Rotterdam classification of the CT scan introduced by Maas and collaborators in 2005 seems to have a stronger predictive value than the Marshall classification (Maas et al. 2005). It also allows for the comparison of the CT scans over time.

Magnetic resonance tomography: MR imaging might have an important role in prognostication after severe head injury. The method is complicated to use in an intensive care setting. In almost all of the studies reporting on MR findings, the investigation has been done at 1 week or later after trauma. Thus, the findings will have little consequence on the early prognostication. The timing of the MR investigation seems to have an influence on the use of the results for prognostication (Moen et al. 2012; Skandsen et al. 2011). On the other hand, it can be a useful tool in understanding the process of the disease.

20.3.5 Clinical Course

Intracranial pressure: Intuitively, one would assume that ICP should be a strong prognostic factor. Some treatment concepts are focused on reducing the ICP (ICP targeted therapy). Most authors report correlations between, e.g. the highest observed ICP and outcome and the mean ICP over at certain time or the "delivered" ICP over time (Farahvar et al. 2011; Vik et al. 2008). The majority of authors do present a prognostic value of ICP (Balestreri et al. 2005; Farahvar et al. 2011; Vik et al. 2008; Marmarou et al. 1991). Strictly, the prognostic value of ICP is difficult to interpret.

Cerebral perfusion pressure: Intuitively, the CPP should be a prognostic factor. The same applies for the CPP as for the ICP; there have been many different ways trying to establish a prognostic correlation. Authors have reported the prognostic value of CPP (Clifton et al. 2002; Juul et al. 2000; Kirkness et al. 2005), and others have reported of the non-prognostic value of the CPP (Balestreri et al. 2006). Strictly the prognostic value of the CPP is difficult to interpret.

Periods of hypotension and hypoxia: There are reports stating that the number and duration of episodes with hypotension and/or hypoxia during the course of treatment correlates negatively to the outcome (Chesnut et al. 1993a, b; Sarrafzadeh et al. 2001).

Autoregulation, Pressure reactivity—PR index and PR_x: The PR, which is the regression coefficient of several MAP/ICP points, can be regarded as a surrogate measure for the autoregulative state of the brain, with a negative to zero value of the PR regarded as indicator of intact autoregulation. A disturbed autoregulation has been reported to correlate with or even predict poor outcome (Balestreri et al. 2005; Adams et al. 2017; Hiler et al. 2006; Howells et al. 2005; Sorrentino et al. 2012; Zweifel et al. 2008).

20.4 Prognostic Models: To Make a Prognosis

During the last decade, several attempts to construct a prognosis model based on different prognostic factors have been done. One has used pooled data from large series of patients, e.g. from the prospective trials. These data have then been analysed using advanced statistics to produce models of prognostication. One of the goals has been to try to find a model allowing for individualised prognostication.

Some of these attempts have resulted in prognostic formulas or calculators of which some are available on the Internet (see Table 20.1).

Several of these prognostic models have been validated using external data. These validations have found a fairly good reliability (Castano-Leon et al. 2016; Han et al. 2014; Majdan et al. 2014; Olivecrona and Koskinen 2012; Olivecrona and Olivecrona 2013). On attempts to validate these prognostic tools, several authors found a tendency to an overestimation of the risk for poorer outcomes. None of the instruments are good enough to allow for prognostication and thus not allowing for treatment decisions in an individual case. The user of these prognostic tools has to be aware of the limitations of the prognostication.

Table 20.1 Prognostic calculators available on-line

Name	Factors used	Link	Predicts for
IMPACT (Marmarou et al. 2007b)	Clinical data CT findings Laboratory data	http://www.tbi-impact.org/?p=impact/calc	Mortality and unfavourable outcome at 6 months
CRASH (MRC CRASH Trial Collaborators et al. 2008)	Clinical data CT findings	http://www.crash.lshtm.ac.uk/Risk%20calculator/index.html	Mortality at 14 days Unfavourable outcome at 6 months
Nijmegen (Jacobs et al. 2013)	Clinical data CT findings	http://www.tbi-prognosis.com	Mortality at 6 months Unfavourable outcome at 6 months
Helsinki score (Raj et al. 2014)	Clinical data CT findings	http://links.lww.com/NEU/A676	Mortality at 6 months Unfavourable outcome at 6 months
Stockholm score (Nelson et al. 2010)	CT findings Clinical data	Probability score for unfavourable outcome: $1/1 + e^{(3,5\text{-}1,1*\text{tally})}$ Tally = midline-shift (mm)/10 + SAH/IVH-score/2–1 (if EDH) + 1 if DAI + 1(if dual-sided SDH) + 1	Best outcome at 1 year
Stockholm rule of thumb (Nelson et al. 2010)		Probability for unfavourable outcome: Age—3 *GCS + mid-line shift (mm) + 10 rule 10 rule = +10 if non-responsive pupils; +10 if SAH/ÌVH; +10 if DAI; −10 if EDH	Best outcome at 1 year

20.5 To Treat or Not to Treat: Does the Knowledge About Prognosis Help?

When the unconscious trauma victim, i.e. the person with a severe head injury, arrives in the A&E, the receiving physician or surgeon is put to a challenge. She or he has relatively limited information to make difficult decisions, the basic question being to initiate treatment or not.

First of the questions is if diagnostic procedures should be initiated or if the patient e.g. has fixed and dilated pupils upon arrival, the decision to just say that the prognosis is so bad that there is no indication for any kind of diagnostic measures. As the author has tried to outline above, there are so many factors to take into consideration in this decision.

Irrespective of later decisions, one should even in this acute situation try to gather as much information as possible.

To manage this would, in the opinion of the author, be to (if so needed) secure the airway and progress to doing a CT scan, preferable a "trauma CT" including not only the head but also the main part of the body. In this time, there is an opportunity to gather more information about the history of the patient, the circumstances surrounding the accident, and primary clinical and neurological status. This together with the information attained from the CT scan gives valuable information for the decision-making process.

Even though several markers for poor prognosis might be present, we also know that the exactness of the prognosis is not very good at the individual level.

Not to initiate treatment in a young, otherwise healthy person, with an isolated blunt severe head injury, even if the person presents with bilateral, dilated fixed pupils, is a doubtful decision. On the other hand, not to initiate treatment in a person 85 years of age, with bilateral fixed and dilated pupils, would most probably be wise.

The clinical outcome learns, in this author's opinion, that a primary aggressive initiation of treatment is preferable. A good help in early treatment decisions is the use of aggressive ICP monitoring, as it at least to some extent gives information about the risk of cerebral hypoperfusion/ischaemia.

If one starts with an aggressive treatment approach, one also has to be open for continuous re-evaluation of this treatment decision. It is in this process of a continuing re-evaluation of treatment that the knowledge about certain factors' influence on prognosis comes to use. This in a synthesis with clinical experience, local experience, and knowledge about the attitudes of the stricken and its relatives, will build a ground on which the treating physician or surgeon can make decisions about the treatment ambitions, level of treatment, or even withdrawal of treatment.

20.6 Specific Paediatric Concerns

There are relatively few studies of severe traumatic brain injury in the paediatric population. Generally, one can assume the severely injured child has a better prognosis than the adult with a corresponding injury. This might be due to several factors, such as greater plasticity of the young brain, a general better healing capacity, and fewer concomitant diseases.

One recent publication indicates that PR_x has a prognostic value for children (Hockel et al. 2017).

Generally, the recommendation must be to treat a child with severe traumatic brain injury aggressively.

References

Adams H, Donnelly J, Czosnyka M, Kolias AG, Helmy A, Menon DK, et al. Temporal profile of intracranial pressure and cerebrovascular reactivity in severe traumatic brain injury and association with fatal outcome: an observational study. PLoS Med. 2017;14(7):e1002353. https://doi.org/10.1371/journal.pmed.1002353.

Alexander S, Kerr ME, Kim Y, Kamboh MI, Beers SR, Conley YP. Apolipoprotein E4 allele presence and functional outcome after severe traumatic brain injury. J Neurotrauma. 2007;24(5):790–7. https://doi.org/10.1089/neu.2006.0133.

Arango-Lasprilla JC, Rosenthal M, Deluca J, Cifu DX, Hanks R, Komaroff E. Functional outcomes from inpatient rehabilitation after traumatic brain injury: how do Hispanics fare? Arch Phys Med

Rehabil. 2007a;88(1):11–8. https://doi.org/10.1016/j.apmr.2006.10.029.

Arango-Lasprilla JC, Rosenthal M, Deluca J, Komaroff E, Sherer M, Cifu D, et al. Traumatic brain injury and functional outcomes: does minority status matter? Brain Inj. 2007b;21(7):701–8. https://doi.org/10.1080/02699050701481597.

Arbabi S, Jurkovich GJ, Wahl WL, Franklin GA, Hemmila MR, Taheri PA, et al. A comparison of prehospital and hospital data in trauma patients. J Trauma. 2004;56(5):1029–32.

Baker SP, O'Neill B, Haddon W Jr, Long WB. The injury severity score: a method for describing patients with multiple injuries and evaluating emergency care. J Trauma. 1974;14(3):187–96.

Balestreri M, Czosnyka M, Steiner LA, Hiler M, Schmidt EA, Matta B, et al. Association between outcome, cerebral pressure reactivity and slow ICP waves following head injury. Acta Neurochir Suppl. 2005;95:25–8.

Balestreri M, Czosnyka M, Hutchinson P, Steiner LA, Hiler M, Smielewski P, et al. Impact of intracranial pressure and cerebral perfusion pressure on severe disability and mortality after head injury. Neurocrit Care. 2006;4(1):8–13. https://doi.org/10.1385/NCC:4:1:008.

Butcher I, Maas AI, Lu J, Marmarou A, Murray GD, Mushkudiani NA, et al. Prognostic value of admission blood pressure in traumatic brain injury: results from the IMPACT study. J Neurotrauma. 2007;24(2):294–302. https://doi.org/10.1089/neu.2006.0032.

Castano-Leon AM, Lora D, Munarriz PM, Cepeda S, Paredes I, de la Cruz J, et al. Predicting outcomes after severe and moderate traumatic brain injury: an external validation of impact and crash prognostic models in a large Spanish cohort. J Neurotrauma. 2016;33(17):1598–606. https://doi.org/10.1089/neu.2015.4182.

Chamoun RB, Robertson CS, Gopinath SP. Outcome in patients with blunt head trauma and a Glasgow Coma Scale score of 3 at presentation. J Neurosurg. 2009;111(4):683–7. https://doi.org/10.3171/2009.2.JNS08817.

Chesnut RM, Marshall LF, Klauber MR, Blunt BA, Baldwin N, Eisenberg HM, et al. The role of secondary brain injury in determining outcome from severe head injury. J Trauma. 1993a;34(2):216–22.

Chesnut RM, Marshall SB, Piek J, Blunt BA, Klauber MR, Marshall LF. Early and late systemic hypotension as a frequent and fundamental source of cerebral ischemia following severe brain injury in the Traumatic Coma Data Bank. Acta Neurochir Suppl. 1993b;59:121–5.

Clifton GL, Miller ER, Choi SC, Levin HS. Fluid thresholds and outcome from severe brain injury. Crit Care Med. 2002;30(4):739–45.

Clusmann H, Schaller C, Schramm J. Fixed and dilated pupils after trauma, stroke, and previous intracranial surgery: management and outcome. J Neurol Neurosurg Psychiatry. 2001;71(2):175–81.

Combes P, Fauvage B, Colonna M, Passagia JG, Chirossel JP, Jacquot C. Severe head injuries: an outcome prediction and survival analysis. Intensive Care Med. 1996;22(12):1391–5.

Edwin Smith Surgical Papyrus. http://archive.nlm.nih.gov/proj/ttp/flash/smith/smith.html (n.d.) Accessed 20190331.

Ellenberg JH, Levin HS, Saydjari C. Posttraumatic amnesia as a predictor of outcome after severe closed head injury. Prospective assessment. Arch Neurol. 1996;53(8):782–91.

Farahvar A, Gerber LM, Chiu YL, Hartl R, Froelich M, Carney N, et al. Response to intracranial hypertension treatment as a predictor of death in patients with severe traumatic brain injury. J Neurosurg. 2011;114(5):1471–8. https://doi.org/10.3171/2010.11.JNS101116.

Haller CS. Twelve-month prospective cohort study of patients with severe traumatic brain injury and their relatives: coping, satisfaction with life and neurological functioning. Brain Inj. 2017;31(13–14):1903–9. https://doi.org/10.1080/02699052.2017.1346295.

Han J, King NK, Neilson SJ, Gandhi MP, Ng I. External validation of the CRASH and IMPACT prognostic models in severe traumatic brain injury. J Neurotrauma. 2014;31(13):1146–52. https://doi.org/10.1089/neu.2013.3003.

Healey C, Osler TM, Rogers FB, Healey MA, Glance LG, Kilgo PD, et al. Improving the Glasgow Coma Scale score: motor score alone is a better predictor. J Trauma. 2003;54(4):671–8. https://doi.org/10.1097/01.TA.0000058130.30490.5D; discussion 8–80.

Helmy A, Timofeev I, Palmer CR, Gore A, Menon DK, Hutchinson PJ. Hierarchical log linear analysis of admission blood parameters and clinical outcome following traumatic brain injury. Acta Neurochir. 2010;152(6):953–7. https://doi.org/10.1007/s00701-009-0584-y.

Hiler M, Czosnyka M, Hutchinson P, Balestreri M, Smielewski P, Matta B, et al. Predictive value of initial computerized tomography scan, intracranial pressure, and state of autoregulation in patients with traumatic brain injury. J Neurosurg. 2006;104(5):731–7. https://doi.org/10.3171/jns.2006.104.5.731.

Hippocrates. On wounds in the head. Cambridge/London: Hippocrates/Harvard University Press; 1999. p. 7–51.

Hockel K, Diedler J, Neunhoeffer F, Heimberg E, Nagel C, Schuhmann MU. Time spent with impaired autoregulation is linked with outcome in severe infant/paediatric traumatic brain injury. Acta Neurochir. 2017;159(11):2053–61. https://doi.org/10.1007/s00701-017-3308-8.

Howells T, Elf K, Jones PA, Ronne-Engstrom E, Piper I, Nilsson P, et al. Pressure reactivity as a guide in the treatment of cerebral perfusion pressure in patients with brain trauma. J Neurosurg. 2005;102(2):311–7. https://doi.org/10.3171/jns.2005.102.2.0311.

Hukkelhoven CW, Steyerberg EW, Rampen AJ, Farace E, Habbema JD, Marshall LF, et al. Patient age and outcome following severe traumatic brain injury: an analysis of 5600 patients. J Neurosurg. 2003;99(4):666–73. https://doi.org/10.3171/jns.2003.99.4.0666.

Hukkelhoven CW, Steyerberg EW, Habbema JD, Farace E, Marmarou A, Murray GD, et al. Predicting outcome after traumatic brain injury: development and validation of a prognostic score based on admission characteristics. J Neurotrauma. 2005;22(10):1025–39. https://doi.org/10.1089/neu.2005.22.1025.

Husson EC, Ribbers GM, Willemse-van Son AH, Verhagen AP, Stam HJ. Prognosis of six-month functioning after moderate to severe traumatic brain injury: a systematic review of prospective cohort studies. J Rehabil Med. 2010;42(5):425–36. https://doi.org/10.2340/16501977-0566.

Jacobs B, Beems T, van der Vliet TM, van Vugt AB, Hoedemaekers C, Horn J, et al. Outcome prediction in moderate and severe traumatic brain injury: a focus on computed tomography variables. Neurocrit Care. 2013;19(1):79–89. https://doi.org/10.1007/s12028-012-9795-9.

Jennett B, Bond M. Assessment of outcome after severe brain damage. Lancet. 1975;1(7905):480–4.

Juul N, Morris GF, Marshall SB, Marshall LF. Intracranial hypertension and cerebral perfusion pressure: influence on neurological deterioration and outcome in severe head injury. The Executive Committee of the International Selfotel Trial. J Neurosurg. 2000;92(1):1–6. https://doi.org/10.3171/jns.2000.92.1.0001.

Kirkness CJ, Burr RL, Cain KC, Newell DW, Mitchell PH. Relationship of cerebral perfusion pressure levels to outcome in traumatic brain injury. Acta Neurochir Suppl. 2005;95:13–6.

Maas AI, Hukkelhoven CW, Marshall LF, Steyerberg EW. Prediction of outcome in traumatic brain injury with computed tomographic characteristics: a comparison between the computed tomographic classification and combinations of computed tomographic predictors. Neurosurgery. 2005;57(6):1173–82; discussion −82.

Maas AI, Steyerberg EW, Butcher I, Dammers R, Lu J, Marmarou A, et al. Prognostic value of computerized tomography scan characteristics in traumatic brain injury: results from the IMPACT study. J Neurotrauma. 2007;24(2):303–14. https://doi.org/10.1089/neu.2006.0033.

Majdan M, Lingsma HF, Nieboer D, Mauritz W, Rusnak M, Steyerberg EW. Performance of IMPACT, CRASH and Nijmegen models in predicting six month outcome of patients with severe or moderate TBI: an external validation study. Scand J Trauma Resusc Emerg Med. 2014;22:68. https://doi.org/10.1186/s13049-014-0068-9.

Marmarou A, Anderson RL, Ward JD, Choi SC, Young HF, Eisenberg HM, et al. Impact of ICP instability and hypotension on outcome in patients with severe head trauma. J Neurosurg. 1991;75(Supplement November):s59–66.

Marmarou A, Lu J, Butcher I, McHugh GS, Murray GD, Steyerberg EW, et al. Prognostic value of the Glasgow Coma Scale and pupil reactivity in traumatic brain injury assessed pre-hospital and on enrollment: an IMPACT analysis. J Neurotrauma. 2007a;24(2):270–80. https://doi.org/10.1089/neu.2006.0029.

Marmarou A, Lu J, Butcher I, McHugh GS, Mushkudiani NA, Murray GD, et al. IMPACT database of traumatic brain injury: design and description. J Neurotrauma. 2007b;24(2):239–50. https://doi.org/10.1089/neu.2006.0036.

Marshall LF, Marshall SB, Klauber MR, van Berkum Clark M, Eisenberg HM, Jane JA, et al. A new classification of head injury based on compurerized tomography. J Neurosurg. 1991;75:S14–20.

Mauritz W, Leitgeb J, Wilbacher I, Majdan M, Janciak I, Brazinova A, et al. Outcome of brain trauma patients who have a Glasgow Coma Scale score of 3 and bilateral fixed and dilated pupils in the field. Eur J Emerg Med. 2009;16(3):153–8. https://doi.org/10.1097/MEJ.0b013e32832a0864.

McHugh GS, Engel DC, Butcher I, Steyerberg EW, Lu J, Mushkudiani N, et al. Prognostic value of secondary insults in traumatic brain injury: results from the IMPACT study. J Neurotrauma. 2007;24(2):287–93. https://doi.org/10.1089/neu.2006.0031.

Miller JD, Sweet RC, Narayan R, Becker DP. Early insults to the injured brain. JAMA. 1978;240(5):439–42.

Moen KG, Skandsen T, Folvik M, Brezova V, Kvistad KA, Rydland J, et al. A longitudinal MRI study of traumatic axonal injury in patients with moderate and severe traumatic brain injury. J Neurol Neurosurg Psychiatry. 2012;83(12):1193–200. https://doi.org/10.1136/jnnp-2012-302644.

MRC CRASH Trial Collaborators, Perel P, Arango M, Clayton T, Edwards P, Komolafe E, et al. Predicting outcome after traumatic brain injury: practical prognostic models based on large cohort of international patients. BMJ. 2008;336(7641):425–9. https://doi.org/10.1136/bmj.39461.643438.25.

Murray GD, Butcher I, McHugh GS, Lu J, Mushkudiani NA, Maas AI, et al. Multivariable prognostic analysis in traumatic brain injury: results from the IMPACT study. J Neurotrauma. 2007;24(2):329–37. https://doi.org/10.1089/neu.2006.0035.

Mushkudiani NA, Engel DC, Steyerberg EW, Butcher I, Lu J, Marmarou A, et al. Prognostic value of demographic characteristics in traumatic brain injury: results from the IMPACT study. J Neurotrauma. 2007;24(2):259–69. https://doi.org/10.1089/neu.2006.0028.

Nelson DW, Nystrom H, MacCallum RM, Thornquist B, Lilja A, Bellander BM, et al. Extended analysis of early computed tomography scans of traumatic brain injured patients and relations to outcome. J Neurotrauma. 2010;27(1):51–64. https://doi.org/10.1089/neu.2009.0986.

Norup A, Kristensen KS, Poulsen I, Mortensen EL. Evaluating clinically significant changes in health-related quality of life: a sample of relatives of patients with severe traumatic brain injury. Neuropsychol Rehabil. 2017;27(2):196–215. https://doi.org/10.1080/09602011.2015.1076484.

Nylen K, Ost M, Csajbok LZ, Nilsson I, Hall C, Blennow K, et al. Serum levels of S100B, S100A1B and S100BB are all related to outcome after severe traumatic brain injury. Acta Neurochir. 2008;150(3):221–7. https://doi.org/10.1007/s00701-007-1489-2; discussion 7.

Olivecrona M, Koskinen LO. The IMPACT prognosis calculator used in patients with severe traumatic brain injury treated with an ICP-targeted therapy. Acta Neurochir. 2012;154(9):1567–73. https://doi.org/10.1007/s00701-012-1351-z.

Olivecrona M, Olivecrona Z. Use of the CRASH study prognosis calculator in patients with severe traumatic brain injury treated with an intracranial pressure-targeted therapy. J Clin Neurosci. 2013;20(7):996–1001. https://doi.org/10.1016/j.jocn.2012.09.015.

Olivecrona M, Rodling-Wahlström M, Naredi S, Koskinen L-OD. Prostacylin treatment in severe traumatic brain injury—a microdialysis and outcome study. J Neurotrauma. 2009a;26(8):1251–62. https://doi.org/10.1089/neu.2008.0605.

Olivecrona M, Rodling-Wahlstrom M, Naredi S, Koskinen LO. S-100B and neuron specific enolase are poor outcome predictors in severe traumatic brain injury treated by an intracranial pressure targeted therapy. J Neurol Neurosurg Psychiatry. 2009b;80(11):1241–7. https://doi.org/10.1136/jnnp.2008.158196.

Ostermann RC, Joestl J, Tiefenboeck TM, Lang N, Platzer P, Hofbauer M. Risk factors predicting prognosis and outcome of elderly patients with isolated traumatic brain injury. J Orthop Surg Res. 2018;13(1):277. https://doi.org/10.1186/s13018-018-0975-y.

Patel HC, Bouamra O, Woodford M, Yates DW, Lecky FE. Clinical article: mortality associated with severe head injury in the elderly. Acta Neurochir. 2010;152(8):1353–7. https://doi.org/10.1007/s00701-010-0666-x; discussion 7.

Perrin PB, Krch D, Sutter M, Snipes DJ, Arango-Lasprilla JC, Kolakowsky-Hayner SA, et al. Racial/ethnic disparities in mental health over the first 2 years after traumatic brain injury: a model systems study. Arch Phys Med Rehabil. 2014;95(12):2288–95. https://doi.org/10.1016/j.apmr.2014.07.409.

Rainey T, Lesko M, Sacho R, Lecky F, Childs C. Predicting outcome after severe traumatic brain injury using the serum S100B biomarker: results using a single (24h) time-point. Resuscitation. 2009;80(3):341–5. https://doi.org/10.1016/j.resuscitation.2008.11.021.

Raj R, Siironen J, Skrifvars MB, Hernesniemi J, Kivisaari R. Predicting outcome in traumatic brain injury: development of a novel computerized tomography classification system (Helsinki computerized tomography score). Neurosurgery. 2014;75(6):632–46. https://doi.org/10.1227/NEU.0000000000000533; discussion 46–7.

Rating the Severity of Tissue Damage: I. The Abbreviated Scale. JAMA. 1971;215(2):277–280. https://doi.org/10.1001/jama.1971.03180150059012.

Rothoerl RD, Woertgen C, Brawanski A. S-100 serum levels and outcome after severe head injury. Acta Neurochir Suppl. 2000;76:97–100.

Sarrafzadeh AS, Peltonen EE, Kaisers U, Kuchler I, Lanksch WR, Unterberg AW. Secondary insults in severe head injury—do multiply injured patients do worse? Crit Care Med. 2001;29(6):1116–23.

Servadei F, Murray GD, Penny K, Teasdale GM, Dearden M, Iannotti F, et al. The value of the "worst" computed tomographic scan in clinical studies of moderate and severe head injury. European Brain Injury Consortium. Neurosurgery. 2000;46(1):70–5; discussion 5–7.

Shafi S, Marquez de la Plata C, Diaz-Arrastia R, Shipman K, Carlile M, Frankel H, et al. Racial disparities in long-term functional outcome after traumatic brain injury. J Trauma. 2007;63(6):1263–8. https://doi.org/10.1097/TA.0b013e31815b8f00; discussion 8–70.

Skandsen T, Kvistad KA, Solheim O, Lydersen S, Strand IH, Vik A. Prognostic value of magnetic resonance imaging in moderate and severe head injury: a prospective study of early MRI findings and one-year outcome. J Neurotrauma. 2011;28(5):691–9. https://doi.org/10.1089/neu.2010.1590.

Sorani MD, Lee M, Kim H, Meeker M, Manley GT. Race\ethnicity and outcome after traumatic brain injury at a single, diverse center. J Trauma. 2009;67(1):75–80. https://doi.org/10.1097/TA.0b013e31818234e8.

Sorrentino E, Diedler J, Kasprowicz M, Budohoski KP, Haubrich C, Smielewski P, et al. Critical thresholds for cerebrovascular reactivity after traumatic brain injury. Neurocrit Care. 2012;16(2):258–66. https://doi.org/10.1007/s12028-011-9630-8.

Stocchetti N, Pagan F, Calappi E, Canavesi K, Beretta L, Citerio G, et al. Inaccurate early assessment of neurological severity in head injury. J Neurotrauma. 2004;21(9):1131–40. https://doi.org/10.1089/neu.2004.21.1131.

Teasdale GM, Nicoll JA, Murray G, Fiddes M. Association of apolipoprotein E polymorphism with outcome after head injury. Lancet. 1997;350(9084):1069–71. https://doi.org/10.1016/S0140-6736(97)04318-3.

Teasdale GM, Murray GD, Nicoll JA. The association between APOE epsilon4, age and outcome after head injury: a prospective cohort study. Brain. 2005;128(Pt 11):2556–61. https://doi.org/10.1093/brain/awh595.

The Brain Trauma Foundation. The American Association of Neurological Surgeons. The Joint Section on Neurotrauma and Critical Care. Computed tomography scan features. J Neurotrauma. 2000;17(6–7):597–627. https://doi.org/10.1089/neu.2000.17.597.

Van Beek JG, Mushkudiani NA, Steyerberg EW, Butcher I, McHugh GS, Lu J, et al. Prognostic value of admission laboratory parameters in traumatic brain injury: results from the IMPACT study. J Neurotrauma. 2007;24(2):315–28. https://doi.org/10.1089/neu.2006.0034.

van Leeuwen N, Lingsma HF, Perel P, Lecky F, Roozenbeek B, Lu J, et al. Prognostic value of major extracranial injury in traumatic brain injury: an individual patient data meta-analysis in 39,274 patients. Neurosurgery. 2012;70(4):811–8. https://doi.org/10.1227/NEU.0b013e318235d640; discussion 8.

Vik A, Nag T, Fredriksli OA, Skandsen T, Moen KG, Schirmer-Mikalsen K, et al. Relationship of "dose" of intracranial hypertension to outcome in severe traumatic brain injury. J Neurosurg. 2008;109(4):678–84. https://doi.org/10.3171/JNS/2008/109/10/0678.

Vos PE, Jacobs B, Andriessen TM, Lamers KJ, Borm GF, Beems T, et al. GFAP and S100B are biomarkers of traumatic brain injury: an observational cohort study. Neurology. 2010;75(20):1786–93. https://doi.org/10.1212/WNL.0b013e3181fd62d2.

Walia S, Sutcliffe AJ. The relationship between blood glucose, mean arterial pressure and outcome after severe head injury: an observational study. Injury. 2002;33(4):339–44.

Wan X, Zhao K, Wang S, Zhang H, Zeng L, Wang Y, et al. Is it reliable to predict the outcome of elderly patients with severe traumatic brain injury using the IMPACT prognostic calculator? World Neurosurg. 2017;103:584–90. https://doi.org/10.1016/j.wneu.2017.04.069.

Wilson JT, Pettigrew LE, Teasdale GM. Structured interviews for the Glasgow Outcome Scale and the extended Glasgow Outcome Scale: guidelines for their use. J Neurotrauma. 1998;15(8):573–85.

Zweifel C, Lavinio A, Steiner LA, Radolovich D, Smielewski P, Timofeev I, et al. Continuous monitoring of cerebrovascular pressure reactivity in patients with head injury. Neurosurg Focus. 2008;25(4):E2. https://doi.org/10.3171/FOC.2008.25.10.E2.

21 Potential Organ Donor: Organ Donor Management

Pia Löwhagen Hendén

Recommendations

Level I

There are mostly insufficient data to support Level I recommendations for this topic. Randomized controlled trials on active lung treatment, including lung protective ventilation, have shown increased number of eligible and transplanted lungs with unchanged recipient survival rates.

Level II

Active donor management according to "bundle" protocols is associated with more organs transplanted per donor. Hormone replacement therapy (HRT) and strict blood glucose control are both associated with more organs transplanted per donor.

Level III

Active donor management according to "bundle" protocols is associated with more organs transplanted per donor.

P. Löwhagen Hendén (✉)
Department of Anesthesiology and Intensive Care, Sahlgrenska University Hospital, Gothenburg, Sweden
e-mail: pia.lowhagen@vgregion.se

21.1 Introduction

The primary aim in the critical care of severe TBI is to provide full neurointensive care until treatment is regarded futile. If all objective signs indicate complete loss of brain function, procedures leading to the diagnosis of death are initiated. For the potential organ donor, the critical care is changed toward maintenance of organ function and investigation of donation will. Potential organ donor, according to the terminology recommended by the WHO 2010, is "a person whose clinical condition is suspected to fulfill brain death criteria" (Dominguez-Gil et al. 2011).

Diagnosis of death is regulated in national legal documents and is subjected to modifications. The basis of diagnosis of death is, in most western countries, the irreversible cessation of all functions of the entire brain, including the brainstem (Citerio and Murphy 2015). We emphasize that organ donation from diseased persons is regulated by each country's legislation.

Death due to brain-related criteria leads to circulatory, pulmonary, renal, hepatic, and metabolic consequences that need attention in order to maintain sufficient organ function. The treatment strategies should aim at normalization of organ physiology as far as possible (Maciel and Greer 2016; Kotloff et al. 2015; McKeown and Ball 2014).

© Springer Nature Switzerland AG 2020
T. Sundstrøm et al. (eds.), *Management of Severe Traumatic Brain Injury*, https://doi.org/10.1007/978-3-030-39383-0_21

21.2 Organ Donor Management Goals

Rigorous organ donor management is a major determinant of outcome after organ transplantation. The use of an organ donor management protocol with physiological goals is mandatory. Several studies have shown that achieving organ donor physiological goals before the organ donation surgery results in a higher number of available organs per donor and better organ outcomes (Patel et al. 2014, 2017; Abuanzeh et al. 2015; Marshall et al. 2014). Common organ donor physiological goals are presented in Table 21.1. However, management strategies for the treatment of the organ donor and preservation of organ function are based on sparse scientific evidence.

21.3 Pathophysiology of Brainstem Herniation and Death

With increasing intracranial pressure, the brainstem herniation into foramen magnum leads to pathophysiological changes explained by the rostral to caudal brainstem ischemia evolution. The faster the herniation process, the more aggravating pathophysiological signs are seen. Initial parasympathetic stimulation with profound bradycardia is followed by a sympathetic storm with hypertension and tachycardia. Finally, loss of sympathetic tone causes peripheral vasodilation and hypotension.

Both the hypertension and the hypotension have the potential to result in end-organ damage during and after the brainstem herniation process.

Table 21.1 Organ donor management goals

Parameter	Goal	Commentary
Systolic blood pressure Mean arterial pressure	>100 mmHg >60 mmHg	Maintain normovolemia with sufficient fluids and use vasopressor support
Cardiac output	>2.5 L/min/m^2	Maintain normovolemia with sufficient fluids and use vasopressor support Inotropic drugs as needed
Lactate	<2 mmol/L	Maintain normovolemia with sufficient fluids and use vasopressor support
Urinary output	>1 mL/kg/h	Maintain normovolemia with sufficient fluids and use vasopressor support
Hemoglobin	>70 g/L	Transfusion of red blood cells
PaO_2	>10 kPa	Use lung protective ventilation, avoid atelectasis and aspiration
$PaCO_2$	4.5–6.0 kPa	Normoventilation
Central venous pressure (CVP)	<10 mmHg	Maintain normovolemia. Too high PEEP will impede venous return
Body temperature	>35 °C	Warming blankets, warm fluids
Blood glucose	<5–10 mmol/L	Short-acting insulin
Sodium	<155 mmol/L	Desmopressin, restricted use of sodium-containing fluids
Potassium-magnesium-calcium	Normal	Electrolyte supplement
pH	7.35–7.45	Maintaining normovolemia, normoventilation, sodium bicarbonate
Platelet count	>50 × 10^9/L	Transfusion of platelets if hemorrhage
PT/INR[a]	>1.5	Transfusion of fresh frozen plasma if hemorrhage

[a]Prothrombin time/International Normalised Ratio

Cessation of the cerebral blood flow leads to hypothalamic and hypophysis insufficiency, resulting in lost thermoregulation, hypothermia, and lack of hypophysis hormones. The sympathetic storm triggers the inflammatory system as well as the coagulation system and leads to peripheral insulin resistance.

Not all patients experience all the described effects. Diabetes insipidus, for example, as a sign of posterior hypophysis insufficiency, is described in 65–90% of brain-dead persons (McKeown and Ball 2014; Essien et al. 2017; Smith 2004).

Tips, Tricks, and Pitfalls

Be prepared for the pathophysiological changes after brainstem herniation with the following:

- Vasopressor infusion
- Desmopressin
- Warming blankets

By these measures, the most common problems, i.e., profound hypotension, hypovolemia, hypernatremia, and hypothermia, can be avoided.

21.4 Circulatory Considerations

Hypertension during brainstem herniation is most often self-limiting. The sympathetic storm results in increased preload and afterload for the heart with an obvious risk of cardiac ischemia, arrhythmia, and pulmonary edema. Treatment with short-acting agents (i.e., esmolol, labetalol, metoprolol) might be necessary to protect the heart.

Bradycardia in this setting cannot be treated with atropine as the vagus nerve is not active. If bradycardia has to be treated, beta-receptor-stimulating drugs can be used (isoprenaline).

Subsequent hypotension, due to loss of vasomotor tone, is the major problem in the care of an organ donor. Hypotension caused by vasodilation can be aggravated by hypovolemia due to diabetes insipidus or pre-existing hypovolemia before herniation, caused by hemorrhage and cerebral edema treatment (i.e., mannitol and negative fluid balance).

To achieve the organ donor goals, blood pressure should be kept at an acceptable level using sufficient fluids, with balanced salt content to avoid hypernatremia, and in addition, most donors need vasopressor support. Fluid resuscitation should exclude hydroxyethyl starch solutions due to the possibility of negative effects on kidney function (Patel et al. 2015). No scientific evidence exists regarding the use of crystalloids versus albumin or plasma.

The preferable first-line vasopressor is, in most guidelines, arginine vasopressin (antidiuretic hormone). Another commonly used vasopressor is norepinephrine. Arginine vasopressin might be in favor of norepinephrine for hemodynamically instable patients and patients with cardiac failure, due to the lack of adrenergic receptor stimulation (Kotloff et al. 2015). The vasopressin analogue desmopressin has no significant vasopressor activity.

In case of increasing vasopressor support, hemodynamic monitoring (PICCO, PA catheter, repeated echocardiography) should be instituted to differ between vasoplegia, hypovolemia, and cardiac failure and to tailor the treatment and avoid coronary, renal, and splanchnic vasoconstriction.

Dopamine, milrinone, dobutamine, or epinephrine may be used in primary cardiac pump dysfunction. Hypothermal myocardial depression must be avoided. Repeated echocardiography examinations should be performed in assessment for heart donation, as myocardial hypokinesia occurring during brainstem herniation might be reversible.

Recommended doses for vasoactive drugs are as follows:

- Norepinephrine <0.2 mcg/kg/min
- Arginine vasopressin 0.5–4 U/h
- Dopamine <10 mcg/kg/min
- Dobutamine <10 mcg/kg/min

If recommended doses are exceeded, a combination of vasoactive drugs should be considered.

Bolus dose of methylprednisolone is included in most protocols for its effect on hemodynamic stabilization, although the scientific evidence is weak (D'Aragon et al. 2017; Dupuis et al. 2014). The recommendation is methylprednisolone 15 mg/kg IV as a bolus in conjunction with the brain death declaration.

In several protocols, a combined hormone replacement therapy (HRT) is recommended if hemodynamic goals are not met despite vasopressor treatment and/or if left ventricular ejection fraction remains less than 45% (Kotloff et al. 2015). HRT includes arginine vasopressin, thyroid hormone (T3 or T4), methylprednisolone, and insulin. HRT is in retrospective studies associated with improved number of organs transplanted per donor and improved graft function (Buchanan and Mehta 2018; Novitzky et al. 2014). Recommended doses for thyroid hormones are as follows: T3 bolus dose 4 mcg followed by infusion 3 mcg/h or T4 bolus dose 20 mcg followed by infusion 10–40 mcg/h (Buchanan and Mehta 2018). T4 is converted to T3 in target tissues.

Aggressive hemodynamic support prevents cardiovascular collapse before a planned organ donation operation. Without vigorous treatment, 25–40% of the organ donors will have a circulatory arrest within the first few days (McKeown and Ball 2014).

21.5 Central Diabetes Insipidus

Diabetes insipidus, caused by decreased secretion of antidiuretic hormone (ADH), leads to polyuria, and if left uncorrected, it will quickly lead to severe hypovolemia and hypernatremia. Clinically manifest diabetes insipidus (urinary output >300 mL/h, serum sodium >150 mmol/L, urinary sodium <20 mmol/L, urinary specific gravity ≤1.005) can threaten organ donation due to the profound hypovolemia.

Treatment is by bolus dose of the vasopressin analogue desmopressin (1-deamino-8-D-arginine vasopressin, DDAVP) or by infusion of arginine vasopressin (8-arginine vasopressin, AVP). Arginine vasopressin is an exact synthetic protein of antidiuretic hormone (ADH).

Recommended doses are as follows: for desmopressin titrated bolus doses of 0.25–1 mcg IV and for arginine vasopressin infusion 0.6–2.4 U/h (Kotloff et al. 2015). It is important to remember that the terminal half-life of desmopressin is around 3 h in patients without renal impairment. Administration of desmopressin and arginine vasopressin does not negatively affect the kidney graft.

Drug administration is most often combined with administration of intravenous fluids and/or pure water administration via the nasogastric tube. The urinary losses of magnesium, phosphate, and potassium must be replaced if profound polyuria persists.

21.6 Pulmonary Considerations

The lungs have the highest risk of being unsuitable for transplantation, and historically a low rate of suitable lungs has been identified among organ donors. Intensified lung donor management in the intensive care unit (ICU) increases the number of lungs recovered and transplanted (Minambres et al. 2014, 2013; Kirschbaum and Hudson 2010; Venkateswaran et al. 2008; Angel et al. 2006).

During the brainstem herniation, the sympathetic storm can result in both a neurogenic and a cardiogenic lung edema. The use of colloids together with meticulous fluid balance has shown to be beneficial in minimizing the development of pulmonary edema (Dictus et al. 2009).

The lungs are also most susceptible to the systemic inflammatory response caused by the sympathetic storm, and they might furthermore be harmed following blunt trauma and/or aspiration. There is also a risk of ventilator-associated pneumonia in the ICU. Every effort should be made to prevent further exacerbation of pre-existing lung injury. Antibiotics should be liberally administered after a bronchoscopy has been performed (to obtain material for bacterial examination and culture).

Most donor management protocols include administration of corticosteroids (methylprednisolone 15 mg/kg) moderating the release of pro-inflammatory molecules and, in animal models, improving alveolar fluid clearance (Folkesson et al. 2000). Clinically, improved donor oxygenation, lung utilization, and graft outcomes are described (Naik and Angel 2011; Follette et al. 1998).

The lung donor management protocols include:

- Methylprednisolone
- Lung protective ventilation
  - Low tidal volumes (6–8 mL/kg predicted body weight)
  - Normoventilation ($PaCO_2$ 4.5–6.0 kPa)
  - Plateau inspiratory pressure <30 cm H_2O
  - PEEP of (5–)10 cm H_2O

  In one RCT, lung protective ventilation resulted in 54% of the lungs being utilized for transplantation compared to 27% in the control group (Mascia et al. 2010).
- Neutral fluid balance
- Avoiding atelectasis by
  - Adequate, individualized PEEP titration
  - Regularly turning the patient
  - Humidification of inspired air/oxygen
  - Appropriate bronchoscopies if necessary to avoid mucous plugs
  - Careful recruitment maneuvers with subsequent adequate PEEP setting
- Avoiding gastric aspiration by
  - Elevation of the head of the bed
  - Oral care
  - Assessing for a cuff leak

21.7 Renal and Hepatic Considerations

The kidneys and liver are affected both by the sympathetic storm and by the following hypotensive situation. Hemodynamic optimization is of uttermost importance for possible donation. The urinary output should be kept >1 mL/kg/h. This is primarily achieved by adequate fluid administration and vasopressor support. Expert opinions differ regarding which vasopressor agent should be first line in a kidney donor; both norepinephrine and vasopressin are used. As earlier mentioned, fluid resuscitation should exclude hydroxyethyl starch solutions due to the possibility of negative effects on kidney function (Patel et al. 2015). In a multicenter RCT, low-dose dopamine (4 mcg/kg/min) reduced the need for dialysis after kidney transplantation with no effect on graft survival (Schnuelle et al. 2017, 2018).

21.8 Metabolic Considerations

Hypophysis insufficiency includes hormones from both posterior and anterior hypophysis as vasopressin, oxytocin, ACTH, GH, LH, FSH, and TSH. Administration of the vasopressin analogue desmopressin, in order to treat diabetes insipidus, is considered standard procedure in organ donor management (Maciel and Greer 2016; Kotloff et al. 2015; McKeown and Ball 2014), and replacement with corticosteroids is included in most organ donor management protocols although the scientific evidence is scarce (D'Aragon et al. 2017; Dupuis et al. 2014).

Thyroid hormone replacement might be of benefit in therapy-resistant hemodynamic instability (Buchanan and Mehta 2018; Novitzky et al. 2014).

Hypothalamic insufficiency leads to dysregulation of body temperature, most often resulting in hypothermia. Hypothermia can cause numerous complications such as decreased cardiac contractility, cardiac arrhythmia, and coagulation disorders and must be prevented by warm blankets, external warming devices, and warm fluids. The body temperature should be kept >35 °C.

Hyperglycemia is considered to be a consequence of elevated levels of catecholamines, infusion of glucose, administration of corticosteroids, and peripheral insulin resistance. Blood glucose ≤180 mg/dL (10 mmol/L) was an independent predictor of number of organs transplanted per donor and better graft outcome in a retrospective study (Sally et al. 2014). Normoglycemia should be maintained and insulin infusion is most often needed.

Lingering respiratory alkalosis as a result of hyperventilation for treatment of imminent brainstem herniation should be corrected and results in normalization of arterial pH in order to promote tissue oxygen delivery. Hyperlactatemia and metabolic acidosis as a result of hypoperfusion must be avoided.

Coagulopathies, e.g., disseminated intravascular coagulation (DIC), as well as dilution coagulopathy and hypothermia are not uncommon after brain death. Appropriate blood components are transfused if clinically significant hemorrhage occurs.

21.9 Specific Pediatric Concerns

Scientific data concerning donor management strategies are limited in adults and even more limited when it comes to children (Mallory et al. 2009; Finfer et al. 1996). Pediatric organ donors are rare in most hospitals. The diagnosis of death due to brain-related criteria is the same in pediatric patients as in adults, although the confirmation of death in infants may require specially trained staff. Consultation of specific expertise for advice and support should be liberally used, both for diagnosis of death and for management of the organ donor. The level of physiological and laboratory parameters must be adjusted for age, especially levels for blood pressure. A cuffed endotracheal tube is recommended even in young children due to the risk of aspiration (Mallory et al. 2009).

References

Abuanzeh R, Hashmi F, Dimarakis I, Khasati N, Machaal A, Yonan N, et al. Early donor management increases the retrieval rate of hearts for transplantation in marginal donors. Eur J Cardiothorac Surg. 2015;47(1):72–7; discussion 7.

Angel LF, Levine DJ, Restrepo MI, Johnson S, Sako E, Carpenter A, et al. Impact of a lung transplantation donor-management protocol on lung donation and recipient outcomes. Am J Respir Crit Care Med. 2006;174(6):710–6.

Buchanan IA, Mehta VA. Thyroid hormone resuscitation after brain death in potential organ donors: a primer for neurocritical care providers and narrative review of the literature. Clin Neurol Neurosurg. 2018;165:96–102.

Citerio G, Murphy PG. Brain death: the European perspective. Semin Neurol. 2015;35(2):139–44.

D'Aragon F, Belley-Cote E, Agarwal A, Frenette AJ, Lamontagne F, Guyatt G, et al. Effect of corticosteroid administration on neurologically deceased organ donors and transplant recipients: a systematic review and meta-analysis. BMJ Open. 2017;7(6):e014436.

Dictus C, Vienenkoetter B, Esmaeilzadeh M, Unterberg A, Ahmadi R. Critical care management of potential organ donors: our current standard. Clin Transplant. 2009;23(Suppl 21):2–9.

Dominguez-Gil B, Delmonico FL, Shaheen FA, Matesanz R, O'Connor K, Minina M, et al. The critical pathway for deceased donation: reportable uniformity in the approach to deceased donation. Transpl Int. 2011;24(4):373–8.

Dupuis S, Amiel JA, Desgroseilliers M, Williamson DR, Thiboutot Z, Serri K, et al. Corticosteroids in the management of brain-dead potential organ donors: a systematic review. Br J Anaesth. 2014;113(3):346–59.

Essien EO, Fioretti K, Scalea TM, Stein DM. Physiologic features of brain death. Am Surg. 2017;83(8):850–4.

Finfer S, Bohn D, Colpitts D, Cox P, Fleming F, Barker G. Intensive care management of paediatric organ donors and its effect on post-transplant organ function. Intensive Care Med. 1996;22(12):1424–32.

Folkesson HG, Norlin A, Wang Y, Abedinpour P, Matthay MA. Dexamethasone and thyroid hormone pretreatment upregulate alveolar epithelial fluid clearance in adult rats. J Appl Physiol (Bethesda, Md: 1985). 2000;88(2):416–24.

Follette DM, Rudich SM, Babcock WD. Improved oxygenation and increased lung donor recovery with high-dose steroid administration after brain death. J Heart Lung Transplant. 1998;17(4):423–9.

Kirschbaum CE, Hudson S. Increasing organ yield through a lung management protocol. Prog Transplant (Aliso Viejo, Calif). 2010;20(1):28–32.

Kotloff RM, Blosser S, Fulda GJ, Malinoski D, Ahya VN, Angel L, et al. Management of the potential organ donor in the ICU: Society of Critical Care Medicine/American College of Chest Physicians/Association of Organ Procurement Organizations Consensus Statement. Crit Care Med. 2015;43(6):1291–325.

Maciel CB, Greer DM. ICU management of the potential organ donor: state of the art. Curr Neurol Neurosci Rep. 2016;16(9):86.

Mallory GB Jr, Schecter MG, Elidemir O. Management of the pediatric organ donor to optimize lung donation. Pediatr Pulmonol. 2009;44(6):536–46.

Marshall GR, Mangus RS, Powelson JA, Fridell JA, Kubal CA, Tector AJ. Donor management parameters and organ yield: single center results. J Surg Res. 2014;191(1):208–13.

Mascia L, Pasero D, Slutsky AS, Arguis MJ, Berardino M, Grasso S, et al. Effect of a lung protective strategy for organ donors on eligibility and availability of lungs for transplantation: a randomized controlled trial. JAMA. 2010;304(23):2620–7.

McKeown DW, Ball J. Treating the donor. Curr Opin Organ Transplant. 2014;19(2):85–91.

Minambres E, Ballesteros MA, Rodrigo E, Garcia-Miguelez A, Llorca J, Ruiz JC, et al. Aggressive lung donor management increases graft procurement without increasing renal graft loss after transplantation. Clin Transplant. 2013;27(1):52–9.

Minambres E, Coll E, Duerto J, Suberviola B, Mons R, Cifrian JM, et al. Effect of an intensive lung donor-management protocol on lung transplantation outcomes. J Heart Lung Transplant. 2014;33(2):178–84.

Naik PM, Angel LF. Special issues in the management and selection of the donor for lung transplantation. Semin Immunopathol. 2011;33(2):201–10.

Novitzky D, Mi Z, Sun Q, Collins JF, Cooper DK. Thyroid hormone therapy in the management of 63,593 brain-dead organ donors: a retrospective analysis. Transplantation. 2014;98(10):1119–27.

Patel MS, Zatarain J, De La Cruz S, Sally MB, Ewing T, Crutchfield M, et al. The impact of meeting donor management goals on the number of organs transplanted per expanded criteria donor: a prospective study from the UNOS Region 5 Donor Management Goals Workgroup. JAMA Surg. 2014;149(9):969–75.

Patel MS, Niemann CU, Sally MB, De La Cruz S, Zatarain J, Ewing T, et al. The impact of hydroxyethyl starch use in deceased organ donors on the development of delayed graft function in kidney transplant recipients: a propensity-adjusted analysis. Am J Transplant. 2015;15(8):2152–8.

Patel MS, De La Cruz S, Sally MB, Groat T, Malinoski DJ. active donor management during the hospital phase of care is associated with more organs transplanted per donor. J Am Coll Surg. 2017;225(4):525–31.

Sally MB, Ewing T, Crutchfield M, Patel MS, Raza S, De La Cruz S, et al. Determining optimal threshold for glucose control in organ donors after neurologic determination of death: a United Network for Organ Sharing Region 5 Donor Management Goals Workgroup prospective analysis. J Trauma Acute Care Surg. 2014;76(1):62–8; discussion 8–9.

Schnuelle P, Schmitt WH, Weiss C, Habicht A, Renders L, Zeier M, et al. Effects of dopamine donor pretreatment on graft survival after kidney transplantation: a randomized trial. Clin J Am Soc Nephrol. 2017;12(3):493–501.

Schnuelle P, Benck U, Yard BA. Dopamine in transplantation: written off or comeback with novel indication? Clin Transplant. 2018;32(7):e13292.

Smith M. Physiologic changes during brain stem death—lessons for management of the organ donor. J Heart Lung Transplant. 2004;23(Suppl 9):S217–22.

Venkateswaran RV, Patchell VB, Wilson IC, Mascaro JG, Thompson RD, Quinn DW, et al. Early donor management increases the retrieval rate of lungs for transplantation. Ann Thorac Surg. 2008;85(1):278–86; discussion 86.

22 Ethical Aspects and Communication

Christina Rosenlund

Recommendations

Level I

Data are insufficient to support Level I recommendations for this subject.

Level II

Data are insufficient to support Level II recommendations for this subject.

Level III

Effective communication is an essential nontechnical skill for all intensive care clinicians.

Training, practice, preparation, and reflective review may improve performance when conducting family meetings and lead to better outcomes for patients and families.

Decision-making regarding organ donation depends heavily on the family's trust in the healthcare professionals, on the professional's communicative skills, and on the family's understanding of (brain) death.

C. Rosenlund (✉)
Department of Neurosurgery, Odense University Hospital, Odense, Denmark
e-mail: christina.rosenlund2@rsyd.dk

Tips, Tricks, and Pitfalls

- The decision to limit or withdraw treatment is clinically based and is always the medical doctor's responsibility, never the relatives.
- When treatment is withdrawn, the healthcare professionals should avoid making decisions on behalf of the relatives. The patient's last hours or days belong to the family and they should be informed and, if they want to, also involved in interventions.
- Organ donation is an option and not a burden. Present the relatives with the possibility for organ donation when this is an option.
- Be honest about what you know and what you don't know.
- Be true.

22.1 Overview

The aim of this chapter is to overview considerations regarding communication with relatives and surrogate decision-makers in the ICU setting. A recommendation is to undergo regular training of nontechnical skills.

Patients with severe TBI need, by definition, both acute and intensive care. The situation is

© Springer Nature Switzerland AG 2020
T. Sundstrøm et al. (eds.), *Management of Severe Traumatic Brain Injury*,
https://doi.org/10.1007/978-3-030-39383-0_22

often more or less chaotic, and we, as healthcare providers, are busy saving the patient's life and minimizing the evolvement of secondary injuries. Finding time to inform the relatives is important, but challenging in the acute phase. Prioritizing the patient is number 1 at all times, something that the relatives expect. Nevertheless, they have some basic needs we should consider:

- What has happened?
- Is he/she going to survive?
- Are you doing everything you can?
- Can we see him/her?
- Can I trust you?

Communicating is a multidisciplinary task. Informal communication is as important as formal. The nurse talking with the relatives while nursing the patient is the typical example of an informal situation. It is, however, important to initiate and maintain the formal communication in a formal setting. Preparation is crucial:

- Be sure to have a thorough overview of the patient's history.
- Know what has been done and what is going to be done.
- Know what the nurse knows about the relatives, the way they are related to each other, what they may have expressed concerns about, etc.
- Prepare for the dialogue in the multidisciplinary team (anesthetist/intensivist, neurosurgeon/neurologist, patient-responsible ICU nurse): Who does what/who leads the dialogue? Where are we? What is the short-term plan?

Good/effective communication, especially in the acute phase and in the situation where treatment is withdrawn, depends primarily on:

- Trust.
- Sensitivity overrules effectivity.
- The patient is a *person* (son/daughter/brother etc.), not a complex traumatic brain injury case.
- Thorough information, understandable/simple and in small portions.
- Physical surroundings, tidy room, closed door (not standing around the ICU bed or in the hallway).
- Honesty - not creating false hope, tell what you know and be honest about what you do not know.
- Competence. Everything is done to save the patient's life.
- Leaving room for the relatives to react and speak their minds.
- Time to consume the information and a possibility to have a talk again.
- Keeping your personal opinion apart from the ethics. What is right for you is not necessarily right for this patient and this family. Decisions involving beliefs, feelings, rituals, etc. are for the relatives to make.
- The medical doctor decides to end the treatment. The relatives are to be informed and heard. They are not the ones responsible for ending their relative's life.
- Be present. Turn off your phone or let somebody else outside the room hold it and take notes for you.

It is important to document a summary of the dialogue in the patient journal. It helps your colleagues to take over, and it is crucial for the relatives' impression of coherence that the next dialogue is a continuation of the former. Official documentation of specific treatment limitations should be made, including that relatives have been informed of these decisions.

Consider to offer counseling to the relatives. The chaplain or psychologist has the advantage of not being part of the team treating their relative and can help them to deal with their thoughts and concerns. This is not only helpful in cases, where the patient is going to die, but also in other situations where a patient is critically ill, the family structure is complex, children are involved, etc.

22.2 Background

Understanding the relatives' needs and what they understand are not something that is in every medical doctor's genes. Effective communication is an essential nontechnical skill for all intensive care clinicians, and there is a still growing acknowledgement for the importance of this (Quinn et al. 2017). Interviewing the experts, i.e., the relatives, has revealed that they go to the clinician primarily for the truth and to seek hope elsewhere (Quinn et al. 2017; Apatira et al. 2008). When treating TBI patients, it is seldom possible to say anything definite about the future—even in the short term. The uncertainty is the most difficult thing to cope with for the relatives. The only way to help them is to give them insight in our plans for the nearest future and our reasons for choosing this path in this specific case. Especially important is it for parents to an injured child to have insight and a role in care (Roscigno et al. 2013). Avoiding discussions about prognosis is an unacceptable way to maintain hope, and being able to prepare emotionally and logistically for the possibility of a patient's death is essential. To understand that the patient is treated with the highest level of care, both as a trauma patient and as a person, has important consequences for the relatives' ability to cope with the situation here and now, as well as in the future (Jensen 2011; Apatira et al. 2008; Warrillow et al. 2016).

Relatives to a potential organ donor have the same needs as anybody else, but a few important details demand special consideration. Jensen (2011) refers to a series of relatives to organ donors after brain death. They all expressed that it is crucial to understand that the patient is actually dead, even though there is visible breathing movements, heartbeat, warm skin, and not seldom involuntary reflexes. Even if the doctor has explained brain death in understandable terms, the relatives first realize the truth when they see the clinical examination for brain death. It is helpful to give the information about brain death and information about organ donation in two separate occasions, as it is important to understand that the patient is going to die before the relatives can consider what to do when death has occurred. Some relatives will, however, mention the possibility themselves during the first dialogue. In the same study, the relatives mentioned that it was important for them to see the organ donation as a gift and that the healthcare professionals remembered to treat the patient with respect as a dying person and not simply as an organ donor (Jensen 2011).

References

Apatira L, Boyd EM, Evans L, Luce JL, White D. Hope, truth, and preparing for death: perspectives of surrogate decision makers. Ann Intern Med. 2008;149(12):861–8.

Jensen AB. Orchestrating an exceptional death: donor family experiences and organ donation in Denmark. Ph.D. Series no. 69. Department of Anthropology, University of Copenhagen (abstract vedlagt som bilag 2); 2011.

Quinn T, Moskowitz J, Khan MW, Shutter L, Goldberg R, Col N, et al. What families need and physicians deliver: contrasting communication preferences between surrogate decision-makers and physicians during outcome prognostication in critically ill TBI patients. Neurocrit Care. 2017;27(2):154–62.

Roscigno CI, Savage TA, Grant G, Philipsen G. How healthcare provider talk with parents of children following severe traumatic brain injury is perceived in early acute care. Soc Sci Med. 2013;90:32–9.

Warrillow S, Farley K, Jones D. How to improve communication quality with patients and relatives in the ICU. Minerva Anestesiol. 2016;82(7):797–803.

Part V

Acute Surgical Treatment

Terje Sundstrøm

23 Basic Trauma Craniotomy

Terje Sundstrøm, Eirik Helseth, and Knut Gustav Wester

Recommendations

Level I

There are insufficient data to support a Level I recommendation for this topic.

Level II

There are insufficient data to support a Level II recommendation for this topic.

Level III

A basic trauma craniotomy is a large frontotemporoparietal craniotomy that provides access to the most common intracranial haematomas and bleeding sites.

Patients requiring surgery for brain trauma should be operated as soon as possible.

23.1 Overview

A basic trauma craniotomy is a large craniotomy (Bullock et al. 2006; Greenberg 2016; Quiñones-Hinojosa 2012; Winn 2017). This allows the surgeon to remove the most common types of acute intracranial haematomas, such as epidural, subdural and intracerebral haematomas and cerebral contusions. It also provides access to the most usual sources of bleeding. These include large draining veins near the superior sagittal sinus as well as contused tissue in the subtemporal and subfrontal areas and the temporal and frontal poles.

The fundamentals of surgical treatment have not changed much the last decades (Valadka and Robertson 2007). Basic trauma craniotomies should be large, and mass lesions should be evacuated without undue delay. Early surgical intervention is preferable to awaiting clinical deterioration, because the degree of ischemic brain damage is dependent on the duration of ischemia.

A basic trauma craniotomy, as described here, will easily facilitate primary or secondary decompressive craniectomy. However, the neurosurgeon

T. Sundstrøm (✉)
Department of Neurosurgery, Haukeland University Hospital, Bergen, Norway

Department of Clinical Medicine, University of Bergen, Bergen, Norway
e-mail: tjsu@helse-bergen.no

E. Helseth
Institute of Clinical Medicine, University of Oslo, Oslo, Norway

Department of Neurosurgery, Oslo University Hospital, Oslo, Norway
e-mail: EHELSETH@ous-hf.no

K. G. Wester
Department of Clinical Medicine, University of Bergen, Bergen, Norway
e-mail: Knut.Wester@uib.no

© Springer Nature Switzerland AG 2020
T. Sundstrøm et al. (eds.), *Management of Severe Traumatic Brain Injury*,
https://doi.org/10.1007/978-3-030-39383-0_23

must in each case consider what is best for the patient and tailor the surgical approach to the identified pathology.

Tips, Tricks and Pitfalls
- Always look at the patient.
- Do not hesitate if there is indication for surgery.
- The best treatment for patients with very severe injuries can be to withhold surgery.
- Remember that cervical instability must be ruled out before positioning.
- Always remember: skin flap > bone flap.
- Make sure that scalp injuries do not interfere with the blood supply of your planned skin flap.
- If you believe that you have to remove the bone flap, make sure it is large enough to yield sufficient decompression.

23.2 How to Perform a Basic Trauma Craniotomy

Up to 25% of hospital-admitted TBI patients with reduced consciousness can have a concomitant cervical injury. It is therefore important to rule out cervical instability before positioning. The head of the patient is placed on a doughnut or similar headrest (Mayfield head holder can also be used, but be aware of cranial fractures), turned almost 90° to the opposite side and slightly elevated above the level of the heart. The craniotomy opening should be in the horizontal plane. A sandbag or pillow under the ipsilateral shoulder helps to prevent positional obstruction of cranial venous outflow. Such obstruction can be visualised by venous stasis on the neck. The patient should be placed in the lateral position if the cervical spine is not radiologically cleared. Unless deterioration is rapid, the scalp is shaved and prepared as for a standard operative procedure.

Scalp injuries and potential interference with circulation of the skin should always be considered. The skin incision is started 1 cm in front of the tragus at the zygomatic arch, then curved posteriorly and superiorly above the helix of the ear to the midline in the parietal region, further along the midline to the frontal region and, if possible, ending at the hairline. Generally, the exposed cranial area must be sufficiently large to accommodate a craniotomy with 14–16 cm anteroposterior diameter (always remember: skin flap larger than bone flap).

Haemostasis of the skin margins is obtained with plastic clips or multiple curved forceps applied to the galea. The superficial temporal fascia and the temporalis muscle are incised down to the bone, close to the margin of the skin opening. The myocutaneous flap is reflected and secured.

Multiple burr holes (≥2; more holes in older patients) are placed in the parietal and frontal regions, preferably over suture lines. The burr holes are undermined, gently separating the dura and skull, and joined to form a large free bone flap. Special care is advised when operating near the superior sagittal sinus and in case of fractures crossing the sinus. The medial margin of the bone flap should be approximately 2 cm from the midline to avoid arachnoid granulations and large dural and cortical veins. The lateral sphenoid wing and temporal bone can be resected using Leksell rongeurs under direct visual control, thereby securing adequate exposure of the middle fossa. The temporal exposure should extend all the way to the skull base.

Intracranial injuries may evolve during the surgical procedure, and the neurosurgeon should not rely only on the preoperative imaging. Subdural inspection should therefore be considered after evacuation of an epidural haematoma even if only epidural haemorrhage was anticipated.

The dural opening is performed in a controlled manner to avoid massive external herniation, and care must be taken to avoid cortical lacerations. The opening begins over the area of maximal clot thickness or in the anterior temporal region, because relatively silent cortex will be affected here if the brain starts to herniate through the opening. The dura can be opened in a U-shaped manner going low over the frontal and temporal regions with the base towards the superior sagittal sinus, carefully avoiding damage to parasagittal bridging veins. This ensures safe access to the areas along the midline, as well as the middle and frontal fossa. There are also other ways to open the dura, for example, in a cruciate manner or by multiple individual slits. Subdural and intracerebral haematomas are evacuated, and careful haemostasis is obtained by bipolar electrocautery (caution is advised with respect to bridging veins) and haemostatic agents.

The dura is closed primarily when there is no present or anticipated significant brain swelling. The brain is otherwise simply covered with a dura substitute (artificial or periosteum) and sutureless adaptation of the dura. We do not recommend leaving the dura open with exposed brain if a craniectomy is indicated. If primary dural closure is performed, multiple dural tacking sutures are placed around the craniotomy margin, and one or two are placed centrally in the bone flap to prevent a postoperative epidural haematoma.

The bone flap is replaced and fixed, and the scalp is closed in two layers. Placement of a subgaleal drain can be considered. The wound is dressed, and a circular head bandage is placed.

Considerations on primary and secondary decompressive craniectomy are described in another section.

23.3 Specific Paediatric Concerns

A three-pin skull fixation device should not be used in infants as the cranium is thin and sutures are not closed. Bone flaps in infants and small children should preferably be fixed with resorbable material (sutures or plates/screws). Replacement of small bone flaps in infants can also be omitted, as new bone will fill the defect spontaneously.

A craniotomy for the evacuation of an epidural or subdural haematoma in small children entails a risk of significant blood loss. A continuous and meticulous haemostasis must therefore be exercised throughout the procedure. The anaesthesiologist in charge should keep the neurosurgeon continuously informed about the extent of blood loss and be prepared for blood transfusion.

References

Bullock MR, Chesnut R, Ghajar J, Gordon D, Hartl R, Newell DW, Servadei F, Walters BC, Wilberger JE, Surgical Management of Traumatic Brain Injury Author Group. Surgical management of traumatic brain injury. Neurosurgery. 2006;58:S2-1–S2-62.

Greenberg MS. Handbook of neurosurgery. 8th ed. New York: Thieme Medical Publishers, Inc.; 2016.

Quiñones-Hinojosa A. Schmidek & Sweet operative neurosurgical techniques: indications, methods, and results. 6th ed. Philadelphia: Saunders, an imprint of Elsevier; 2012.

Valadka AB, Robertson CS. Surgery of cerebral trauma and associated critical care. Neurosurgery. 2007;61:203–20.

Winn HR. Youmans & Winn neurological surgery. 7th ed. Philadelphia: Elsevier; 2017.

Surgical Management of Traumatic Intracranial Haematomas

24

Terje Sundstrøm, Eirik Helseth, and Knut Gustav Wester

Recommendations

Level I

There are insufficient data to support a Level I recommendation for this topic.

Level II

There are insufficient data to support a Level II recommendation for this topic.

Level III

Patients with intracranial haematomas and indications for surgery should be operated as soon as possible.

Patients with devastating brain injuries and/or high probability of a poor outcome should generally not be subjected to surgical treatment. In all other patients with intracranial haematomas, surgery should be considered.

Indications and methods for surgery based on the Brain Trauma Foundation (BTF) guidelines (Bullock et al. 2006) and the expert opinion of the Scandinavian Neurotrauma Committee (SNC):

- Epidural haematoma (EDH)
  - Volume >30 cm^3
  - GCS <9 and anisocoria.
  - Can observe if volume <30 cm^3, <15 mm thickness, <5 mm midline shift and GCS >8 without focal neurological deficits—but, consider surgery in all patients with a GCS <14 and/or symptoms attributable to the haematoma.
  - *Methods*: tailored craniotomy preferably providing complete exposure of the EDH and the bleeding source.
- Acute subdural haematoma (ASDH)
  - Thickness >10 mm or midline shift >5 mm, regardless of GCS score.

T. Sundstrøm (✉)
Department of Neurosurgery, Haukeland University Hospital, Bergen, Norway

Department of Clinical Medicine, University of Bergen, Bergen, Norway
e-mail: tjsu@helse-bergen.no

E. Helseth
Institute of Clinical Medicine, University of Oslo, Oslo, Norway

Department of Neurosurgery, Oslo University Hospital, Oslo, Norway
e-mail: EHELSETH@ous-hf.no

K. G. Wester
Department of Clinical Medicine, University of Bergen, Bergen, Norway
e-mail: Knut.Wester@uib.no

© Springer Nature Switzerland AG 2020
T. Sundstrøm et al. (eds.), *Management of Severe Traumatic Brain Injury*,
https://doi.org/10.1007/978-3-030-39383-0_24

  - Thickness <10 mm and midline shift <5 mm, if a GCS <9 drops ≥2 points, and/or anisocoria and/or ICP >20 mmHg, but consider surgery if GCS <14.
  - *Methods*: large craniotomy with adequate exposure of the frontal and temporal poles and the area along the superior sagittal sinus.
- Traumatic intracerebral haematoma (TICH) and cerebral contusions
  - Volume >50 cm^3
  - GCS 6–8 with frontal or temporal contusions >20 cm^3, midline shift ≥5 mm and/or cisternal compression
  - Neurological dysfunction or deterioration referable to the lesion or refractory high ICP
  - *Methods*: large craniotomy because these lesions are frequently associated with extracerebral haematomas
- Posterior fossa mass lesions
  - Mass effect on CT scan, neurological dysfunction or deterioration referable to the lesion (even a small volume can have profound effects)
  - *Methods*: midline suboccipital craniotomy with access to the midline and both hemispheres (consider placing an EVD, either as an initial or closing manoeuvre)

24.1 Overview

One of the most important complications of a traumatic brain injury (TBI) is the development of an intracranial haematoma. Secondary brain injury can result and reduce the likelihood of a good outcome. An effective trauma care system with high-quality neurosurgery is therefore essential, as intracranial haematomas occur in 25–45% of severe TBI patients, 3–12% of moderate TBI patients and approximately 1/500 patients with mild TBI (Bullock et al. 2006).

Rates of mortality and morbidity after an acute subdural haematoma (ASDH) are the highest of all traumatic mass lesions, with an overall mortality rate of 40–60% (Bullock et al. 2006). This poor outcome results largely from associated parenchymal lesions and subsequent intracranial hypertension. About 50% of ASDHs have associated lesions (Bullock et al. 2006).

Patients with epidural haematomas (EDH) generally have a favourable prognosis, and the overall mortality rate is about 10% (Bullock et al. 2006). It is not infrequent to observe excellent outcomes even in patients with ipsilateral mydriasis. However, less than one-third of patients present with a GCS score below 9, and in the subgroup of patients with a GCS score of 3–5, mortality rates can approach 40% (Bullock et al. 2006).

The key factors in deciding whether to proceed with surgery of an intracranial haematoma are the overall clinical condition of the patient, the neurological status (including neurological deterioration) and the CT findings. Patients with a potential surgical lesion on the initial CT scan should, as a general rule, have a follow-up CT scan within 6–8 h or sooner if clinically indicated.

There are different attitudes towards indications for surgery of posttraumatic intracranial haematomas and decompressive craniectomy both in Europe (Compagnone et al. 2005) and in the USA (Bulger et al. 2002). Some of the most difficult questions are whether moderate-sized haematomas or contusions should be evacuated or simply observed (Valadka and Robertson 2007). Several courses of action are possible, and the decisions are often based on the judgement and experience of the responsible physicians.

The evidence-based guidelines for the surgical management of brain injuries published by the Brain Trauma Foundation (BTF) in 2006 provide us with some directions (Bullock et al. 2006). All the recommendations are at the option level, supported by Class III scientific evidence. The guidelines are, however, logical and clinically useful, and the recommendations on surgical indications, timing of operative treatment and choice of operative methods are presented here.

The indications for surgery provided by the BTF are slightly modified, based on the expert opinion of the Scandinavian Neurotrauma Committee (SNC). This especially applies to patients with EDH or ASDH and a GCS <14. For these patients, it is good clinical practice to consider surgery if the neurosurgeon believes that this can provide symptomatic relief and possibly shorten hospital stay and improve prognosis. This is the expert opinion of the Scandinavian Neurotrauma Committee, and not recommended in the BTF surgical guidelines.

The objective of the Scandinavian Neurotrauma Committee (SNC) with these guidelines is to give the young neurosurgeon a practical and basic manual of acute surgical management of brain injuries. Details on trauma surgery per se are not extensively covered in the otherwise comprehensive surgical guidelines from the BTF (Bullock et al. 2006). Our descriptions of relevant surgical techniques are therefore based on the expert opinion of the SNC and acknowledged textbooks in neurosurgery (Greenberg 2016; Narayan et al. 1995; Quiñones-Hinojosa 2012; Winn 2017).

Rigorous surgical guidelines are difficult, perhaps impossible, to define due to the diversity of intracranial lesions, the complexity of multitraumatised patients and a variety of individual patient characteristics. But, when doubt exists and consciousness is depressed, the neurosurgeon should always monitor intracranial pressure (ICP) and remove significant mass lesions without undue delay.

Tips, Tricks and Pitfalls

- Always utilise all the information provided by the CT scan in the operative planning (e.g. scout view, fractures, reconstructions).
- Withhold surgery in futile cases; consider surgery in all other patients with reduced consciousness.
- Exploratory burr holes are not recommended.
- In general, place burr holes outside fracture lines.
- Cervical injuries are prevalent in patients with severe traumatic brain injuries.
- Practise a lower threshold for evacuation of epidural haematomas in children than in adults.
- Intracranial haematomas in neonates and infants may present with symptoms of blood loss-hypotension.
- A craniotomy for the evacuation of an epidural or subdural haematoma in small children entails a risk of significant blood loss.
- In the absence of an adequate head trauma, always look for other injuries in infants with intracranial haematomas—child abuse?
- Adults and children with temporal arachnoid cysts are prone to get subdural haematomas, even after minor head traumas.

24.2 Background

24.2.1 Epidural Haematoma

24.2.1.1 Pathogenesis

Epidural haematomas (EDHs) are primarily located in the temporal and temporoparietal regions (Fig. 24.1). The bleeding is often caused by a tear in an anterior or posterior branch of the middle meningeal artery and is frequently associated with a linear cranial fracture. The fracture is thought to initiate dural stripping, and as the EDH enlarges, the dura is progressively stripped from the inner table of the skull. The haematoma typically has a biconvex shape and is limited by cranial sutures. EDHs have a peak incidence in the second decade of life. Due to the stronger dural adherence to the skull with increasing age, EDHs are a rare entity among older patients. Injuries to the middle meningeal veins, the diploic veins or the venous sinuses are other possible sources of bleeding, and venous origin is not as infrequent as thought for many years. Venous bleeding is reported to be accountable for approximately one-third of EDHs in both adult and paediatric patients (Mohanty et al. 1995). An arterial focus is more often identified as a source of bleeding among adult than paediatric patients. Notably, up to 50% of EDH patients display a so-called free interval,

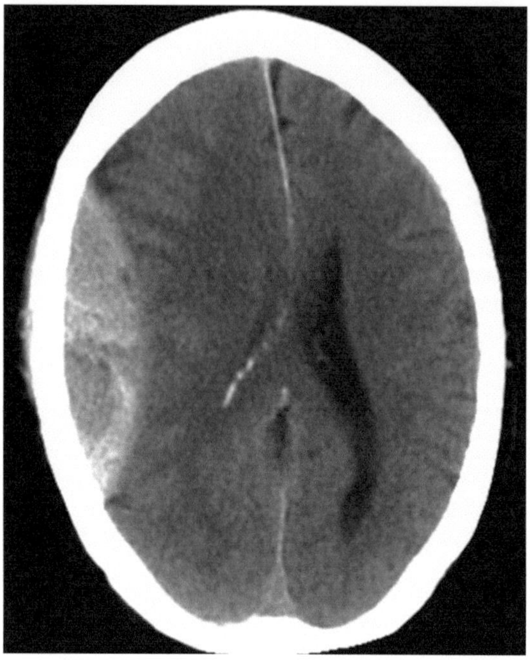

Fig. 24.1 Epidural haematoma with a typical biconvex appearance. This patient had a very rapid clinical deterioration. The *slightly darker area* in the posterior region of the haematoma is a sign of ongoing bleeding

where they wake up after the injury and then, as the bleeding increases, deteriorate with headache and eventually depressed consciousness.

24.2.1.2 Treatment

An EDH greater than 30 cm^3 should be evacuated regardless of the Glasgow Coma Scale (GCS) score.

It is strongly recommended that patients with an EDH, GCS of less than 9 and anisocoria undergo immediate surgical evacuation (Bullock et al. 2006).

An EDH less than 30 cm^3, with less than 15 mm thickness, and with less than a 5 mm midline shift, in patients with a GCS score greater than 8 without focal deficits can be managed conservatively with serial CT scans and close neurological observation in a neurosurgical centre (Bullock et al. 2006). However, it is good clinical practice to consider surgery in all patients with a GCS <14 and/or other symptoms attributable to the EDH.

There are insufficient data to support one surgical treatment method (Bullock et al. 2006). However, a craniotomy facilitates a more complete evacuation of the haematoma.

24.2.1.3 Surgical Considerations

A tailored craniotomy preferably providing complete exposure of the haematoma and the bleeding source is carried out using the preoperative CT scan and anatomical landmarks as guides (Fig. 24.2). After the information on the extent of the haematoma is visualised on the scout view, it can readily be transferred to the patient's head, and the scalp incision and craniotomy can be planned and carried out accordingly. Bony landmarks, such as the coronal suture, superior temporal line and ear, are also helpful in localising the position and extent of the haematoma. The EDH is usually clotted and removed with irrigation, suction and cup forceps.

If the neurological deterioration has been very rapid, it has previously been recommended to place an initial burr hole with or without a small craniectomy over or near the area of maximal clot thickness and evacuate accessible haematoma before continuing with the craniotomy. The rationale has been to rapidly reduce ICP and decompress the midbrain at the tentorial incisura, but this strategy has been largely abandoned since a complete craniotomy can today be performed expeditiously without undue loss of time.

Thorough haemostasis is obtained by using bipolar electrocautery, haemostatic agents, bone wax and tacking sutures. Bleeding from a branch of the middle meningeal artery can usually be controlled with bipolar electrocautery. EDHs arising from a tear in the main trunk of the middle meningeal artery in relation to a petrous bone fracture may necessitate packing of the foramen spinosum with haemostatic material (including bone wax). Bleeding from beyond the bony exposure may require additional bone removal but can often be controlled with dural tacking sutures. When haemostasis eventually is achieved in the epidural space, peripheral and bone flap tacking sutures are placed. An epicranial vacuum drain should be considered.

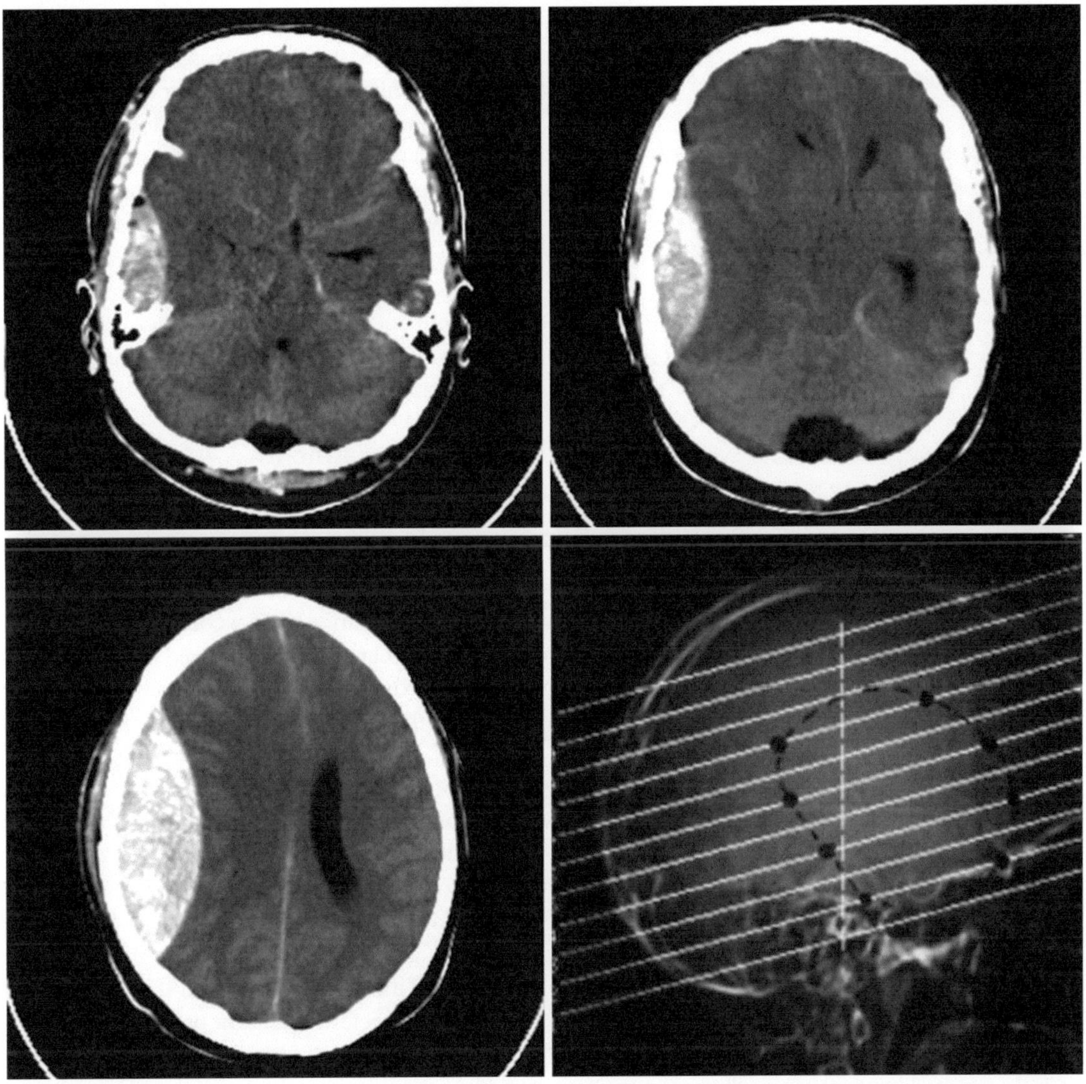

Fig. 24.2 Right-sided epidural haematoma with the equivalent extent delineated on a corresponding scout view. When planning the craniotomy, print the scout view and go through the series slice by slice, plotting the anterior and posterior margins of the haematoma on the skin

If the dura remains tense or has a bluish colour suggestive of intradural bleeding, and this was not expected from the preoperative CT scan, the subdural space should be inspected. A limited dural incision is initially made and expanded if necessary. Alternatively, intraoperative ultrasound can be used to look for underlying pathology.

24.2.2 Acute Subdural Haematoma

24.2.2.1 Pathogenesis

Acute subdural haematomas (ASDHs) may arise from cortical contusions or lacerations or from torn surface or bridging veins (Fig. 24.3). With the latter, primary brain damage may be less severe. Approximately 50% of all patients have associated

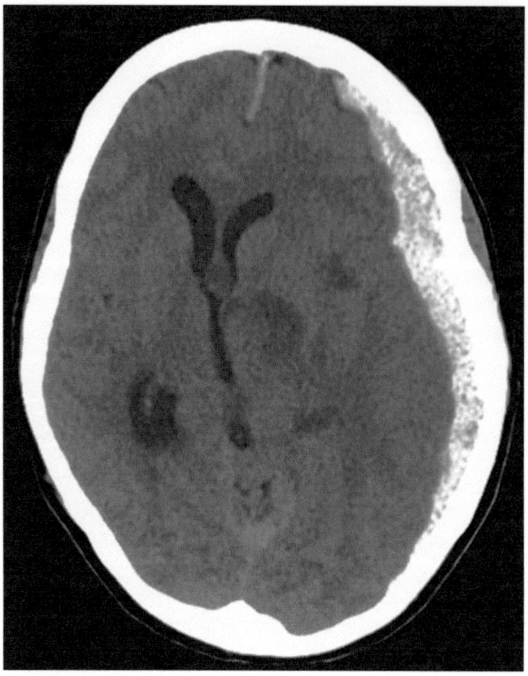

Fig. 24.3 Left-sided acute subdural haematoma with midline shift to the right. The patient herniated during transport to the hospital. Surgery required a large frontotemporoparietal craniotomy

lesions, including contusions, haematomas or cortical lacerations, with the majority occurring in the frontal and temporal lobes. Thus, patients with ASDHs more frequently have persistently depressed consciousness as compared to patients with EDHs. ASDHs are typically crescent-shaped over the cerebral hemisphere, as they are only limited by the falx cerebri and tentorium cerebelli.

An increased incidence of subdural haematomas appears to be associated with the increased use of antithrombotic drugs in the population, especially the use of vitamin K antagonists among older patients (Gaist et al. 2017). The use of vitamin K antagonists (e.g. warfarin) alone or in combination with clopidogrel is associated with a significantly increased risk of subdural haematomas. In general, there is significant risk related to concomitant use of more than one antithrombotic drug and moderate risk increase with novel oral anticoagulants (NOACs) or clopidogrel as monotherapies, whereas low-dose aspirin only carries a small risk increase.

Other risk factors for ASDH are alcohol abuse or high age with brain atrophy, shunt-treated hydrocephalus or temporal arachnoid cysts (Wester and Helland 2008). Subdural haematomas most frequently occur in patients over 75 years of age and are twice as common in men than in women. The mortality rate of ASDH in the elderly is high (70–80%), and only a minority of those who survive will be independent (Benedetto et al. 2017). Hence, critical judgement should be exercised when it comes to surgical indication.

24.2.2.2 Treatment

An ASDH with a thickness greater than 10 mm, or with a midline shift greater than 5 mm on a CT scan, should be evacuated, regardless of the GCS score (Bullock et al. 2006).

A patient with a GCS score less than 9, an ASDH less than 10 mm thick and a midline shift less than 5 mm should undergo evacuation of the lesion if the GCS score decreased between the time of injury and hospital admission by two or more points and/or the patient presents with anisocoria and/or the ICP exceeds 20 mmHg (Bullock et al. 2006).

From clinical experience, it is recommended to consider surgery in all patients with a GCS less than 14 and/or other symptoms that can be ascribed to the ASDH. However, it is judicious to maintain a stricter indication practice for ASDH than for EDH.

If surgical evacuation of an ASDH is indicated, it should be performed using a large trauma craniotomy with or without bone flap removal and duraplasty.

24.2.2.3 Surgical Considerations

A large frontotemporoparietal craniotomy, as described in Chap. 23, is typically required to remove an ASDH and to address associated parenchymal lesions. Adequate exposure of the temporal and frontal poles and the area along the superior sagittal sinus is essential.

The blood clot is removed with irrigation, suction and cup forceps. Care must be taken not to provoke any additional bleeding (especially towards the midline). The subdural space is widely inspected for additional haematoma, active bleeding and surface contusions. Expansion of the craniotomy margins is sometimes needed. Small amounts of clot that are not properly visualised and require undue brain retraction should be left undisturbed. Cortical bleeding points and avulsed bridging veins are coagulated with bipolar electrocautery, and haemostatic agents are used to control more diffuse cortical bleeding. Bleeding from the sinus wall should not be cauterised, as this will only enlarge the dural opening. Haemostatic agents combined with cottonoids should instead be used. A fibrin sealant or muscle patch may be needed if other measures prove inadequate.

Management of coexistent cortical contusions and intracerebral haematomas is described in the next section.

Dural closure is considered when the haematoma is evacuated and haemostasis is obtained. If the dura can be closed easily and future brain swelling is deemed unlikely, the dura is sutured watertight following placement of multiple dural tacking sutures, and the bone flap is replaced. However, a duraplasty is often required, and replacement of the bone flap should then be avoided (see Chap. 26).

24.2.3 Intracerebral Haematomas and Cerebral Contusions

24.2.3.1 Pathogenesis

Traumatic intracerebral haematomas (TICH) and cerebral contusions are often associated with epidural or subdural haematomas (Fig. 24.4). They occur most frequently in the frontal and temporal lobes, due to the brain impact against the irregular cranial surface. The areas most prone to haemorrhagic contusions are the inferior orbital aspects of the gyrus rectus and inferior frontal gyrus in the frontal lobes and the tips of the temporal lobes. Parietal and occipital lesions are less common and usually directly associated with the impact.

Such lesions are seen in almost all patients with severe head injury and up to 40% of those with moderate head injuries (Einarsen et al. 2018). However, only about 25% of trauma craniotomies are performed primarily for cerebral contusions or TICHs (Winn 2017).

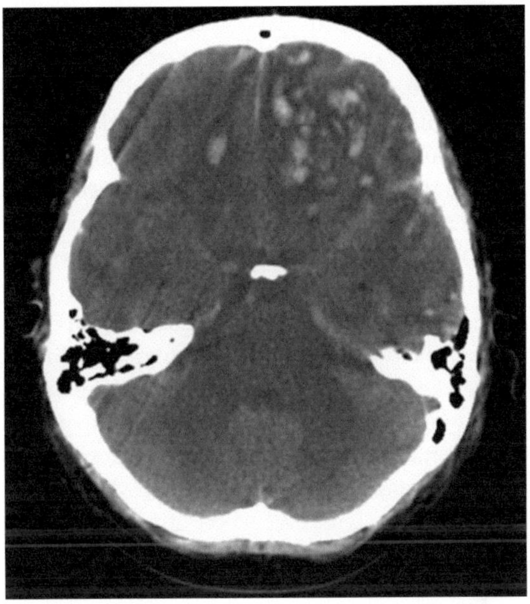

Fig. 24.4 Extensive cerebral contusions especially in the left frontal lobe. The patient also had a small acute subdural haematoma (not visualised on this image) and was operated with evacuation of the subdural haematoma followed by a duraplasty and craniectomy

The role of surgery and its timing remains undefined. In a randomised controlled trial on TICHs, early surgery was found to be beneficial as compared to conservative management (Mendelow et al. 2015). The authors found a significant survival benefit and a non-significant benefit on functional outcome. Early surgery seemed most advantageous in patients with a GCS of 9–12; above or below this interval, there was more uncertainty. However, this study was underpowered and geographically skewed towards resource-poor centres, and further research is warranted.

Subacute surgery may be required if TICHs or contusions diagnosed by the initial CT scan evolve with perifocal oedema and/or enlargement of bleeding. Please refer to the chapter on subacute surgery in Part VIII-Chap. 57.

24.2.3.2 Treatment

Patients with parenchymal mass lesions and signs of progressive neurological deterioration referable to the lesion, medically refractory intracranial hypertension or signs of mass effect on CT scan should be treated operatively.

Patients with GCS scores of 6–8 with frontal or temporal contusions greater than 20 cm^3 in volume with a midline shift of at least 5 mm and/or cisternal compression on CT scan, and patients with any lesion greater than 50 cm^3 in volume should be treated operatively.

Patients with parenchymal mass lesions who do not show evidence of neurological compromise, who have controlled ICP and no significant signs of mass effect on CT scan, may be managed non-operatively with intensive monitoring and serial imaging (Bullock et al. 2006).

Craniotomy with evacuation of mass lesions is recommended for those patients who have focal lesions, and the surgical indications as listed above.

24.2.3.3 Surgical Considerations

A standard trauma craniotomy is usually indicated because TICHs and cerebral contusions are frequently associated with extra-axial haematomas. Special surgical considerations as specified for EDH or ASDH should therefore be remembered.

Sizeable areas (>1–2 cm) of cerebral contusions with irreparably damaged brain, appearing purplish and mottled, can be removed. Ultrasound can be helpful in localising a TICH at considerable depth from the cortex. The pia and bleeding superficial vessels are cauterised over the most traumatised area or in an otherwise non-eloquent area. A pial incision is made, and a subpial plane is established. Blood clots and adjacent contused brain are removed with gentle aspiration and bipolar electrocautery. A more limited resection of parenchymal lesions is prudent in eloquent areas, such as along the dominant superior temporal gyrus and the central sulcus. Avoid sacrificing arteries and veins that traverse a traumatised area and that supply or drain healthy cortex.

Haemostasis after removal of a TICH or cerebral contusions can be achieved by bipolar electrocautery, gentle tamponade with cottonoids soaked in saline and lining the cavity with haemostatic agents. This is followed by routine closure.

A minimalistic approach through a small burr hole should only be considered in patients with an isolated TICH and no other associated lesions.

24.2.4 Posterior Fossa Mass Lesions

24.2.4.1 Pathogenesis

Traumatic lesions in the posterior fossa are rare and occur in less than 3% of all head injuries (Karasawa et al. 1997). The vast majority of published series deal with epidural haematomas. Subdural and intraparenchymal lesions are less frequent, but the more dangerous, as patients with mass lesions in the posterior fossa can undergo rapid clinical deterioration because of the limited space available and close relationship to vital centres in the brainstem. Timely recognition and surgical evacuation are therefore especially warranted. It is particularly important to monitor the respiration if the patient is not already on a ventilator, as impaired lung ventilation will cause hypercapnia with vasodilatation and subsequently a rapidly developing vicious circle due to increased pressure on respiration regulating areas in the brainstem. The neurosurgeon must also be aware of any complicating hydrocephalus and be prepared to put in an external drainage.

24.2.4.2 Treatment

Patients with mass effect on the CT scan, neurological dysfunction or deterioration referable to the lesion should undergo operative intervention. Mass effect on the CT scan is defined as distortion, dislocation or obliteration of the fourth ventricle; compression or loss of visualisation of the basal cisterns; or the presence of obstructive supratentorial hydrocephalus. Close observation including respiration and serial imaging can be considered in patients with no significant mass effect on the CT scan and without signs of neurological dysfunction (Bullock et al. 2006).

In patients with indications for surgical intervention, evacuation should be performed as soon as possible because patients can deteriorate rapidly, thus worsening their prognosis (Bullock et al. 2006).

A suboccipital craniotomy is recommended for evacuation of posterior fossa mass lesions.

24.2.4.3 Surgical Considerations

The patient is usually placed in the Concorde position, and a midline suboccipital craniotomy is performed. Access to the midline and both cerebellar hemispheres is ensured. The traumatic mass lesion is evacuated, and haemostasis is obtained. Standard supratentorial ventricular drainage should be considered if there is a risk of the patient developing hydrocephalus, as an initial or closing manoeuvre.

Traumatic lesions in the posterior fossa are so infrequent that a detailed surgical description is not warranted in these basic guidelines on trauma surgery. The reader is referred to neurosurgical textbooks on operative procedures for further information.

24.3 Specific Paediatric Concerns

Most of the foundation for the medical and surgical treatment of children with severe head injuries is based on adult studies. This is a result of the lack of scientific data primarily dealing with children. Children generally have a better overall outcome than adults, but younger children fare worse than older children with respect to both mortality and long-term disability (Adelson 2000; Anderson et al. 2005; Garg et al. 2017). Moreover, the long-term deficits are often persistent and severe, even with aggressive management. Notably, the younger brain has better potential for reorganisation after focal injuries, but the negative consequences of diffuse injuries can be more extensive than in adults (Dennis et al. 2018).

Young children have a more compressible brain and flexible skull than older children and adults. Because of this, there are fewer intracranial mass lesions and more white matter shear injuries in young children (Hahn et al. 1988; Zimmerman and Bilaniuk 1994). As the child gets older, the incidence of ASDH and TICH becomes more similar to that of the adult (Luerssen et al. 1988; Zimmerman and Bilaniuk 1994). EDHs are more frequent among older children and adolescents than among neonates and infants. This is due to the relatively stronger attachment between the dura and the cranium, but also because of a smaller risk of bony injury to the middle meningeal artery. A lower threshold for surgical treatment of EDH should be practised in children than in adults; only neurologically intact patients with a GCS score of 15 with or without headache should be considered candidates for observation.

In the absence of an adequate head trauma, always look for other injuries in infants with intracranial haematomas with respect to abusive head trauma. This also applies to CT findings of interhemispheric ASDH or subdural blood of varying ages over one or both convexities, potentially combined with traumatic subarachnoid haemorrhage and/or cerebral contusions. Keep at the same time in mind that young children or even infants harbouring a temporal arachnoid cyst are especially prone to get subdural haematomas even after minor head traumas (Wester and Helland 2008). These haematomas may be of different ages and thus raise unjustified suspicion of child abuse. The same applies to infants with external hydrocephalus (Lee et al. 2018).

References

Adelson PD. Pediatric trauma made simple. Clin Neurosurg. 2000;47:319–35.

Anderson V, Catroppa C, Morse S, Haritou F, Rosenfeld J. Functional plasticity or vulnerability after early brain injury? Pediatrics. 2005;116:1374–82.

Benedetto N, Gambacciani C, Montemurro N, Morganti R, Perrini P. Surgical management of acute subdural haematomas in elderly: report of a single center experience. Br J Neurosurg. 2017;31:244–8.

Bulger EM, Nathens AB, Rivara FP, Moore M, MacKenzie EJ, Jurkovich GJ, Foundation BT. Management of severe head injury: institutional variations in care and effect on outcome. Crit Care Med. 2002;30:1870–6.

Bullock MR, Chesnut R, Ghajar J, Gordon D, Hartl R, Newell DW, Servadei F, Walters BC, Wilberger JE, Surgical Management of Traumatic Brain Injury Author Group. Surgical management of trau matic brain injury. Neurosurgery. 2006;58:S2-1–S2-62.

Compagnone C, Murray GD, Teasdale GM, Maas AI, Esposito D, Princi P, D'Avella D, Servadei F. The management of patients with intradural post-trau matic mass lesions: a multicenter survey of current approaches to surgical management in 729 patients coordinated by the European Brain Injury Consortium. Neurosurgery. 2005;57:1183–92.

Dennis EL, Babikian T, Giza CC, Thompson PM, Asarnow RF. Neuroimaging of the injured pediatric brain: methods and new lessons. Neuroscientist. 2018;24:652–70.

Einarsen CE, van der Naalt J, Jacobs B, Follestad T, Moen KG, Vik A, Håberg AK, Skandsen T. Moderate Traumatic brain injury: clinical characteristics and a prognostic model of 12-month outcome. World Neurosurg. 2018;114:e1199–210. https://doi.org/10.1016/j.wneu.2018.03.176.

Gaist D, García Rodríguez LA, Hellfritzsch M, Poulsen FR, Halle B, Hallas J, Pottegård A. Association of antithrombotic drug use with subdural hematoma risk. JAMA. 2017;317(8):836–46. https://doi.org/10.1001/jama.2017.0639.

Garg K, Sharma R, Gupta D, Sinha S, Satyarthee GD, Agarwal D, Kale SS, Sharma BS, Mahapatra AK. Outcome predictors in pediatric head trauma: a study of clinicoradiological factors. J Pediatr Neurosci. 2017;12:149–53.

Greenberg MS. Handbook of neurosurgery. 8th ed. New York: Thieme Medical Publishers, Inc.; 2016.

Hahn YS, Chyung C, Barthel MJ, Bailes J, Flannery AM, McLone DG. Head injuries in children under 36 months of age. Demography and outcome. Childs Nerv Syst. 1988;4:34–40.

Karasawa H, Furuya H, Naito H, Sugiyama K, Ueno J, Kin H. Acute hydrocephalus in posterior fossa injury. J Neurosurg. 1997;86:629–32.

Lee HC, Chong S, Lee JY, Cheon JE, Phi JH, Kim SK, Kim IO, Wang KC. Benign extracerebral fluid collection complicated by subdural hematoma and fluid collection: clinical characteristics and management. Childs Nerv Syst. 2018;34:235–45.

Luerssen TG, Klauber MR, Marshall LF. Outcome from head injury related to patient's age. A longitudi nal prospective study of adult and pediatric head injury. J Neurosurg. 1988;68:409–16.

Mendelow AD, Gregson BA, Rowan EN, Francis R, McColl E, McNamee P, Chambers IR, Unterberg A, Boyers D, Mitchell PM, STITCH(Trauma) Investigators. Early surgery versus initial conservative treatment in patients with traumatic intracerebral hemorrhage (STITCH[Trauma]): the first randomized trial. J Neurotrauma. 2015;32:1312–23.

Mohanty A, Kolluri VR, Subbakrishna DK, Satish S, Mouli BA, Das BS. Prognosis of extradural haematomas in children. Pediatr Neurosurg. 1995;23:57–63.

Narayan RK, Wilberger JE, Povlishock JT. Neurotrauma. New York: McGraw Hill; 1995.

Quiñones-Hinojosa A. Schmidek & Sweet operative neurosurgical techniques: indications, methods, and results. 6th ed. Philadelphia: Saunders, an imprint of Elsevier; 2012.

Valadka AB, Robertson CS. Surgery of cerebral trauma and associated critical care. Neurosurgery. 2007;61:203–20.

Wester K, Helland CA. How often do chronic extracerebral haematomas occur in patients with intracranial arachnoid cysts? J Neurol Neurosurg Psychiatry. 2008;79:72–5.

Winn HR. Youmans & Winn neurological surgery. 7th ed. Philadelphia: Elsevier; 2017.

Zimmerman RA, Bilaniuk LT. Pediatric head trauma. Neuroimaging Clin N Am. 1994;4:349–66.

Surgical Management of Penetrating Brain Injuries

25

Terje Sundstrøm, Eirik Helseth, and Knut Gustav Wester

Recommendations

Level I

There are insufficient data to support a Level I recommendation for this topic.

Level II

There are insufficient data to support a Level II recommendation for this topic.

Level III

Patients with penetrating brain injuries that are otherwise stabilized and demonstrate neurological function or deterioration referable to a mass lesion should be considered for surgery.

25.1 Overview

Penetrating brain injuries (PBIs) have high fatality rates. Patients who survive the initial phase can however demonstrate favourable outcomes. The primary injuries can entail a combination of scalp lesions, cranial fractures, intracranial haematomas and cerebral lacerations. High energy PBIs frequently encompass distant lesions and are often followed by a detrimental increase in intracranial pressure (ICP).

There is no defined threshold for whom surgery should be withheld, but the patient must have a possibility of a reasonable functional outcome. Patients with devastating brain injuries and/or high probability of a poor outcome should generally not be subjected to surgical treatment.

Tips, Tricks and Pitfalls

- Consider ICP monitoring and/or EVD.
- Carefully plan the way in and out (vascularity, exposure, wound closure).
- If you plan a skin flap, you have to take the wound into consideration: is it most suitable to incorporate the wound in the skin incision or is it better to place the

T. Sundstrøm (✉)
Department of Neurosurgery, Haukeland University Hospital, Bergen, Norway

Department of Clinical Medicine, University of Bergen, Bergen, Norway
e-mail: tjsu@helse-bergen.no

E. Helseth
Institute of Clinical Medicine, University of Oslo, Oslo, Norway

Department of Neurosurgery, Oslo University Hospital, Oslo, Norway
e-mail: EHELSETH@ous-hf.no

K. G. Wester
Department of Clinical Medicine, University of Bergen, Bergen, Norway
e-mail: Knut.Wester@uib.no

© Springer Nature Switzerland AG 2020
T. Sundstrøm et al. (eds.), *Management of Severe Traumatic Brain Injury*,
https://doi.org/10.1007/978-3-030-39383-0_25

incision around it, with a broad base to ensure a sufficient blood supply to the entire flap?
- Perform a thorough debridement of all tissue layers.
- If possible, do not add foreign material.
- Antibiotics and antiepileptic medication should be liberally applied.

25.2 Background

25.2.1 Pathogenesis

The majority of PBIs in the civilian setting are caused by low-velocity gunshot wounds to the head (GSWH) (Potapov et al. 2001). These injuries have a mortality rate of more than 90% (Aarabi et al. 2014). However, survivors may experience a favourable recovery. Significant factors related to outcome in PBI are admission Glasgow Coma Scale (GCS) score, missile trajectory, pupillary status and patency of basal cisterns (Aarabi et al. 2014).

Shrapnel (fragments thrown out by an exploding bomb or shell), and not GSWH, is the major cause of PBIs in military conflicts. The overall mortality rate is therefore lower; it is generally reported to be around 20% (Potapov et al. 2001).

A combination of soft tissue injuries, fractures and parenchymal lesions may constitute the primary injuries from GSWH. The impact velocity of a projectile reflects the true wounding potential, and deformation and fragmentation of the missile enhance energy delivery to the tissue. Comminute fractures may injure the directly underlying structures, and bone fragments may be driven into the brain as secondary projectiles. Brain injuries can occur along the path of the projectile(s), as well as in more distant locations, due to pressure waves and coup/contrecoup lesions. A rapid rise in ICP may follow a GSWH.

25.2.2 Treatment Options

No surgical intervention is generally warranted for patients with a post-resuscitation GCS score of 3, dilated and nonreactive pupils and no significant mass lesion on the CT scan. Patients that are otherwise stabilized and demonstrating some neurological function (motor or brain stem) or deterioration referable to a mass lesion should be considered for urgent surgical treatment.

Small entrance bullet wounds to the head can be treated with local wound care and closure if the scalp is not devitalized and there are no surgical intracranial lesions. Treatment of more extensive wounds requires extensive debridement before primary closure to secure a watertight wound. In the presence of significant mass effect, debridement of necrotic brain tissue and safely accessible bone fragments, together with evacuation of intracranial haematomas with significant mass effect, is recommended. A minimal invasive approach is prudent in the absence of significant mass effect (Potapov et al. 2001).

If possible, any protruding part of a foreign body should not be removed before the patient is in the operating room.

Infection is an important secondary complication, and liberal use of antibiotics is recommended.

Seizures in the acute phase are unfavourable and liberal use of antiepileptic drugs (AEDs) is recommended. About 50% of survivors will suffer seizures and require antiepileptic medication.

The neurosurgeon must carefully consider the need for intracranial pressure measurement and/or external ventricular drainage, in addition to the primary surgical treatment.

25.2.3 Surgical Considerations

The cranium is examined for external injuries. Thorough irrigation of the wound site(s) is performed. Consultation with a plastic surgeon may be warranted in selected cases. The skin incision must be carefully planned in order to, first, ensure vascularity and enable wound closure following excision of devitalized tissue and, second, to secure sufficient exposure of the bony defect and underlying haematomas. The cranial opening should extend well beyond the visible bone injury until intact dura is visualized.

Herniated brain tissue and the intracerebral penetration tract are flushed through the dural lesion, and accessible necrotic tissue, bone fragments and foreign bodies are gently removed.

The dural opening may need to be enlarged to accommodate adequate debridement and haematoma evacuation. A thorough exploration must be performed, but preservation of viable brain tissue supersedes removal of deeply located fragments (Potapov et al. 2001). Haemostasis is preferably ensured by bipolar electrocautery and dural repair by autologous grafts (e.g. temporalis fascia or pericranium).

Bone replacement should be performed in case of no present or anticipated future significant brain swelling. High-velocity injuries are often associated with substantial oedema development, and it may be wise not to replace the bone in these cases. Before replacement of the bone flap or fragments, ample debridement and cleaning must be secured. Foreign materials must be utilized at a minimum, but miniplates, titanium wires and craniofix devices are often needed to assemble multiple bony fragments. The importance of meticulous scalp closure is previously stated.

25.3 Specific Paediatric Concerns

There are no specific paediatric concerns. Please refer to Chaps. 23 and 24 for supplementary information.

References

Aarabi B, Tofighi B, Kufera JA, Hadley J, Ahn ES, Cooper C, Malik JM, Naff NJ, Chang L, Radley M, Kheder A, Uscinski RH. Predictors of outcome in civilian gunshot wounds to the head. J Neurosurg. 2014;120:1138–46.

Potapov AA, Shahinian GG, Kravtchouk AD. Surgical management of penetrating brain injury. J Trauma. 2001;51:16–25.

26 Decompressive Craniectomy

Jussi P. Posti and Pål A. Rønning

Recommendations

Level I

Decompressive craniectomy does not improve the rate of patients surviving with favourable functional outcome. Decompressive craniectomy effectively lowers intracranial pressure (ICP) and reduces mortality rate following severe diffuse traumatic brain injury and diffuse traumatic brain injury with surgical intracranial lesions.

Level II

There are insufficient data to support a Level II recommendation for this topic.

Level III

Decompressive craniectomy is a surgical option to control ICP in patients with refractory ICP not responding to first tier of therapy.

J. P. Posti (✉)
Clinical Neurosciences, Department of Neurosurgery and Turku Brain Injury Centre, Turku University Hospital and University of Turku, Turku, Finland
e-mail: jussi.posti@utu.fi

P. A. Rønning
Department of Neurosurgery, Oslo University Hospital, Oslo, Norway

Tips, Tricks and Pitfalls

- Decompressive craniectomy effectively lowers intracranial pressure and reduces the mortality rate following severe diffuse TBI and intractable intracranial pressure.
- Major randomised trials indicate that the benefits are translated almost directly into survival with severe disability.
- The temporal bone should be removed to the floor of the middle fossa to prevent upper brainstem compression.
- The dura should always be opened and closed without sutures.

26.1 Background

26.1.1 Overview

According to the Monroe-Kelly doctrine, the intracranial volume is constant and dictated by the confines of the skull, brain tissue, cerebrospinal fluid (CSF) and intracranial blood (Wilson 2016):

$$V_{IC} = V_{BR} + V_{BL} + V_{CSF}$$

where V_{IC} is intracranial volume, V_{BR} is brain tissue volume, V_{BL} is blood volume and V_{CSF} is CSF volume.

© Springer Nature Switzerland AG 2020
T. Sundstrøm et al. (eds.), *Management of Severe Traumatic Brain Injury*,
https://doi.org/10.1007/978-3-030-39383-0_26

The volume of these compartments is rigorously regulated, and cerebral perfusion pressure (CPP) is maintained by cerebral autoregulation. When the physiological equilibrium is disturbed by expansion in some of these volumes, compensatory mechanisms are activated in order to keep ICP constant (Stocchetti and Maas 2014).

Traumatic brain injury (TBI) is a complex continuum, which causes both cerebral and systemic events. These events may exacerbate an already sustained brain injury, often referred to as secondary brain injury. Brain injury might disturb the Monroe-Kellie equation by increased volumes on the right-hand side of the equation due to (1) focal pathologies such as contusions, intracerebral haematomas and hydrocephalus or (2) diffuse brain swelling from oedema (Unterberg et al. 2004), hyperaemia and microvascular injury (congestive brain swelling) (Kelly et al. 1996; Logsdon et al. 2015). Systemic responses include, e.g. pro-inflammatory responses (Bulstrode et al. 2014), coagulopathy (Maegele et al. 2017) and fever. In severe TBI, these phenomena appear in innumerable combinations.

Due to the rigidness of the skull after closing of the sutures, an intracranial volume increase causes increased pressure when the compensatory mechanisms of reduced CSF and intracranial blood have been exhausted. When the standard measures for decreasing ICP have failed, an alternative option is to increase the intracranial volume (V_{IC}) utilising decompressive craniectomy (DC). DC is a neurosurgical emergency procedure in which a large bone flap is removed and the underlying dura mater is left open in order to allow brain tissue expansion and thus to lower ICP (Timofeev et al. 2012).

Primary DC refers to the decompression procedure combined with the evacuation of a space-occupying intracranial lesion or, in case of an initial diffuse hemispheric swelling, the decompression alone. A secondary DC refers to an intervention that is a part of tiered therapeutic protocol in the intensive care setting in order to reduce intractable ICP and ensure adequate CPP (Kolias et al. 2016). Along with medically refractory elevated ICP due to severe TBI, other indications for DC are intractable brain swelling due to, e.g. stroke, subarachnoid haemorrhage and intracerebral haemorrhage.

26.1.2 Major Randomised Controlled Trials

Increased ICP following TBI is correlated with poor outcome and death in several studies (Sahuquillo and Arikan 2006). Although not supported by Level I evidence (Carney et al. 2017), ICP monitoring and administration of ICP lowering measures are widely utilised in the intensive care unit setting. In some patients, brain swelling may result in refractory intracranial hypertension despite tiered medical treatment (Grindlinger et al. 2016).

The current evidence leaves little uncertainty about the lifesaving effect of DC in patients with severe TBI and refractory ICP. However, there is a risk that survival from injury following DC may come at the expense of severe functional disability and dependency on others. So far, two major clinical randomised controlled trials (RCTs) have investigated survival and neurological outcome of patients with TBI and refractory ICP following DC.

The international multicentre DECRA study investigated the role of early bi-frontotemporoparietal DC in patients with intractable ICP following TBI (Cooper et al. 2011). Out of 3478 evaluated patients, 155 patients with TBI with either Glasgow Coma Score (GCS) <8 or CT demonstrating moderate diffuse brain injury were considered eligible and enrolled. Patients with refractory ICP, defined as having ICP > 20 mmHg for 15 min within a 1-h period, were randomly assigned to the following groups: 73 underwent early bi-frontotemporoparietal DC and 82 received standard medical care. DC decreased ICP in patients belonging to the surgical group, but the intervention did not result in improved neurological outcome: 70% of patients in the DC group had an unfavourable outcome vs. 51% of patients in the standard care group at 6-month follow-up.

The ensuing international multicentre RESCUEicp study involved 409 eligible patients from 2008 assessed patients (Hutchinson et al. 2016). The inclusion criteria for the RESCUEicp study differed from the DECRA study in two important aspects: the ICP threshold was higher (25 mmHg for 1–12 h despite maximal medical treatment excluding barbiturates) and included patients who had previously undergone evacuation of an earlier intracranial space-occupying lesion without DC. Two hundred and two eligible patients were randomly assigned to undergo DC with medical therapy, and 196 patients were assigned to receive continued medical therapy with an option for barbiturates. The surgical technique was either a large unilateral frontotemporoparietal DC or a bifrontal craniectomy depending on the imaging characteristics and the discretion of the surgeon. DC resulted in reduced ICP and mortality rate, higher incidence of vegetative state, lower severe disability and upper severe disability (independent at home) when compared with medical therapy at 6 months. Because upper severe disability (Glasgow Outcome Scale Extended 4) (Wilson et al. 1998) was included in favourable outcome, 43% of the patients in the DC group had favourable outcome vs. 35% of the patients in the medical care group.

There are issues that should be considered when translating the findings of these two studies into clinical practice. First, the aims of the studies were different. The DECRA study examined the role of early DC in moderate ICP elevation, which can be considered under a prophylactic neuroprotective perspective, whereas the RESCUEicp study applied DC as the last tier of intervention, which can be considered rescue or salvage therapy. In the DECRA study, the trial enrolment ICP threshold (>20 mmHg for 15 min as recruitment criterion) is criticised to be unjustified as any potential improvement obtained by DC was offset by surgical morbidity. It should be noted that the DECRA study enrolled more patients with fixed pupils in the DC group (27%) than in the standard care group (12%), but after adjustment, there were no differences in the rate of unfavourable outcome in these groups. Third, in both studies, there was substantial crossover of patients from the medical care group to the DC group: 23% and 37% in the DECRA and RESCUEicp studies, respectively. Fourth, the surgical procedures in the studies were different. The RESCUEicp trial allowed both bifrontotemporoparietal (bifrontal) and frontotemporoparietal (hemicraniectomy) craniectomies, in contrast to DECRA that only allowed bifrontal craniectomies. Patients with surgical lesions were not included in the DECRA study, but in the RESCUEicp trial, patients with intracranial haematoma accounted for nearly 20% of cases.

26.1.3 Other Randomised Controlled Trials

Along with the major randomised trials (DECRA and RESCUEicp), another RCT has examined the effect of DC on ICP following TBI. Qiu et al. conducted a RCT including 74 adult patients divided into unilateral DC following medical therapy and medical therapy alone (Qiu et al. 2009): mean ICP was lower at all assessed time points in the patients in the DC group.

Similar to DECRA and RESCUEicp, the smaller RCT indicated that DC by and large halved the risk for death (Cooper et al. 2011; Hutchinson et al. 2016; Qiu et al. 2009). In that particular study, favourable outcome was reported in 32% of the patients in the medical therapy group vs. 57% in the DC group ($p = 0.035$) (Qiu et al. 2009).

26.1.4 Conclusion

RCTs in patients with severe TBI face a number of problems such as lack of clinical equipoise, lack of patient consent, strong clinician preference, imbalance in surgical expertise, crossover of patients, difficulty with blinding and problems in translating the findings into clinical practice due to the uncontrollable heterogeneity in practice of study centres (Ergina et al. 2009; Kolias et al. 2016).

Results from these four clinical randomised trials imply that DC effectively lowers ICP and reduces the mortality rate but that these benefits are translated almost directly into survival with severe disability (DECRA and RESCUEicp). There are some aspects to consider when interpreting these results. In most clinical situations, DC is usually carried out once medical therapy has failed, especially in young patients with TBI. The validated prognostic models (MRC CRASH Trial Collaborators et al. 2008; Steyerberg et al. 2008) demonstrated that young age is an important prognostic factor for favourable outcome after TBI. Hence, in young patients suffering from intractable ICP after failed medical therapy, neurosurgeons need to assess and balance the chance of survival with an acceptable level of disability with the possibility of permanent severe neurological disability.

26.2 Operative Technique

The goal of surgery is to provide the brain with room for expansion. Therefore, a large craniectomy is preferred (De Bonis et al. 2013; Güresir et al. 2009) (Fig. 26.1). Usually, DCs are divided into hemicraniectomies (frontotemporoparietal) or bifrontal (bifrontotemporoparietal) craniectomies. The indications are unilateral or bifrontal expansion, respectively. The authors advocate only the use of hemicraniectomy, and hence, only its operative technique is described.

26.2.1 Incision

The shape and placement for the skin incision depends on the localisation of DC. For hemicraniectomies, generally three variants are utilised. We prefer using the expanded trauma flap (Fig. 26.2a) or the reversed question mark (Fig. 26.2b), because the incisions can be placed outside the craniectomy margins in order to minimise wound problems related to cranioplasty. Another option is the T-incision (Fig. 26.2c). All the aforementioned incisions provide room for temporal decompression in order to prevent upper brainstem compression (Fig. 26.2d). There are pros and cons for all the incisions in terms of preservation of the vascu-

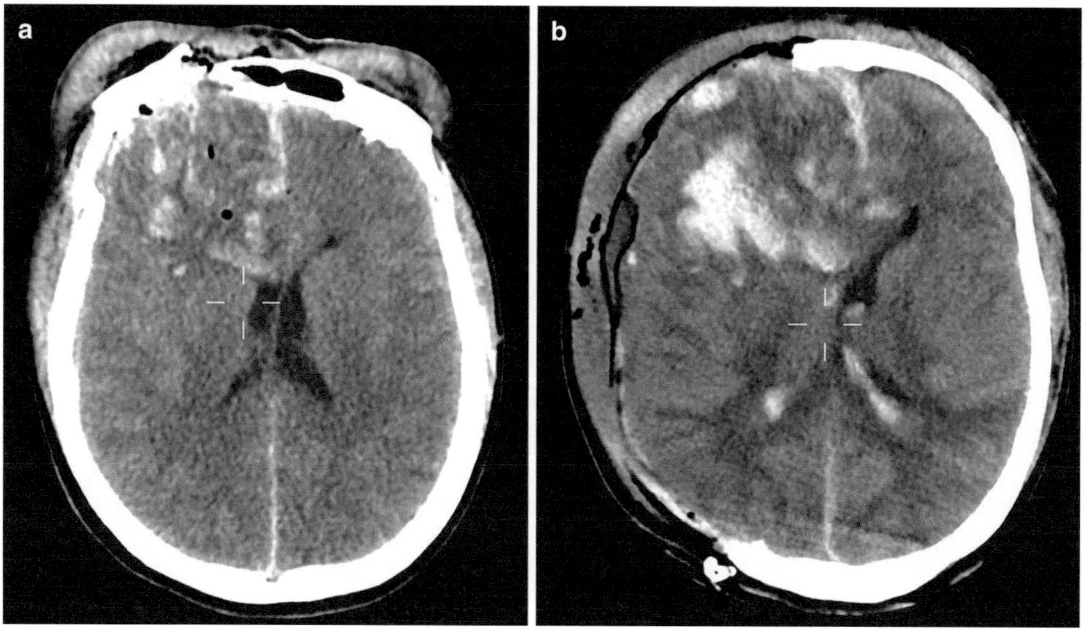

Fig. 26.1 (**a**) Severe diffuse right-sided TBI with complex frontal bone fracture in a 37-year-old male patient, fall from height accident, (**b**) blossoming of the haemorrhages causing diffuse swelling seen on postoperative head CT after DC. The patient survived and became independent with upper moderate disability (Glasgow Outcome Scale Extended 6/8)

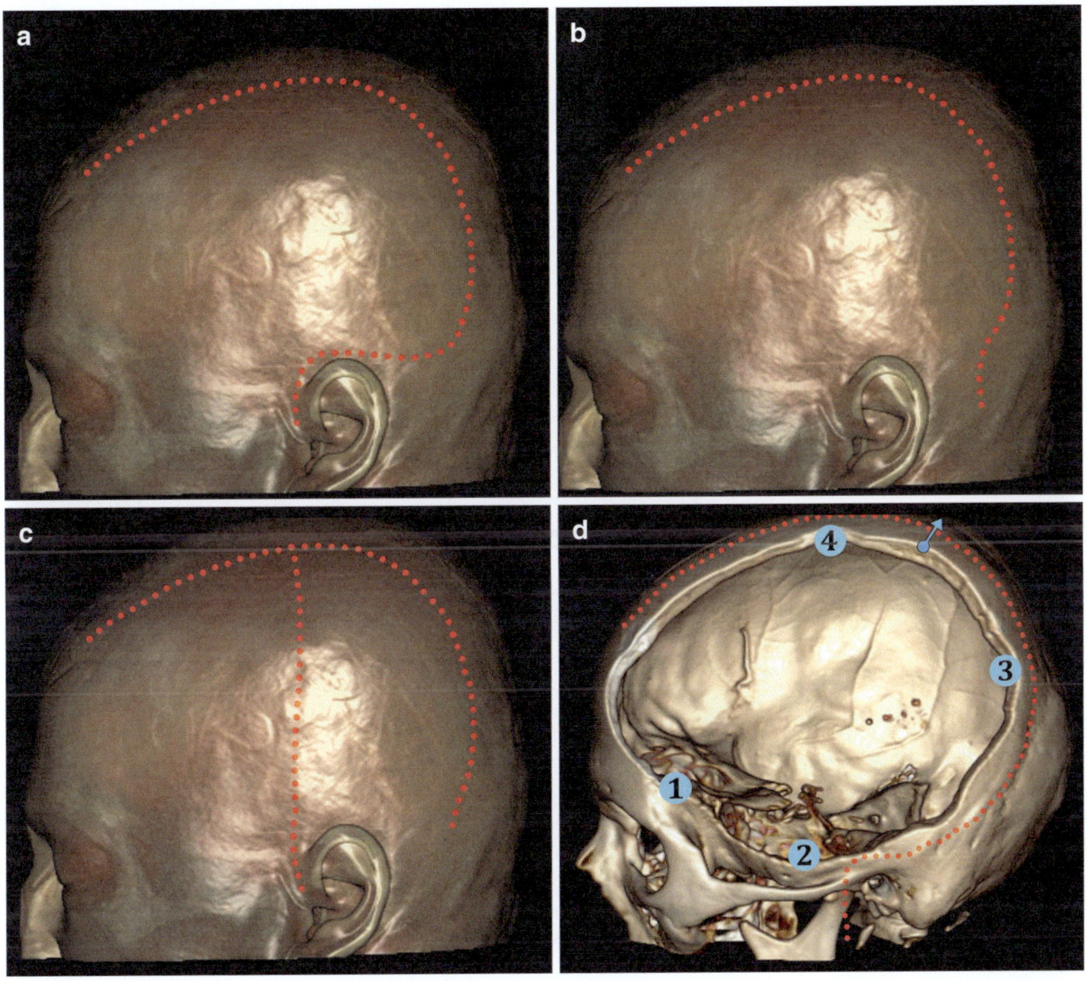

Fig. 26.2 (**a**) Extended trauma flap, (**b**) reversed question mark, (**c**) T-shaped incision, and (**d**) hemicraniectomy after extended trauma flap incision; numbers in the cyan spheres denote the burr holes; note that the head is tilted differently in the panel **d**

lature. The superficial temporal artery, including both frontal and parietal branches, is preserved using the expanded trauma flap and the reversed question mark incisions, while the posterior auricular artery and the occipital artery with its branches may be sacrificed depending on the inferior and posterior extension of the incisions. The T-incision is a modification of the reversed question mark incision. It usually preserves the posterior auricular artery and the occipital artery, while it sacrifices the parietal branch of the superficial temporal artery (Kurzbuch 2015). In both extended trauma flap and T-incision, the incision should be placed close to the ear in order to provide protection of temporal and zygomatic branches of the facial nerve (Fig. 26.2a and c). Dissecting the scalp and temporal muscle en bloc helps to avoid injuries to vascular and neural structures.

26.2.2 Craniectomy

The size of the craniotomy is of paramount importance. If the bone flap is too small, the swelling brain can herniate during the procedure causing severe strangulation. A bone flap with a diameter of 12–15 cm is considered adequate (De Bonis et al. 2013; Güresir et al. 2009). It is imperative to decompress the middle fossa; hence, the hemicraniectomy should be extended caudally so that the floor of the middle fossa is exposed (Fig. 26.2d). The cranio-caudal and anteroposterior dimensions determine the size of the DC. The anatomical landmarks for the DC are anteriorly the superior area above the orbital rim and the sinus of the frontal bone, posteriorly the lambdoid suture, cranially the superior sagittal sinus and inferiorly the zygomatic arch. We recommend placing the first burr hole behind the zygomatic process of the frontal bone (Fig. 26.2d, burr hole (1), the second as close to the zygomatic arch as possible (Fig. 26.2d, burr hole (2), the third on the lambdoid suture approximately 3–4 cm from the midline (Fig. 26.2d, burr hole (3) and an optional fourth behind the coronal suture not closer than 2.5–3 cm to the midline in order to avoid lesions of superior sagittal sinus and large bridging veins (Fig. 26.2d, burr hole (4). Additionally, the cranial border of the craniectomy should not be closer than 2.5 cm to the midline in order to decrease a possible risk of postoperative subdural hygroma and hydrocephalus (Fig. 26.2d, the cyan arrow). The temporal decompression is important, and the bony decompression must be flushed with the floor of the middle fossa. Thus, any remaining temporal bone should be removed with a small rongeur or a rose burr bit. We advocate the use of bone wax to seal the exposed cancellous bone in the temporal area in order to prevent CSF leak.

The middle meningeal artery may bleed following fracture of the temporal bone due to trauma or surgical decompression. The bleeding can be controlled by using bipolar, bone wax or placing tenting sutures between the dura and skull edges in order to eliminate the dead space.

26.2.3 Durotomy and Duraplasty

Durotomy is a key element in DC as it decreases ICP substantially (Yoo et al. 1999). There are a multitude of techniques for opening the dura when performing hemicraniectomy. In the absence of hard evidence on the efficacy of the different techniques, we consider that an inverse T-shaped dural incision centred on the temporal lobe is preferable to other incisions centred more superiorly due to the increased decompression of the temporal region. Haematomas that can be easily accessed should be evacuated.

Regarding the duraplasty, the gold standard is a synthetic sutureless, non-adhesive, on-lay dura patch of variable materials. It is claimed that the on-lay collagen dural substitutes produce less tissue reaction and easier dissection of the dura-galea interface when the time has come to perform cranioplasty (Biroli et al. 2008; Horaczek et al. 2008). The use of double dural patch has been advocated by some neurosurgeons. In this technique, a second dural sheet is positioned to separate the inner dural patch from the temporal muscle in order to facilitate safe surgical dissection of the temporal muscle in the subsequent cranioplasty (Missori et al. 2008).

26.2.4 Closure

Due to the large surface area of the skin flap, an epidural drain is recommended in selected cases if there is concern about haemostasis (coagulopathy is common in trauma patients). The drain should be removed within 24 h. Suturing the temporal fascia should not be done due to the restrictive effect this can have on brain expansion. Instead, the skin is closed by subcutaneous sutures followed by cutaneous staples or sutures.

26.2.5 Bone Storage

Synthetic implants should be preferred in cranioplasty (Malcolm et al. 2018; van de Vijfeijken et al. 2018). Autologous bone should not be used in young patients and smokers or in case of a fracture in the bone flap (Dünisch et al. 2013; Korhonen et al. 2018). However, if cranioplasty using autologous bone is planned, the bone flap can be frozen, or it can be stored autologously. In the case of freezing, the bone flap is immediately dried off, marked and deep-frozen (at least −70 °C). We recommend obtaining swab sample before storage and discarding flaps with positive culture. Otherwise, the bone can be implanted in the subcutaneous tissue of the abdomen.

26.3 Acute-Phase Complications

An early postoperative CT should be performed to assess blossoming of contusions (Fig. 26.1b) and contralateral injuries that often increase (Fig. 26.3a) postoperatively due to the tamponading effect of preoperative intracranial hypertension. In case of a contralateral mass lesion following DC, a subsequent lesion evacuation is recommended if the prognosis of the patient is not futile. Furthermore, the CSF circulation is often influenced resulting in convexity hygromas (Fig. 26.3b) and ventriculomegaly. Usually these CSF abnormalities should be left untreated if possible, since cranioplasty usually rectifies the problem (Stiver, 2009). However, in some patients, CSF diversion is recommended with an adjustable valve to prevent excessive sinking flap syndrome (Timofeev et al. 2012).

Cerebral autoregulation may be compromised after DC resulting in hyperaemia, possibly contributing to brain swelling and worsening of the secondary injury.

26.4 Decompressive Craniectomy in Paediatric Patients

The current Guidelines for the Management of Pediatric Severe Traumatic Brain Injury reports Level III evidence for DC for controlling ICP in paediatric patients with severe TBI. More specifically, the evidence suggests DC in treating neurologic deterioration, brain herniation or intracranial hypertension refractory to conservative management (Kochanek et al. 2019).

In a systematic review, Ardissino et al. reported a possible benefit in the use of DC in paediatric patients with TBI for reducing high ICP (>25 mmHg) that is refractory to medical treatment. The authors reported that the quality of evidence remains extremely low, and the findings from RCTs exhibit substantial uncertainty in translating the benefits of DC into long-term neurological outcome (Ardissino et al. 2019). The only RCT included in the systematic review by Ardissino et al. was an older study by Taylor

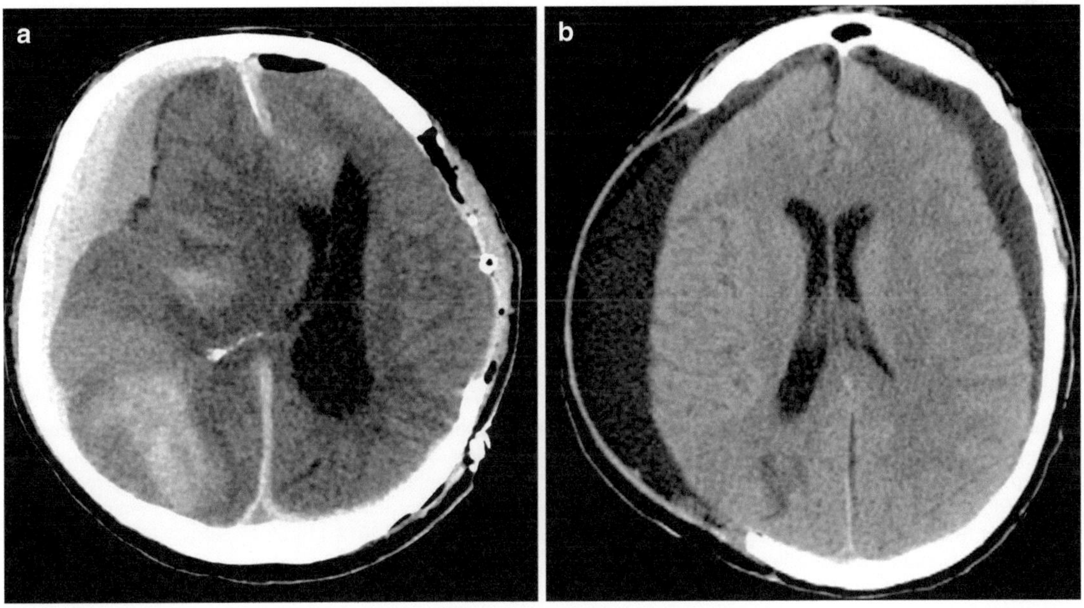

Fig. 26.3 (**a**) Severe contralateral postoperative subdural haematoma following DC (note too small decompression), (**b**) postoperative convexity hygroma that resolved after cranioplasty

et al. who studied the role of very early DC in paediatric patients with elevated ICP following TBI (Taylor et al. 2001). Altogether 27 patients were divided into (unconventional) bi-temporal DC following medical therapy and medical therapy alone groups. The results demonstrated reduced ICP and fewer episodes of intracranial hypertension in the DC group than in the conventional medical treatment group.

References

Ardissino M, Tang A, Muttoni E, Tsang K. Decompressive craniectomy in paediatric traumatic brain injury: a systematic review of current evidence. Childs Nerv Syst. 2019;35(2):209–16. https://doi.org/10.1007/s00381-018-3977-5.

Biroli F, Fusco M, Bani GG, Signorelli A, Esposito F, De Divitiis O, et al. Novel equine collagen-only dural substitute. Neurosurgery. 2008;62(3 Suppl 1):273–4. https://doi.org/10.1227/01.neu.0000317404.31336.69.

Bulstrode H, Nicoll JAR, Hudson G, Chinnery PF, Di Pietro V, Belli A. Mitochondrial DNA and traumatic brain injury. Ann Neurol. 2014;75(2):186–95.

Carney N, Totten AM, O'Reilly C, Ullman JS, Hawryluk GWJ, Bell MJ, et al. Guidelines for the Management of Severe Traumatic Brain Injury, Fourth Edition. Neurosurgery. 2017;80(1):6–15. https://doi.org/10.1227/NEU.0000000000001432.

Collaborators MRCCT, Perel P, Arango M, Clayton T, Edwards P, Komolafe E, et al. Predicting outcome after traumatic brain injury: practical prognostic models based on large cohort of international patients. BMJ (Clinical Research Ed). 2008;336:425–9.

Cooper DJ, Rosenfeld JV, Murray L, Arabi YM, Davies AR, D'Urso P, et al. Decompressive craniectomy in diffuse traumatic brain injury. N Engl J Med. 2011;364(16):1493–502. https://doi.org/10.1056/NEJMoa1102077.

De Bonis P, Sturiale CL, Anile C, Gaudino S, Mangiola A, Martucci M,et al. Decompressive craniectomy, interhemispheric hygroma and hydrocephalus: A timeline of events? Clin Neurol Neurosurg. 2013.

Dünisch P, Walter J, Sakr Y, Kalff R, Waschke A, Ewald C. Risk factors of aseptic bone resorption: a study after autologous bone flap reinsertion due to decompressive craniotomy. J Neurosurg. 2013;118(5):1141–7. https://doi.org/10.3171/2013.1.JNS12860.

Ergina PL, Cook JA, Blazeby JM, Boutron I, Clavien PA, Reeves BC, Seiler CM. Challenges in evaluating surgical innovation. Lancet. 2009;374(9695):1097–104. https://doi.org/10.1016/S0140-6736(09)61086-2.

Grindlinger G, Skavdahl D, Ecker R, Sanborn M. Decompressive craniectomy for severe traumatic brain injury: clinical study, literature review and meta-analysis. SpringerPlus. 2016;5:1605.

Güresir E, Schuss P, Vatter H, Raabe A, Seifert V, Beck J. Decompressive craniectomy in subarachnoid hemorrhage. Neurosurg Focus. 2009;26(6):E4. https://doi.org/10.3171/2009.3.FOCUS0954.

Horaczek JA, Zierski J, Graewe A. Collagen matrix in decompressive hemicraniectomy. Neurosurgery. 2008;63(1 Suppl):ONS176–81. https://doi.org/10.1227/01.NEU.0000312707.25073.CB.

Hutchinson PJ, Kolias AG, Timofeev IS, Corteen EA, Czosnyka M, Timothy J, et al. Trial of decompressive craniectomy for traumatic intracranial hypertension. N Engl J Med. 2016;375:1119–30. https://doi.org/10.1056/NEJMoa1605215.

Kelly DF, Kordestani RK, Martin NA, Nguyen T, Hovda DA, Bergsneider M, et al. Hyperemia following traumatic brain injury: relationship to intracranial hypertension and outcome. J Neurosurg. 1996;85:762–71. https://doi.org/10.3171/jns.1996.85.5.0762.

Kochanek P, Tasker R, Carney N, Totten A, Adelson P, Selden N, et al. Guidelines for the management of pediatric severe traumatic brain injury, Third Edition: update of the Brain Trauma Foundation guidelines. Pediatr Crit Care Med. 2019;20:S1–S82.

Kolias AG, Adams H, Timofeev I, Czosnyka M, Corteen EA, Pickard JD, et al. Decompressive craniectomy following traumatic brain injury: developing the evidence base. Br J Neurosurg. 2016;30(2):246–50. https://doi.org/10.3109/02688697.2016.1159655.

Korhonen TK, Tetri S, Huttunen J, Lindgren A, Piitulainen JM, Serlo W, et al. Predictors of primary autograft cranioplasty survival and resorption after craniectomy on behalf of the Finnish National Cranial Implant Registry (FiNCIR) study group. J Neurosurg. 2018;130:1409–788. https://doi.org/10.3171/2017.12.jns172013.

Kurzbuch AR. Does size matter? Decompressive surgery under review. Neurosurg Rev. 2015;38(4):629–40. https://doi.org/10.1007/s10143-015-0626-2.

Logsdon AF, Lucke-Wold BP, Turner RC, Huber JD, Rosen CL, Simpkins JW. Role of microvascular disruption in brain damage from traumatic brain injury. Compr Physiol. 2015;5(3):1147–60. https://doi.org/10.1002/cphy.c140057.

Maegele M, Schöchl H, Menovsky T, Maréchal H, Marklund N, Buki A, Stanworth S. Coagulopathy and haemorrhagic progression in traumatic brain injury: advances in mechanisms, diagnosis, and management. Lancet Neurol. 2017;16(8):630–47. https://doi.org/10.1016/S1474-4422(17)30197-7.

Malcolm JG, Mahmooth Z, Rindler RS, Allen JW, Grossberg JA, Pradilla G, Ahmad FU. Autologous cranioplasty is associated with increased reoperation rate: a systematic review and meta-analysis. World Neurosurg. 2018;116:60–8. https://doi.org/10.1016/j.wneu.2018.05.009.

Missori P, Polli FM, Peschillo S, D'Avella E, Paolini S, Miscusi M. Double dural patch in decompressive craniectomy to preserve the temporal muscle: technical note. Surg Neurol. 2008;70(4):437–9. https://doi.org/10.1016/j.surneu.2007.03.029.

Qiu W, Guo C, Shen H, Chen K, Wen L, Huang H, et al. Effects of unilateral decompressive craniectomy on patients with unilateral acute post-traumatic brain swelling after severe traumatic brain injury. Crit Care (London, England). 2009;13(6):R185. https://doi.org/10.1186/cc8178.

Sahuquillo J, Arikan F. Decompressive craniectomy for the treatment of refractory high intracranial pressure in traumatic brain injury. Cochrane Database Syst Rev. 2006;12:CD003983. https://doi.org/10.1002/14651858.CD003983.pub2.

Steyerberg EW, Mushkudiani N, Perel P, Butcher I, Lu J, McHugh GS, et al. Predicting outcome after traumatic brain injury: development and international validation of prognostic scores based on admission characteristics. PLoS Med. 2008;5:e165; discussion e165.

Stocchetti N, Maas A. Traumatic intracranial hypertension. N Engl J Med. 2014;371(10):972. https://doi.org/10.1056/NEJMra1208708.

Taylor A, Butt W, Rosenfeld J, Shann F, Ditchfield M, Lewis E, et al. A randomized trial of very early decompressive craniectomy in children with traumatic brain injury and sustained intracranial hypertension. Childs Nerv Syst. 2001;17(3):154–62. https://doi.org/10.1007/s003810000410.

Timofeev I, Santarius T, Kolias AG, Hutchinson PJA. Decompressive craniectomy - operative technique and perioperative care. Adv Tech Stand Neurosurg. 2012;38:115–36.

Unterberg AW, Stover J, Kress B, Kiening KL. Edema and brain trauma. Neuroscience. 2004;129(4):1019–27. https://doi.org/10.1016/j.neuroscience.2004.06.046.

van de Vijfeijken SECM, Münker TJAG, Spijker R, Karssemakers LHE, Vandertop WP, Becking AG, et al. Autologous bone is inferior to alloplastic cranioplasties: safety of autograft and allograft materials for cranioplasties, a systematic review. World Neurosurg. 2018;117:443–452.e8. https://doi.org/10.1016/j.wneu.2018.05.193.

Wilson MH. Monro-Kellie 2.0: the dynamic vascular and venous pathophysiological components of intracranial pressure. J Cereb Blood Flow Metab. 2016;36(8):1338–50. https://doi.org/10.1177/0271678X16648711.

Wilson JT, Pettigrew LE, Teasdale GM. Structured interviews for the Glasgow Outcome Scale and the extended Glasgow Outcome Scale: guidelines for their use. J Neurotrauma. 1998;15:573–85.

Yoo DS, Kim DS, Cho KS, Huh PW, Park CK, Kang JK. Ventricular pressure monitoring during bilateral decompression with dural expansion. J Neurosurg. 1999;91(6):953–9. https://doi.org/10.3171/jns.1999.91.6.0953.

27 Skull Fractures

Pål André Rønning and Tor Brommeland

Recommendations

Level I

There are insufficient data to support a Level I recommendation for this topic.

Level II

There are insufficient data to support a Level II recommendation for this topic.

Level III

Open fractures, vault fractures depressed more than one bone width and cosmetically disfiguring fractures should be operated.

27.1 Overview

Fractures of the skull can be divided into fractures of the vault or the base of the skull. Such fractures are quite common and are important to acknowledge because they are associated with a risk of intracranial haematomas, CSF leakage and meningitis. Open fractures or fractures through the sinuses predispose to intracranial infections and they can be cosmetically disfiguring.

P. A. Rønning (✉)
Department of Neurosurgery, Oslo University Hospital Rikshospitalet, Oslo, Norway

T. Brommeland
Department of Neurosurgery, Oslo University Hospital Ullevål, Oslo, Norway
e-mail: torbro@ous-hf.no

27.2 Background

27.2.1 Vault Fractures

Vault fractures are common. They can be further divided into open or closed and depressed or non-depressed fractures. Fractures of the vault have a tendency to cause epidural haemorrhage which may be arterial or venous in nature. Usually, the arterial haematomas are caused by a bony spicula tearing the middle meningeal artery. The venous haematomas are usually secondary to oozing from the fracture edges and have a tendency to expand slower than the arterial haematomas.

Tips, Tricks and Pitfalls

- The skin incision must provide good exposure of the fracture.
- The dura should be inspected for lacerations, and a watertight dura seal should be attempted in case of CSF leakage. In case of rhinorrhea and anterior skull base fracture, we advise a multilayer

© Springer Nature Switzerland AG 2020
T. Sundstrøm et al. (eds.), *Management of Severe Traumatic Brain Injury*,
https://doi.org/10.1007/978-3-030-39383-0_27

reconstruction including a vascularized autologous pericranium layer.
- Minimize the use of synthetic substitutes in patients with open fractures to prevent infection.
- Tack-up sutures surrounding the fracture site should be placed to prevent postoperative epidural haematomas.

Fracture lines crossing a venous sinus may cause complete or partial thrombosis of the vein (Slasky et al. 2017). This may be demonstrated with a CT venography. In some instances, antithrombotic treatment with low-molecular-weight heparin may be indicated.

The indications for surgery of vault fractures are based on the following (Bullock et al. 2006):

1. *Infection*: open fractures expose dura and/or the brain to microorganisms.
2. *Cosmetics*: fractures depressed more than one bone width have a tendency for disfiguration.
3. *Function*: depressed fractures (or haematomas secondary to the fracture) may cause symptoms such as epileptic seizures and neurological deficits.

27.2.1.1 Operative Technique

Plan the incision to fully expose the fractured area. After exposure, accessing the dura is essential; this can be obtained by elevating the bone fragment with a periosteal elevator. If the fragments are wedged, a burr hole is placed clearly outside the fractured area and a craniotomy surrounding the fracture complex is performed. The fragments are carefully collected and saved. Any epidural haematoma is evacuated, and we also advise a small durotomy if there is bluish discoloration or a more tense dura than anticipated to rule out a subdural haematoma. Next, the dura is sewn watertight before tack-up sutures are placed between the dura and the bone edges (and centrally if the bone flap is large.) Fracture fragments can be reassembled into a large bone flap by using plates and multiple microscrews or similar devices. The assembled bone flap is then reattached in a normal fashion.

In case of an open fracture, the skin edge needs thorough debridement before closure, and we advise for proper antibiotic prophylaxis.

In the case of comminute fractures where it is impossible to reassemble the bone, there are several options: make a split bone graft utilizing the contralateral skull with a similar curvature or use a material for bone replacement, e.g. bone cement, prefabricated bone substitutes, etc. (Kakar et al. 2009).

27.2.2 Skull Base Fractures

Clinical signs of skull base fractures may be haematotympanum, racoon eyes, Battle's sign, otorrhoea, rhinorrhoea or cranial nerve dysfunction. Fractures through the base of the skull are divided into fractures through the anterior, middle and posterior fossa. The latter entity will not be further discussed. The important factors to consider when dealing with skull base fractures are:

- *CSF leakage:* this can manifest as rhinorrhoea and/or otorrhoea. The fluid leak results from dural and arachnoid lacerations with fistula formation.
- *Infection*: CSF leaks represent a corridor for bacteria to gain access to the CSF space.
- *Vessel and nerve injury*: vessels and nerves have an intimate relationship with the skull base; hence, fractures through the base of the skull can manifest with cranial nerve deficits (I, II, VI, VII and VIII most often) and vessel injury. Notably, temporal bone fractures may cause both sensorineural and conductive hearing loss.

The diagnosis of CSF leakage can be made by detecting clear discharge from the nose or ear in the presence of a known skull base fracture with pneumocephalus. When the leak is minimal, the diagnosis can be much more difficult. CSF contains 60% of serum glucose; however, nasal discharge also has glucose present and discharge with a positive glucose test has a high sensitivity, but low specificity for CSF leakage. Differentiating CSF from mucosal discharge can be made by the presence of beta-2-transferrin or beta-trace protein in the discharge, but the tests are not always readily available (Davies and Teo 1995). After verifying that the leaking fluid indeed is CSF, the site of leakage must be identified. If there is pneumocephalus and obvious fracture fragments tearing the dura, the leak site can usually be identified rather easily. It can, however, be difficult to pinpoint the exact location of the CSF leakage. Usually, CT with thin cuts can provide a plausible leak site; further diagnosis requires either MR or CT cisternography.

In most cases of CSF leakage associated with skull base fractures, the leak spontaneously ceases within the first 10–12 days. Within this time frame, the risk of developing meningitis is rather low. The use of prophylactic antibiotics in patients with posttraumatic CSF leakage is not indicated (Ratilal et al. 2011). We recommend lumbar drainage and bed rest in order to accelerate the resolution of leakage. The amount of CSF drained must be balanced with respect to leakage resolution, and the patient must be clinically monitored for symptoms of overdrainage.

Treatment of cranial nerve deficits secondary to skull base fractures and their management have a poor evidence base. Some advocate the use of steroids, whilst others recommend decompression of the affected nerve (Samii and Tatagiba 2002). The complexity of the anatomy also plays an important role, and decompressive temporal bone facial nerve surgery is rarely indicated, whilst decompression of the optic nerve has better documentation and is easier to perform.

In the acute setting, indications for surgery are:

1. CSF leaks and fractures where the prospect of resolution is deemed very unlikely
2. CSF leaks that do not resolve within 14 days
3. Cranial nerve deficits in progression

In the chronic setting, recurrent meningitis is also an indication for surgery.

27.2.2.1 Operative Technique

The basic goal is to achieve reasonable bony continuity, decompress neural structures and patch the dura defect. In the case of a large comminute anterior skull base fracture with CSF leakage, a bi-coronal incision is planned. The periosteum is left intact with a vascularized pedicle so that it can be used later as a dura patch. Burr holes are placed over the superior sagittal sinus, and a large bi-frontal craniotomy is made, ensuring adequate access to the floor of the anterior fossa. If the frontal sinus is opened, the mucosa should be removed. Instruments used for this purpose are contaminated by nasal pathogens and should be resterilized before further use. Next, the dura is dissected free from the anterior skull base (as far posterior as the planum sphenoidale), and the bony skull base is reconstructed if necessary. Most likely, this will entail tearing both olfactory nerves at the thin lamina cribrosa. Next, the dura is opened, and the sagittal sinus and falx is ligated and cut at the anteriormost end. Subfrontal dissection then allows basofrontal contusions to be removed, and the intradural floor can be carpeted using a dura substitute (artificial or fascia lata). Next, the dura is closed, and the epidural skull base can be glued with the pedicled periosteum flap or another dura substitute for a sandwich reconstruction of the basofrontal dura. Finally, the bone flap is reattached, and the skin is closed (Scholsem et al. 2008).

Postoperatively, care must be taken with respect to positive pressure ventilation to prevent pneumocephalus. The patient should be covered prophylactically for upper respiratory tract microorganisms for the ensuing 5 days.

27.3 Specific Paediatric Concerns

Particular attention should be paid to children who sustain a diastatic fracture. Rarely, these fractures have a dural tear that subsequently can provide the nidus for a growing skull fracture whereby a leptomeningeal cyst with or without brain parenchyma protrudes through the bony opening. Symptoms and signs indicative of a growing fracture include a diastatic fracture that fails to fuse, progressive neurological symptoms and/or seizures. Particularly patients under the age of 3 with a cephalohaematoma and a diastatic fracture should be followed up closely.

A "ping-pong fracture" is a localized bony impression of the skull vault caused by a direct, focal trauma to the head. It resembles the look of a ping-pong ball after compression with a finger. If cosmetically disfiguring, these fractures should be operated. A craniotomy around the fracture complex with remodelling of the bone and reattachment using small plates and screws may be performed. In the very young child, the skull bone has considerable plasticity, and the depressed fracture may be elevated by a small periosteal elevator passed under the bone through a burr hole lateral to the injury.

References

Bullock MR, Chesnut R, Ghajar J, Gordon D, Hartl R, Newell DW, Servadei F, Walters BC, Wilberger J. Surgical management of depressed cranial fractures. Neurosurgery. 2006;58:S56–60.

Davies MA, Teo C. Management of traumatic cerebrospinal fluid fistula. J Craniomaxillofac Trauma. 1995;1:9–17.

Kakar V, Nagaria J, John KP. The current status of decompressive craniectomy. Br J Neurosurg. 2009;23:147–57.

Ratilal BO, Costa J, Sampaio C, Pappamikail L. Antibiotic prophylaxis for preventing meningitis in patients with basilar skull fractures. Cochrane Database Syst Rev. 2011;(8):CD004884. https://doi.org/10.1002/14651858.CD004884.pub3.

Samii M, Tatagiba M. Skull base trauma: diagnosis and management. Neurol Res. 2002;24:147–56.

Scholsem M, Scholtes F, Collignon F, Robe P, Dubuisson A, Kaschten B, Lenelle J, Martin D. Surgical management of anterior cranial base fractures with cerebrospinal fluid fistulae: a single-institution experience. Neurosurgery. 2008;62:463–9.

Slasky SE, Rivaud Y, Suberlak M, Tairu O, Fox AD, Ohman-Strickland P, et al. Venous sinus thrombosis in blunt trauma: incidence and risk factors. J Comput Assist Tomogr. 2017;41:891–7.

28 Vessel Injuries

Pål André Rønning and Tor Brommeland

Recommendations

Level I

There are insufficient data to support a Level I recommendation for this topic.

Level II

There are insufficient data to support a Level II recommendation for this topic.

Level III

The radiological investigation of choice is CT angiography. The goal of therapy is to prevent further neurological injury by maintaining sufficient cerebral blood flow and preventing embolic incidents.

28.1 Overview

Vessel injuries are uncommon but potentially devastating to the patient. Both blunt and penetrating trauma to the head can result in vessel injury. We will here divide vessel injuries into extracranial and intracranial vessel injuries.

They are both difficult to diagnose without special contrast-enhanced radiological investigations, and a high index of suspicion must be entertained (Vertinsky et al. 2008). The vessel pathology itself can be divided into:

- Dissection—a tear in the intima leaves a highly thrombogenic intimal flap in the vessel lumen and a haematoma can develop in the vessel wall. Hence, blood flow can be impeded by both thrombosis and mural haematoma. Distal blood flow can be influenced due to embolic phenomena from the local thrombosis.
- True aneurysms—focal outpouching from an injured vessel where at least one layer of the vessel wall is intact.
- Pseudoaneurysms—focal outpouching from an injured vessel where all vessel wall layers are compromised, leaving just an organized haematoma as the barrier to further bleeding.

Both true aneurysms and pseudoaneurysms have turbulent blood flow and can serve as a nidus for thrombosis and subsequent embolization.

P. A. Rønning (✉) · T. Brommeland
Department of Neurosurgery, Oslo University Hospital Rikshospitalet, Oslo, Norway

Department of Neurosurgery, Oslo University Hospital Ullevål, Oslo, Norway
e-mail: torbro@ous-hf.no

© Springer Nature Switzerland AG 2020
T. Sundstrøm et al. (eds.), *Management of Severe Traumatic Brain Injury*,
https://doi.org/10.1007/978-3-030-39383-0_28

Tips, Tricks and Pitfalls

- Maintain a high index of suspicion for vessel injury when there is:
  - Discrepancy between plain CT findings and the clinical state of the patient
  - Subarachnoid haemorrhage in the interhemispheric fissure
  - Fractures in close proximity to vessels

28.2 Background

28.2.1 Extracranial Vessel Injury

The incidence of blunt carotid or vertebral injury (BCVI) in hospitalized trauma patients is 1–2% (Weber et al. 2018; Esnault et al. 2017). In patients with severe head injury (initial GCS < 9), the incidence may be as high as 9% and BCVI is also clearly associated with major facial injury, as well as cervical spine fractures. The usual mechanism of injury is dissection with formation of a thrombus, wall hematoma or pseudoaneurysm. These processes may narrow the vessel lumen or shed an embolus to a more peripheral brain artery and result in a stroke.

The true risk of a stroke in patients with extracranial vessel injury is unknown, but the literature indicates around 11% with a mortality rate of approximately 26% (Weber et al. 2018). The time interval from injury to onset of cerebral ischemia itself is difficult to pinpoint, but from 1 to 72 h has been documented. Penetrating injuries more often transect the vessel or parts of the vessel and thereby expose the patient to compromised blood flow and significant blood loss. Explosions and ballistic injuries can cause dissections due to the shock wave resulting in an intima tear.

Several screening criteria have been developed for the detection of BCVI of which we recommend the expanded Denver criteria (Table 28.1) (Geddes et al. 2016). The most important risk factor for BCVI is a high-energy trauma mechanism in combination with severe TBI (GCS < 9), cervical spine fracture, severe

Table 28.1 The expanded Denver screening criteria for BCVI

Signs/symptoms of BCVI
Arterial haemorrhage from the neck/nose/mouth
Cervical bruit in patients <50 years
Expanding cervical haematoma
Focal neurological deficit
Neurological exam incongruous with head CT findings
Stroke on secondary CT scan
Risk factors for BVCI High-energy transfer mechanism with:
Le Fort II or III
Mandible fracture
Complex skull fracture/basilar skull fracture/occipital condyle fracture
Severe traumatic brain injury (TBI) with GCS < 6
Cervical spine fracture, subluxation or ligamentous injury at any level
Near-hanging with anoxic brain injury
Seat belt abrasion with significant swelling, pain or altered mental status
TBI with thoracic injury
Scalp degloving
Thoracic vascular injury
Blunt cardiac rupture
Upper rib fracture

CT angiography is indicated if one or more of the criteria are present

facial injury (Le Fort 2 and 3) or skull base fractures.

The radiological investigation of choice is CT angiography (CTA) (Roberts et al. 2013). It is readily available, fast and easily performed in a trauma setting. Usually, this is sufficient to exclude extracranial vessel injury, but MRI can provide further confirmation and also information on possible infarction.

The goal of therapy is to prevent further neurological injury by maintaining sufficient cerebral blood flow and preventing embolic incidents. Therapeutic options are anticoagulation/platelet inhibition or endovascular intervention. Both heparin/low-molecular-weight heparin (LMWH) and platelet inhibitors are options for preventing further thrombosis and embolic events. There is insufficient documentation to recommend one over the other, but a reasonable algorithm is to start with medical therapy such as LMWH with transition to acetylsalicylic acid (Harrigan et al.

2013; Brommeland et al. 2018). Endovascular intervention is usually reserved for cases with embolic events despite medical therapy. The natural history of these lesions shows a strong tendency towards spontaneous healing within the first couple of months. Treatment length for traumatic dissections has not been determined, but 3 months may be sufficient. A control CTA should be performed before stopping medical therapy.

Less often, patients present with an extracranial carotid or vertebral aneurysm. They can demonstrate symptoms secondary to embolization, rupture or local volume effect. Therapy is controversial; their natural history shows a clear tendency towards regression, but anticoagulation is often indicated to prevent embolization. However, they should be subject to repeated radiological investigations. Enlargement, embolization and severe compressive symptoms should mandate consultation with expertise proficient in either flow-sparing therapy (suturing the aneurysm sac, resection and anastomosis or endovascular stent therapy) or flow-stopping therapy (balloon occlusion test with subsequent ligation/coiling or bypass).

28.2.2 Intracranial Vessel Injury

These are divided into arteriovenous fistulas (AVF), traumatic aneurysms, thrombosis and sinus injuries.

28.2.2.1 Arteriovenous Fistulas

The most common traumatic AVF is the carotid-cavernous fistula. Symptoms are related to arterialization, volume and increased venous pressure and include headache, chemosis, ptosis, ophthalmoplegia and visual loss. CTA can give hints to the presence of an AVF (arterialized cavernous sinus and increased size of ophtalmic vein), but digital subtraction angiography (DSA) is mandatory to further elucidate the flow pattern. If it is a direct carotid-cavernous fistula (direct connection between ICA and the cavernous sinus), occlusion of the fistula is warranted to prevent neurological deterioration; however, if it is an indirect fistula (a fistula within the leaves of the cavernous sinus that are fed by intracavernous branches of the internal and/or external carotid artery), spontaneous thrombosis of the fistula can occur and conservative treatment may be sufficient. Usually, endovascular embolization of the fistula is the method of choice in treating both direct and indirect carotid cavernous fistulas.

28.2.2.2 Traumatic Aneurysms

These are rare, comprising less than 1% of all intracranial aneurysms (Semple 2004). Compared with 'spontaneous' aneurysms, they have a larger propensity for bleeding: 50% rupture within the first week. This can be explained by the fact that these aneurysms are pseudoaneurysms. They also have a clear predilection for more distal localizations than spontaneous aneurysms, especially the A3 + 4 segments of the anterior cerebral arteries. They also show a clear tendency for rapid growth, and regular controls are warranted if indications for surgery have not already been made. A high index of suspicion must be maintained in patients admitted with penetrating injuries, where the offending object has been in close vicinity of the vessel; in patients with localized subarachnoid clots; in patients with large bleeds in the basal cisterns; in patients with fractures of the clivus, sphenoid sinus or medial temporal bone; and in patients exposed to shock waves. Data on the sensitivity of CTA compared with DSA is lacking with regards to traumatic aneurysms. However, if there are any irregularities on the CTA, we recommend DSA, as it better reveals the hallmarks of traumatic aneurysms: delayed emptying and filling of the aneurysm, irregular contours and absence of a neck. Obliteration of these aneurysms is usually recommended.

The method of choice has traditionally been open surgery due to the lack of a neck and the poor strength of the aneurysm wall making traumatic aneurysms poor candidates for endovascular treatment. However, there are now several reports claiming good results using combined endovascular stentassisted coiling (Cohen et al. 2008). During surgery, these aneurysms have been notorious for their intraoperative tendency for rupture and difficult clip reconstruction, necessitating wrapping, ligation or trapping with or without bypass (Semple 2004).

28.2.2.3 Traumatic Occlusion

The most common intracranial vessel to be occluded is the proximal intracranial ICA where the vessel is in intimate contact with bone. Fractures in the vicinity of the ICA should arouse concern and mandate an angiographic examination. CTA is usually sufficient, but if there are any irregularities, we advocate DSA. The occlusion is usually secondary to dissection with subsequent mural haematoma and thrombosis. Rates of 70–85% suffering from massive hemispheric infarction have been reported. However, the patency of the circle of Willis clearly plays a role, and previous reports are hampered by obvious selection bias. We advocate anticoagulation and perfusion studies to elucidate whether the cross-flow is adequate. In case of perfusion asymmetry, we recommend increasing the blood pressure and preferably utilize some form of metabolic monitoring in the affected hemisphere. There are also case reports on vascular augmentation procedures. In case the patient has already sustained a massive infarction, we generally discourage decompressive hemicraniectomy.

28.2.2.4 Dural Sinus Injury

Fractures extending across major dural sinuses can potentially tear the vessel wall and produce an extracerebral haemorrhage, usually an epidural haematoma. If an indication for evacuation is found, one should make arrangements for a potentially large haemorrhage when the bone flap is raised. Usually, the sinus tear is found and can be plugged with a finger while contemplating the next move. Depending on the size of the tear, a small piece of Tachosil® or similar material and slight pressure might be sufficient, but if large parts of the sinus are torn, reconstruction is recommended. Temporary occlusion using aneurysm clips to visualize the rent while reconstructing the vessel using sutures and an overlay of dura can be done, but depending on the sinus involved, occlusion can increase the pressure with subsequent herniation. A few case reports indicate that if the patient does not tolerate temporary sinus occlusion, a Fogarty® catheter can be inserted and used as a bypass vehicle while the sinus is reconstructed.

28.3 Specific Paediatric Concerns

There are no specific paediatric concerns for this subject.

References

Brommeland, et al. Best practice guidelines for the management of cerebrovascular injury. Scand J Trauma Resusc Emerg Med. Scand J Trauma Resusc Emerg Med. 2018;26(1):90. https://doi.org/10.1186/s13049-018-0559-1.

Cohen, et al. Results of endovascular treatment of traumatic intracranial aneurysms. Neurosurgery. 2008;63:476–85; discussion 485–6. https://doi.org/10.1227/01.NEU.0000324995.57376.79.

Esnault, et al. Blunt cerebrovascular injuries in severe traumatic brain injury: incidence, risk factors, and evolution. J Neurosurg. 2017;127(1):16–22.

Geddes, et al. Expanded screening criteria for blunt cerebrovascular injury: a bigger impact than anticipated. Am J Surg. 2016;212(6):1167–74.

Harrigan, et al. Management of vertebral artery injuries following non-penetrating cervical trauma. Neurosurgery. 2013;72(Suppl 2):234–43.

Roberts, et al. Diagnostic accuracy of computed tomographic angiography for blunt cerebrovascular injury detection in trauma patients: a systematic review and meta-analysis. Ann Surg. 2013;257(4):621–32.

Semple P. Traumatic aneurysms. In: LeRoux PD, Winn H, Newell DW, editors. Management of cerebral aneurysms. Philadelphia: Saunders; 2004. p. 397–408.

Vertinsky, AT et al. Comparison of multidetector CT angiography and MR imaging of cervical artery dissection. AJNR Am J Neuroradiol. 2008;29(9):1753–60. https://doi.org/10.3174/ajnr.A1189.

Weber, et al. Blunt cerebrovascular injury and stroke in severely injured patients: an international multi center analysis. World J Surg. 2018;42(7):2043–53.

Insertion of Intracranial Monitoring Devices

29

Zandra Olivecrona and Bo-Michael Bellander

Recommendations

Level I

Data are insufficient to support a Level I recommendation for this topic.

Level II

A measuring device for intracranial pressure should be inserted in salvageable TBI patients with an abnormal computed tomography scan and a GCS score of 3–8.

Management of severe TBI patients using information from ICP monitoring is recommended to reduce in-hospital and 2-week post-injury mortality.

Level III

Intracranial pressure should be measured in all unconscious patients with a severe TBI and normal CT scan if two of the following features are noted at admission: age over 40 years, unilateral or bilateral motor posturing (GCS M < 4), and/or systolic blood pressure less than 90 mmHg.

ICP monitoring should be considered in TBI patients who require urgent surgery for extracranial injuries, who need mechanical ventilation because of extracranial injuries, or who evidence progression of pathology on CT imaging or clinical deterioration.

Brain tissue oxygen monitoring can help to guide treatment towards improved brain oxygenation.

Brain temperature measurement can help to guide treatment towards normothermia.

Cerebral microdialysis is a reliable and safe technique that is used in the clinical management of neurocritical care patients and in particular those with severe TBI.

Tips, Tricks, and Pitfalls

- When the map is different from the landscape, the landscape is right! Be aware of technical malfunction, and do not trust monitoring values blindly.
- Two monitors telling the same story are more convincing than just one.

Z. Olivecrona (✉)
Department of Medical Sciences, Faculty of Medicine, Örebro University, Örebro, Sweden

Section for Neurosurgery, Department of Anaesthesia and Intensive Care, University Hospital, Örebro, Sweden
e-mail: zandra.olivecrona@regionorebrolan.se

B.-M. Bellander
Department of Clinical Neuroscience, Karolinska Institutet, Stockholm, Sweden

Department of Neurosurgery, Karolinska University Hospital, Stockholm, Sweden
e-mail: bo-michael.bellander@sll.se

© Springer Nature Switzerland AG 2020
T. Sundstrøm et al. (eds.), *Management of Severe Traumatic Brain Injury*,
https://doi.org/10.1007/978-3-030-39383-0_29

- Always consider inserting an EVD in the early phase of treatment.
- When ICP monitoring is indicated, also consider adding brain tissue oximetry and microdialysis.
- It is not the values but what you do with the values that improves outcome.

29.1 Overview

There are two main methods of measuring ICP: via parenchymal ICP probes or external ventricular drains (EVD). ICP data can indicate progress of intracranial pathology and can be used to calculate and manage cerebral perfusion pressure (CPP). ICP monitoring through an EVD also permits therapeutic drainage of CSF. Cerebral blood flow (CBF) probes, oxygen tension catheters and microdialysis can be used to assess regional events but may fail to detect harmful events in other parts of the brain. Conversely, more global approaches (venous oxygen saturation) fail to detect regional abnormalities (Maas et al. 2008). Multimodal monitoring is generally considered state-of-the-art, including ICP, $P_{BT}O_2$ and microdialysis.

Intracranial monitoring is not without risk of complications. Obstruction and subsequent malfunction of an EVD occur in approximately 6% of patients (Bavetta et al. 1996). The risk of infection is higher with EVDs (up to 10%) compared to intraparenchymal ICP catheters (close to 0%) (Hagel et al. 2014; Koskinen and Olivecrona 2005). The risk of haemorrhagic complications is between 1 (Bratton et al. 2007a, b) and 5% (Kakarla et al. 2008) with EVDs, but very low (3 out of approximately 1000 patients) with intraparenchymal ICP catheters (Koskinen and Olivecrona 2005; Koskinen et al. 2013). Clinically significant infections and haemorrhage associated with ICP devices are relatively rare and should not deter the decision to monitor ICP.

29.2 Background

29.2.1 Intracranial Pressure (ICP) and Cerebral Perfusion Pressure (CPP)

The main objective of neurointensive monitoring is to maintain adequate cerebral perfusion and oxygenation to ensure an optimal balance between cerebral blood flow and metabolism and to avoid secondary insults while the brain recovers.

Elevated ICP may be the first indicator of progressive intracranial pathology. Intracranial hypertension is found in 30–75% of patients with severe TBI (Narayan et al. 1982; Eisenberg et al. 1990) and is an independent predictor of mortality (Badri et al. 2012). Preventive treatment of an unknown, perhaps increased ICP, is not without risks (Bratton et al. 2007a, b).

The recommendations regarding ICP monitoring in the third edition of the Brain Trauma Foundation (BTF) guidelines were mainly based on observational studies (Bratton et al. 2007a, b). The recommendations were:

- “Intracranial pressure (ICP) should be monitored in all salvageable patients with severe traumatic brain injury (TBI; Glasgow Coma Scale (GCS) of 3–8 after resuscitation) and an abnormal computed tomography (CT) scan”.
- “ICP monitoring is indicated in patients with TBI with normal CT scan if two or more of the following features are noted at admission: age over 40, unilateral or bilateral motor posturing, or systolic blood pressure (BP) < 90 mmHg”.

In a recent trial, Chesnut and colleagues failed to detect a statistical difference between patients randomized to ICP monitoring versus no ICP monitoring (Chesnut et al. 2012). Based on this study, the BTF changed their recommendations to Level IIB in the fourth edition of the BTF guidelines:

- "Management of severe TBI patients using information from ICP monitoring is recommended to reduce in-hospital and 2-week post-injury mortality".

ICP monitoring is still the gold standard for guiding therapy and is considered in all patients with severe TBI. It is also necessary for calculation of CPP. Systemic hypotension and intracranial hypertension reduce CPP, and this has a negative impact on outcome especially when autoregulation is impaired (Guiza et al. 2017).

CPP is an indirect measure of cerebral perfusion that incorporates mean arterial blood pressure (MAP) and ICP: CPP = MAP – ICP. Both MAP and ICP are dependent on the choice of zero-points. Blood pressure is, according to the new BTF guidelines, by convention calibrated to the level of the right atrium of the heart (Carney et al. 2017). This contrasts the seminal paper from Rosner and co-workers, where the MAP was measured in supine patients at the level of the middle cranial fossa to estimate transcranial perfusion (Rosner et al. 1995). In a recent UK study, it was found that the heart was used as zero-point for MAP in 58% of the participating neurosurgical intensive care units, while 42% used the tragus a zero-point. As 84% nurse their patients in 30° head-up position, the difference in CPP can be substantial between centres (Thomas et al. 2015). In a similar survey from Scandinavia, it was estimated that CPP differed up to 23 mmHg between centres, based on differences in patient positioning and zero-points for MAP (Stubhaug et al. 2003). Thus, this is important to keep in mind when using CPP-targeted therapy and when reading or writing scientific literature on CPP measurements.

However, ICP and CPP monitoring provides limited information regarding other important factors in TBI pathophysiology, such as cerebral blood flow (CBF) and metabolism. Further, it does not eliminate the risk of cerebral hypoxia (Gracias et al. 2004; Okonkwo et al. 2017).

29.2.2 Brain Tissue Oximetry ($P_{BT}O_2$)

To prevent secondary brain injuries, the brain is reliant of adequate supply of oxygen and metabolic substrates. This is a function of the oxygen content, as well as the glucose level of the blood reaching the brain (Fox et al. 1988). Development of monitoring systems that can provide information on CBF and metabolism has been a long-standing goal in neurocritical care. Notably, the depth and duration of tissue hypoxia is an independent predictor of unfavourable outcome and death (van den Brink et al. 2000).

Several brain tissue oxygen monitoring systems that continuously monitor brain oxygen partial pressure ($P_{BT}O_2$) are available. Jugular bulb measurement of oxygen content in the cerebral venous outflow can be used to estimate brain oxygen saturation, and this technique has been around for many years. Furthermore, methods to monitor cerebral perfusion bed side have been developed, including thermal diffusion probes, transcranial Doppler, near-infrared spectroscopy and jugular venous saturation monitors.

Studies indicate that directing treatment to improve brain oxygenation might benefit the patient more than conventional ICP-/CPP-targeted treatment. Most of these studies conclude that low $P_{BT}O_2$ (<10–15 mmHg over 30 min) increases both mortality and morbidity (Bardt et al. 1998; Valadka et al. 1998; Van den Brink et al. 2000; Stiefel et al. 2005; Narotam et al. 2009; Spiotta et al. 2010; Okonkwo et al. 2017). However, other studies have not been able to confirm these findings (Martini et al. 2009; Green et al. 2013; McCarthy et al. 2009), and the BTF therefore downgraded the recommendations for brain tissue oxygen monitoring in the fourth edition (Carney et al. 2017).

29.2.3 Intracerebral Microdialysis

Monitoring of regional cerebral metabolism is possible to perform using intracerebral microdialysis, and this is a reliable and safe technique.

A decreasing level of glucose together with increasing lactate/pyruvate ratio (LPR) warns of a developing metabolic crisis. LPR can be used to differentiate ischaemic from non-ischaemic causes of energy dysfunction and is an important complement to classical intracranial monitors (Hutchinson et al. 2015).

Microdialysis allows the chemistry of the extracellular interstitial fluid to be monitored continuously. Microdialysis is a complementary technique to ICP, CPP and $P_{BT}O_2$, providing additional information on substrate delivery and metabolism at the cellular level. At a consensus meeting on the use of microdialysis in TBI in 2015, the following recommendations were provided (Hutchinson et al. 2015):

- In diffuse TBI, placing the catheter in the right (non-dominant) frontal lobe is recommended.
- In focal TBI, there are different options for catheter placement that depend on whether the goal is to monitor tissue at risk or normal brain, e.g. to guide systemic glucose treatment.
- Where there is a focal lesion, catheter placement ipsilateral to the lesion and in radiographically normal brain is recommended if feasible.
- Multiple catheters are an option in focal TBI, e.g. placed at craniotomy for a focal lesion into perilesional brain with a contralateral "bolt" catheter in radiographically normal brain.
- Stereotactic placement is an option but rarely practical.

Assessment of microdialysis is thoroughly described elsewhere in this book, but as a rule of thumb, glucose >1 mmol/L and lactate/pyruvate ratio <30 indicate that the regional metabolic state is normal.

29.3 Insertion of Monitoring Devices

29.3.1 Intraparenchymal Devices

Insertion of an intraparenchymal device is a quick and easy procedure. The operation can be done in the ICU or in theatre. It is also possible to insert an ICP catheter after evacuation of a haematoma through the craniotomy opening.

29.3.1.1 Insertion of an Intraparenchymal ICP Measuring Device Using a Bolt

Application of the different monitors is described in respective manuals and should be followed rigorously. The following are general recommendations:

- The monitor is placed in the right or left prefrontal area, allowing the patient's head to be rotated without interfering with the monitor's function. Select the most injured side in a focal injury. In diffuse injury, the right hemisphere is generally recommended.
- Localize and mark the insertion point, corresponding to Kocher's point: 2–3 cm anterior to the coronal suture and 2 cm lateral to the midline. This point is chosen because it minimizes the involvement of eloquent brain through which the catheter must pass and facilitates nursing care.
- Shave or cut the hair and mark a 0.5 cm skin incision.
- Sterilize the area using chlorhexidine or povidone-iodine.
- Inject local anaesthesia (adrenalin-lidocaine mixture) in a radial fashion around the planned incision site.
- Drape the operation area.
- A 0.5 cm linear incision is made and carried down to the bone.
- Use a small skin retractor to expose the bone and achieve haemostasis of the skin edges.
- Drill a hole through the outer and inner tables of the skull. Ensure the drill guard is in place to avoid penetration of the dura or trauma to the brain.
- Remove the drill and irrigate the hole with sterile saline to remove any bone or soft tissue debris.
- Manually screw the bolt into the skull.
- Insert the stylet through the bolt to penetrate the dura.

- Remove the catheter from the package and attach it to the monitor. Zero the catheter if required, according to the manufacturer's instructions.
- Insert the catheter through the strain-relief protective sheath and then into the bolt so that it extends 0.5–1 cm beyond the end of the bolt into the brain parenchyma (any significant resistance usually results from non-penetration of both tables of the skull and the dura).
- If using a fibre-optic catheter, pull back on the catheter a millimetre or two so that it is not under tension against a blood vessel or brain parenchyma. Then, turn the compression cap clockwise to secure the monitor in place. Place a dressing or a suture to secure the strain-relief protective sheath to the fibre-optic cable.
- Check for a pressure waveform and record the initial ICP. In order to see that the catheter is in place, you might lower the head rest or perform Queckenstedt's test, both should result in a rise in ICP.

29.3.1.2 External Ventricular Drainage (EVD)

EVD is the most accurate, low-cost and reliable method of monitoring ICP as well as allowing therapeutic drainage of CSF. It is always possible to recalibrate it in situ, which is not always the case with intraparenchymal catheters. The external transducer must be constantly maintained at a fixed reference point relative to the patient's head to avoid measurement errors. Correct placement of an EVD into the lateral ventricle at the level of the foramen of Monro requires skill and training. Patients likely to develop intracranial hypertension should be considered for an EVD in the first place instead of an intraparenchymal ICP catheter, if it is suitable according to the CT findings and coagulation status. It is often difficult to place the EVD in a TBI patient because of midline shift or slit ventricles. If so, a neuronavigation system can help to place the EVD in the correct position (for neuronavigation, see below). Be aware not to bend the catheter too tightly, and be cautious not to put sutures that obstruct or puncture the EVD when closing the incision. Potential risks of EVD placement include intraparenchymal haematoma and infection/ventriculitis. The operation must be carried out under rigorous sterile conditions, preferably in the operating room. To prevent infections, it is also recommended to tunnel the drain at least 5 cm under the skin, unless using a bolt.

Insertion of an EVD

- In the absence of contraindications, the right prefrontal region is chosen for insertion of an EVD.
- Mark a 3–4 cm curvilinear incision centred around Kocher's point. Other approaches include Keens point, 2.5 cm posterior and superior to the top of the ear, and the occipital parietal, 6 cm above the inion, 4 cm from the midline.
- The incision should be performed with a scalpel and carried down to the skull. Ensure haemostatic control of bleeding skin arteries.
- The skull should be cleared of the periosteum and a small retractor placed.
- A burr hole is made, perpendicular to the skull.
- Perform haemostasis in the burr hole. Use bone wax if needed.
- Use a hook and a Kerrison to clean the burr hole if necessary.
- The dura is opened using either cautery or a scalpel.
- The arachnoid and cortex are cautiously coagulated and a small corticotomy is performed.
- The ventricular catheter, with the mandrel, stylet or the metal wire in place, should be directed in a plane towards the medial canthus of the ipsilateral side in the sagittal plane and towards a point 0–1 cm anterior to the tragus in the coronal plane, essentially aiming towards the foramen of Monro.
- The catheter should be advanced to 5 cm below the dura, which is 6–7 cm below the skull surface. This will place the tip of the catheter just above the ipsilateral foramen of Monro.
- Usually, a "pop" or a "give in" is felt at about 3–4 cm, indicating entry into the ventricle. Advance the catheter without the mandrel so it

remains 6 cm at skull. This ensures that all the holes in the ventricular catheter are within the ventricle.

- Immediate egress of clear or haemorrhagic (depending on the pathology) CSF is seen. Care must be taken not to lose too much CSF at this point, as the brain may not tolerate sudden decompression of the ventricles.
- The catheter should be secured externally by tunnelling under the scalp to prevent infection (>5 cm). The drain may then be looped and secured with 2-0 nylon suture and stitched into place using three suture points. Make sure that the catheter is firmly attached and not easily removable.
- Close the wound, preferably in two layers.
- A sterile dressing is then placed, and the EVD is connected to the external collection system and ICP measuring transducer.
- Check that the EVD is still working properly.

The EVD is calibrated at the level of the tragus, i.e. the tragus is the zero-point for the ICP. The drain can either be kept closed and opened at a certain level of ICP (intermittent drainage) or be kept open as an overflow drain at a defined height (e.g. 15 cm H_2O; continuous drainage).

Remember that an open EVD does not warn for herniation as the open drain cannot measure higher levels than the distance between the zero point and the level of drainage!

Weaning of External Ventricular Drainage

Once the ICP is normalized, it is essential to determine whether the patient's own intrinsic CSF absorption pathways maintain an equilibrium between CSF production and absorption. In this case, the EVD weaning protocol is instituted.

- The height of the EVD is gradually increased from the actual level of drainage, e.g. in steps of 5–10 mmHg up to a height of 20 mmHg, for a certain time, e.g. 24 h.
- If the patient's neurology and ICP remain stable, the EVD is clamped to allow the patients intrinsic CSF pathways to assume full control of the CSF equilibrium.
- If, after 24 h of clamping the EVD, the patient remains neurologically stable with normal ICP and head CT scanning demonstrates stable ventricular size, the EVD is removed and a single stitch placed at the skin entry site.

Stereotactic Placement of an EVD by Neuronavigation

Neuronavigation is a tool that provides numerous advantages to the neurosurgeon (AlAzri et al. 2017), including high-precision intraoperative localization of anatomical structures. There are several suppliers of neuronavigation today, but they are principally very similar. An EVD stylet (akin to an ordinary mandrel) is typically linked to the preoperative CT images. This can support intraoperative control, especially if the ventricles are small.

29.3.2 Intracerebral Microdialysis

29.3.2.1 Insertion of an Intracerebral Microdialysis Catheter

A multi-lumen bolt could be preferable if it is desirable to monitor ICP, microdialysis and $P_{BT}O_2$ simultaneously.

When using a bolt, it is important to make sure that the dura, arachnoid and cortex are open for passage of the sensible microdialysis membrane. It is also important that the membrane (the 10 mm white tip of the probe) is not damaged during handling, which often is the reason why the perfusate does not reach the microvial ("empty microvial") for analysis. When attaching the microdialysis pump, it is also necessary to ensure that there are no air bubbles in the perfusion fluid.

It is possible to install a microdialysis probe without a bolt, e.g. after evacuation of a haematoma. In that case, the catheter should be tunnelled under the skin and fixed with sutures.

29.3.3 Parenchymal $P_{BT}O_2$ Catheter

Indications for installing $P_{BT}O_2$ catheters are no different from regular ICP measurement. The $P_{BT}O_2$ catheter should preferably be positioned in a non-lesioned area in the white matter to gain reliable O_2 information. The $P_{BT}O_2$ catheter is more expensive than a regular ICP catheter and the cost-effectiveness is still unknown. The $P_{BT}O_2$ catheter is more prone to dysfunctions than regular ICP catheters, but it gives valuable information on brain oxygenation. Most catheters also offer information on the brain temperature.

29.3.3.1 Insertion of $P_{BT}O_2$_ Catheter

The procedure should be performed as indicated for the microdialysis catheter. See also 31.3.1.1. for surgical instructions and the manufacturer's manual for the applied device. It is generally recommended to use a multi-lumen bolt.

- Note that it is possible that $P_{BT}O_2$ is not initially correct (in case of blood around the tip of the catheter), but it should read correctly after a possible blood clot has absorbed.
- Test the $P_{BT}O_2$ response to 80–100% oxygen in the ventilator for a couple of minutes to ensure adequate readings.

29.4 Specific Paediatric Concerns

The EVD enables therapeutic CSF drainage, but an intraparenchymal ICP monitor is also an accurate and reliable alternative in children (Adelson et al. 2003). Notably, children have practically no extra intracranial space allowing room for haematomas or brain swelling after TBI, and ICP can rapidly reach dangerous levels with poor response to pressure-reducing medical therapy. Initial insertion of an EVD instead of a regular ICP catheter should therefore be considered before the ventricles are obliterated due to oedema. Implantation of a $P_{BT}O_2$ and microdialysis catheters are other options that should be considered, preferably in conjunction with an ICP monitor.

References

Adelson PD, Bratton SL, Carney NA, Chesnut RM, du Coudray HE, Goldstein B, et al. Guidelines for the acute medical management of severe traumatic brain injury in infants, children, and adolescents. Chapter 7. Intracranial pressure monitoring technology. Pediatr Crit Care Med. 2003;4(3 Suppl):S28–30.

AlAzri A, et al. Placement accuracy of external ventricular drain when comparing freehand insertion to neuronavigation guidance in severe traumatic brain injury. Acta Neurochir (Wien). 2017;159(8):1399–411.

Badri S, et al. Mortality and long-term functional outcome associated with intracranial pressure after traumatic brain injury. Intensive Care Med. 2012;38(11):1800–9.

Bardt TF, Unterberg AW, et al. Monitoring of brain tissue PO2 in traumatic brain injury: effect of cerebral hypoxia on outcome. Acta Neurochir Suppl. 1998;71:153–6.

Bavetta S, et al. A prospective comparison of fibre-optic and fluid-filled single lumen bolt subdural pressure transducers in ventilated neurosurgical patients. Br J Neurosurg. 1996;10(3):279–84.

Bratton SL, et al. Guidelines for the management of severe traumatic brain injury. VI. Indications for intracranial pressure monitoring. J Neurotrauma. 2007a;24(Suppl 1):S37–44.

Bratton SL, et al. Guidelines for the management of severe traumatic brain injury. VII. Intracranial pressure monitoring technology. J Neurotrauma. 2007b;24(Suppl 1):S45–54.

Carney N, Totten AM, O'Reilly C, Ullman JS, Hawryluk GW, Bell MJ, Bratton SL, Chesnut R, Harris OA, Kissoon N, Rubiano AM, Shutter L, Tasker RC, Vavilala MS, Wilberger J, Wright DW, Ghajar J. Guidelines for the management of severe traumatic brain injury, Fourth Edition. Neurosurgery. 2017;80(1):6–15.

Chesnut RM, et al. A trial of intracranial-pressure monitoring in traumatic brain injury. N Engl J Med. 2012;367(26):2471–81.

Eisenberg HM, et al. Initial CT findings in 753 patients with severe head injury. A report from the NIH Traumatic Coma Data Bank. J Neurosurg. 1990;73(5):688–98.

Fox PT, et al. Nonoxidative glucose consumption during focal physiologic neural activity. Science. 1988;241(4864):462–4.

Gracias VH, Guillamondegui OD, Stiefel MF, Wilensky EM, Bloom S, Gupta R, et al. Cerebral cortical oxygenation: a pilot study. J Trauma. 2004;56(3):469–72; discussion 472–4

Green JA, et al. Goal directed brain tissue oxygen monitoring versus conventional management in traumatic brain injury: an analysis of in hospital recovery. Neurocrit Care. 2013;18(1):20–5.

Guiza F, Meyfroidt G, Piper I, Citerio G, Chambers I, Enblad P, et al. Cerebral perfusion pressure insults and associations with outcome in adult traumatic brain injury. J Neurotrauma. 2017;34(16):2425–31.

Hagel S, et al. External ventricular drain infections: risk factors and outcome. Interdiscip Perspect Infect Dis. 2014;2014:708531.

Hutchinson PJ, Jalloh I, Helmy A, Carpenter KL, Rostami E, Bellander BM, et al. Consensus statement from the 2014 International Microdialysis Forum. Intensive Care Med. 2015;41(9):1517–28.

Kakarla UK, et al. Safety and accuracy of bedside external ventricular drain placement. Neurosurgery. 2008;63(1 Suppl 1):ONS162–6; discussion ONS166-167.

Koskinen LO, Olivecrona M. Clinical experience with the intraparenchymal intracranial pressure monitoring Codman MicroSensor system. Neurosurgery. 2005;56(4):693–8; discussion 693–8.

Koskinen LO, et al. The complications and the position of the Codman MicroSensor ICP device: an analysis of 549 patients and 650 Sensors. Acta Neurochir (Wien). 2013;155(11):2141–8; discussion 2148.

Maas A, Stocchetti N, et al. Moderate and severe traumatic brain injury in adults. Lancet Neurol. 2008;7:728–41.

Martini RP, et al. Management guided by brain tissue oxygen monitoring and outcome following severe traumatic brain injury. J Neurosurg. 2009;111(4):644–9.

McCarthy MC, et al. Neurologic outcomes with cerebral oxygen monitoring in traumatic brain injury. Surgery. 2009;146(4):585–90; discussion 590–1.

Narayan RK, et al. Intracranial pressure: to monitor or not to monitor? A review of our experience with severe head injury. J Neurosurg. 1982;56(5):650–9.

Narotam PK, et al. Brain tissue oxygen monitoring in traumatic brain injury and major trauma: outcome analysis of a brain tissue oxygen-directed therapy. J Neurosurg. 2009;111(4):672–82.

Okonkwo DO, Shutter LA, Moore C, Temkin NR, Puccio AM, Madden CJ, et al. Brain oxygen optimization in severe traumatic brain injury phase-II: a phase II randomized trial. Crit Care Med. 2017;45(11):1907–14.

Rosner MJ, Rosner SD, Johnson AH. Cerebral perfusion pressure: management protocol and clinical results. J Neurosurg. 1995;83:949–62.

Spiotta AM, et al. Brain tissue oxygen-directed management and outcome in patients with severe traumatic brain injury. J Neurosurg. 2010;113(3):571–80.

Stiefel MF, Spiotta A, et al. Reduced mortality rate in patients with severe traumatic brain injury treated with brain tissue oxygen monitoring. J Neurosurg. 2005;103:805–11.

Stubhaug A, et al. Hvordan måles cerebralt perfusjonstrykk i Skandinavia? Norsk anestesiologisk forening – Høstmøtet 2003. Rikshospitalet, Oslo, Norway. Tidskrift for Norsk anestesiologisk förening NAForum. 16:65. 2003.

Thomas E, et al. Calculation of cerebral perfusion pressure in the management of traumatic brain injury: joint position statement by the councils of the Neuroanaesthesia and Critical Care Society of Great Britain and Ireland (NACCS) and the Society of British Neurological Surgeons (SBNS). Br J Anaesth. 2015;115(4):487–8.

Valadka AB, Gopinath SP, et al. Relationship of brain tissue PO2 to outcome after severe head injury. Crit Care Med. 1998;26:1576–81.

Van den Brink WA, Van Santbrink H, et al. Brain oxygen tension in severe head injury. Neurosurgery. 2000;46:868–78.

30 Maxillofacial Fractures

Ann Hermansson

Recommendations

Level I

There are insufficient data to support a Level I recommendation for this topic.

Level II

There are insufficient data to support a Level II recommendation for this topic.

Level III

The outcome of white blowout fractures (greenstick fractures of the orbit) in children is better if the entrapped soft tissue is freed within 48 h.

30.1 Overview

Many facial fractures do not need surgical reconstruction. If needed, it can often be performed after the acute phase. A thorough planning and investigation with imaging and control of the function and the mobility of the eyes, jaws and teeth should be undertaken. Some fractures lead to troublesome bleedings and/or airway problems that have to be addressed immediately. Airway problems and surgical timing should be discussed at an early stage between neurosurgeons, anaesthesiologists and facial surgeons to decide upon thc bcst approach.

Tips, Tricks and Pitfalls

- Facial fractures might cause troublesome bleedings and airway obstruction.
- Skin lacerations in the face should be carefully stitched with consideration of structures under the skin that might be injured. Be aware of the facial nerve, the tear canals, the parotid glands and the structures in the eyelids and lips.
- Try to remove asphalt stains and dust from excoriations to avoid 'tattoos' after healing. A toothbrush might be helpful!
- Special considerations have to be made regarding timing of surgery and imaging in children.
- Early evaluation of eye movements and if possible function is important.
- Antibiotic treatment should be considered.
- Tetanus vaccination should be considered.

A. Hermansson (✉)
ENT Department, University Hospital, Lund, Sweden

Department of Otorhinolaryngology, Lund University Hospital, Lund, Sweden
e-mail: ann.hermansson@med.lu.se

© Springer Nature Switzerland AG 2020
T. Sundstrøm et al. (eds.), *Management of Severe Traumatic Brain Injury*,
https://doi.org/10.1007/978-3-030-39383-0_30

- Evaluation of sight and hearing is important and should be carried out as soon as possible.
- Paediatric fractures, with the exception of white blowout fractures, can often be treated conservatively with good results.

30.2 Background

Trauma to the skull often results in more or less obvious fractures extending into the facial bones. These will often result in disfiguration and, perhaps, disturbances in function in the orbit, midface and/or teeth and jaws and might be obvious already in the emergency room. However, some fractures are not that obvious and might be overlooked initially. It is therefore important to evaluate both functional and aesthetic aspects of facial trauma. Below follows more detailed information on diagnosis, timing of surgery and follow-up. Especially interested readers are referred to textbooks (Zide 2006; Hammer 1995; Perry 2011).

30.2.1 Diagnostics

CT scans of the facial bones (including the mandible) with or without 3D reconstructions can often be made from the initial trauma CT, but if not, it should be obtained. In some cases, mainly in children, an MRI might be helpful to map soft tissue in the orbit when white blowout fractures are suspected.

In some cases, one can see fractures in the mid-face, but with very little dislocation. In most of these cases, no intervention is needed if there is no impaired function. Therefore, an early evaluation of eye movements and function will often be needed to decide whether to operate or not. Special considerations also have to be given to the function of the teeth and yaws.

30.2.2 Timing of Surgery

In most cases, facial fractures do not have to be addressed immediately, although this is often advantageous. If needed, they might be operated within 10–14 days or even later with good results. However, some fractures need to be addressed earlier. The naso-orbito-ethmoidal (NOE) fractures should be repositioned as soon as possible (Sargent and Rogers 1999). If a regular operation is not possible immediately, a closed reduction lifting the naso-orbito-ethmoidal complex in place should be considered as a first step to later reconstruction and is often effective.

The most obvious fractures needing immediate intervention are those causing airway obstruction and/or life-threatening bleedings. In some cases, endotracheal intubation is not possible, and a coniotomy with a cannula placed through the cricothyroid membrane has to be performed early on, while in other cases, a regular tracheostomy should be considered both to facilitate the later reduction and osteosynthesis of facial fractures and the rehabilitation. If this is needed perioperatively, it is often wise to perform the tracheostomy as soon as possible to facilitate patient care (Holmgren et al. 2007).

Skull base fractures can cause both bleeding and CSF leakage. While most leakages from the ear will cease spontaneously, liquorrhea from the nose must in many cases be patched operatively. This can be done either by open or endoscopic approaches.

In most cases, it is thus wise to plan the surgery of maxillofacial trauma when appropriate evaluation has been made, often as a collaboration between ENT and plastic surgeons, maxillofacial surgeons and ophthalmologists. In some cases, the surgery has to be planned according to neurosurgical interventions, for instance, to address CSF leakages, which of course should be done *after* surgery including reposition of a NOE fracture! In most cases, surgery is best planned in one session.

30.2.3 Follow-Up

All cases of maxillofacial fractures have to be carefully followed. Not only must the aesthetic aspects be considered, but it is also important to assess function. Both eyesight and hearing should be checked, and teeth and jaws should be evaluated by a dentist or a maxillofacial surgeon. It is often wise to inform the patient and his or her family that additional operations or reconstructions are frequently needed over the ensuing years after a craniofacial trauma.

30.3 Specific Paediatric Concerns

Facial fractures are rare in children; when they do occur, special considerations have to be made. Fractures of the skull bones are much more common but might involve the mid-face and jaws. However, most of these fractures will not show much dislocation and will heal without intervention. To keep radiation doses low, especially to the eyes, is even more important in children than in adults. In some instances, MRI might be useful. Greenstick fractures in the orbit, so-called white blowout fractures or trapdoor fractures, pose a special problem since they might cause entrapment of the periorbital structures and severely restricted eye movements. These fractures are often difficult to visualise both on CT scans and MRI. If there are clinical signs of entrapment, it is mandatory to explore the orbit even if imaging does not show a fracture. Thus, a forced duction test (testing the eye movements by trying to move the eye when gripping the muscles with a pair of forceps) might be needed to decide whether to operate or not. It has been shown that the outcome of these fractures is better if the entrapped soft tissue is freed within 48 h (Grant et al. 2002). Delay may result in permanent problems with double vision. Fractures of the maxilla and mandible in children should be given special consideration, keeping the possible damage to non-erupted teeth in mind.

References

Grant JH III, Patrinely JR, Weiss AH, Kierney PC, Gruss JS. Trapdoor fracture of the orbit in a pediatric population. Plast Reconstr Surg. 2002;109(2):482–9; discussion 490–5.

Hammer B. Orbital fractures: diagnosis, operative treatment, secondary corrections. Seattle: Hogrefe & Huber Publishers; 1995.

Holmgren EP, Bagheri S, Bell RB, Bobek S, Dierks EJ. Utilization of tracheostomy in craniomaxillofacial trauma at a level-1 trauma center. J Oral Maxillofac Surg. 2007;65(10):2005–10.

Perry M. Fractures of the facial bones. Oxford: Wiley and Blackwell; 2011.

Sargent LA, Rogers GF. Nasoethmoid orbital fractures: diagnosis and management. J Craniomaxillofac Trauma. 1999;5(1):19–27.

Zide BM. Surgical anatomy around the orbit: the system of zones. Philadelphia: Lippincott Williams & Wilkins; 2006.

31 Considerations in Patients with Concomitant Cervical Spine Injury

Tor Brommeland and Terje Sundstrøm

Recommendations

Level I

There are insufficient data to support a Level I recommendation for this topic.

Level II

There are insufficient data to support a Level II recommendation for this topic.

Level III

All patients with a severe TBI should have a CT scan of the cervical spine.

Patients with documented cervical spine injury should have a supplementary CT angiography.

The cervical collar may be removed in obtunded adult trauma patients after a negative, high-quality CT scan of the cervical spine.

Surgery in the prone position should be postponed until the ICP is manageable.

Tips, Tricks, and Pitfalls

- Cervical spine injury is rare in TBI patients, but TBI is frequent in patients with cervical spine injuries.
- Protection from hypoxia and hypotension is equally important for the injured brain and spine.
- Surgery of cervical spine injuries should be preceded by an MRI.
- Vascular injuries in relation to cervical spine injuries are more frequent than previously thought.
- Posterior cervical spine surgery should be delayed until the ICP is stable/manageable.

31.1 Overview

Severe TBI is often part of a multi-trauma setting. Due to the biomechanical relationship between the head and neck, there is a clear association between TBI and cervical spine injury: The prevalence of concomitant cervical spine injury in patients with TBI is around 6.5% (12% for patients injured in motor vehicle accidents). Vice versa, the prevalence of concomitant TBI in

T. Brommeland (✉)
Department of Neurosurgery, Oslo University Hospital Ullevål, Oslo, Norway

T. Sundstrøm
Department of Neurosurgery, Haukeland University Hospital, Bergen, Norway

Department of Clinical Medicine, University of Bergen, Bergen, Norway
e-mail: tjsu@helse-bergen.no

© Springer Nature Switzerland AG 2020
T. Sundstrøm et al. (eds.), *Management of Severe Traumatic Brain Injury*, https://doi.org/10.1007/978-3-030-39383-0_31

patients with cervical spine injury is approximately 40% (Pandrich et al. 2018). Blunt cerebrovascular injury occurs at a rate of about 9% in patients with severe TBI (Esnault et al. 2017).

Hypotension and hypoxia are two important parameters that predict a poorer outcome in patients with TBI. This may occur in multi-traumatized patients due to haemorrhagic shock, thoracic injury or non-patent airways. Notably, spinal cord injury with neurogenic shock can produce severe haemodynamic derangements, which are particularly dangerous for patients with a concomitant TBI. A high cervical cord injury (from C5 and above) may affect respiratory function and create hypoxia. Rapid identification and treatment of hypotension and hypoxia are key to successful management of patients with traumatic brain and spine injuries.

Please refer to Chaps. 15 and 18 Radiological Evaluation of Cervical Spine Trauma for considerations related to admission, diagnostics and planning and Chaps. 28 and 34 for considerations related to acute surgical treatment.

31.1.1 TBI and Concomitant Spine Injury

Care for TBI patients with concomitant injuries is often characterized by conflicts of interests: Rigid cervical collars may compress the jugular veins, which in turn may compromise venous return from the brain and increase ICP (Kolb et al. 1999). Restrictions of mobilization are often required before unstable spinal, pelvic, or extremity fractures have been appropriately managed, while TBI patients benefit from early mobilization. Immobilized trauma patients require low-molecular-weight heparin for thrombus prophylaxis, which again may worsen intracranial haemorrhage.

Cervical spine clearance is a challenge in consciously depressed trauma patients. Neurologic deficits, neck pain, and radiculopathy may be revealed by clinical examinations in awake patients, while this is not so straightforward in obtunded trauma victims. Though CT scanning of the cervical spine reveals bony fractures and misalignment, MRI is needed to visualize traumatic disc herniations, ligamentous injuries, haematomas within the spinal canal, or spinal cord injury. Some institutions therefore advocate the use of MRI before the cervical spine is finally cleared in TBI patients that are intubated and anesthetized. However, transporting such a patient from the intensive care unit to perform an MRI is associated with risks related to compromised airway patency and oxygenation, circulatory monitoring, and fluctuations in ICP. In a recent review of cervical spine clearance in obtunded adult trauma patients, cervical collar removal was recommended after a negative high-quality CT scan of the cervical spine: 100% negative predictive value of finding an unstable cervical spine injury among 1718 patients in 11 studies (Patel et al. 2015).

31.1.2 Timing of Surgery for Concomitant C-spine Injuries

Timing of surgery for extra-cranial injuries is similarly difficult. Injuries causing derangements of circulation or respiration must be dealt with immediately. Early surgical management in the form of orthopaedic damage control (i.e. external fixation) of extremity fractures does not seem to negatively affect the outcome in patients with concurrent TBI. In general, definitive treatment should be postponed until the ICP is manageable and stable (Cryer et al. 2015).

Positioning of a TBI patient on the operating table is crucial in cases where the ICP is in the upper normal range or displays unstable trends. The prone position is known to increase ICP due to reduced venous return and/or increased intra-thoracic/abdominal pressures. Thus, posterior spinal procedures should not be undertaken until the ICP is manageable in this position.

31.2 Specific Paediatric Concerns

Data on this topic within the paediatric population is very limited. The recommendations for children therefore generally follow adult protocols.

References

Cryer et al. Best practices in the management of traumatic brain injury. American College of Surgeons. 2015.

Esnault, et al. Blunt cerebrovascular injuries in severe traumatic brain injury: incidence, risk factors, and evolution. J Neurosurg. 2017;127(1):16–22.

Kolb, et al. Cervical collar induced changes in intracranial pressure. Am J Emerg Med. 1999;17(2):135–7.

Pandrich, et al. Prevalence of concomitant traumatic cranio-spinal injury: a systematic review and meta-analysis. Neurosurg Rev. 2018; https://doi.org/10.1007/s10143-018-0988-3.

Patel, et al. Cervical spine collar clearance in the obtunded adult blunt trauma patient: a systematic review and practice management guideline from the Eastern Association for the Surgery of Trauma. J Trauma Acute Care Surg. 2015;78(2):430–41.

Soft Tissue Injuries

32

Daniel Isacson and Daniel Nowinski

Recommendations

Level I

Wounds should be thoroughly irrigated.

Removal of sutures in the face should be done within 5–7 days to avoid track marks.

Level II

Tap water is as efficient as sterile water with no difference in infection rates.

Antibiotics may have benefits in contaminated wounds.

Level III

Layered closure leads to restoration of muscle and reduces dead space with less scarring.

Timing is of importance in suspected nerve injuries, as after approximately 48–72 h, the distal nerve end can no longer be stimulated.

Tips, Tricks, and Pitfalls

- Meticulous wound irrigation is the most important aspect of treatment of soft tissue injuries.
- There is no evidence for antibiotic prophylaxis except for contaminated wounds.
- Lip repair requires meticulous attention to details, as a misalignment of the vermillion border of only 1 mm is clearly noticeable at conversational distance.
- Staples saves time and reduces alopecia. Pay attention to hair-bearing areas when closing the scalp.
- Always consider wound irrigation in sedation in the pediatric consideration.

32.1 Overview

Soft tissue injuries in the head and neck area are commonly encountered in trauma patients. Their early identification and treatment is important to prevent hemorrhage, infections, and later deformity. Minor lacerations may usually be adequately treated in the emergency room. However, more complex injuries should be managed in an operating room setting with access to surgical assistance and instruments. Soft tissue injury should always alert to the presence of deeper

D. Isacson (✉)
Department of Plastic and Maxillofacial Surgery, Uppsala University Hospital, Uppsala, Sweden
e-mail: daniel.isacson@akademiska.se

D. Nowinski
Department of Plastic and Maxillofacial Surgery, Uppsala University Hospital, Uppsala, Sweden

Department of Surgical Sciences, Plastic Surgery, Uppsala University, Uppsala, Sweden
e-mail: daniel.nowinski@akademiska.se

© Springer Nature Switzerland AG 2020
T. Sundstrøm et al. (eds.), *Management of Severe Traumatic Brain Injury*,
https://doi.org/10.1007/978-3-030-39383-0_32

injuries to the bone or vital structures, and a thorough understanding of the mechanism of trauma is of paramount importance.

Management of soft tissue injuries should be performed in a systematic way following the sequence of hemorrhage control, wound assessment, irrigation, and repair. Depending on the anatomical region consultation with plastic surgery, ENT or ophthalmology should be considered.

32.2 Hemorrhage Control

Hemorrhage from superficial soft tissues may usually be controlled by local compression. Scalp injuries that disrupt major vessels may result in hypovolemic shock and may need ligation in the emergency setting. Bleeding in the nasal cavity that cannot be controlled by direct pressure requires packing. Packing is usually effective and rarely requires a transnasal balloon catheter. If massive hemorrhage is present, the airway should be managed first by emergent intubation, followed by packing and direct pressure. Control of the source bleed, usually a branch from the external carotid artery, is best done by angiographic embolization. Surgical ligation of the external carotid is not adequate and will not control bleeding (Thorne et al. 2013).

32.3 Wound Assessment

Once hemorrhage control is achieved, a thorough wound assessment should be made. Location, size, and extent of defect all determine the extent of further treatment. The location of the wound may lead to suspicion of nerve damage, muscular injury, or underlying fractures. The size of the wound, large soft tissue avulsion, or areas of necrosis may not allow for primary closure and require consultation with a plastic surgeon.

Fractures to the supporting facial bones should be excluded by clinical exam and computer tomography. A recent large study from the US national trauma database found the incidence of facial fractures to be 13.5% in patients with a cervical spine injury, 21.7% in patients with a head injury, and 24.0% in patients with a combined cervical spine and head trauma. Furthermore, about 5–8% of isolated and 7–11% of multiple facial fracture cases are associated with cervical spine injury, and appropriate care should always be taken to stabilize the neck before ruling out these injuries (Mulligan et al. 2010).

32.4 Irrigation

Thorough irrigation and removal of any foreign bodies is essential before closure. Irrigation reduces the risk of infection, and foreign bodies are a cause of prolonged inflammation which may ultimately lead to infection. Devitalized tissue should be removed with sharp debridement. Debris must be removed from the dermis or may result in permanent tattooing. Freshening the wound margins contributes to rapid healing and improves final outcome (Thorne et al. 2013). Cleansing is best performed with a mild surgical soap and the light use of a scrub brush. Extensive and contaminated wounds should be irrigated with a pulsed lavage system (Thorne et al. 2013). The role of irrigation cannot be overemphasized and should not be delayed. A Cochrane review and several RCTs support the role of tap water to be as efficient as sterile water with no difference in infection rates (Fernandez and Griffiths 2012; Moscati et al. 2007; Weiss et al. 2013). The head and neck's rich vascularity increases resistance to infection (Adalarasan et al. 2010; Hollander et al. 2001); however, the risk increases the longer a wound is open (Waseem et al. 2012).

32.5 Repair

Primary closure is usually the preferred treatment. Wounds may heal by secondary intention but have increased risk of scarring and infection which will generally result in inferior final appearance compared with other reconstructive options. Absolute contraindications to closure are signs of inflammation(Hollander and Singer 1999).

Layered closure of the muscles and skin is preferred to restore muscle function and reduce dead space. Further, by placing the tension of the closure deep to the skin with excellent approximation of the dermal layer, the resulting scar is improved. Layered suturing does unfortunately lead to increased risk of infection. Select monofilament sutures small enough to minimize the risk of tissue damage and suture marks but strong enough to avoid wound dehiscence. Good choices include 5-0 for face and 6-0 in the eyelid. Local flaps should be avoided in the acute setting.

Noninfected wounds in the scalp and face caused by clean objects may undergo primary closure up to 24 h after injury (Berk et al. 1988). Factors that may increase the likelihood of infection include wound contamination, laceration length greater than 5 cm, laceration located on the lower extremities, extensive soft tissue contusion, and diabetes mellitus (Quinn et al. 2014).

Delayed primary closure should be considered for complicated wounds that present after 24 h. It involves cleaning and debridement followed by a 4–5 day of waiting period. This allows the host defense system to decrease bacterial load and initialize wound healing. Antibiotics may be administered. Additional debridement and granulation tissue trimming back to wound margins may be needed at time of closure (Marion 2018). Other indications for healing by secondary intention are deep wounds that cannot be adequately irrigated, contaminated wounds, small non-cosmetic animal bites, abscess cavities, and presentation after significant delay (Berk et al. 1988).

32.5.1 Scalp

The scalp consists of five layers: the skin, subcutaneous tissue, galea aponeurotica, loose areolar tissue, and pericranium. The scalp's blood vessels, lymphatic system, and nerves run superficially to the galea aponeurotica in the subcutaneous tissues. The galea is continuous with the frontalis muscle anteriorly, the occipitalis posteriorly, and temporoparietal fascia laterally. The galea is very inelastic, but where the galeal edges blend into the temporoparietal fascia and scalp musculature fascia, there is better mobility (Desai et al. 2015).

The blood supply to the scalp arises from both the internal and external carotid arteries. The arteries form a collateralization in the subcutaneous tissue. The paired supraorbital and supratrochlear arteries arise anteriorly. The superficial temporal artery supplies the lateral portion. It branches into an anterior-frontal and posterior-parietal division at the superior helix of the ear. The posterior scalp is supplied by the occipital artery superior to the nuchal line, and inferior to this, perforating branches form the trapezius and splenic capitis muscle. This rich blood supply may lead to hemorrhagic shock in scalp injuries. Shock, if present, is usually associated with underlying complex facial fractures or intracranial injury and delayed control of hemorrhage or other injuries such as abdominal trauma or long bone fractures (Fonseca 2013).

The dense galea and underlying loose areolar tissue predispose to large avulsion or degloving of tissue, with maintained blood supply in the avulsion flaps. Scalp lacerations without tissue loss should be closed with 3.0 or 4.0 interrupted nonabsorbable sutures. Alternatively, a layered closure with absorbable sutures in the galea and staples in the skin can be used. The hair does not need removal unless it interferes with wound closure (Howell and Morgan 1988; Tang et al. 2001). Staples are faster and more cost-effective than using sutures (Edlich et al. 1990; Bennett 1988). Staples may cause less alopecia on the scalp than other forms of closure. Cautery should be used with caution for similar reasons (Ritchie and Rocke 1989).

Large shearing injuries, where there is tissue loss that does not allow for primary closure, may need flap reconstruction. This should not be done in the acute phase. When considering reconstruction of the scalp, the unique characteristics of scalp skin and its hair-bearing nature must be considered to provide an aesthetically pleasing reconstruction. Consultation with a plastic surgeon is therefore recommended (Fig. 32.1).

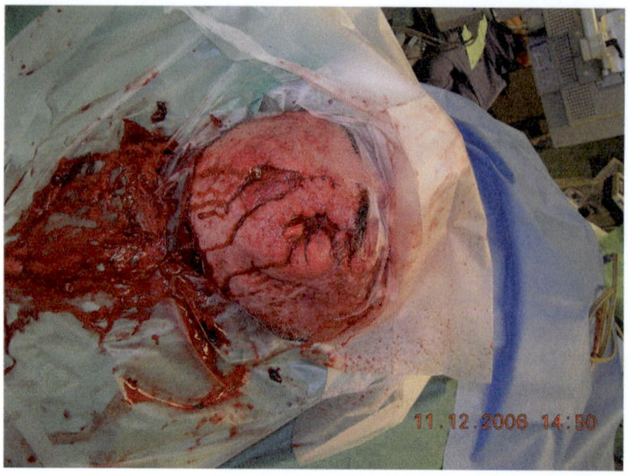

Fig. 32.1 Crush injury of the scalp with underlying fractures

32.5.2 Face

Soft tissue injuries to the face require consideration of several important aspects. Besides the obvious and clearly visible scars that may result, special consideration should also be taken to the examination of the eye and lacrimal apparatus, the external auditory meatus, the facial nerve, and the parotid duct. If the patient is awake, motor and sensory innervation should be evaluated before local anesthetic is administered. Testing should include eyebrow elevation, forced closure of the eyes, voluntary smile, and eversion of the lower lip. Deficits in the presence of a penetrating injury likely represent transection of a facial nerve branch and require operative exploration. Timing is of importance, as after approximately 48–72 h, the distal nerve end can no longer be stimulated, making it difficult to identify and repair it during microscopic surgery. Nerve regeneration typically occurs at a rate of 1 mm/day after a 1-month lag (Thorne et al. 2013).

If open fractures are present, meticulous, early wound treatment is of paramount importance to prevent deep infection and enable subsequent fracture treatment at a later stage.

Forehead lacerations may injure the temporal (frontal) branch of the facial nerve or the frontalis muscle causing brow ptosis. The temporal branch of the facial nerve and the superficial temporal artery lies within the deep temporoparietal fascia. Its course is consistent from 0.5 cm below the tragus to 1.5 cm above the lateral brow (Pitanguy's line). The eyebrow should be preserved. Attention should be paid to alignment, as misalignment is aesthetically obvious. The frontalis is repaired with interrupted absorbable sutures. The skin is closed with nonabsorbable monofilament sutures.

With trauma to the eye or eyelid, the most important aspect is to ensure that there is no globe injury. An ophthalmologist should be consulted. The most important aspect of eyelid repair is placement of an everting suture along the lid margin gray line. This facilitates proper alignment and makes notching of the lid margin less likely. All layers of the eyelid—inner, middle, and outer lamella—should be repaired.

With ear injuries, hematomas should be evacuated as they may cause cartilage resorption and ultimately a reactive chondrogenesis, which will lead to cauliflower ears. Hematomas are usually drained with an incision through the overlying skin. A bolster dressing is then required to avoid re-accumulation of the hematoma. Through-and-through sutures may be used for this. Skin laceration can usually be closed in one layer. It is unnecessary to place sutures in the cartilage as the skin adheres firmly to it and allows for proper alignment.

The nose consists of three lamella: the skin and soft tissue, cartilaginous framework, and mucosa. Intranasal examination is required to rule out septal hematomas and mucosal lacerations. Once hemorrhage control is established, evaluation of the soft tissue injury is important. In contrast to the ear, damage to the underlying nose cartilage requires repair of all layers, after appropriate anatomic reduction. Skin lacerations may be sutured with nonabsorbable 5-0 sutures. Deeper injuries require consultation with a plastic or ENT surgeon.

Lip repair requires meticulous attention to details, as a misalignment of the vermillion border of only 1 mm is clearly noticeable at conversational distance (Thorne et al. 2013). Prior to infiltration of local anesthetic, the location of the vermillion border on either side of the laceration should be marked out. The lip is sutured in all three layers: the skin, orbicularis oris, and mucosa. Failure to reapproximate the orbicularis oris muscle separately will result in bunching of the mus-

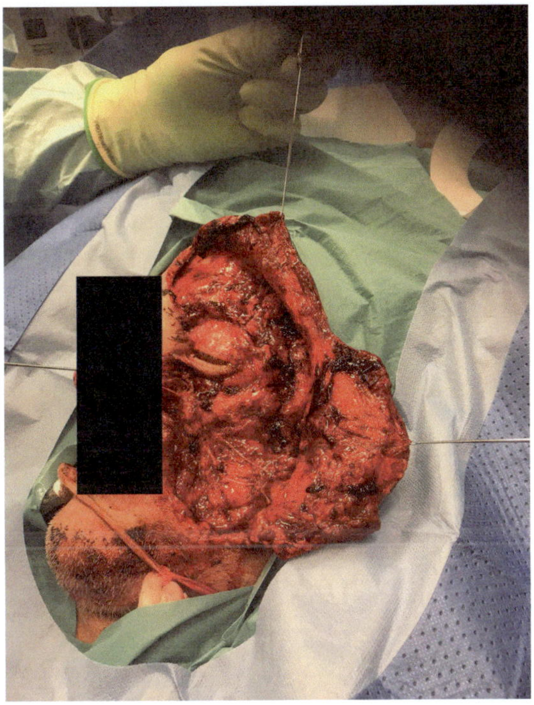

Fig. 32.2 Facial laceration and degloving injury of the left face with the facial nerve exposed

cle with animation and shortened scar, with an exaggerating notching of the lip. Use resorbable 6-0 sutures for the two inner layers and nonabsorbable 5-0 or 6-0 suture for the skin (Fig. 32.2).

32.5.3 Aftercare

Scalp wounds should be left open to air unless they require a pressure dressing. After 24–48 h, they can be let to air and cleansed with soap and water. Staples and nonabsorbable sutures should be removed after 7–10 days, but large and deeper wounds warrant removal at 10–14 days. Highly contaminated wounds should be seen for follow-up within 48–72 h. Removal of sutures in the face should be done within 5–7 days.

32.5.4 Antibiotics

Prophylactic antibiotics have little benefit in healthy patients with clean wounds. A meta-analysis of seven RCTs with simple wounds found that those who received systematic antibiotics did not have a significantly lower incidence of infection compared with untreated patients (Cummings and Del Beccaro 1995). Antibiotics may provide benefit in grossly contaminated wounds, immunocompromised patients, open fractures, wounds contaminated with oral secretion, or delayed closure (Abubaker 2009).

Bites may be associated with polymicrobial infection. These are most common after feline bites because of the deep, puncture-type wounds and virulent bacteria. The most common bacterium is *Pasteurella multocida* (Jaindl et al. 2016).

A tetanus booster dose should be given to patients who have had (1) three vaccine doses and whose last injection is >10 years ago or <10 years ago if the wound is deep or (2) four vaccine doses and their last injection is >20 years ago. Patients who have had less than three vaccine doses should complete a basic scheme with pure tetanus vaccine and diphtheria vaccine (Ljungberg 2019).

32.6 Specific Pediatric Concerns

Soft tissue injuries occur in the pediatric population and are usually caused by accidents related to sports and play. The same fundamental principles of wound care outlined above for adults hold true in the pediatric age group. However, there are also special considerations to be made. In the case of vascular injury, children have less margin for blood loss, and it may also be more difficult to control hemorrhage by compression in the awake child. Vascular access for resuscitation should therefore be promptly ascertained when indicated. Physical examination of nerve injuries may not be as reliable as in adults; that is why proper nerve exploration should be performed if there is reason to suspect injuries to the facial nerve.

Children have less skin laxity and redundancy, and tissue loss through avulsion is usually not manageable by direct wound edge approximation. On the other hand, children heal efficiently with low risk for infection; that is why some minor avulsion injuries may be primarily managed by healing through secondary intention.

Facial fractures are generally rare in the pediatric population. There are also differences in the typical fracture patterns compared to adults due to less developed paranasal sinuses, a more elastic and immature bony framework, and a relatively less prominent facial skeleton compared to the cranium. In general, pediatric facial fractures can be managed more conservatively compared to adults, and the future, expected growth has to be considered in the planning of surgical reduction and fixation.

Depending on the age and maturity of the child, general anesthesia will frequently be indicated to ascertain adequate wound assessment and treatment while preventing psychological trauma. If local anesthetic is used, the physician needs to be familiar with dosing. Topical anesthetic should be used to prepare the area of injection, and sodium bicarbonate should be added in a 1:10 ratio to the local anesthetic to neutralize the solution and reduce pain when injected. Topical local anesthetic (EMLA) can also be applied in advance to reduce sensation to needle injections.

Children often heal quickly, but increased collagen deposition also increases the tendency for hypertrophic scars. Rapidly absorbable sutures are best utilized to avoid general anesthesia for suture removal. Permanent sutures, if used, should be removed within 5 days and wound support dressings applied for 10–14 days to remove tension from the wound bed.

When the wound is well epithelialized, usually within 7–10 days, silicone sheeting or topical gels can be applied for 3 months to minimize scar formation.

It is always important to remember that if the wound or presentation seems suspicious, child health services should be contacted to avoid potential further harm to the child.

References

Abubaker AO. Use of prophylactic antibiotics in preventing infection of traumatic injuries. Dent Clin North Am. 2009;53(4):707–15, vi. https://doi.org/10.1016/j.cden.2009.08.004. PubMed PMID: 19958907.

Adalarasan S, Mohan A, Pasupathy S. Prophylactic antibiotics in maxillofacial fractures: a requisite? J Craniofac Surg. 2010;21(4):1009–11. https://doi.org/10.1097/SCS.0b013e3181e47d43. PubMed PMID: 20613562.

Bennett RG. Selection of wound closure materials. J Am Acad Dermatol. 1988;18(4 Pt 1):619–37. PubMed PMID: 3286691.

Berk WA, Osbourne DD, Taylor DD. Evaluation of the 'golden period' for wound repair: 204 cases from a Third World emergency department. Ann Emerg Med. 1988;17(5):496–500. PubMed PMID: 3364832.

Cummings P, Del Beccaro MA. Antibiotics to prevent infection of simple wounds: a meta-analysis of randomized studies. Am J Emerg Med. 1995;13(4):396–400. https://doi.org/10.1016/0735-6757(95)90122-1. PubMed PMID: 7605521.

Desai SC, Sand JP, Sharon JD, et al. Scalp reconstruction: an algorithmic approach and systematic review. JAMA Facial Plast Surg. 2015;17(1):56–66. https://doi.org/10.1001/jamafacial.2014.889. PubMed PMID: 25375669.

Edlich RF, Becker DG, Thacker JG, et al. Scientific basis for selecting staple and tape skin closures. Clin Plast Surg. 1990;17(3):571–8. PubMed PMID: 2199146.

Fernandez R, Griffiths R. Water for wound cleansing. Cochrane Database Syst Rev. 2012;15(2):CD003861. https://doi.org/10.1002/14651858.CD003861.pub3. PubMed PMID: 22336796.

Fonseca R. Oral and maxillofacial trauma. Philadelphia: Elsevier; 2013. English.

Hollander JE, Singer AJ. Laceration management. Ann Emerg Med. 1999;34(3):356–67. PubMed PMID: 10459093.

Hollander JE, Singer AJ, Valentine SM, et al. Risk factors for infection in patients with traumatic lacerations. Acad Emerg Med. 2001;8(7):716–20. PubMed PMID: 11435186.

Howell JM, Morgan JA. Scalp laceration repair without prior hair removal. Am J Emerg Med. 1988;6(1):7–10. PubMed PMID: 3334801.

Jaindl M, Oberleitner G, Endler G, et al. Management of bite wounds in children and adults-an analysis of over 5000 cases at a level I trauma centre. Wien Klin Wochenschr. 2016;128(9–10):367–75. https://doi.org/10.1007/s00508-015-0900-x. PubMed PMID: 26659907.

Ljungberg B. [Bett av hund och katt - handläggning]. www.internetmedicin.se. Accessed 8 March 2019.

Marion D. Minor wound preparation and irrigation. UpToDate, Waltham, MA. Accessed 10 Oct 2018. (Post T, editor.).

Moscati RM, Mayrose J, Reardon RF, et al. A multicenter comparison of tap water versus sterile saline for wound irrigation. Acad Emerg Med. 2007;14(5):404–9. https://doi.org/10.1197/j.aem.2007.01.007. PubMed PMID: 17456554.

Mulligan RP, Friedman JA, Mahabir RC. A nationwide review of the associations among cervical spine injuries, head injuries, and facial fractures. J

Trauma. 2010;68(3):587–92. https://doi.org/10.1097/TA.0b013e3181b16bc5. PubMed PMID: 19996802.

Quinn JV, Polevoi SK, Kohn MA. Traumatic lacerations: what are the risks for infection and has the 'golden period' of laceration care disappeared? Emerg Med J. 2014;31(2):96–100. https://doi.org/10.1136/emermed-2012-202143. PubMed PMID: 23314208; PubMed Central PMCID: PMCPMC3797169.

Ritchie AJ, Rocke LG. Staples versus sutures in the closure of scalp wounds: a prospective, double-blind, randomized trial. Injury. 1989;20(4):217–8. PubMed PMID: 2592097.

Tang K, Yeh JS, Sgouros S. The Influence of hair shave on the infection rate in neurosurgery. A prospective study. Pediatr Neurosurg. 2001;35(1):13–7. https://doi.org/10.1159/000050379. PubMed PMID: 11490185.

Thorne CH, Chung KC, Gosain AK, et al. Grabb and Smith's plastic surgery. 7th ed. Phliadelphia: Wolters Kluwer Health/Lippincott Williams & Wilkins; 2013

Waseem M, Lakdawala V, Patel R, et al. Is there a relationship between wound infections and laceration closure times? Int J Emerg Med. 2012;5(1):32. https://doi.org/10.1186/1865-1380-5-32. PubMed PMID: 22835090; PubMed Central PMCID: PMCPMC3414831.

Weiss EA, Oldham G, Lin M, et al. Water is a safe and effective alternative to sterile normal saline for wound irrigation prior to suturing: a prospective, double-blind, randomised, controlled clinical trial. BMJ Open. 2013;3(1) https://doi.org/10.1136/bmjopen-2012-001504. PubMed PMID: 23325896; PubMed Central PMCID: PMCPMC3549228.

Surgery Outside Neurosurgical Units

33

Per Enblad

Recommendations

Level I

There are insufficient data to support a Level I recommendation for this topic.

Level II

There are insufficient data to support a Level II recommendation for this topic.

Level III

Acute neurosurgery on vital indications can be initiated by surgeons at local hospitals after consultation with the regional neurosurgeon on call.

Appropriate education, training and support should be provided by the regional neurosurgical unit.

33.1 Overview

The national organizations of trauma care have historically been dependent on demographic factors, availability, economic factors, local interests and traditions. Historically, trauma cases have been referred also to smaller hospitals, and life-saving evacuations of extracerebral haematomas have been done by non-neurosurgeons in many countries. A survey regarding the distribution of acute traumatic head injury operations at Nordic hospitals in the year 2000 using data from administrative registries revealed that the patients were operated in local or central hospitals in 33% of the cases in Sweden, 19% of the cases in Norway and 15% of the cases in Finland, while all patients were operated in neurosurgical departments in Denmark (Sollid et al. 2009). It has been considered important to organize the trauma care into more centralized trauma care systems where patients are referred acutely only to trauma centres better equipped for multi-specialized advanced trauma care. This development occurs at different speeds in different countries. The smallest hospitals are usually excluded in the trauma care organizations. However, due to demographic reasons in many countries, trauma centres without neurosurgical expertise need to be included in the trauma systems. One important topic to discuss is whether it is desirable at all, or under certain conditions today, that non-neurosurgeons continue to perform life-saving operations outside neurosurgical units?

P. Enblad (✉)
Department of Neuroscience/Neurosurgery, Section of Neurosurgery, Uppsala University Hospital, Uppsala University, Uppsala, Sweden
e-mail: per.enblad@neuro.uu.se

© Springer Nature Switzerland AG 2020
T. Sundstrøm et al. (eds.), *Management of Severe Traumatic Brain Injury*,
https://doi.org/10.1007/978-3-030-39383-0_33

> **Tips, Tricks and Pitfalls**
> - Neurosurgery should preferably be done at designated neurosurgical units, but emergency procedures on vital indication can be taught to surgeons at local hospitals.
> - The neurosurgical unit should have regular communication about TBI management, continuous further education and mutual development of trauma care with local hospitals.
> - The neurosurgical unit should provide round-the-clock telephone neurosurgical consultant service, and electronic transmission of radiology examinations should be mandatory.
> - The neurosurgeon on call decides if urgent haematoma evacuation is indicated at the local hospital, and the neurosurgical unit should be able to send a neurosurgeon to support the local surgeon.
> - The patient should be transferred to the neurosurgical department for neurointensive care following surgery at a local hospital.

33.2 Background

33.2.1 Bypassing the Nearest Hospital for More Specialized Care

It has been recommended in international guidelines in, e.g. Scotland, the USA and New Zealand (Lecky et al. 2017) that patients with suspected severe TBI at the scene of the accident should be transferred immediately to trauma centres with neurosurgery, bypassing nearer trauma centres without neurosurgery. Concerns have been expressed regarding the potential risk of delaying the stabilization of ABC (Lecky et al. 2008) and the risk of overtriage of patients not needing neurosurgery (Lecky et al. 2017). A recent cluster randomized controlled trial, including 74 English ambulance stations, evaluated whether direct transport of TBI patients to specialist neuroscience centres bypassing the nearest non-specialist acute hospitals could improve outcome, found an overtriage (false positive) ratio of 13:1 for neurosurgical intervention (<10%) and 4:1 for the diagnosis of TBI (<25%) (Lecky et al. 2017). The criteria for inclusion (head injury, GCS < 13–14 and stable ABC) fitted with major trauma bypass criteria (Lecky et al. 2017). One suggested explanation for the overtriage was that the criteria have been extrapolated from the findings in TBI patients at admission to the hospital which may not be comparable (Lecky et al. 2017). Thus, further research is required to assess which patients in the prehospital setting would benefit from direct transportation to trauma centres with neurosurgery.

Trauma centres without neurosurgery will probably also exist in the future due to demographic reasons. In this context, it is important to consider that patients arriving with a GCS 15 may develop a life-threatening intracranial haematoma requiring acute evacuation. There may also be situations when patients with signs of severe head injury and unstable ABC are admitted to the nearest local hospital and an extracerebral haematoma needs to be treated after stabilization or the patient is too unstable for transfer to the neurosurgical unit. Thus, in the future and in selected cases, non-neurosurgeons may need to perform life-saving neurosurgical operations.

33.2.2 Primary-Secondary Brain Injury and the Time Factor

Patients with extra cerebral haematomas who have a free lucid interval after the trauma may have none or very mild primary brain injury. A later impairment is usually caused by uncal herniation and a fast increase of ICP when the ability to compensate for additional intracranial volume is exhausted. The properties of the intracranial pressure-volume interaction in itself indicate that a delay of neurosurgical intervention may be disastrous because of progressive brain herniation and the development of secondary brain injury. It is difficult in individual patients to assess a precise time limit for the development of irreversible secondary brain injury, but the available time to react is very restricted. The adverse effects of delaying treatment of extracerebral haematomas have been clearly demonstrated in older keynote studies (Mendelow et al. 1979; Seelig et al. 1981). Mendelow and colleagues showed in 1979 that if a delay in surgical evacuation of extradural haematomas exceeded 2 h from deterioration of consciousness (not from the time of injury), the morbidity and mortality became unacceptably high (Mendelow et al. 1979). They argued that the neurosurgeons should teach and train general surgeons, have round-the-clock telephone consultant service and provide a flying squad assistance to support the local surgeon evacuating a clot when needed (Mendelow and Gillingham 1979). Seelig and colleagues reported similar results for acute subdural haematomas in 1981, showing that patients who had a delay of more than 4 h from injury to operation had a 90% mortality rate as compared to 30% in those who had less than 4 h of delay (Seelig et al. 1981).

33.2.3 Reported Experiences of Surgery Outside Neurosurgical Units in Norway and Sweden

In 1999, Wester and colleagues analysed the surgical activity outside of neurosurgical units in Norway by collecting data from a nationwide survey and from the records of all patients with a severe head injury treated in one central hospital (Wester et al. 1999). In the survey, the Norwegian county central hospitals performed 2.5–3 surgical evacuations of intracranial haematomas per year. The operations were in general performed by orthopaedic or general surgeons. In the central hospital, 16 of 31 operated patients (52%) had favourable outcome, and 15 of 31 operated patients (48%) had unfavourable outcome after evacuation of extracerebral haematomas. Only 45% of the operations (14 of 31) were judged to be urgent. One-third of the operations (10 of 31) were classified as inadequate. In the neurosurgical unit, 19 of 23 (83%) had favourable outcome, and 4 of 23 (17%) had unfavourable outcome after evacuation of extracerebral haematomas (n = 14), traumatic intracerebral haematomas (n = 5) and cerebral contusions (n = 4). In extracerebral haematomas, the difference in outcome between the central hospital and the neurosurgical unit was significant for acute subdural haematomas only. It was discussed whether one explanation for the poorer results in the local hospital could be transfer selection bias. However, the conclusion was that patients in need of surgical decompression should be transferred to neurosurgical units for surgery. This study was also the foundation for the recommendation in the guidelines for prehospital care of severe traumatic brain injury from the Scandinavian Neurotrauma Committee in 2008, saying that no patient with acute brain injury should be operated on county hospitals without neurosurgical expertise (Bellander et al. 2008).

In 2014, Fischerstrom and colleagues published a study on how often acute decompressive neurosurgery occurred outside the neurosurgical department in the Uppsala-Örebro region in Sweden (Fischerstrom et al. 2014). They also looked into whether there was a vital indication and assessed the outcome of patients. Notably, there has been a long tradition in the Uppsala-Örebro region of education and training of general surgeons in neurosurgery, round-the-clock telephone neurosurgical consultant service and possibility to send a neurosurgeon to support the local surgeon evacuating a haematoma. The decision to perform acute life-saving decompressive neurosurgery outside the neurosurgical unit in Uppsala is always made after consultation with the neurosurgeon on call. Over a 6-year period, a total of 49 patients were operated in local hospitals (mean 8 patients per year; 17 epidural haematomas and 32 acute subdural haematomas). The operation was judged to have been performed on vital indication in all cases, according to the presence of five evaluated severe preoperative characteristics (free lucid interval, unconsciousness, pupillary dilatation, haematoma width >10 mm and midline shift >5 mm); 8 (16%) patients had all five characteristics, 17 (35%) had

4 and no patient had less than 2. After surgery, there was improvement on the postoperative CT scan in 92% of the patients, and the reaction level and the pupillary reactions were also significantly improved. Long-term outcomes showed favourable outcome in 51% of patients, unfavourable outcome in 33% and unknown outcome in 16%. Overall, considering that all operations appeared to have been performed on vital indication, the results were judged to be favourable, and it was concluded that the regional policy to perform life-saving decompressive neurosurgery in local hospitals by general surgeons should not be changed.

33.2.4 What Is in the Bowls of the Scale?

Is it best for the patient to be operated immediately by a general surgeon with less neurosurgical experience or to be operated later by an experienced neurosurgeon? It is not easy to answer this question, but it is possible to get a relative indication of the need for immediate surgery based on theoretical knowledge regarding volume-pressure relationships and clinical experience. The following factors speak in favour of immediate evacuation without delay: free lucid interval with impairment, rapidly falling consciousness, low GCS at the time of deciding, pupillary dilatation, haematoma width >10 mm and midline shift >5 mm.

33.2.5 Neurosurgical Training Program for General Surgeons

In regions where it may be relevant to perform life-saving evacuations of extracerebral haematomas, it is desirable that a few of the general surgeons in local hospitals receive education and training in the neurosurgical unit (Fischerstrom et al. 2014). According to Fischerstrom and colleagues, the training program should have to following focus areas (Fischerstrom et al. 2014):

1. Ability to trepanate and evacuate chronic subdural haematomas
2. Ability to evacuate extracerebral haematomas via a bone flap
3. Master acute pre- and postoperative evaluation and management of TBI
4. Knowledge of coma scales
5. Knowledge of the interpretation of CT scans
6. Knowledge of basic neurointensive care principles
7. Knowledge of neurosurgical instruments, e.g. trephines
8. Knowledge of neurosurgical haemostasis principles
9. Knowledge about principles for antibiotic and thromboembolic prophylaxis
10. Knowledge of acute epilepsy therapy
11. Knowledge of management of skull fractures

However, it is important to emphasize that the purpose is not to train surgeons to independently perform emergency neurosurgical procedures, but prepare them to initiate acute management of severe TBI in consultation with the neurosurgeon on call.

33.3 Specific Paediatric Concerns

It is important to keep in mind that small children tolerate very little blood loss, and therefore the haemostasis must be meticulous. In case of bleeding problems, the child should liberally receive blood substitution, thrombocytes and coagulation factors. Compression according to damage control principles is recommended to make it possible for the anaesthesiology team to keep up with the transfusions.

Children with closed skull sutures have in general less ability to compensate for an added intracranial volume compared to adults; i.e. time factor is even more important to consider when deciding to whether do immediate decompressive surgery or transport the patient to the neurosurgical unit.

References

Bellander BM, Sollid S, Kock-Jensen C, Juul N, Eskesen V, Sundstrom T, Wester K, Romner B. [Prehospital management of patients with severe head injuries. Scandinavian guidelines according to Brain Trauma Foundation]. Lakartidningen. 2008;105:1834–1838.

Fischerstrom A, Nyholm L, Lewen A, Enblad P. Acute neurosurgery for traumatic brain injury by general surgeons in Swedish county hospitals: a regional study. Acta Neurochir (Wien). 2014;156:177–85.

Lecky F, Bryden D, Little R, Tong N, Moulton C. Emergency intubation for acutely ill and injured patients. Cochrane Database Syst Rev. 2008;(2):CD001429.

Lecky FE, Russell W, McClelland G, Pennington E, Fuller G, Goodacre S, Han K, Curran A, Holliman D, Chapman N, Freeman J, Byers S, Mason S, Potter H, Coats T, Mackway-Jones K, Peters M, Shewan J. Bypassing nearest hospital for more distant neuroscience care in head-injured adults with suspected traumatic brain injury: findings of the head injury transportation straight to neurosurgery (HITS-NS) pilot cluster randomised trial. BMJ Open. 2017;7:e016355.

Mendelow AD, Gillingham FJ. Extradural haematoma: effect of delayed treatment. Br Med J. 1979;2:134.

Mendelow AD, Karmi MZ, Paul KS, Fuller GA, Gillingham FJ. Extradural haematoma: effect of delayed treatment. Br Med J. 1979;1:1240–2.

Seelig JM, Becker DP, Miller JD, Greenberg RP, Ward JD, Choi SC. Traumatic acute subdural hematoma: major mortality reduction in comatose patients treated within four hours. N Engl J Med. 1981;304:1511–8.

Sollid S, Sundstrom T, Ingebrigtsen T, Romner B, Wester K. Organisation of traumatic head injury management in the Nordic countries. Emerg Med J. 2009;26:769–72.

Wester T, Fevang LT, Wester K. Decompressive surgery in acute head injuries: where should it be performed? J Trauma. 1999;46:914–9.

Planning of Cranial and Extracranial Surgery in Multitraumatised Patients

34

Aqeel Chaudhry and Thomas Geisner

Recommendations

Level I

There are insufficient data to support a Level I recommendation for this topic.

Level II

There are insufficient data to support a Level II recommendation for this topic.

Level III

Oxygenation and blood pressure should be monitored, and hypotension (systolic blood pressure < 90 mmHg) and hypoxia ($SaO_2 < 90\%$) should be avoided.

Multitraumatised patients should be managed according to the well-established ABCDE criteria.

The risk of secondary brain injuries can be reduced by adhering to the ABCDE criteria.

In the multitrauma setting, there are no isolated head injuries, and optimal treatment of injuries in other organ systems is crucial for better head injury and overall outcome.

34.1 Overview

Surgical management of traumatic brain injuries should as a general rule be performed as soon as possible. However, management must always be individualised and contextualised. Guidelines for the surgical management of intracranial haematomas provide recommendations primarily based on haematoma characteristics (e.g. type, volume), mass effect and clinical signs, but age, comorbidity, clinical deterioration and concomitant injuries are other important factors that must be considered. An intracranial haematoma in a young person may give rise to more severe clinical signs than in an older patient with significant brain atrophy. Old age and severe comorbidity may contraindicate surgery that is otherwise indicated in a young patient. Clinical deterioration suggestive of haematoma expansion requires more expeditious assessment and management than mass effect per se. In multitraumatised patients, there is not only a head injury to consider, but possibly several critical injuries in need of acute and appropriate treatment, either serially or in parallel.

A. Chaudhry (✉)
Department of Neurosurgery, Haukeland Trauma Center, Haukeland University Hospital, Bergen, Norway
e-mail: aeec@helse-bergen.no

T. Geisner
Department of Vascular Surgery, Haukeland Trauma Center, Haukeland University Hospital, Bergen, Norway
e-mail: tgei@helse-bergen.no

© Springer Nature Switzerland AG 2020
T. Sundstrøm et al. (eds.), *Management of Severe Traumatic Brain Injury*,
https://doi.org/10.1007/978-3-030-39383-0_34

Tips, Tricks and Pitfalls

- Mortality is up to three times higher in multitraumatised patients with head injuries than without head injuries.
- The primary goal of neurosurgical intervention is to prevent secondary brain injuries.
- If the brain does not get a sufficient supply of blood and oxygen, it does not matter what the neurosurgeon has to offer.
- Minor neurosurgery, such as insertion of an ICP monitor or external ventricular drain, can be done at the same time as damage control surgery.

34.2 Background

Severe traumatic brain injury (TBI) is the strongest predictor of overall outcome for multitraumatised patients, and mortality rates are up to three times higher in patients with TBI than in patients without TBI. Clinical assessment and timing of acute neurosurgery in multitraumatised patients with head injuries can be very challenging. TBI-specific treatment is often complementary or adjunctive to treatment of the trauma patient without neurological injury. The basic principles of trauma resuscitation should be followed: rapid assessment and maintenance of airways, breathing and circulation.

34.2.1 The ABCDEs of Major Trauma

Treatment of trauma patients is prioritised based on their vital signs, injuries and the injury mechanism. Vital functions must be assessed quickly and efficiently. Management consists of a rapid primary survey with simultaneous resuscitation of vital functions, a more detailed secondary survey and the initiation of definitive care. The primary survey encompasses the ABCDEs of trauma care and identifies life-threatening conditions by adhering to this sequence:

Airway maintenance with restriction of cervical spine motion.

- A definitive airway must be established if there is any doubt about the patient's ability to maintain airway integrity.
- Clear the airway; inspect for foreign bodies; identify facial/mandibular/tracheal fractures that may result in airway obstruction, suctioning, supplemental oxygen or intubation if needed; or establish an airway surgically if intubation is contraindicated or cannot be accomplished.
- Manual in-line stabilisation (MILS), neck collar or other forms of spinal immobilization should be applied.

Breathing and ventilation require adequate function of the lungs, chest wall and diaphragm.

- Assessment of tracheal position, jugular venous distention, visual inspection, auscultation and percussion of the chest wall and following chest decompression if needed (tension pneumothorax/haemothorax).
- A chest X-ray should be performed.

Circulation.

- Identifying and quickly controlling haemorrhage/blood loss (level of consciousness, skin perfusion and pulse). Identify any source of bleeding by chest X-ray, pelvic X-ray, FAST (focused assessment with sonography for trauma) or diagnostic peritoneal lavage (DPL).
- Definitive bleeding control is essential, along with appropriate replacement of intravascular volume.
- Vascular access is established; typically, two large-bore peripheral venous catheters are

placed to administer whole blood or balance transfusion of blood components.

- In severe cases, laparotomy (major abdominal bleeding) or thoracotomy (cardiac tamponade, uncontrollable bleeding distal to the intrathoracic part of the descending aorta) may be indicated.

When the ABCs are assessed and under control, even if it means performing haemodynamically stabilising surgery in the trauma room, you may move on to D, *disability*:

- Rapid neurologic evaluation (GCS, pupillary examination, lateralizing signs)

Exposure and environment is the last component of the primary survey.

- Undressing the patient for a thorough examination of the skin and then covering up with warm blankets to avoid hypothermia

It is critical to adhere to the ABCDE sequence, as different injuries kill in certain reproducible time frames. The loss of an airway kills more quickly than the loss of the ability to breathe, which again kills more quickly than a depleted circulating blood volume. The presence of an expanding intracranial mass lesion is the next most lethal problem. The mnemonic ABCDE defines the specific order of evaluations and interventions that should be followed in all injured patients, as the primary goal is to keep the patient alive and the secondary goal is to prevent any secondary injury.

The secondary survey is performed only when and if the patient is haemodynamically stable. The survey includes a complete examination from top to bottom: head, face, neck, upper extremities, axilla, thorax, abdomen, pelvis, genitals and lower extremities.

The next step will typically be to run a trauma CT scan to visualise the extent of injuries and any ongoing bleeding. Next, the trauma team can plan further examinations, treatments or observation.

34.2.2 Traumatic Brain Injury in Multitraumatised Patients: Prioritisation and Timing

In multitraumatised patients with concurrent injuries, the trauma team may need to perform rapid prioritisations of timing and sequence of various required surgical procedures. The undebatable principle remains that the patient needs to be haemodynamically stable before performing neurosurgery. Open airways, breathing with sufficient gas exchange and adequate circulation are prerequisites to keep the brain alive. When the patient is stable, with or without stabilising surgery or fluid resuscitation, the neurosurgeon may be called to action. No matter how severe the brain injury, or clear the indication for immediate neurosurgery, the patient needs to be stabilised in terms of ABC first. This might include performing a laparotomy and/or a thoracotomy in the trauma room or the operating theatre (OR) before neurosurgery. Prioritising like this will secure adequate oxygenation and blood flow to the brain and hence reduce or avoid secondary brain injuries. Even though the brain injury may be addressed with quick and accurate surgery, it is of little help if the rescued brain suffers because of lack of oxygenation/perfusion due to compromised ABCs. Compromised airways, breathing and circulation are more life-threatening for the trauma patient than any coexisting head injury.

The whole scale of injuries is often unknown until the patient has undergone a trauma CT scan. If a traumatic head injury needs immediate surgery, and the patient is stable, neurosurgery has priority. If the CT scan reveals a traumatic intracranial haematoma and the indication for surgery is clear, it must generally be performed as soon as possible. Other concurring injuries (abdominal, thoracic and orthopaedic) will have to wait, as long as those injuries do not affect the haemodynamic status of the patient. If there is indication for minor surgery of other body parts (e.g. relieving a pneumothorax with a chest tube), this can be performed immediately before the neurosurgery, but without interfering or delaying the planned neurosurgical intervention. When the neurosurgeon has finished surgery, concomitant injuries can be handled surgically in the same OR, with the necessary change of setup, or the patient may be brought to another OR more suitable for the next surgical intervention.

Occasionally the patient needs to undergo stabilising surgery in the OR after the CT scan is performed and the source of bleeding is clear (ruptured spleen or liver, damage to the heart or aorta). In this case, if there also is an intracranial haematoma, the patient needs to undergo stabilising surgery first. This is necessary even if the patient shows signs of herniation (both clinically and radiologically). The neurosurgeon must optimise the conservative management as much as possible until it is time for decompressive neurosurgery. No matter how frustrating, this is the logical sequence of prioritisation, so that secondary injury to the brain can be minimised or avoided. The neurosurgeon should, however, be ready to commence immediately after, or by the closing up of, the latter surgery.

Minor neurosurgery, which doesn't interfere with the timing of stabilising surgery, e.g. insertion of an ICP probe or external ventricular drain, might be done simultaneously with damage control surgery in the thorax, abdomen or pelvis. You will only need access to the patient's head, requiring a small amount of space. Moreover, the equipment needed may be easily transferred to the OR of choice and may even be done in the ICU.

As already mentioned, it might be very frustrating for neurosurgeons not to be able to perform immediate surgery when indicated. Nevertheless, it is crucial to realise that decision-making in a multitraumatised patient with severe injuries to other organs in addition to the brain is more challenging. The prioritising sequence must, however, be clear and not up for discussion during critical minutes in the trauma room. A haemodynamically unstable patient needs to be stabilised so that secondary brain injuries can be reduced or avoided; in this way, patients will have a better chance of survival and better outcome.

34.3 Specific Paediatric Concerns

Head injuries in children due to, for example, traffic accidents, child abuse or falls can be associated with injuries in other organ systems. Hypotension and hypoxia ("the evil duo") from associated injuries adversely affect the outcome from head injuries.

The priorities for assessing and managing paediatric trauma patients are the same as for adults. However, the unique anatomical and physiological characteristics of children produce distinct injury patterns. The most serious paediatric trauma is blunt trauma that involves the brain. As a result, hypoventilation, apnoea and hypoxia occur up to five times more often than hypovolemia with hypotension in multitraumatised children. Consequently, treatment protocols emphasise aggressive management of the airway and breathing in children.

Children are particularly susceptible to the effects of secondary brain injury. Although the combined effect of hypovolemia and hypoxia is devastating, hypotension from hypovolemia is the most serious single risk factor. Therefore, any bleeding source causing hypovolemia needs to be addressed. Hence, a rapid ABCDE assessment and management is just as crucial as in adults.

Suggested Readings[1]

American College of Surgeons Committee on Trauma. Resources for optimal care of the injured patient. Chicago: American College of Surgeons Committee on Trauma; 2006.

Atkinson JLD. The neglected prehospital phase of head injury: apnea and cathecolamine surge. Mayo Clin Proc. 2000;75(1):37–47.

Brain Trauma Foundation; American Association of Neurological Surgeons; Congress of Neurological Surgeons; Joint Section on Neurotrauma and Critical Care; AANS/CNS. Pediatrics 2009;124(1):e166–71.

[1] In addition to the below list of references, this chapter is heavily based on expert opinion and local experience.

Carney N, Totten AM, O'Reilly C, Ullman JS, et al. Guidelines for the management of severe traumatic brain injury. Neurosurgery. 2017;80(1):6–13.

Chestnut RM, Marshall LF, Klauber MR, et al. The role of secondary brain injury in determining outcome from severe head injury. J Trauma. 1993;34:216–22.

Chesnut RM, Ghajar J, Maas AIR, et al. Early indicators of prognosis in severe traumatic brain injury. Brain Trauma Foundation: New York; 2000.

Esposito TJ, Kuby A, Unfred C, et al. General surgeons and the advanced trauma life support course. American College of Surgeons: Chicago; 2008.

Manser T. Teamwork and patient safety in dynamic domains of healthcare: a review of the literature. Acta Anaesthesiol Scand. 2009;53:143–51.

McHugh GS, Engel DC, Butcher I, et al. Prognostic value of secondary insults in traumatic brain injury: results from the IMPACT study. J Neurotrauma. 2007;24:287–93.

McSwain NE Jr, Salmone J, Pons P, et al., editors. PHTLS: prehospital trauma life support. 7th ed. St. Louis: Mosby/Jems; 2011.

Neugebauer EAM, Waydhas C, Lendemans S, et al. Clinical practice guideline: the treatment of patients with severe and multiple traumatic injuries. Dtsch Arztebl Int. 2012;109(6):102–8.

Robertson CS, Valadka AB, Hannay HJ, et al. Prevention of secondary ischemic insults after severe head injury. Crit Care Med. 1999;27:2086–95.

Valadka AB, Narayan RK. Emergency room management of the head-injured patient. In: Narayan RK, Wilberger JE, Povlishock JT, editors. Neurotrauma. New York: McGraw- Hill; 1996. p. 120.

Zink BJ. Traumatic brain injury outcome: concepts for emergency care. Ann Emerg Med. 2001;37:318–32.

Part VI

Perioperative Anaesthesia

Bent Lob Dahl

Choice of Anaesthesia, Drugs and Medications

35

Christian Sigvald Langfrits and Bent Lob Dahl

Recommendations

Level I

There are insufficient data to support a Level I recommendation for this topic.

Level II

Prophylactic administration of barbiturates to induce burst suppression EEG is not recommended.

High-dose barbiturate administration is recommended to control elevated ICP refractory to maximum standard medical and surgical treatment. Hemodynamic stability is essential before and during barbiturate therapy.

Propofol is recommended for the control of ICP but not for improvement in mortality or 6-month outcome. High-dose propofol can produce significant morbidity.

Level III

There are many Level III recommendations for the topics dealt with in this chapter.

35.1 Overview

The most important in the treatment of patients with brain injury is to maintain oxygenation and blood pressure while securing airway and circulation in order to ensure the best outcome for the patients.

All procedures should be aimed at preserving a normal ICP, cerebral circulation and oxygenation. Use the drugs that you are familiar with. Titrate drugs carefully to avoid hypotension and changes in PaO_2 and $PaCO_2$. Head should be in neutral position and elevated 10–15° to increase cerebral venous drainage without compromising CBF. It must be checked whether the venous drainage is compromised by a cervical collar.

Sedatives and analgesics are widely used to treat pain and agitation in prehospital setting as well as during operative procedures and intensive care. The most widely used drugs are:

C. S. Langfrits (✉)
Department of Anesthesia and Intensive Care, Aalborg University Hospital, Aalborg, Denmark
e-mail: c.langfrits@rn.dk

B. L. Dahl
Department of Anesthesia and Intensive Care, Silkeborg Regional Hospital, Silkeborg, Denmark
e-mail: bentdahl@rm.dk

© Springer Nature Switzerland AG 2020
T. Sundstrøm et al. (eds.), *Management of Severe Traumatic Brain Injury*,
https://doi.org/10.1007/978-3-030-39383-0_35

Sedatives	Thiopental, propofol, midazolam, dexmedetomidine, ketamine, etomidate, clonidine
Analgesics	Morphine, fentanyl, remifentanil, sufentanil, alfentanil
Volatile anaesthetics	Sevoflurane, isoflurane, nitrous oxide
Muscle relaxants	Succinylcholine, mivacurium, atracurium, cisatracurium, vecuronium, rocuronium
Inotropics	Dopamine, dopexamine, noradrenaline, phenylephrine, epinephrine, adrenaline
Weak analgesics	Ketorolac, paracetamol (acetaminophen)

Tips, Tricks and Pitfalls

- Use the drug you are most familiar with.
- A decrease in blood pressure, or an unexpected high or low CO_2, may create more havoc in the injured brain than the use of a suboptimal anaesthetic drug since the differences between the drugs detected in clinical trials are minor.
- Titrate your drugs to avoid hypotension and changes in PaO_2 and $PaCO_2$. Remember many of the severely head-injured patients have additional injuries and are prone to be hypovolemic and will require smaller doses of drugs.
- The acute patient has decreased intracranial compliance and hence decreased compensative ability for even minor changes in ICP. Anaesthesia and intubation should be performed according to this. All procedures should aim at maintaining normal ICP. The head should be in neutral position and elevated 10–15° to increase cerebral venous drainage without compromising CBF. It must be checked whether the venous drainage is compromised if a cervical collar is used.
- For acute intubation in a cardiorespiratory stable patient, propofol or thiopental can be used for sedation. Ketamine or etomidate can be used in cardiorespiratory unstable patients. All analgesics can be used. If relaxation is needed, succinylcholine can be used for rapid sequence intubation, unless there is recent spinal cord injury or severe burns. Mivacurium, atracurium, cisatracurium and vecuronium or rocuronium can also be used according to local instructions.
- 'Inotropics' such as norepinephrine, dopamine, dopexamine, phenylephrine and ephedrine can be used according to the clinical situation. Most TBI patients have a normal to increased cardiac output and vasodilatation and may benefit from norepinephrine infusion (0.02–0.20 μg/kg body weight/min).

35.2 Background

35.2.1 Propofol

Propofol has become widely used because of its rapid onset and short duration, facilitating neurologic examination. Propofol has been shown to reduce cerebral metabolism and oxygen consumption, thereby providing a potential neuroprotective effect. One double-blind randomized controlled clinical trial (RCT) comparing morphine and propofol failed to show a significant difference in GOS or mortality. In a post hoc analysis, a significant increase in neurological outcome was observed in patients receiving high-dose propofol (Kelly et al. 1999).

Propofol infusion syndrome is a safety concern. The clinical features are hyperkalaemia, hepatomegaly, lipaemia, metabolic acidosis, myocardial failure, rhabdomyolysis and renal failure resulting in death. Doses exceeding 5 mg/kg/h, or any dose for more than 48 h, should be avoided.

35.2.2 Midazolam

Midazolam, a relatively short-acting benzodiazepine, is frequently used in neurointensive care units. Its use carries a significant risk of a decrease in MAP and a sustained increase in ICP resulting in a decrease in CPP. Midazolam can be reversed by flumazenil.

35.2.3 Barbiturates

Barbiturates have been used in two different situations: prophylactically and for treatment of refractory intracranial hypertension. Prophylactic use of barbiturates was investigated in two RCTs (Schwartz et al. 1984; Ward et al. 1985), which failed to demonstrate significant clinical benefit. In patients with diffuse injury, Swartz et al. observed a mortality of 77% compared with 43% in the mannitol control group. In both studies, an undesirable decrease in blood pressure was observed. Prophylactic use of barbiturates is not recommended.

The use of barbiturates for treatment of refractory intracranial hypertension was investigated by Eisenberg et al. (1988) in an RCT. The likelihood of survival for those patients whose ICP responded to barbiturates was 92% compared to 17% in non-responders. In patients with hypotension before randomization, barbiturates provided no benefit.

A Cochrane review (Roberts and Sydenham 2012) concluded: 'There is no evidence that barbiturate therapy in patients with acute severe head injury improves outcome. Barbiturate therapy results in a fall in blood pressure in one of four treated patients. The hypotensive effect will offset any ICP lowering effect on cerebral perfusion pressure'.

35.2.4 Ketamine

Ketamine has previously been contraindicated because of fear of increase in CBF and ICP as shown in older studies (Sharma and Vavilala 2012). However, this effect may have been caused by an increase in $PaCO_2$, since all recent studies show no relevant signs of increased ICP during or after ketamine infusion. Some studies even show signs of a decrease in ICP and increase in CPP after ketamine administration (Zeiler 2014). Also the major difference between older and more recent studies is the fact that older studies were based on sedated patients with spontaneous respiration, whereas all later studies are made on anesthetized, mechanically ventilated patients.

It is important to maintain blood pressure and oxygenation in these patients. The advantage of ketamine is that blood pressure and ventilation are better preserved.

In the prehospital and emergency department settings, ketamine has been compared to etomidate for rapid sequence intubation (RSI), with no difference in mortality or patient outcome. Ketamine can, for this reason, be used in patients with TBI, with a recommended dose of 1–2 mg/kg for RSI, but is not recommended for sedation without mechanical ventilation.

35.2.5 Dexmedetomidine

Dexmedetomidine is an alpha-2 adrenergic receptor agonist with rapidly titratable sedative, sympatholytic and some analgesic effects (both per- and postoperative), but only minor respiratory depression. Dexmedetomidine produces a decrease in CBF. The effect on cerebral metabolism in humans is unknown (Pasternak and Lanier 2009). In a small series of healthy persons, an uncoupling of supply and demand in the brain was not found (Drummond et al. 2008). How it influences the injured brain is unknown. The possible benefit of attenuating the sympathetic response (decrease in heart rate and blood pressure to noxious stimuli and reduction in stress response and pulmonary vascular permeability) remains to be investigated.

Recent meta-analysis found a reduction of inflammatory mediators and neuroendocrine hormones postoperatively with dexmedetomidine compared to placebo. However, due to the heterogeneity of the studies, the actual outcomes as regards to brain protection are inconclusive (Jiang et al. 2017).

When compared to propofol, dexmedetomidine has shown a noninferiority as regards to cerebral blood flow velocity and brain oxygenation (Farag et al. 2017).

35.2.6 Etomidate

Etomidate is a short-acting intravenous anaesthetic agent whose primary effects of sedation and amnesia are mediated through the γ-aminobutyric acid (GABA) inhibitory neurotransmitter system. Beneficial effects on the CNS include a decrease in cerebral metabolic rate for oxygen, in cerebral blood flow and in ICP.

A great concern with etomidate is the inhibition of the enzyme 11-β hydroxylase and thereby reduction in cortisol production. Etomidate is not to be used as a continuous infusion, but is largely used in several countries as an induction agent in the prehospital setting and in the ICU, due to its rapid onset and favourable hemodynamic effect.

According to Cochrane (Bruder et al. 2015), there is no evidence of increased mortality, ICU lengths of stay or time with mechanical ventilation related to a single-dose administration. It does however increase the risk of adrenal gland dysfunction.

35.3 Analgesics

35.3.1 Spontaneous Ventilation

Morphine and analogue drugs should be administered with extreme caution in the spontaneously breathing patient with exhausted intracranial compliance. Careful monitoring of conscious state, respiration, blood pressure and eventually arterial blood gas analysis (PaO_2, $PaCO_2$), or capnometry/oximetry, is mandatory. Even a small dose of morphine (e.g. 3 mg IV) might provoke a decrease in $AVDO_2$, suggesting a state of hyperaemia.

35.3.2 Controlled Ventilation

35.3.2.1 Morphine, Fentanyl and Remifentanil

In the ventilator-treated patient, morphine and fentanyl do not increase CBF or ICP. On the contrary, a decrease in ICP is observed. This is caused by the sedative effect giving rise to a decrease in CO_2 production and a decreased level of circulating catecholamines. An additive effect of hypnotics and analgesics on cerebral oxygen uptake may also play a role.

35.3.2.2 Sufentanil and Alfentanil

Comparative studies of fentanyl, alfentanil and sufentanil in patients subjected to craniotomy indicate that the use of the two latter drugs was accompanied by a decrease in CPP and an increase in CSF pressure. Cerebral autoregulation may play a role because correction of blood pressure normalized ICP. Both sufentanil and alfentanil elicit a decrease in blood pressure. As a consequence, a decrease in CVR and an increase in CBV may occur. Under these circumstances, an increase in ICP is observed.

In a systematic review (Roberts et al. 2011) of agents used for postoperative sedation (propofol, etomidate, ketamine, opioids, benzodiazepine, α-2 agonist and antipsychotics), no differences in neurological outcome or mortality between drugs were found.

35.4 Volatile Anaesthetics

Neuroprotection vs. brain cell apoptosis is discussed, but mainly in infants, volatile anaesthetics are widely used.

35.5 Muscular Relaxation

Muscular relaxation can be necessary for intubation and to facilitate ventilatory support, but the latter should be restricted because of a risk of hypoxaemia in case of extubation, masking of seizures, association to myopathy and increased length of stay in ICU.

The neuromuscular blockade of rocuronium and vecuronium can be reversed by sugammadex.

In experimental as well as human studies, succinylcholine increases ICP shortly. The rise in ICP is caused by activation from peripheral impulses from the muscles. Nondepolarizing agents such as rocuronium, vecuronium, mivacurium, atracurium and cisatracurium do not increase ICP during controlled ventilation.

Succinylcholine should not be used for patients with major burns or spinal cord injury from 24 h after injury to at least 6 months due to upregulation of acetylcholine receptors and risk of life-threatening hyperkalaemia.

Nondepolarizing neuromuscular blockers may have advantages on short-term effects on ICP as compared to succinylcholine, but no evidence of differences in long-term outcome are found (Sanfilippo et al. 2015).

35.6 Inotropics

A sufficient blood pressure is important for outcome. If hypotension is observed and hypovolemia is excluded or treated, inotropics should be used. The effect of inotropics on CBF, $CMRO_2$ and ICP is not fully understood as there seems to be relatively few such receptors in cerebral vessels. The effect might depend on whether the BBB is broken or not. Inotropics can be used according to the clinical situation.

35.7 Weak Analgesics

Paracetamol (acetaminophen) might decrease the demand for morphine, and it lowers the body temperature. Ketorolac might also decrease the need for morphine. Often, it is not used because of adverse effects (bleeding and inhibition of bone healing). In a study by Casanelli et al. (2008) of 25 patients undergoing spine surgery, no bleeding was observed in the ketorolac group as compared to 3 patients in the placebo group.

Indomethacin decreases CBF and ICP very effectively and should be used very cautiously for pain management. It is regarded as an experimental drug for reduction of ICP (Sader et al. 2015).

35.8 Specific Pediatric Concerns

Propofol anaesthesia is widely used for paediatric patients. Adverse effects of propofol (increased mortality and the propofol infusion syndrome) have restricted the use of propofol for sedation and ICP control in paediatric patients with or without TBI, which are not recommended by the US FDA. Propofol for anaesthesia can be used according to local rules.

Ketamine has, in a single study, shown a decrease in ICP and increase in CCP after a single-dose administration, in a paediatric population with increased ICP and unresponsiveness to first- and second-tier interventions.

In a small study of paediatric patients with traumatic brain injury and ICP over 20 mmHg, a decrease in ICP and CPP was found without a decrease in MAP (Bramwell et al. 2006). Single dose of etomidate is to be used with caution as regards to children due to the possible worsening of outcome in the septic child.

Sedatives, analgesics and neuromuscular blockers are widely used in children and infants with TBI. Apoptotic effects of anaesthesia and surgery observed in animals are discussed, and an association between anaesthesia and an increased risk of brain damage in human infants is found. However, the evidence is considered inconclusive due to methodological difficulties. Further research of dosing thresholds, (age, number and duration of anaesthesia) is necessary (Noguchi et al. 2017).

There are few studies on the paediatric consequences of sedatives, analgesics and neuromuscular blockers. For this reason, their use is left to the treating doctor (Adelson et al. 2003; Ketharanathan et al. 2017; Kochanek et al. 2019). The use of bolus doses of midazolam and/or fentanyl during ICP crisis should be avoided due to the risk of cerebral hypoperfusion (Kochanek et al. 2019).

References

Adelson PD, Bratton SL, Carney NA, et al. Guidelines for the acute medical management of severe traumatic brain injury in infants, children and adolescents. Pediatr Crit Care Med. 2003;4(3 Suppl):S1–S491. http://tbiguidelines.org/glHome.aspx.

Bramwell KJ, Haizlip J, Pribble C, et al. The effect of etomidate on intracranial pressure and systolic blood pressure in pediatric patients with severe traumatic brain injury. Pediatr Emerg Care. 2006;22(2):90–3.

Bruder EA, Ball IM, Stacy R, William P, Corinne H. Single induction dose of etomidate versus other induction agents for endotracheal intubation in critically ill patients. Cochrane Database Syst Rev. 2015;1:CD010225. https://doi.org/10.1002/14651858.CD010225.pub2.

Casanelli EH, Dean CL, Garcia RM, et al. Ketorolac use for postoperative pain management following lumbar decompression surgery: a prospective, randomized, double-blinded, placebo-controlled trial. Spine. 2008;33(12):1313–7.

Drummond JC, Dao AV, Roth DM, et al. Effect of dexmedetomidine on cerebral flow velocity, cerebral metabolic rate and carbon dioxide response in normal humans. Anesthesiology. 2008;108:225–32.

Eisenberg HM, Frankowski RF, Contant CF, et al. High-dose barbiturate control of elevated intracranial pressure in patients with severe head injury. J Neurosurg. 1988;69:15–23.

Farag E, Kot M, Podolyak A, et al. The relative effects of dexmedetomidine and propofol on cerebral blood flow velocity and regional brain oxygenation: a randomised noninferiority trial. Eur J Anaesthesiol. 2017;34(11):732–9. https://doi.org/10.1097/EJA.0000000000000662.

Jiang L, Hu M, Lu Y, Cao Y, Chang Y, Dai Z. The protective effects of dexmedetomidine on ischemic brain injury: a meta-analysis. J Clin Anesth. 2017;40(2017):25–32. https://doi.org/10.1016/j.jclinane.2017.04.003.

Kelly PF, Goodale LA, Williams J, et al. Propofol in the treatment of moderate and severe head injury: a randomized double-blinded pilot trial. J Neurosurg. 1999;90:1042–57.

Ketharanathan N, Yamamoto Y, Rohlwink U, et al. Analgosedation in pediatric severe traumatic brain injury (TBI): practice, pittfalls and possibilities. Childs Nerv Syst. 2017;33(10):1703–10.

Kochanek PM, Tasker RC, Carney N, et al. Guidelines for the management of pediatric severe traumatic brain injury, third edition: update of the brain trauma foundation guidelines. Pediatr Crit Care Med. 2019;20:S1–S82.

Noguchi KK, Johnson SA, Dissen GA, et al. Isoflurane exposure for three hours triggers apoptotic cell death in neonatal macaque brain. Br J Anaesth. 2017;119(3):524–31.

Pasternak JJ, Lanier WL. Neuroanesthesiology update. J Neurosurg Anesthesiol. 2009;21:73–97.

Roberts I, Sydenham E. Barbiturates for acute traumatic brain injury (review). Cochrane Database Syst Rev. 2012;12:CD000033. https://doi.org/10.1002/14561858.CD000033.pub2.

Roberts DJ, Hall RI, Kramer AH, et al. Sedation for critically ill adults with severe traumatic brain injury: a systematic review of randomized controlled trials. Crit Care Med. 2011;39:2743–51.

Sader N, Zeiler FA, Gillman LM, et al. Indomethacin for control of ICP. Neurocrit Care. 2015;22(3):437–49.

Sanfilippo F, Santonovito C, Veenith T, et al. The role of neuromuscular blockade in patients with traumatic brain injury: a systematic review. Neurocrit Care. 2015;22:325–34.

Schwartz M, Tator C, Towed D, et al. The University of Toronto head injury treatment study: a prospective randomized comparison of pentobarbital and mannitol. Can J Neurol Sci. 1984;11:434–40.

Sharma D, Vavilala MS. Perioperative management of adult traumatic brain injury. Anesthesiol Clin. 2012;30(2):333–46.

Ward JD, Becker DP, Miller JD, et al. Failure of prophylactic barbiturate coma in the treatment of severe head injury. J Neurosurg. 1985;62:383–8.

Zeiler FA, Teitelbaum J, West M, et al. The Ketamine Effect on ICP in Traumatic Brain Injury. Neurocritical Care 2014;21(1):163–173.

36 Blood Pressure, CO_2, and Oxygen Saturation

Kristian Dahl Friesgaard and Bent Lob Dahl

Recommendations

Level I

There are insufficient data to support a Level I recommendation for blood pressure, oxygenation, and hyperventilation.

Level II

Blood pressure should be monitored and hypotension (systolic blood pressure <100 mmHg) avoided. Individualization of BP minimum according to age and CPP should be considered. Prolonged prophylactic hyperventilation with $PaCO_2$ is not recommended.

Level III

Normal oxygenation is recommended. Oxygenation should be monitored and hypoxemia (PaO_2 < 60 mmHg (8 kPa) or O_2 saturation < 90%) avoided.

Hyperventilation is recommended for acute treatment of impending transtentorial herniation resistant to other treatments, such as sedation and osmotherapy.

36.1 Overview

Experimental studies indicate that cerebral hypoxia after traumatic brain injury is related to cerebral hypoperfusion as well as low arterial blood oxygen tension (PaO_2). As the injured brain probably is more prone to ischemia because of insufficient cellular oxygen delivery, secondary insults after traumatic brain injury should be avoided by ensuring adequate blood pressure and oxygen saturation. Measurement of cerebral oxygenation has either temporal or spatial limitations (Table 36.1) especially in the initial acute treatment of TBI patients where such measurements may have marginal value. The best possible way to ensure sufficient cerebral oxygenation in the acute setting is therefore to control blood pressure and blood oxygen saturation and to maintain normocapnia.

Retrospective data of 717 patients with GCS < 9 from the Traumatic Coma Data Bank showed that hypoxemia (PaO_2 < 60 mmHg) and hypotension (SBP < 90 mmHg) were independently associated with a significant increase in morbidity and mortality from severe head injury in the prehospital setting (Chesnut et al. 1993).

K. D. Friesgaard (✉)
Department of Anesthesiology and Intensive Care, Aarhus University Hospital, Aarhus, Denmark

B. L. Dahl
Department of Anesthesia and Intensive Care, Silkeborg Regional Hospital, Silkeborg, Denmark
e-mail: bentdahl@rm.dk

© Springer Nature Switzerland AG 2020
T. Sundstrøm et al. (eds.), *Management of Severe Traumatic Brain Injury*,
https://doi.org/10.1007/978-3-030-39383-0_36

Table 36.1 Advanced measures of cerebral oxygenation and its limitations in acute management of traumatic brain injury

Temporal limitation	MRI
	Xe-CT
Spatial limitation	Jugular bulb oxygen saturation—$SjvO_2$
	Brain tissue partial pressure of oxygen—$PtiO_2$
	Microdialysis
	Near-infrared spectroscopy—NIRS
	Transcranial Doppler—TCD

Hypotension was associated with a doubling in mortality. For ethical reasons, prospective controlled studies of the effect of hypoxemia and oxygenation have never been done and will probably never be done. However, clinical intuition and observational data indicate that correction of hypotension and hypoxia improves outcome. Observational data of 13,151 patients with moderate or severe traumatic brain from the Excellence in Prehospital Injury Care (EPIC) study showed that hypoxemia (oxygen saturation < 90%) and hypotension (SBP < 90 mmHg) in the prehospital setting were independently associated with a significant increase in mortality. Also, the effect of combined hypoxemia and hypotension more than doubles mortality compared with either hypoxemia or hypotension (Spaite et al. 2017a, b).

36.2 Background

TBI is divided in two separate events. The primary injury is the result of mechanical forces at the time of injury, resulting in damage to neurons, glia cells, and vascular tissue. This leads to disruption of cell membranes and disturbance of ionic homeostasis (Stiefel et al. 2005) causing a neurotoxic cascade. Only preventive measures can avoid this. The secondary injury is the result of ischemia and possibly an acceleration of the initial events and calls for immediate and appropriate treatment. Hypotension and hypoxia might influence outcome in a negative direction. As it is unethical to perform randomized, prospective trials on the effect of hypotension and hypoxia, our recommendations are based on Level II and III evidence.

36.3 Hypoxemia

The oxygen consumption of the brain ($CMRO_2$) is approximately 3–3.5 mL/100 g/min or 40–50 mL oxygen per minute. The oxygen reserve of the brain is very limited, and cessation of blood flow will lead to unconsciousness in 10–15 s.

In prospectively collected data from the prehospital EPIC study, hypoxemia among 13,151 patients with moderate or severe traumatic brain injury was significantly associated with mortality. The impact of combined hypoxemia and hypotension raises mortality considerably (Spaite et al. 2017a, b). The same result was found in a meta-analysis of pooled data from seven randomized controlled trials (McHugh et al. 2007). In the classical prehospital study by Chesnut and colleagues, hypoxemia occurred in 22.4% of severe TBI patients and was significantly associated with increased morbidity and mortality (Chesnut et al. 1993). Duration of hypoxemia was studied in a subgroup of 71 inhospital patients with TBI of varying degrees of severity. Duration of hypoxemia (defined as SaO_2 < 90%; median duration ranging from 11.5 to 20 min) was found to be an independent predictor of mortality, but not morbidity (Jones et al. 1994). In patients with severe head injury (GCS 3–8), it is therefore important to administer high-flow oxygen, secure the airway under C-spine control, and ventilate the patient as soon as possible. Always consider the possibility of pneumo- or hemothorax in trauma patients.

The effect of positive end-expiratory pressure (PEEP) has been controversial (see Chap. 37 - Intracranial pressure reduction) as it might decrease MAP and increase ICP leading to a reduction in CPP. However, Mascia et al. (2005) found no increase in ICP during alveolar recruitment. In a recent observational study (n = 341), no significant clinical effect of PEEP on ICP and CPP was shown (Boone et al. 2017).

Tips, Tricks, and Pitfalls

- Vigorous evaluation and stabilization of the patient according to ABC principles (Advanced Trauma Life Support 2013).
- Start with noninvasive monitoring of blood pressure, oxygen saturation, and $ETCO_2$ and, when suitable, arterial blood gas and invasive measurement of blood pressure.
- Maintain SBP > 100 mmHg.
- Maintain oxygen saturation > 95 or PaO_2 > 10 kPa.
- PEEP = 2–5 mmHg or higher according to clinical situation.
- Avoid hypotonic solutions (isotonic glucose).
- Hypertonic saline might correct hypotension (see individual chapter).
- Maintain normocapnia ($PaCO_2$ = 4.5–5.0 kPa).
- Maintain normothermia (36.5–38 °C).
- In case of clinical signs of increased ICP (decrease in GCS ≥ 2, pupil abnormalities, or paralysis of extremities), immediately start hyperventilation ($PaCO_2$ = 3.5–4.0 kPa), perhaps supplemented with hypertonic saline (7.2%, 100–200 mL) or mannitol (0.5–1 g/kg).
- In patients with possible hypovolemia, hypertonic saline is preferable to mannitol to avoid osmotic diuresis and worsening of hypovolemia.
- Reverse Trendelenburg position 0–15°.
- Head in neutral position.
- Indwelling catheter with the goal of a diuresis of 1 mL/kg/h.
- If volume treatment of the trauma patient only transiently or not at all stabilizes vital parameters, ongoing bleeding must be suspected.
- Naso- or orogastric tube (nasogastric tube is contraindicated in suspicion of skull base fracture).

36.4 Hypotension

In patients with TBI, cerebral autoregulation, which normally secures CBF within a certain range of blood pressure, is compromised, leading to a linear correlation between blood pressure and CBF. Low blood pressure therefore might decrease CBF. In the study from TCDB, a single episode of SBP < 90 mmHg was an independent predictor of outcome and in fact was associated with increased morbidity and a doubling of mortality (Chesnut et al. 1993). Other studies show similar results (Gentleman 1992; Hill et al. 1993; Jeffreys and Jones 1981; Kohi et al. 1984; Miller and Becker 1982; Miller et al. 1978; Narayan et al. 1982; Pietropaoli et al. 1992; Rose et al. 1977; Seelig et al. 1986; Struchen et al. 2001). Duration and number of hypotensive events might also influence outcome. Duration of episodes of hypotension was a significant, independent factor of mortality and morbidity (Jones et al. 1994). Recent studies have questioned the classical threshold for hypotension of SBP < 90 mmHg, and a higher cutoff might be beneficial for improving outcome (Bullock et al. 2007; Berry et al. 2012; Brenner et al. 2012; Fuller et al. 2014; Spaite 2016).

In trauma patients, hypotension is caused by hypovolemia until proven otherwise. However, one must always consider tension pneumothorax and cardiac tamponade. Other forms of shock in trauma patients are rare, but might be the primary reason for the trauma (allergic, cardiogenic, neurogenic, or septic shock). Two IV lines must be inserted with rapid infusion of normotonic saline. Visible bleeding must be stopped immediately. Internal bleeding must be excluded or treated as soon as possible. According to ATLS, the response to volume treatment must be monitored continuously to guide volume therapy as well as the stability of the patient. If volume treatment only transiently or not at all stabilizes vital parameters, ongoing bleeding must be suspected. Until now, a positive effect of hypothermia as a neuroprotective measure in TBI patients has failed to be proven (Lewis et al. 2017). In order to minimize hemorrhagic diathesis, it is important to avoid hypothermia.

Table 36.2 Beneficial and detrimental effects of induced hyperventilation (Cold 1990)

Induced hyperventilation	
Beneficial effect • Decrease in ICP • Respiratory alkalosis neutralizing metabolic acidosis • Normalization of cerebral autoregulation • Inverse steal phenomenon (Robin Hood) • Reduction of CSF formation	Detrimental effect • Cerebral oligemia in focal or watershed areas • Decrease in diastolic filling and cardiac output • Decrease in MABP and CPP • Water and salt retention • Inhibition of oxygen delivery to the tissues (Bohr effect) • Barotrauma

36.5 CO_2

$ETCO_2$ should be monitored continuously, at least after intubation, and should be evaluated by serial arterial blood gas analyses. CO_2 reactivity averages a change in CBF of 2.5 mL/100 g/min/mmHg change in $PaCO_2$ (Cold 1990). The theoretical effects of hyperventilation are summarized in Table 36.2. Hyperventilation is discussed in detail in Chap. 60. Prophylactic hyperventilation ($PaCO_2$ of 25 mmHg or less) is not recommended (Muizelaar et al. 1991). Hyperventilation is recommended only as a temporary measure for the reduction of elevated intracranial pressure (ICP). Hyperventilation should be avoided during the first 24 h after injury when cerebral blood flow (CBF) often is critically reduced. If hyperventilation is used, jugular venous oxygen saturation (SjO_2) or brain tissue oxygen tension ($PbrO_2$) measurements can be used to monitor oxygen delivery.

36.6 Specific Pediatric Concerns

Resuscitation and stabilization of the cardiovascular and respiratory systems in the field, during transfer, and in the hospital need to be emphasized in an effort to optimize outcome from severe pediatric brain injury (Adelson et al. 2003). Children are more susceptible to trauma. They differ from adults in that they have shorter trachea, softer epiglottis, large occiput, and a soft chest wall and abdomen. The spleen and liver are not protected by costae, and children have a large body surface area compared to body mass; this leads easily to hypothermia.

Table 36.3 Lower limits of normal systolic blood pressure at different ages

Age	Minimal systolic blood pressure
0–28 days	>60 mmHg
1–12 months	>70 mmHg
1–10 years	>70 + 2× age in years mmHg
>10 years	> 100 mmHg

Hypotension (Table 36.3) and hypoxemia should be avoided in children as well as in adults. Hypotension is a late sign of shock in children (>45% blood loss). Tachycardia, decreased urinary output, and skin manifestations (cold, clammy, cyanotic, pale skin or increased capillary filling time (>2 s)) are earlier signs of hypovolemia (Advanced Trauma Life Support 2013).

If ICP is measured, CPP between 40 and 50 mmHg, but not lower, is recommended. The thresholds for infants may be at the lower end of this range and for adolescents at or above the upper end (Kochanek et al. 2019).

Hypoxia in children is defined as $PaO_2 < 60–65$ mmHg (8–8.7 kPa) or O_2 saturation <90%. Desaturation occurs more rapidly in children than in adults; therefore, oxygen saturation >95 or $PO_2 > 10$ kPa is recommended. Priorities in evaluation and treatment for traumatized patients (ABCDE) are the same for children and adults (Advanced Trauma Life Support 2013).

Prophylactic severe hyperventilation to a $PaCO_2$ below 30 mmHg (4 kPa) in the initial 48 h after injury is not recommended. If hyperventilation is used in the management of refractory intracranial hypertension, advanced neuromonitoring for evaluation of cerebral ischemia is suggested (Hardcastle et al. 2012; Godoy et al. 2017; Kochanek et al. 2019). If transtentorial herniation is suspected, it is considered a medical disaster and hyperventilation to $PaCO_2$ 4–4.5 kPa may temporarily (minutes) be used.

References

Adelson PD, Bratton SL, Carney NA, et al. Guidelines for the acute medical management of severe traumatic brain injury in infants, children and adolescents. Pediatr Crit Care Med. 2003;4(3 Suppl):S1–S491. http://tbiguidelines.org/glHome.aspx.

Advanced Trauma Life Support. 2013. https://www.ncbi.nlm.nih.gov/pubmed/23609291.

Berry C, Ley EJ, Bukur M, et al. Redefining hypotension in traumatic brain injury. Injury. 2012;43(11):1833–7.

Boone. 2017. https://www.ncbi.nlm.nih.gov/pubmed/27848125.

Brenner M, Stein DM, HU PF, et al. Traditional systolic blood pressure targets underestimate hypotension-induced secondary brain injury. J Trauma Acute Care Surg. 2012;72(5):115–9.

Bullock I, Maas AI, Marmarou A, et al. Prognostic value of admission blood pressure in traumatic brain injury: results from the IMPACT study. J Neurotrauma. 2007;24(2):294–302.

Chesnut RM, Marshall LF, Klauber MR, et al. The role of secondary brain injury in determining outcome from severe head injury. J Trauma. 1993;34:216–22.

Cold GE. Cerebral blood flow in acute head injury. The regulation of cerebral blood flow and metabolism during the acute phase of head injury and its significance for therapy. Acta Neurochir Suppl. 1990;49:1–66.

Fuller G, Hasler RM, Mealing N, et al. The association between admission systolic blood pressure and mortality in significant traumatic brain injury: a multicentre cohort study. Injury. 2014;45(3):612–7.

Gentleman D. Causes and effects of systemic complications among severely head-injured patients transferred to a neurosurgical unit. Int Surg. 1992;77:297–302.

Godoy DA, Seifi A, Garza D, et al. Hyperventilation therapy for the control of posttraumatic intracranial hypertension. Front Neurol. 2017;8:250.

Hardcastle N, Benzon HA, Valvila MS. Update on the 2012 guidelines for the management of pediatric traumatic brain injury—information to the anesthesiologist. Pediatr Anaesth. 2012;24:703–10.

Hill DA, Abraham KJ, West RH. Factors affecting outcome in the resuscitation of severely injured patients. Aust N Z J Surg. 1993;63:604–9.

Jeffreys RV, Jones JJ. Avoidable factors contributing to the death of head injury patients in general hospitals in Mersey region. Lancet. 1981;2:459–61.

Jones PA, Andrews PJD, Midgely S, et al. Measuring the burden of secondary insults in head injured patients during intensive care. J Neurosurg Anesthesiol. 1994;6:4–14.

Kochanek PM, Tasker RC, Carney N, et al. Guidelines for the management of pediatric severe traumatic nrain injury, third edition: update of the brain trauma foundation guidelines. Pediatr Crit Care Med. 2019;20:S1–S82.

Kohi YM, Mendelow AD, Teasdale GM, et al. Extracranial insults and outcome in patients with acute head injury – relationship to the Glasgow Coma Scale. Injury. 1984;16:25–9.

Lewis SR, Evans DJW, Butler AR, et al. Hypothermia for traumatic brain injury. Cochrane Database Syst Rev. 2017;9:CD001048. https://doi.org/10.1002/14651858.CD001048.pub5.

Mascia. 2005. https://www.ncbi.nlm.nih.gov/pubmed/15668765.

McHugh GS, Engel DC, Butcher I, et al. Prognostic value of secondary insults in traumatic brain injury: results from the IMPACT study. J Neurotrauma. 2007;24(2):287–93.

Miller JD, Becker DP. Secondary insults to the injured brain. J R Coll Surg Edinb. 1982;27:292–8.

Miller JD, Sweet RC, Narayan R, et al. Early insults to the injured brain. JAMA. 1978;240:439–42.

Muizelaar JP, Marmarou A, Ward JD, et al. Adverse effects of prolonged hyperventilation in patients with severe head injury: a randomized clinical trial. J Neurosurg. 1991;75(5):731–9.

Narayan R, Kishore P, Becker D, et al. Intracranial pressure: to monitor or not to monitor? A review of our experience with head injury. J Neurosurg. 1982;56:650–9.

Pietropaoli JA, Rogers FB, Shackford SR, et al. The deleterious effects of intraoperative hypotension on outcome in patients with severe head injuries. J Trauma. 1992;33:403–7.

Rose J, Valtonen S, Jennett B. Avoidable factors contributing to death after head injury. Br Med J. 1977;2:615–8.

Seelig JM, Klauber MR, Toole BM, et al. Increased ICP and systemic hypotension during the first 72 hours following severe head injury. In: Miller JD, Teasdale GM, Rowan JO, et al., editors. Intracranial pressure VI, vol. 40. Berlin: Springer; 1986. p. 764–7.

Spaite. 2016. https://www.ncbi.nlm.nih.gov/pubmed/27926759.

Spaite DW, Hu C, Bobrow BJ, et al. Mortality and prehospital blood pressure in patients with major traumatic brain injury: implications for the hypotension threshold. JAMA Surg. 2017a;152(4):360–8.

Spaite DW, Hu C, Bobrow BJ, et al. The effect of combined out of hospital hypotension and hypoxia on mortality in major traumatic brain injury. Ann Emerg Med. 2017b;69(1):62–72.

Stiefel MF, Tomita Y, Marmarou A. Secondary ischemia impairing the ion homeostasis following traumatic brain injury. J Neurosurg. 2005;103:707–14.

Struchen MA, Hannay HJ, Contant CF, et al. The relation between acute physiological variables and outcome on the Glasgow outcome scale and disability rating scale following severe traumatic brain injury. J Neurotrauma. 2001;18:115–25.

Intracranial Pressure Reduction

37

Bent Lob Dahl and Kristian Dahl Friesgaard

Recommendations

The Brain Trauma Foundation guidelines (2016) do not specifically deal with the perioperative period. In this chapter however, the recommendations from the Brain Trauma Foundation concerning indications for intracranial pressure monitoring, intracranial pressure monitoring technology, and intracranial pressure thresholds are incorporated for the perioperative period also.

37.1 Overview

ICP hypertension should be anticipated in patients with traumatic brain injury. Perioperatively, ICP should be measured on wide indications, and treatment should be instituted if ICP increases to more than 20 mmHg. The control of intracranial hypertension (ICP > 20 mmHg) is based on the control of intracranial blood volume via either control of cerebral venous distension (central venous pressure, neck compression) or control by neurophysiologic mechanisms including the chemical ($PaCO_2$, PaO_2, indomethacin, theophyllamine), neurogenic or hormonal (catecholamine), metabolic (hypnotics, analgesics, hypothermia), and autoregulatory control of cerebral circulation. Control of cerebral tissue water content is possible by osmotic acting drugs like hypertonic saline (HTS) and mannitol.

During anaesthesia, it is important to have and to apply a thorough understanding of the intracranial pathophysiology in order to avoid and treat intracranial hypertension in adults as well as in children.

B. L. Dahl (✉)
Department of Anesthesia and Intensive Care, Silkeborg Regional Hospital, Silkeborg, Denmark
e-mail: bentdahl@rm.dk

K. D. Friesgaard
Department of Anesthesiology and Intensive Care, Aarhus University Hospital, Aarhus, Denmark

Tips, Tricks, and Pitfalls

ICP control calls for preoperative planning and careful perioperative management in order to avoid ICP hypertension and a treatment plan in case of ICP hypertension.

Anaesthesia planning:

- Planning of anaesthesia for patients with severe traumatic brain injury must always be in close collaboration with the neurosurgeon.
- Anticipate that increased intracranial pressure might occur during surgery.
- Measure ICP, if possible. Ask the neurosurgeon if the dura is tense before opening.
- Use trauma mechanism, clinical examination, age, GCS, motor posturing, and CT findings to evaluate the risk of

© Springer Nature Switzerland AG 2020
T. Sundstrøm et al. (eds.), *Management of Severe Traumatic Brain Injury*,
https://doi.org/10.1007/978-3-030-39383-0_37

increased intracranial pressure if actual measurement is not possible.

- Consider measurement of ICP during anaesthesia for acute surgery in trauma patients, even for patients with normal cerebral CT scan.

Anaesthesia basics:

- Normoventilation $PaCO_2$ = 4.5–5.5 kPa (35–40 mmHg).
- Avoid hypo- and hyperoxia.
- Always head in neutral position if possible.
- Always check cervical collar for neck pressure.
- Always reverse Trendelenburg position (rTP) 0–15° elevation of head.
- Keep ICP below 20 mmHg and CPP over 60 mmHg.
- If ICP/CPP is not measured, keep systolic blood pressure > 100 mmHg (Pts 50–69 years old) or >110 mmHg (Pts 15–49 and +70 years old).
- Dura tension should be evaluated by the surgeon or actually measured before opening of dura.
- Treatment of high dura tension or ICP should immediately be instituted before dura opening to avoid herniation through the craniotomy.

Anaesthesia ICP problems:

- Treatment if ICP is above 20 mmHg.
- Is anaesthesia deep enough?
- Keep head in neutral position.
- Increase rTP to 15°.
- Increase ventilation to CO_2 approximately 4 kPa (30 mmHg) or 3.5 kPa (26 mmHg) very shortly.
- Hypertonic saline 7.2%. 20–100 ml in repeated doses (beware of hyponatraemia). In our intensive care setting, small doses of 20–100 mL 7.2% NaCl usually control ICP.
- Mannitol 0.25–1 g/kg (beware of osmotic diuresis, especially in hypovolaemic patients).
- Ask surgeon for surgical possibility to remove mass lesion.

37.2 Background

In the analysis of perioperative anaesthesia and ICP control, the guidelines from the Brain Trauma Foundation are of much value, although these guidelines do not have anaesthesia as its primary aim. The basis of this chapter has to rely on scientific evidence, basic physiology, experience, and common sense in the absence of Level I evidence. Therefore, it is imperative to understand the relationship between cerebral blood flow (CBF), mean arterial blood pressure (MABP), cerebral perfusion pressure (CPP), intracranial pressure (ICP), and the clinical examination.

The Monro-Kellie doctrine, formulated in the 1820s, indicates that the cranium is a nonexpandable box containing the brain, cerebrospinal fluid (CSF), and arterial and venous blood volume. CSF is formed at a rate of 0.3 mL/min. The total amount of CSF is 140–200 mL with 25–35 mL in the ventricular system and the rest in the cranial and spinal subarachnoid spaces. ICP is fairly constant, as it is regulated by changes mainly in blood and CSF volumes. In traumatic brain injury, an intracranial haemorrhage or oedema may develop. If the compensatory changes in blood volume and CSF are exhausted, ICP may increase rapidly even with minor changes in intracranial volume, as indicated in the pressure-volume curve (Fig. 37.1).

CPP is the difference between mean arterial blood pressure and ICP (CPP = MABP − ICP). Normally cerebral autoregulation (Fig. 37.2) insures CBF of 50 mL/100 g brain/min (750 mL/min) within a range of MABP of approximately 50 and 160 mmHg. Below this value, CBF declines rapidly and EEG becomes isoelectric. At CBF 5 mL/100 g/min, irreversible cell death hap-

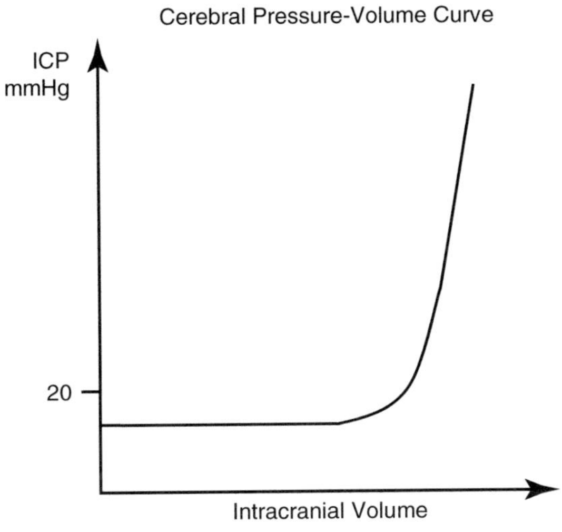

Fig. 37.1 Relationship between intracranial volume and intracranial pressure (ICP). During the initial intracranial volume increase, ICP is fairly constant because of compensatory mechanisms. When these mechanisms are exhausted, even small increases in volume lead to a marked increase in ICP

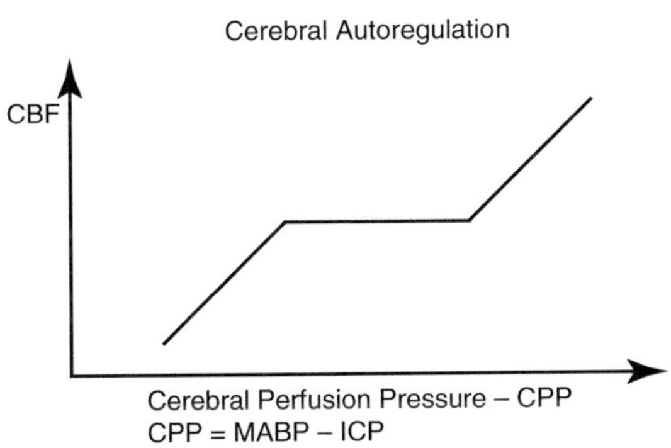

Fig. 37.2 Cerebral autoregulation. CBF of 50 mL/100 g/min are maintained in a range of MABP between 50 and 160 mmHg. Below 50 mmHg, CBF decreases and above 160 mmHg CBF increases

pens. MABP above 160 leads to an increase in CBF which again increases cerebral blood volume and increases ICP and possibly adds to the formation of cerebral oedema.

In the injured brain, cerebral autoregulation may be abolished globally or regionally. As a consequence, there will be a direct correlation between blood pressure and cerebral blood flow.

As a result of increased ICP, brain herniation might occur leading to further arterial compromise and pressure on brain tissue and nerves leading to a decline in GCS, pupillary abnormalities, and/or paralysis. Cushing's response (increase in blood pressure and bradycardia in order to maintain CPP) is, compared to clinical changes, a late sign of high ICP.

Anaesthesiologists dealing with trauma patients, no matter if it is for neurosurgery or surgery for other lesions, must be aware that an increase in ICP might occur even though CT scan is normal. In a prospective study of comatose patients with abnormal CT scans, the incidence of intracranial hypertension was 53–63%. If patients with normal CT scans demonstrated 2 or 3 adverse features (age > 40 years, unilateral or bilateral posturing, or systolic blood pressure < 90 mmHg), the risk of intracranial hypertension was similar to that of patients with abnormal CT scans. In patients with normal CT scans, intracranial hypertension was found in 13% of patients (Narayan et al. 1982). Before performing anaesthesia in a trauma patient, the demand for monitoring ICP must be evaluated. If there are signs of brain injury or intracranial hypertension, ICP must be monitored during surgery. In a retrospective study, Miller et al. (2004) found that even midline shift, basal cisterns, ventricular effacement, sulci compression, and grey/white matter contrast did not correlate with the initial ICP.

Intracranial hypertension is closely correlated to death in severe TBI. A randomized clinical trial of ICP monitoring with and without treatment will probably never be done; however, data suggest that normalization of ICP improves outcome. It is generally accepted that intracranial hypertension must be treated regardless of whether it is actually monitored or diagnosed on clinical suspicion alone. Not monitoring ICP while treating for intracranial hypertension can be deleterious and result in poor outcome. This concept has been challenged. No difference in outcome was found whether treatment was based on measurement of ICP or clinical and radiological examination (Chestnut et al. 2012). How to measure ICP is described in Chaps. 29 and 40. A ventricular catheter connected to an external strain gauge transducer is the most accurate method of monitoring ICP. Parenchymal transducers are good alternatives, while subarachnoid or subdural fluid-coupled devices and epidural devices are less accurate. The threshold for ICP is 20–25 mmHg, above which treatment to lower ICP generally is recommended.

37.2.1 Perioperative Management of ICP

Neuroanaesthesia is different from anaesthesia for other procedures in the way that both the surgeon and the anaesthesiologist work on the same organ—the brain. Removal of mass lesions might reduce the risk of intracranial hypertension. Operative approach for correction of intracranial hypertension may be restricted, if the main reason for intracranial hypertension is cerebral swelling as a consequence of brain oedema or increased cerebral blood volume. The control of intracranial hypertension under such circumstances is based on the control of intracranial blood volume via either control of cerebral venous distension (central venous pressure, neck compression, dihydroergotamine) or control by neurophysiologic mechanisms including the chemical ($PaCO_2$, PaO_2 indomethacin, theophyllamine), neurogenic, hormonal (catecholamine), metabolic (hypnotics, analgesics, hypothermia), and autoregulatory control of the cerebral circulation. Control of cerebral tissue water content is possible by osmotically acting drugs like hypertonic saline and mannitol.

Studies from1994 to 2008 of mainly tumour patients and patients with subarachnoid haemorrhage in a total of 1833 patients might indicate how intracranial hypertension is treated (Cold 2008). The ICP-reducing procedures most frequently used were (Table 37.1):

Only 0.8% of the patients were treated for traumatic brain injury (TBI). However, there is no reason to believe that the treatment modalities are different in TBI. It is important to avoid hypotension, hypoxia, and ICP hypertension during the pre-, per-, and the postoperative period.

Table 37.1 In a study of 1833 patients, the most frequently used measures to reduce ICP hypertension were reverse Trendelenburg position, hyperventilation, cyst puncture, and mannitol (Cold 2008)

Procedure	Number of patients	Percent of total
Reverse Trendelenburg position (rTP)	188	10.3
Hyperventilation	168	9.2
Decompression (drainage or cyst puncture)	74	4.0
Mannitol	56	3.1

37.2.2 Pre- and Postoperative Period

In the pre- and postoperative period, it is important to anticipate ICP problems when planning premedication and pain management, as sedation might induce hypoventilation leading to hypercapnia and increase in ICP. If ICP is not monitored, clinical symptoms and CT findings are used for evaluation of the risk of ICH.

37.2.3 Positive End-Expiratory Pressure (PEEP)

Adult respiratory distress syndrome develops in up to 20% of patients with severe head injury. Positive end-expiratory pressure (PEEP) is often required to maintain oxygenation; however, PEEP might influence ICP through decreased venous outflow as well as venous return and reduced arterial blood pressure. The effect of PEEP is mainly investigated in the ICU setting and the results are conflicting. Coughing, Valsalva manoeuvre, application of PEEP and CPAP, and neck compression are supposed to increase ICP. Even application of a cervical collar for immobilization might increase ICP (Raphael and Chotai 1994).

When patients are maintained in the 30-degree head-up position (reverse Trendelenburg position—rTP), PEEP improves arterial oxygenation without increasing ICP (Frost 1977). In a study including patients with head injury, SAH, or hydrocephalus, PEEP at 5 cmH_2O did not alter ICP, and the clinical relevance of ICP increase at PEEP levels of 10 and 15 cmH_2O was questionable, as CPP did not change and remained

Table 37.2 The effect of application of 5 and 10 cmH_2O PEEP on BP, ICP, and CPP (Duch and Cold 2008)

	5 cmH_2O		10 cmH_2O	
	Before	After	Before	After
BP	70.9	68.2	75.3	72.3
ICP	5.7	6.7	5.1	8.2
CPP	65.4	61.5	70.2	65.1

>60 mmHg. Application of PEEP at 10 and 15 cmH_2O has been shown to produce an increase in ICP without significant effect on CPP (Videtta et al. 2002). Generally, PEEP is considered as a valuable therapy for the comatose patient with pulmonary disorders such as pneumonia or pulmonary oedema (Frost 1977). Perioperatively, the effect of PEEP 5 and 10 cmH_2O on BP, ICP, and CPP has been investigated mainly in tumour patients ($N = 13$) (Table 37.2).

The application of PEEP had a minor negative effect on BP, ICP, and CPP (Duch and Cold 2008). In a retrospective study of 341 patients with 28,644 paired observations of PEEP and ICP and CPP, an increase in PEEP of 1 cmH20 resulted in a minor increase in ICP of 0.31 mmHg. This result suggests that PEEP can be applied safely (Boone et al. 2017). The magnitude of these changes in ICP has to be weighted against the possibly positive effect of PEEP on atelectasis and oxygenation.

37.2.4 Patient Position

37.2.4.1 Head Elevation

In one study, the decrease in ICP during head elevation was smaller than the decline in blood pressure resulting in a decrease in CPP (Rosner and Coley 1986). In another study, head elevation was not accompanied by a change in CPP because the decrease in ICP corresponded to the decrease in BP (Feldman et al. 1992). In comatose patients, CBF decreases gradually with head elevation from 0 to 45°, from 46 to 29 mL/min/100 g. During head elevation, the difference between arterial pressure and jugular pressure was the major determinant of CBF regardless of head position (Moraine et al. 2000).

37.2.4.2 Head Flexion, Rotation, and Tilting

Changes in head position, including maximal flexion and lateral rotation, lead to an increase in ICP, and elevation of the head induces a fall in ICP. The most alarming increase in ICP is observed during head-down position (Schneider et al. 1993; Mavrocordatos et al. 2000). The mechanisms are intracranial venous distension and an increase in cerebral blood volume (Mchedlishvili 1988; Schreiber et al. 2002). Some studies indicate that moderate flexion of the head 15–30° is associated with a decrease in ICP due to the improved venous drainage (Kanter et al. 1991).

37.2.4.3 Reverse Trendelenburg Position (rTP)

If ICP is not already monitored during craniotomy, subdural pressure can be measured after opening the cranium, but before opening the dura (Cold et al. 1996). An i.v. needle is introduced under the dura and connected to a pressure monitor. Repeated measurements of subdural pressure and CPP at neutral position and at varying degrees of rTP between 5 and 15° can thus be obtained within a few minutes, and a decision concerning optimal position, as regards the level of both ICP and CPP, can be drawn. The optimal position is defined as the position in which subdural ICP was as low as possible, with CPP remaining above 60 mmHg or as high as possible. In patients operated for cerebral aneurysms, a considerable individual variation in the optimal position from 0 to 15° rTP was found. The optimal position was 10–15° rTP (Juul and Cold 2008). It is recommended to optimize the position in trauma patients as well. During craniotomy for tumour or haematoma, opening of the dura represents a critical moment. In order to avoid herniation of the brain tissue when the dura is opened, and to secure optimal condition for the neurosurgeon, the same method was used. In a study of 692 tumour patients, subdural ICP was the strongest predictor of intraoperative brain swelling. It was possible to define thresholds of cerebral swelling. At a subdural ICP < 5 mmHg, brain swelling rarely occurred (5% probability). At ICP > 13 mmHg, brain swelling occurred with 95% probability (Rasmussen et al. 2004).

37.2.4.4 Hyperventilation

Hyperventilation lowers subdural ICP significantly independent of anaesthetic method, but the effect differs between different medications. It is effective during propofol-fentanyl, propofol-remifentanil, isoflurane-fentanyl, and sevoflurane-fentanyl anaesthesia. The effect was most pronounced during isoflurane/sevoflurane-fentanyl anaesthesia and less effective during propofol-remifentanil/fentanyl anaesthesia. The reason for the low CO_2 reactivity during propofol anaesthesia might be that CPP in propofol anaesthesia is lower and close to the reflection point on the pressure-volume curve where compensatory mechanisms are exhausted (Juul and Cold 2008). However, even though jugular bulb oxygen tension ($SvjO_2$) was significantly lower during propofol anaesthesia, ischemia has never been described, probably because of the neuroprotective properties of propofol. For more detailed information on hyperventilation, see Chap. 60.

37.2.4.5 Mannitol or Hypertonic Saline (HS)

Mannitol is effective in reducing ICP in the management of traumatic intracranial hypertension in doses of 0.25–1.0 g/kg body weight. Current evidence on the effect on outcome is not strong enough to make recommendations on the use, concentration, and method of administration of hypertonic saline for the treatment of traumatic intracranial hypertension. However, osmotherapy seems effective when treating elevated ICP during surgery.

Which of mannitol and hypertonic saline are more effective is debatable. Mangat et al. (2020) found that the effect of bolus doses of hypertonic saline was superior to mannitol on the duration of increased ICP and decreased CPP during intensive care.

Pre-existing hyponatraemia should be excluded before administration of HS to avoid neurological symptoms as central pontine myelinolysis.

Osmotherapy is discussed in detail in Chap. 61.

37.3 Specific Paediatric Concerns

The general threshold of ICP is 20 mmHg. The approach to the treatment of intracranial pressure should be individualized and modified by the response. The treatment modalities are in principal much the same as in adults. The patients should be properly sedated and positioned with the head in neutral position. $PaCO_2$ should be aimed at the lower end of eucapnia ($PaCO_2$ 4.5 kPa (35 mmHg)) and CPP should be maintained according to age.

If intracranial hypertension occurs in spite of this, apply RTP of up to 30° in normovolaemic patients under ICP and CPP control (40–50 mmHg). Consider neuromuscular blockade. Proceed to CSF drainage and hyperosmolar therapy hypertonic saline (se-sodium <170 mEq/L) or mannitol (<320 mOsm/L). If surgery and ICP-reducing therapy are still ineffective, apply further hyperventilation ($PaCO_2$ = 4–4.5 kPa (30–35 mmHg)). Treatment should now be guided with CBF, $SjvO_2$, or tissue partial pressure of oxygen ($PtiO_2$) in the brain. If ICP is not normalized, you must proceed to second-tier therapy, at the discretion of the treating physicians (hyperventilation to CO_2 = 30 mmHg (4 kPa), barbiturate coma, decompressive craniectomy) (Kochanek et al. 2019).

References

Boone MD, Jinadasa SP, Mueller A, et al. The effect of positive end-expiratory pressure and cerebral hemodynamics. Neurocrit Care. 2017;26(2):174–81. https://doi.org/10.1007/s12028-016-0328-9.

Chestnut RM, Temkin N, Carney N, et al. A trial of intracranial-pressure monitoring in traumatic brain injury. N Engl J Med. 2012;367(26):2471–81.

Cold GE. Material included in the database. In: Cold GE, Juul N, editors. Monitoring of cerebral and spinal haemodynamics during neurosurgery. Berlin: Springer; 2008. p. 59–66.

Cold GE, Tange M, Jensen TM, Ottesen S. Subdural pressure measurement during craniotomy. Correlation with tactile estimation of dural tension and brain herniation after opening of dura. Br J Neurosurg. 1996;10(1):69–75.

Duch B, Cold GE. Effect of positive end-expiratory pressure on subdural intracranial pressure in patients undergoing supratentorial craniptomy. In: Cold GE, Juul N, editors. Monitoring of cerebral and spinal haemodynamics during neurosurgery. Berlin: Springer; 2008. p. 255–72.

Feldman Z, Kanter MJ, Robertson CS, et al. Effect of head elevation on intracranial pressure, cerebral perfusion pressure, and cerebral blood flow in head-injured patients. J Neurosurg. 1992;76:207–11.

Frost EA. Effects of positive end-expiratory pressure on intracranial pressure and compliance in brain-injured patients. J Neurosurg. 1977;47:195–200.

Guidelines for the acute medical management of severe traumatic brain injury in infants, children and adolescents. Brain Trauma Foundation 2016.

Juul N, Cold GE. In: Cold GE, Juul N, editors. Monitoring of cerebral and spinal haemodynamics during neurosurgery. Berlin: Springer; 2008. p. 70.

Kanter MJ, Robertson CS, Sheinberg MA, et al. Changes in cerebral haemodynamics with head elevated vs. head flat. Intracranial pressure. 1991;8, abstract 079.

Kochanek PM, Tasker RC, Carney N, et al. Guidelines for the management of pediatric severe traumatic brain injury, third edition: update of the brain trauma foundation guidelines. Pediatr Crit Care Med. 2019;20:S1–S82.

Mangat HS, Wu X, Gerber LM, et al. Hypertonic saline is superior to mannitol for the combined effect on intracranial pressure and cerebral perfusion pressure burdens in patients with evere traumatic brain injury Neurosurgery. 2020;86:221–30.

Mavrocordatos P, Bissonnette P, Ravussion P. Effects of neck position and head elevation on intracranial pressure in anaesthetized neurosurgical patients: preliminary results. J Neurosurg Anesthesiol. 2000;12:10–4.

Mchedlishvili G. Pathogenetic role of circulatory factors in brain oedema development. Neursurg Rev. 1988;11:7–13.

Miller MT, Pasquale M, Kurek S, et al. Initial head computerized tomographic scan characteristics have a linear relationship with intracranial pressure after trauma. J Trauma. 2004;56:967–72.

Moraine J-J, Berré J, Mélot C. Is cerebral perfusion pressure a major determinant of cerebral blood flow during head elevation in comatose patients with severe intracranial lesions? J Neurosurg. 2000;92:606–14.

Narayan RK, Kishore PR, Becker DP, et al. Intracranial pressure: to monitor or not to monitor? A review of our experience with severe head injury. J Neurosurg. 1982;56:650–9.

Raphael JH, Chotai R. Effects of cervical collar on cerebrospinal fluid pressure. Anaesthesia. 1994;49:437–9.

Rasmussen M, Bundgaard H, Cold GE. Craniotomy for supratentorial tumours: risk factors for brain swelling after opening the dura mater. Anaesthesia. 2004;59:229–36.

Rosner MJ, Coley IB. Cerebral perfusion pressure, intracranial pressure, and head elevation. J Neurosurg. 1986;65:636–41.

Schneider GH, von Helden GH, Franke R, Lanksch WR, Unterberg A. Influence of body position and cerebral perfusion pressure. Acta Neurochir. 1993;59:107–12.

Schreiber SJ, Lambert UKW, Doepp F, Valdueza JM. Effects of prolonged head-down tilt on internal jugular vein cross-sectional area. Br J Anaesth. 2002;89:769–71.

Videtta W, Villarejo F, Cohen M, et al. Effects of positive end-expiratory pressure on intracranial pressure and cerebral perfusion pressure. Acta Neurochir Suppl. 2002;81:93–7.

Part VII

Monitoring in Neurointensive Care

Christina Rosenlund
and Bo-Michael Bellander

38 Secondary Clinical Assessment

Jacob Bertram Springborg
and Christina Rosenlund

Tips, Tricks, and Pitfalls
- Always take into consideration the current medication of the patient when evaluating the neurological state.
- The brainstem can anatomically be considered as a three floor structure.
- Detailed motor and sensory examinations are most often not possible or necessary in the neurointensive care unit.
- Correlate neurological findings to information from the more technical physiological monitoring.

Recommendations

Level I

Data are insufficient to support Level I recommendations for this subject.

Level II

Data are insufficient to support Level II recommendations for this subject.

Level III

Repeated evaluation of consciousness and neurological status should be conducted. Clinical changes in neurointensive care patients should be correlated with the more advanced monitoring systems.

38.1 Overview

Repeated neurological examinations should be performed as part of monitoring neurological dysfunction in the neurointensive care unit, taking into consideration the pharmacological treatment of the patient. Deteriorations should be correlated to changes in the supplementary physiological monitoring, and together these observations should guide clinical decisions.

38.2 Background

Patients with severe TBI are as part of their treatment in the neurointensive care unit frequently under the influence of various analgesics, sedatives, and/or muscle relaxants. Moreover, many

J. B. Springborg (✉)
Department of Neurosurgery, University Clinic of Neurosurgery, Copenhagen University Hospital, Copenhagen, Denmark
e-mail: jacob.springborg@rh.regionh.dk

C. Rosenlund
Department of Neurosurgery, Odense University Hospital, Odense, Denmark
e-mail: Christina.rosenlund2@rsyd.dk

© Springer Nature Switzerland AG 2020
T. Sundstrøm et al. (eds.), *Management of Severe Traumatic Brain Injury*,
https://doi.org/10.1007/978-3-030-39383-0_38

of these patients are intubated and mechanically ventilated. Together, these conditions limit the clinical examination normally used to evaluate neurological function. Nevertheless, some form of basic clinical monitoring should, together with the more technical, physiological monitoring described in the next chapters, be initiated in the neurointensive care unit, and these repeated observations should guide clinical decisions.

38.3 Measures of Consciousness

Neurons of the reticular formation, particularly those of the ascending reticular activating system, play a crucial role in maintaining behavioural arousal and consciousness. The level of consciousness should repeatedly be evaluated to appreciate clinical improvement or deterioration, of course taking into consideration the level of analgesia and sedation (Table 38.1). The Glasgow Coma Scale (GCS) was originally designed to evaluate the severity of brain dysfunction in the early posttraumatic period in patients with TBI and not as a monitoring tool (Teasdale and Jennett 1974). Nevertheless, the three components tested are useful to monitor the depth and duration of impaired consciousness, but should however always be reported with the three separate scores to appreciate in which components the patient has deficits (King et al. 2000). In intubated patients, the verbal score is untestable and the summed GCS score is not directly applicable. Models have been designed to estimate the verbal score from the eye opening score and the motor score (Rutledge et al. 1996; Meredith et al. 1998), but the use of such models has been questioned (Chesnut 1997). A recent study recommends a multidimensional use of the three-component GCS, describing floor and ceiling effects of the individual components. In the range 3–7, the sum score is primarily determined by the motor component. In the range 8–12, the effect of the motor component attenuates and the sum score is mainly influenced by the verbal and eye components. The motor, eye, and verbal scores reach their ceiling effects at sum 13, 14, and 15, respectively. The prognostic value of the three components combined, was consistently higher than that of the sum score alone (Reith et al. 2017).

Table 38.1 Site of lesion and relevant clinical test with abnormal findings on neurological examination in the neurointensive care unit

Finding	Site of lesion	Test
Loss of consciousness	Reticular formation	Glasgow Coma Scale
Pupillary dilation	Oculomotor nerve or upper brainstem (midbrain)	Pupillary light reaction and diameter
Pinpoint pupils	Middle brainstem (pons)	Pupillary light reaction and diameter
Eye deviation (towards lesion)	Frontal cortical or upper brainstem (midbrain) gaze centres	Eye examination
Eye deviation (away from lesion)	Middle brainstem (pontine) gaze centre	Eye examination
Fixed eyes on head rotation	Upper and middle brainstem	Oculocephalic reflex
Absent ciliary and/or cornea reflex	Middle brainstem	Ciliary and cornea reflexes
Absent gag and/or cough reflex	Lower brainstem	Gag and cough reflexes

38.4 Symptoms and Signs Involving the Eyes and the Brainstem

More comprehensive evaluations of the brainstem function should also be conducted, and for didactic reasons, the brainstem can be considered a three floor structure consisting of the midbrain (mesencephalon), pons, and medulla oblongata (Table 38.1).

A detailed examination of the pupils and eyes should be repeated, and changes in the pupil light reaction or diameter should be considered a warning sign of pathology close to or in the midbrain or oculomotor nerve. Be aware that irregular/oval pupils may be the first sign of a third nerve palsy, and thus indicate an imminent transtentorial herniation. The distinct pupillary abnormalities seen in lesions in or near the midbrain (dilated fixed pupils) and pons (pinpoint pupils) should be recognized, as should the different horizontal eye deviation patterns seen in lesions in the frontal cortical (deviation towards lesion), midbrain (deviation towards lesion), and pontine (deviation away from lesion) gaze centres. Lesions in the medial longitudinal fasciculus cause internuclear ophthalmoplegia, which in the comatose patient is only assessable by testing the oculocephalic reflexes. Vertical eye deviation (downwards) can be seen with lesions in the mesencephalon and in more pronounced brainstem lesions, which may also cause skew deviation. Vertical gaze paresis can also be seen as a sign of increased ICP or a lesion in the pretectal area. In the unconscious patient, spontaneous roving eye movements may be present if the upper and middle brainstem is intact, as they depend on normal function of the oculomotor nuclei and connections from these. Different forms of nystagmus can be seen with lesions in the cerebellum and brainstem.

The oculocephalic and oculovestibular reflexes are anatomically complex, but mainly driven by signals from the semicircular canals via the vestibular nuclei located between the pons and medulla oblongata. From here, signals extend to the abducens and oculomotor nuclei in the pons and mesencephalon and from these to the lateral and medial rectus muscles of the eyes. In the unconscious patient with a preserved oculocephalic reflex, the eyes will move in the orbit in the opposite direction of head movements, apparently "looking" at the same spot in the surroundings ('doll's eyes phenomenon'), whereas with an absent reflex, the eyes don't move and just passively follow when the head is turned. The reflex is suppressed in a conscious adult with normal neurological function. An absent reflex is found in patients with upper and middle brain stem lesions. Caloric testing of the oculovestibular reflex with cold water is a strong stimulus, which in the unconscious patient results in conjugated eye movements towards the ear that is rinsed. Ice water is normally only used as part of the diagnosis of brain death - no eye movements then indicate lack of neural activity in this reflex loop, compatible with brain death.

Middle brainstem (pontine) impairment can be further tested by examining the ciliary and cornea reflexes, which have an afferent limb in the trigeminal nerve and an efferent limb in the facial nerve with a relay in the middle brainstem. The reflexes disappear in deep coma and with lesions in the pons.

Lower brainstem dysfunction can be tested by an examination of the gag reflexes with an afferent limb in the glossopharyngeal nerve and an efferent limb in the vagus nerve and the cough reflex with both an afferent and efferent limb in the vagus nerve. A formal assessment of lower brainstem dysfunction in the unconscious patient is often reserved for patients where brain death is suspected.

Finally, evaluation of respiratory function is also a test of brainstem function, as the respiratory regulatory centre is anatomically located in this area (reticular formation). However, with controlled mechanical ventilation, the spontaneous respiratory pattern is not recognizable.

38.5 Motor and Sensory Function

When evaluating the best motor response during GCS assessment, a brief evaluation of the motor function of all four extremities should be performed and recorded. Abnormal flexion implies that the lesion is located in the cerebral hemispheres or internal capsule with disinhibition above the midbrain, and abnormal extension implies midbrain to upper pontine dysfunction (Matis and Birbilis 2008). The muscle tone, deep tendon reflexes, and plantar reflexes are of less importance in the unconscious patient, but assessment may serve as baseline for later comparison. Especially side differences are important to recognize, as they are indicative of focal pathology. Hyperactive reflexes together with sympathetic storms (e.g. hypertension, tachycardia, etc.) can be caused by paroxystic sympathetic hyperactivity which should be addressed (see separate chapter). Moreover, repetitive testing of these modalities may reveal spinal cord or peripheral nerve lesions not appreciated in the initial evaluation of the patient or disclose improvements or deteriorations in such lesions.

A comprehensive examination of sensory modalities is most often not possible or necessary in the neurointensive management of patients with severe traumatic brain injury, but should of course be performed in patients with coexistent spinal cord or peripheral nerve lesions as soon as the patient is able to cooperate. Sensory stimulation is on the other hand important to apply as a part of the ultra-early rehabilitation, and included in the everyday monitoring of the patient will secure this even if the patient doesn't respond to the examination (Padilla and Domina 2016).

Neurointensive care unit nurses should be trained in GCS scoring and evaluation of the pupils and motor response. Instructions for the actions that should be taken when deterioration is observed, should be available. How often the different examinations should be performed depends on the clinical condition of the patient, the time from injury, and the current treatment of the patient, e.g. extensive stimulation is not meaningful in a patient deeply sedated as part of intracranial pressure management.

38.6 Specific Paediatric Concerns

Standard GCS scoring of non-verbal children is inapplicable. The paediatric modification of the GCS is described in previous chapters. Take into consideration the normal development of the central nervous system in children when evaluating the current neurological state.

References

Chesnut RM. Appropriate use of the Glasgow Coma Scale in intubated patients: a linear regression prediction of the Glasgow verbal score from the Glasgow eye and motor scores. J Trauma. 1997;42:345.

King BS, Gupta R, Narayan RK. The early assessment and intensive care unit management of patients with severe traumatic brain and spinal cord injuries. Surg Clin North Am. 2000;80:855–70.

Matis G, Birbilis T. The Glasgow Coma Scale—a brief review. Past, present, future. Acta Neurol Belg. 2008;108:75–89.

Meredith W, Rutledge R, Fakhry SM, Emery S, Kromhout-Schiro S. The conundrum of the Glasgow Coma Scale in intubated patients: a linear regression prediction of the Glasgow verbal score from the Glasgow eye and motor scores. J Trauma. 1998;44:839–44.

Padilla R, Domina A. Effectiveness of sensory stimulation to improve arousal and alertness of people in coma or persistent vegetative state after traumatic brain injury: a systematic review. Am J Occup Ther. 2016;70(3):7003180030p1–8.

Reith FCM, Lingsma HF, Gabbe BJ, Lecky FE, Roberts I, Maas AIR. Differential effects of the Glasgow Coma Scale Score and its components: an analysis of 54,069 patients with traumatic brain injury. Injury. 2017;48(9):1932–43.

Rutledge R, Lentz CW, Fakhry S, Hunt J. Appropriate use of the Glasgow Coma Scale in intubated patients: a linear regression prediction of the Glasgow verbal score from the Glasgow eye and motor scores. J Trauma. 1996;41:514–22.

Teasdale G, Jennett B. Assessment of coma and impaired consciousness. A practical scale. Lancet. 1974;2:81–4.

A Wake-Up Test in the Neurointensive Care Management of Severe TBI: Pros and Cons

39

Niklas Marklund

Recommendations

Level I

There is a lack of Level I evidence to use, or to avoid using, the Neurological Wake-up Test (NWT) in the neurocritical care monitoring of TBI patients.

Level II

Results from one randomized trial of a small cohort of TBI patients indicated that the NWT led to nonsignificantly shorter neurocritical care stay and time on ventilator.

In the majority of evaluated studies, the NWT is associated with a systemic stress response that is highly variable in severity.

Level III

The NWT remains the best clinical monitoring tool in the neurocritical care unit. However, the added value of the NWT over multimodality monitoring and neuroimaging has not been established.

39.1 Overview

Traumatic brain injury (TBI) may have a dynamic and unpredictable clinical course. In the 1970s, a large number of TBI patients, who on admission to the hospital were awake and able to talk later died. The entity "talk-and-die" was coined (Reilly et al. 1975), describing TBI patients with relatively mild initial, primary injuries who later had a fatal outcome due to secondary, and presumably "avoidable", factors. These findings, among others, led to improved organization of TBI care as well as the introduction of the Glasgow Coma Scale (GCS) score (Teasdale and Jennett 1974). The risk factors for neurological worsening in the mild-moderate TBI population have been addressed in numerous previous publications and guidelines (Astrand et al. 2016; Babl et al. 2017; Undén et al. 2013), although rapid exacerbation of the neurological condition of the patient may be observed in all forms and severities of TBI. In patients with severe TBI, e.g. ongoing hemorrhage or increased brain swelling (Morris et al. 1998; Juul et al. 2000), may lead to clinical deterioration that may go unnoticed in intubated and sedated patients. The use of pre-hospital sedation, paralysis, and intubation at the scene of the accident (Pakkanen et al. 2016) makes a neurological assessment difficult, although it is recommended that a post-resuscitation GCS score is obtained (Carney et al. 2017; Smith and Weingart 2012) to achieve a TBI severity grading and to enable clinical decisions (Garvin et al.

N. Marklund (✉)
Department of Clinical Sciences Lund, Neurosurgery, Lund University, Skåne University Hospital, Lund, Sweden
e-mail: niklas.marklund@med.lu.se

© Springer Nature Switzerland AG 2020
T. Sundstrøm et al. (eds.), *Management of Severe Traumatic Brain Injury*, https://doi.org/10.1007/978-3-030-39383-0_39

2015). Most severe TBI patients require continued care in a neurocritical care (NCC) unit where the basic management protocols include controlled ventilation, stress reduction using continuous sedation, neuroimaging, and multimodality monitoring. Continuous sedation is an integral component of NCC management; it prevents pain and anxiety, controls agitation, and enables endotracheal tube tolerance (Barr et al. 2013; Patel and Kress 2012; Oddo et al. 2016). In addition, continuous sedation reduces cerebral energy metabolism and oxygen consumption, attenuates the risk of seizure, and facilitates ICP and temperature control (Rhoney and Parker Jr 2001). Obviously, continuous sedation can mask important changes in the neurological condition of the patients (Helbok and Badjatia 2009), and excessive sedation may lead to significant morbidity (Girard et al. 2008; Pinhu et al. 2003; Kollef et al. 1998). Since neurological worsening, commonly defined as a decrease of ≥ two points on the motor component of the Glasgow Coma Scale (GCS-M) score, may occur in up to 40% of TBI patients during NCC within the first 48 h post-injury (Maas et al. 2006; Iaccarino et al. 2014)), clinical monitoring is also warranted. However, clinical examinations in NCC are controversial and are not mentioned in any recent guidelines, since they require sedation interruption which commonly elicits an undesired stress response.

Thus, in the era of multimodal NCC monitoring, is there an additional benefit of using the neurological examination (here named the neurological wake-up test, NWT), a test which requires sedation interruption? Furthermore, does the NWT lead to changed management of the patient with severe TBI, and what are its associated risks?

Advocates for using the NWT in TBI argue that this test is the only monitoring tool that can reliably detect clinically important neurological improvement or deterioration (Maas et al. 2008), and the obtained information can be useful in clinical decision-making. In the present overview, the rather scarce literature on neurological evaluation [here named the neurological wake up test, NWT (Skoglund et al. 2009)] is presented. Although the term "wake-up test" is used, the response should be considered more comparable to an arousal reaction (Stover 2012). Several terms to describe interruption of sedation strategies during NCC are in use and include spontaneous awakening trials, spontaneous breathing trials, daily interruption of sedation (DIS or IS) trials, and lightening of sedation.

To date, there are only scarce reports evaluating the NWT in NCC, and there are no clinical guidelines for using, or avoiding, the NWT. Surprisingly, systematic analyses of the information achieved by the NWT in TBI, and what clinical decisions are made based on this information, are rare. The NWT in NCC and its use may predominantly be based on personal preferences and/or experience as well as locally adopted guidelines and traditions.

An obvious goal in the management of severe TBI is the reduction of cerebral energy metabolic demands in severe TBI, for which continuous sedation is mandatory. The NWT, by definition, requires interruption of sedation although at present there are no robust data showing that the NWT-induced stress response results in a significant secondary brain injury. On the other hand, there are no strong arguments for a clinical benefit of the NWT, although when it is used by personnel experienced in the test, useful clinical information such as neuroworsening or neuro-improvement is commonly obtained. This remains the main argument for implementing the NWT in management protocols for those TBI patients with a stable intracranial situation. There are also well-founded reasons for not using the NWT, including a fear of a NWT-induced stress response and uncertainty about the added value of the NWTs in view of the possibilities for multimodality monitoring and modern neuroimaging. In this chapter, the pros and cons of the NWT are summarized.

Tips, Tricks and Pitfalls

- Propofol sedation is ideal when using the neurological wake-up test in TBI patients on continuous sedation and mechanical ventilation.
- Although modern multimodality monitoring and neuroimaging provide

valuable information on the injured brain, the neurological wake-up test remains a useful clinical monitoring tool in medically stable TBI patients

- The neurological wake-up test elicits a stress response and should only be attempted in TBI patients with stable ICP, $PtiO_2$, and/or CPP levels.
- The choice may not be between multi-modality monitoring and the NWT; TBI management strategies may include a combination of both.
- When performing the test, stop the sedation and examine the patient in the supine position. When the patient is sufficiently awake, evaluate if the patient obeys simple commands, and score the response according to the motor component of the GCS. If the patient does not obey commands, deliver a painful stimulus at the angle of the jaw and note the best motor response. In addition, the presence of focal neurological deficits and pupillary abnormalities is also evaluated.

39.2 Background

Sedation and systemic as well as intracranial monitoring are key components of the NCC of TBI patients. TBI induces *per se* a marked systemic biochemical stress response with the release of e.g., cortisol and the catecholamines norepinephrine and epinephrine. Continuous sedation attenuates the TBI-induced stress response, helps achieving ICP and CPP control and reduces the cerebral energy metabolic demands (Rhoney and Parker Jr 2001).

Furthermore, sedation facilitates mechanical ventilation. Importantly, heavy sedation may increase the risk of ventilator-associated pneumonias, prolong mechanical ventilation, and lead to a higher mortality. Thus, protocols using daily interruption of sedation and spontaneous breathing trials were associated with reduced duration of mechanical ventilation and length of stay in general intensive care (Girard et al. 2008; Wittbrodt 2005). Importantly, no significant adverse effects were noted by these procedures (Girard et al. 2008; Wittbrodt 2005; Jackson et al. 2010; Schweickert et al. 2004). Although these protocols can be combined with a neurological exam, the NWT, it was not the aim of these studies. In the NCC, there are several sedatives for use in the NCC where the most commonly used ones are propofol and midazolam although others, such as the selective α_2-adrenergic agonist dexmedetomidine (Pajoumand et al. 2016; Schomer et al. 2019; Humble et al. 2016) or the *N*-methyl-d-aspartate receptor antagonist ketamine (Oddo et al. 2016), are gaining popularity. The selected sedative obviously influences the possibility of using the NWT in the NCC setting.

In the only randomized controlled trial addressing a daily interruption of continuous sedation (DIS) protocol in TBI, 21 TBI patients were compared to 17 TBI controls in whom continuous sedation was used. The sedation interruption resulted in a nonsignificant reduction in the duration of mechanical ventilation and NCC stay (7.7 days in TBI/DIS patients vs. 11.6 days in controls and 14 vs. 17 days, respectively) (Anifantaki et al. 2009).

There are numerous neuromonitoring possibilities in modern NCC, such as ICP, CPP, intracerebral microdialysis, brain tissue oxygen ($PbtiO_2$), and jugular venous oxygen saturation ($SjvO_2$) monitoring, among others. One important limitation of ICP monitoring is that although ICP elevations and brain herniation are commonly linked, they can occur independently. As examples, in temporal contusions or following decompressive craniectomy, worsening of the intracranial situation may occur without distinctly increased ICP but be detected by an NWT. Thus, the NWT remains the gold standard for the detection of neurological deterioration even in the presence of advanced neuromonitoring (Helbok and Badjatia 2009).

For the NWT to be considered, it is imperative that the patient shows stable ICP, CPP and $PbtiO_2$ values at baseline, during continuous sedation and NWT should not be used in patients with marked hyperthermia, status epilepticus, and/ or barbiturate treatment (Oddo et al. 2016; Marklund 2017). When an NWT is planned, the continuous infusion of sedatives is interrupted, although a low dose of analgesics may be maintained (Marklund 2017; Beretta et al. 2011). The technique used to perform the NWT is described elsewhere (Marklund 2017), although in brief the patient should be placed in the supine position and be sufficiently awakened from the sedation to enable further assessment. Then, the patient is requested to obey simple commands, and if he/she does not, a painful stimulus is delivered at the angle of the jaw and the best GCS-M response is noted. In addition, the presence of focal neurological deficits as well as the pupil diameter, the presence of anisocoria, and the direct and indirect pupillary light reflexes must be evaluated in each NWT.

The potential benefits or risks associated with the NWT have only been studied in a few reports. In an initial report, 127 NWTs in 12 TBI and 9 subarachnoid hemorrhage (SAH) patients were evaluated (Skoglund et al. 2009). In all NWTs, a stress response was observed including transient increases in pulse rate and increased mean arterial blood pressure (MABP). The ICP increased by a mean of 69%, from 13 to 23 mmHg, in TBI patients, while the CPP showed a nonsignificant 5% increase during the NWTs. In 9 TBI patients, the ICP levels reached >30 mmHg, and the CPP levels decreased to <50 mmHg in 4 patients. These ICP increases and/or CPP changes were predominately brief and transient (Skoglund et al. 2009). In a subsequent study (Skoglund et al. 2014), $PbtiO_2$, $SjvO_2$, and interstitial neurochemistry as measured by cerebral microdialysis were evaluated in 17 severe TBI patients. The $PbtiO_2$ remained unaltered during 51 NWTs, and no jugular venous catheter readings were exacerbated by the tests. Furthermore, the NWT did not alter interstitial glucose, lactate, glycerol, glutamate, or the lactate/pyruvate ratio as measured by microdialysis. These data argue that despite an NWT-induced stress response, no evidence of an additional brain injury was observed (Skoglund et al. 2014). Severe TBI is *per se* accompanied by a systemic biochemical stress response including the release of stress-related hormones such as cortisol and the catecholamines norepinephrine and epinephrine. NWT- induced changes in plasma adrenocorticotrophic hormone (ACTH), as well as serum norepinephrine and epinephrine levels, were evaluated and compared to baseline samples drawn during continuous sedation and prior to NWT. In addition, saliva cortisol was collected by a sublingual swab (Skoglund et al. 2012). In eight TBI patients, the catecholamines epinephrine and norepinephrine levels were increased by 87.5 and 40.4%, respectively. For ACTH and cortisol, the NWT-induced increases were 72.5 and 30.7%, respectively. Although these stress hormone levels were all increased by the NWT, their increases in absolute numbers were minor. This study provided evidence for a rather mild stress response induced by the NWT. In contrast, in a mixed cohort of brain-injured patients of which only four had a severe TBI, interruption of sedation was not performed in 47% of patients due to increased ICP levels, hemodynamic instability, and sedation requirements (Helbok et al. 2012). The authors then performed 54 interruption of sedation trials of which a third could not be completed due to ICP crisis, agitation, desaturation, or a combination of these factors. In addition, reduced $PbtiO_2$ levels were commonly observed. Importantly, in only one trial was a clinical worsening observed. Although there were only few TBI patients, these results argue for careful risk stratifications and individualized assessments prior to initiating an NWT (Stover 2012; Helbok et al. 2012; Prisco and Citerio 2012).

Surprisingly, there are only limited data available showing how often the NWT alters clinical decisions and patient management or detects neuroworsening. In the previously mentioned study, evidence of a new focal neurological deficit was found only in one SAH patient and none in TBI patient (Helbok et al. 2012). If the NWT does not provide information needed for important clinical decisions, its use cannot be justified. However, if the NWT leads to more active management, detection of relevant causes for neuroworsening and/or improvement, and guides clinical decisions, then the stress response can be tolerated if the patient is carefully monitored during the NWT (Stocchetti et al. 2017). Such studies could be crucial in interpreting the role of NWTs in TBI.

Another important question is how detrimental the NWT-induced stress response is to the injured brain. Although sedation *per se* has never been shown to positively influence outcome, it facilitates ICP and CPP control, reduces stress, and attenuates cerebral energy metabolism. Arguably, the NWT-induced stress response is likely to increase cerebral metabolism and oxygen consumption, factors not desirable in the vulnerable TBI patient (Rhoney and Parker Jr 2001; Stover 2012). Only when the ICP, CPP, and/or $PbtiO_2$ recordings are within accepted limits at baseline, the NWT may be considered. Another valid argument against the routine implementation of the NWT is the exclusion of unstable patients, since these individuals may be those in whom the NWT could add the most important information.

Such concerns may explain the variability of the use of the NWT. In Scandinavia, ca 50% of neurosurgical departments never used the NWT, with a marked variation in the frequency of NWTs used in the other 50% of centers (Skoglund et al. 2013). One reason for this variability may be the use of midazolam in many neurosurgical departments, but presumably the fear of inducing a NWT-induced stress response, and the questioned additional value of NWTs in modern multimodality NCC, may be a more common reason. A reasonable approach may be combining the use of modern multimodal monitoring and NWT, and in particular use these monitoring tools to define in what TBI patients it is safe, or unsafe, to perform an NWT. Since important information of the clinical condition of the patient can be obtained using the NWT, more research is needed to establish the benefits or risks associated with this procedure.

39.3 Summary

From a scientific perspective, there is evidence neither against the use of the NWT nor in its favor. The NWT is associated with a stress response, the consequences of which have not been firmly established. Local management traditions, experience of the nursing staff, or the choice of sedatives appears to decide the use of the NWT. An individualized assessment based on neuromonitoring and neuroimaging parameters is recommended. A study systematically evaluating the NWT appears feasible and could define the role of the NWT in modern NCC and help and determine its future role in the management of severe TBI patients. The pros and cons of the NWT may be summarized as follows (modified from (Marklund 2017)).

Pros	Cons
Clinical decision-making (e.g., extubation, neuroimaging, surgery, tracheostomy, etc.)	A stress response, including increased ICP and/or CPP, is elicited
More active management and detection of clinically important neurological changes (including a dilated pupil or emerged focal neurological deficit)	No proven added value over modern multimodality monitoring
Sedation interruption reduces ventilation-associated adverse event and shortens time on ventilator (?)	Increased brain metabolism and oxygen consumption

References

Anifantaki S, Prinianakis G, Vitsaksaki E, Katsouli V, Mari S, Symianakis A, et al. Daily interruption of sedative infusions in an adult medical-surgical intensive care unit: randomized controlled trial. J Adv Nurs. 2009;65(5):1054–60.

Astrand R, Rosenlund C, Unden J, Scandinavian Neurotrauma C. Scandinavian guidelines for initial management of minor and moderate head trauma in children. BMC Med. 2016;14:33.

Babl FE, Borland ML, Phillips N, Kochar A, Dalton S, McCaskill M, et al. Accuracy of PECARN, CATCH, and CHALICE head injury decision rules in children: a prospective cohort study. Lancet. 2017;389(10087):2393–402.

Barr J, Fraser GL, Puntillo K, Ely EW, Gelinas C, Dasta JF, et al. Clinical practice guidelines for the management of pain, agitation, and delirium in adult patients in the intensive care unit. Crit Care Med. 2013;41(1):263–306.

Beretta L, De Vitis A, Grandi E. Sedation in neurocritical patients: is it useful? Minerva Anestesiol. 2011;77(8):828–34.

Carney N, Totten AM, O'Reilly C, Ullman JS, Hawryluk GW, Bell MJ, et al. Guidelines for the management of severe traumatic brain injury, fourth edition. Neurosurgery. 2017;80(1):6–15.

Garvin R, Venkatasubramanian C, Lumba-Brown A, Miller CM. Emergency neurological life support: traumatic brain injury. Neurocrit Care. 2015;23(Suppl 2):S143–54.

Girard TD, Kress JP, Fuchs BD, Thomason JW, Schweickert WD, Pun BT, et al. Efficacy and safety of a paired sedation and ventilator weaning protocol for mechanically ventilated patients in intensive care (awakening and breathing controlled trial): a randomised controlled trial. Lancet. 2008;371(9607):126–34.

Helbok R, Badjatia N. Is daily awakening always safe in severely brain injured patients? Neurocrit Care. 2009;11(2):133–4.

Helbok R, Kurtz P, Schmidt MJ, Stuart MR, Fernandez L, Connolly SE, et al. Effects of the neurological wake-up test on clinical examination, intracranial pressure, brain metabolism and brain tissue oxygenation in severely brain-injured patients. Crit Care. 2012;16(6):R226.

Humble SS, Wilson LD, Leath TC, Marshall MD, Sun DZ, Pandharipande PP, et al. ICU sedation with dexmedetomidine after severe traumatic brain injury. Brain Inj. 2016;30(10):1266–70.

Iaccarino C, Schiavi P, Picetti E, Goldoni M, Cerasti D, Caspani M, et al. Patients with brain contusions: predictors of outcome and relationship between radiological and clinical evolution. J Neurosurg. 2014;120(4):908–18.

Jackson DL, Proudfoot CW, Cann KF, Walsh T. A systematic review of the impact of sedation practice in the ICU on resource use, costs and patient safety. Crit Care. 2010;14(2):R59.

Juul N, Morris GF, Marshall SB, Marshall LF. Intracranial hypertension and cerebral perfusion pressure: influence on neurological deterioration and outcome in severe head injury. The Executive Committee of the International Selfotel Trial. J Neurosurg. 2000;92(1):1–6.

Kollef MH, Levy NT, Ahrens TS, Schaiff R, Prentice D, Sherman G. The use of continuous i.v. sedation is associated with prolongation of mechanical ventilation. Chest. 1998;114(2):541–8.

Maas AI, Murray G, Henney H 3rd, Kassem N, Legrand V, Mangelus M, et al. Efficacy and safety of dexanabinol in severe traumatic brain injury: results of a phase III randomised, placebo-controlled, clinical trial. Lancet Neurol. 2006;5(1):38–45.

Maas AI, Stocchetti N, Bullock R. Moderate and severe traumatic brain injury in adults. Lancet Neurol. 2008;7(8):728–41.

Marklund N. The neurological wake-up Test-A role in neurocritical care monitoring of traumatic brain injury patients? Front Neurol. 2017;8:540.

Morris GF, Juul N, Marshall SB, Benedict B, Marshall LF. Neurological deterioration as a potential alternative endpoint in human clinical trials of experimental pharmacological agents for treatment of severe traumatic brain injuries. Executive Committee of the International Selfotel Trial. Neurosurgery. 1998;43(6):1369–72. discussion 72-4

Oddo M, Crippa IA, Mehta S, Menon D, Payen JF, Taccone FS, et al. Optimizing sedation in patients with acute brain injury. Crit Care. 2016;20(1):128.

Pajoumand M, Kufera JA, Bonds BW, Devabhakthuni S, Boswell S, Hesselton K, et al. Dexmedetomidine as an adjunct for sedation in patients with traumatic brain injury. J Trauma Acute Care Surg. 2016;81(2):345–51.

Pakkanen T, Virkkunen I, Kamarainen A, Huhtala H, Silfvast T, Virta J, et al. Pre-hospital severe traumatic brain injury—comparison of outcome in paramedic versus physician staffed emergency medical services. Scand J Trauma Resusc Emerg Med. 2016;24:62.

Patel SB, Kress JP. Sedation and analgesia in the mechanically ventilated patient. Am J Respir Crit Care Med. 2012;185(5):486–97.

Pinhu L, Whitehead T, Evans T, Griffiths M. Ventilator-associated lung injury. Lancet. 2003;361(9354):332–40.

Prisco L, Citerio G. To wake-up, or not to wake-up: that is the Hamletic neurocritical care question! Crit Care. 2012;16(6):190.

Reilly PL, Graham DI, Adams JH, Jennett B. Patients with head injury who talk and die. Lancet. 1975;2(7931):375–7.

Rhoney DH, Parker D Jr. Use of sedative and analgesic agents in neurotrauma patients: effects on cerebral physiology. Neurol Res. 2001;23(2-3):237–59.

Schomer KJ, Sebat CM, Adams JY, Duby JJ, Shahlaie K, Louie EL. Dexmedetomidine for refractory intracranial hypertension. J Intensive Care Med. 2019;34(1):62–6.

Schweickert WD, Gehlbach BK, Pohlman AS, Hall JB, Kress JP. Daily interruption of sedative infusions and complications of critical illness in mechanically ventilated patients. Crit Care Med. 2004;32(6):1272–6.

Skoglund K, Enblad P, Hillered L, Marklund N. The neurological wake-up test increases stress hormone levels in patients with severe traumatic brain injury. Crit Care Med. 2012;40(1):216–22.

Skoglund K, Enblad P, Marklund N. Effects of the neurological wake-up test on intracranial pressure and cerebral perfusion pressure in brain-injured patients. Neurocrit Care. 2009;11(2):135–42.

Skoglund K, Enblad P, Marklund N. Monitoring and sedation differences in the management of severe head injury and subarachnoid hemorrhage among neurocritical care centers. J Neurosci Nurs. 2013;45(6):360–8.

Skoglund K, Hillered L, Purins K, Tsitsopoulos PP, Flygt J, Engquist H, et al. The neurological wake-up test does not alter cerebral energy metabolism and oxygenation in patients with severe traumatic brain injury. Neurocrit Care. 2014;20(3):413–26.

Smith WS, Weingart S. Emergency Neurological Life Support (ENLS): what to do in the first hour of a neurological emergency. Neurocrit Care. 2012;17(Suppl 1):S1–3.

Stocchetti N, Carbonara M, Citerio G, Ercole A, Skrifvars MB, Smielewski P, et al. Severe traumatic brain injury:

targeted management in the intensive care unit. Lancet Neurol. 2017;16(6):452–64.
Stover JF. Arousal from sedation in wake-up tests requires careful risk stratification. Crit Care Med. 2012;40(1):338–40.
Teasdale G, Jennett B. Assessment of coma and impaired consciousness. A practical scale. Lancet. 1974;2(7872):81–4.
Unden J, Ingebrigtsen T, Romner B, Scandinavian Neurotrauma C. Scandinavian guidelines for initial management of minimal, mild and moderate head injuries in adults: an evidence and consensus-based update. BMC Med. 2013;11:50.
Wittbrodt ET. Daily interruption of continuous sedation. Pharmacotherapy. 2005;25(5 Pt 2):3S–7S.

40 Intracranial Pressure (ICP): Theoretical and Practical Aspects

Peter Reinstrup

Recommendations

Level I

There are insufficient data to support a Level I recommendation for this topic.

Level II

There are insufficient data to support a Level II recommendation for this topic.

Level III

ICP monitoring is recommended and even mandatory when manipulating the cerebral perfusion pressure (CPP) following traumatic brain injury (TBI) as well as in patients with subarachnoidal haemorrhage (SAH) and suspected hydrocephalus. On the other hand, there is one report claiming that the use of an ICP device by itself reduces outcome; this finding can, however, be due to the treatment in the ICP monitored group.

P. Reinstrup (✉)
Department of Intensive and Perioperative Care, Skånes University Hospital, Lund, Sweden
e-mail: peter.reinstrup@med.lu.se

40.1 Overview

Monitoring brain functions is difficult in comatose patients. Continuous ICP recording is of value in cases of severe head trauma, since the therapy of head-injured patients aims at preventing secondary injuries due to an elevated ICP and/or a low cerebral blood flow (CBF) due to low cerebral perfusion pressure (CPP), and ICP monitoring has been found to improve outcome (Alali et al. 2013). However, it must be noted that a randomised controlled study evaluating outcome in severe TBI patients with and without ICP devices, found no benefit in outcome in the ICP monitored group (Chesnut et al. 2012). Furthermore, one study concluded that placement of an ICP device worsens outcome (Piccinini et al. 2017). Notwithstanding this, insertion of an ICP device should be considered following intracranial surgery, if complications are estimated as probable, and in a limited number of cases also for evacuation of CSF, as well as for the differentiation between normal and low-pressure states. In cases of a subarachnoid bleeding, it is recommended to insert a ventricular catheter, not only as a means for ICP measurements, but also since it might become necessary to drain ventricular fluid. Under normal circumstances, the pressure is isobaric throughout the intrathecal fluid system, when measured at a similar level, i.e. with the patient in a supine position. Pathological conditions like foramina

© Springer Nature Switzerland AG 2020
T. Sundstrøm et al. (eds.), *Management of Severe Traumatic Brain Injury*,
https://doi.org/10.1007/978-3-030-39383-0_40

Monroi cysts or obstructed flow through the aqueduct may lead to differences between ventricular and spinal pressures. Local changes may exist between the supratentorial and infratentorial parenchyma and even between different sites in the same compartment.

The gold standard at our department in Lund for continuous ICP measurement is a ventricular catheter connected to an external pressure transducer placed at the highest point of the head with a 6 mmHg addition of the registered pressure in order to achieve a reference point at the supratentorial origo of the brain in all clinical situations, with the alternative being a parenchymatous pressure device with its zero reference at the tip of the catheter. Readings from the latter might, however, deviate from the true ICP values and the fact that even small changes in ICP can have a dramatic impact on the patient, these deviations may have clear consequences on the outcome if allowed to guide therapy.

Tips, Tricks and Pitfalls

- If the ventricles are visible on the CT scan, insertion of a ventricular ICP device should always be considered.
- If a parenchymatous device is to be used, always assess the credibility of the readings by comparing with a recent CT scan.
- While most departments agree on an upper limit for a normal ICP of 20 mmHg, inter-centre differences in ICP catheter zero point choice will influence this limit and hence the estimated CPP.
- Ventricular ICP recording curves should always oscillate. Should the amplitude diminish, the following causes have to be excluded: misplacement of the catheter tip, air in the tubings, clotting of the catheter or a collapse of the entire ventricular system (Fig. 40.1).
- Is an elevated ICP as such deleterious for the brain? An upper limit for damages solely related to an elevated ICP has not been possible to establish, but it is generally accepted that an ICP higher than 20 mmHg is abnormal. An ICP above 40 mmHg is always associated with neurological symptoms such as impaired consciousness accompanied by abnormal electrical activity (EEG), as well as pupillary dilatation. A persisting pressure above 60 mmHg bears a high risk of being fatal.
- ICP and brain death? Supratentorial blood flow comes to an arrest when mean ICP approaches the systolic arterial blood pressure. Since clinical brain death criteria are based on the loss of function of the cranial nerves emanating from the infratentorial space, it is possible to have a supratentorial ICP indicating abolished circulation with preserved functions in these nerves.
- Transcranial Doppler (TCD), optic nerve sheet diameter (ONSD) or tympanic membrane displacement (TMD) can be an aid in the decision of whether an ICP device is necessary or not since these parameters correlate to some extent with the ICP.
- It is generally recommended to place the ICP device in the non-dominant hemisphere, but in cases of acute subdural hematomas, the highest and therefore most relevant pressure is found in the affected hemisphere (Chambers et al. 1998).

40.2 Background

Magendie observed in 1842 that the pressure in a meningocele sac in infants with spina bifida was transmitted to the fontanel and that high pressure in this system caused loss of consciousness. Key and Retzius (1875) were the first to measure and Knoll (1886) to record ICP in animals. Quincke

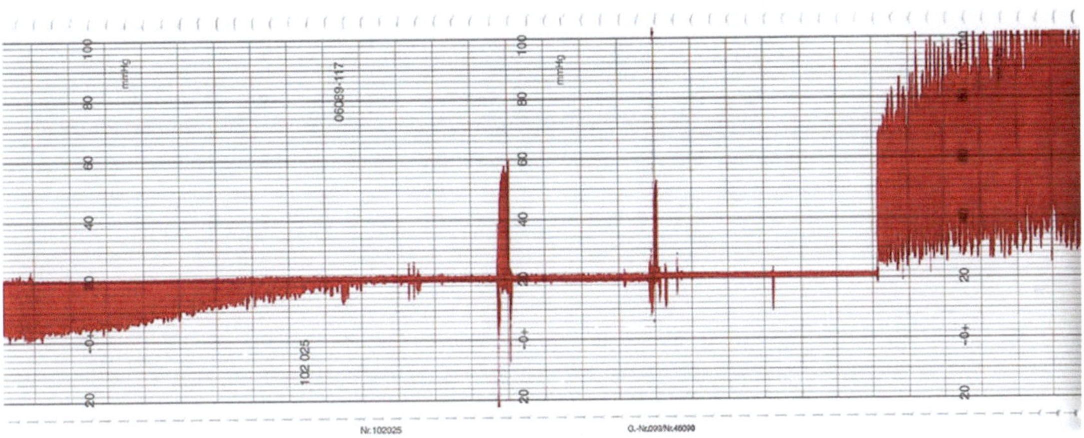

Fig. 40.1 ICP registration from a patient with an open ventricular pressure device as shown in mmHg and with a 5-min resolution, events going from *left to right*. The amplitude of the ICP diminishes to zero around the drainage level of 20 mmHg. The drainage is closed on three occasions. During the closure the correct ICP is registered. Following the two first closures, the drainage is again opened and the ICP curve follows the drainage level of 20 mmHg, whereas at the third closure (on the *right side* of the registration) the line is kept closed and registered mean ICP approaches 60 mmHg

(1891) introduced lumbar puncture to the clinical tools, opening up for studies of ICP using this route. Our present knowledge of brain physiology and pathophysiology is to a large extent based on continuous measurements of ICP. Under normal circumstances, the intrathecal fluid is isobaric in the cerebrospinal fluid (CSF) system (Lenfeldt et al. 2007) when measured at similar levels. However, local changes can exist in the parenchyma, and differences in ICP exist between the infratentorial and supratentorial compartments, and this discrepancy is changing over time (Slavin and Misra 2003). ICP correlates to changes in tissue oedema (intracellular and/or interstitial) and changes in the amount of liquor and/or cerebral blood volume (CBV) (including bleedings) to a certain degree.

40.2.1 Ventricular ICP Monitoring

The ventricular pressure was first measured in humans by Hodgson in 1928. Guillaume and Janny (1951) reported the first cannulations of the ventricular system in order to measure ICP. Lundberg (1960) developed the equipment for continuous measurements of ventricular ICP in the late 1950s, and this is the technique still utilised for ventricular pressure measurements and drainage. This is considered the gold standard for measuring ICP, using tubing from the ventricular system to an extracranial pressure transducer, which must be positioned at a fixed anatomical reference point on the head. Whereas the chosen reference point for the zero level of this pressure device differs between centres, the technique originally described by Lundberg builds on a reference zero point at the highest point of the head, simply for practical reasons. With such a set-up, the true ICP value at the supratentorial origo or brain centre needs to be corrected by adding 5.9 mmHg resulting in a maximum deviation from the ideal brain centre of ≤1.8 mmHg in all clinical head positions. If the Monro reference point is warranted as zero reference point, 6.3 mmHg is added giving an exact Monro-ICP deviating of ≤0.9 mmHg in all clinical head positions (Reinstrup et al. 2019). Different centres dealing with ICP measurements often use Monro or Meatus-Glabella as reference points. However, Monro is not an externally identifiable anatomical reference point, and its location is indeed described differently in different centres. Meatus and Glabella are external anatomical reference points that have been introduced, but have yet to be evaluated. Although this

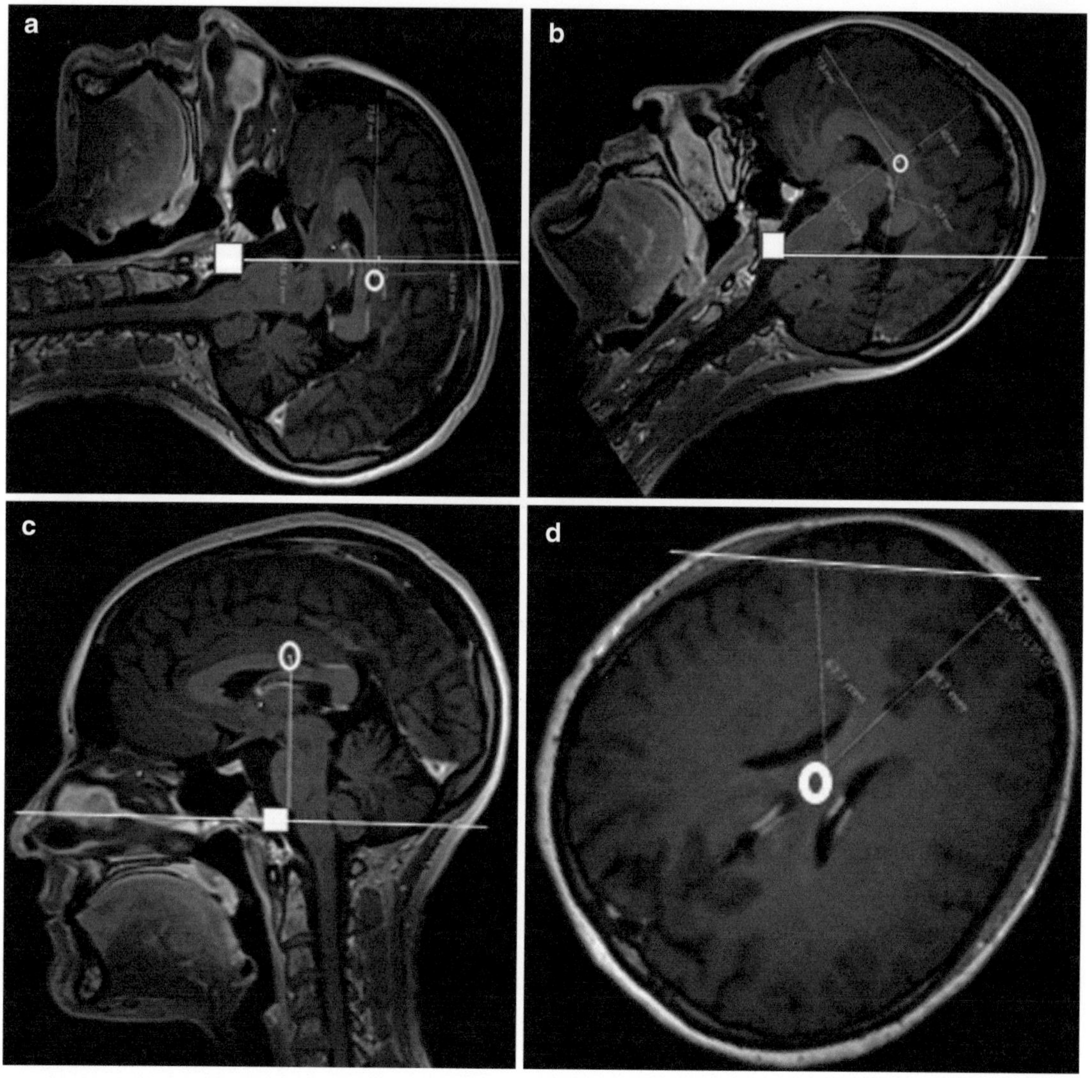

Fig. 40.2 Deviation from supratentorial brain centre (BC) using meatus-glabella as external anatomical reference points. O BC; ■ meatus projected to a midsagittal image. The white line represents the zero reference point ICP with the transducer placed at the external auditory meatus. (**a**) Sagittal image with the head in supine position. (**b**) With a 45° head elevation. (**c**) Upright. (**d**) White line with the transducer at glabella-nose tip with placement in 45° lateral position. Published in a Springer journal (Acta Neurochirurgica) - permission obtained

approach seems ideal with the patient lying strict supine or lateral, it shows huge deviations (app ±6 mmHg) from brain centre in clinical practice (Fig. 40.2) (Reinstrup et al. 2019). Parenchymatous devices all have their zero points at the tip of the catheter. The parenchymatous ICP readings may, therefore, vary within approximately 0–10 mmHg depending on the placement of the catheter tip and position of the head.

40.2.2 Complications with ICP Devices

The risk of infection is approximately 1% per day with an intraventricular ICP catheter. It has been suggested that it is the drainage of liquor per se that causes the ventriculitis (Rossi et al. 1998). Since drainage is most common in patients with blood in the ventricular system, the blood itself could act as a bacterial growth substrate. Though rare, the insertion procedure of these catheters might also give rise to complications such as intraparenchymal bleedings and cerebrospinal fluid leakage (Guyott et al. 1998; Rossi et al. 1998). Hence, a normal coagulation screening test should ideally be obtained before inserting a catheter.

In an attempt to overcome the drawbacks associated with ventricular ICP measurements, a variety of extraventricular devices has been developed including subdural devices based on saline-filled transducers, e.g. Richmond screw or Leeds bolt, as well as extradural devices based on electrical impedance, e.g. Gaeltec and Ladd. Each of these devices is hampered by problems associated with blockage of the lumen if the brain swells, as well as baseline measurement drifts over time.

40.2.3 Parenchymatous ICP Monitoring

In the early 1990s, microsensors opened up for catheters to be placed within the brain parenchyma for measurement of ICP. They were based on either fibre optics (Camino) or electrical impedance (Codman 'Microsensor', Spiegelberg). The readings are comparable with those of the intraventricular catheters; they are minimally invasive and have minimal baseline drift, but this drift, unfortunately, increases with time and can in rare cases reach 10 mmHg (Al-Tamimi et al. 2009). Hence, in order to circumvent this drawback, Raumedic made a catheter with an air duct to the tip, but even these catheters have, so far, drift over time (Citerio et al. 2008). Despite these shortcomings, microcatheters have become the standard method for measuring ICP in many neurosurgical centres worldwide. It is vital though to note that a number of neurosurgical centres have reported on cases where these devices have given false values (Fernandes et al. 1998).

40.2.4 Lumbar Versus Supratentorial ICP Monitoring

There is a good correlation between mean lumbar and ventricular pressures in the supine patient with a mean difference of 10 mmH_2O (0.75 mmHg) (Lenfeldt et al. 2007). However, wave amplitudes have been found to be 2 mmHg smaller in lumbar recordings, possibly due to inertia of the spinal canal or smaller catheter bore (Eide and Brean 2006).

40.2.5 Infratentorial Versus Supratentorial Intracranial Pressure

Hitherto, the infratentorial volume down to the foramen magnum has not been thoroughly investigated. In one attempt, Slavin and Misra (2003) used external ventricular drainage placed in a lateral ventricle together with infratentorial ICP measurement using an intraparenchymal sensor inserted into the cerebellum. In patients with various infratentorial pathologies, a difference in ICP was found between the infratentorial and supratentorial compartments, a difference which also changed over time.

Following posterior fossa surgery, a parenchymatous pressure transducer was placed in the cerebellum and a Richmond bolt in the frontal area. During the first 12 h, the posterior fossa pressure was 50% higher than that in the supratentorial compartment in all patients. Over the next 12 h, the supratentorial pressures were 10–15% higher than those measured in the posterior fossa, but following 48 h of monitoring, the pressures had equilibrated (Rosenwasser et al. 1989).

40.2.6 Non-invasive Methods for Assessing ICP

ICP cannot be measured exactly by non-invasive means, but crude estimates can be made to give the clinician a hint as to what the ICP is likely to be. Such assessments are based on case history, clinical symptoms (headache, vomiting, nausea), and radiological investigations. It must be emphasised that a normal morphology of the brain, as visualised by a CT or even an MR scan, never can exclude an elevated ICP; consequently, a physician cannot rely solely on radiological features to interpret ICP. An MR imaging-derived elastance index, on the other hand, correlates with ICP over a wide range of ICP values (Alperin et al. 2000). This method as such is unfortunately hampered with such a low sensitivity that it allows for differentiation only between normal and elevated ICP notwithstanding it being complicated to perform.

Bedside technologies for estimation of ICP exist and may give a hint as to whether ICP is high or normal. All techniques require training and can have intra and inter-observer variance, and one has to be aware of coexisting disorders affecting the measurement. It is a good idea to measure during a craniectomy or when a reliable ICP device is present as a calibration tool and then use the techniques to detect ICP variations rather than the absolute numbers—these should never be interpreted in isolation, but ideally be a part of a holistic evaluation of the patients' intracranial situation. There are a lot of upcoming new techniques, and the below-mentioned are only the most frequently used.

Tympanic membrane displacement (TMD) is a technique that builds on the communication of the CSF via the perilymphatic duct, such that an increase in ICP is directly transmitted to the footplate of the stapes, thereby changing its initial position and affecting the direction and magnitude of the acustic or stapedes displacement of the eardrum in response to sound. This TMD correlates to ICP to some extent, but merely in younger persons (Shimbles et al. 2005).

Optic nerve sheath diameter (ONSD) expands during increased ICP as the subarachnoid space surrounding the nerve communicates with the intracranial subarachnoid space. ONSD can be visualised using transocular ultrasound, CT or MRI (Sahu and Swain 2017). Measurements of the outer ONSD are performed 3 mm behind the optic globe or sclera, and an increased ONSD correlates to a high ICP, although with reservations (Robba et al. 2018). The cut-off diameter indicating an ICP > 20 mmHg differs from 4.8 to 5.9 mm between studies that indicate the method's problems in clinical use (Rajajee et al. 2011; Robba et al. 2018).

Transcranial Doppler (TCD) can be used to estimate ICP. The calculations in a mathematical model using arterial blood pressure and cerebral flow velocity should predict ICP with good accuracy (Schmidt et al. 2002). A more straightforward method utilises the correlation between pulsatility index (PI) and ICP where $ICP = 10.9 \times PI - 1.3$ or $ICP \sim 10 \times PI$. This correlates well with ICP from 0 to 120 mmHg, but is imprecise in the clinically relevant area around 20 mmHg (Bellner et al. 2004). However, the technique can be used to follow changes in ICP.

40.2.7 When to Monitor ICP

Monitoring brain functions is difficult in comatose patients. Since one aim of the therapy of head-injured patients is to prevent secondary injuries to the brain due to high ICP and/or low cerebral perfusion pressure, continuous recording of ICP has been found to be of value in cases of severe head trauma. Thus, in head-injured patients with intracranial mass lesions on the admission CT, a persistent high ICP was observed in 60% as compared to 13% in those with a normal CT, while the presence of at least two or more of the following factors increased the incidence of high ICP up to 60% in the group with a normal CT: age above 40, systolic blood pressure below 90 mmHg, and motor posturing (Narayan et al. 1982).

Insertion of an ICP device should be considered following intracranial surgery if complications are estimated as probable, in the presence of establishing elevated intracranial pressure, in a limited number of cases for the evaluation of CSF shunts and for the purpose of differentiating between normal and low-pressure states. Treatment of intracranial hypertension is also best guided by continuous intracranial pressure monitoring (Johnston and Jennet 1973). In cases of subarachnoid bleeding, it is recommended to insert a ventricular catheter not only as a means for ICP measurements, but also because drainage of ventricular fluid might be necessary (Sakowitz et al. 2006).

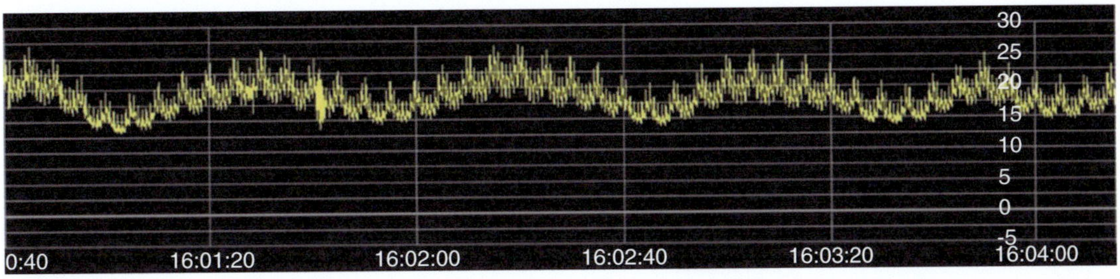

Fig. 40.3 An ICP tracing in a TBI patient during sedation and artificial ventilation. The pressure is shown in mmHg and between *vertical lines* passes 40 s. The fast undulation is due to the arterial pulse pressure and the slow part (12/min) the Lundberg C-waves (43 peaks in the picture) due to the ventilation. A slower wave (four peaks in the picture) of approx. 1/min, the so-called Lundberg B-wave, is seen in sedated or sleeping patients

40.2.8 ICP Waveform Analysis

Mean ICP has until recently been the sole information of interest obtained from the ICP devices, but an ICP recording contains additional information. ICP can be a stable parameter, but may often fluctuate over time due to mainly cerebrovascular changes. The ICP curve has variations superimposed on the arterial pulse pressure curve, one of which has respiratory synchronicity and which is referred to as the Lundberg C or the Traube-Hering-Mayer waves (Lundberg 1960) (Fig. 40.3). During respiration, mainly during mechanical ventilation and hypovolemia, the cardiac filling pressure varies with the ventilation creating ABP changes, also described as pulse pressure variations (PPV) or systolic pressure variations (SPV). A completely functioning cerebrovascular reactivity tries to keep the CBF constant and should be able to cope with these PPV and create a constant ICP curve. If the cerebrovascular tree is malfunctioning, the PPV might also create covariations in ICP. The covariation between ICP and mean ABP variations is described as the cerebrovascular pressure reactivity index (PRx). A negative PRx reflects intact cerebrovascular reactivity, whereas a positive PRx reflects impaired response (Czosnyka et al. 2017). The PRx index might reflect cerebral autoregulation (Brady et al. 2008). PRx might be utilised as a tool to estimate the optimal CPP (CPPopt) (Steiner et al. 2001), CPPopt is the CPP where PRx displays the best vascular reactivity. In TBI there us an uncoupling of the CMR-CBF, why a CPPopt is not equivalent to an optimal CPP for the brain tissue. Similar entities like PRx are PAx (correlation between ICP amplitude and mean ABP variations) and RAC or (ICP amplitude variations with CPP).

Beside these ICP variations with ventilation ABP, there are other variants with a lower frequency of 0.5–2/min and described by Lundberg (1960) as B-waves and seen during sedation or sleep and might represent a sleep pattern, but otherwise of unknown origin (Fig. 40.3). There is agreement on B-waves being indicative of reduced intracranial compliance and an indicator for intact autoregulation (Spiegelberg et al. 2016).

On top of this, some TBI patients develop plateau waves or A-waves as described by Lundberg (1960), but still of unidentified origin even though one might suspect rapid changes in arterial CBV (Fig. 40.4). Plateau waves have been considered a malignant sign, but have been shown not to be associated with a worse outcome (Castellani et al. 2009) if they are of reasonable duration.

During rising ICP, the arterial pulse pressure wave of the ICP curve increases in amplitude as a sign of the decreased compliance in the CNS (Fig. 40.5), while conversely, the ICP curve oscillations become minute after a craniectomy.

The introduction of digital registration has facilitated analysis of the single cardiac curve itself, but until recently it was mainly the amplitude which was used to interpret the status of the brain (Eide and Kerty 2011).

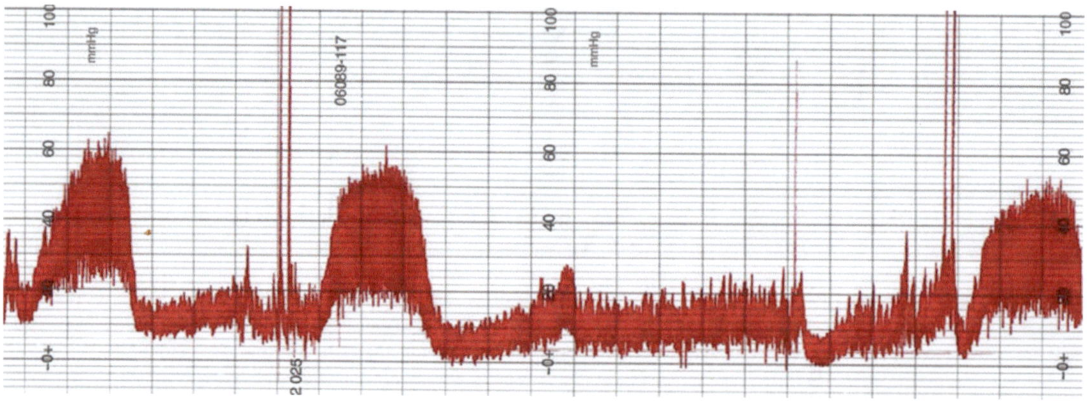

Fig. 40.4 ICP recording in a TBI patient showing plateau waves. The pressure is shown in mmHg; and there is 5 min between *vertical lines*, events going from *left* to *right*

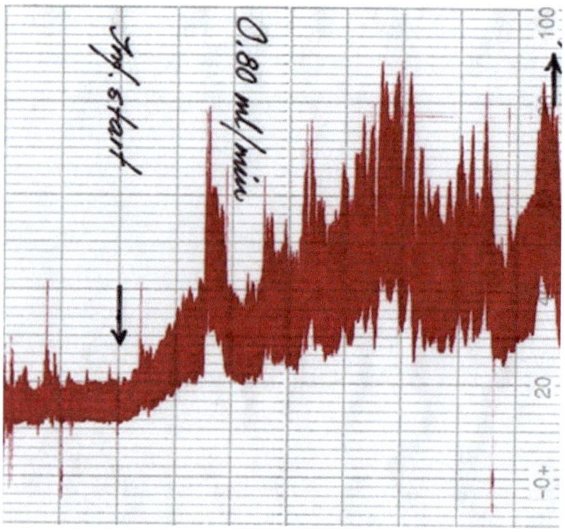

Fig. 40.5 ICP recording from a patient during a lumbar infusion of fluid (0.8 mL/min) showing a concomitant rise both in ICP and amplitude. The pressure is shown in mmHg, and there is 5 min between *vertical lines*, events going from *left* to *right*

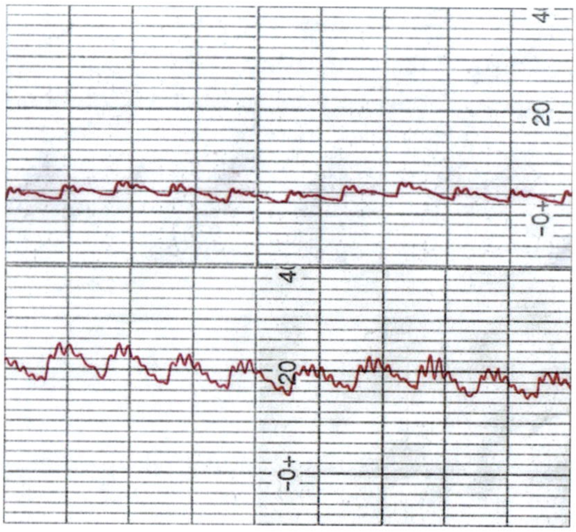

Fig. 40.6 Typical curve forms at normal (*upper panel*) and slightly elevated (*lower panel*) ICP from the same patient. The pressure is shown in mmHg, and the paper speed gives 1 s per *vertical line*, events going from *left* to *right*. The ICP curve created by the systolic pulse is usually tetrahumped, and the individual waves are called p_1–p_4. This can be seen very vaguely on the *left side of the panel*, whereas in the *right side of the panel* up to six humps can be identified. The *curve* during low ICP has a prominent p_1 (*upper panel*), but a prominent p_2 is seen in the *lower panel* where the ICP is higher

The ICP curve is usually tetrahumped and the individual waves are called P1–P4, respectively.

The appearance of the curve differs; under conditions of normal ICP, the P1 has the greatest amplitude, whereas during states of elevated ICP, the P2 waves often, but not always, become the highest (Fan et al. 2008) (Fig. 40.6). Using phase contrast MRI just below the skull base, flow in the arteries and veins to and from the brain can be measured as cardiac cycle CBF (ccCBF) on the arterial and venous side, as well as CSF flow back and forth at the foramen of magnum with high time resolution sampling. With concomitant registration of the ICP curve, it is possible to elucidate the source of the cardiac cycle ICP curve. The difference between the arterial inflow and venous outflow equals the cardiac cycle change in CBV (ccCBV). ccCBV correlates to the P2 P3

P4 part of the area under the ICP curve even at different configurations of the curve (Unnerbäck et al. 2019). As the venous outflow from the brain is rather constant and with knowledge of the cerebrovascular tree, where the highest resistance is in the precapillary-capillary segments, this increase in CBV must equal the input on the arterial side, and an increase in P2 P3 P4 (see Fig. 40.6) must be due to a lost cerebrovascular tension in the large cerebral arteries, or in other words it might present a malfunctioning cerebral autoregulation. Hence, in the future, the curve form can be utilised to guide treatment in order to optimise cerebral circulation. When the ICP curve is converted to a volume-converted area under the curve, this curve is explained by the pulsatile part of the arterial ccCBF (Unnerbäck 2018). In the near future, there is therefore a possibility to translate an ICP curve into a CBF_{ICP} (see Chap. 44).

40.2.9 Cerebral Perfusion Pressure (CPP)

Cerebral perfusion pressure (CPP), as introduced by Lassen (1959), is the difference between mean arterial pressure (MAP) and intracranial pressure (ICP) with both transducers at the same level. CPP is used as a surrogate for online cerebral blood flow (CBF). An extremely low CPP results in hypoperfusion, while a high CPP causes hyperperfusion leading to cerebral oedema during normal conditions as well as in TBI. Keeping the CPP within certain limits should secure for a sufficient CBF. The optimal CPP parameter could have been settled by the scientific community a long way back, but the CPP parameter has been mistreated in such a way that it has become confusing. First of all, the optimal CPP differs between brain pathologies and over time age, vessel status and brain metabolism, which has to be accounted for when evaluating optimal CPP. However, this is not the main problem, but rather the inconsistency in the placement of the transducers between various centres (for details of the ICP transducer, see Sect. 40.2.1). If meatus-glabella is used as the ICP reference point, this value may deviate approximately ±6 mmHg from the correct brain centre ICP in clinical practice (Reinstrup et al. 2019). This error is not seen in the calculated CPP, even if the ABP transducer is at the same level. On top of this, the ABP transducer is at the same level as the ICP transducer in only 36% of the centres dealing with TBI (Rao et al. 2013). At many centres, the ABP transducer is positioned in the bed resulting in huge differences in calculated CPP differences that are not accounted for in the literature (Rao et al. 2013; Reinstrup et al. 2019). As an example, the procedure in Lund is to align the ICP transducer at the highest point of the head and the ABP transducer in the bed at the atrium level. The Lund therapy concept aims to lower CPP down to 50 mmHg, and if corrected for the transducer placement, it would be approximately 35 mmHg. Such a CPP has been extensively evaluated with microdialysis in the TBI patients' penumbra zones and has been found to be sufficient in deeply sedated patients (Nordström et al. 2003). Each centre using CPP to guide therapy is familiar with their own way of dealing with this parameter, but in articles presenting CPP concepts, it is really a challenge to determine the placement of the ICP and ABP transducers, if mentioned at all, as well as the position of the patient in order to get an opinion of the actual used CPP. ICP monitoring is found to both improve and worsen outcome, which can be based on the divergent way ICP-ABP-CPP are measured.

40.2.10 MR Compatibility

Provided no metal is used in connection with the ventricular ICP device, an MR scan can be performed without risks. Many centres have dedicated equipment for ABP monitoring in the scanning room, and these systems can be used also for ICP monitoring, provided the pressure transducer is situated well away from the scanning site.

Generally, all parenchymatous ICP devices should be disconnected, and if placed via a bolt, this must be non-magnetic. The Raumedic catheter is claimed to be approved for the use in the

MR environment. The Codman sensor is approved for MR scanners of up to 1.5 T and with a radiofrequency below 1 SAR, provided the catheter is coiled and taped to the head in a special way to minimise thermogenesis (Newcombe et al. 2008).

40.3 Specific Paediatric Concerns

In infants, ICP can be assessed by measuring the head circumference and palpating the fontanel, a method that is no longer available after closure of the cranial sutures, leaving fundoscopy as the remaining bedside non-invasive method. It is important to bear in mind that the lack of papilloedema does not exclude an elevated ICP.

Neonates have slightly lower ICP, i.e. between 0 and 10 mmHg, as compared to 0 and 15 mmHg in grown-ups. On the other hand, the pressure-volume curve of a normal infant shows less ability to buffer increments of volume, resulting in a steeper volume ICP slope as a sign of lower total compliance (Shapiro et al. 1994). Very high intracranial pressures are usually fatal if prolonged, but children, in general, can tolerate higher pressures for longer periods.

References

Alali AS, Fowler RA, Mainprize TG, Scales DC, Kiss A, de Mestral C, Ray JG, Nathens AB. Intracranial pressure monitoring in severe traumatic brain injury: results from the American College of Surgeons Trauma Quality Improvement Program. J Neurotrauma. 2013;30:1737–46.

Alperin NJ, Lee SH, Loth F, Raksin PB, Lichtor T. MR–Intracranial pressure (ICP): a method to measure intracranial elastance and pressure noninvasively by means of MR imaging: baboon and human study. Radiology. 2000;217(3):877–85.

Al-Tamimi YZ, Helmy A, Bavetta S, Price SJ. Assessment of zero drift in the Codman intracranial pressure monitor: a study from 2 neurointensive care units. Neurosurgery. 2009;64(1):94–8.

Bellner J, Romner B, Reinstrup P, Kristiansson KA, Ryding E, Brandt L. Transcranial Doppler sonography pulsatility index (PI) reflects intracranial pressure (ICP). Surg Neurol. 2004;62(1):45–51.

Brady KM, Lee JK, Kibler KK, Easley RB, Koehler RC, Shaffner DH. Continuous measurement of autoregulation by spontaneous fluctuations in cerebral perfusion pressure. Stroke. 2008;39(9):2531–37.

Castellani G, Zweifel C, Kim DJ, Carrera E, Radolovich DK, Smielewski P, Hutchinson PJ, Pickard JD, Czosnyka M. Plateau waves in head injured patients requiring neurocritical care. Neurocrit Care. 2009;11:143–50.

Chambers IR, Kane PJ, Signorini DF, Jenkins A, Mendelow AD. Bilateral ICP monitoring: its importance in detecting the severity of secondary insults. Acta Neurochir Suppl. 1998;71:42–3.

Chesnut RM, Temkin N, Carney N, Dikmen S, Rondina C, Videtta W, Petroni G, Lujan S, Pridgeon J, Barber J, Machamer J, Chaddock K, Celix JM, Cherner M, Hendrix T. A trial of intracranial-pressure monitoring in traumatic brain injury. N Engl J Med. 2012;367(26):2471–81.

Citerio G, Piper I, Chambers IR, Galli D, Enblad P, Kiening K, Ragauskas A, Sahuquillo J, Gregson B, BrainIT Group. Multicenter clinical assessment of the Raumedic Neurovent-P intracranial pressure sensor: a report by the BrainIT group. Neurosurgery. 2008;63(6):1152–8.

Czosnyka M, Czosnyka Z, Smielewski P. Pressure reactivity index: journey through the past. Acta Neurochir. 2017;159(11):2063–5.

Eide PK, Brean A. Lumbar cerebrospinal fluid pressure waves versus intracranial pressure waves in idiopathic normal pressure hydrocephalus. Br J Neurosurg. 2006;20(6):407–14.

Eide PK, Kerty E. Static and pulsatile intracranial pressure in idiopathic intracranial hypertension. Clin Neurol Neurosurg. 2011;113:123–8.

Fan JY, Kirkness C, Vicini P, Burr R, Mitchell P. Intracranial pressure waveform morphology and intracranial adaptive capacity. Am J Crit Care. 2008;17(6):545–54.

Fernandes HM, Bingham K, Chambers IR, Mendelow AD. Clinical evaluation of the Codman microsensor intracranial pressure monitoring system. Acta Neurochir Suppl. 1998;71:44–6.

Guillaume J, Janny P. Continous intracranial manometry; importance of the method and first results. Rev Neurol (Paris). 1951;84(2):131–42.

Guyott LL, Dowling C, Diaz FG, Michael DB. Cerebral monitoring devices: analysis of complications. Acta Neurochir Suppl. 1998;71:47–9.

Johnston IH, Jennet B. The place of continuous intracranial pressure monitoring in neurosurgical practice. Acta Neurochir. 1973;29:53–63.

Key A, Retzius G. Studies in der Anatomie des Nerven system und der Bindesgewebes. Stockholm: Bd. I. Samson & Wallin; 1875.

Knoll PH. Uber die Druckschwankungen in der Cerebrospinalflussigkeit und den Wechsel in der Blutfulle des centralen Nervensystems. Sitzungs-berichte der Kaiserlichen Akademie der Wissenschaften; 1886. p. 217–246.

Lassen NA. Cerebral blood flow and oxygen consumption in man. Physiol Rev. 1959;39:183–38.

Lenfeldt N, Koskinen LO, Bergenheim AT, Malm J, Eklund A. CSF pressure assessed by lumbar puncture agrees with intracranial pressure. Neurology. 2007;68(2):155–8.

Lundberg N. Continuous recording and control of ventricular fluid pressure in neurosurgical practice. Acta Psychiatr Neurol Scand. 1960;1(Supplement 149):193.

Narayan RK, Kishore PR, Becker DP, Ward JD, Enas GG, Greenberg RP, Domingues Da Silva A, Lipper MH, Choi SC, Mayhall CG, Lutz HA 3rd, Young HF. Intracranial pressure: to monitor or not to monitor? A review of our experience with severe head injury. J Neurosurg. 1982;56(5):650–9.

Newcombe VFJ, Hawkes RC, Harding SG, Willcox R, Brock S, Hutchinson PJ, Menon DK, Carpenter TA, Coles JP. Potential heating caused by intracranial pressure transducers in a 3-Tesla magnetic resonance imaging system using a body radiofrequency resonator: assessment of the Codman MicroSensor transducer. J Neurosurg. 2008;109:159–64.

Nordström CH, Reinstrup P, Xu W, Gärdenfors A, Ungerstedt U. Assessment of the lower limit for cerebral perfusion pressure in severe head injuries by bedside monitoring of regional energy metabolism. Anesthesiology. 2003;98(4):809–14.

Piccinini A, Lewis M, Benjamin E, Aiolfi A, Inaba K, Demetriades D. Intracranial pressure monitoring in severe traumatic brain injuries: a closer look at the level 1 trauma centers in the United States. Injury. 2017;48(9):1944–50.

Quincke HI. Verhandlungen des Congresses für Innere Medizin, Zehnter Congress. Wiesbaden. 1891;10:321–31.

Rajajee V, Vanaman M, Fletcher JJ, Jacobs TL. Optic nerve ultrasound for the detection of raised intracranial pressure. Neurocrit Care. 2011;15:506–15.

Rao V, Klepstad P, Kristian Losvik O, Solheim O. Confusion with cerebral perfusion pressure in a literature review of current guidelines and survey of clinical practise. Scandinavian Journal of Trauma, Resuscitation and Emergency Medicine 2013;21(1).

Reinstrup P, Unnerbäck M, Marklund N, Schalen W, Cabrera Arrocha J, Bloomfield EL, Sadegh V, Hesselgard K. Best zero level for external ICP transducer. Acta Neurochir. 2019;161(4):635–42.

Robba C, Santori G, Czosnyka M, Corradi F, Bragazzi N, Padayachy L, Taccone FS, Citerio G. Optic nerve sheath diameter measured sonographically as non-invasive estimator of intracranial pressure: a systematic review and meta-analysis. Intensive Care Med. 2018;44:1284–94.

Rosenwasser RH, Kleiner LI, Krzeminski JP, Buchheit WA. Intracranial pressure monitoring in the posterior fossa: a preliminary report. J Neurosurg. 1989;71(4):503–5.

Rossi S, Buzzi F, Paparella A, Mainini P, Stocchetti N. Complications and safety associated with ICP monitoring: a study of 542 patients. Acta Neurochir Suppl. 1998;71:91–3.

Sahu S, Swain A. Optic nerve sheath diameter: a novel way to monitor the brain. J Neuroanaesthesiol Crit Care. 2017;4(Suppl S1):13–8.

Sakowitz OW, Raabe A, Vucak D, Kiening KL, Unterberg AW. Contemporary management of aneurysmal subarachnoid hemorrhage in Germany: results of a survey among 100 neurosurgical departments. Neurosurgery. 2006;58(1):137–45.

Schmidt B, Czosnyka M, Klingelhöfer J. Clinical applications of a non-invasive ICP monitoring method. Eur J Ultrasound. 2002;16(1–2):37–45.

Shapiro K, Morris WJ, Teo C. Intracranial hypertension: mechanisms and management. In: Cheek WR, Marlin AE, McLone DG, et al., editors. Pediatric neurosurgery: surgery of the developing nervous system. 3rd ed. Philadelphia: Saunders; 1994. p. 307–19.

Shimbles S, Dodd C, Banister K, Mendelow AD, Chambers IR. Clinical comparison of tympanic membrane displacement with invasive intracranial pressure measurements. Physiol Meas. 2005;26(6):1085–92.

Slavin KV, Misra M. Infratentorial intracranial pressure monitoring in neurosurgical intensive care unit. Neurol Res. 2003;25(8):880–4.

Spiegelberg A, Preuss M, Kurtcuoglu V. B-waves revisited. Interdicip Neurosurg. 2016;6:13–7.

Steiner LA, Czosnyka M, Piechnik SK, Smielewski P, Chatfield D, Menon DK, Pickard JD. Continuous monitoring of cerebrovascular pressure reactivity allows determination of optimal cerebral perfusion pressure in patients with traumatic brain injury. Critical Care Medicine. 2001;30(4):733–8.

Unnerbäck M, Bloomfield E, Söderström S, Reinstrup P. The intracranial pressure curve correlates to the pulsatile component of cerebral blood flow. J Clin Monit Comput. 2019;33(1):77–83. https://doi.org/10.1007/s10877-018-0129-0.

Unnerbäck M, Ottesen J, Reinstrup P. ICP curve morphology and intracranial flow-volume changes: a simultaneous ICP and cine phase contrast MRI study in humans. Acta Neurochirurgica (Wien). 2018;160:219–24.

41 Brain Tissue Oxygen Monitoring

Troels Halfeld Nielsen and Jon Axel Forsse

Recommendations

Level I

There are insufficient data to support a Level I recommendation for this topic.

Level II

There are insufficient data to support a Level II recommendation for this topic.

Level III

Brain tissue oxygen below 5–15 mmHg is associated with higher mortality after severe TBI. Brain tissue oxygen monitoring is recommended as a part of a multimodal monitoring context in patients at risk of cerebral ischemia and/or hypoxia.

41.1 Overview

Monitoring of brain tissue oxygenation represents one of an array of regional cerebral monitors including microdialysis for measurements of regional metabolism, thermal diffusion probes for measurements of CBF, and near-infrared spectroscopy that also measures brain tissue oxygenation. Common for all modalities is that they comprise a supplement to the routinely used ICP monitoring. These regional monitors have gained increasing interest because they open up possibilities to develop treatment strategies aiming at optimizing not only ICP, but also cerebral blood flow, oxygenation, and metabolism.

In the last two decades, direct measurement of brain tissue oxygen tension ($PbtO_2$) has become the most frequently used technique for monitoring brain oxygenation because of its ease of use and continuous measurement. It is used in concert with ICP monitoring, most often placed in the least affected frontal lobe's subcortical white matter, to best reflect global cerebral oxygenation and provide information regarding interventions such as ventilator adjustments, fluid balance, positioning, and ultimately surgical intervention.

In spite of the wide distribution of the technique, there has been some debate as to exactly what brain tissue oxygen monitors measure. $PbtO_2$ is influenced by changes in FiO_2, PaO_2, $PaCO_2$ and MAP among others (Maloney-Wilensky and Le Roux 2010). Rosenthal et al. demonstrated that $PbtO_2$ primarily represents the product of CBF and the arteriovenous oxygen tension difference (Rosenthal et al. 2009), suggesting that $PbtO_2$ reflects the diffusion of

T. H. Nielsen (✉) · J. A. Forsse
Department of Neurosurgery, Odense University Hospital, Odense, Denmark
e-mail: troels.halfeld.nielsen@rsyd.dk; troels.nielsen@rsyd.dk; jon.axel.forsse@rsyd.dk

© Springer Nature Switzerland AG 2020
T. Sundstrøm et al. (eds.), *Management of Severe Traumatic Brain Injury*,
https://doi.org/10.1007/978-3-030-39383-0_41

oxygen across the blood-brain barrier and delivery, rather than cerebral oxygen metabolism.

Quite a few studies have tried to determine the normal values and ischemic values of $PbtO_2$. Normal values range between 23 and 48 mmHg, but values as low as 9 mmHg have been observed in uninjured human brain (Meixensberger et al. 1993; Pennings et al. 2008). Ischemic values range from 10 to 25 mmHg in different studies (Chang et al. 2009; Doppenberg et al. 1998; Kiening et al. 1996; Valadka et al. 1998; van den Brink et al. 2000; van Santbrink et al. 1996; Zauner et al. 1997; Veenith et al. 2016). The wide range of both normal and ischemic values makes it difficult to establish an ischemic threshold, but an intervention threshold at 20 mmHg is supported by current expert opinion (Le Roux et al. 2014).

Studies have been conducted to assess both the relationship between $PbtO_2$ levels and mortality after severe TBI (Chang et al. 2009; Doppenberg et al. 1998; Kiening et al. 1996; Valadka et al. 1998; van den Brink et al. 2000; van Santbrink et al. 1996; Zauner et al. 1997; Bardt et al. 1998) and the effect of a $PbtO_2$-guided therapy on outcome (Chang et al. 2009; van den Brink et al. 2000; Fletcher et al. 2010; Martini et al. 2009; Meixensberger et al. 2003, 2004; Tolias et al. 2004; Okonkwo et al. 2017). Observational studies support that episodes with hypoxia are associated with increased mortality, and a recent phase II RCT supports evidence of a positive effect of $PbtO_2$-guided therapy on outcome after severe TBI, although the level of efficacy is yet to be determined (Okonkwo et al. 2017).

41.2 Background

A relatively large number of clinical studies have suggested a relation between measured $PbtO_2$ levels and mortality following TBI (Chang et al. 2009; Doppenberg et al. 1998; Kiening et al. 1996; Valadka et al. 1998; van den Brink et al. 2000; van Santbrink et al. 1996; Zauner et al. 1997; Bardt et al. 1998). In a prospective study of 22 patients with severe TBI, van Santbrink et al. demonstrated that episodes with $PbtO_2 < 5$ mmHg for at least 0.5 h were correlated to significantly increased mortality (van Santbrink et al. 1996). In a prospective study including 34 patients, Bardt et al. reported a higher mortality rate after TBI in patients with $PbtO_2 < 10$ mmHg for more than 30 min (56% vs. 9%) (Bardt et al. 1998). In 1998, Valadka et al. reported in a prospective observational study an increased mortality after TBI with $PbtO_2$ values less than 15 mmHg (Valadka et al. 1998). Similarly, van den Brink et al. found in a prospective observational study of 101 patients with TBI an increasing mortality after TBI with $PbtO_2$ values less than 15 mmHg, with the likelihood of death increasing with rising duration of time below 15 mmHg (van den Brink et al. 2000). Accordingly, there is Level III evidence that brain tissue oxygen below 5–15 mmHg is associated with increased mortality.

The association between $PbtO_2$ levels after severe TBI and outcome raises the question whether a therapy focused on optimizing $PbtO_2$ ($PbtO_2$-guided therapy) can improve outcome. In 2004, Tolias et al. reported the effect of treatment of 52 patients with severe TBI with a FiO_2 of 1.0 and compared the results with a cohort of 112 matched historical controls (Tolias et al. 2004). All patients were monitored with $PbtO_2$ probes along with microdialysis to study cerebral metabolism. Although they found a decreased brain lactate and lactate/pyruvate ratio in the treatment group, no improvement in outcome in this group could be demonstrated. In total, Stiefel et al., Narotam et al. and Spiotta et al. studied 234 patients with severe TBI managed according to a $PbtO_2$ optimizing protocol and compared them to a control group managed with ICP-/CPP-guided therapy only (Narotam et al. 2009; Spiotta et al. 2010; Stiefel et al. 2004). The three studies reported quite similar results with decreasing mortality from around 44% in the control group to around 25% in the treatment group. Additionally Narotam et al. found a significantly higher GOS in the treatment group compared to the control group (3.55 vs. 2.71). These three studies, however, relied on historical controls with a significant mortality compared to today's standard. In 2017 a multicentre phase II RCT of 119 patients concluded that time with hypoxia could be reduced through a tiered intervention protocol based on $PbtO_2$ and that the results were consistent with reduced mortality and more favourable outcomes than ICP-only management. The study was not powered for efficacy (Okonkwo et al. 2017). Contrary to these findings, Martini et al. showed, in a retrospective study comparing 506 patients managed by ICP-/CPP-guided therapy with 123 patients managed with $PbtO_2$-guided therapy, a higher mortality rate in the $PbtO_2$ group, correcting for baseline differences in severity of brain injury (Martini et al. 2009). In a similar, but smaller retrospective study by Green et al., there were no outcome improvements at discharge using additional $PbtO_2$-guided therapy (Green et al. 2013). Noteworthy is that $PbtO_2$-guided therapy can be associated with complications: in a retrospective study of 41 patients, $PbtO_2$-guided therapy was associated with increased cumulative fluid balance, use of vasopressors and increased rates of refractory intracranial hypertension and pulmonary oedema (Fletcher et al. 2010).

In conclusion, a high-level evidence-based recommendation regarding $PbtO_2$-guided therapy cannot be given.

41.3 Specific Paediatric Concerns

Studies of brain oxygen tension in paediatric TBI have shown that low $PbtO_2$ and the amount of time with low $PbtO_2$ are associated with poor outcome in children with severe TBI. The thresholds seem to be identical to those in the adult population. Further, episodes with reduced $PbtO_2$ may be seen without significant changes in normal physiological values (i.e. ICP, CPP, SaO_2, PaO_2, etc.) (Figaji and Adelson 2009; Figaji et al. 2008, 2009a, b). The numbers of included patients in paediatric studies are small.

Tips, Tricks and Pitfalls

- A low or decreasing $PbtO_2$ can reflect low or decreasing CBF as a result of high ICP/low CPP, hyperventilation, or low PaO_2. Also, a low or decreasing $PbtO_2$ can reflect cerebral oedema and therefore diffusion-limited delivery of oxygen (diffusion limited hypoxia).
- Always allow at least 1 h after implantation of the $PbtO_2$ catheter for stabilization. To ensure that the $PbtO_2$ probe is functioning correctly, always do an 'oxygen challenge test'. That is, $PbtO_2$ should increase threefold when increasing FiO_2 to 1.0 for 2–5 min.
- Bear in mind that $PbtO_2$ is a regional measurement, and the interpretation of the values should always be based on the location of the probe; the probe could be placed in a traumatic contusion, infarcted tissue, etc.

References

Bardt TF, Unterberg AW, Hartl R, Kiening KL, Schneider GH, Lanksch WR. Monitoring of brain tissue PO2 in traumatic brain injury: effect of cerebral hypoxia on outcome. Acta Neurochir Suppl. 1998;71:153–6.

Chang JJ, Youn TS, Benson D, Mattick H, Andrade N, Harper CR, Moore CB, Madden CJ, Diaz-Arrastia RR. Physiologic and functional outcome correlates of brain tissue hypoxia in traumatic brain injury. Crit Care Med. 2009;37:283–90.

Doppenberg EM, Zauner A, Watson JC, Bullock R. Determination of the ischemic threshold for brain oxygen tension. Acta Neurochir Suppl. 1998;71:166–9.

Figaji AA, Adelson PD. Does ICP monitoring in children with severe head injuries make a difference? Am Surg. 2009;75:441–2.

Figaji AA, Fieggen AG, Argent AC, Leroux PD, Peter JC. Does adherence to treatment targets in children with severe traumatic brain injury avoid brain hypoxia? A brain tissue oxygenation study. Neurosurgery. 2008;63:83–91; discussion 91–92.

Figaji AA, Zwane E, Thompson C, Fieggen AG, Argent AC, Le Roux PD, Peter JC. Brain tissue oxygen tension monitoring in pediatric severe traumatic brain injury. Part 1: relationship with outcome. Childs Nerv Syst. 2009a;25:1325–33.

Figaji AA, Zwane E, Thompson C, Fieggen AG, Argent AC, Le Roux PD, Peter JC. Brain tissue oxygen tension monitoring in pediatric severe traumatic brain injury. Part 2: relationship with clinical, physiological, and treatment factors. Childs Nerv Syst. 2009b;25:1335–43.

Fletcher JJ, Bergman K, Blostein PA, Kramer AH. Fluid balance, complications, and brain tissue oxygen tension monitoring following severe traumatic brain injury. Neurocrit Care. 2010;13:47–56.

Green JA, Pellegrini DC, Vanderkolk WE, Figueroa BE, Eriksson EA. Goal directed brain tissue oxygen monitoring versus conventional management in traumatic brain injury: an analysis of in hospital recovery. Neurocrit Care. 2013;18:20–5.

Kiening KL, Unterberg AW, Bardt TF, Schneider GH, Lanksch WR. Monitoring of cerebral oxygenation in patients with severe head injuries: brain tissue PO2 versus jugular vein oxygen saturation. J Neurosurg. 1996;85:751–7.

Le Roux P, Menon DK, Citerio G. The international multidisciplinary consensus conference on multimodality monitoring in neurocritical care: a list of recommendations and additional conclusions. Neurocrit Care. 2014;21(2):282–96.

Maloney-Wilensky E, Le Roux P. The physiology behind direct brain oxygen monitors and practical aspects of their use. Childs Nerv Syst. 2010;26:419–30.

Martini RP, Deem S, Yanez ND, Chesnut RM, Weiss NS, Daniel S, Souter M, Treggiari MM. Management guided by brain tissue oxygen monitoring and outcome following severe traumatic brain injury. J Neurosurg. 2009;111:644–9.

Meixensberger J, Dings J, Kuhnigk H, Roosen K. Studies of tissue PO2 in normal and pathological human brain cortex. Acta Neurochir Suppl (Wien). 1993;59:58–63.

Meixensberger J, Jaeger M, Vath A, Dings J, Kunze E, Roosen K. Brain tissue oxygen guided treatment supplementing ICP/CPP therapy after traumatic brain injury. J Neurol Neurosurg Psychiatry. 2003;74:760–4.

Meixensberger J, Renner C, Simanowski R, Schmidtke A, Dings J, Roosen K. Influence of cerebral oxygenation following severe head injury on neuropsychological testing. Neurol Res. 2004;26:414–7.

Narotam PK, Morrison JF, Nathoo N. Brain tissue oxygen monitoring in traumatic brain injury and major trauma: outcome analysis of a brain tissue oxygendirected therapy. J Neurosurg. 2009;111:672–82.

Okonkwo D, Shutter L, Moore C. Brain oxygen optimization in severe traumatic brain injury phase-II: a phase II randomized trial. Crit Care Med. 2017;45(11):1907–14.

Pennings FA, Schuurman PR, van den Munckhof P, Bouma GJ. Brain tissue oxygen pressure monitoring in awake patients during functional neurosurgery: the assessment of normal values. J Neurotrauma. 2008;25:1173–7.

Rosenthal G, Hemphill JC 3rd, Manley G. Brain tissue oxygen tension is more indicative of oxygen diffusion than oxygen delivery and metabolism in patients with traumatic brain injury. Crit Care Med. 2009;37:379–80.

Spiotta AM, Stiefel MF, Gracias VH, Garuffe AM, Kofke WA, Maloney-Wilensky E, Troxel AB, Levine JM, Le Roux PD. Brain tissue oxygen-directed management and outcome in patients with severe traumatic brain injury. J Neurosurg. 2010;113(3):571–80.

Stiefel MF, Heuer GG, Smith MJ, Bloom S, MaloneyWilensky E, Gracias VH, Grady MS, LeRoux PD. Cerebral oxygenation following decompressive hemicraniectomy for the treatment of refractory intracranial hypertension. J Neurosurg. 2004;101:241–7.

Tolias CM, Reinert M, Seiler R, Gilman C, Scharf A, Bullock MR. Normobaric hyperoxia–induced improvement in cerebral metabolism and reduction in intracranial pressure in patients with severe head injury: a prospective historical cohort-matched study. J Neurosurg. 2004;101:435–44.

Valadka AB, Gopinath SP, Contant CF, Uzura M, Robertson CS. Relationship of brain tissue PO2 to outcome after severe head injury. Crit Care Med. 1998;26:1576–81.

van den Brink WA, van Santbrink H, Steyerberg EW, Avezaat CJ, Suazo JA, Hogesteeger C, Jansen WJ, Kloos LM, Vermeulen J, Maas AI. Brain oxygen tension in severe head injury. Neurosurgery. 2000;46:868–76; discussion 76–78.

van Santbrink H, Maas AI, Avezaat CJ. Continuous monitoring of partial pressure of brain tissue oxygen in patients with severe head injury. Neurosurgery. 1996;38:21–31.

Veenith TV, Carter E, Geeraerts T, Grossac J, Newcombe V, Outtrime J, Gee G, Lupson V, Smith R, Aigbirhio F, Fryer T, Hong Y, Menon DK, Coles JP. Pathophysiologic mechanisms of cerebral ischemia and diffusion hypoxia in traumatic brain injury. JAMA Neurol. 2016;73(5):542–50.

Zauner A, Doppenberg EM, Woodward JJ, Choi SC, Young HF, Bullock R. Continuous monitoring of cerebral substrate delivery and clearance: initial experience in 24 patients with severe acute brain injuries. Neurosurgery. 1997;41:1082–91; discussion 91–93.

Monitoring Microdialysis

42

Peter Reinstrup and Carl-Henrik Nordström

Recommendations

Level I

There are insufficient data to support a Level I recommendation for this topic.

Level II

There are insufficient data to support a Level II recommendation for this topic.

Level III

With intracerebral microdialysis, it is possible to detect upcoming ischemia, mitochondrial dysfunction and cell death.

42.1 Overview

Microdialysis is an invasive technique based on the placement of a small catheter into the brain parenchyma where the distal end of the catheter is a dialysis membrane. The lumen is perfused with a fluid with a composition of electrolytes similar to normal CSF. By osmosis from the surrounding tissue, molecules are taken up into the perfusion fluid through the dialysis membrane and collected in microvials. The irrigation fluid can then be analysed online bedside (most commonly) or later at some convenient time. With the current technique, approximately 70% of the parenchymal substances most commonly analysed will be recovered in the perfusion fluid.

The variables analysed routinely are glucose, lactate, pyruvate, glycerol and glutamate. The lactate/pyruvate ratio is a sensitive marker for the detection of compromised oxidative metabolism (e.g. during ischemia), whereas glycerol is considered to reflect the degradation of cell membranes. By positioning the catheter in an area of interest, e.g. the penumbra zone surrounding a contused area, the method can provide an early warning of impending tissue damage before it is reflected in global physiological variables or clinical state.

It is recommended to use intracerebral microdialysis as a complement to intracranial pressure (ICP) and cerebral perfusion pressure (CPP) monitoring in severe cases of TBI, subarachnoid haemorrhage and other severe cerebral conditions treated during neurocritical care.

P. Reinstrup (✉)
Department of Intensive and Perioperative Care, Skånes University Hospital, Lund, Sweden
e-mail: peter.reinstrup@med.lu.se

C.-H. Nordström
Department of Neurosurgery, Odense University Hospital, Odense, Denmark
e-mail: chnorstrom@health.sdu.com

© Springer Nature Switzerland AG 2020
T. Sundstrøm et al. (eds.), *Management of Severe Traumatic Brain Injury*,
https://doi.org/10.1007/978-3-030-39383-0_42

Tips, Tricks and Pitfalls

- The microdialysis catheter can be placed either during a craniotomy in the operating theatre or at the neurointensive care unit using local anaesthetics (Poca et al. 2006).
- As the microdialysis catheter reflects the biochemical composition of a very narrow zone surrounding the semipermeable membrane, it is important to document its position in relation to focal brain lesions, e.g. by a CT or an MR scanning.
- If the catheter is placed in the especially vulnerable penumbra zone surrounding a focal lesion, the microdialysis may give an early warning of impending deterioration before the risk is detected by global cerebral monitoring or clinical state.

Interpretation of bedside results

- In neurocritical care, microdialysis is primarily used to evaluate cerebral energy metabolism by measuring the sole normal substrate (glucose) and the efficacy of oxidative metabolism, i.e. the lactate/pyruvate (LP) ratio. Disintegration of phospholipids of cell membrane is revealed by an increase in interstitial glycerol concentration.
- The results obtained should be compared with the levels described in normal human brain by utilizing identical analytical techniques.
- Ischemia is characterized by an increased level of lactate accompanied by marked decreases in the concentrations of pyruvate and glucose. As a result, the LP ratio is usually very high.
- Mitochondrial dysfunction is characterized by a marked increase in lactate concentration at a normal or elevated level of pyruvate. As a result, the LP ratio is only moderately elevated while glucose concentrations often are within normal limits.
- Degradation of cell membranes is reflected in a marked increase in interstitial glycerol levels irrespective of the underlying pathophysiological mechanism.

42.2 Background

Microdialysis (Gr. *mikros* small + *dia* through + *lysis* dissolution) is primarily a technique for extracting substances from a tissue in order to analyse the chemical composition of extracellular fluids, but the technique may be used also to deliver chemical substances to tissues (e.g. drugs). The microdialysis method was developed almost 40 years ago for monitoring chemical events in the animal brain and is since long regarded as a reliable scientific technique. In the late 1980s, techniques for using microdialysis for the monitoring of the human brain were explored. In 1995 CMA Microdialysis (Stockholm, Sweden) introduced a sterile microdialysis catheter together with a robust microdialysis pump and a bedside biochemical analyser adapted to clinical conditions. The instrumentation was originally intended for subcutaneous and intramuscular use, but with a slight modification of the microdialysis catheter, it has mainly been used intracerebrally as an integrated part of routine multimodality brain monitoring (Hillered et al. 2006; Nordström et al. 2017). Since microdialysis is a technique permitting sampling of stable biochemical compounds that traverse the dialysis membrane, it has rapidly been accepted for research purposes.

The currently used equipment is manufactured by M Dialysis AB, Stockholm, Sweden. The perfusion fluid is a Ringer solution adjusted to be iso-osmolar to the composition of cerebral interstitial fluid. As a standard, a small pump delivering a continuous flow of 0.3 μL/min is utilized. From the pump, the fluid is lead through thin tubing to the 10-mm-long microdialysis membrane at the end of the catheter. The diameter of the microdialysis probe is approximately 0.6 mm. At the tip of the probe, a small gold thread is implanted in order to be identifiable on CT or MR scanning but small enough not to obscure the images. After having passed the microdialysis membrane, the perfusion fluid continues into a thin inner tube positioned within the tip of the microdialysis catheter (*c.f.* Fig. 42.1). Finally, the microdialysis perfusate is collected into microvials which are routinely exchanged every 30 or 60 min to be analysed bedside utilizing enzymatic techniques (*c.f.* Fig. 42.1). The chemical variables usually monitored during routine neurocritical care are glucose, pyruvate, lactate, glutamate and glycerol. The analysis of the four biochemical variables usually takes 6–10 min. When the technique is used as clinical routine—with a perfusion rate of 0.3 μL/min, a membrane length of 10 mm and membrane permeability cut-off set at 20 kDa—a recovery of approximately 70% of the true interstitial concentrations is obtained. When microdialysis is performed as a routine clinical technique, this difference from the true interstitial levels is without clinical relevance. For scientific purposes, it is possible to obtain true interstitial concentration levels by performing online estimation of relative recovery.

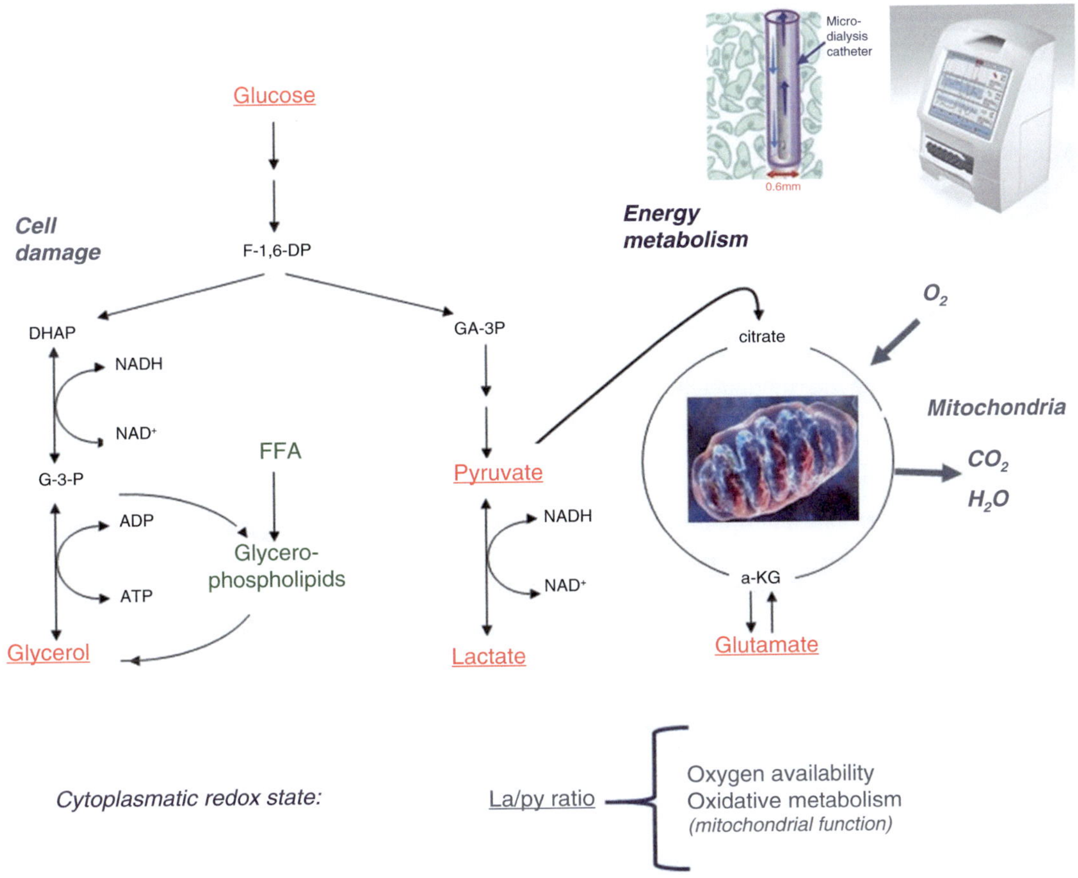

Fig. 42.1 Schematic diagram of cerebral intermediary metabolism with focus on the glycolytic chain and its relation to glycerol and glycerophospholipids and to the citric acid cycle. *F-1,6-DP* fructose-1,6-diposphate, *DHAP* dihydroxyacetone-phosphate, *GA-3P* glyceraldehyde-3-phosphate, *G-3-P* glycerol-3-phosphate, *FFA* free fatty acids, *α-KG* α-ketoglutarate. Underlined metabolites in red colour are measured at the bedside with enzymatic techniques. Upper right corner shows the tip of the microdialysis catheter and the analyser

42.3 Chemical Variables Monitored During Routine Clinical Microdialysis

A simplified diagram of the biochemical variables and their relations is shown in Fig. 42.1. Under normal conditions, glucose is the sole substrate for cerebral energy metabolism. In the cellular cytoplasm, it is degraded to pyruvate which enters into the mitochondria and—in the citrate cycle and in the presence of oxygen—is completely metabolized to CO_2 and H_2O. In the citrate cycle, the majority of the energy in the glucose molecule is recovered and transferred into the formation of ATP from ADP. Under normal circumstances, approximately 5% of pyruvate is converted to lactate in the cytoplasm. This is a reversible equilibrium reaction in which NADH is re-oxidized to NAD^+ (Fig. 42.1). The calculated LP ratio reflects the efficacy of cerebral oxidative energy metabolism (i.e. oxygen availability and mitochondrial function) in relation to tissue energy demands.

In routine microdialysis, glutamate may also be analysed. Glutamate is the main excitatory neurotransmitter in the brain. After its release, the interstitial glutamate level is during normal conditions closely controlled by reuptake into the astrocytes through an energy demanding mechanism. Hence, an increase in the interstitial level of glutamate may indicate insufficient energy supplies.

When the glycerophospholipids of cerebral cellular membranes is decomposed, free fatty acids and glycerol are released (Fig. 42.1). An increase in cerebral interstitial glycerol concentration is generally considered to be a marker of cell membrane degradation in the brain (Hutchinson et al. 2015; Nordström et al. 2017).

By utilizing the technique described above, the following reference values have been obtained in normal human brain tissue (Reinstrup et al. 2000) (mean ± SD): glucose 1.7 ± 0.9 mmol/L, lactate 2.9 ± 0.9 mmol/L, pyruvate 166 ± 47 μmol/l, LP ratio 23 ± 4, glutamate 16 ± 16 μmol/L and glycerol 80 ± 40 μmol/L.

42.4 Bedside Diagnosis of Cerebral Ischemia and Mitochondrial Dysfunction

Since the brain is completely dependent on oxidative energy metabolism, the LP ratio is a sensitive indicator of compromised energy metabolism in many pathological situations. Figure 42.2 compares the biochemical patterns in cerebral ischemia and mitochondrial dysfunction.

In severe ischemia, impaired blood supply causes an insufficient delivery of oxygen as well as glucose. The instantaneous increase in LP ratio is pronounced due to a concomitant increase in lactate and a decrease in pyruvate concentrations. Mitochondrial dysfunction may occur due to compromised mitochondrial uptake of pyruvate (e.g. in bacterial meningitis) or a block in one or more steps in the citrate cycle. This may occur during recirculation after transient cerebral ischemia or as an effect of various toxins (Nordström et al. 2017). Figure 42.3 illustrates the variations in lactate, pyruvate and LP ratio in ischemia and mitochondrial dysfunction. In cerebral ischemia, a marked increase of the LP ratio and a very low pyruvate level are noticed, while mitochondrial dysfunction is characterized by a moderate increase in LP ratio and a normal or increased level of pyruvate.

From a clinical point of view, it is important to separate cerebral ischemia and mitochondrial dysfunction, since the two conditions demand different therapy, n.b. to such a degree that the efficacy of the therapeutic interventions may be evaluated directly from the effects on the biochemical pattern obtained from microdialysis.

The biochemical pattern obtained when energy utilization rate exceeds the capacity of the oxidative metabolism (e.g. during generalized epileptic seizures) also exhibits the characteristics of mitochondrial dysfunction. For bedside diagnosis of ischemia and mitochondrial dysfunction, it is necessary to relate the level of the biochemical variables obtained to their normal reference values (*c.f.* above).

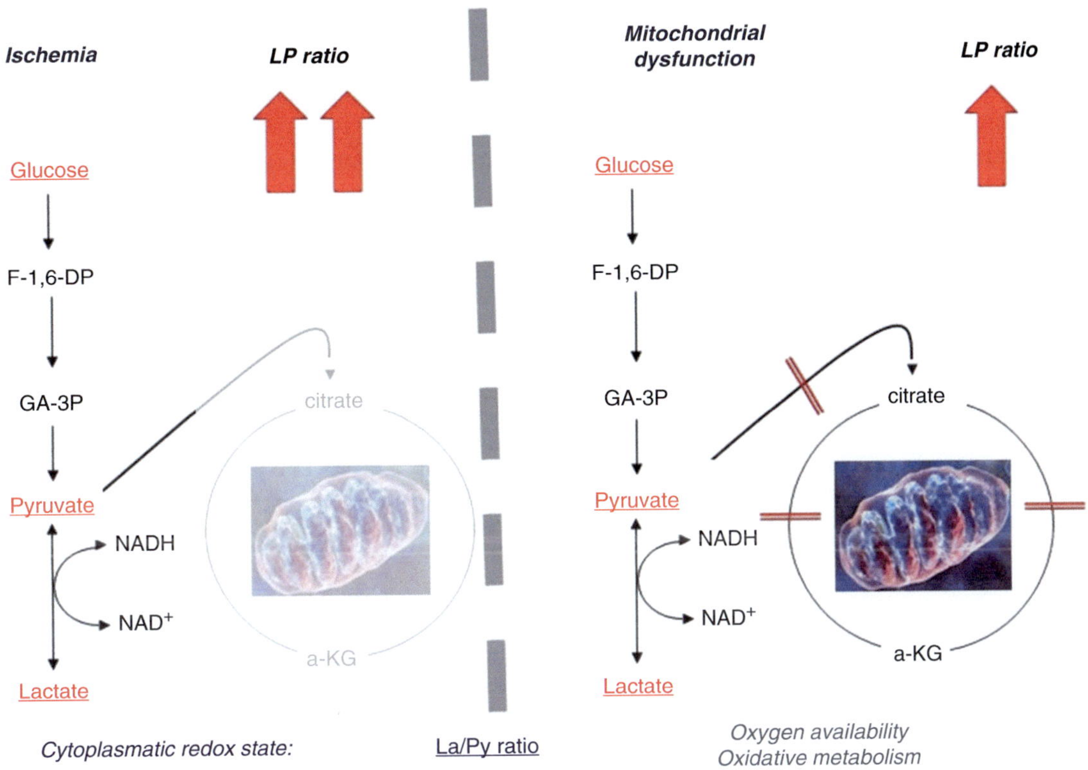

Fig. 42.2 Schematic illustration of the biochemical patterns during cerebral ischemia and mitochondrial dysfunction. The arrows indicate the change due to the various conditions, and the text size represents the resulting concentration. For explanation of abbreviations, see Fig. 42.1

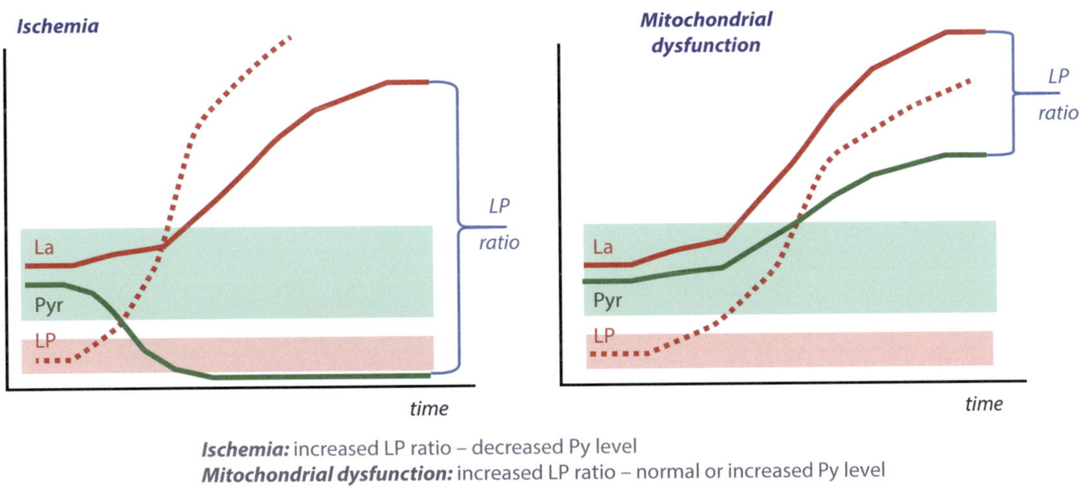

Fig. 42.3 Schematic diagrams of the changes in the intracerebral levels of lactate, pyruvate and the LP ratio during ischemia and mitochondrial dysfunction

42.5 Clinical Microdialysis: Possibilities and Limitations

The microdialysis catheter recovers the chemical composition of a very narrow interstitial zone surrounding the semipermeable membrane. Accordingly, it is necessary to document where the catheter is located in relation to a focal cerebral lesion (e.g. from CT or MR scanning) (Engström et al. 2005). Figure 42.4 illustrates the biochemical information obtained from three intracerebral microdialysis probes in a patient with an extracerebral haematoma. In two microdialysis catheters inserted into the penumbra of the focal lesion, a marked increase in LP ratio is measured, while the catheter positioned in intact brain tissue in the opposite hemisphere records a normal LP ratio.

The information obtained from the penumbra zone gives an early warning of deterioration before it is detected by global techniques or clinical signs. When the microdialysis catheter is positioned in such a way, the local technique provides for improved therapeutic interventions. The limitations of a local technique are related to the fact that the biochemical pattern obtained is often not representative for the whole cerebral hemisphere (Nordström et al. 2017).

Presently, the main limitation of microdialysis from being used as a clinical routine is due to the fact that the perfusion fluid is collected into microvials before its transfer to the analyser. During rou-

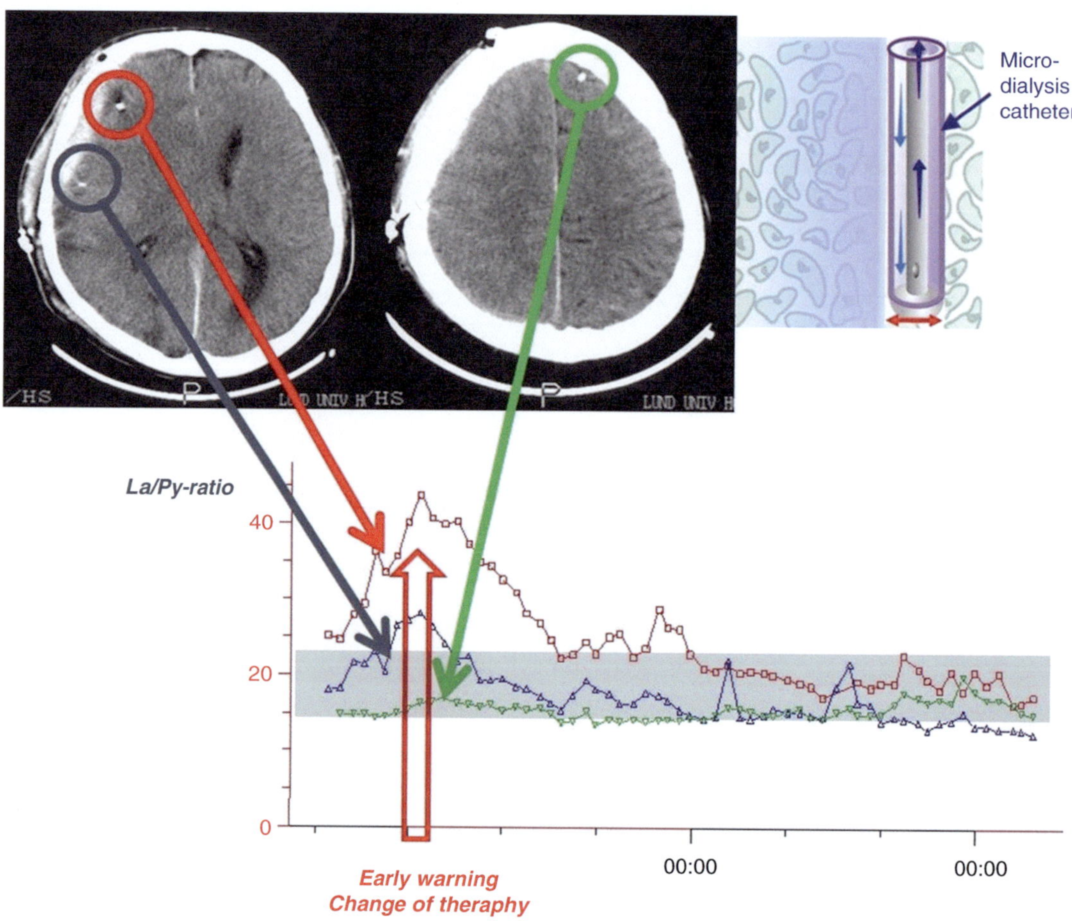

Fig. 42.4 Comparison of the changes in LP ratio detected by microdialysis catheters positioned in the penumbra zone of a focal brain lesion and, in the opposite, normal hemisphere. Upper right corner presents a microdialysis catheter with its measuring zone

tine intensive care, this procedure is sometimes regarded as too labour-intensive. Further, the biochemical pattern is obtained at relatively long intervals (usually 60 min). Techniques based on microsensors for bedside online analyses of glucose, lactate and pyruvate have recently been presented and will presumably soon be available as a clinical routine tool. Accordingly, we will in the near future probably have the possibility to analyse the key variables reflecting cerebral oxidative energy metabolism (glucose, pyruvate, lactate, LP ratio) continuously online and to display the patterns obtained on a bedside monitor.

42.6 Specific Paediatric Concerns

Children generally tolerate a lower CPP than adults. However, the lowest acceptable limit for normal brain functions has not been determined in children and probably also varies with age and between individuals. Hence, in anti-oedema therapy utilizing a lowering of the CPP (e.g. the Lund concept), it is valuable to guide therapy by using results from intracerebral microdialysis analysis (Nordström 2003). Few studies have been directed specifically to cerebral microdialysis in children suffering from TBI (Tolias et al. 2002; Charalambides et al. 2010). There is however no reason to believe that the basic principles differ between children and adults regarding cerebral energy metabolism.

References

Charalambides C, Sgouros S, Sakas D. Intracerebral microdialysis in children. Childs Nerv Syst. 2010;26(2):215–20.

Engström M, Polito A, Reinstrup P, Romner B, Ryding E, Ungerstedt U, Nordström CH. Intracerebral microdialysis in severe brain trauma: the importance of catheter location. J Neurosurg. 2005;102(3):460–9.

Hillered L, Persson L, Nilsson P, Ronne-Engstrom E, Enblad P. Continuous monitoring of cerebral metabolism in traumatic brain injury: a focus on cerebral microdialysis. Curr Opin Crit Care. 2006;12(2):112–8.

Hutchinson PJ, Jalloh I, Helmy A, et al. Consensus statement from the 2014 international microdialysis forum. Intensive Care Med. 2015;41(9):1517–28.

Nordström CH. Assessment of critical thresholds for cerebral perfusion pressure by performing bedside monitoring of cerebral energy metabolism. Neurosurg Focus. 2003;15(6):E5.

Nordström CH, Koskinen LO, Olivecrona M. Aspects on the physiological and biochemical foundations of neurocritical care. Front Neurol. 2017;19(8):274.

Poca MA, Sahuquillo J, Vilalta A, de los Rios J, Robles A, Exposito L. Percutaneous implantation of cerebral microdialysis catheters by twist-drill craniostomy in neurocritical patients: description of the technique and results of a feasibility study in 97 patients. J Neurotrauma. 2006;23(10):1510–7.

Reinstrup P, Ståhl N, Mellergård P, Uski T, Ungerstedt U, Nordström CH. Intracerebral microdialysis in clinical practice: baseline values for chemical markers during wakefulness, anesthesia, and neurosurgery. Neurosurgery. 2000;47(3):701–9.

Tolias CM, Richards DA, Bowery NG, Sgouros S. Extracellular glutamate in the brains of children with severe head injuries: a pilot microdialysis study. Childs Nerv Syst. 2002;18(8):368–74.

Jugular Bulb Measurements ($SJVO_2$)

43

Bo-Michael Bellander and Peter Reinstrup

Recommendations

Level I

There are insufficient data to support a Level I recommendation for this topic.

Level II

There are insufficient data to support a Level II recommendation for this topic.

Level III

Jugular venous saturation measurements can be used to monitor cerebral oxygenation where a jugular venous saturation ($SjvO_2$) below 50% should be considered as a treatment threshold (Bratton et al. 2007). Jugular bulb monitoring of arteriovenous oxygen content difference ($AVDO_2$), as a source of information for management decisions, may be considered to reduce mortality and improve outcome at 3 and 6 months post-injury (Carney et al. 2017; Cruz 1998; Le Roux et al. 1997; Robertson 1993; Robertson et al. 1995)

B.-M. Bellander (✉)
Department of Clinical Neuroscience, Karolinska Institutet, Stockholm, Sweden

Department of Neurosurgery, Karolinska University Hospital, Stockholm, Sweden
e-mail: bo-michael.bellander@sll.se

P. Reinstrup
Department of Intensive and Perioperative Care, Skånes University Hospital, Lund, Sweden
e-mail: peter.reinstrup@med.lu.se

43.1 Overview

Jugular bulb venous oxygen saturation ($SjvO_2$) is the percentage of oxygen bound to haemoglobin in the blood returning from the brain. This reflects the residue of oxygen in the blood having passed the brain tissue. Measuring $SjvO_2$ can provide information about global hypoperfusion or hypoxemia, but there are many pitfalls when looking at focal brain pathologies.

Tips, Tricks and Pitfalls

- Global $SjvO_2$ does not necessarily unmask focal or even regional ischemia.
- The jugular venous blood is not truly mixed, and hence an ischemic area might be drained by the opposite jugular vein.
- Tissue with limited capacity for oxygen extraction, e.g. re-perfused infarcted tissue or tissue with mitochondrial dysfunction, will give false normal or even high $SjvO_2$.

© Springer Nature Switzerland AG 2020
T. Sundstrøm et al. (eds.), *Management of Severe Traumatic Brain Injury*,
https://doi.org/10.1007/978-3-030-39383-0_43

- The tip of the catheter has to be situated in the jugular bulb in order to avoid contamination from extracerebral blood (Fig. 43.1).
- A radiographic check, lateral skull X-ray or CT, is mandatory before jugular venous samples are used. The tip of the catheter should be located slightly medial to the mastoid bone at the level of the mastoid base.
- Rapid evacuation ($\geq$10 mL/min) from a jugular bulb catheter increases the risk for contamination of extracerebral blood in the sample.
- A rapid injection of fluid in the retrograde catheter does not affect the brain. Even in situations of low CBF, a rapid injection of contrast only reaches up to the sinus confluens and drains again through the contralateral sinus transversus (Fig. 43.1).

43.2 Background

Sixty-seven percent (range 22–97) of the cerebral blood flow (CBF) leaves through the internal jugular veins. The blood from the left and right transverse sinuses draining into the two internal jugular veins is not evenly distributed (Fig. 43.1). Most persons have a dominant flow in one of the internal jugular veins, and 5% show a no flow situation in one vein. It is important to emphasise that the blood leaving the brain through one internal jugular vein can, but does not necessarily, emanate from the ipsilateral hemisphere; it may more or less be "polluted" from the contralateral side (Fig. 43.1). An ischemic area might therefore to varying degrees be drained by the opposite jugular vein.

Access to the jugular bulb, the conjunction between the transverse sinus and the intern jugular vein, offers a method to analyse blood leaving the brain. Blood chemistry from this site provides an insight into the correlation between the global cerebral blood flow (CBF_{global}) and the cerebral metabolic rate of O_2 ($CMRO_2$). The measuring is based on the insertion of a catheter in a retrograde direction into the internal jugular vein up to the jugular bulb (Fig. 43.2). The ideal set-up is using a catheter which can provide continuous measurements in real time.

The method was introduced in the mid-1980s (Garlick and Bihari 1987) and is today regarded as an important part of modern multimodal monitoring in the NICU (Gopinath et al. 1994), even though contradictory opinions have been presented (Latronico et al. 2000).

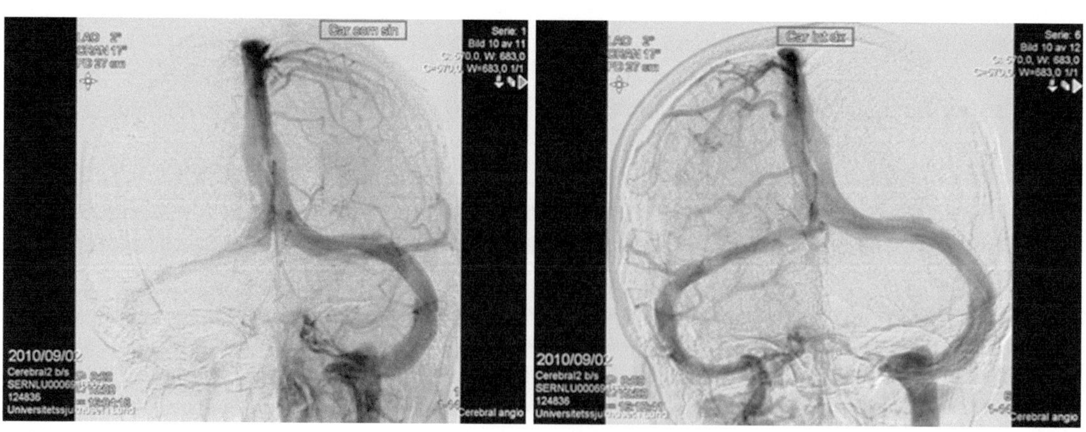

Fig. 43.1 Cerebral angiograms showing the sinuses and the internal jugular veins. The *left picture* is taken after injection in the left internal carotid artery (ICA), and in this patient the blood from the left hemisphere leaves mainly through the left internal jugular vein. The *right picture*, from the same patient, is taken after injection of contrast in the right ICA. The blood from this hemisphere leaves through both internal jugular veins

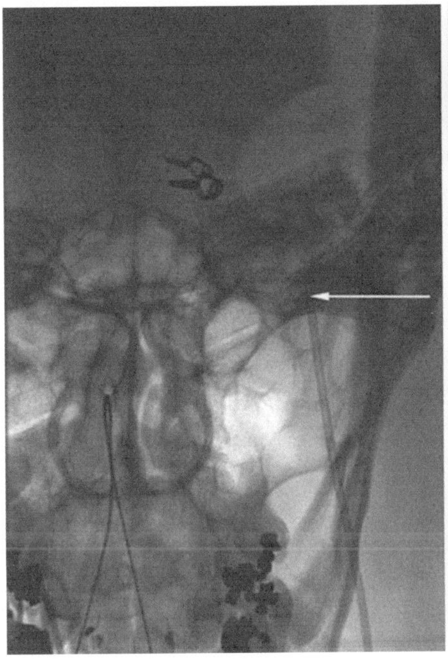

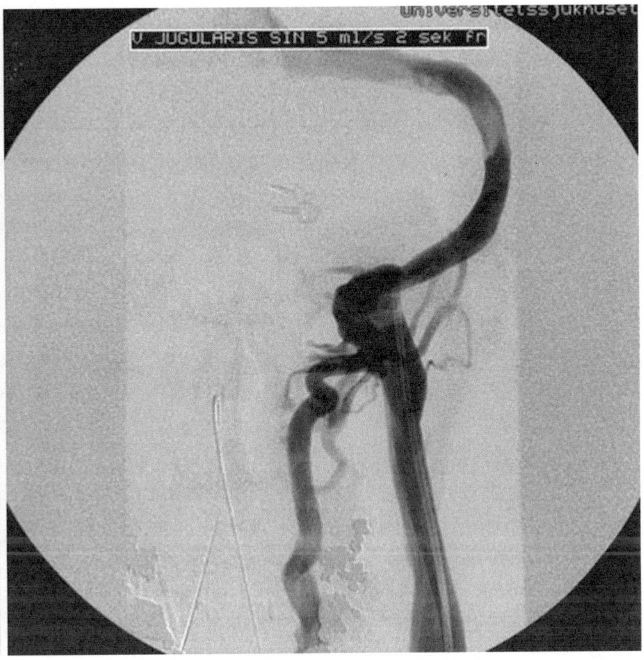

Fig. 43.2 Both pictures are from the same patient. On the *left side* is a plain X-ray of the skull where the *arrow* is pointing at the tip of the catheter. On the *right side* is a plain X-ray during a 5 mL/s contrast injection, thereby visualising the sinus transverses up to sinus confluens and the bulb in the middle of the picture,and the internal jugular vein going down out of the picture. A catheter is seen in the internal jugular vein and just below the jugular bulb are the extracerebral veins

43.2.1 Adequate Catheter Positioning

The catheter is threaded in a retrograded fashion to the jugular bulb, at which point a resistance will be felt approximately 15 cm from the skin puncture, after which the catheter is withdrawn 1 cm. A radiographic check, either a skull X-ray (Fig. 43.2) or a CT scan is necessary before jugular venous samples are collected. The tip of the catheter should be located slightly medial to the mastoid bone at the level of the mastoid base (Jakobsen and Enevoldsen 1989).

43.2.2 Contamination with Extracerebral Blood

Approximately 2.7% (0–6.6%) of the blood in the internal jugular vein is of extracerebral in origin (Shenkin et al. 1948). A jugular bulb catheter that is retracted more than 2 cm below the skull base shows an increase in $SjvO_2$ of more than 10% in 33% of the patients (Jakobsen and Enevoldsen 1989), indicating increased contamination. Rapid evacuation (10 mL/min) of jugular venous blood tends to present with higher $SjvO_2$ values than slow evacuation (2 mL/min), again indicating contamination with extracerebral blood (Matta and Lam 1997). Furthermore, a decrease in CBF and thereby reduced flow out through the internal jugular vein may lead to an increased proportion of extracerebral blood and a false high $SjvO_2$.

43.2.3 Normal Values of $SjvO_2$

Normal values for $SjvO_2$ were established by Gibbs and co-workers as early as in 1942 (Gibbs et al. 1942), reporting on average values of 62% (range between 55 and 71%) (Woodman and Robertson 1995). In a recent report, the average $SjvO_2$ was 61% with the upper limit at 71%

(Henson et al. 1998), even though others have used 75% as an upper limit (Cormio et al. 1999). A lower limit for $SjvO_2$ has been suggested to be 55% (Cormio et al. 1997; Cruz 1993), but lower limits - down to 45% - has also been suggested (Chieregato et al. 2003; Chan et al. 2005).

43.2.4 Factors Lowering $SjvO_2$

Decreased Oxygen Delivery: One reason for a decreased oxygen delivery is a reduced CBF. There are several factors attenuating CBF, one being increased cerebral vascular resistance (CVR) as during increased ICP, hyperventilation and vasospasm (Schneider et al. 1995), or by endogenous or exogenous cerebral vasoconstrictors. A decrease in oxygen delivery can also be of extracerebral origin as in hypotension, hypoxia or anaemia (Robertson et al. 1995).

Increased Cerebral Metabolism: Fever and seizures increase oxygen consumption. Fever increases the body's metabolic rate by 10–13% per centigrade. In piglets, a rise in temperature from 38 to 42 °C increases CBF by 97% and $CMRO_2$ by 65% (Busija et al. 1988). The uncoupling between CMR and CBF with an increased CBF will in this situation counteract a lowering of the $SjvO_2$. Seizures in rats increase $CMRO_2$ by 150–250% (Meldrum and Nilsson 1976), and it is often difficult for the circulation to cope with such an increase, resulting in a lowering of $SjvO_2$.

43.2.5 Factors Increasing $SjvO_2$

Decreased Cerebral Metabolism: Hypothermia decreases $CMRO_2$ by approximately 5% per centigrade (Woodman and Robertson 1995). Barbiturate coma treatment may reduce cerebral oxygen consumption up to 50% (Pierce et al. 1962). With the CBF-CMR coupling $SjvO_2$ might not be changed, but since barbiturates have a vasoconstrictive effect in low concentrations, and in high concentrations act as vasodilators, the $SjvO_2$ can change in unpredictable directions. Anaemia has been shown to result in low $SjvO_2$ values underestimating the reduction in CBF (Cruz et al. 1993).

43.2.6 $SjvO_2$ Versus CBF

If CMR, as well as arterial blood pressure, arterial oxygen saturation and haemoglobin content are stable, changes in $SjvO_2$ correspond to changes in CBF (Robertson et al. 1989). However, alkalosis as e.g. induced by hyperventilation, makes the tissue less able to extract oxygen; thus, a normal $SjvO_2$ might occur despite a low tissue pO_2 and an ischemic cerebral metabolism. However, provided pH is <7.6, tissue extraction of O_2 is not impaired, resulting in a $SjvO_2$ that adequately reflects a tissue pO_2 (Cruz et al. 1992). The multitude of factors involved makes this an unreliable method to estimate CBF except for special cases.

43.2.7 TBI Patients

In head trauma, patients' $SjvO_2$ has been reported to average 68% (range: 32–96%) (Woodman and Robertson 1995).

43.2.8 Jugular Venous Desaturation ($SjvO_2 \leq 50\%$)

Jugular venous desaturation has been shown to occur on at least one occasion during the observation time in 39% of severely brain-injured patients. Approximately half of the episodes were due to cerebral causes (intracranial hypertension or vascular spasm), and the rest had systemic causes (hypotension, hypoxia, hypocarbia or anaemia) (Robertson et al. 1995). Microdialysis of the injured brain tissue in concert with jugular bulb measurements has shown increased concentrations of lactate and glutamate to occur in conjunction with $SjvO_2 < 50\%$ in 7 out of 22 patients (Robertson et al. 1995).

43.2.9 Early Episodes of Desaturation

Jugular venous desaturation was identified in six out of eight patients during evacuation of a traumatic intracranial hematoma in the emergency operating room. In all six cases, $SjvO_2$ increased from 47 ± 10% to 63 ± 5% after the evacuation of the hematoma (Robertson et al. 1995). Spontaneous episodes of desaturation have been shown to occur frequently during the acute phase (<48 h) of TBI, SAH and ICH (Schneider et al. 1995). Approximately one-third of patients with severe TBI present with cerebral desaturation on admission (Vigue et al. 1999). Many episodes of desaturation are attributed to hyperventilation, insufficient cerebral perfusion pressure (CPP) and severe therapy-resistant vasospasm (Schneider et al. 1995). In a study including 25 patients with severe TBI, a total of 42 episodes of jugular bulb oxygen desaturation (<50% >10 min) were observed. The majority of incidences, 83%, occurred within 48 h following injury. Of the major associated secondary insults, hypocapnia was involved in 45% of the episodes, hypoperfusion in 22%, raised ICP in 9% and a combination of the above in 24% (Lewis et al. 1995).

43.2.10 $SjvO_2 \leq 50\%$ and Outcome

Episodes of desaturation among patients suffering from severe TBI (GCS ≤ 8) have a strong association to poor outcome (Robertson et al. 1995). Mortality rate 3 months post-trauma increased from 21% in the group of no incidence of desaturation to 37% if one episode of desaturation occurred and 69% if multiple episodes of desaturation occurred during the NICU stay (Robertson et al. 1995). In accordance, good recovery or moderate disability (GOS 4–5) was found with incidences of desaturation at 44%, 30% and 15%, respectively.

43.2.11 $SjvO_2 \geq 75\%$ and Outcome

In a study including 450 severely head-injured patients, increased mortality 6 months post-trauma was found among those presenting with $SjvO_2 > 75\%$ (Cormio et al. 1999). Patients with high SjvO due to O_2 extraction problems or regional ischemia was found to present with unfavourable outcome, while patients with high $SjvO_2$ due to excessive cerebral blood flow in relation to the metabolic demands, hyperaemia, had a favourable outcome (Cormio et al. 1999).

43.2.12 $AVD_{lactate}$

An arteriovenous difference in lactate exceeding 0.3 mmol/L, with the higher lactate in the jugular bulb, indicates ischemia as long as the peripheral serum level of lactate is <2.1 mmol/L (Artru et al. 2004).

43.3 Specific Paediatric Concerns

There are no specific paediatric concerns due to lack of specific paediatric data.

References

Artru F, Dailler F, Burel E, Bodonian C, Grousson S, Convert J, et al. Assessment of jugular blood oxygen and lactate indices for detection of cerebral ischemia and prognosis. J Neurosurg Anesthesiol. 2004;16:226–31.

Bratton SL, Chestnut RM, Ghajar J, McConnell Hammond FF, Harris OA, Hartl R, Manley GT, Nemecek A, Newell DW, Rosenthal G, Schouten J, Shutter L, Timmons SD, Ullman JS, Videtta W, Wilberger JE, Wright DW. Guidelines for the management of severe traumatic brain injury. J Neurotrauma. 2007;24:S65–70.

Busija DW, Leffler CW, Pourcyrous M. Hyperthermia increases cerebral metabolic rate and blood flow in neonatal pigs. Am J Phys. 1988;255:H343–6.

Carney N, et al. Guidelines for the management of severe traumatic brain injury, 4th edition. Neurosurgery. 2017;80(1):6–15.

Chan MT, Ng SC, Lam JM, Poon WS, Gin T. Re-defining the ischemic threshold for jugular venous oxygen saturation—a microdialysis study in patients with severe head injury. Acta Neurochir Suppl. 2005;95:63–6.

Chieregato A, Calzolari F, Trasforini G, Targa L, Latronico N. Normal jugular bulb oxygen saturation. J Neurol Neurosurg Psychiatry. 2003;74:784–6.

Cormio M, Robertson CS, Narayan RK. Secondary insults to the injured brain. J Clin Neurosci. 1997;4:132–48.

Cormio M, Valadka AB, Robertson CS. Elevated jugular venous oxygen saturation after severe head injury. J Neurosurg. 1999;90:9–15.

Cruz J. On-line monitoring of global cerebral hypoxia in acute brain injury. J Neurosurg. 1993;79:228–33.
Cruz J. The first decade of continuous monitoring of jugular bulb oxyhemoglobinsaturation: management strategies and clinical outcome. Crit Care Med. 1998;26(2):344–51.
Cruz J, Gennarelli TA, Hoffstad OJ. Lack of relevance of the Bohr effect in optimally ventilated patients with acute brain trauma. J Trauma. 1992;33:304–10.
Cruz J, Jaggi JL, Hoffstad OJ. Cerebral blood flow rate of oxygen consumption? Crit Care Med. 1993;21:1218–24.
Garlick R, Bihari D. The use of intermittent and continuous recordings of jugular venous bulb oxygen saturation in the unconscious patient. Scand J Clin Lab Invest Suppl. 1987;188:47–52.
Gibbs EL, Lennox WG, Nims LF, Gibbs FA. Arterial and cerebral venous blood: arterial-venous differences in man. J Biol Chem. 1942;144:325–32.
Gopinath SP, Robertson CS, Contant CF, Hayes C, Feldman Z, Narayan RK, et al. Jugular venous desaturation and outcome after head injury. J Neurol Neurosurg Psychiatry. 1994;57:717–23.
Henson LC, Calalang C, Temp JA, Ward DS. Accuracy of a cerebral oximeter in healthy volunteers under conditions of isocapnic hypoxia. Anesthesiology. 1998;88:58–65.
Jakobsen M, Enevoldsen E. Retrograde catheterization of the right internal jugular vein for serial measurements of cerebral venous oxygen content. J Cereb Blood Flow Metab. 1989;9:717–20.
Latronico NMD, Beindorf AEMD, Rasulo FAMD, Febbrari PMD, Stefini RMD, Cornali CMD, et al. Limits of intermittent jugular bulb oxygen saturation monitoring in the management of severe head trauma patients. Neurosurgery. 2000;46:1131–9.
Le Roux PD, et al. Cerebral arteriovenous oxygen difference: a predictor of cerebral infarction and outcome in patients with severe head injury. J Neurosurg. 1997;87(1):1–8.
Lewis SB, Myburgh JA, Reilly PL. Detection of cerebral venous desaturation by continuous jugular bulb oximetry following acute neurotrauma. Anaesth Intensive Care. 1995;23:307–14.
Matta BF, Lam AM. The rate of blood withdrawal affects the accuracy of jugular venous bulb. Oxygen saturation measurements. Anesthesiology. 1997;86:806–8.
Meldrum BS, Nilsson B. Cerebral blood flow and metabolic rate early and late in prolonged epileptic seizures induced in rats by bicuculline. Brain. 1976;99:523–42.
Pierce EC Jr, Lambertsen CJ, Deutsch S, Chase PE, Linde HW, Dripps RD, et al. Cerebral circulation and metabolism during thiopental anesthesia and hyperventilation in man. J Clin Invest. 1962;41:1664–71.
Robertson C. Desaturation episodes after severe head injury: influence on outcome. Acta Neurochir Suppl (Wien). 1993;59:98–101.
Robertson CS, Narayan RK, Gokaslan ZL, Pahwa R, Grossman RG, Caram P Jr, et al. Cerebral arteriovenous oxygen difference as an estimate of cerebral blood flow in comatose patients. J Neurosurg. 1989;70:222–30.
Robertson CS, Gopinath SP, Goodman JC, Contant CF, Valadka AB, Narayan RK. SjvO2 monitoring in head-injured patients. J Neurotrauma. 1995;12:891–6.
Schneider GH, von Helden A, Lanksch WR, Unterberg A. Continuous monitoring of jugular bulb oxygen saturation in comatose patients–therapeutic implications. Acta Neurochir. 1995;134:71–5.
Shenkin HA, Harmel MH, Kety SS. Dynamic anatomy of the cerebral circulation. Arch Neurol Psychiatr. 1948;60:240–52.
Vigue B, Ract C, Benayed M, Zlotine N, Leblanc PE, Samii K, et al. Early SjvO2 monitoring in patients with severe brain trauma. Intensive Care Med. 1999;25:445–51.
Woodman T, Robertson SC. Jugular venous oxygen saturation monitoring. In: Narayan RK, Wilberger Jr JE, Povlishock JT, editors. Neurotrauma. New York: McGraw-Hill; 1995. p. 519–53.

44 Cerebral Blood Flow (CBF) and Cerebral Metabolic Rate (CMR)

Peter Reinstrup, Eric L. Bloomfield, and Elham Rostami

Recommendations

Level I

There are insufficient data to support a Level I recommendation for this topic.

Level II

There are insufficient data to support a Level II recommendation for this topic.

Level III

Individualized treatment of traumatic brain injury (TBI) can be guided by cerebral blood flow (CBF) measurements.

P. Reinstrup (✉)
Department of Intensive and Perioperative Care, Skånes University Hospital, Lund, Sweden
e-mail: peter.reinstrup@med.lu.se

E. L. Bloomfield
Department of Anesthesiology, Mayo Clinic, Rochester, MN, USA
e-mail: bloomfield.eric@mayo.edu

E. Rostami
Department of Neurosurgery, Uppsala University Hospital, Uppsala, Sweden

Department of Neuroscience, Karolinska Institutet, Stockholm, Sweden
e-mail: Elham.rostami@neuro.uu.se

44.1 Overview

Over time, we have come to understand the concepts of cerebral blood flow and its relationship to pH changes and metabolism of the brain.

Current evidence from the research field of CNS injuries and pathologies tells us that insufficient cerebral blood flow can lead to ischaemic regions of the brain with poor clinical outcome. The challenge today is to find a non-invasive economical hands-on method to measure CBF continuously at bedside. With such techniques, one could hope to foster better outcome for patients with TBI. Many of the present methods still remain in the research realm; however, bedside Xenon-CT is currently a method which can be used on daily basis in the neurointensive care unit and fulfils some of the criteria mentioned above, but not all. Hopefully, the future will see new avenues for CBF measurements that will fill in the gap and give us continuous bedside CBF measurements.

Tips, Tricks and Pitfalls

- Measurement of CBF and CMR in TBI patients can give information about how to optimize the cerebral circulation.
- MR, CT and some of the SPECT techniques are not accurate in absolute blood

© Springer Nature Switzerland AG 2020
T. Sundstrøm et al. (eds.), *Management of Severe Traumatic Brain Injury*,
https://doi.org/10.1007/978-3-030-39383-0_44

flow values, but gives excellent information regarding the relative distribution.

- A crude estimation of the absolute blood flow can be obtained by comparing the relative CBF picture with the blood flow through the cerebellum. Cerebellum does under normal circumstances have a constant high flow.
- Appropriate safety measures must be taken to minimize radiation exposure to medical staff and patients. In handling ^{133}Xe, care should be taken to avoid direct contact with any part of the body. Our safety rules involve 0.6 rad/min of exposure time for the surgeon and less than 5 µrad/min exposure to surrounding personnel.
- Concerning information about ^{133}Xenon, the emitted photons from ^{133}Xenon are of low energy and can be absorbed by 0.1 mm of lead to reduce exposure by 90%. The physical half-life of ^{133}Xe is 5.27 days.

44.2 Background

44.2.1 Normal Brain

The brain weight is only 2% of body mass, but it receives 20% of the cardiac output. The reason for this is the high cerebral metabolic rate (CMR) that demands a constant delivery of oxygen and nutrients as well as removal of waste products such as CO_2. CMR changes with activity and during deep sleep and sedation; anaesthesia can reduce O_2 consumption down to 50% from the normal (3.3 mL O_2/100 g brain/min or 29 mmol glucose/100 g brain/min) (Reinstrup et al. 2008; Alkire et al. 1995, 1997; Madsen et al. 1991; Kaisti et al. 2002). Metabolism increases in areas with increased neuronal activity as in normal movement-thinking (Ingvar and Philipson 1977; Paradiso et al. 1999; Buxton 2002; Qiu et al. 2008). During pathological circumstances, as in epilepsy, O_2 metabolism can increase up to 200%. In these local areas with elevated metabolism, there will be a concomitant increase in the local CBF. Under normal circumstances, this coupling upholds the constant relationship between the CMR and CBF (Qiu et al. 2008; Buxton 2002). The CBF_{global} through the brain is determined by the CPP and the cerebrovascular resistance (CVR) with CBF = CPP/CVR. Within normal limits of mean arterial blood pressure - MAP - (60–150 mmHg), the CPP does not affect the CBF due to the cerebral auto-regulation (Fog 1938; Paulson et al. 1990).

CVR is under neuronal and chemical control. The reason for the increase in CBF during increased metabolism is mainly due to the increased CO_2 production lowering the perivascular pH (Kontos et al. 1977; Reinstrup et al. 1992). A relaxation of the cerebral arteries can also be attained due to the small extracellular potassium increase as a result of the neuronal membrane depolarization. The cerebral arteries also react to global changes in CO_2, with uniform changes in CBF such as during hyperventilation (Reinstrup et al. 1994), the normal response being 1–2 mL/100 g brain/mmHg change in $pACO_2$ or 7–10 mL/100 g brain/kPa change in $pACO_2$, depending on the measurement technique. The Kety and Schmidt (1948) technique, which investigates global CBF, describes a CO_2 response of 1 mL/100 g brain/min. Another investigation, looking at the response in the cortical grey substance, reports a CO_2 response of 1.8 mL/100 g brain/min (Messeter et al. 1986). Lowering the CO_2, as in hypocapnic hyperventilation, therefore results in a vasoconstriction with a lowering of the CBF. If the CMR and hence the CO_2 production is constant, such a lowering of the blood flow results in a gradual increase in the perivascular CO_2. The concomitant lowering of the perivascular pH may thus counteract the effect of the arterial hypocapnia, resulting in a reduced vasoconstrictive effect over time.

The neuronal tropic centres for metabolism are in the cell bodies situated in the grey substance of the brain. With the strict coupling between CMR and CBF (Buxton 2002; Qiu et al. 2008), local differences in CMR create a similar uneven, but geographically correlated distribution of the CBF (see Fig. 44.1).

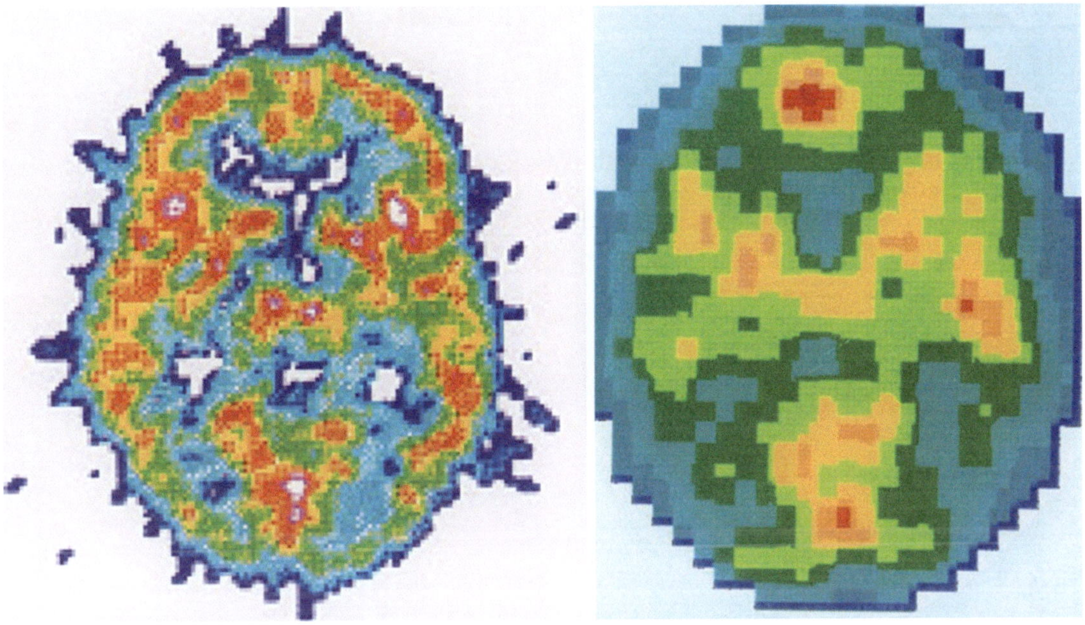

Fig. 44.1 A slice 2 cm above the orbitomeatal line representing the brain metabolism on the left and the corresponding CBF (right [133]Xenon SPECT). The $CMR_{glu\text{-}Global}$ was 27 mmol/100 g brain/min, and the CBF_{global} was 55 mL/100 g brain/min (The *left picture* (CMR-PET) has been published in *Br J Anaesthesiol.* The *right* (CBF-SPECT) has been published in *Anesthesiology*)

44.2.2 CMR and CBF

44.2.3 Traumatic Brain Injury

Traumatic brain injury (TBI) affects the cerebral circulation. The metabolic reactions to brain trauma fuel the production and liberation of a variety of biochemical substances, including vasoactive ones (Golding et al. 1999). This might be the reason for the change in CBF_{global} over time. Generally after a brain trauma, CMR_{global} is reduced up to 50%; the reduction on CMR seems to correlate to the severity of the brain trauma (Obrist et al. 1984). Not all, but many patients follow a specific pattern (Obrist et al. 1984). In the hyper-acute phase after the injury, CMR_{global} is low with a similar reduction as the CBF_{global}. After approximately 12 h, the hyperaemic phase starts, and CBF_{global} increases to normal awake values. If there is a low CMR, one could invoke relative hyperaemia. Three days after the trauma, the CBF_{global} is back to the same low level as in the immediate phase after the trauma, but now there may be signs of vasospasm in many patients (Martin et al. 1997). Besides this, auto-regulation (Enevoldsen and Jensen 1978; Jünger et al. 1997) and the CO_2 response (Obrist et al. 1984; Enevoldsen and Jensen 1978; Schalén et al. 1991) may be impaired, which can lead to hyperaemia. The 3D picture of CMR and, even more pronounced, the 3D CBF picture, do often show a patchy pattern due to local changes in metabolism and vasoactive substances (Fig. 44.2). In TBI patients, 3D investigations have indeed revealed that ischaemia occurs at a local level (Von Oettingen et al. 2002; Abate et al. 2008; Werner and Engelhard 2007; Bouma et al. 1992; Coles et al. 2004; Inoue et al. 2005), and that the presence of such ischaemia is associated with poor neurological outcome (Werner and Engelhard 2007; Bouma et al. 1992).

44.2.4 Measuring CBF

For many neurologic or neurosurgical patients, an ideal brain monitoring would be a non-invasive, continuous 3D measurement of cerebral blood

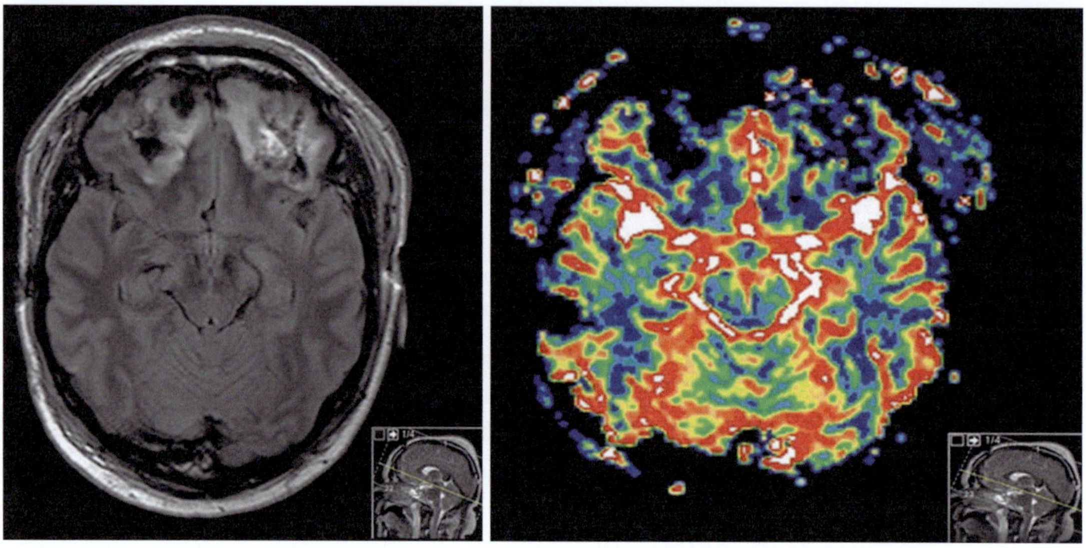

Fig. 44.2 A traumatic brain injury with frontal contusions seen on the MR FLAIR on the *left image*. On the *right image* is the corresponding CBF showing low perfusion in and adjacent to the frontal contusions

flow and metabolism in real time, but our present monitoring capacity is far from this situation. CBF measurements are still cumbersome and involve remedies limiting such investigations in daily usage. Prior to the Kety–Schmidt method, attempts to get information of the CBF were based on probes placed into the jugular vein to detect physiologic changes in cerebral blood flow. Over the years, a number of techniques have been utilized to measure blood flow in the arteries of the neck. The measurement of cerebral venous outflow can include heat clearance techniques in blood vessels and in brain tissue, hydrogen clearance, angiography, ultrasonography, diffusible and non-diffusible tracer-based measurements of cerebral flow, laser Doppler, positron emission tomography (PET), magnetic resonance imaging (MRI), and computerized tomography (CT). One has to be aware of the accuracy of the different techniques. Perfusion-weighted MRI, CT perfusion and stable Xenon-CT CBF are in principle based on the same technology and might under- or overestimate CBF values where PET CBF shows low or high values, respectively (Heiss and Sobesky 2008; Shinohara et al. 2010; Bergholt et al. 2000). Some of the important methods are briefly described below.

44.2.5 Measuring the Global CBF (CBF_{global}) (Kety-Schmidt)

The Fick principle is used to calculate blood flow through different organs where blood flow is equal to the quantity of a substance removed or added in time, divided by the difference between arterial and venous concentrations of the substance. This method for measuring organ blood flow was first applied to the brain in 1944 by C. F. Schmidt and S. S. Kety.

They used inhalation of a highly diffusible, inert gas (nitrous oxide (N_2O)) and frequent measurements of the arterial N_2O. To represent output of blood leaving the brain, N_2O concentration is measured in the jugular bulb. N_2O uptake in the brain per unit time is equal to the amount of N_2O brought to the brain by the arterial blood minus the amount carried away in the cerebral venous blood. Thus, at a time when the N_2O content of the brain and its cerebral venous blood reached equilibrium in approximately 10–15 min, the brain content of nitrous oxide and CBF could be estimated. Kety and Schmidt (1946) found that the CBF_{global} was 54 mL/100 g brain/min in young healthy males.

44.2.6 Measuring Global CMR (CMR_{global})

By combining the CBF measurements with arterial and jugular venous oxygen measurements, it was possible to calculate the CMRO by the following equation:

$CMRO = CBF \times (CaO_2 - CjvO_2)$

CaO_2 is the arterial content of O_2, and $CjvO_2$ is the O_2 content from the blood leaving the brain at the jugular bulb.

The arterial or venous content of O_2 (C_xO_2) is dependent on the O_2 amount dissolved in plasma and the O_2 bound to haemoglobin. Since PaO_2 reflects only free oxygen molecules dissolved in plasma and not those bound to haemoglobin, PaO_2 alone does not give the C_xO_2 in the blood; for that, you need also to know how much oxygen is bound to haemoglobin. The SaO_2 and haemoglobin give this. Many factors influence on these amounts, but in general:

$C_xO_2/100\,mL = O_{2\,-\,plasma} + O_{2\,-\,haemoglobin} = (K_{plasma} \times pO_2) + (Hb \times K_{haemoglobin} \times SO_2)$

- If pO_2 is in mmHg, $K_{plasma} = 0.003$.
- If pO_2 is in kPa, $K_{plasma} = 0.023$.
- If Hb is in g/100 mL, $K_{haemoglobin} = 1.36$.
- If Hb is in mmol/l, $K_{haemoglobin} = 2.18$.

44.2.7 Alternative Methods to Measure CBF_{global}

44.2.7.1 Double-Indicator Dilution Technique

The transcerebral double-indicator dilution technique is a rather new method to measure CBF_{global}.

It is based on bolus injection of ice-cold indocyanine green dye with a simultaneous recording of thermo- and dye-dilution curves in the aorta and the jugular bulb using combined fibre-optic thermistor catheters. CBF was calculated from the mean transit times of the dye and thermal indicator through the brain. However, the authors conclude that, as of yet, the accuracy and resolution of this technique is not high enough to detect the effect of minor changes of physiological variables (Mielck et al. 2004). This method has been compared with Xenon-CT and showed a high failure rate with consistent overestimation of perfusion compared to Xenon-CT (Schutt et al. 2001).

44.2.8 Ultrasound

This method is a simple technique performing Doppler ultrasound examination of the extracranial arteries in the neck. Several articles describe flow and flow volume measurements in the internal carotid artery and vertebral artery (Scheel et al. 2000; Albayrak et al. 2007; Yazici et al. 2005). The examination is performed in supine position with the head slightly to the opposite side. The vessel lumen diameter is measured at systole, and the cross-sectional area of each vessel is calculated. Angle-corrected blood flow velocity is measured with the pulsed Doppler and sample volume expanded to encompass the entire vessel diameter (Fig. 44.3). The volume of blood flow in each artery is calculated as time-averaged maximum flow velocity and multiplied with the area. In theory it is a simple technique, though not in practice; it has never been evaluated against the classic standard techniques previously described.

44.2.9 Local–Regional CBF

Kety proceeded in his laboratory and developed techniques to present local CBF in animals by inhalation of a diffusible radioactive gas (trifluoroiodomethane). Kety could obtain post mortem slices of the brain showing relative CBF in different brain regions, and this is in fact the beginning of the later 3D CMR–CBF visualizations.

In 1961, Lassen and Ingvar (1961) introduced the intra-carotid ^{85}Krypton method introducing radioisotopes into CBF measurements in vivo. By rapid injection of this radioactive ß-emitter and multiple (Geiger–Müller) ionization detec-

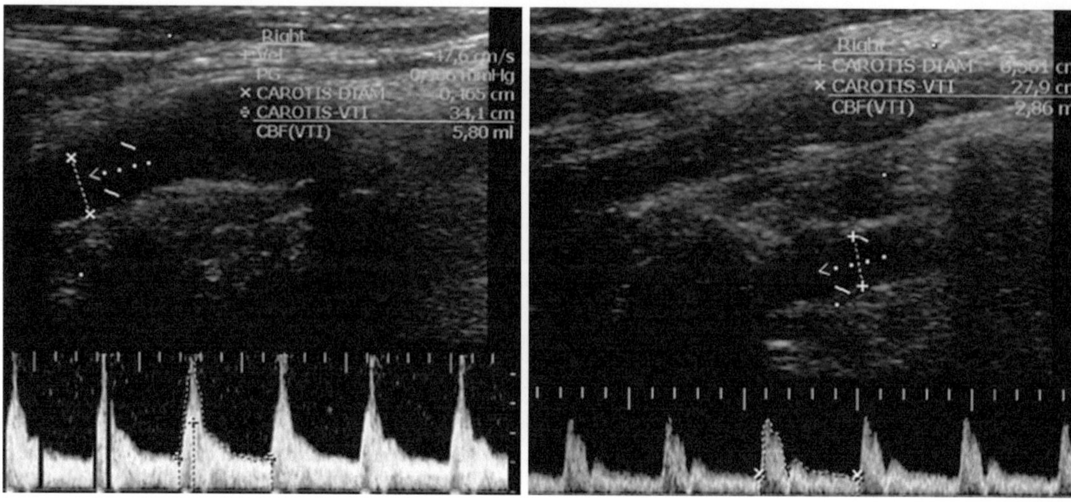

Fig. 44.3 Measurement of CBF with ultrasound at the neck. *Left picture* is measurement in the internal carotid artery, and *right* is the vertebral artery (even though the text in the picture states it should be carotid artery). The vertebral artery is found in between two vertebras that can be seen as *dark shadows* on each side

tors placed directly on the brain surface, they were able to look at regional CBF in animals. The washout curves of ^{85}Krypton recorded on the different detectors were predominantly influenced by the CBF in the tissue closest to the detectors. In order to penetrate the skull bone, Harper et al. (1964) substituted ^{85}Krypton for ^{133}Xenon and started to use collimators for a higher resolution. Mallett and Veall (1963) started with the inhalation of ^{133}Xenon, thereby making the method less invasive. Obrist (Obrist et al. 1975) applied the Kety–Schmidt equations so that intravenously injected ^{133}Xenon became a clinical method for investigating CBF and CMR. These methods gave excellent information of the cortical structures, but there is no information of deeper structures warranting 3D systems.

44.2.10 Thermal Diffusion Flow Probes

This is an invasive procedure that measures flow by estimating the temperature gradient between two plates on the surface of the brain. It measures the blood flow only in the one area of cortex underlying it. The technique yields continuous values and has been used intraoperatively. The microprobe provides a sensitive, continuous and real-time assessment of intraparenchymal regional cerebral blood flow (rCBF) in absolute flow values that is in good agreement with sXe-rCBF measurements (Vajkoczy et al. 2000). However, it can yield false estimations if it is even slightly displaced.

44.2.10.1 3D Brain Investigations

Positron emission tomography (PET) and single-photon emission computed tomography (SPECT). In PET, the radioisotope decay creates emission of positrons resulting in production of gamma photons moving in opposite directions. This fact makes it possible to pinpoint the exact location of the decay of the radioisotope. In SPECT, the tracer emits gamma rays making it more difficult to determine its exact origin, and the spatial resolution is therefore much better with PET. This can be seen in the figure above (see Fig. 44.1). The left picture being a CMR-PET study and the right a CBF-SPECT study presenting slices through the same brain areas. The basic technique requires injection of a radioisotope (radionuclide) where individual differences in binding sites and attachments allow for investigations of different brain structures and brain functions. The foundation of these techniques is based on the detection of radioisotopes emitted by an emission-computed tomography. A computer calculates the three dimensions of the isotope distribution, which allows for imaging of the investigated volume into thin slices. In modern scanners, the correlation to brain structures is often accomplished with the aid of a CT X-ray scan performed on the patient during the same session.

The concept of emission tomography was started in the late 1950s, and clinically useful apparatus came in the 1970s and 1980s. The scanners are based on the placement of multiple scintillation detectors in a ring around the head.

44.2.11 Stable Xenon-CT

Development of the stable Xenon-CT method came shortly after the introduction of the CT in the mid-1970s. Xenon, with its high atomic number, attenuates X-rays, and thus in the CT scan, one can directly measure its concentration in the brain. Determination of the outflow or venous concentration is therefore not required when utilizing the Fick principle. The input or arterial concentration was established by Kelcz et al. (1978), determining the solubility of xenon in tissue and blood; this was the basis for converting end-tidal xenon values to arterial concentrations. The concentration of xenon in arterial blood could therefore be determined from end-tidal xenon measured by a thermo-conductivity analyser. Now, by measuring the concentration of xenon in the blood and brain and the time for which xenon has been administered and knowing the blood–brain partition coefficient for xenon, the CBF can be calculated, using a modified Kety–Schmidt formula for xenon.

Xenon in high concentrations is an anaesthetic, and in the beginning, it was necessary to inhale it in such high concentrations, but the improvements in CT scan technology in combination with the modern computer capabilities have made the process of Xe/CBF more user-friendly. The risks of side effects are very low using Xenon-CT, and no permanent morbidity or sequela has been detected (Carlson et al. 2011). The Xe/CBF measurement can be repeated after an interval of 20 min, making it useful for investigating also autoregulation and CO_2 response. Xenon-CT is fast and provides quantitative measurements of CBF. The big advantage is that by using a mobile CT scanner, CBF can be measured at bedside with no need of transport of the patient to a different setting. The connection to a CT scan also provides a CBF map coupled to the anatomical location. Currently bedside Xenon-CT emerges as an economical and more accessible imaging technique with few adverse effects that can be used in the routine NICU to measure CBF following TBI (Rostami et al. 2014). However, it provides a snapshot of CBF with low resolution compared to PET. Xenon-CT has been combined with cerebral microdialysis showing association between loss of CO_2 reactivity with increased ICP and increased lactate, glutamate and glycerol and a fatal outcome (Doppenberg et al. 1999). Combining with brain tissue pO2, Valadka et al. showed a linear relationship between $pbrO_2$ and CBF (Valadka et al. 2002). It has also been compared to PET (Bergholt et al. 2000). Xe-CT/CBF showed greater differences between high and low flow areas than PET CBF. Correlation was found within subjects between ROIs, but no agreement or correlation between the methods could be demonstrated.

44.2.12 CT Perfusion

CT perfusion was first described by Axel (1980, 1983), but it has taken many years to develop the technique to be used in clinical practice. To obtain information about cerebral blood flow with the CT, an amount of intravenous contrast medium is injected. The CT scanning and contrast injection is started simultaneously. The CT scanner runs the same slices over and over again, while the contrast medium passes the brain. The examination is based on the indicator dilution theory. Following administration of the intravenous bolus of contrast medium, the X-ray density of the vessels and brain temporarily increases. In basic terms, the method is based on the determination of the speed by which the blood is traversing the brain or in other words, the mean transit time (MTT) as well as the cerebral blood volume (CBV). Conclusions about these parameters are drawn from the extent and course over time of the increase in density due to the contrast medium over time. These estimations require the use of software-employing complex deconvolution algorithms, but when the MTT and CBF is found, the CBF = CBV/MTT (Hoeffner et al. 2004). Some controversies exist concerning the accuracy of the quantitative results and their reproducibility. Despite this, many clinics use CT perfusion in evaluating their neurological patients as it is the most convenient method, and some correlation to the PET methodology has been found (Shinohara et al. 2010).

44.2.13 MR Perfusion

The way of measuring CBF with MR is essentially the same as the CT perfusion method. The use of dynamic susceptibility contrast magnetic resonance imaging (DSC-MRI) for assessment of perfusion-related parameters is promising (Wirestam et al. 2009), but the concept is hampered by a number of methodological complications. For example, an accurate registration of the arterial input function, i.e. the concentration versus time curve in an appropriate tissue-feeding artery, is interfered by different factors (Østergaard et al. 1996; Wirestam et al. 2009). Attempts to achieve absolute quantification of perfusion parameters by standard DSC-MRI have typically been characterized by overestimated values of CBV and CBF (Knutsson et al. 2007; Wirestam et al. 2009), which is due to a correspondingly underestimated arterial concentration time integral. Hence, the majority of existing implementations of DSC-MRI provide only relative perfusion values (Kaneko et al. 2004), even though it clearly reflects absolute changes due to CO_2 variations (Wirestam et al. 2009).

In 1992, Williams et al. (1992) found an alternative to the above method using contrast, called arterial spin labelling. Arterial spin labelling uses magnetically labelled water protons as an endogenous tracer. The overall goal of all-existing arterial spin labelling is to produce a flow-sensitized image or 'labelled' image and a 'control' image, in which the static tissue signals are identical. At the same time, one has to see that the magnetization of the inflowing blood differs. Despite the remarkable progress in this technique, arterial spin labelling has still not replaced traditional invasive methods (Petersen et al. 2006).

44.2.14 MR and CBF_{global}

There are four arteries (carotids and vertebrals) that supply blood to the brain. With a flow-sensitive slice just under the skull base, the sum of these flows represents the global CBF. Phase-contrast MRI applying a brief magnetic field gradient in the direction of flow and the phase shift in the magnetization created by the flowing material, can provide such information. The phase shift is proportional to the flow velocity given in pixels, and the flow velocity curve over the cardiac cycle provides the flow (Enzmann et al. 1994). The technique has a maximum error below 10% (Bryant et al. 1984; Marks et al. 1992). So far, there is no correlation study comparing it to conventional CBF methods, but the global CBF findings with the technique (Marks et al. 1992; Spilt et al. 2002; Zarrinkoob et al. 2015; Unnerbäck et al. 2019a, b) are in accordance to the normal CBF range (50–60 mL/100 g/min) when the global MR-CBF findings are divided with the approximate brain weight.

44.2.15 CBF from the ICP Curve (CBF_{ICP})

Mosso (1881) found stronger brain pulsations during brain stimulation as a sign of increased CBF. In 1953 Ryder presented the commencement of the correlation between change in volume and ICP opening up for the pressure–volume relationship (Ryder et al. 1953). A lot of efforts has been made to find the ICP–CBF correlation. The first real correlations were made by Hu et al. (2010) looking at the ICP curve morphology, where different ICP appearances correlate to low

CBF, as measured with a traditional ^{133}Xenon CBF method. One reason is that the area under the pulsatile part of the ICP curve represents only the pulsatile part of the CBF, while traditional CBF measurements provide the total CBF value in mL/100 g/min. The first correlation between the pulsatile ICP and the pulsatile CBF was found by Unnerbäck et al. (2019a, b), using the MR-CBF described above (Sect. 44.2.14), where the CBF can be divided into a pulsatile and non-pulsatile part. Unnerbäck et al. (2019a, b) converted the ICP curve into a volume curve using a compliance–elastance measurement, and this converted curve correlated by 68% to the pulsatile CBF (R^2 = 0.68). This correlation can be improved and even include the non-pulsatile part by creating a mathematical model to translate the ICP curve morphology into the different flows (Unnerbäck et al. 2019a, b).

44.3 Specific Paediatric Concerns

At birth, cortical rCBFs are lower than in adults. CBF increases and reaches a maximum at the fifth year of 50–85% higher than those for adults and thereafter decreased, reaching adult levels after 15 years. The time needed to reach normal adult values differed for each cortical region. The shortest time was found for the primary cortex and, the longest, for the associative cortex. Cognitive development of the child seems to be related to changes in blood flow of the corresponding brain regions (Chiron et al. 1992). There is only one report on CBF measurement in severe TBI using Xenon-CT (Adelson et al. 1997) and a few others that report on mild TBI using advanced arterial spin labelling (ASL) MRI.

References

Abate MG, Trivedi M, Fryer TD, Smielewski P, Chatfield DA, Williams GB, Aigbirhio F, Carpenter TA, Pickard JD, Menon DK, Coles JP. Early derangements in oxygen and glucose metabolism following head injury: the ischemic penumbra and pathophysiological heterogeneity. Neurocrit Care. 2008;9:319–25.

Adelson PD, Clyde B, Kochanek PM, Wisniewski SR, Marion DW, Yonas H. Cerebrovascular response in infants and young children following severe traumatic brain injury: a preliminary report. Pediatr Neurosurg. 1997;26(4):200–7.

Albayrak R, Degirmenci B, Acar M, Haktanır A, Colbay M, Yaman M. Doppler sonography evaluation of flow velocity and volume of the extracranial internal carotid and vertebral arteries in healthy adults. J Clin Ultrasound. 2007;35:27–33.

Alkire MT, Haier RJ, Barker SJ, Shah NK, Wu JC, Kao YJ. Cerebral metabolism during propofol anesthesia in humans studied with positron emission tomography. Anesthesiology. 1995;82:393–403.

Alkire MT, Haier RJ, Shah NK, Anderson CT. Positron emission tomography study of regional cerebral metabolism in humans during isoflurane anesthesia. Anesthesiology. 1997;86:549–57.

Axel L. Cerebral blood flow determination by rapid-sequence computed tomography. Radiology. 1980;137:679–86.

Axel L. Tissue mean transit time from dynamic computed tomography by a simple deconvolution technique. Invest Radiol. 1983;18:94–9.

Bergholt B, Ostergaard L, von Oettingen G, Johannsen P, Poulsen PH, Bundgaard H, et al. Cerebral blood flow in volunteers measured by PET and Xe CT/CBF. A comparison. Keio J Med. 2000;49(Suppl 1):A55–7.

Bouma GJ, Muizelaar JP, Stringer WA, Choi C, Fatouros P, Young HF. Ultra-early evaluation of regional cerebral blood flow in severely head-injured patients using xenon-enhanced computerized tomography. J Neurosurg. 1992;77:360–8.

Bryant DJ, Payne JA, Firmin DN, Longmore DB. Measurement of flow with NMR imaging using a gradient pulse and phase difference technique. J Comput Assist Tomogr. 1984;8:588–93.

Buxton RB. Coupling between CBF and CMRO2 during neuronal activity. Int Congr Ser. 2002;1235:23–32.

Carlson AP, Brown AM, Zager E, Uchino K, Marks MP, Robertson C, et al. Xenon-enhanced cerebral blood flow at 28% xenon provides uniquely safe access to quantitative, clinically useful cerebral blood flow information: a multicenter study. AJNR Am J Neuroradiol. 2011;32(7):1315–20.

Chiron C, Raynaud C, Maziere B, Zilbovicius M, Laflamme L, Masure MC, Dulac O, Bourguignon M, Syrota A. Changes in regional cerebral blood flow during brain maturation in children and adolescents. J Nucl Med. 1992;33:696–703.

Coles JP, Fryer TD, Smielewski P, et al. Defining ischemic burden after traumatic brain injury using 15O PET imaging of cerebral physiology. J Cereb Blood Flow Metab. 2004;24:191–201.

Doppenberg EM, Reinert M, Zauner A, Massie TS, Bullock R. Determinants of cerebral extracellular potassium after severe human head injury. Acta Neurochir Suppl. 1999;75:31–4.

Enevoldsen EM, Jensen FT. Autoregulation and CO2 responses of cerebral blood flow in patients with acute severe head injury. J Neurosurg. 1978;48(5):689–703.

Enzmann DR, Ross MR, Marks MP, Pelc NJ. Blood flow in major cerebral arteries measured by phase-contrast cine MR. Am J Neuroradiol. 1994;15:123–9.

Fog M. The relationship between the blood pressure and the tonic regulation of the pial arteries. J Neurol Psychiatry. 1938;1:187–97.

Golding EM, Robertson CS, Bryan RM Jr. The consequences of traumatic brain injury on cerebral blood flow and autoregulation: a review. Clin Exp Hypertens. 1999;21(4):299–332.

Harper AM, Glass HI, Steven JL, Granat AH. The measurement of local blood flow in the cerebral cortex from the clearance of xenon. J Neurol Neurosurg Psychiatry. 1964;27:255.

Heiss WD, Sobesky J. Comparison of PET and DW/PW-MRI in acute ischemic stroke. Keio J Med. 2008;57(3):125–31.

Hoeffner EG, Case I, Jain R, Gujar SK, Shah GV, Deveikis JP, Carlos RC, Thompson BG, Harrigan MR, Mukherji SK. Cerebral perfusion CT: technique and clinical applications. Radiology. 2004;231(3):632–44, Epub 2004 Apr 29.

Hu X, Glenn T, Scalzo F, Bergsneider M, Sarkiss C, Martin N, et al. Intracranial pressure pulse morphological features improved detection of decreased cerebral blood flow. Physiol Meas. 2010;31:679–95.

Ingvar DH, Philipson L. Distribution of cerebral blood flow in the dominant hemisphere during motor ideation and motor performance. Ann Neurol. 1977;2:230–7.

Inoue Y, Shiozaki T, Tasaki O, et al. Changes in cerebral blood flow from the acute to the chronic phase of severe head injury. J Neurotrauma. 2005;22:1411–8.

Jünger EC, Newell DW, Grant GA, Avellino AM, Ghatan S, Douville CM, Lam AM, Aaslid R, Winn HR. Cerebral autoregulation following minor head injury. J Neurosurg. 1997;86:425–32.

Kaisti KK, Metsähonkala L, Teräs M, Oikonen V, Aalto S, Jääskeläinen S, Hinkka S, Scheinin H. Effects of surgical levels of propofol and sevoflurane anesthesia on cerebral blood flow in healthy subjects studied with positron emission tomography. Anesthesiology. 2002;96(6):1358–70.

Kaneko K, Kuwabara Y, Mihara F, Yoshiura T, Nakagawa M, Tanaka A, Sasaki M, Koga H, Hayashi K, Honda H. Validation of the CBF, CBV, and MTT values by perfusion MRI in chronic occlusive cerebrovascular disease: a comparison with 15O-PET. Acad Radiol. 2004;11(5):489–97.

Kelcz F, Hilal SK, Hartwell P, Joseph PM. Computed tomography measurement of the xenon brain–blood partition coefficient and implications for the regional cerebral blood flow: a preliminary report. Radiology. 1978;127:358–92.

Kety SS, Schmidt CF. Measurement of cerebral blood flow and cerebral oxygen consumption in man. Fed Proc. 1946;5:264.

Kety SS, Schmidt CF. The effect of altered arterial tension of carbon dioxide and oxygen on cerebral oxygen consumption of normal young men. J Clin Invest. 1948;27:484–92.

Knutsson L, Börjesson S, Larsson EM, Risberg J, Gustafson L, Passant U, Ståhlberg F, Wirestam R. Absolute quantification of cerebral blood flow in normal volunteers: correlation between Xe-133 SPECT and dynamic susceptibility contrast MRI. J Magn Reson Imaging. 2007;26:913–20.

Kontos HA, Wei EP, Jarrel Raper A, Patterson JL. Local mechanism of CO2 action on cat pial arterioles. Stroke. 1977;8:226–9.

Lassen NA, Ingvar DH. The blood flow of the cerebral cortex determined by radioactive krypton. Experientia. 1961;17:42–3.

Madsen PL, Schmidt JF, Wildschiødtz G, Friberg L, Holm S, Vorstrup S, Lassen NA. Cerebral O2 metabolism and cerebral blood flow in humans during deep and rapid-eye-movement sleep. J Appl Physiol. 1991;70(6):2597–601.

Mallett BL, Veall N. Investigation of cerebral blood-flow in hypertension, using radioactive-xenon inhalation and extracranial recording. Lancet. 1963;1(7290):1081–2.

Marks MP, Pelc NJ, Ross MR, Enzmann DR. Determination of cerebral blood flow with a phase-contrast cine MR imaging technique: evaluation of normal subjects and patients with arteriovenous malformations. Radiology. 1992;182:467–76.

Martin NA, Patwardhan RV, Alexander MJ, Africk CZ, Lee JH, Shalmon E, Hovda DA, Becker DP. Characterization of cerebral hemodynamic phases fol- lowing severe head trauma: hypoperfusion, hyperemia, and vasospasm. J Neurosurg. 1997;87(1):9–19.

Messeter K, Nordström CH, Sundbärg G, Algotsson L, Ryding E. Cerebral hemodynamics in patients with acute severe head trauma. J Neurosurg. 1986;64(2):231–7.

Mielck F, Bräuer A, Radke O, Hanekop G, Loesch S, Friedrich M, Hilgers R, Sonntag H. Changes of jugular venous blood temperature associated with measurements of cerebral blood flow using the transcerebral double-indicator dilution technique. Eur J Anaesthesiol. 2004;21(4):289–95.

Mosso A. Ueber den Kreislauf des Blutes im menschlichen Gehirn. Leipzig: Verlag von Veit; 1881.

Obrist WD, Thompson HK, Wang HS, Wilkinson WE. Regional cerebral blood flow estimated by 133Xenon inhalation. Stroke. 1975;6:245–56.

Obrist WD, Langfitt TW, Jaggi JL, Cruz J, Gennarelli TA. Cerebral blood flow and metabolism in comatose patients with acute head injury. J Neurosurg. 1984;61:241–53.

Østergaard L, Weisskoff RM, Chesler DA, Gyldensted C, Rosen BR. High resolution measurement of cerebral blood flow using intravascular tracer bolus passages. Part I: mathematical approach and statistical analysis. Magn Reson Med. 1996;36:715–25.

Paradiso S, Johnson DL, Andreasen NC, O'Leary DS, Watkins GL, Boles Ponto LL, Hichwa RD. Cerebral blood flow changes associated with attribution of emotional valence to pleasant, unpleasant, and neutral visual stimuli in a PET study of normal subjects. Am J Psychiatry. 1999;156:1618–29.

Paulson OB, Strandgaard S, Edvinsson L. Cerebral autoregulation. Cerebrovasc Brain Metab Rev. 1990;2(2):161–92.

Petersen ET, Zimine I, Ho Y-CL, Golay X. Non-invasive measurement of perfusion: a critical review of arterial spin labelling techniques. Br J Radiol. 2006;79:688–701.

Qiu M, Ramani R, Swetye M, Rajeevan N, Constable RT. Anesthetic effects on regional CBF, BOLD, and the coupling between task-induced changes in CBF and BOLD: an fMRI study in normal human subjects. Magn Rcson Mcd. 2008;60(4):987–96.

Reinstrup P, Uski T, Messeter K. Modulation by carbon dioxide and pH of the contractile response to potassium and prostaglandin F2α in isolated pial arteries. Br J Anaesth. 1992;69:615–20.

Reinstrup P, Ryding E, Algotsson L, Berntman L, Uski T. Effects of nitrous oxide on human regional cerebral blood flow and isolated pial arteries. Anesthesiology. 1994;81(2):396–402.

Reinstrup P, Ryding E, Ohlsson T, Sandell A, Erlandsson K, Ljunggren K, Salford LG, Strand S, Uski T. Regional cerebral metabolic rate (positron emission tomography) during inhalation of nitrous oxide 50% in humans. Br J Anaesth. 2008;100(1):66–71, Epub 2007 Nov 23.

Rostami E, Engquist H, Johnson U, Howells T, Ronne-Engstrom E, Nilsson P, et al. Monitoring of cerebral blood flow and metabolism bedside in patients with subarachnoid hemorrhage—a Xenon-CT and microdialysis study. Front Neurol. 2014;5:89.

Ryder HW, Espey FF, Kimbell FD, Penka EJ, Rosenauer A, Podolsky B, et al. The mechanism of the change in cerebrospinal fluid pressure following an induced change in the volume of the fluid space. J Lab Clin Med. 1953;41:428–35.

Schalén W, Messeter K, Nordström CH. Cerebral vasoreactivity and the prediction of outcome in severe traumatic brain lesions. Acta Anaesthesiol Scand. 1991;35(2):113–22.

Scheel P, Ruge C, Schoning M. Flow velocity and flow volume measurements in the extracranial carotid and vertebral arteries in healthy adults: reference data and the effects of age. Ultrasound Med Biol. 2000;26:1261–6.

Schutt S, Horn P, Roth H, Quintel M, Schilling L, Schmiedek P, et al. Bedside monitoring of cerebral blood flow by transcranial thermo-dye-dilution technique in patients suffering from severe traumatic brain injury or subarachnoid hemorrhage. J Neurotrauma. 2001;18(6):595–605.

Shinohara Y, Ibaraki M, Ohmura T, Sugawara S, Toyoshima H, Nakamura K, Kinoshita F, Kinoshita T. Whole-brain perfusion measurement using 320-detector row computed tomography in patients with cerebrovascular steno-occlusive disease: comparison with 15O-positron emission tomography. J Comput Assist Tomogr. 2010;34(6):830–5.

Spilt A, Box FM, van der Geest RJ, et al. Reproducibility of total cerebral blood flow measurements using phase contrast magnetic resonance imaging. J Magn Reson Imaging. 2002;16:1–5.

Unnerbäck M, Bloomfield EL, Söderström S, Reinstrup P. The intracranial pressure curve correlates to the pulsatile component of cerebral blood flow. J Clin Monit Comput. 2019a;33(1):77–83.

Unnerbäck M, Ottesen J, Reinstrup P (2019b) Validation of a mathematical model for understanding the intracranial pressure curve morphology. J Clin Monit Comput. Submitted.

Vajkoczy P, Roth H, Horn P, Lucke T, Thomé C, Hubner U, Martin GT, Zappletal C, Klar E, Schilling L, Schmiedek P. Continuous monitoring of regional cerebral blood flow: experimental and clinical validation of a novel thermal diffusion microprobe. J Neurosurg. 2000;93:265–74.

Valadka AB, Hlatky R, Furuya Y, Robertson CS. Brain tissue PO2: correlation with cerebral blood flow. Acta Neurochir Suppl. 2002;81:299–301.

Von Oettingen G, Bergholt B, Gyldensted C, Astrup J. Blood flow and ischemia within traumatic cerebral contusions. Neurosurgery. 2002;50(4):781–8.

Werner C, Engelhard K. Pathophysiology of traumatic brain injury. Br J Anaesth. 2007;99:4–9.

Williams DS, Detre JA, Leigh JS, Koretsky AP. Magnetic resonance imaging of perfusion using spin inversion of arterial water. Proc Natl Acad Sci U S A. 1992;89:212–6.

Wirestam R, Engvall C, Ryding E, Holtås S, Ståhlberg F, Reinstrup P. Change in cerebral perfusion detected by dynamic susceptibility contrast magnetic resonance imaging: normal volunteers examined during normal breathing and hyperventilation. J Biomed Sci Eng. 2009;2:210–5.

Yazici B, Erdoğmuş B, Tugay A. Cerebral blood flow measurements of the extracranial carotid and vertebral arteries with Doppler ultrasonography in healthy adults. Diagn Interv Radiol. 2005;11:195–8.

Zarrinkoob L, Ambarki K, Wahlin A, Birgander R, Eklund A, Malm J. Blood flow distribution in cerebral arteries. J Cereb Blood Flow Metab. 2015;35:648–54.

45 Transcranial Doppler (TCD)

Peter Reinstrup and Jan Frennström

Recommendations

Level I

There are insufficient data to support a Level I recommendation for this topic.

Level II

There are insufficient data to support a Level II recommendation for this topic.

Level III

TCD is useful for the detection of vasospasm and cerebral haemodynamic impairment following spontaneous and traumatic subarachnoid haemorrhage. TCD gives an indication as to whether the ICP is normal or high.

45.1 Overview

By using a 1–2 MHz pulsed transcranial Doppler (TCD), it is possible to penetrate the skull bone at special sites (windows) and register the flow velocity (FV) in the insonated artery at well-defined depths. In this way, the FV can be registered in the central arteries as well as in some of the veins. As a rule, a normal FV in an artery indicates an adequate circulation to the territory it supplies. High and low FV does not necessarily have correlations to the CBF, since the diameter of the measured vessel is unknown. If the FV is high, a differentiation between hyperaemia and vasospasm can be obtained by performing a Lindegaard index (LI), which is the correlation between the FV in the middle cerebral artery and the internal carotid artery.

The shape of the FV curve can in addition give an indication of increased intracranial pressure.

> **Tips, Tricks and Pitfalls**
> - For a TCD investigation, it is best to stand on the patient's right side. Let the left wrist rest on the patient's forehead and insonate the MCA through the posterior temporal window. By this approach, you will have your right hand free to adjust the equipment.
> - The normally high CBF is to a great extent due to a low mean resistance in the cerebral circulation. This is reflected as a high FV during diastole as compared to noncerebral arteries of similar size (Fig. 45.1).
> - Start insonating the middle cerebral artery at a depth of 50 mm, and proceed

P. Reinstrup (✉)
Department of Intensive and Perioperative Care, Skånes University Hospital, Lund, Sweden
e-mail: peter.reinstrup@med.lu.se

J. Frennström
Department of Neurosurgery, Skåne University Hospital, Lund, Sweden

© Springer Nature Switzerland AG 2020
T. Sundstrøm et al. (eds.), *Management of Severe Traumatic Brain Injury*,
https://doi.org/10.1007/978-3-030-39383-0_45

inwards until you find a flow which moves away from the probe at which point you have reached the anterior communicating artery (ACA). This finding strengthens that it is the MCA. Then follow the vessel out again, and register the highest FV value.

45.2 Background

Ultrasound is sound waves with frequencies greater than the upper limit of the human hearing, i.e. above 20 kHz. Within medicine, ultrasound has been utilized during the last 50 years to penetrate into the human body measuring the reflections that can be used for the imaging of soft tissues in the body. Superficial structures are visualized at frequencies ranging from 7 to 18 MHz, but in order to penetrate into deeper structures such as the liver or the kidneys, the frequency has to be lowered down to between 1 and 6 MHz.

Unfortunately, the lower the frequency you use, the lower resolution of the picture you get. Also, the higher the density of a tissue, the less the penetration of the sound wave, and the mature skull bone is indeed obstructing ultrasound to penetrate freely into the brain. After the age of 1 year, it is already impossible to identify individual structures within the brain with this technique. However, in a brain-traumatized patient upon whom a craniectomy has been performed, there is an artificial window through which it is possible to investigate the brain rather than using a CT scan. On youngsters, the fontanel can be utilized in a similar manner for improved resolution (Fig. 45.2).

There are many advantages of utilizing TCD. It is non-invasive and inexpensive, can be performed bedside, is easily repeated and can be used for continuous monitoring. TCD ultrasound was introduced in 1982 by Aaslid et al. (1982). A Doppler ultrasound beam of 2 MHz produced from a piezoelectric crystal is bounced back from the erythrocytes in an individual artery. The ultrasound examination of a blood vessel by these means is referred as to insonate the vessel. The TCD probe is placed over different 'acoustic windows', i.e. specific areas of the skull where the bone layer is thin, or through the foramen magnum. In order to help the investigator to insonate the artery, the signal is presented as a sound through a loudspeaker as well. The reflected signal is received by the transducer and converted to an electric

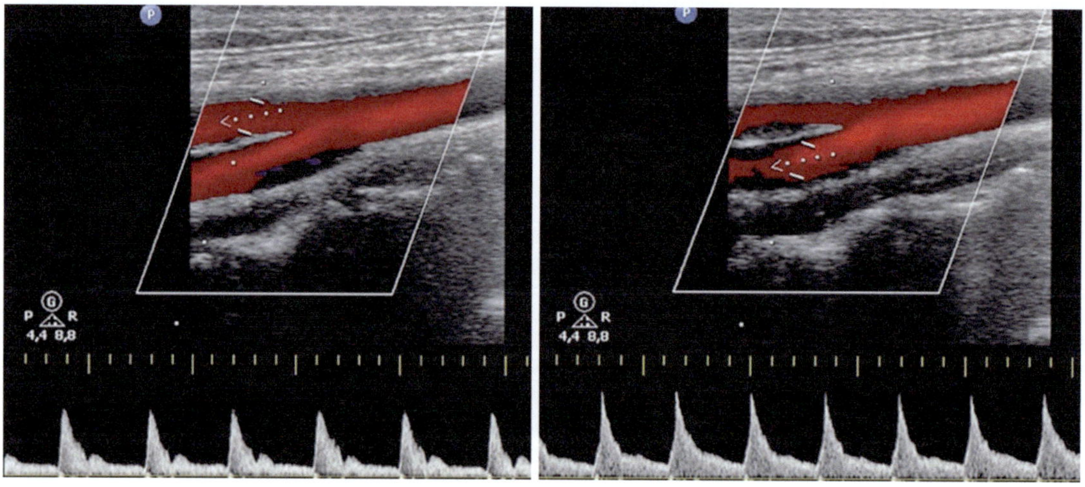

Fig. 45.1 Pictures of the carotid arteries in the neck. The common carotid artery is seen to the *right* in both pictures, and the FV curves at the *bottom*. The *left curve* shows the FV in the external carotid artery (ECA), whereas the internal carotid artery (ICA) is on the *right*

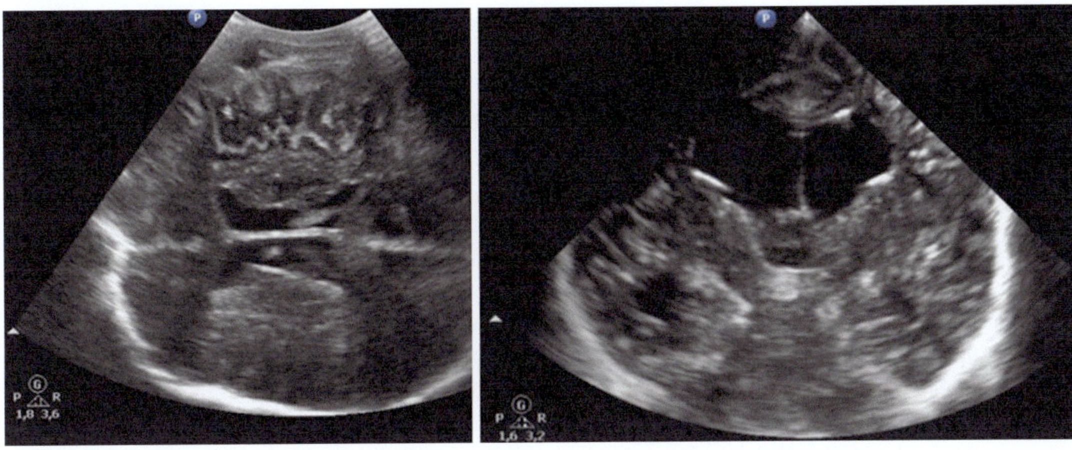

Fig. 45.2 Ultrasound images of the brain. On the *left hand* is an axial slice showing highly detailed brain anatomy in a craniotomized patient. On the *right hand* is a similar detailed coronary view through the fontanel in a 6-month-old child with hydrocephalus

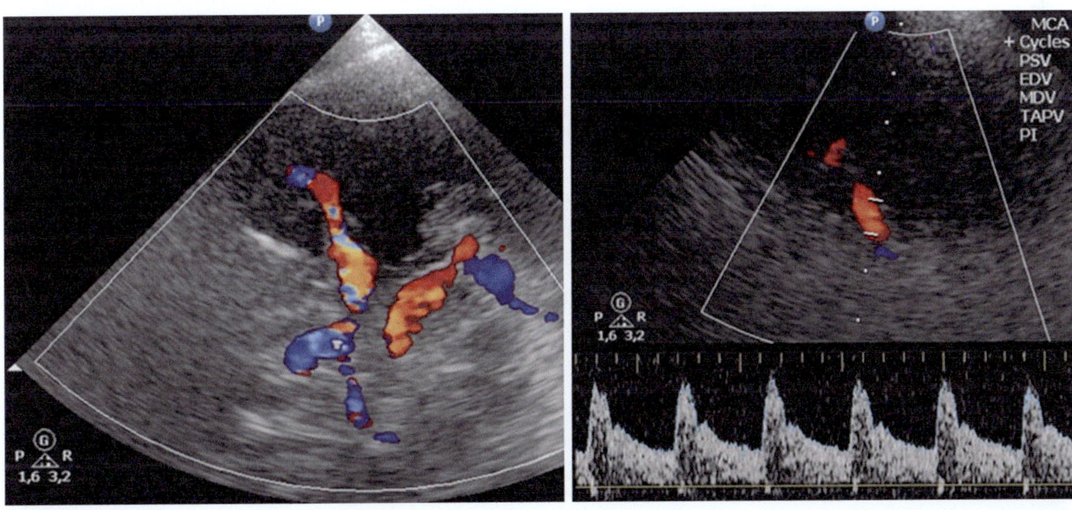

Fig. 45.3 *Left picture* is a colour Doppler visualization of the cerebral arteries showing the middle cerebral artery (MCA) pointing upward towards the Doppler probe, the anterior cerebral artery (ACA) in the *left side* of the picture and the posterior cerebral artery (PCA) in the *right side*. Blue colours code for a flow direction away from the probe, whereas red/orange code for flow towards the probe. The *right picture* shows a TCD recording in the MCA

signal after the subtraction of the original emission. The signal is pulsed, making it possible to register from different distances or depths from the probe. A computer converts the resulting signal into a graph that provides information about the speed and direction of blood flow through the blood vessel being examined (Fig. 45.3).

45.2.1 Temporal Window

Finding the thin bony layer of the temporal bone, 'the temporal window', can be difficult; it varies in size and location with each patient and may also differ individually from the one side to the other. Furthermore, such a transtemporal window is absent in up to 10% of the adult population, and it is most difficult to find in older individuals, females and black people. There are usually two possible sites to penetrate with the ultrasound wave in the temporal window: one situated approximately 1 cm behind the corner of the eye and the other one a cm up and in front of the ear meatus (Fig. 45.4). The transducer's orientation should be pointed in a slightly upward direction, pointing in between these two centres. The transducer should be tilted and moved slowly over the skin to pinpoint the best signal and highest flow velocity. The temporal window can be used to insonate the middle cerebral artery (MCA), the anterior cerebral artery (ACA), the posterior cerebral artery (PCA) and the terminal portion of the internal carotid artery (ICA) just prior to its bifurcation.

45.2.2 Transorbital Window

The transorbital window gives access to the ophthalmic artery (OA) as well as the internal carotid artery at the siphon level. The transducer is gently placed on the closed eyelid. The transducer should be pointed slightly medially (Figs. 45.4 and 45.5). Damage to the eye has never been reported, but not every equipment is approved for the use of this approach, and it is important to start the investigation at a low power setting.

45.2.3 Suboccipital Window

The occipital or foraminal window allows for insonating the distal vertebral arteries (VA) and the basilar artery (BA). When evaluating the vertebrobasilar system, the best results are obtained with the patient lying on the side with the head extended forward to open up the gap between the atlas and the cranium. The transducer is placed in the nuchal crest (Fig. 45.5). The orientation should be towards the bridge of the patient's nose. The BA is found in the midline and the VA slightly at each side. The depth of the anatomic structures will vary with each patient depending upon the thickness of the suboccipital soft tissue.

Depths to investigate the cerebral arteries together with their respective typical flow velocities (FV (cm/s))

3–6 cm	Middle cerebral artery	*MCA*	55 ± 12
6–8 cm	Anterior cerebral artery	*ACA*	50 ± 11
6–7 cm	Posterior cerebral artery	*PCA*	40 ± 10
3.5–7 cm	Vertebral artery	*VA*	40 ± 10
7.5–12 cm	Basilar artery	*BA*	40 ± 10

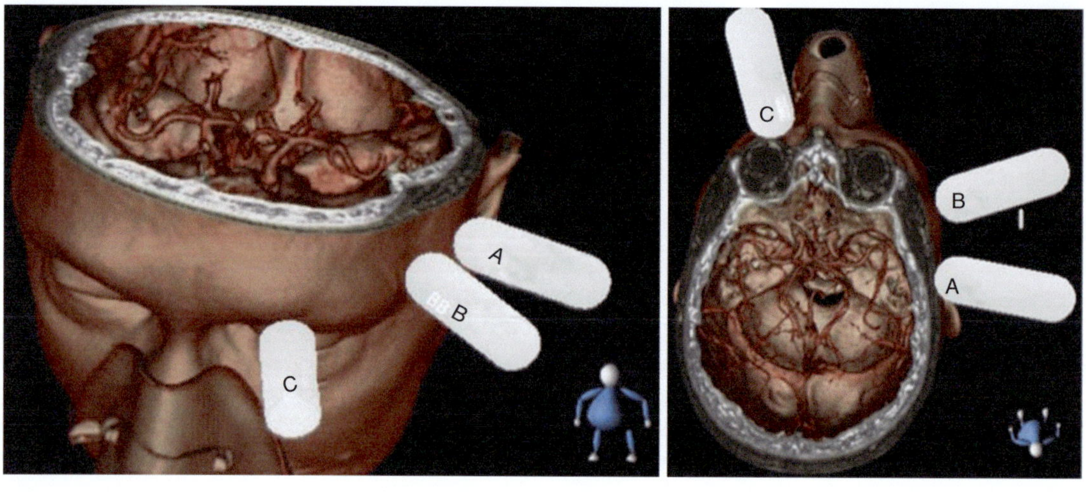

Fig. 45.4 The figures indicate the position and angle to insonate the MCA and ACA. *A* is the posterior temporal window, and *B* is the anterior. MCA signal is found 3–6 cm below the skin. Following the MCA inward, the bifurcation with the anterior and posterior artery is eventually found as an additional flow directed away from the probe, i.e. a negative curve component. *C* anterior cerebral artery is found at a depth of 6–8 cm

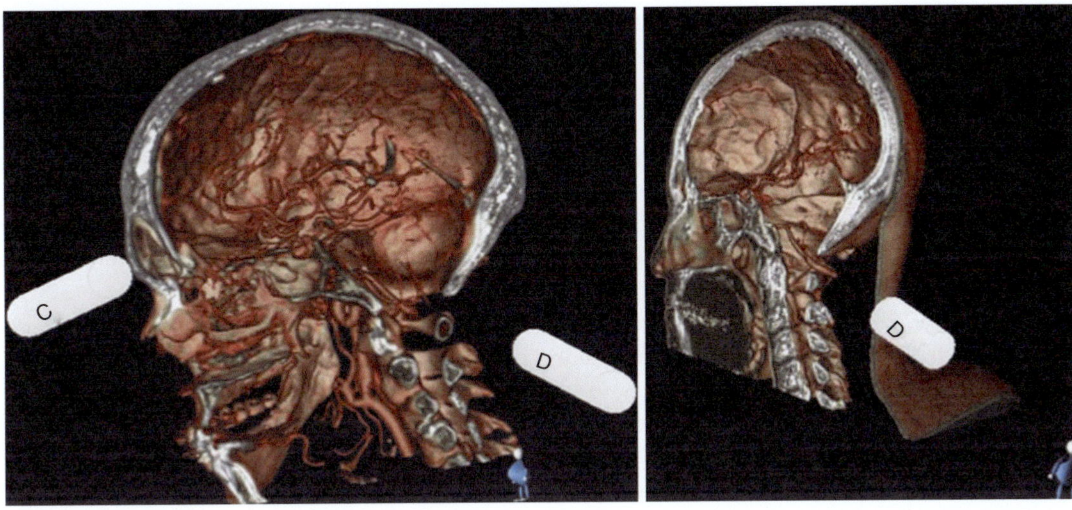

Fig. 45.5 In the *left* picture *C* shows the horizontal angle to insonate the ophthalmic artery (OA), the anterior cerebral artery (ACA) and the internal carotid artery (ICA), whereas *D* indicates the angle by which to investigate the vertebral artery (VA) and basilar artery (BA). *Right* picture shows the placement of the probe on the skin in the nuchal crest

45.2.4 TCD Flow Velocity (FV) Correlation to Cerebral Blood Flow (CBF)

TCD FV is measured in the basal arteries of the brain. If CBF is altered with an unchanged tone in these large arteries, i.e. by changing the tone only in the peripheral pial resistance arteries, there should be a direct positive correlation between the FV in the basal arteries and the CBF. However, this direct correlation will be altered if similar changes are taking place simultaneously in basal arteries and peripheral resistance arteries. If the CBF regulating change in arterial tone only occurs in the basal arteries, there is a direct negative correlation between CBF and TCD FV readings, as described by Giller et al. (1998) in the formula FV = cerebral blood flow/vessel diameter in the insonated artery. Unfortunately, no general correlation has been found between absolute CBF and FV (Bishop et al. 1986; Clark et al. 1996). However, despite the limitation of the above-mentioned assumption, the simplicity of the TCD technique and its lack of invasiveness warrant for further evaluations to determine whether it can replace considerably more complicated CBF measurements for the evaluation of the cerebral circulation.

45.2.5 CO_2 Response

In healthy individuals, blood flow velocities in the large intracranial arteries are in direct relation to the arterial CO_2 concentrations ($pACO_2$), reflecting global cerebral vasoconstriction and relaxation due to changes in $pACO_2$ (Markwalder et al. 1984). Despite this, no correlation was found between the absolute values of CBF and FV during CO_2 provocation (Bishop et al. 1986; Clark et al. 1996). Furthermore, this TCD/CBF correlation is absent also in patients with various brain pathologies, such as after subarachnoid haemorrhage (Romner et al. 1991) or following traumatic brain injury (Reinstrup et al. 2011).

45.2.6 Cerebrovascular Autoregulation

Cerebral autoregulation is the self-adjustments of the cerebrovascular tree in order to maintain a sufficient cerebral blood flow during alterations in mean arterial blood pressure (MAP). TCD is valid for determination of the lower limit of CBF autoregulation, and changes in CBF can be evaluated by TCD during changes in cerebral perfusion pressure in normal subjects (Larsen et al. 1994). TCD measurements of FV and pulsative index (PI) before and during pharmacological or mechanical manipulation of MAP and hence autoregulation, can be used to monitor the reactivity of the intracranial vasculature tree (Aaslid et al. 1989; Mahony et al. 2000). The easiest and now widely used approach is the transient hyperaemic response (THR) test first described in 1991 by Giller (1991). It involves a continuous recording of the MCA FV during which a 3- to 10-s compression of the ipsilateral common carotid artery is performed. This results in a sudden reduction in the MCA FV, which in turn provokes a vasodilatation in the vascular bed distal to the MCA if the autoregulation is intact (Fig. 45.6). Thus, following the release of the compression, a transient increase, well above the previous base level, is seen in MCA FV due to the autoregulatory compensatory dilatation, while later, this response will return to normal.

45.2.7 High Flow Velocity (FV) and the Lindegaard Index (LI)

Increased FV is found in vasospastic parts of an artery. The vasospasm can be very local, affecting only millimetre-long segments of the artery; hence, it is important to investigate as much of the artery as possible. High FV can also be caused by hyperaemia, and there is nothing in the curve form that can be used to differentiate between these two sources for a high FV. The ICA feeds the MCA, ACA and PCA. In case of vasospasm in MCA, ACA and PCA, resulting in a reduced flow through some or all of them, the effect in the feeding artery is a reduced flow as measured on the neck in the ICA. Contrary to this, the flow through the ICA increases during hyperaemia. The ICA lumen is usually unchanged during different intracranial pathologies resulting in a direct relationship between FV and flow.

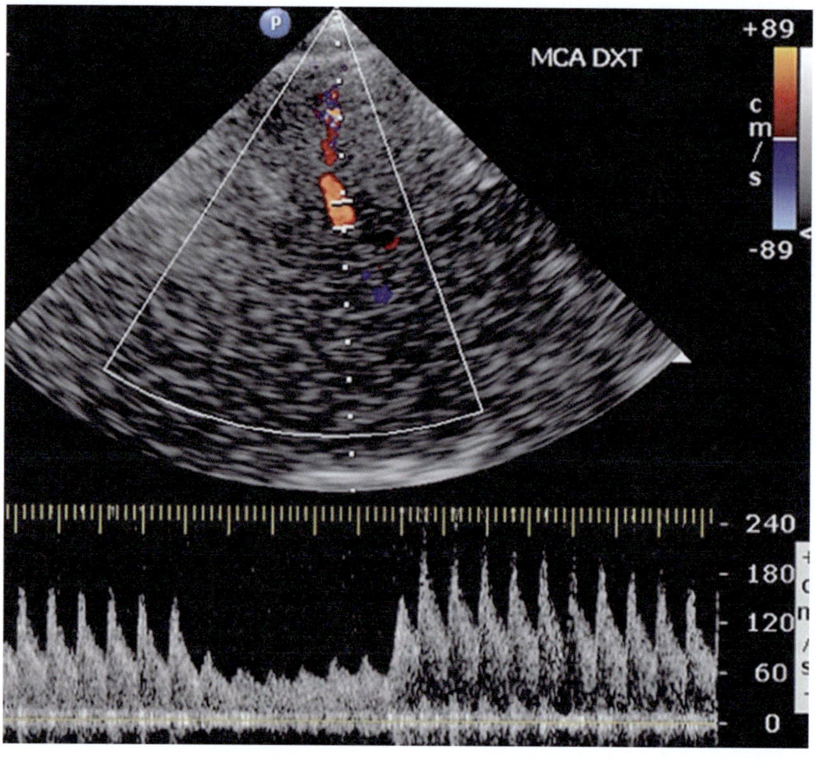

Fig. 45.6 Test of the cerebral vasoreactivity during TCD of the MCA. Following onset of the carotid artery compression, there is an immediate fall in ipsilateral MCA FV followed by a gradual rise due to autoregulation. On release, there is a brief overshoot due to the compensatory vasodilation

Lindegaard et al. (1988) used the MCA/ICA FV relationship to discriminate between hyperaemia and vasospasm and to assess the severity of vasospasm. The MCA/ICA ratio is normally around 2 with some age and sex variations (Krejza et al. 2005).

Generally, a flow velocity above 120 cm/s is indicative of a vasospasm. However, if the FV increases slowly over days to this level, it seldom gives rise to clinical symptoms.

If MCA FV rises to between 120 and 150 cm/s with a LI at 3–5, the vasospasm is considered moderate.

If MCA FV is 150–220 cm/s and LI is >6, the vasospasm is generally severe, and if MCA increases above 200 cm/s with LI > 6, the vasospasm is usually critical.

Hyperaemia increases flow velocities in both MCA and ICA keeping LI unchanged <3, whereas in cases of escalating vasospasm, FV is increased in the intracranial arteries with a reduced FV in the ICA, showing up as an elevated LI.

In order to evaluate the flow in the BA, one has to look at the intracranial/extracranial FV ratio in the posterior circulation, i.e. the ratio between BA and one of the vertebral arteries measured extracranially on the neck in analogy with the MCA/ICA ratio. An FV threshold of 80 cm/s is indicative of BA vasospasm. A normative value of a BA/extracranial VA FV ratio (BA/EVA) is 1.7. The BA/EVA is >2 in all patients with BA vasospasm and generally <2 in patients without. Furthermore, the BA/EVA ratio shows a close correlation with BA diameter and is >3 in all patients with severe vasospasm (Soustiel et al. 2002). EVA should be insonated at depths ranging from 45 to 55 mm.

45.2.8 TCD, ICP and Pulsative Index (PI)

Pulsative index PI = systFV – diastFV/meanFV was originally thought to describe the cerebrovascular resistance, but this is probably not the case, since hyperventilation with vasoconstriction does not increase PI (Czosnyka et al. 1996). However, an artificially increased ICP brought about by increasing the pressure in the epidural space brings about a more pronounced reduction of flow velocities in the diastolic phase than in the systolic phase, i.e. increasing the pulse peak between systole and diastole. Furthermore, there is a lowering of the mean FV (Nagai et al. 1997). Looking at the PI equation, it should therefore be sensitive to increases in ICP, and such a correlation has indeed been found in children with hydrocephalus (Goh and Minns 1995; Govender et al. 1999; Nadvi et al. 1994), even though not all findings have been positive (Hanlo et al. 1995; Figaji et al. 2009). In adults with various brain pathologies and equipped with ventricular ICP devices with a reference zero at the forehead level, a strong relationship was found between ICP and PI, with ICP = 10.93 × PI − 1.28 or ICP ≈ 10 × PI (Bellner et al. 2004). It must be emphasized, however, that PI cannot be used as a substitute for an ICP device, but rather may be utilized as one additional tool in the evaluation of patients with suspected brain pathologies, in the guidance whether the patient might gain from an ICP device.

45.3 Brain Trauma

45.3.1 Absolute FV

In comatose TBI patients, cerebral metabolic rate (CMR) is reduced with up to 50%, and compared to the normal coupling between CMR and CBF, these patients have normal to supranormal CBF values (Obrist et al. 1984). Most patients present with CBF changes over time, starting with low CBF values shortly after the trauma (Bouma and Muizelaar 1992) evolving to a hyperaemic phase, again substituted for a state of low CBF, but now due to vasospasm. It takes around 3 weeks before the CBF returns to normal (Inoue et al. 2005). This development would be expected to show up as changes in the TCD FV, but the FV starts initially at normal values with a normal LI and hence does not reflect the low absolute CBF. The FV typically rises during the following 3 days up towards 100 cm/s and stays elevated for the next

14 days (Martin et al. 1997). LI remains low, and thus the first increase in FV is due to hyperaemia. LI increases slowly over time indicating that the reason for the high FV goes from hyperaemia to vasospasm.

The infratentorial vascular territory is seldom investigated following TBI, despite the fact that Soustiel and Shik found that one third of such patients presented with high FV in the BA as a sign of vasospasm (2004).

45.3.2 CO_2 Response

Arterial reactivity in brain-damaged areas is impaired so that a reduced CO_2 reactivity as measured with CBF correlates not only to the extent of damaged tissue and thereby to the severity of the brain injury, but also to outcome (Cold et al. 1977; Schalén et al. 1991; Poon et al. 2005). In healthy subjects, blood flow velocities in the basal intracranial arteries are directly related to the $pACO_2$ (Markwalder et al. 1984). However, this correlation is absent in patients with subarachnoid haemorrhage (Romner et al. 1991). On the other hand, following TBI there is a more pronounced change in TCD FV than in CBF upon changes in $pACO_2$ (Reinstrup et al. 2011). A relationship of individual reactivity indices between the two parameters concerning CO_2 reactivity is therefore not established, and CBF and mean FV are hence not exchangeable in patients with severe brain trauma.

45.3.3 Autoregulation

The correlation between CBF, as measured indirectly with changes in arteriovenous oxygen difference ($AVDO_2$), and TCD during autoregulation provocations has been established in healthy volunteers (Larsen et al. 1994). However, the classic correlation between CBF and TCD autoregulation has so far not been investigated for TBI patients. Autoregulatory capacity, as measured simultaneously in the basal arteries by TCD FV and in the pial arteries by laser Doppler flowmetry, was more severely impaired in the cortex than in the MCA during conditions of rising ICP and falling CPP. However, providing CPP was kept above 60 mmHg, cortical autoregulatory capacity was on level with that of the MCA (Zweifel et al. 2010). In an investigation of TCD-measured autoregulation in TBI patients, a correlation between the impaired autoregulation and outcome was found (Sorrentino et al. 2011). In patients with minor head injuries, autoregulation is impaired in 28% (Jünger et al. 1997).

45.3.4 Brain Death (Cerebral Circulatory Arrest)

TCD FV measurement is not a legally approved method to establish cerebral circulatory arrest, but it can give some useful information of the status of circulation. In this context; it is mandatory to investigate both the supratentorial and the infratentorial compartments. As described above, an increasing ICP brings about a reduction in flow velocity mainly in the diastolic phase, finally leaving only a flow at the systolic peak in the basal arteries of the brain (Petty et al. 1990). Further elevation of the ICP leads to a reverberating FV, or it is oscillating around zero, ending up with a brief peak in systole, called the 'systolic spike', and with a close to zero net flow through the brain (Langfitt et al. 1964). The final stage in intracranial hypertension is a no-flow situation revealing no Doppler signal as investigated in animals (Nagai et al. 1997).

When using TCD to guide the appropriate time for performing a four-vessel angiogram in cases where clinical diagnostics are inappropriate, we usually start the angiography procedure when the FV is reverberating or only showing a systolic spike both supra- and infratentorially, and so far, all angiograms have shown total cerebral circulatory arrest using such an approach. However, hitherto no investigation has been conducted in order to correlate the TCD with angiography during upcoming circulatory arrest.

45.4 Specific Paediatric Concerns

Children between the age of 2 and 10 years have a mFV of 95 cm/s and a PI of 0.95. After the tenth year, the mFV are declining over the years to finally reach 85 cm/s and the PI to 0.80 at the age of 20. Girls do generally have a higher mFV than boys (Brouwers et al. 1990).

References

Aaslid R, Markwalder TM, Nornes H. Noninvasive transcranial Doppler ultrasound recording of flow velocity in basal cerebral arteries. J Neurosurg. 1982;57:769–74.

Aaslid R, Lindegaard KF, Sorteberg W, Nornes H. Cerebral autoregulation dynamics in humans. Stroke. 1989;20:45–52.

Bellner J, Romner B, Reinstrup P, Kristiansson KA, Ryding E, Brandt L. Transcranial Doppler sonography pulsatility index (PI) reflects intracranial pressure (ICP). Surg Neurol. 2004;62:45–51.

Bishop CC, Powell S, Rutt D, Browse NL. Transcranial Doppler measurement of middle cerebral artery blood flow velocity: a validation study. Stroke. 1986;17:913–5.

Bouma GJ, Muizelaar JP. Cerebral blood flow, cerebral blood volume, and cerebrovascular reactivity after severe head injury. J Neurotrauma. 1992;9(Suppl 1):S333–48.

Brouwers PJAM, Vries EM, Musbach M, Wieneke GH, Van Huffelen AC. Transcranial pulsed doppler measurements of blood flow velocity in the middle cerebral artery: reference values at rest and during hyper- ventilation in healthy children and adolescents in relation to age and sex. Ultrasound Med Biol. 1990;16(1):1–8.

Clark JM, Skolnick BE, Gelfand R, Farber RE, Stierheim M, Stevens WC, Beck G Jr, Lambertsen CJ. Relationship of 133Xe cerebral blood flow to middle cerebral arterial flow velocity in men at rest. J Cereb Blood Flow Metab. 1996;16:1255–62.

Cold GE, Jensen FT, Malmros R. The effects of pACO2 reduction on regional cerebral blood flow in the acute phase of brain injury. Acta Anaesthesiol Scand. 1977;21:359–67.

Czosnyka M, Richards HK, Whitehouse HE, Pickard JD. Relationship between transcranial Doppler- determined pulsatility index and cerebrovascular resistance: an experimental study. J Neurosurg. 1996;84:79–84.

Figaji AA, Zwane E, Fieggen AG, Siesjo P, Peter JC. Transcranial Doppler pulsatility index is not a reliable indicator of intracranial pressure in children with severe traumatic brain injury. Surg Neurol. 2009;72:389–94.

Giller CA. A bedside test for cerebral autoregulation using transcranial Doppler ultrasound. Acta Neurochir. 1991;108:7–14.

Giller CA, Hatab MR, Giller AM. Estimation of vessel flow and diameter during cerebral vasospasm using transcranial Doppler indices. Neurosurgery. 1998;42:1076–81.

Goh D, Minns RA. Intracranial pressure and cerebral arterial flow velocity indices in childhood hydrocephalus: current review. Childs Nerv Syst. 1995;11:392–6.

Govender PV, Nadvi SS, Madaree A. The value of transcranial Doppler ultrasonography in craniosynostosis. J Craniofac Surg. 1999;10:260–3.

Hanlo PW, Gooskens RH, Nijhuis IJ, Faber JA, Peters RJ, van Huffelen AC, Tulleken CA, Willemse J. Value of transcranial Doppler indices in predicting raised ICP in infantile hydrocephalus. A study with review of the literature. Childs Nerv Syst. 1995;11:595–603.

Inoue Y, Shiozaki T, Tasaki O, Hayakata T, Ikegawa H, Yoshiya K, Fujinaka T, Tanaka H, Shimazu T, Sugimoto H. Changes in cerebral blood flow from the acute to the chronic phase of severe head injury. J Neurotrauma. 2005;22:1411–8.

Jünger EC, Newell DW, Grant GA, Avellino AM, Ghatan S, Douville CM, Lam AM, Aaslid R, Winn HR. Cerebral autoregulation following minor head injury. J Neurosurg. 1997;86:425–32.

Krejza J, Szydlik P, Liebeskind DS, Kochanowicz J, Bronov O, Mariak Z, Melhem ER. Age and sex variability and normal reference values for the V(MCA)/V(ICA) index. AJNR Am J Neuroradiol. 2005;26:730–5.

Langfitt TW, Weinstein JD, Kassell NF. Cerebral vasomotor paralysis as a cause of brain swelling. Trans Am Neurol Assoc. 1964;89:214–5.

Larsen FS, Olsen KS, Hansen BA, Paulson OB, Knudsen GM. Transcranial Doppler is valid for determination of the lower limit of cerebral blood flow autoregulation. Stroke. 1994;25:1985–8.

Lindegaard KF, Nornes H, Bakke SJ, Sorteberg W, Nakstad P. Cerebral vasospasm after subarachnoid haemorrhage investigated by means of transcranial Doppler ultrasound. Acta Neurochir Suppl (Wien). 1988;42:81–4.

Mahony PJ, Panerai RB, Deverson ST, Hayes PD, Evans DH. Assessment of the thigh cuff technique for measurement of dynamic cerebral autoregulation. Stroke. 2000;31:476–80.

Markwalder TM, Grolimund P, Seiler RW, Roth F, Aaslid R. Dependency of blood flow velocity in the middle cerebral artery on end-tidal carbon dioxide partial pressure—a transcranial ultrasound Doppler study. J Cereb Blood Flow Metab. 1984;4:368–72.

Martin NA, Patwardhan RV, Alexander MJ, Africk CZ, Lee JH, Shalmon E, Hovda DA, Becker DP. Characterization of cerebral hemodynamic phases following severe head trauma: hypoperfusion, hyperemia, and vasospasm. J Neurosurg. 1997;87:9–19.

Nadvi SS, Du Trevou MD, Van Dellen JR, Gouws E. The use of transcranial Doppler ultrasonography as a method of assessing intracranial pressure in hydrocephalic children. Br J Neurosurg. 1994;8:573–7.

Nagai H, Moritake K, Takaya M. Correlation between transcranial Doppler ultrasonography and regional cerebral blood flow in experimental intracranial hypertension. Stroke. 1997;28:603–37.

Obrist WD, Langfitt TW, Jaggi JL, Cruz J, Gennarelli TA. Cerebral blood flow and metabolism in comatose patients with acute head injury. Relationship to intracranial hypertension. J Neurosurg. 1984;61:241–53.

Petty GW, Mohr JP, Pedley TA, Tatemichi TK, Lennihan L, Duterte DI, Sacco RL. The role of transcranial Doppler in confirming brain death: sensitivity, specificity, and suggestions for performance and interpretation. Neurology. 1990;40:300–3.

Poon WS, Ng SC, Chan MT, Lam JM, Lam WW. Cerebral blood flow (CBF)-directed management of ventilated head-injured patients. Acta Neurochir Suppl. 2005;95:9–11.

Reinstrup P, Ryding E, Asgeirsson B, Hesselgard K, Unden J, Romner B. Cerebral blood flow (CBF) and transcranial doppler sonography (TCD) measurements of cerebrovascular CO2-reactivity in patients with acute severe head injury. J Cereb Blood Flow Metab. 2011;20(1):54–9.

Romner B, Brandt L, Berntman L, Algotsson L, Ljunggren B, Messeter K. Simultaneous transcranial Doppler sonography and cerebral blood flow measurements of cerebrovascular CO2-reactivity in patients with aneurysmal subarachnoid haemorrhage. Br J Neurosurg. 1991;5:31–7.

Schalén W, Messeter K, Nordström CH. Cerebral vasoreactivity and the prediction of outcome in severe traumatic brain lesions. Acta Anaesthesiol Scand. 1991;35:113–22.

Sorrentino E, Budohoski KP, Kasprowicz M, Smielewski P, Matta B, Pickard JD, Czosnyka M. Critical thresholds for transcranial Doppler indices of cerebral autoregulation in traumatic brain injury. Neurocrit Care. 2011;14:188–93.

Soustiel JF, Shik V. Posttraumatic basilar artery vasospasm. Surg Neurol. 2004;62:201–6.

Soustiel JF, Shik V, Shreiber R, Tavor Y, Goldsher D. Basilar vasospasm diagnosis: investigation of a modified "Lindegaard Index" based on imaging studies and blood velocity measurements of the basilar artery. Stroke. 2002;33:72–7.

Zweifel C, Czosnyka M, Lavinio A, Castellani G, Kim DJ, Carrera E, Pickard JD, Kirkpatrick PJ, Smielewski P. A comparison study of cerebral autoregulation assessed with transcranial Doppler and cortical laser Doppler flowmetry. Neurol Res. 2010;32:425–8.

46 Near-Infrared Spectroscopy (NIRS) or Cerebral Oximetry

Peter Reinstrup

Recommendations

Level I

There are insufficient data to support a Level I recommendation for this topic.

Level II

There are insufficient data to support a Level II recommendation for this topic.

Level III

NIRS can be used to detect upcoming intra- and extracerebral haematomas.

46.1 Overview

Near-infrared spectroscopy (NIRS) measures the oxygenation of the haemoglobin in the cerebral tissue lying just underneath a probe. The probe is most often placed on the forehead, since hair follicles affect the readings. Some doubts have been raised whether NIRS specifically measures the cerebral tissue or is contaminated by signals from extracerebral tissues. Furthermore, as haemoglobin absorbs infrared light, NIRS is affected by underlying blood of extravascular origin, such as in subdural haematomas, contusions, subarachnoid blood, as well as changes in intravascular cerebral blood volume (CBV). These factors are difficult to decipher, and at present, the use of NIRS in TBI patients is controversial. However, by using more than one sensor and by focusing on trends, NIRS readings might be of value in this patient group.

Tips, Tricks and Pitfalls

- NIRS probes can be placed over hair follicles, but the melatonin in the hair affects the absorption of infrared light.
- NIRS from one single probe is too difficult to interpret.
- In patients with unilateral brain pathologies, a symmetrically placed contralateral probe should be used as reference.
- Never use the NIRS reading as the only monitoring device; changes in a NIRS reading should be controlled with other techniques.
- Keep in mind that patients with total brain infarctions can still have a normal NIRS value.

P. Reinstrup (✉)
Department of Intensive and Perioperative Care, Skånes University Hospital, Lund, Sweden
e-mail: peter.reinstrup@med.lu.se

© Springer Nature Switzerland AG 2020
T. Sundstrøm et al. (eds.), *Management of Severe Traumatic Brain Injury*,
https://doi.org/10.1007/978-3-030-39383-0_46

46.2 Background

Oximetry is a method for monitoring the oxygenation of haemoglobin. With near-infrared spectroscopy (NIRS) it is possible to measure oxygen saturation (SO_2). Jobsis (1977) was the first to report on this, and in 1985 came the first report on cerebral oximetry in humans (Ferrari et al. 1985). A proportion of the near-infrared light passing through tissues is absorbed. The absorption of light relates to the amount and properties of the material through which the light is passing based on the Beer–Lambert law. Tissues such as skin, bone and brain are transparent to the near-infrared spectrum, whereas the two chromophores oxy- and deoxyhaemoglobin are not. Since the absorption characteristics of oxy- and deoxy-haemoglobin are different at different wavelengths, it is possible to quantify the cerebral oxygenation of the blood with its venous/arterial relationship of 70%/30%, by choosing two or more wavelengths where the absorption of oxy- and deoxyhaemoglobin is maximally and minimally separated, i.e. between 700 and 850 nm (wavelength - nanometers).

At 810 nm, the absorption of NIR is equal for oxy- and deoxyhaemoglobin, and hence it is theoretically possible to measure the total amount of haemoglobin at this wavelength. With knowledge of the amount of haemoglobin, it is possible to calculate the CBV continuously when knowing the haemoglobin concentration. However, so far this technique is too unstable to be used in clinical practice (Canova et al. 2011).

An infrared beam penetrating into a tissue scatters in such a way that some of it is reflected back to the surface from where it is emitted. To this end, most apparatuses use reflectance-mode NIRS in which the optical sensors are placed ipsilateral to the transmitter; they exploit the fact that photons transmitted through a sphere will traverse an elliptical path in which the mean depth of penetration is proportional to the separation of the transmitter and the optical sensor.

Though small, some absorption does occur both in normal cerebral and extracerebral tissues. Extracerebral tissue is not a homogenous layer, but a composite of all the layers of the scalp, bone and dura. Each of these layers with individual optical absorption characteristics may affect the results in a non-foreseeable manner. Especially melatonin, in hair and hair follicles, absorbs near-infrared light to a high degree. The effect on the oximeter reading from these extracerebral layers is hence poorly understood (Young et al. 2000), and in adults, the infrared beam has to pass a thick layer of extracranial tissue twice. In order to minimize the influence of the extracerebral tissue and extracerebral circulation, different algorithms have been applied, and a number of techniques have been developed, but still without complete success (Al-Rawi and Kirkpatrick 2006).

46.2.1 Normal Values of NIRS

The normal value for cerebral oximetry or cerebral regional oxygen saturation (rSO_2) is 58–82% (Kim et al. 2000). The wide normal range makes it more optimal to follow the trend in the particular patient rather than absolute values, and compare with contralateral measurements.

46.2.2 Factors Affecting NIRS

An oximeter reading using NIRS is highly influenced by the venous blood since 70% of the normal cerebral blood volume (CBV) is of venous origin. A venous saturation is giving an indication of the relationship between cerebral blood flow (CBF) and cerebral metabolism (CMR). The change in cerebral venous oxygenation is described in detail in Sects. 43.2.4 and 43.2.5. An increased ICP will compromise CBF, thereby lowering NIRS. But with a normal venous outflow, an increased ICP will compress the thin-walled veins reducing the venous part of the CBV. As a result, the NIRS reading should theoretically increase as it would be more influenced by the arterial side. In fact Zuluaga et al. (2010) found NIRS during increased ICP to generally decline, but dispersed to both higher and lower values.

46.2.3 TBI and Pathologic Brain

A major problem with NIRS is the diverse influence of underlying brain pathologies. In dead or non-metabolizing tissue, the NIRS can show either high or low values (Dunham et al. 2002), depending on the status of the sequestered blood. Extravasated blood can contain a varying degree of oxyhaemoglobin, whereas in cerebral contusions, the non-metabolizing tissue does not affect the oxyhaemoglobin content even though the flow through such a region is low (see Fig. 46.1). In fact, NIRS has been used to detect the development of intra- and extracerebral haematomas using a wavelength of 760 nm, at which the absorption is increased at the haematoma side compared to the normal side (Gopinath et al. 1995), resulting in an increased NIRS reading at the haematoma side. In TBI the different underlying pathologies, haemoglobin level, manipulation with CMR and CBF and differences in ICP are factors that make a NIRS reading difficult to interpret and therefore problematic to use in TBI patients (Weigl et al. 2016).

46.2.4 CBF Measurements with NIRS

By using a contrast medium and looking at its passage and amount, it is possible to calculate the mean transit time (MTT) and CBV and thereby calculate the local CBF under the probe. Indocyanine green is an ideal contrast medium in conjunction with NIRS, as it has an absorption peak at 805 nm. However, a correlation to CBF has been found in some (Kuebler et al. 1998; Keller et al. 2003), but not all studies (Newton et al. 1997), and the method is not widely used.

46.3 Specific Paediatric Concerns

In healthy children, the normal range for cerebral oximetry is 60–80% (95% confidence interval, average is 68%). There are no studies investigating NIRS and TBI in children.

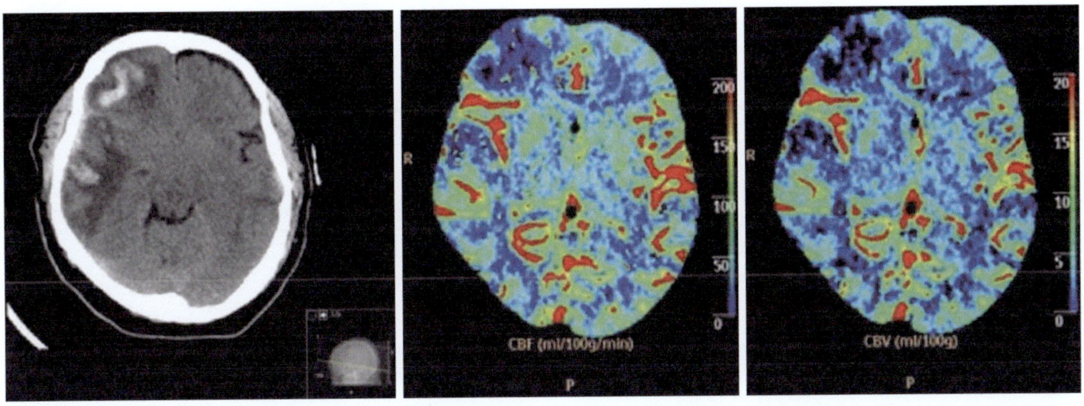

Fig. 46.1 A CT scan showing contusions in the right frontal and temporal regions (*left picture*). CBF (*middle picture*) and CBV (*right picture*) were measured simultaneously with CT perfusion. Cerebral oximetry probes were placed in a symmetrical manner bifrontally where the right sensor was placed over the frontal contusion (*left picture*). The reading was 94% over the contusion and 71% over the left side. The local CBF was low in the contused area (*middle picture*) as was the CBV (*right picture*). The reason for the high saturation in the contusion is most probably due to the extravasated blood, but can also be influenced by the non-metabolizing tissue in the contusioned area, even though both CBF and CBV were low

References

Al-Rawi PG, Kirkpatrick PJ. Tissue oxygen index: thresholds for cerebral ischemia using near-infrared spectroscopy. Stroke. 2006;37:2720–5.

Canova D, Roatta S, Bosone D, Micieli G. Inconsistent detection of changes in cerebral blood volume by near infrared spectroscopy in standard clinical tests. J Appl Physiol. 2011;110(6):1646–55, Epub 2011 Apr 7.

Dunham CM, Sosnowski C, Porter JM, Siegal J, Kohli C. Correlation of noninvasive cerebral oximetry with cerebral perfusion in the severe head injured patient: a pilot study. J Trauma. 2002;52:40–6.

Ferrari M, Giannini I, Sideri G, Zanette E. Continuous noninvasive monitoring of human brain by near infrared spectroscopy. Adv Exp Med Biol. 1985;191:873–82.

Gopinath SP, Robertson CS, Contant CF, Narayan RK, Grossman RG, Chance B. Early detection of delayed traumatic intracranial hematomas using near- infrared spectroscopy. J Neurosurg. 1995;83(3):438–44.

Jobsis FF. Noninvasive infrared monitoring of cerebral and myocardial oxygen sufficiency and circulatory parameters. Science. 1977;198:1264–7.

Keller E, Nadler A, Alkadhi H, Kollias SS, Yonekawa Y, Niederer P. Noninvasive measurement of regional cerebral blood flow and regional cerebral blood volume by near-infrared spectroscopy and indo- cyanine green dye dilution. Neuroimage. 2003;20:828–39.

Kim MB, Ward DS, Cartwright CR, Kolano J, Chlebowski S, Henson LC. Estimation of jugular venous O2 saturation from cerebral oximetry or arterial O2 saturation during isocapnic hypoxia. J Clin Monit Comput. 2000;16(3):191–9.

Kuebler WM, Sckell A, Habler O, Kleen M, Kuhnle GE, Welte M, Messmer K, Goetz AE. Noninvasive measurement of regional cerebral blood flow by near-infrared spectroscopy and indocyanine green. J Cereb Blood Flow Metab. 1998;18:445–56.

Newton CR, Wilson DA, Gunnoe E, Wagner B, Cope M, Traystman RJ. Measurement of cerebral blood flow in dogs with near infrared spectroscopy in the reflectance mode is invalid. J Cereb Blood Flow Metab. 1997;17(6):695–703.

Weigl W, Milej D, Janusek D, Wojkiewicz S, Sawosz P, Kacprzak M, Gerega A, Maniewski R, Liebert A. Application of optical methods in the monitoring of traumatic brain injury: a review. J Cereb Blood Flow Metab. 2016;36(11):1825–43.

Young AER, Germon TJ, Barnett NJ, Manara AR, Nelson RJ. Behaviour of near-infrared light in the adult human head: implications for clinical near-infra red spectroscopy. Br J Anaesth. 2000;84:38–42.

Zuluaga MT, Esch ME, Cvijanovich NZ, Gupta N, McQuillen PS. Diagnosis influences response of cerebral NIRS to intracranial hypertension in children. Pediatr Crit Care Med. 2010;11(4):514–22.

47 Clinical Neurophysiology: Evoked Potentials

Birger Johnsen

Recommendations

Level I

There are insufficient data to support a Level I recommendation for this topic.

Level II

The presence of event-related potentials (ERPs) (P300 or MMN) in comatose TBI patients predicts a favourable prognosis and justifies continuation of intensive therapy. Bilateral absent somatosensory evoked potentials (SSEPs) indicate only 5% awakening, which may be considered in the decision on continuation of intensive therapy.

Level III

Results from evoked potentials (EPs) should always be interpreted in the actual clinical setting and combined with clinical findings.

B. Johnsen (✉)
Department of Clinical Neurophysiology, Aarhus University Hospital, Aarhus, Denmark
e-mail: birgjohn@rm.dk

47.1 Overview

Evoked potentials (EPs) are objective, non-invasive tests that may assess brainstem damage and detect cognitive functions in comatose patients; EPs are therefore of predictive value in TBI patients.

EPs are electrical signals recorded from the brain in response to different kinds of sensory stimuli, for example, auditory or somatosensory stimuli. These responses directly track the afferent volleys and appear with latencies less than 25 ms and are therefore also named short-latency EPs. Event-related potentials (ERPs) are EPs with longer latencies (up to 300 ms), and these EPs reflect higher cortical functions (Duncan et al. 2009).

EPs assess functional aspects of brain damage in addition to the clinical examination and in addition to the assessment of structural lesions by imaging techniques.

EPs of different modalities are of prognostic value in TBI patients, with some modalities predictive for a favourable prognosis and others predictive for an unfavourable prognosis. Absence of short-latency EPs predicts an unfavourable outcome (Guérit et al. 2009), while the strongest predictor for a good prognosis is the presence of ERPs (Daltrozzo et al. 2007).

© Springer Nature Switzerland AG 2020
T. Sundstrøm et al. (eds.), *Management of Severe Traumatic Brain Injury*,
https://doi.org/10.1007/978-3-030-39383-0_47

Tips, Tricks, and Pitfalls

- EPs performed too early may show over-optimistic results due to the risk of secondary damage in TBI patients (Guérit et al. 2009).
- Drugs may have a pronounced influence on ERPs (Duncan et al. 2009).
- EPs should be performed by experienced neurophysiology technicians and be interpreted by clinical neurophysiologists.
- The predictive power of EPs should, together with clinical findings and results of imagining techniques, be taken into consideration in the handling of TBI patients.

47.2 Background

The different EP modalities are easily performed, often in less than 15 min in comatose patients. Significant abnormalities of EPs include the absence of responses, increases in latencies, or increases in inter-peak latencies. The absence of responses or the presence of normal responses is the most reliable predictors, although an increase in latencies, an increase in inter-peak latencies, or amplitude changes may also be valuable.

47.2.1 BAEP

Brainstem auditory evoked potentials (BAEPs) are signals generated in the brainstem and recorded by scalp electrodes in response to click stimulation of the ears. Responses from the ear and the neural pathways in the pons are recorded with latencies less than 10 ms. BAEPs are present in about 50% of TBI patients (Guérit 2005). There are some controversies about the prognostic ability of BAEPs, and some of these controversies are probably caused by differences in timing of the examinations and differences in criteria for BAEP abnormalities. There is, however, rather good agreement on the fact that absence of BAEPs is a bad prognostic sign; for example, in a study of 64 TBI patients, Tsubokawa et al. (1980) found that all 23 cases with absence of the later BAEP waves died or went into a permanent vegetative state. On the other hand, the presence of BAEPs in TBI patients is not a useful predictor for a favourable outcome, as damage to brain regions outside the brainstem will not affect the BAEPs.

47.2.2 SSEP

Somatosensory evoked potentials (SSEPs) are recorded after electrical stimulation of the skin over a peripheral nerve of the limbs. When used as a prognostic tool in comatose patients, the most used technique is to stimulate the median nerve at the wrist while recording responses from the peripheral nerve at the elbow or at Erb's point, over the spine at level C7 and over the primary sensory cortex. A systematic review of 41 articles on SSEP as a prognostic marker for awakening from coma in TBI patients showed only 5% awakening in case of bilateral absent SSEPs, 70% awakening in case of present, but abnormal SSEPs, and 89% awakening in case of normal SSEPs (Robinson et al. 2003). Amantini et al. (2005) found that SSEP showed a good predictive value both for good and bad prognoses. Graded SSEP at day 3 after head trauma was found to correlate with functional and cognitive outcome (Houlden et al. 2010).

47.2.3 VEP

Visual evoked potentials (VEPs) are recorded after visual light stimuli. VEPs are only rarely used as a prognostic tool in comatose patients (Guérit 2005).

47.2.4 ERP

Event-related potentials (ERPs), also called cognitive evoked potentials, reflect higher cortical functions. ERPs are elicited by occasional different stimuli within a repetitive standard stimulation, the so-called oddball paradigm. P300 is a positive response with a latency of about 300 ms that can be measured as a response to infrequent, randomly presented stimuli, for example, a different tone in a sequence of frequently presented tones. Some attention or vigilance is required in order to obtain a P300 response, and it cannot be elicited in all normal subjects, which limits its sensitivity in predicting coma outcome. Another kind of ERP, the mismatch negativity (MMN) potential, is the brain's automatic response to change in auditory stimulation, and it has the great advantage of not being dependent on patient attention, as it can be recorded in comatose patients (Näätänen 2000). The MMN response occurs as a negative peak in the ERP 100–250 ms after stimulation change. Kane et al. (1996) reported that the presence of a MMN response in serial studies of TBI patients has a specificity of 100% and a sensitivity of 89.7% for awakening.

In a meta-analysis, very high positive predictive values for a favourable outcome were found for P300 (89%) and MMN (93%) when present. However, the sensitivity was not very high (76% for P300 and 34% for MMN) (Daltrozzo et al. 2007). This meta-analysis showed equal predictive power of P300 and MMN, and both techniques are recommended (Daltrozzo et al. 2007). On the other hand, the absence of ERPs has no predictive value for a bad prognosis, as these components are not always present in normal subjects and they are sensitive to other factors, e.g. sedatives.

47.2.5 Combinations of EP Modalities

Some authors combine findings from different EP modality studies in indices for global cortical function and for brainstem conduction, which is of prognostic value (Guérit 2005). Kane et al. (1996) suggest that when short-latency EPs are normal, ERPs may be performed in order to directly check brain function related to cognitive processes.

47.2.6 Influence of Drugs

Drugs interfering with EEG do also interfere with EPs, and drugs may have large influence on EPs, in particular ERPs. Halogenated gases, propofol, and thiopental (membrane interference) may cause latency increase due to interference with subcortical conduction. In contrast, short-latency EPs are very resistant.

47.2.7 Timing of Examinations

EPs performed too early after the trauma may give false optimistic results if secondary brain damage occurs, and some authors suggest serial examinations. Facco et al. (1988) suggest that EPs have the best predictive value when performed 3–6 days post injury.

47.3 Specific Paediatric Concerns

There are only sparse results regarding the use of EPs in children. Robinson et al. (2003) found a higher chance for awakening and less disability in children with absent SSEPs compared with adults. Carter and Butt (2005) found that bilateral absent SSEPs had a specificity of 92% for an unfavourable outcome in 40 children with TBI. In general, there is insufficient evidence of an age limit above which the same interpretation criteria can be used as those used in adults (Guérit et al. 2009), and interpretations should therefore be made more cautiously in children.

References

Amantini A, Grippo A, Fossi S, Cesaretti C, Piccioli A, Peris A, Ragazzoni A, Pinto F. Prediction of 'awakening' and outcome in prolonged acute coma from severe traumatic brain injury: evidence for validity of short latency SEPs. Clin Neurophysiol. 2005;116:229–35.

Carter BG, Butt W. A prospective study of outcome predictors after severe brain injury in children. Intensive Care Med. 2005;31(6):840–5. Epub 2005 Apr 28. PubMed PMID: 15864546.

Daltrozzo J, Wioland N, Mutschler V, Kotchoubey B. Predicting coma and other low responsive patients outcome using event-related brain potentials: a meta-analysis. Clin Neurophysiol. 2007;118:606–14.

Duncan CC, Barry RJ, Connolly JF, Fischer C, Michie PT, Näätänen R, Polich J, Reinvang I, Van Petten C. Event-related potentials in clinical research: guidelines for eliciting, recording, and quantifying mismatch negativity, P300, and N400. Clin Neurophysiol. 2009;120:1883–908.

Facco E, Munari M, Casartelli Liviero M, Caputo P, Martini A, Toffoletto F, Giron G. Serial recordings of auditory brainstem responses in severe head injury: relationship between test timing and prognostic power. Intensive Care Med. 1988;14:422–8.

Guérit JM. Evoked potentials in severe brain injury. Prog Brain Res. 2005;150:415–26.

Guérit JM, Amantini A, Amodio P, Andersen KV, Butler S, de Weerd A, Facco E, Fischer C, Hantson P, Jäntti V, Lamblin MD, Litscher G, Péréon Y. Consensus on the use of neurophysiological tests in the intensive care unit (ICU): electroencephalogram (EEG), evoked potentials (EP), and electroneuromyography (ENMG). Neurophysiol Clin. 2009;39:71–83.

Houlden DA, Taylor AB, Feinstein A, Midha R, Bethune AJ, Stewart CP, Schwartz ML. Early somatosensory evoked potential grades in comatose traumatic brain injury patients predict cognitive and functional outcome. Crit Care Med. 2010;38(1):167–74 . PubMed PMID: 19829103. https://doi.org/10.1097/CCM.0b013e3181c031b3.

Kane NM, Curry SH, Rowlands CA, Manara AR, Lewis T, Moss T, Cummins BH, Butler SR. Event-related potentials—neurophysiological tools for predicting emergence and early outcome from traumatic coma. Intensive Care Med. 1996;22:39–46.

Näätänen R. Mismatch negativity (MMN): perspectives for application. Int J Psychophysiol. 2000;37:3–10.

Robinson LR, Micklesen PJ, Tirschwell DL, Lew HL. Predictive value of somatosensory evoked potentials for awakening from coma. Crit Care Med. 2003;31:960–7.

Tsubokawa T, Nishimoto H, Yamamoto T, Kitamura M, Katayama Y, Moriyasu N. Assessment of brain- stem damage by the auditory brainstem response in acute severe head injury. J Neurol Neurosurg Psychiatry. 1980;43:1005–11.

48 Clinical Neurophysiology: Continuous EEG Monitoring

Birger Johnsen

Recommendations

Level I

There are insufficient data to support a Level I recommendation for this topic.

Level II

There are insufficient data to support a Level II recommendation for this topic.

Level III

Continuous EEG monitoring is recommended in TBI patients with unexplained altered consciousness to detect epileptic seizures, in particular non-convulsive seizures.

48.1 Overview

Electroencephalography (EEG) is the standard diagnostic tool when there is clinical suspicion of epileptic seizures, in particular non-convulsive seizures (NCSs), which most often can only be diagnosed by EEG. By the use of continuous EEG (cEEG) monitoring performed over one to several days, it has been found that 11–18% of TBI patients had NCSs and 8% non-convulsive status epilepticus (NCSE) (Claassen et al. 2004; Vespa 2005). Prolonged seizure activity may be harmful by causing secondary brain damage. The aim of cEEG is to diagnose these subclinical seizures and to guide the clinician in the antiepileptic treatment. Based on expert opinion from 42 studies, it is recommended to do EEG in TBI patients with unexplained and persistent altered consciousness (Claassen et al. 2013).

Tips, Tricks, and Pitfalls

- Neurointensivists should be trained in detection of suspect EEG patterns and recognizing usual EEG artefacts. Clinical neurophysiologists should perform further analyses remotely by use of telemedicine.
- Without cEEG, the neurointensivists should be aware of subtle signs of NCSs: lowering of level of consciousness, myoclonia, nystagmus, eye deviation, pupil abnormalities, autonomic instability, or confusion (Friedman et al. 2009).
- Drugs, especially sedatives, may have profound effect on the EEG.

B. Johnsen (✉)
Department of Clinical Neurophysiology, Aarhus University Hospital, Aarhus, Denmark
e-mail: birgjohn@rm.dk

© Springer Nature Switzerland AG 2020
T. Sundstrøm et al. (eds.), *Management of Severe Traumatic Brain Injury*,
https://doi.org/10.1007/978-3-030-39383-0_48

48.2 Background

48.2.1 EEG Diagnosis

EEG is used in TBI patients to diagnose NCS, to differentiate epileptic and non-epileptic movements, to identify other toxic or metabolic concurrent factors in coma, and to diagnose locked-in state. EEG is most often the only way to diagnose NCSs and NCSE (Friedman et al. 2009). cEEG monitoring in different groups of neurointensive patient has shown that a large fraction of patients suffers from NCS or NCSE, which could only be diagnosed by EEG.

48.2.2 Incidence of Seizures

Out of 13 TBI patients, 5 (38%) showed NCE and 2 of those were in NCSE (Bergsneider et al. 1997). Convulsive seizures within the first week of TBI have been estimated to occur in 4–14% of untreated patients (Annegers et al. 1980; Temkin et al. 1990; Lee et al. 1995), and if NCSs are also taken into consideration, the incidence of seizures is higher (Friedman et al. 2009). Claassen et al. (2004) found NCSs in 18% of 51 TBI patients, of which 8% were NCSE. Vespa (2005) found 22% of patients with seizures, of which half were NCSs. These figures may have been affected by prophylactic anticonvulsant treatment. In a study by Aquino et al. (2017), subclinical seizures were found in only 3.8% of the patients, probably because prophylactic anticonvulsant treatment was used. Sutter et al. (2011) showed that cEEG monitoring increases the frequency of NCSE diagnosis in ICU patients. The use of continuous sedation with e.g. midazolam may have further impact on the incidence of seizure activity (Olivecrona et al. 2009).

48.2.3 Are Non-convulsive Seizures Harmful?

Data from human (Lowenstein and Alldredge 1993; Towne et al. 1994; Young et al. 1996; Vespa et al. 2010) and animal studies (Meldrum et al. 1973; Krsek et al. 2004; DeGiorgio et al. 1992, 1996) suggest that prolonged seizure activity may cause damage to the brain. An association between duration of status epilepticus and an unfavourable prognosis has been found (Young et al. 1996), and the chance of successful treatment is higher, and mortality is lower if immediate treatment is instituted (Lowenstein and Alldredge 1993; Towne et al. 1994). Wang et al. (2008) found that the presence of early seizures in TBI patients is an independent risk factor for poor outcome. Other studies have shown that seizures in TBI patients result in increases in intracranial pressure and microdialysis lactate/pyruvate ratio (Vespa et al. 2007). Furthermore, NCSs and periodic discharges on EEG have been shown associated with the development of secondary brain injury (Vespa et al. 2016). On the other hand, aggressive antiepileptic treatment is not without risk, as shown in a population of critically ill elderly patients (Litt et al. 1998), emphasizing that a correct diagnosis is important. Controlled outcome studies of the effects of cEEG and subsequent antiepileptic treatment of NCSs and NCSE have, however, not been done.

48.2.4 Technical Aspects

Sedatives, such as propofol cause EEG changes including progressive slowing, burst suppression, and suppression. Neurophysiology technicians should be available for applying the electrodes and starting the monitoring. Bedside nurses and neurointensivists should be trained in detection of suspicious EEG patterns and recognition of usual artefacts and be able to prevent some of these, for example, by fixating an electrode. Clinical neurophysiologists can perform further analyses remotely by use of telemedicine at another department or at home. Analyses of the raw EEG from the huge amount of data generated by days of monitoring are not possible, and data analysing methods presenting compressed data in the time or frequency domain are necessary. These methods should allow the clinical neurophysiologist to detect suspicious areas and subsequently analyse the raw EEG of that area.

48.3 Specific Paediatric Concerns

NCSs and NCSE have also been described in children with TBI (Jette et al. 2006). In a more recent study, cEEG identified seizures in 30% of 144 children with TBI, and more than half of these had NCSE (O'Neil et al. 2015).

References

Annegers JF, Grabow JD, Groover RV, Laws ER Jr, Elveback LR, Kurland LT. Seizures after head trauma: a population study. Neurology. 1980;30:683–9.

Aquino L, Kang CY, Harada MY, Ko A, Do-Nguyen A, Ley EJ, Margulies DR, Alban RF. Is routine continuous EEG for traumatic brain injury beneficial? Am Surg. 2017;83(12):1433–7. PubMed PMID: 29336768.

Bergsneider M, Hovda DA, Shalmon E, Kelly DF, Vespa PM, Martin NA, Phelps ME, McArthur DL, Caron MJ, Kraus JF, Becker DP. Cerebral hyperglycolysis following severe traumatic brain injury in humans: a positron emission tomography study. J Neurosurg. 1997;86:241–51.

Claassen J, Mayer SA, Kowalski RG, Emerson RG, Hirsch LJ. Detection of electrographic seizures with continuous EEG monitoring in critically ill patients. Neurology. 2004;62:1743–8.

Claassen J, Taccone FS, Horn P, Holtkamp M, Stocchetti N, Oddo M, Neurointensive Care Section of the European Society of Intensive Care Medicine. Recommendations on the use of EEG monitoring in critically ill patients: consensus statement from the neurointensive care section of the ESICM. Intensive Care Med. 2013;39(8):1337–51 . Epub 2013 May 8. Review. PubMed PMID: 23653183. https://doi.org/10.1007/s00134-013-2938-4.

DeGiorgio CM, Tomiyasu U, Gott PS, Treiman DM. Hippocampal pyramidal cell loss in human status epilepticus. Epilepsia. 1992;33:23–7.

DeGiorgio CM, Gott PS, Rabinowicz AL, Heck CN, Smith TD, Correale JD. Neuron-specific enolase, a marker of acute neuronal injury, is increased in complex partial status epilepticus. Epilepsia. 1996;37:606–9.

Friedman D, Claassen J, Hirsch LJ. Continuous electroencephalogram monitoring in the intensive care unit. Anesth Analg. 2009;109:506–23.

Jette N, Claassen J, Emerson RG, Hirsch LJ. Frequency and predictors of nonconvulsive seizures during continuous electroencephalographic monitoring in critically ill children. Arch Neurol. 2006;63:1750–5.

Krsek P, Mikulecká A, Druga R, Kubová H, Hlinák Z, Suchomelová L, Mares P. Long-term behavioral and morphological consequences of nonconvulsive status epilepticus in rats. Epilepsy Behav. 2004;5:180–91.

Lee ST, Lui TN, Wong CW, Yeh YS, Tzaan WC. Early seizures after moderate closed head injury. Acta Neurochir. 1995;137:151–4.

Litt B, Wityk RJ, Hertz SH, Mullen PD, Weiss H, Ryan DD, Henry TR. Nonconvulsive status epilepticus in the critically ill elderly. Epilepsia. 1998;39:1194–202.

Lowenstein DH, Alldredge BK. Status epilepticus at an urban public hospital in the 1980s. Neurology. 1993;43:483–8.

Meldrum BS, Vigouroux RA, Brierley JB. Systemic factors and epileptic brain damage. Prolonged seizures in paralyzed, artificially ventilated baboons. Arch Neurol. 1973;29:82–7.

Olivecrona M, et al. Absence of electroencephalographic seizure activity in patients treated for head injury with an intracranial pressure-targeted therapy. J Neurosurg. 2009;110(2):300–5.

O'Neill BR, Handler MH, Tong S, Chapman KE. Incidence of seizures on continuous EEG monitoring following traumatic brain injury in children. J Neurosurg Pediatr. 2015;16(2):167–76. https://doi.org/10.3171/2014.12.PEDS14263. Epub 2015 May 8. PubMed PMID: 25955809.

Sutter R, Fuhr P, Grize L, Marsch S, Rüegg S. Continuous video-EEG monitoring increases detection rate of nonconvulsive status epilepticus in the ICU. Epilepsia. 2011;52:453–7.

Temkin NR, Dikmen SS, Wilensky AJ, Keihm J, Chabal S, Winn HR. A randomized, double-blind study of phenytoin for the prevention of post-traumatic seizures. N Engl J Med. 1990;323:497–502.

Towne AR, Pellock JM, Ko D, DeLorenzo RJ. Determinants of mortality in status epilepticus. Epilepsia. 1994;35:27–34.

Vespa P. Continuous EEG monitoring for the detection of seizures in traumatic brain injury, infarction, and intracerebral hemorrhage: "to detect and protect". J Clin Neurophysiol. 2005;22:99–106.

Vespa PM, Miller C, McArthur D, Eliseo M, Etchepare M, Hirt D, Glenn TC, Martin N, Hovda D. Nonconvulsive electrographic seizures after traumatic brain injury result in a delayed, prolonged increase in intracranial pressure and metabolic crisis. Crit Care Med. 2007;35:2830–6.

Vespa PM, McArthur DL, Xu Y, Eliseo M, Etchepare M, Dinov I, Alger J, Glenn TP, Hovda D. Nonconvulsive seizures after traumatic brain injury are associated with hippocampal atrophy. Neurology. 2010;75(9):792–8 . PubMed PMID: 20805525; PubMed Central PMCID:PMC2938965. https://doi.org/10.1212/WNL.0b013e3181f07334.

Vespa P, Tubi M, Claassen J, Buitrago-Blanco M, McArthur D, Velazquez AG, Tu B, Prins M, Nuwer M. Metabolic crisis occurs with seizures and periodic discharges after brain trauma. Ann Neurol. 2016;79(4):579–90 . Epub 2016 Feb 28. PubMed PMID: 26814699. https://doi.org/10.1002/ana.24606.

Wang HC, Chang WN, Chang HW, Ho JT, Yang TM, Lin WC, Chuang YC, Lu CH. Factors predictive of outcome in posttraumatic seizures. J Trauma. 2008;64:883–8.

Young GB, Jordan KG, Doig GS. An assessment of nonconvulsive seizures in the intensive care unit using continuous EEG monitoring: an investigation of variables associated with mortality. Neurology. 1996;47:83–9.

49 Imaging of Severe Traumatic Brain Injury in the Neurointensive Care Unit

Leif Hovgaard Sørensen and Kent Gøran Moen

Recommendations

Level I

There is insufficient data to support a level I recommendation for this topic.

Level II

There is insufficient data to support a level II recommendation for this topic.

Level III

Non-contrast-enhanced computer tomography (NECT) is the preferred initial imaging modality in severe traumatic brain injury (TBI). Follow-up NECT should be based on results of the initial scan and clinical course instead of routine serial imaging.

Early clinical MRI is important for prognostication, and if practically possible, all patients with severe TBI should be examined with MRI within 2–4 weeks post injury.

When traumatic cerebrovascular injury is suspected, a CT angiography should be performed immediately.

49.1 Overview

In severe traumatic brain injury (TBI), imaging is mandatory for visualizing the degree of injury as well as the nature and location of the lesions in the acute phase and in later phases as well (Duhaime et al. 2010). Imaging is important in triaging patients for acute intervention, for follow-up, and for evaluation of the long-term outcome. In the acute phase, imaging with non-contrast-enhanced computer tomography (NECT) is still recommended as the most important modality. However, early clinical MRI is recommended during the first 2–4 weeks after a severe TBI, for a more detailed injury evaluation and for better prognostication and planning of rehabilitation. If a traumatic cerebrovascular injury is suspected, a CT angiography (CTA) should be performed immediately. Digital subtraction angiography (DSA) is first considered when a CTA is non-conclusive or if endovascular therapy (EVT) is indicated.

L. H. Sørensen (✉)
Department of Neuroradiology, Aarhus University Hospital, Aarhus, Denmark
e-mail: leisoere@rm.dk

K. G. Moen
Faculty of Medicine and Health Sciences, Department of Neuromedicine and Movement Science, Norwegian University of Science and Technology (NTNU), Trondheim, Norway

Department of Radiology, Nord-Trøndelag Hospital Trust, Levanger Hospital, Levanger, Norway
e-mail: kent.g.moen@ntnu.no

© Springer Nature Switzerland AG 2020
T. Sundstrøm et al. (eds.), *Management of Severe Traumatic Brain Injury*,
https://doi.org/10.1007/978-3-030-39383-0_49

Tips, Tricks, and Pitfalls

- NECT is still the primary imaging modality for severe TBI in the acute phase.
- Early follow-up NECT should be guided by the severity of the initial trauma, results of the initial NECT, and serial clinical examinations. Routine serial NECTs only have therapeutic consequences for a minority of the patients and seldom cause changes in treatment strategy.
- In severe TBI, a clinical MRI is recommended during the 2–4 first weeks after the injury.
- If a traumatic vascular injury is suspected, a CT angiography should be performed immediately. DSA should be reserved for cases where EVT is or may be indicated.
- Pitfalls
  - Not all acute extracerebral haematomas are of high density on CT: in severely anaemic patients and patients with disseminated intravascular coagulation, subdural (SDH) and epidural (EDH) haematoma can be iso- or hypodense relative to the brain.

49.2 Background

TBI is defined as an alteration in brain function, or other evidence of brain pathology, caused by an external force (Menon et al. 2010). TBI is a heterogeneous disease and span from primary to secondary pathologies (Saatman et al. 2008). The primary injury happens at the time of accident (i.e. focal contusions, haematomas, lacerations, fractures), while secondary pathologies develop over minutes, hours, or days after the primary impact (i.e. hypoxic/hypotensive injury, brain oedema, hydrocephalus, ischaemic lesions, secondary haemorrhages, infections, or leakage of cerebrospinal fluid). Secondary injuries are potentially reversible or preventable if triage and proper treatment is initiated. Dividing injuries in primary and secondary lesions is in many ways arbitrary, as TBI rather should be seen as a dynamic process (Gean and Fischbein 2010).

Today, NECT is still the primary imaging modality for TBI, due to widespread accessibility, compatibility with monitoring equipment, and fast scanning times with a quick clarification on whether neurosurgery is necessary or not. Findings in the acute NECT are also known to predict outcome in severe TBI (Englander et al. 2003; Nelson et al. 2010). NECT can precisely identify primary injuries and also early signs of secondary injuries. But clinical MRI has a higher sensitivity and specificity for detecting diffuse axonal injuries (DAI), lesions in the brainstem, non-haemorrhagic contusions, small extra-axial haematomas, and lesions adjacent to bony structures. Today's literature supports that all patients who have suffered a severe TBI should be imaged with a clinical MRI during 2–4 weeks post injury due to the prognostic value and the fact that NECT only shows "the tip of the iceberg" of all injuries after a TBI (Mutch et al. 2016; Cicuendez et al. 2018; Moen et al. 2014).

If a traumatic vascular injury is suspected, a CTA should be performed immediately since medical treatment should be initiated early and the indication for urgent DSA and possible acute EVT must be clarified (Brommeland et al. 2018).

49.2.1 Skull Radiographs in TBI

Skull radiographs give no additional information in the clinical management of acute TBI, and most trauma centres no longer use skull x-rays as a primary radiological modality since conventional radiographs cannot give precise information on the intracranial injury (Parizel et al. 2005). Even in the initial assessment of paediatric mild TBI, skull x-rays have been abandoned (Astrand et al. 2016). However, they are still used in some centres in suspected non-accidental injuries as a part of the skeletal survey (Mutch et al. 2016).

49.2.2 Initial and Serial Non-contrast Computer Tomography and Typical Findings in Severe TBI

NECT is still the primary initial imaging modality of choice in both moderate and severe TBI patients in the acute phase, due to rapid scanning times and efficient clarification of whether immediate neurosurgical intervention is necessary (Mutch et al. 2016; Parizel et al. 2005). NECT is also sensitive to skeletal injuries and foreign bodies and is today accessible 24/7 in most hospitals. Imaging findings from NECT have also shown to be useful in predicting clinical outcomes (Wintermark et al. 2015), and are important components in the IMPACT prognostic models (Steyerberg et al. 2008). If the clinical evaluation or initial scan suggests an ischaemic event or a spontaneous aneurysmal rupture, the NECT should be followed by an immediate CTA.

A cerebral contusion is a focal area of brain parenchymal disruption due to acute mechanical deformation. This is often due to impact of the brain parenchyma towards bony structures inside the skull, and the bulk of these lesions will frequently be against the surface of the brain. In NECT, cerebral contusions are reported in up to 35% of patients with severe TBI (Iaccarino et al. 2014). Cerebral contusions are classified as "coup" injuries when localized at the site of direct impact or "contrecoup" injuries when localized on the opposite surface of the brain (Hijaz et al. 2011). "Contrecoup" injuries are typically larger in size than the "coup" injuries (Lolli et al. 2016). Cerebral contusions can be haemorrhagic or non-haemorrhagic and often scattered with normal tissue in between. Traumatic parenchymal haemorrhage or intracerebral haemorrhage can sometimes be difficult to differ from cerebral contusions, but are often defined as a collection of confluent, relatively homogeneous blood within the brain parenchyma, typically with a more deep location in the brain. Cerebral contusions are most often located in the anteroinferior frontal and temporal lobes and gyri near the Sylvian fissures. Cerebral contusions may not be seen on the initial NECT, and follow-up scans are important if the patient deteriorates or after decompression of a mass lesion, since haemorrhagic contusions may grow significantly (Parizel et al. 2005).

Traumatic subarachnoid haemorrhage (tSAH) is seen in approximately 60–80% of severe TBI and is mainly located in sulci adjacent to contusions, but may also be found in the basal cisterns as in aneurysmal SAH (Fukuda et al. 1998). In these situations, it is important to find out whether the SAH is secondary to an aneurysm rupture or is a true tSAH by performing a cerebral CTA. The potential complications after tSAH are the same as for SAH following aneurysm rupture, such as vascular spasms and hydrocephalus.

Subdural haematoma (SDH) is a bleeding in the space between the dura and the arachnoid, most commonly after rupture of bridging veins. SDH is reported in 12–29% of severe TBI patients (Bullock et al. 2006). SDH can cross the cranial sutures but not dural attachments, and thus a SDH can never cross the midline. SDH is typically crescent shaped and hyperdense relative to the brain cortex in the acute phase (Kim and Gean 2011). At follow-up NECT after days to a few weeks, it becomes increasingly isodense with the cerebral cortex, and in weeks to months, it becomes hypodense and will eventually reach attenuation values close to cerebrospinal fluid. Subdural collections with different ages in one patient are not an uncommon finding (Fig. 49.1). Large SDHs with mass effect and midline shift are usually removed as soon as possible with a control NECT typically the following day. Small SDH with limited mass effect will often be treated conservatively, where follow-up scans must be considered due to risk of rebleeding or increment in size over time.

Epidural haematoma (EDH) is a bleeding between the skull and dura, most often from a lacerated meningeal artery, and is reported in up to 22% of severe TBI patients (Leitgeb et al. 2013). EDHs are nearly always associated with a skull fracture and most often seen in the frontotemporal regions. They are typically biconcave and do not cross cranial sutures but can cross the midline. In the acute phase, EDHs are hyperdense, but if NECT is performed in the hyperacute phase with an ongoing bleeding, the fresh blood will appear dark known as the "swirl sign" (Parizel et al. 2005). EDH can expand to a life-threatening size within a short time, and close observation is necessary with a liberal appreciation for follow-up NECT (Fig. 49.2).

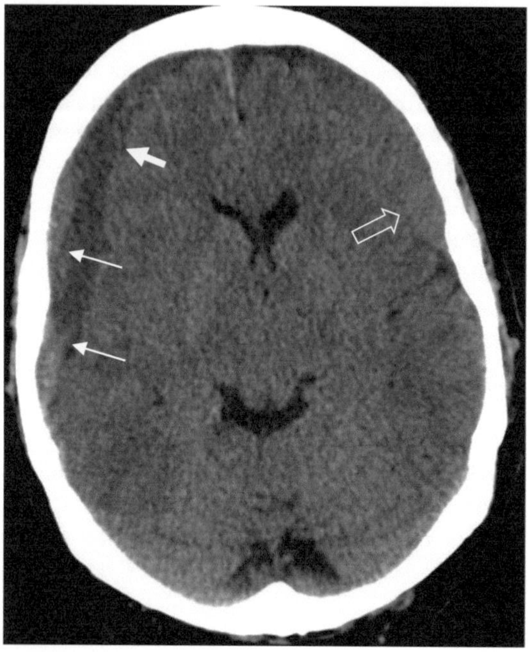

Fig. 49.1 NECT image showing subdural haematomas (SDHs) with different age with acute SDH (thin arrows), chronic SDH (fat arrow), and subacute SDH (open arrow)

Also remember that not all acute extracerebral haematomas are of high density on NECT: in severely anaemic patients and patients with disseminated intravascular coagulation, SDH or EDH can be iso- or hypodense relative to the brain.

Repeat head NECT is a standard practice for TBI patients at many trauma centres, but so far there is lack of consensus in the literature regarding indications and at what time point(s) the follow-up scans should be done (Wang et al. 2006). Instead of routinely performing serial NECT, it is recommended that follow-up imaging should be based on the results of the initial scan and the clinical course (Smith et al. 2007). Routine use of CT follow-up without a clear indication should be avoided, as transportation from the ICU will expose these often critically ill patients to a significant risk for complications like haemodynamic changes, desaturation, and increased intracranial pressure (Lee et al. 1997). A recent systematic review with subgroup analyses based on injury severity also concluded that repeat head NECT caused a change in management only for a

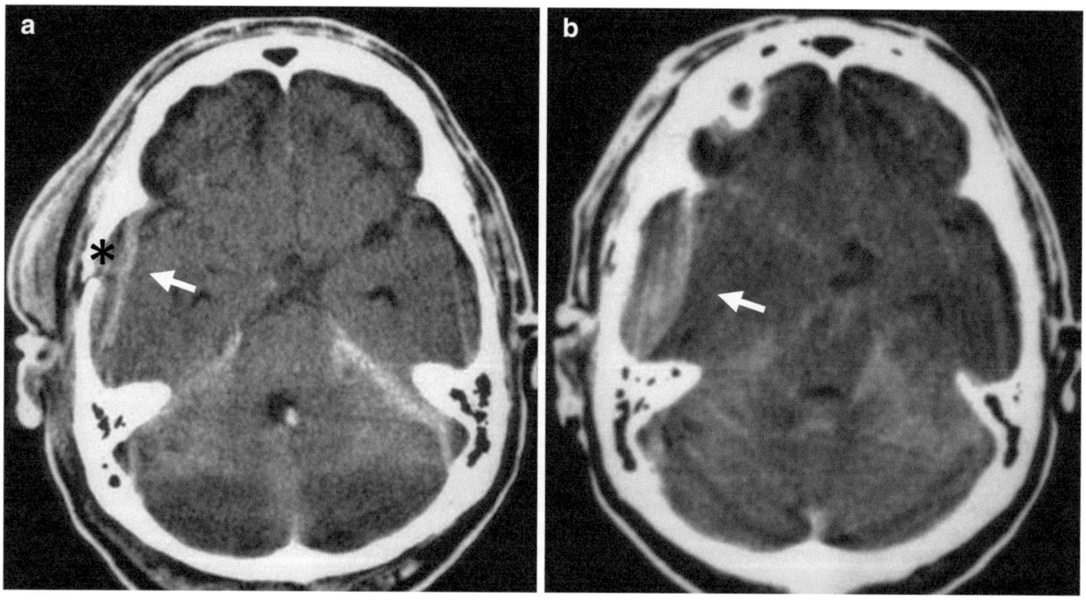

Fig. 49.2 Acute epidural haematoma (EDH), (**a**): NECT 35 min after injury. (**b**): NECT 10 min after the initial scan showing significantly increased size of the EDH. Also note the skull fracture (asterisk)

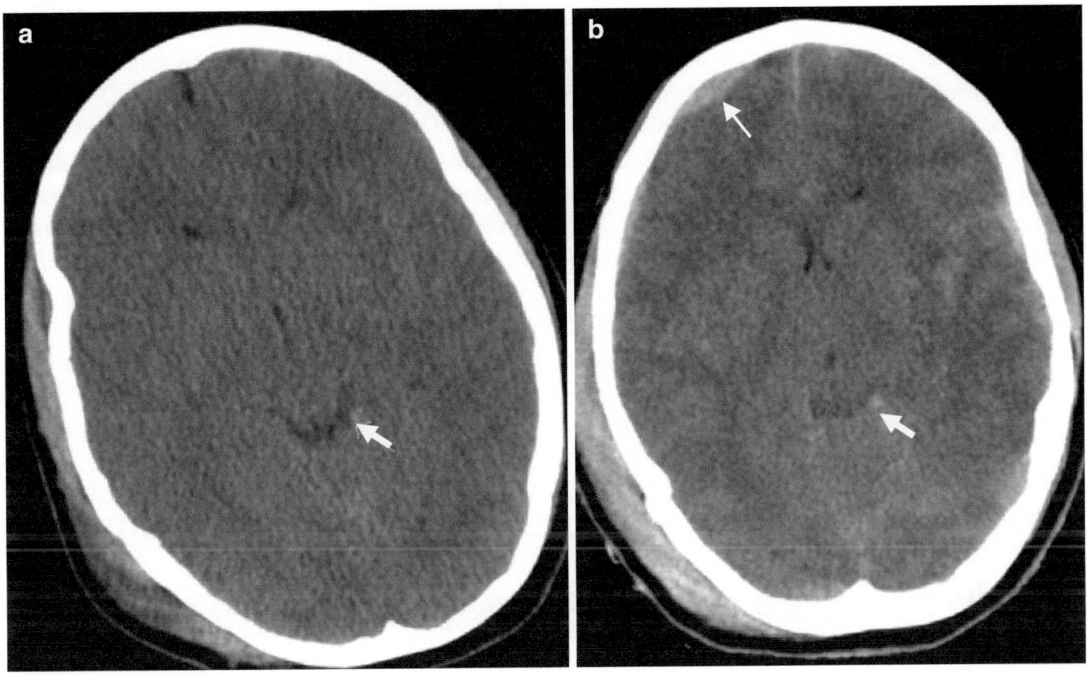

Fig. 49.3 (**a**) CT 1 h after a severe head injury. (**b**) 12 h later. The basal cistern is increasingly compressed (fat arrows). Note occurrence of a small EDH (thin arrow)

minority of the patients (Reljic et al. 2014), indicating that serial, predetermined NECT may not be as important as earlier thought. However, a follow-up scanning is mandatory whenever the clinical status of a TBI patient is worsening, as this might be due to increased intracranial pressure due to an expanding haematoma, increased cerebral oedema, development of hydrocephalus, or other conditions that might need urgent neurosurgical intervention (Fig. 49.3).

49.2.3 Computer Tomography Perfusion (CTP) in Severe TBI

CT perfusion (CTP) imaging is a bolus tracking technique, which can provide valuable information in the evaluation of tissue viability, as it can help to distinguish areas with preserved and impaired autoregulation. This technique has shown to predict long-term outcome in severe TBI and characterize traumatic ischaemic consequences or clarify differential diagnoses of ischaemic nature also with regard to guiding stroke therapy (Bendinelli et al. 2013). CTP can visualize both focal and diffuse brain injuries and help in the prediction of progressing brain contusions and outline areas of risk of secondary injuries (Soustiel et al. 2008). In cerebral contusions, cerebral blood flow (CBF) and cerebral blood volume (CBV) are typically low, while mean transit time (MTT) is significantly prolonged. For more details on CTP, we refer to Chap. 44 in this book (Fig. 44.1).

49.2.4 Clinical MRI and Timing of MRI in Severe TBI

Already in 1986, Jenkins et al. proved that even low-field MRI can visualize nearly twice as many abnormalities as NECT after TBI (Jenkins et al. 1986), e.g. DAI and small extra-axial collections. Because of a better spatial and contrast resolution, MRI is far more sensitive than NECT, especially in detection of DAI, lesions in the brainstem, non-haemorrhagic contusions, small extra-axial haematomas, and lesions adjacent to bony structures that can be obscured by bony artefacts on NECT (Parizel et al. 2005; Gentry 1994). MRI in general gives a better overview over all parenchymal injuries in the brain, where NECT sometimes is normal or only shows the "tip of the iceberg" of lesions (Fig. 49.4).

A clinical MRI protocol in TBI should at least consist of T1-weighted, T2-weighted (T2W), T2W fluid-attenuated inversion recovery (FLAIR), diffusion-weighted imaging (DWI), and T2∗ gradient echo (GRE) or SWI (susceptibility-weighted imaging) sequences. T2∗GRE and SWI are gradient echo sequences, both of which are sensitive for paramagnetic and diamagnetic substances, such as methaemoglobin, deoxyhaemoglobin, haemosiderin, and other blood products (Fig. 49.5).

SWI is a high-resolution, velocity-compensated, 3D gradient echo sequence based on both magnitude and phase data. SWI is highly sensitive and can reveal four to six times more microhaemorrhages than T2∗GRE, mainly because SWI include phase information (Gean and Fischbein 2010; Sehgal et al. 2005; Tong et al. 2003). FLAIR and DWI are sequences sensitive for depicting non-haemorrhagic lesions. The FLAIR sequence is a spin echo sequence where the high signal from the cerebrospinal fluid (CSF) is suppressed by use of long inversion time so that lesions adjacent to the CSF will be easier to detect (Ashikaga et al. 1997). White matter hyperintensities (WMHs) or non-haemorrhagic lesions depicted in FLAIR follow-

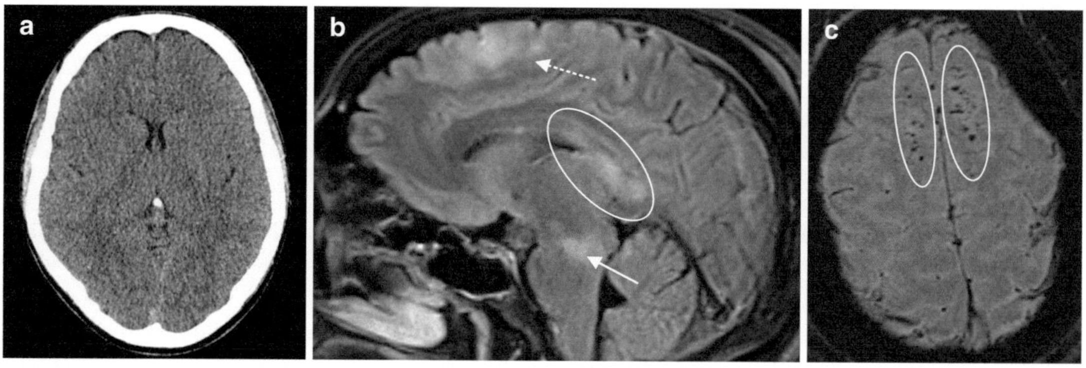

Fig. 49.4 A young male admitted with severe TBI after a road traffic accident. CT at admission (**a**) showed no trauma-related pathology, but early clinical MRI within 1 week after the injury showed extensive diffuse axonal injury, classified as grade 3. In the sagittal FLAIR sequence (**b**), hyperintense lesions are shown in the subcortical white matter (dashed arrow), in the corpus callosum (marked with ring), and in the mesencephalon (arrow). In the transversal SWI sequence (**c**), multiple microhaemorrhages are shown bifrontally (marked with rings)

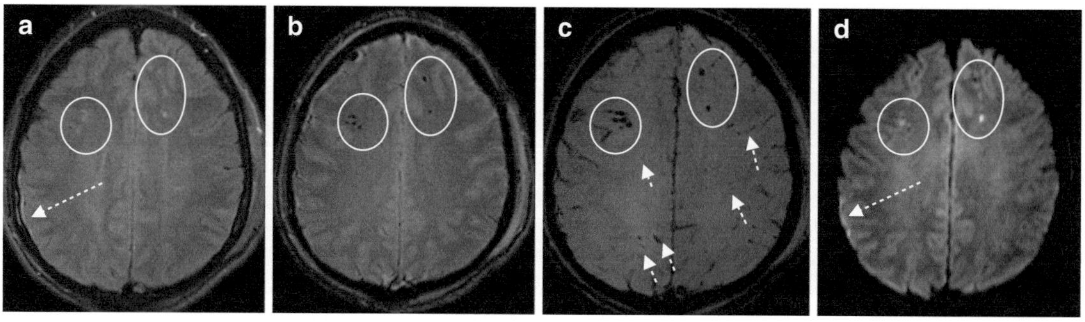

Fig. 49.5 MRI after a severe TBI with Glasgow Coma Scale score of 4. (**a**) T2 FLAIR image. (**b**) T2∗GRE image. (**c**) SWI image. (**d**) DWI image. DAI, which are visible on all of the shown MR sequences, are marked with rings. On the SWI image (**c**), additional DAI are marked with small arrows. Note the small SDH (dashed arrows) which was not visible on NECT

ing TBI, represent oedema in the acute stage and encephalomalacia or gliosis due to scarring in the chronic stage (Parizel et al. 2005). Diffusion-weighted imaging (DWI) is based on changes in the Brownian movements of water molecules in the brain, quantified by applying different amounts of diffusion weighting, thereby creating a map that indicates if there are areas in the brain with restricted or increased diffusion (Schaefer 2001). This method was first used in stroke imaging but has also shown to be important for prognostication in TBI (Huisman et al. 2003; Shakir et al. 2016). For more details on the clinical MRI protocol and details on the different sequences and prognostication, we refer to Chap. 85 in this book.

As mentioned, clinical MRI outperforms NECT in detection of parenchymal lesions, and clinical MRI has also for many years been recommended as the primary imaging modality in subacute and chronic stages of TBI due to this higher sensitivity (Parizel et al. 2005; Hesselink et al. 1988). However, clinical MRI has first been recommended when symptoms or findings could not be explained by the NECT. A recent systematic review concludes that early assessment of deep cerebral structures with MRI in moderate and severe TBI is important for prognostication (Haghbayan et al. 2017). Since some prognostically important lesions may disappear during the first weeks post injury, imaging in the early phase has been regarded important (Brandstack et al. 2006; Moen et al. 2012). Microhaemorrhagic lesions also to some degree attenuate in the chronic stages, even though one study suggests that lesions in SWI actually may grow between 1 and 7 days after the trauma (Toth et al. 2016). Due to these dynamic processes, recent studies indicate that if it is practically possible, a clinical MRI should routinely be performed within 2–4 weeks after the trauma in all patients with moderate to severe TBI (Mutch et al. 2016; Cicuendez et al. 2018; Moen et al. 2014). MRI has also shown to depict a significantly larger number of clinically meaningful lesions compared to NECT in the general ICU population (Algethamy et al. 2015). Besides the important prognostic role of an early MRI, there are also other important advantages: The TBI patient is typical young with hopefully many years ahead, they have injured the most important and complex organ in the body, and a thorough injury evaluation with the most optimal modality seems justified. An early MRI can contribute to a more tailored discharge planning and rehabilitation (Wintermark et al. 2015), give a more correct or precise diagnosis, and thus be important for economical/insurance issues. An early MRI will better explain symptoms, signs, and/or findings that cannot be clarified with NECT. Another advantage with MRI is the lack of ionizing radiation, opposed to NECT, which in particular is beneficial for this patient group with many young adults and children.

We acknowledge that early clinical MRI in ICU patients is demanding since it is difficult to observe and treat critically injured patients in the MR scanner. Even with modern equipment, MRI is more time-consuming than NECT; a complete whole body NECT can be completed in less than a minute. On the other hand, an MRI with all the relevant sequences will usually take between 30 and 45 min (Maas et al. 2017). This longer imaging time can be a significant problem in ICU patients. These patients often have equipment for monitoring and treatment, and to be able to perform early MRI, it is crucial that all equipment is MRI compatible. This also applies to other metallic foreign bodies (i.e. shrapnel), devices, or implants (i.e. old aneurysm clip and pacemakers). MRI is contraindicated until MRI compatibility is clarified. Early clinical MRI is challenging for the neuroanaesthesiologist, and imaging and accordingly time point for imaging must therefore be arranged in close collaboration.

49.2.5 Advanced MRI Methods and the Role of Artificial Intelligence (AI) in TBI

More advanced MRI techniques like MR spectroscopy, diffusion tensor imaging, diffusion kurtosis imaging, and functional MRI are seldom indicated in the acute or ICU phase of TBI and therefore not further described in this chapter. However, these techniques can be indicated in the subacute or chronic stages after TBI or in research protocols (Hunter et al. 2012; Hulkower et al. 2013). We refer to later chapters for more information on some of these techniques and their applicability in severe TBI.

In the future, also artificial intelligence (AI) will probably be more important in the image evaluation in TBI. Since AI methods currently are not routinely in use, they will not be further described, but methods are under development for both cerebral microbleeds (van den Heuvel et al. 2016) and white matter hyperintensities (Stone et al. 2016) in TBI research.

49.2.6 Traumatic Cerebrovascular Injuries and Endovascular Therapy (EVT) in Severe TBI

Traumatic cerebrovascular injuries are divided into blunt cerebrovascular injuries (BCVIs) and penetrating cerebrovascular injuries. The latter will not be further described in this chapter. BCVI has traditionally been considered as rare, but in severe TBI, the incidence is reported to be over 9% (Esnault et al. 2017). A recent clinical guideline suggests using the expanded Denver screening criteria (Geddes et al. 2016), and for those fulfilling these criteria, an immediate CT angiography (CTA) is recommended (Brommeland et al. 2018). CTA should be an option in all trauma centres, since it is fast and easy to perform. The scan should include carotid and vertebral arteries from the aortic arch through the base of the skull including the circle of Willis. If BCVI is shown in the CTA, early antithrombotic treatment is advised as soon as considered safe in addition to a re-examination with CTA at 7 days, either to confirm or to discard the diagnosis. The antithrombotic therapy should be continued for at least 3 months, and a final CTA control at 3 months should be performed. Further treatment will be individually dependent on the follow-up imaging.

In the above mentioned guideline, CTA is recommended as a screening tool since CTA detects almost all clinically significant BCVIs and very few strokes have been observed when CTA is normal. Catheter angiography or DSA is still considered the gold standard in BCVI, but it is impractical as a primary screening tool, since the expanded Denver criteria also make more patients eligible for imaging and DSA is time-consuming and only accessible at larger trauma centres and carries a higher risk for procedure-related complications (Brommeland et al. 2018). MRI technology and availability have also greatly improved over the last decades with a comparable sensitivity and specificity to CTA (Fig. 49.6). But MR angiography is too impractical and time-consuming as an initial screening tool in this patient group (Brommeland et al. 2018).

Arterial dissection is the most frequent cerebrovascular lesion after head and neck trauma followed by vascular transections, arteriovenous fistulas, formation of pseudoaneurysms, incarcerations with a vessel trapped between bony fragments, and thrombosis. Dissection is defined as an intramural haematoma mainly associated with an intimal tear allowing the arterial blood to pass under the intima and propagate distally resulting in stenosis, irregularity of the vessel lumen, and in some cases arterial dilatation (Zhao et al. 2007). On CTA and DSA, the typical dissection will present as a stenosis followed by a

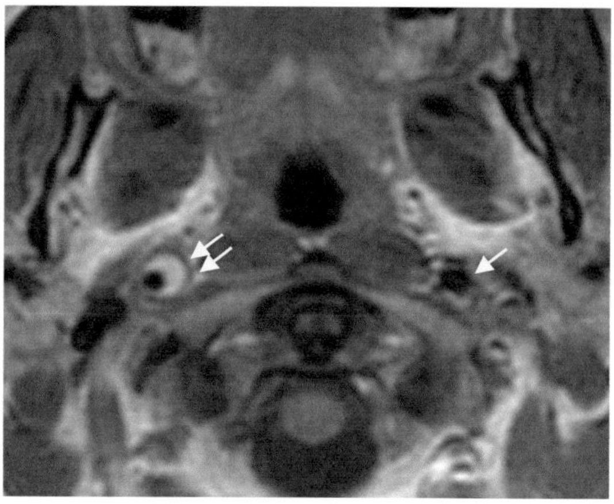

Fig. 49.6 Internal carotid artery (ICA) dissection. On this axial T1-weighted image, the false lumen is visible as a crescent-shaped, white structure (double arrow). The left ICA is normal (single arrow)

tapering of the vessel lumen. Sometimes an intimal flap indicating a true and a false lumen is visible. Traumatic arterial dissection will improve or resolve spontaneously in only 55% compared with 85% in spontaneous dissections (Sturzenegger 1995). There is a risk of total occlusion in 20% (Rao et al. 2011). The primary treatment is anticoagulation therapy in order to avoid thromboembolic complications. It is also important to preserve the patency of the vessel. Endovascular therapy (EVT) with stenting, vessel occlusion, or surgery is indicated in patients that remain symptomatic on medical therapy or where anticoagulation is contraindicated; the latter might be the case in trauma patients.

Traumatic aneurysms represent only 1% of all intracranial aneurysms (20% in paediatric cases) with internal carotid artery (ICA) aneurysms in the cavernous segment as the most frequent type, representing nearly 50%; they are often associated with skull base fractures (Krings et al. 2008). An aneurysm can give rise to compression of the cranial nerves running in the cavernous sinus – most often the abducens nerve, as it is located in the same compartment as ICA (Fig. 49.7).

If the aneurysm ruptures, it can give rise to a carotid-cavernous fistula (CC fistula), which is a direct communication between the intracavernous part of the ICA and the venous cavernous sinus. This can happen immediately or after a delay of days to weeks. The clinical findings are related to increased venous pressure with pulsating exophthalmos, vascular bruit, impaired motility of the eye, glaucoma, dilated veins, and chemosis. DSA can give the definitive diagnosis as it will show early opacification of the cavernous sinus and dilated draining veins. If an aneurysm ruptures into the sphenoid sinus, it can result in a life-threatening epistaxis (Fig. 49.8).

EVT is the preferred method in treatment of traumatic aneurysms. One possibility is trapping of the aneurysm using coils or balloons, thereby sacrificing the parent artery. This is an effective and fairly safe procedure, provided that there are sufficient collaterals. ICA aneurysms in the cavernous sinus can be treated using a closed stent, as that segment of ICA is without branches. A CC fistula may also be treated with EVT by placing coils or balloons in the fistula. If the embolic material cannot be placed safely, trapping of the fistula can treat the lesion.

49.3 Specific Paediatric Concerns

The general imaging recommendations indicated above are also valid in paediatric severe TBI. NECT is still regarded the modality of choice in the acute phase (Suskauer and Huisman 2009), even though there are some small studies

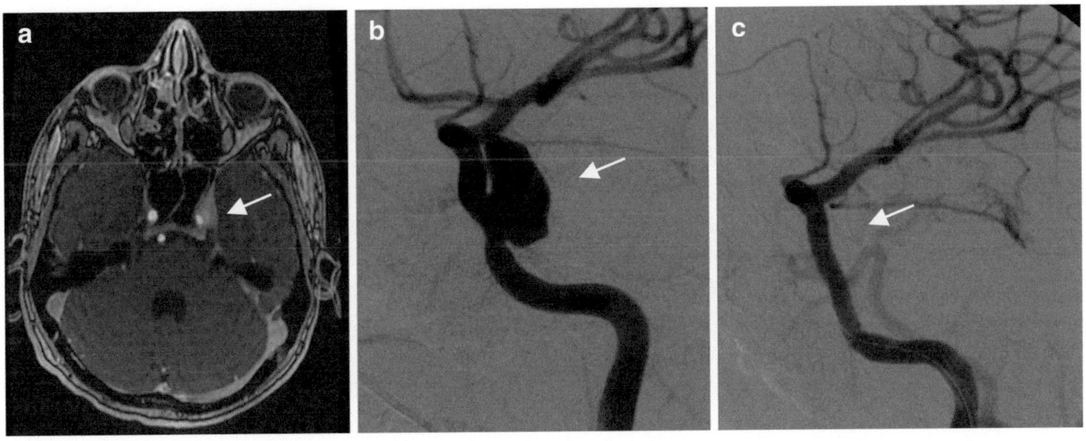

Fig. 49.7 Pseudoaneurysm following a severe TBI. The patient presented with right-sided abducens palsy. (**a**) MRA showing a pseudoaneurysm (arrow). (**b**) DSA before EVT and (**c**) after treatment with a closed stent. The patient is without any symptoms post stenting

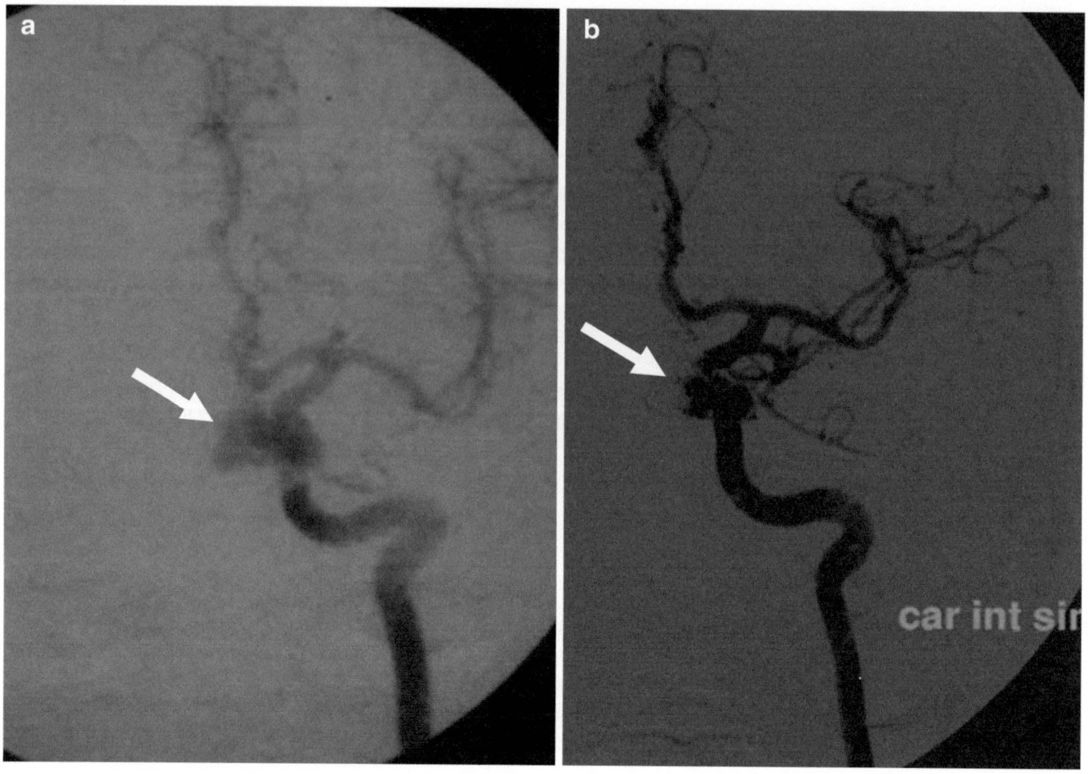

Fig. 49.8 A traumatic intracavernous aneurysm presenting with severe epistaxis 2 weeks after a traffic accident. (**a**) before EVT (arrow). (**b**) after coiling

with acute MRI in the paediatric TBI population without any clear recommendations (Cohen et al. 2015; Sheridan et al. 2017). A drawback regarding NECT is of course the radiation exposure in prone brains under development. When repeated scans are necessary, clinical MRI should be considered instead of NECT also in the ICU phase. Since early MRI is prognostically important in paediatric TBI (Smitherman et al. 2016), children with severe TBI are also recommended an early clinical MRI during the first weeks post injury. Since the incidence of BCVI in traumatized children is identical to that of the adult population, the extended Denver criteria are recommended also in the paediatric population, still with CTA as the primary screening modality (Brommeland et al. 2018).

References

Algethamy HM, Alzawahmah M, Young GB, Mirsattari SM. Added value of MRI over CT of the brain in intensive care unit patients. Can J Neurol Sci. 2015;42(5):324–32.

Ashikaga R, Araki Y, Ishida O. MRI of head injury using FLAIR. Neuroradiology. 1997;39(4):239–42.

Astrand R, Rosenlund C, Unden J, Scandinavian Neurotrauma C. Scandinavian guidelines for initial management of minor and moderate head trauma in children. BMC medicine. 2016;14:33.

Bendinelli C, Bivard A, Nebauer S, Parsons MW, Balogh ZJ. Brain CT perfusion provides additional useful information in severe traumatic brain injury. Injury. 2013;44(9):1208–12.

Brandstack N, Kurki T, Tenovuo O, Isoniemi H. MR imaging of head trauma: visibility of contusions and other intraparenchymal injuries in early and late stage. Brain Inj. 2006;20(4):409–16.

Brommeland T, Helseth E, Aarhus M, Moen KG, Dyrskog S, Bergholt B, et al. Best practice guidelines for blunt cerebrovascular injury (BCVI). Scand J Trauma Resusc Emerg Med. 2018;26(1):90.

Bullock MR, Chesnut R, Ghajar J, Gordon D, Hartl R, Newell DW, et al. Surgical management of acute subdural hematomas. Neurosurgery. 2006;58(3 Suppl):S16–24; discussion Si-iv.

Cicuendez M, Castano-Leon A, Ramos A, Hilario A, Gomez PA, Lagares A. The added prognostic value of magnetic resonance imaging in traumatic brain injury: The importance of traumatic axonal injury when performing ordinal logistic regression. J Neuroradiol. 2018;46(5):299–306.

Cohen AR, Caruso P, Duhaime AC, Klig JE. Feasibility of "rapid" magnetic resonance imaging in pediatric acute head injury. Am J Emerg Med. 2015;33(7):887–90.

Duhaime AC, Gean AD, Haacke EM, Hicks R, Wintermark M, Mukherjee P, et al. Common data elements in radiologic imaging of traumatic brain injury. Arch Phys Med Rehabil. 2010;91(11):1661–6.

Englander J, Cifu DX, Wright JM, Black K. The association of early computed tomography scan findings and ambulation, self-care, and supervision needs at rehabilitation discharge and at 1 year after traumatic brain injury. Arch Phys Med Rehabil. 2003;84(2):214–20.

Esnault P, Cardinale M, Boret H, D'Aranda E, Montcriol A, Bordes J, et al. Blunt cerebrovascular injuries in severe traumatic brain injury: incidence, risk factors,and evolution. J Neurosurg. 2017;127(1):16–22.

Fukuda T, Hasue M, Ito H. Does traumatic subarachnoid hemorrhage caused by diffuse brain injury cause delayed ischemic brain damage? Comparison with subarachnoid hemorrhage caused by ruptured intracranial aneurysms. Neurosurgery. 1998;43(5):1040–9.

Gean AD, Fischbein NJ. Head trauma. Neuroimaging Clin N Am. 2010;20(4):527–56.

Geddes AE, Burlew CC, Wagenaar AE, Biffl WL, Johnson JL, Pieracci FM, et al. Expanded screening criteria for blunt cerebrovascular injury: a bigger impact than anticipated. Am J Surg. 2016;212(6):1167–74.

Gentry LR. Imaging of closed head injury. Radiology. 1994;191(1):1–17.

Haghbayan H, Boutin A, Laflamme M, Lauzier F, Shemilt M, Moore L, et al. The prognostic value of MRI in moderate and severe traumatic brain injury: a systematic review and meta-analysis. Crit Care Med. 2017;45(12):e1280–e8.

Hesselink JR, Dowd CF, Healy ME, Hajek P, Baker LL, Luerssen TG. MR imaging of brain contusions: a comparative study with CT. AJR AmJRoentgenol. 1988;150(5):1133–42.

Hijaz TA, Cento EA, Walker MT. Imaging of head trauma. Radiol Clin North Am. 2011;49(1):81–103.

Huisman TA, Sorensen AG, Hergan K, Gonzalez RG, Schaefer PW. Diffusion-weighted imaging for the evaluation of diffuse axonal injury in closed head injury. J Comput Assist Tomogr. 2003;27(1):5–11.

Hulkower MB, Poliak DB, Rosenbaum SB, Zimmerman ME, Lipton ML. A decade of DTI in traumatic brain injury: 10 years and 100 articles later. AJNR Am J Neuroradiol. 2013;34(11):2064–74.

Hunter JV, Wilde EA, Tong KA, Holshouser BA. Emerging imaging tools for use with traumatic brain injury research. J Neurotrauma. 2012;29(4):654–71.

Iaccarino C, Schiavi P, Picetti E, Goldoni M, Cerasti D, Caspani M, et al. Patients with brain contusions: predictors of outcome and relationship between radiological and clinical evolution. J Neurosurg. 2014;120(4):908–18.

Jenkins A, Teasdale G, Hadley MD, Macpherson P, Rowan JO. Brain lesions detected by magnetic resonance imaging in mild and severe head injuries. Lancet. 1986;2(8504):445–6.

Kim JJ, Gean AD. Imaging for the diagnosis and management of traumatic brain injury. Neurotherapeutics. 2011;8(1):39–53.

Krings T, Geibprasert S, Lasjaunias PL. Cerebrovascular trauma. Eur Radiol. 2008;18(8):1531–45.

Lee TT, Aldana PR, Kirton OC, Green BA. Follow-up computerized tomography (CT) scans in moderate and severe head injuries: correlation with Glasgow Coma Scores (GCS), and complication rate. Acta Neurochir (Wien). 1997;139(11):1042–7; discussion 7-8.

Leitgeb J, Mauritz W, Brazinova A, Majdan M, Wilbacher I. Outcome after severe brain trauma associated with epidural hematoma. Arch Orthop Trauma Surg. 2013;133(2):199–207.

Lolli V, Pezzullo M, Delpierre I, Sadeghi N. MDCT imaging of traumatic brain injury. Br J Radiol. 2016;89(1061):20150849.

Maas AIR, Menon DK, Adelson PD, Andelic N, Bell MJ, Belli A, et al. Traumatic brain injury: integrated approaches to improve prevention, clinical care, and research. Lancet Neurol. 2017;16(12):987–1048.

Menon DK, Schwab K, Wright DW, Maas AI, Demographics, Clinical Assessment Working Group of the I, et al. Position statement: definition of traumatic brain injury. Arch Phys Med Rehabil. 2010;91(11):1637–40.

Moen KG, Skandsen T, Folvik M, Brezova V, Kvistad KA, Rydland J, et al. A longitudinal MRI study of traumatic axonal injury in patients with moderate and severe traumatic brain injury. J Neurol Neurosurg Psychiatry. 2012;83(12):1193–200.

Moen KG, Brezova V, Skandsen T, Haberg AK, Folvik M, Vik A. Traumatic axonal injury: the prognostic value of lesion load in corpus callosum, brain stem, and thalamus in different magnetic resonance imaging sequences. J Neurotrauma. 2014;31(17):1486–96.

Mutch CA, Talbott JF, Gean A. Imaging evaluation of acute traumatic brain injury. Neurosurg Clin N Am. 2016;27(4):409–39.

Nelson DW, Nystrom H, MacCallum RM, Thornquist B, Lilja A, Bellander BM, et al. Extended analysis of early computed tomography scans of traumatic

brain injured patients and relations to outcome. J Neurotrauma. 2010;27(1):51–64.
Parizel PM, Van Goethem JW, Ozsarlak O, Maes M, Phillips CD. New developments in the neuroradiological diagnosis of craniocerebral trauma. Eur Radiol. 2005;15(3):569–81.
Rao AS, Makaroun MS, Marone LK, Cho JS, Rhee R, Chaer RA. Long-term outcomes of internal carotid artery dissection. J Vasc Surg. 2011;54(2):370–4; discussion 5.
Reljic T, Mahony H, Djulbegovic B, Etchason J, Paxton H, Flores M, et al. Value of repeat head computed tomography after traumatic brain injury: systematic review and meta-analysis. J Neurotrauma. 2014;31(1):78–98.
Saatman KE, Duhaime AC, Bullock R, Maas AI, Valadka A, Manley GT. Classification of traumatic brain injury for targeted therapies. J Neurotrauma. 2008;25(7):719–38.
Schaefer PW. Applications of DWI in clinical neurology. J Neurol Sci. 2001;186(Suppl 1):S25–35.
Sehgal V, Delproposto Z, Haacke EM, Tong KA, Wycliffe N, Kido DK, et al. Clinical applications of neuroimaging with susceptibility-weighted imaging. J Magn Reson Imaging. 2005;22(4):439–50.
Shakir A, Aksoy D, Mlynash M, Harris OA, Albers GW, Hirsch KG. Prognostic value of quantitative diffusion-weighted MRI in patients with traumatic brain injury. J Neuroimaging. 2016;26(1):103–8.
Sheridan DC, Newgard CD, Selden NR, Jafri MA, Hansen ML. Quick brain MRI for the detection of acute pediatric traumatic brain injury. J Neurosurg Pediatr. 2017;19(2):259–64.
Smith JS, Chang EF, Rosenthal G, Meeker M, von Koch C, Manley GT, et al. The role of early follow-up computed tomography imaging in the management of traumatic brain injury patients with intracranial hemorrhage. J Trauma. 2007;63(1):75–82.
Smitherman E, Hernandez A, Stavinoha PL, Huang R, Kernie SG, Diaz-Arrastia R, et al. Predicting outcome after pediatric traumatic brain injury by early magnetic resonance imaging lesion location and volume. J Neurotrauma. 2016;33(1):35–48.
Soustiel JF, Mahamid E, Goldsher D, Zaaroor M. Perfusion-CT for early assessment of traumatic cerebral contusions. Neuroradiology. 2008;50(2):189–96.
Steyerberg EW, Mushkudiani N, Perel P, Butcher I, Lu J, McHugh GS, et al. Predicting outcome after traumatic brain injury: development and international validation of prognostic scores based on admission characteristics. PLoS Med. 2008;5(8):e165; discussion e.
Stone JR, Wilde EA, Taylor BA, Tate DF, Levin H, Bigler ED, et al. Supervised learning technique for the automated identification of white matter hyperintensities in traumatic brain injury. Brain Inj. 2016;30(12):1458–68.
Sturzenegger M. Spontaneous internal carotid artery dissection: early diagnosis and management in 44 patients. J Neurol. 1995;242(4):231–8.
Suskauer SJ, Huisman TA. Neuroimaging in pediatric traumatic brain injury: current and future predictors of functional outcome. Dev Disabil Res Rev. 2009;15(2):117–23.
Tong KA, Ashwal S, Holshouser BA, Shutter LA, Herigault G, Haacke EM, et al. Hemorrhagic shearing lesions in children and adolescents with posttraumatic diffuse axonal injury: improved detection and initial results. Radiology. 2003;227(2):332–9.
Toth A, Kovacs N, Tamas V, Kornyei B, Nagy M, Horvath A, et al. Microbleeds may expand acutely after traumatic brain injury. Neurosci Lett. 2016;617:207–12.
van den Heuvel TL, van der Eerden AW, Manniesing R, Ghafoorian M, Tan T, Andriessen TM, et al. Automated detection of cerebral microbleeds in patients with traumatic brain Injury. Neuroimage Clin. 2016;12:241–51.
Wang MC, Linnau KF, Tirschwell DL, Hollingworth W. Utility of repeat head computed tomography after blunt head trauma: a systematic review. J Trauma. 2006;61(1):226–33.
Wintermark M, Sanelli PC, Anzai Y, Tsiouris AJ, Whitlow CT. Imaging evidence and recommendations for traumatic brain injury: conventional neuroimaging techniques. J Am Coll Radiol. 2015;12(2):e1–14.
Zhao WY, Krings T, Alvarez H, Ozanne A, Holmin S, Lasjaunias P. Management of spontaneous haemorrhagic intracranial vertebrobasilar dissection: review of 21 consecutive cases. Acta Neurochir (Wien). 2007;149(6):585–96; discussion 96.

Serum Protein Biomarkers in the Management of Severe Traumatic Brain Injury

50

Eric Peter Thelin, David W. Nelson, Johan Undén, Ramona Åstrand, and Bo-Michael Bellander

Recommendations

Level I

There is insufficient data to support Level 1 recommendations for this topic.

Level II

Retrospective and prospective clinical studies, using S100B in the management of severe traumatic brain injury (TBI), have indicated a robust capability to monitor ongoing injury and to predict

E. P. Thelin (✉)
Department of Clinical Neuroscience, Karolinska Institutet, Stockholm, Sweden

Division of Neurosurgery, Department of Clinical Neurosciences, University of Cambridge, Cambridge, UK
e-mail: Eric.thelin@ki.se

D. W. Nelson
Department of Physiology and Pharmacology, Section of Perioperative Medicine and Intensive Care, Karolinska Institutet, Stockholm, Sweden
e-mail: david.nelson@ki.se

J. Undén
Department of Anaesthesia and Intensive Care, Hallands Hospital, Halmstad, Sweden

Department of Operation and Intensive Care, Hallands Hospital, Halmstad, Sweden

Lund University, Lund, Sweden

R. Åstrand
Department of Neurosurgery, Rigshospitalet, Copenhagen University Hospital, Copenhagen, Denmark

B.-M. Bellander
Department of Clinical Neuroscience, Karolinska Institutet, Stockholm, Sweden

Department of Neurosurgery, Karolinska University Hospital, Stockholm, Sweden
e-mail: bo-michael.bellander@sll.se

© Springer Nature Switzerland AG 2020
T. Sundstrøm et al. (eds.), *Management of Severe Traumatic Brain Injury*,
https://doi.org/10.1007/978-3-030-39383-0_50

outcome. Furthermore, there is evidence from prospective trials of improved outcome prediction using glial fibrillary acidic protein (GFAP), ubiquitin carboxy-terminal hydrolase L1 (UCH-L1), neuron-specific enolase (NSE), and neurofilament light (NF-L) in the management of severe TBI.

Level III

Several other protein biomarkers show encouraging results in outcome prediction and injury stratification and to monitor injury processes and may thus act as a secondary endpoint to determine clinical efficacy in clinical trials, but more controlled, prospective, and randomized trials are needed.

Tips, Tricks, and Pitfalls

- Serum levels of protein biomarkers are potent outcome predictors - but kinetics are important, as first day samples are usually stronger in outcome models.
- Serial sampling of protein biomarkers in neurocritical care TBI patients act as a global marker for novel brain lesions.
- While brain enriched, some proteins like S100B and UCH-L1 seem to be released from extracranial tissues as well.
- A panel of brain biomarkers increases outcome prediction - use markers of different cellular origin and temporal dynamics.

50.1 Overview

Traumatic brain injury (TBI) is one of the most common causes of death and acquired disability, increasing in frequency worldwide causing vast burdens on the affected as well as on society (Hyder et al. 2007; Roozenbeek et al. 2013). The mainstay diagnostics for admitted severe TBI patients remains to be radiological imaging, preferably computerized tomography (CT), to rule out space-occupying mass lesions which may require surgical evacuation. While current TBI guidelines exist (Carney et al. 2017), they provide little solid evidence as how to monitor the brain, and there are few metrics used apart from intracranial pressure (ICP) monitoring. The ongoing pathophysiology in the aftermath of severe TBI is complex, and development of secondary injuries is common. Additional methods, such as partial brain oxygen pressure and microdialysis catheters only monitor focal brain regions and measurements from them, which may be difficult to extrapolate to the entire brain. Because of this, there is a need for more readily available objective markers of brain tissue fate after severe TBI, in order to predict injury severity and functional outcome, monitor deterioration, and determine treatment efficacy.

50.2 Background

Organ-enriched proteins as markers of tissue fate ("biomarkers") in serum are used in several medical specialties, such as cardiology (troponin) and gastroenterology (pancreas amylase). Similarly, by measuring proteins in serum that are specifically brain enriched, i.e., not present to any greater extent in other tissues, one could in theory assess the amount of brain parenchyma that is affected following TBI. Unlike focal monitors, brain biomarkers are "global" monitors and are currently not able to discriminate where in the CNS the injury is located, other than that of different cellular origins and possibly lesion types. However, this lack of regional specificity may be mitigated by their sensitivity to capture lesion development.

Leading authors in the field have identified the desired properties of an ideal brain biomarker (Bakay and Ward 1983; Kleindienst et al. 2007; Papa et al. 2008), e.g., a passive release from the injured central nervous system (CNS) to blood, an unlimited passage through the blood-brain barrier, the ability to demonstrate both sensitivity and specificity for CNS injury, a lack of effect on cells in the

CNS, and a rapid appearance in accessible biological fluids. Currently in the biomarker literature, none of the introduced candidates fulfill all proposed criteria. However, extensive research in the last decade has greatly increased the understanding of these proteins and improved their clinical utility (Thelin et al. 2016a, 2017a; Brophy et al. 2011). Because of this, several protein biomarker candidates have been introduced and are currently used locally in the management of TBI patients.

In severe TBI, there are several areas where biomarkers could be of use, including when differentiating between different types of injury, patient stratification in trials, detecting and monitoring secondary injury when sampling the biomarker serially, outcome prediction, as well as acting as a surrogate endpoint in drug trials where higher levels would assume more affected brain tissue. All these areas will be addressed in this chapter for the clinically most used protein biomarkers today. While some of these proteins have been shown to provide relevant information if measured in cerebrospinal fluid, this chapter will focus exclusively on the utility of serum levels. However, serum levels are more likely to be influenced by extracranial injuries, especially in poly-/multitrauma situations, which will be highlighted. A summary of some characteristics for the biomarkers presented in this chapter is available in Table 50.1.

Table 50.1 An overview of the protein biomarkers presented in this chapter and some of their characteristics

Protein biomarker	Predominant cellular origin in the central nervous system	Other tissue expressing protein (according to the Human Protein Atlas) (Sjostedt et al. 2015)	Estimated effective serum half-life in severe TBI (Thelin et al. 2017a)	Properties as a biomarker in moderate-to-severe TBI
S100B	Perivascular astrocytes	Colon (ganglion), breast (myoepithelial cells), adipose tissue, peripheral nerves, skin	About 24 h	– Most studied protein biomarker in TBI – Extracranial contribution in serum early after injury – Rapid clinical assays available
NSE	Neurons	Pancreas (islets of Langerhans), erythrocytes, colon (ganglion), peripheral nerves	About 48 h	– Well-studied biomarker – Hemolysis in sample should be adjusted for (as well as extracranial trauma) – Rapid clinical assays available
GFAP	Astrocyte cytoskeleton	Not detected	About 48 h	– Brain-enriched biomarker – Lacks rapid clinical assays
UCH-L1	Neurons	Pancreas (islets of Langerhans), colon (ganglion), kidney, testis, peripheral nerves	About 10 h	– Few studies – Lacks rapid clinical assays
NF-L	Neurons and axons	Not detected	>2 weeks	– Few studies – Seem to present a different pathophysiology with constantly increasing levels – Lacks rapid clinical assays

50.3 Clinically Used Protein Biomarkers in TBI

50.3.1 S100B

S100B is a relatively small protein (9–14 kDa) primarily present in perivascular astrocytes in the CNS. It belongs to a family of intracellular, calcium-binding proteins and has a range of intra- and extracellular properties, both potentially beneficial and detrimental (Donato et al. 2009). S100B is used as a marker for malignant melanoma treatment efficacy (Egberts et al. 2009), but has attracted a lot of interest for its role as a screening tool to rule out lesions in mild TBI (Unden et al. 2013) and is the most studied protein biomarker in severe TBI in terms of publications.

50.3.1.1 Extracranial Contribution

The protein S100B is extensively expressed by non-CNS tissue; S100B mRNA is expressed only 1.44 times more in the cerebral cortex than in adipose tissue (Sjostedt et al. 2015) but also expressed in cells such as chondrocytes, Schwann cells, melanocytes, and myocytes (Haimoto et al. 1987). This is probably why trauma patients without brain injury also may have high serum levels of S100B (Unden et al. 2005a; Anderson et al. 2001; Thelin et al. 2016b; Pfortmueller et al. 2016). However, it has been shown that the extracerebral contribution of S100B is relatively low (Pham et al. 2010) and likely affects the total levels of S100B primarily the first 12 h after injury (Thelin et al. 2016a).

50.3.1.2 Outcome Prediction

In a systematic review article from 2013 (Mercier et al. 2013), it was concluded that S100B was associated with outcome in TBI, but that adequate cutoff levels to discriminate mortality/unfavorable outcome were difficult to determine. Research from our own group shows similar results (Thelin et al. 2013, 2016a), but also highlights that the predictive accuracy of S100B varies significantly over time after brain trauma. Levels acquired in the range of 12–36 h after trauma exhibit a clearly increased correlation with outcome, as compared to earlier levels (Thelin et al. 2016a). Presumably, but not decisively, this is due to an influence of the extracranial contribution early after trauma and a better discrimination between patients with and without secondary brain injury development at about 24 h post trauma (Thelin et al. 2017b).

50.3.1.3 Serial Sampling to Monitor Secondary Injury Development

Serial sampling of S100B is often performed in studies of NCCU TBI patients. The true serum half-life of S100B is relatively short; in post-cardiac surgery patients, the half-life has been shown to be as short as 25 min (Jonsson et al. 2000). This contrasts severe TBI patients, where the assumed ongoing injury and multi-compartmental release results in a slow release and an effective half-life of about 24 h (excluding that sampled immediately after trauma) (Thelin et al. 2017a). Studies have shown that serial sampling of S100B is useful to detect any secondary lesion development in patients with severe TBI (Thelin et al. 2014; Unden et al. 2007; Korfias et al. 2007; Raabe et al. 2004; Raabe and Seifert 1999; Olivecrona et al. 2015). In a cohort of $n = 250$ NCCU TBI patients, it was found that if S100B is sampled every 12 h, a secondary increase of even 0.05 μg/L is 89% specific and 80% sensitive of CNS lesion development on future CT scans (Thelin et al. 2014). This could not be detected using conventional NCCU monitoring. Similarly, Raabe et al. found in a cohort of severe TBI and SAH patients that in 21% of cases, a secondary increase of S100B was the first sign of developing neurological complications, prompting further diagnostic work-up (Raabe et al. 2004).

50.3.1.4 Injury Differentiation

Different intracranial lesions result in different temporal profiles of S100B in serum (Herrmann et al. 2000). The highest levels of S100B are seen in large parenchymal lesions or damages where more brain is affected, as well as in escalating contusion size (Thelin et al. 2013; Herrmann et al. 2000; Raabe et al. 1998). In comparison, epidural hematomas and diffuse axonal injury with limited parenchymal involvement usually present with limited levels (Unden et al. 2005b; Ljungqvist et al. 2017). S100B has also been shown to be associated with higher degree of disruption of functional resting-state connectivity measured using functional magnetic resonance imaging (fMRI) (Thompson et al. 2016). Moreover, it has been shown that higher Rotterdam (Maas et al. 2005) and Stockholm (Nelson et al. 2010) computerized tomography (CT) scores are related to higher levels of S100B (Thelin et al. 2016a), exemplifying its utility as a marker for injury differentiation.

50.3.1.5 Surrogate Endpoint in Clinical Studies

Studies have investigated S100B as a secondary endpoint metric (i.e., as a marker of brain tissue fate). For example, in two randomized trials of erythropoietin (EPO), TBI patients in one trial showed lower levels in the treatment group as compared to placebo, indicative of the treatment efficacy (Li et al. 2016), while the other did not show any significant difference between treatment groups (Nirula et al. 2010). These studies corroborated biomarker levels with the functional outcome reported by the studies. This suggests possible utility for S100B to act as a surrogate endpoint for treatment efficacy in clinical trials.

50.3.2 Neuron-Specific Enolase (NSE)

NSE is a 46 kDa phosphopyruvate hydratase, an enzyme of glycolysis, present in, among other cells, the neuronal soma. Apart from being used to assess the severity of TBI, it is also a marker for neuro-endocrinal tumors and is a metric to assess outcome following cardiac arrest (Cronberg et al. 2011; Herman et al. 1989). It is the second most studied biomarker in severe TBI following S100B.

Despite its name, NSE is expressed not only in neurons, but to a large extent in other tissues, such as endocrine and gastro-intestinal (Sjostedt et al. 2015). In TBI patients, extracranial injuries have been shown to influence levels of NSE up to 48 h post trauma (Thelin et al. 2016a). Another extracranial source of NSE is erythrocytes, and hemolysis may complicate interpretation in clinical scenarios as it leads to increasing levels of NSE in serum (Gao et al. 1997; Johnsson et al. 2000). An equation, involving red blood cell count and free hemoglobin, has been suggested in order to adjust for the "false" increase contributed by hemolysis (Tolan et al. 2013), but modern clinical assays usually discard the sample if the free hemoglobin levels have increased above a certain threshold (Rundgren et al. 2014).

50.3.2.1 Outcome Prediction

In a systematic review article from 2016, it was concluded that serum NSE levels were associated with outcome and mortality in TBI; however no clear thresholds could be identified (Mercier et al. 2016). Furthermore, outcome prediction seems less sensitive by the timing of sampling after trauma (at least within 48 h after TBI) (Thelin et al. 2016a), as compared to S100B. Moreover, if NSE is added to multivariable outcome prediction models also including S100B, it provides limited additional information (Thelin et al. 2016a), suggesting that, despite their differing cellular origins, they represent a similar pathophysiology.

50.3.2.2 Serial Sampling to Monitor Secondary Injury Development

The effective serum half-life of NSE is longer than for S100B, suggested to be 30 h in extracorporeal circulation patients without ongoing brain injury (Johnsson et al. 2000). In moderate-to-severe TBI patients, where there might be a continued release of NSE from the injured brain, a systematic review indicated that the effective half-life is somewhere closer to 48 h (Thelin et al. 2017a). This makes it more difficult to correlate secondary increases of NSE with imminent neurological deterioration. However, patients with secondary brain injuries have been shown to present more increasing trajectories of NSE in serum (Woertgen et al. 1997; McKeating et al. 1998), but there is still insufficient data to suggest a threshold for secondary injury development.

50.3.2.3 Injury Differentiation

Different trajectories have been suggested for different types of intracranial pathologies (Herrmann et al. 2000), with more elevated levels in more "diffuse" injuries as classified by Marshall CT classification (Raabe et al. 1998; McKeating et al. 1998; Marshall et al. 1991). We have shown that with escalating levels of intracranial severity, based on Rotterdam and Stockholm CT scoring systems, NSE significantly increases, albeit this was not as robust as with S100B (Thelin et al. 2016a).

50.3.2.4 Surrogate Endpoint in Clinical Studies

Similar to S100B, NSE has been used as a surrogate marker of treatment effect in both trials of EPO and saline dextran fluid resuscitation (vs. crystalloid fluids) (Li et al. 2016; Baker et al. 2009), suggesting its utility as a marker of brain tissue fate in TBI trials.

50.3.3 Glial Fibrillary Acidic Protein (GFAP)

GFAP is an intermediate filament protein (50–55 kDa), present almost exclusively in astrocytes in the adult CNS. Except for brain injury research and management, there are no other current areas of serum GFAP levels in clinical medicine.

50.3.3.1 Extracranial Contribution

GFAP is one of the most brain-enriched proteins, expressing mRNA levels in cortex that are 374.81 times more common in the brain compared to the second most enriched tissue (adipose tissue) (Sjostedt et al. 2015). However, studies have shown that both severe and mild TBI patients with extracranial trauma exhibit increased levels of GFAP in blood compared to isolated TBI patients (Papa et al. 2014; Pelinka et al. 2004), supported by a recent study that indicated elevated levels in orthopedic trauma patients (Posti et al. 2017). Nevertheless, the extracranial contribution seems limited if compared with S100B and NSE.

50.3.3.2 Outcome Prediction

According to a meeting abstract from 2012 presenting a systematic review of 7 studies (Laroche et al. 2012), higher levels of GFAP are associated with less favorable outcome. More recent prospective studies have shown similar results (Takala et al. 2016; Lei et al. 2015), but no definitive cutoffs for unfavorable outcome have been suggested.

50.3.3.3 Serial Sampling to Monitor Secondary Injury Development

Similar to NSE, the effective half-life for GFAP in serum is longer than for S100B, close to 48 h on average (Thelin et al. 2017a). To our knowledge, there are no studies that have looked specifically at the development of secondary injuries by monitoring GFAP, albeit prolonged increases of serum GFAP levels seem to be associated with a more unfavorable outcome and increased ICP (Thelin et al. 2017a; Pelinka et al. 2004). In a cohort of milder TBI, Papa et al. noted that patients in need of neurosurgical interventions had higher levels of GFAP (peaking at 4.0–6.0 ng/mL at 8–24 h following injury) and returned to the same levels as the patient that did not need intervention (<1.0 ng/mL) 84 h after trauma (Papa et al. 2016).

50.3.3.4 Injury Differentiation

Several studies indicate that GFAP levels are higher in mass lesions as compared to diffuse injury (according to Marshall CT classifications) (Pelinka et al. 2004; Mondello et al. 2011), see below for comments concerning a "glial/neuronal ratio". An association between escalating CT scoring severity (Stockholm and Rotterdam CT scores) and increasing GFAP serum levels has been shown (Thelin et al. 2019).

50.3.3.5 Surrogate Endpoint in Clinical Studies

To the best of our knowledge, there are no published studies using GFAP to assess treatment efficacy in TBI trials.

50.3.4 Ubiquitin Carboxy-Terminal Hydrolase L1 (UCH-L1)

UCH-L1 is an enzyme (25 kDa) that hydrolyzes small C-terminal adducts of ubiquitin in order to generate the ubiquitin monomer in neurons. While it might have a role to play as a marker for chronic liver disease (Wilson et al. 2015), it is in the field of TBI where most research has been done in the last 10 years.

50.3.4.1 Extracranial Contribution

UCH-L1 has been suggested to be a highly brain-enriched protein, but is expressed to a large degree in the kidney, colon, and testis as well (Sjostedt et al. 2015). Further, there are studies showing increased serum levels of UCH-L1 in response to extracranial trauma (Posti et al. 2017; Papa et al. 2012a). In a recent study of 172 NCCU TBI patients, S100B and UCH-L1 were the two markers where the initial levels could be significantly related to any extracranial multitrauma (Thelin et al. 2019).

50.3.4.2 Outcome Prediction

Only a few studies have focused on serum levels of UCH-L1 to predict outcome in severe TBI, but these show promising results (Brophy et al. 2011; Takala et al. 2016; Mondello et al. 2012a). However, no exact thresholds have yet been suggested concerning serum levels that may differentiate unfavorable outcome and mortality from favorable outcome.

50.3.4.3 Serial Sampling to Monitor Secondary Injury Development

According to Brophy et al., the effective serum half-life of UCH-L1 is about 7 h in mild TBI and up to 10 h in severe TBI (Brophy et al. 2011), the shortest half-life among the biomarkers described in this chapter. While several authors have noted a more increasing trajectory in patients with more unfavorable outcome (Thelin et al. 2017a), none have been able to determine its role in monitoring lesion progression. Papa and co-workers noted that UCH-L1 levels during the first 12 h after trauma were substantially higher in patients that needed neurosurgical intervention than in patients that did not (approximately 5.5 ng/mL vs. <1.0 ng/mL) (Papa et al. 2016).

50.3.4.4 Injury Differentiation

UCH-L1 has been shown to be moderately increased in diffuse brain injury categories, as defined by Marshall CT classification, when compared to more focal injuries (Mondello et al. 2011). Mondello and co-workers have suggested a "glial/neuronal ratio" based on the serum GFAP:UCH-L1 ratio (Mondello et al. 2012b). They hypothesize GFAP to be a "focal" injury marker, which when combined with the marker of diffuse injury, UCH-L1, may be used to create a ratio describing the relation of injury burden between these two pathophysiologies. Recently, however a robust relationship has been established between escalating injury severity as seen on CT scoring systems and levels of UCH-L1 (Thelin et al. 2019), including both diffuse and focal injuries; thus it seems to be elevated in all types of TBI pathologies, depending on the injury severity.

50.3.4.5 Surrogate Endpoint in Clinical Studies

There is currently only one study available investigating UCH-L1 as a surrogate endpoint in TBI trials, thus warranting further studies. UCH-L1 was used as a surrogate marker of treatment efficacy in the Australian EPO-TBI trial studying the effect of EPO in TBI (Hellewell et al. 2017), and similar to the negative results of the trial on outcome, there were no differences in serum UCH-L1 levels between EPO and placebo.

50.3.5 Neurofilament Light (NF-L)

NF-L is the smallest of the three neurofilament subtypes (68 kDa), an intermediate filament present in the cytoplasm in neuronal cells where it forms a part of the cytoskeleton. In CSF, as well as in serum, NF-L is used to diagnose and assess treatment in diseases such as multiple sclerosis (MS) and amyotrophic lateral sclerosis (ALS) (Malmestrom et al. 2003; Gaiottino et al. 2013). In TBI, it is primarily studied in milder TBI, in order to assess trauma severity and potential post-concussion symptoms (Shahim et al. 2018), although there are a few reports from severe TBI cohorts.

50.3.5.1 Extracranial Contribution

There are no studies that report on elevated serum levels of NF-L from extracranial trauma. We studied how NF-L levels were correlated to extracranial multitrauma in NCCU TBI patients, but could not find any correlation with serum NF-L levels (Thelin et al. 2019).

50.3.5.2 Outcome Prediction

Two cohorts of severe TBI found that serum levels of NF-L were correlated with functional outcome (Shahim et al. 2016) and that it added independent information if used in combination with S100B in outcome prediction models (Al Nimer et al. 2015), presumably representing a separate pathophysiology.

50.3.5.3 Serial Sampling to Monitor Secondary Injury Development

The same two cohorts were sampled serially, and it was noted that in a majority of patients, levels of NF-L in serum kept increasing over the first 2 weeks (Shahim et al. 2016; Al Nimer et al. 2015). Therefore, it seems as if there is either an extended production or slow breakdown of the protein leading to late accumulation and a prolonged effective half-life (exceeding 2 weeks). Hence, serial sampling of NF-L suggests that values of NF-L might actually peak at a more chronic phase of TBI than studied thus far.

50.3.5.4 Injury Differentiation

In TBI cohorts with more mixed lesions, there were no correlation between serum levels of NF-L and the presence of diffuse axonal injury (DAI) on MRI (Al Nimer et al. 2015), presumably as other types of intracranial lesions also release NF-L. However, Ljungqvist and co-workers studied NF-L levels in small cohorts of patients with only DAI lesions, as well as low S100B levels (predominantly increased in more focal injuries), and noticed a correlation between NF-L and diffuse tractor imaging abnormalities (Ljungqvist et al. 2017). It has also recently been shown that NF-L is significantly correlated to escalating CT injury severity using Stockholm CT score (Thelin et al. 2019).

50.3.5.5 Surrogate Endpoint in Clinical Studies

To our knowledge, serum NF-L has not been used in TBI studies that assessed treatment efficacy.

50.3.6 Other Fluid Biomarkers of Brain Injury

There are several other markers of TBI in the literature, but many of them are not studied in detail as the ones described in this chapter. The primary Alzheimer proteins amyloid precursor protein (APP) and tau have shown promising results as a serum marker of severe TBI (Thelin et al. 2019; Mondello et al. 2014). Breakdown products of GFAP, as well as spectrin, are also promising markers as they are suggested to be more stable in serum than the initial protein (Berger et al. 2012; Papa et al. 2012b). Other neurofilament proteins, including neurofilament medium (NFM) (Martinez-Morillo et al. 2015) and the phosphorylated neurofilament heavy (pNFH) (Blyth et al. 2011), have also shown utility as markers for more severe TBI. Apart from brain-enriched proteins, metabolite and microRNA levels have also been shown to have diagnostic properties following severe TBI (Oresic et al. 2016; Redell et al. 2010). In summary, there is great interest in fluid biomarker development in TBI that may advance the field in the upcoming years.

50.3.7 Combination of Biomarkers

Several attempts have been made to combine biomarkers to enhance accuracy with mixed results (Thelin et al. 2016a; Mondello et al. 2011; Al Nimer et al. 2015; Vos et al. 2004; Czeiter et al. 2012). Due to a lack of larger trials combining multiple available markers for model selection, it is also difficult to say which biomarkers are "best" at predicting outcome and injury type/severity. In a recent study combining S100B, NSE, GFAP, UCH-L1, NF-L, and tau, it was shown that GFAP was the most robust marker to predict unfavorable outcome, and if NF-L was added, it resulted in most independent information in outcome prediction models (Thelin et al. 2019). Similarly, UCH-L1 was the marker most correlated to mortality. The same study also revealed that many of the proteins are highly inter-correlated, with the exception of NF-L, suggesting that if a panel of different protein biomarkers should be used to predict outcome, then preferably proteins with different cellular origin and temporal dynamics should be combined (Thelin et al. 2019).

50.3.8 Available Assays for Clinical Use

Currently, only S100B and NSE are available as clinical assays (Cobas, Elecsys, Roche Diagnostics), which takes minutes (about 18 min) to run, allowing them to be implemented in clinical decision-making (Smit et al. 2005). GFAP and UCH-L1 are available in tailored ELISAs but take about 3.5–4 h to run which may hamper their utility in clinical management (Bazarian et al. 2018). Point-of-care (POC) devices, being available bedside with a shorter run-time, will probably be available in the upcoming years. For NF-L, there are ELISAs available, but more rapid and sensitive options are available on the SIMOA® (Single Molecule Array) platform (Kuhle et al. 2016), also allowing for multiplexing several biomarkers in a couple of hours.

The price for consumables in clinical assays has also dropped, with a sample of S100B and NSE now costing about 10 USD. If sampled twice daily, this is approximately 150 USD a week, which can be compared with prices for consumables for intracranial pressure (ICP) monitoring (500 USD), microdialysis (650 USD), and brain tissue oxygenation (550 USD).

50.3.9 Use of Protein Biomarkers for Severe Pediatric TBI

Due to varying baseline/reference levels of S100B in pediatric populations, S100B has not been implemented as a screening tool in the emergency room to rule out CT scans, in contrast to adult patients (Piazza et al. 2007; Astrand et al. 2016; Bouvier et al. 2011, 2012). While there are studies suggesting that serum S100B and NSE are useful outcome predictors in the severe pediatric TBI population (Berger et al. 2007), a systematic review from 2014 suggests that UCH-L1 and GFAP are likely better pediatric serum markers for outcome (Daoud et al. 2014). In terms of temporal sampling, a similar principle as can be used in adults may be used in pediatric TBI, where elevated trajectories suggest a more unfavorable outcome with a larger burden of secondary injuries (Berger et al. 2010). In summary, a similar approach to the use of biomarkers in severe TBI in adults could presumably be used in children, though more research is warranted.

50.4 Concluding Remarks

Protein biomarkers are emerging as valuable tools in the management of severe TBI patients. Protein biomarkers should be used in a way so that resources can be utilized optimally and treatment escalated in specific patients. Moreover, secondary increases in temporally sampled biomarkers appear useful tools to monitor TBI, with increases triggering patient review and possibly diagnostic and therapeutic measures. However, they should be corroborated by other multimodal monitoring metrics in order to improve specificity and prevent unnecessary transportation or interventions. As the understanding of biomarker kinetic progresses, our understanding of how levels should be interpreted at different time points increases. Currently, only S100B and NSE represent markers where clinical utility is feasible due to the existence of rapid assays, but more advanced bedside assays will presumably be available in the future. Ideally, markers of different pathophysiology should be combined in order to monitor different processes, but more research is needed in order to fully utilize protein biomarker capabilities in this aspect.

References

Al Nimer F, Thelin E, Nystrom H, Dring AM, Svenningsson A, Piehl F, et al. Comparative assessment of the prognostic value of biomarkers in traumatic brain injury reveals an independent role for serum levels of neurofilament light. PLoS One. 2015;10(7):e0132177.

Anderson RE, Hansson LO, Nilsson O, Dijlai-Merzoug R, Settergren G. High serum S100B levels for trauma patients without head injuries. Neurosurgery. 2001;48(6):1255–8; discussion 8-60.

Astrand R, Rosenlund C, Unden J. Scandinavian guidelines for initial management of minor and moderate head trauma in children. BMC Med. 2016;14:33.

Bakay RA, Ward AA Jr. Enzymatic changes in serum and cerebrospinal fluid in neurological injury. J Neurosurg. 1983;58(1):27–37.

Baker AJ, Rhind SG, Morrison LJ, Black S, Crnko NT, Shek PN, et al. Resuscitation with hypertonic saline-dextran reduces serum biomarker levels and correlates with outcome in severe traumatic brain injury patients. J Neurotrauma. 2009;26(8):1227–40.

Bazarian JJ, Biberthaler P, Welch RD, Lewis LM, Barzo P, Bogner-Flatz V, et al. Serum GFAP and UCH-L1 for prediction of absence of intracranial injuries on head CT (ALERT-TBI): a multicentre observational study. Lancet Neurol. 2018;17(9):782–9.

Berger RP, Beers SR, Richichi R, Wiesman D, Adelson PD. Serum biomarker concentrations and outcome after pediatric traumatic brain injury. J Neurotrauma. 2007;24(12):1793–801.

Berger RP, Bazaco MC, Wagner AK, Kochanek PM, Fabio A. Trajectory analysis of serum biomarker concentrations facilitates outcome prediction after pediatric traumatic and hypoxemic brain injury. Dev Neurosci. 2010;32(5-6):396–405.

Berger RP, Hayes RL, Richichi R, Beers SR, Wang KK. Serum concentrations of ubiquitin C-terminal hydrolase-L1 and alphaII-spectrin breakdown product 145 kDa correlate with outcome after pediatric TBI. J Neurotrauma. 2012;29(1):162–7.

Blyth BJ, Farahvar A, He H, Nayak A, Yang C, Shaw G, et al. Elevated serum ubiquitin carboxy-terminal hydrolase L1 is associated with abnormal blood-brain barrier function after traumatic brain injury. J Neurotrauma. 2011;28(12):2453–62.

Bouvier D, Castellani C, Fournier M, Dauphin JB, Ughetto S, Breton M, et al. Reference ranges for serum S100B protein during the first three years of life. Clin Biochem. 2011;44(10-11):927–9.

Bouvier D, Fournier M, Dauphin JB, Amat F, Ughetto S, Labbe A, et al. Serum S100B determination in the management of pediatric mild traumatic brain injury. Clin Chem. 2012;58(7):1116–22.

Brophy GM, Mondello S, Papa L, Robicsek SA, Gabrielli A, Tepas J 3rd, et al. Biokinetic analysis of ubiquitin C-terminal hydrolase-L1 (UCH-L1) in severe traumatic brain injury patient biofluids. J Neurotrauma. 2011;28(6):861–70.

Carney N, Totten AM, O'Reilly C, Ullman JS, Hawryluk GW, Bell MJ, et al. Guidelines for the management of severe traumatic brain injury, fourth edition. Neurosurgery. 2017;80(1):6–15.

Cronberg T, Rundgren M, Westhall E, Englund E, Siemund R, Rosen I, et al. Neuron-specific enolase correlates with other prognostic markers after cardiac arrest. Neurology. 2011;77(7):623–30.

Czeiter E, Mondello S, Kovacs N, Sandor J, Gabrielli A, Schmid K, et al. Brain injury biomarkers may improve the predictive power of the IMPACT outcome calculator. J Neurotrauma. 2012;29(9):1770–8.

Daoud H, Alharfi I, Alhelali I, Charyk Stewart T, Qasem H, Fraser DD. Brain injury biomarkers as outcome predictors in pediatric severe traumatic brain injury. Neurocrit Care. 2014;20(3):427–35.

Donato R, Sorci G, Riuzzi F, Arcuri C, Bianchi R, Brozzi F, et al. S100B's double life: intracellular regulator and extracellular signal. Biochim Biophys Acta. 2009;1793(6):1008–22.

Egberts F, Hitschler WN, Weichenthal M, Hauschild A. Prospective monitoring of adjuvant treatment in high-risk melanoma patients: lactate dehydrogenase and protein S-100B as indicators of relapse. Melanoma Res. 2009;19(1):31–5.

Gaiottino J, Norgren N, Dobson R, Topping J, Nissim A, Malaspina A, et al. Increased neurofilament light chain blood levels in neurodegenerative neurological diseases. PLoS One. 2013;8(9):e75091.

Gao F, Harris DN, Sapsed-Byrne S, Sharp S. Neurone-specific enolase and Sangtec 100 assays during cardiac surgery: Part III--Dose haemolysis affect their accuracy? Perfusion. 1997;12(3):171–7.

Haimoto H, Hosoda S, Kato K. Differential distribution of immunoreactive S100-alpha and S100-beta proteins in normal nonnervous human tissues. Lab Invest. 1987;57(5):489–98.

Hellewell SC, Mondello S, Conquest A, Shaw G, Madorsky I, Deng JV, et al. Erythropoietin does not alter serum profiles of neuronal and axonal biomarkers after traumatic brain injury: findings from the Australian EPO-TBI Clinical Trial. Crit Care Med. 2017.

Herman MM, Perentes E, Katsetos CD, Darcel F, Frankfurter A, Collins VP, et al. Neuroblastic differentiation potential of the human retinoblastoma cell lines Y-79 and WERI-Rb1 maintained in an organ culture system. An immunohistochemical, electron microscopic, and biochemical study. Am J Pathol. 1989;134(1):115–32.

Herrmann M, Jost S, Kutz S, Ebert AD, Kratz T, Wunderlich MT, et al. Temporal profile of release of neurobiochemical markers of brain damage after traumatic brain injury is associated with intracranial pathology as demonstrated in cranial computerized tomography. J Neurotrauma. 2000;17(2):113–22.

Hyder AA, Wunderlich CA, Puvanachandra P, Gururaj G, Kobusingye OC. The impact of traumatic brain injuries: a global perspective. NeuroRehabilitation. 2007;22(5):341–53.

Johnsson P, Blomquist S, Luhrs C, Malmkvist G, Alling C, Solem JO, et al. Neuron-specific enolase increases in plasma during and immediately after extracorporeal circulation. Ann Thorac Surg. 2000;69(3):750–4.

Jonsson H, Johnsson P, Hoglund P, Alling C, Blomquist S. Elimination of S100B and renal function after cardiac surgery. J Cardiothorac Vasc Anesth. 2000;14(6):698–701.

Kleindienst A, Hesse F, Bullock MR, Buchfelder M. The neurotrophic protein S100B: value as a marker of brain damage and possible therapeutic implications. Prog Brain Res. 2007;161:317–25.

Korfias S, Stranjalis G, Boviatsis E, Psachoulia C, Jullien G, Gregson B, et al. Serum S-100B protein monitoring in patients with severe traumatic brain injury. Intensive Care Med. 2007;33(2):255–60.

Kuhle J, Barro C, Andreasson U, Derfuss T, Lindberg R, Sandelius A, et al. Comparison of three analytical platforms for quantification of the neurofilament light chain in blood samples: ELISA, electrochemiluminescence immunoassay and Simoa. Clin Chem Lab Med. 2016;54(10):1655–61.

Laroche E, Turgeon AF, Boutin A, Mercier E, Lauzier F, Zarychanski R, et al. Predictive value of glial fibrillary acidic protein for prognosis in patients with moderate and severe traumatic brain injury: a systematic review and meta-analysis. ISICEM Crit Care. 2012.

Lei J, Gao G, Feng J, Jin Y, Wang C, Mao Q, et al. Glial fibrillary acidic protein as a biomarker in severe traumatic brain injury patients: a prospective cohort study. Crit Care. 2015;19:362.

Li ZM, Xiao YL, Zhu JX, Geng FY, Guo CJ, Chong ZL, et al. Recombinant human erythropoietin improves functional recovery in patients with severe traumatic brain injury: A randomized, double blind and controlled clinical trial. Clin Neurol Neurosurg. 2016;150:80–3.

Ljungqvist J, Zetterberg H, Mitsis M, Blennow K, Skoglund T. Serum neurofilament light protein as a marker for diffuse axonal injury: results from a case series study. J Neurotrauma. 2017;34(5):1124–7.

Maas AI, Hukkelhoven CW, Marshall LF, Steyerberg EW. Prediction of outcome in traumatic brain injury with computed tomographic characteristics: a comparison between the computed tomographic classification and combinations of computed tomographic predictors. Neurosurgery. 2005;57(6):1173–82; discussion -82.

Malmestrom C, Haghighi S, Rosengren L, Andersen O, Lycke J. Neurofilament light protein and glial fibrillary acidic protein as biological markers in MS. Neurology. 2003;61(12):1720–5.

Marshall LF, Marshall SB, Klauber MR, Clark MV, Eisenberg HM, Jane JA, et al. A new classification of head-injury based on computerized-tomography. J Neurosurg. 1991;75:S14–20.

Martinez-Morillo E, Childs C, Garcia BP, Alvarez Menendez FV, Romaschin AD, Cervellin G, et al. Neurofilament medium polypeptide (NFM) protein concentration is increased in CSF and serum samples from patients with brain injury. Clin Chem Lab Med. 2015;53(10):1575–84.

McKeating EG, Andrews PJ, Mascia L. Relationship of neuron specific enolase and protein S-100 concentrations in systemic and jugular venous serum to injury severity and outcome after traumatic brain injury. Acta Neurochir Suppl. 1998;71:117–9.

Mercier E, Boutin A, Lauzier F, Fergusson DA, Simard JF, Zarychanski R, et al. Predictive value of S-100beta protein for prognosis in patients with moderate and severe traumatic brain injury: systematic review and meta-analysis. BMJ. 2013;f1757:346.

Mercier E, Boutin A, Shemilt M, Lauzier F, Zarychanski R, Fergusson DA, et al. Predictive value of neuron-specific enolase for prognosis in patients with moderate or severe traumatic brain injury: a systematic review and meta-analysis. CMAJ Open. 2016;4(3):E371–E82.

Mondello S, Papa L, Buki A, Bullock MR, Czeiter E, Tortella FC, et al. Neuronal and glial markers are differently associated with computed tomography findings and outcome in patients with severe traumatic brain injury: a case control study. Crit Care. 2011;15(3):R156.

Mondello S, Linnet A, Buki A, Robicsek S, Gabrielli A, Tepas J, et al. Clinical utility of serum levels of ubiquitin C-terminal hydrolase as a biomarker for severe traumatic brain injury. Neurosurgery. 2012a;70(3):666–75.

Mondello S, Jeromin A, Buki A, Bullock R, Czeiter E, Kovacs N, et al. Glial neuronal ratio: a novel index for differentiating injury type in patients with severe traumatic brain injury. J Neurotrauma. 2012b;29(6):1096–104.

Mondello S, Buki A, Barzo P, Randall J, Provuncher G, Hanlon D, et al. CSF and plasma amyloid-beta temporal profiles and relationships with neurological status and mortality after severe traumatic brain injury. Sci Rep. 2014;4:6446.

Nelson DW, Nystrom H, MacCallum RM, Thornquist B, Lilja A, Bellander BM, et al. Extended analysis of early computed tomography scans of traumatic brain injured patients and relations to outcome. J Neurotrauma. 2010;27(1):51–64.

Nirula R, Diaz-Arrastia R, Brasel K, Weigelt JA, Waxman K. Safety and efficacy of erythropoietin in traumatic brain injury patients: a pilot randomized trial. Crit Care Res Prac. 2010;2010.

Olivecrona Z, Bobinski L, Koskinen LO. Association of ICP, CPP, CT findings and S-100B and NSE in severe traumatic head injury. Prognostic value of the biomarkers. Brain Inj. 2015;29(4):446–54.

Oresic M, Posti JP, Kamstrup-Nielsen MH, Takala RSK, Lingsma HF, Mattila I, et al. Human serum metabolites associate with severity and patient outcomes in traumatic brain injury. EBioMedicine. 2016;12:118–26.

Papa L, Robinson G, Oli M, Pineda J, Demery J, Brophy G, et al. Use of biomarkers for diagnosis and management of traumatic brain injury patients. Expert Opin Med Diag. 2008;2(8):937–45.

Papa L, Lewis LM, Silvestri S, Falk JL, Giordano P, Brophy GM, et al. Serum levels of ubiquitin C-terminal hydrolase distinguish mild traumatic brain injury from trauma controls and are elevated in mild and moderate traumatic brain injury patients with intracranial lesions and neurosurgical intervention. J Trauma Acute Care Surg. 2012a;72(5):1335–44.

Papa L, Lewis LM, Falk JL, Zhang Z, Silvestri S, Giordano P, et al. Elevated levels of serum glial fibrillary acidic protein breakdown products in mild and moderate traumatic brain injury are associated with intracranial lesions and neurosurgical intervention. Ann Emerg Med. 2012b;59(6):471–83.

Papa L, Silvestri S, Brophy GM, Giordano P, Falk JL, Braga CF, et al. GFAP out-performs S100beta in detecting traumatic intracranial lesions on computed tomography in trauma patients with mild traumatic brain injury and those with extracranial lesions. J Neurotrauma. 2014;31(22):1815–22.

Papa L, Brophy GM, Welch RD, Lewis LM, Braga CF, Tan CN, et al. Time course and diagnostic accuracy of glial and neuronal blood biomarkers GFAP and UCH-L1 in a large cohort of trauma patients with and without mild traumatic brain injury. JAMA Neurol. 2016.

Pelinka LE, Kroepfl A, Schmidhammer R, Krenn M, Buchinger W, Redl H, et al. Glial fibrillary acidic protein in serum after traumatic brain injury and multiple trauma. J Trauma. 2004;57(5):1006–12.

Pfortmueller CA, Drexel C, Krahenmann-Muller S, Leichtle AB, Fiedler GM, Lindner G, et al. S-100 B concentrations are a predictor of decreased survival in patients with major trauma, independently of head injury. PLoS One. 2016;11(3):e0152822.

Pham N, Fazio V, Cucullo L, Teng Q, Biberthaler P, Bazarian JJ, et al. Extracranial sources of S100B do not affect serum levels. PLoS One. 2010;5(9).

Piazza O, Storti MP, Cotena S, Stoppa F, Perrotta D, Esposito G, et al. S100B is not a reliable prognostic index in paediatric TBI. Pediatr Neurosurg. 2007;43(4):258–64.

Posti JP, Hossain I, Takala RS, Liedes H, Newcombe V, Outtrim J, et al. Glial fibrillary acidic protein and ubiquitin C-terminal hydrolase-L1 are not specific biomarkers for mild ct-negative traumatic brain injury. J Neurotrauma. 2017.

Raabe A, Seifert V. Fatal secondary increase in serum S-100B protein after severe head injury. Report of three cases. J Neurosurg. 1999;91(5):875–7.

Raabe A, Grolms C, Keller M, Dohnert J, Sorge O, Seifert V. Correlation of computed tomography findings and serum brain damage markers following severe head injury. Acta Neurochir. 1998;140(8):787–91; discussion 91-2.

Raabe A, Kopetsch O, Woszczyk A, Lang J, Gerlach R, Zimmermann M, et al. S-100B protein as a serum marker of secondary neurological complications in neurocritical care patients. Neurol Res. 2004;26(4):440–5.

Redell JB, Moore AN, Ward NH 3rd, Hergenroeder GW, Dash PK. Human traumatic brain injury alters plasma microRNA levels. J Neurotrauma. 2010;27(12):2147–56.

Roozenbeek B, Maas AI, Menon DK. Changing patterns in the epidemiology of traumatic brain injury. Nat Rev Neurol. 2013;9(4):231–6.

Rundgren M, Cronberg T, Friberg H, Isaksson A. Serum neuron specific enolase—impact of storage and measuring method. BMC Res Notes. 2014;7:726.

Shahim P, Gren M, Liman V, Andreasson U, Norgren N, Tegner Y, et al. Serum neurofilament light protein predicts clinical outcome in traumatic brain injury. Sci Rep. 2016;6:36791.

Shahim P, Tegner Y, Marklund N, Blennow K, Zetterberg H. Neurofilament light and tau as blood biomarkers for sports-related concussion. Neurology. 2018;90(20):e1780–e8.

Sjostedt E, Fagerberg L, Hallstrom BM, Haggmark A, Mitsios N, Nilsson P, et al. Defining the human brain proteome using transcriptomics and antibody-based profiling with a focus on the cerebral cortex. PLoS One. 2015;10(6):e0130028.

Smit LH, Korse CM, Bonfrer JM. Comparison of four different assays for determination of serum S-100B. Int J Biol Markers. 2005;20(1):34–42.

Takala RS, Posti JP, Runtti H, Newcombe VF, Outtrim J, Katila AJ, et al. Glial fibrillary acidic protein and ubiquitin C-terminal hydrolase-L1 as outcome predictors in traumatic brain injury. World Neurosurg. 2016;87:8–20.

Thelin EP, Johannesson L, Nelson D, Bellander BM. S100B is an important outcome predictor in traumatic brain injury. J Neurotrauma. 2013;30(7):519–28.

Thelin EP, Nelson DW, Bellander BM. Secondary peaks of S100B in serum relate to subsequent radiological pathology in traumatic brain injury. Neurocrit Care. 2014;20(2):217–29.

Thelin EP, Jeppsson E, Frostell A, Svensson M, Mondello S, Bellander BM, et al. Utility of neuron-specific enolase in traumatic brain injury; relations to S100B levels, outcome, and extracranial injury severity. Crit Care. 2016a;20:285.

Thelin EP, Zibung E, Riddez L, Nordenvall C. Assessing bicycle-related trauma using the biomarker S100B reveals a correlation with total injury severity. Eur J Trauma Emerg Surg. 2016b;42(5):617–25.

Thelin EP, Zeiler FA, Ercole A, Mondello S, Buki A, Bellander BM, et al. Serial sampling of serum protein biomarkers for monitoring human traumatic brain injury dynamics: a systematic review. Front Neurol. 2017a;8:300.

Thelin EP, Nelson DW, Bellander BM. A review of the clinical utility of serum S100B protein levels in the assessment of traumatic brain injury. Acta Neurochir. 2017b;159(2):209–25.

Thelin EP, Al Nimer F, Frostell A, Zetterberg H, Blennow K, Nystrom H, et al. A serum protein biomarker panel improves outcome prediction in human traumatic brain injury. J Neurotrauma. 2019;36(20):2850–62.

Thompson WH, Thelin EP, Lilja A, Bellander BM, Fransson P. Functional resting-state fMRI connectivity correlates with serum levels of the S100B protein in the acute phase of traumatic brain injury. Neuroimage Clin. 2016;12:1004–12.

Tolan NV, Vidal-Folch N, Algeciras-Schimnich A, Singh RJ, Grebe SK. Individualized correction of neuron-specific enolase (NSE) measurement in hemolyzed serum samples. Clin Chim Acta. 2013;424:216–21.

Unden J, Bellner J, Eneroth M, Alling C, Ingebrigtsen T, Romner B. Raised serum S100B levels after acute bone fractures without cerebral injury. J Trauma. 2005a;58(1):59–61.

Unden J, Bellner J, Astrand R, Romner B. Serum S100B levels in patients with epidural haematomas. Br J Neurosurg. 2005b;19(1):43–5.

Unden J, Astrand R, Waterloo K, Ingebrigtsen T, Bellner J, Reinstrup P, et al. Clinical significance of serum S100B levels in neurointensive care. Neurocrit Care. 2007;6(2):94–9.

Unden J, Ingebrigtsen T, Romner B, Scandinavian Neurotrauma C. Scandinavian guidelines for initial management of minimal, mild and moderate head injuries in adults: an evidence and consensus-based update. BMC Med. 2013;11:50.

Vos PE, Lamers KJ, Hendriks JC, van Haaren M, Beems T, Zimmerman C, et al. Glial and neuronal proteins in serum predict outcome after severe traumatic brain injury. Neurology. 2004;62(8):1303–10.

Wilson CL, Murphy LB, Leslie J, Kendrick S, French J, Fox CR, et al. Ubiquitin C-terminal hydrolase 1: a novel functional marker for liver myofibroblasts and a therapeutic target in chronic liver disease. J Hepatol. 2015;63(6):1421–8.

Woertgen C, Rothoerl RD, Holzschuh M, Metz C, Brawanski A. Comparison of serial S-100 and NSE serum measurements after severe head injury. Acta Neurochir. 1997;139(12):1161–4; discussion 5.

Cardiopulmonary Aspects

51

Karen-Lise Kobberø Welling, Malin Rundgren, and Kirsten Møller

Abbreviations

CBF	Cerebral blood flow
CO	Cardiac output
CPP	Cerebral perfusion pressure
CRX	Chest X-ray
CVP	Central venous pressure
DBP	Diastolic blood pressure
ECG	Electrocardiogramme
$ETCO_2$	End-tidal CO_2
GCS	Glasgow Coma Scale/Glasgow Coma Score
GOS	Glasgow Outcome Score
HR	Heart rate
ICH	Intracranial hypertension
ICP	Intracranial pressure
LPMV	Lung-protective mechanical ventilation
MAP	Mean arterial pressure
MV	Mechanical ventilation
NIBP	Noninvasive blood pressure
NICU	Neurointensive care unit
PAC	Pulmonary artery catheter
$PbtO_2$	Brain tissue oxygen tension
PPV	Pulse pressure variation
RBC	Red blood cells
RCT	Randomized controlled trial
SaO_2	Arterial oxygen saturation
SBP	Systolic blood pressure
$ScvO_2$	Central venous saturation
SpO_2	Peripheral oxygen saturation (as measured by pulse oximetry)
SV	Stroke volume
TBI	Traumatic brain injury
TEE	Transoesophageal echocardiography
TTE	Transthoracic echocardiography
VILI	Ventilator-induced lung injury

K.-L. K. Welling (✉)
Neurointensive Care Unit, Section 6021, Department of Neuroanaesthesiology, The Neuroscience Centre, Rigshospitalet, University of Copenhagen, Copenhagen, Denmark
e-mail: Karen.lise.kobberoe.welling@regionh.dk

M. Rundgren
Neurointensive Care Unit, Department of Intensive and Preoperative Care, Skåne University Hospital, Lund, Sweden

Department of Clinical Sciences, Anesthesiology and Intensive Care Medicine, Skåne University Hospital, Lund University, Lund, Sweden
e-mail: malin.rundgren@med.lu.se

K. Møller
Department of Neuroanaesthesiology, The Neuroscience Centre, Rigshospitalet, University of Copenhagen, Copenhagen, Denmark

Department of Clinical Medicine, University of Copenhagen, Copenhagen, Denmark
e-mail: kirsten.moeller.01@regionh.dk

© Springer Nature Switzerland AG 2020
T. Sundstrøm et al. (eds.), *Management of Severe Traumatic Brain Injury*,
https://doi.org/10.1007/978-3-030-39383-0_51

Recommendations

Level I

There is insufficient evidence to support a level I recommendation for this topic.

Level II

Prolonged prophylactic hyperventilation ($PaCO_2$ <25 mmHg (3.3 kPa)) is not recommended.

Hyperventilation should be avoided during the first 24 h after traumatic brain injury (TBI), when cerebral blood flow (CBF) is often critically reduced.

Level III

Patients with severe TBI (Glasgow Coma Score (GCS <9)) should undergo prehospital intubation, and hypoxia (PaO_2 <60 mmHg (8 kPa)) should be avoided.

Arterial blood pressure should be continuously monitored in those with severe TBI, and hypotension (mean arterial pressure (MAP) <80 mmHg or systolic blood pressure (SBP) <100–110 mmHg) should be avoided.

Resuscitation with albumin has been associated with higher mortality rates compared with saline.

Central venous pressure (CVP) does not predict preload or blood volume status.

In paediatric patients, cerebral perfusion pressure (CPP) is age dependent and should be in the range between 40 and 50 mmHg, in the low range for infants and in the high range for older children.

Tips, Tricks, and Pitfalls

Circulatory

- Monitoring of blood pressure and heart rate (HR) may aid in predicting a crisis before it becomes clinically overt and may assist in evaluating the response to treatment.
- Assess cardiovascular function by performing a physical examination, measurement of blood pressure, HR, and urine output.
- Central venous pressure (CVP) should not be used for clinical decisions regarding fluid management.
- Monitoring of cardiac output (CO) has not been shown to provide benefit.
- Serial measurements of the central venous oxygen saturation ($ScvO_2$) may provide information on changes in the balance between systemic oxygen delivery and utilization.
- The zero point of the transducer for invasive arterial pressure monitoring should be at the level of the tragus (as opposed to the right atrium) in patients with severe TBI and intracranial pressure (ICP) monitoring.
- While arterial blood gas analysis provides information on systemic aerobic and anaerobic metabolism as well as oxygenation and ventilation, this is not easily translated to the intrathecal environment.
- The optimal haemoglobin threshold is unknown in TBI.

Respiratory

- Protection of the airway and control of oxygenation and ventilation are main goals of mechanical ventilation in TBI patients.
- The optimal level of systemic oxygenation is unknown, but severe hypoxia (<8 kPa) should be avoided, and extreme hyperoxia (>16 kPa) may also be inappropriate.
- Continuous capnography should be used for all intubated and mechanically ventilated patients in the neurointensive care unit (NICU) as well as during intrahospital and inter-hospital transfer. However, it is not a substitute for regular measurement of the arterial carbon dioxide tension ($PaCO_2$).

- Normoventilation ($PaCO_2$ 35–42 mmHg (4.7–5.0 kPa)) is the goal in most TBI patients, and prolonged prophylactic hyperventilation ($PaCO_2$ <25 mmHg (3.3 kPa)) as well as hypoventilation ($PaCO_2$ >45 mmHg (6.0 kPa)) should be avoided because of the risk of critical brain tissue hypoxia, especially in the first 24 h after injury.
- Monitoring of cerebral tissue oxygenation is recommended, in particular for TBI patients who are mechanically hyperventilated, but may also be beneficial for other patients with severe TBI.
- There are no absolute contraindications to the use of lung-protective ventilation in TBI.
- In patients with combined TBI and ARDS, low tidal volumes (6 mL/kg or lower) are recommended and can be safely applied, provided that patients are normoventilated.
- Intracranial pressure (ICP) and, if possible, cerebral tissue oxygenation ($PbtO_2$) should be monitored in patients undergoing permissive hypercapnia.
- Spontaneous breathing modes are not recommended for mechanical ventilation in the early phase of TBI, where hypoventilation may trigger ICP increases. However, such patients are frequently capable of breathing spontaneously with minimal ventilator support in later phases of the NICU stay, despite persistent neurological impairment.
- Extubation success is predicted by younger age, presence of cough, and negative fluid balance rather than by the Glasgow Coma Score (GCS) at extubation.
- Early tracheostomy after severe TBI (0–7 days) is not recommended.

51.1 Overview

51.1.1 Main Goals and Challenges for the Neurointensivist

Cardiopulmonary deterioration in the patient with severe traumatic brain injury (TBI) may result in secondary brain injury (Chesnut et al. 1993) primarily because of hypoxia and hypotension, although hypoventilation with increased arterial CO_2 tension ($PaCO_2$) or iatrogenic hyperventilation with reduced $PaCO_2$ is an additional concern immediately after injury. More recently, the possible detrimental effect of hyperoxia in major trauma with brain injury has also been discussed (Rangel-Castilla et al. 2010). Although there is no general recommendation for the target arterial oxygen tension (PaO_2), there is a general agreement that hypoxia (PaO_2 <60 mmHg (8 kPa)) should be avoided; in most neurointensive care units (NICU), the target PaO_2 is probably between 75 and 100 mmHg (10–14 kPa).

Although many patients with TBI are young with no pre-existing cardiopulmonary problems and sustain isolated brain trauma with no systemic injury, the average age of TBI victims has increased (Brazinova et al. 2016) with a potential increase in the prevalence of pre-existing pulmonary or cardiac disease; others may be affected by multiple trauma including cardiothoracic injury. Moreover, severe brain damage may in itself elicit systemic inflammation as well as excessive sympathetic activation, which may influence both cardiovascular and lung functions (Kalsotra et al. 2018). Thus, the objective of cardiopulmonary monitoring and treatment is (1) to support systemic organ function in general (as in other critically ill patients) and (2) to avoid secondary brain damage.

51.2 Background

51.2.1 Cardiopulmonary Disturbances in TBI

Cardiopulmonary dysfunction is common in patients with severe TBI and may exist as a premorbid condition primarily in elderly patients, may occur concomitantly to TBI, e.g. in multiple trauma, or may develop as a consequence of TBI, e.g. because of sympathetic storm. In either instance, cardiovascular or pulmonary instability may result in hypotension or hypoxia, leading to secondary brain damage. Limited research has been performed on patients suffering from concomitant severe head trauma and cardiovascular problems or the acute respiratory distress syndrome (ARDS) (Bragge et al. 2016). However, the management goals of TBI may conflict in particular with those of severe ARDS.

Even though many TBI patients have stable haemodynamic and respiratory function, the risk of secondary brain injury mandates tight control of cardiovascular as well as pulmonary characteristics. In a prospective observational study of 699 patients with severe TBI who were alive and had a blood pressure and an arterial blood gas measurement on admission, the group without hypoxia (PaO_2 <60 mmHg or definite apnoea or cyanosis) or hypotension (systolic blood pressure (SBP) <90 mmHg) had a mortality of 27%, whereas the mortality was 50% in those with hypoxia alone, 65% in those with hypotension alone, and 75% in those with both hypoxia and hypotension. Hypo- and hypercapnia as well as hypertension may also be associated with unfavourable outcomes; hypocapnia may lead to cerebral ischaemia, whereas both hypercapnia and hypertension may impair outcomes through an aggravation of vasogenic oedema and increased intracranial pressure.

In the severely brain-injured patient, intubation and mechanical ventilation may be life-saving, but is also associated with side effects and life-threatening complications. Intubation and ventilation are mainly done to establish a free and safe airway, prevent hypoxemia, and maintain normocarbia. Despite these beneficial effects, ventilator-induced lung injury (VILI) is a concern even in brain-injured patients with previously healthy lungs. While most patients with TBI do not have a primary respiratory indication for intubation, the brain injury may elicit a systemic inflammatory response (Kalsotra et al. 2018), which may contribute to the subsequent development of ARDS. Thus, a prevalence of ARDS of 8–31% with a threefold increase in the odds of in-hospital mortality has been reported (Rincon et al. 2012). Furthermore, ventilation in TBI patients is particularly challenging in those with concomitant ARDS. This is because the oxygenation and ventilation targets (so-called permissive hypoxia and hypercapnia) as well as restrictive fluid therapy that are recommended for ARDS aim at protecting the injured lung; this may concomitantly trigger hypovolaemia, hypotension, and cerebral arteriolar dilatation with ICP increases and vasogenic oedema, all of which may promote secondary brain injury.

In the later phase of their hospital stay, patients with TBI frequently become capable of breathing spontaneously with minimal ventilator support despite persistent neurological impairment. A systematic approach to weaning and extubation may play a role in improving outcome (Bruni et al. 2017), as may correct timing of tracheostomy (Rizk et al. 2011; Baron et al. 2016; Dunham et al. 2014).

51.3 Physiological Considerations and Monitoring

51.3.1 Circulatory

51.3.1.1 Preload, Contractility, and Afterload

Arterial blood pressure is important to ensure cerebral perfusion both in healthy people and in those with TBI. Mean arterial pressure (MAP) is the product of cardiac output (CO) and the systemic vascular resistance (SVR, also known as the afterload). The arterial pressure curve and heart rate (HR) are routinely monitored in most critically ill patients. In contrast, neither preload, CO, nor SVR is routinely monitored; current methods available for measurement of these variables either use surrogate parameters or have low accuracy (Hadian et al. 2010).

The Frank-Starling law describes the theoretical relationship between cardiac preload and left ventricular stroke volume (SV). This relationship implies that the optimum SV depends on an optimum preload; below and above this optimal preload, cardiac contractility is reduced because of either hypovolaemia or overload. Furthermore, the minute volume of the heart (CO) is calculated by multiplying SV by HR. Thus, preload optimization, which is mainly done by fluid therapy, is considered important for optimal cardiac function. As described above, there is no well-defined target for this procedure. Although most institutions use repeated fluid boluses while simultaneously evaluating cardiovascular parameters such as MAP, central venous pressure (CVP), central venous oxygen saturation ($ScvO_2$), systolic volume variation, or peripheral skin perfusion, none of these markers are reliable markers of circulatory function.

The importance of cardiac function for outcome in TBI was studied in 139 patients without pre-existing cardiac disease; of these, cardiac dysfunction, as diagnosed by echocardiography, occurred in 22% during the first 2 weeks in TBI and was associated with a nine-fold increase in mortality (Prathep et al. 2014). The severity of brain injury emerged as an independent risk factor of cardiac dysfunction and may therefore have "driven" the increased mortality.

51.3.2 Respiratory

51.3.2.1 Oxygenation, Ventilation, and Compliance

In normal individuals, breathing 100% oxygen results in vasoconstriction of the cerebral blood vessels and a subsequent decrease in cerebral blood flow (CBF). The vascular and tissue response to hyperoxia may change in TBI, and relatively little information is available about oxygen reactivity variables in TBI; although hyperoxia may improve cerebral pressure autoregulation (Rangel-Castilla et al. 2010), it may also be associated with augmented ischaemia-reperfusion injury. The use of hyperbaric hyperoxia has been investigated in RCTs, none of which were classified as robust according to a subsequent meta-analysis (Bragge et al. 2016); however, the studies did demonstrate an association between the occurrence of hypoxia and worse outcome. The optimum level of oxygenation is not known, but current guidelines recommend avoidance of arterial oxygen saturation (SaO_2) <90 or PaO_2 <60 mmHg (8.0 kPa) and the maintenance of normoxia (Carney et al. 2017). As hyperoxia has some potential for harm, a careful balance should be sought between benefit and risk when setting the oxygenation targets in individual patients.

In patients with preserved cerebrovascular carbon dioxide reactivity, cerebral resistance arterioles will constrict to changes in arterial carbon dioxide tension ($PaCO_2$) by a pH-dependent mechanism; this will reduce cerebral blood flow, cerebral blood volume, and ICP. Prophylactic extreme hypocarbia was associated with a worse outcome in severe TBI possibly due to cerebral ischaemia ($PaCO_2$ <25 mmHg (3.3 kPa) (Muizelaar et al. 1991); extreme hypercarbia may also be undesirable due to cerebral hyperperfusion with potential increases in cerebral blood volume, ICP, and vasogenic oedema. Although the thresholds for harm are debated (Godoy et al. 2017; Coles et al. 2007), in general, severe hypocapnia ($PaCO_2$ <25 mmHg (3.3 kPa)) is discouraged, whereas normocapnia ($PaCO_2$ 35 mmHg (4.7 kPa)) is encouraged. Thus, optimal ventilation and oxygenation are important in the treatment of TBI; however, normal values do not guarantee protection against cerebral ischaemia, and treatment may have to be individualized (Okonkwo et al. 2017).

Optimal exchange of oxygen and carbon dioxide in the lungs depends on open alveoli, a short alveolar to capillary diffusion distance, and a flow in the pulmonary capillaries that matches the airflow to the individual alveoli (also known as ventilation-perfusion matching). Local ventilation-perfusion mismatch may manifest as a shunt, in which the capillaries are perfused, but the alveoli are hypo- or unventilated (e.g. due to atelectasis caused by obstruction of the bronchioles or external compression), or as increased dead space, in which the alveoli are ventilated, but the capillaries are under- or unperfused (e.g. due to thrombus). Importantly, increasing the inspiratory oxygen fraction will usually not increase arterial oxygenation if hypoxia is caused by a shunt. This is because the blood that perfuses the nonventilated parts will remain nonoxygenated by this intervention, whereas the ventilated parts of the lungs are already fully saturated and will not take up more oxygen. Furthermore, an increased diffusion distance between an alveole and its perfusing capillary (e.g. due to interstitial oedema) will affect oxygen exchange relatively more than carbon dioxide exchange. Finally, an increase in dead space will usually lead to ventilation failure and hypercapnia, because the (effective) alveolar ventilation is reduced, but not necessarily to hypoxia, unless the redistribution of blood leads to severe hyperperfusion in the perfused parts of the lungs.

During mechanical ventilation, inspiration is changed from the normal spontaneous negative intrathoracic pressure inspiration to positive pressure inspiration, which increases intrathoracic pressure and reduces venous return to the heart (preload). As a consequence, many mechanically ventilated patients may become functionally hypovolaemic immediately after intubation and start of mechanical ventilation and may need a fluid load or vasopressors (or both) to compensate for decreased cardiac output. Expiration is passive, but a high positive end-expiratory pressure (PEEP) will offset some of the increase in intrathoracic pressure.

During the respiratory cycle in a mechanically ventilated patient, some alveoli open and some collapse. Cyclic reopening of collapsed alveoli may cause shear or stress injury (atelectrauma) especially in lungs with pre-existing lung damage and is believed to be the main mechanism responsible for VILI, together with volutrauma due to high tidal volumes and barotrauma due to high pulmonary pressures (Definition Task Force et al. 2012; Davies et al. 2015). In healthy lungs, the risk of damage to the pulmonary tissue due to collapse and reexpansion is considered low. Ventilation-perfusion mismatch caused by atelectasis formation is common in mechanically ventilated patients due to mucus plugs, diminished compliance, and pulmonary pathology. It may be reduced with the use of PEEP or reversed with recruitment manoeuvers, during which PEEP is temporarily increased to very high levels; however, intermittent or continuous use of high PEEP levels has both been associated with a risk of increased ICP in the patient with severe brain injury.

Pulmonary compliance (C) is a measure of the ability of the lungs to stretch (distensibility of elastic tissue):

$$C = \Delta V / \Delta P,$$

where V is volume and P is pressure. Low compliance indicates a stiff lung, and high compliance indicates a pliable lung. Compliance is highest at moderate lung volumes and much lower at volumes that are very low or very high. Compliance can be divided into a static (no airflow) and a dynamic (during airflow) compliance. The compliance measured in clinical practice is always *total* pulmonary compliance, which is a function of lung compliance and chest wall (ribcage and diaphragm) compliance. Pneumonia, pulmonary oedema, or ARDS will decrease lung compliance. Chest wall compliance is affected by body position, muscle tonus, and intra-abdominal hypertension (decreased compliance). Decreased compliance can markedly affect the total amount of work required for ventilation and may increase energy expenditure by up to 30% in the spontaneously breathing patient.

51.3.3 Basic Monitoring of the Patient with TBI

Any evaluation of the haemodynamic and respiratory status of a TBI patient starts with a basic clinical examination. Is the skin warm and dry, or does the patient have a cold and clammy hand? Skin colour? Are the peripheral veins visible? Does auscultation reveal a heart murmur? Pulmonary wheezing or rales or decreased breath sounds? Is there jugular vein distension? Peripheral oedema? If possible, obtain the patient's history of pre-existing cardiac or pulmonary problems and medications.

In order to avoid secondary brain injury by correcting hypotension and hypoxia, the question is whether hypotension is caused by hypovolaemia, and, if so, how do we predict fluid responsiveness (Michard and Teboul 2002; Bendjelid and Karim 2003) and how do we detect reasons for respiratory deterioration?

51.3.3.1 Heart Rate and Rhythm

No TBI patient should be without continuous electrocardiography (ECG), usually as a three-lead precordial monitoring, because of the increased risk of significant disturbances in HR or rhythm. However, more than 75% of arrhythmias and ischaemic events have been reported to go undetected by such continuous monitoring. Also, ischaemic episodes commonly occur without significant changes in haemodynamic variables. A standard 12-lead ECG can detect ischaemia. It is usually defined as ST segment depression of more than 0.1 mV. Hypertension or tachycardia is known to elicit ischaemia. Continuous ECG is mainly useful for detecting brady- or tachycardia with accompanying changes in blood pressure.

51.3.3.2 Arterial Blood Pressure

Patients with severe TBI should be monitored with an indwelling arterial line to obtain continuous blood pressure. Arterial pressure provides information on systolic and diastolic pressure as well as arterial waveform but provides little information on flow and oxygen supply. Even so, arterial blood pressure, usually expressed as the mean, MAP (MAP = DBP + 1/3(SBP-DBP)), is often used as a surrogate parameter for organ flow, where SBP is systolic blood pressure and DBP is diastolic blood pressure.

Hypotension increases morbidity and mortality in TBI (Juul et al. 2000; Nordström 2003). The threshold of blood pressure is not known, but current guidelines recommend that maintaining SBP at >100 mmHg for patients 50–69 years old or at >110 mmHg or above for patients 15–49 or >70 years old may be considered to decrease mortality and improve outcomes (Carney et al. 2017). The threshold of hypotension in the patient with TBI is probably dependent on age and pre-existing disease, e.g. hypertension. MAP is used to calculate CPP (MAP-ICP = CPP), and a CPP more than 60 mmHg is recommended in adults and with age-specific goals in children (see chapter on Cerebral Monitoring). In order to calculate CPP, MAP and ICP must be zeroed at the same level, usually at the tragus of the external ear (McNett et al. 2018). If the patient is hypotensive, the main interest is whether the patient is hypovolaemic and responds with an increase in MAP with fluid administration (fluid responsiveness) or, alternatively, if vasopressors or inotropes are needed. MAP should only be increased with vasopressors after cardiac preload assessment and a fluid challenge, most commonly a bolus of crystalloid (Muzevich and Voils 2009) (see chapter on vasopressors), but in clinical practice in the NICU, administration of vasopressor and volume loading initially take place simultaneously in order to avoid even short periods of hypotension.

When the patient is stable, the arterial cannula should be removed due to the risk of thrombosis and embolization. NIBP monitoring is used after the patient has reached definite stabilization or in the rehabilitation period.

51.3.3.3 Urine Output

Except in a few notable situations mentioned below (diuretic treatment including treatment with mannitol and diabetes insipidus), sufficient urine output usually indicates adequate organ perfusion and volume status; and most cases of low urine output are caused by hypovolaemia. Thus, hourly urine output should be monitored in all TBI patients. However, a normal urine output may occur despite hypoperfusion or hypovolaemia, if diuretics (including mannitol) have been administered or in the case of diabetes insipidus; such patients may become severely hypovolaemic and hypotensive, if the fluid deficit is not closely monitored and corrected. In Scandinavia, hyperosmolar therapy with hypertonic saline, which does not lead to osmotic diuresis, has largely replaced mannitol.

51.3.3.4 Pulse Oximetry

Pulse oximetry for the monitoring of peripheral oxygen saturation (SpO_2) is a mainstay in ICU as well as NICU monitoring. SpO_2 is approximately equal to arterial blood saturation (SaO_2) and is thus a marker of PaO_2. It is usually applied to a finger or a toe, but any site allowing proper orientation of the light can be used. If the finger or toe is cold or not well perfused, SpO_2 may be inaccurate. SpO_2 is also unreliable in patients with severe anaemia, skin pigmentation, or jaundice. The major advantage is that it is noninvasive, requires no calibration, and is usually available within seconds. Thus, onset or worsening of conditions resulting in hypoxia can be immediately identified. In otherwise stable patients, procedures such as endotracheal suctioning and positioning may cause desaturation. SpO_2 monitoring detects this and allows the team to prevent and treat these potentially dangerous episodes of hypoxia. The pulse oximeter also acts as a simple perfusion monitor and displays HR. Pulse oximeters typically have an accuracy within 2% in the area of SpO_2 100 to 90 and are less accurate with SpO_2 below 90. However, the clinically relevant distinction lies around a saturation of 90 (corresponding to PaO_2 of 60 mmHg or 8.0 kPa), which definitely is a threshold for intervention (Carney et al. 2017).

51.3.3.5 Monitoring of End-Tidal and Arterial CO_2 Capnography

Continuous monitoring of end-tidal CO_2 ($ETCO_2$) in intubated patients provides information on both ventilation and perfusion. Expired air is sampled from the ventilator tubing as close to the endotracheal tube as possible, and the CO_2 concentration or partial pressure is typically measured continuously in the air by the absorption of infrared light. The CO_2 waveform is displayed on the screen and consists of an inspiratory and an expiratory part. The $ETCO_2$ is the maximal CO_2 level, corresponding to the alveolar air at the end of expiration (which occurs with a delay on the screen compared to the visually observed expiration, as air flows from the alveoles to the capnography equipment). The expiratory component is divided into three phases. Phase I is the start of the phase before CO_2 appears, II is the rapid increase in CO_2, and III (the plateau phase) represents the emptying of alveolar space.

Concomitant measurement of $ETCO_2$ and $PaCO_2$ allows for estimation of the physiologic dead space and total CO_2 production. In patients with normal lung function, $ETCO_2$ is 0.5–1.0 kPa lower than $PaCO_2$, but this difference is affected both by pulmonary and circulatory pathologies; accordingly, capnography cannot substitute for estimation of $PaCO_2$ (Eun and Seo 2011). The shape of the capnography curve also informs on different pathologies; thus, the slope between phases I and II may be reduced (i.e. the curve may be flattened) in bronchospasm or other conditions associated with heterogeneous ventilation-perfusion ratios, such as COPD.

Although capnography is insufficient for the ventilatory management of raised intracranial pressure, it is invaluable for emergency situations, where arterial blood gas sampling and measurement would be too slow and impractical, such as ensuring endotracheal as opposed to oesophageal placement of the tube during intubation, and to detect dislocation of the endotracheal tube. Besides dislocation of the tube, airway obstruction, and severe bronchospasm, a dramatic fall in $ETCO_2$ during controlled ventilation may also indicate impending or manifest cardiac arrest.

51.3.3.6 Central Venous Pressure

For years, central venous pressure (CVP) has been used almost universally to guide fluid therapy in critically ill patients. CVP is at best a poor marker of central blood volume in adults, let alone of the haemodynamic response to a fluid challenge. Accordingly, CVP is not recommended to guide fluid therapy in TBI (Gottlieb and Hunter 2016; Eskesen et al. 2016; Cole 2008).

51.3.3.7 Venous Saturation

Central venous saturation ($ScvO_2$) is determined by CO, the blood haemoglobin concentration, arterial oxygen tension, and total oxygen consumption. A change in $ScvO_2$ theoretically indicates that a change in oxygen transport and/or demand has occurred. An absolute value of 0.68 to 0.77 is considered normal. However, a change in $ScvO_2$ is more important than the absolute value; assuming that haemoglobin, arterial oxygen content, and oxygen consumption are unchanged, $ScvO_2$ reflects cardiac output. A decrease in $ScvO_2$ is easier to interpret than an increase in $ScvO_2$, and in systemic inflammatory response syndrome or sepsis, peripheral shunting or dysfunctional mitochondria may impair oxygen uptake, so that $ScvO_2$ remains high. A low $ScvO_2$ has been associated with increased mortality and, when encountered, should prompt further evaluation of the individual factors influencing oxygen balance, i.e. intravascular volume status, blood haemoglobin, arterial oxygen tension, and cardiac function. As a general guideline, an $ScvO_2$ value greater than 0.66 is considered adequate, 0.50 to 0.65 represents a limited cardiovascular reserve, and less than 0.50 probably reflects inadequate tissue oxygenation (Rivers et al. 2001).

51.3.3.8 Lactate

During glycolysis, glucose is metabolized to pyruvate, which may undergo reduction to lactate or be aerobically degraded in the mitochondria. Increased blood lactate levels may be due to intracellular hypoxia, e.g. caused by tissue hypoperfusion due to reduced aerobic degradation of pyruvate, but may also result from increased glycolytic activity, e.g. because of infusion of sympathomimetics or skeletal muscle activity. While an increase in blood lactate may indicate anaerobic metabolism, the absence of increased blood lactate does not guarantee adequate cellular oxygen supply.

51.3.3.9 Cardiac Output

Previously, haemodynamic monitoring in anaesthesia and intensive care was based on the highly invasive and risk-associated pulmonary artery catheter (PAC), with no proven benefit on outcome (Hadian et al. 2010). Almost no reports on the use of PAC in TBI patients are available (Powner et al. 2005). Today, however, less invasive methods for estimating CO are available, all of which have strengths and limitations. These methods include methods using the Fick principle (thermodilution, dye dilution, lithium dilution) and pulse contour methods as well as ultrasonic methods (transoesophageal echocardiography, oesophageal Doppler monitoring). Electrical bioimpedance is another technique currently evolving.

In general, estimation or measurement of CO is of particular interest in situations where cardiac dysfunction is suspected, or if the patient does not respond to fluid, and there is a therapeutic dilemma between the choice of vasopressors and inotropes. Most studies of individualized goal-directed therapy and protocolled optimization of haemodynamics by measurements of CO and derived parameters have been performed in patients having cardiac or other major surgery, while there are few reports on monitoring of CO and outcome in patients with TBI (Prathep et al. 2014). Beyond a certain minimum, CO is usually not considered to affect CBF; thus, measurement of CO is not recommended as a standard in these patients.

51.3.3.10 Echocardiography and Doppler Techniques

Echocardiography is widely used for evaluating cardiac function, either by the noninvasive transthoracic (TTE) or the semi-invasive transoesophageal (TEE) approach. With the Doppler technique, pressures and blood flow velocities can be measured. The method requires expensive equipment and a trained specialist, but bedside basic critical care echocardiography to assess global ventricular size and systolic function can be taught to and performed by neurointensivists (Lazaridis 2012).

Oesophageal Doppler facilitates a rapid intermittent noninvasive estimation of CO, but is not validated as a tool to replace invasive measurement of CO at present.

51.3.3.11 Pulse Contour Analysis of Arterial Pressure Curve

Analysis of the arterial pressure curve has gained popularity in estimating cardiac output and fluid responsiveness. Analysis of the arterial pressure curve, either invasively or by skin-applied devices, is used to calculate/estimate CO based on HR, MAP, and the arterial waveform. Preload can be evaluated by cyclic respiratory variations in the arterial pressure, and a number of commercially available techniques use derived preload parameters such as pulse pressure variation and stroke volume variation to estimate fluid responsiveness. Recent studies suggest that these indices are the most reliable predictors of fluid responsiveness in different populations.

51.3.3.12 Monitoring of Pulmonary Mechanics and Compliance

Pulmonary compliance is a measure of the lung's ability to stretch, and most modern ventilators display and estimate peak inspiratory pressure, end expiratory pressure, and tidal volume and calculates total static compliance, i.e. both lung and chest wall compliances. Changes (fall) in compliance are important in the TBI patient because of the consequent impact on ventilation and risk of inducing VILI and should lead to clinical examination and reflexion and adjustment of the ventilator.

51.3.3.13 Chest X-Ray (CXR)

CXR provides information on infiltration (aspiration, pneumonia) or lung oedema, pneumothorax, or pleural effusion and placement of tube and catheters. Daily "routine" CXR is not recommended, but CXR is a simple and fast examination for acute respiratory deterioration or in the case of lack of respiratory improvement. Pneumonia occurs frequently in TBI patients and is often due to associated chest trauma or aspiration (Esnault et al. 2017).

51.3.3.14 Bronchoscopy

Bronchoscopy is used in the NICU as a diagnostic or therapeutic tool to clear large amount of secretions, to provide specimens for cultures, and to verify the position of the endotracheal tube or tracheostomy or facilitate replacement of the tracheostomy tube in emergency situations. With the availability of bronchoscopes in most NICU and available expertise, it is easy to perform. However, long bronchoscopy sessions may contribute to hypoventilation and occult hypercarbia, factors known to increase intracranial pressure. Steps to minimize occult hypercarbia, such as using the smallest bronchoscope available, minimizing suctioning, and the length of time the bronchoscopy is in the endotracheal tube, should be undertaken (Reilly et al. 1997).

In conclusion, advanced cardiopulmonary monitoring is not well validated in the TBI patient population, but much information can be gained from basic systemic monitoring. However, even when the patient appears haemodynamically and respiratory stable, there is not guarantee that perfusion in the cerebral microcirculation is sufficient nor that cerebral oxygenation is adequate (see chapter on cerebral monitoring).

51.3.4 Cardiopulmonary Treatment of the TBI Patient

51.3.4.1 Goal-Directed Therapy in Severe TBI: Which Direction?

In most Scandinavian hospitals, the protocolled management of TBI and treatment is based on the American and/or European guidelines. There is good evidence that protocolized care improves outcome. Different principles are used in the "Lund concept", which is a protocol aimed at nonsurgical reduction of increased ICP (Grände 2017). A second aim in the Lund concept is to improve brain perfusion and oxygenation around contusions by antagonizing vasoconstriction through minimizing sympathetic discharge and refraining from vasoconstrictors. As previously stated, the threshold of blood pressure in severe TBI is not known and may be individual, but a single systolic blood pressure of <90 mmHg has been shown to worsen outcomes in brain-injured patients. However, normalization of blood pressure, blood volume, and plasma oncotic pressure as well as general supportive intensive care is an integrated part of the Lund treatment also.

Measurement of ICP and brain oxygen tension; medical management with anaesthetics, analgesics, sedatives, and muscle relaxants; hyperosmolar therapy; management of fever; detection and treatment of infection; treatment of seizures; blood glucose control; deep vein thrombosis; and early nutrition and electrolyte balance are all general critical care issues that are very important after severe head injury and must be taken into account when planning and performing respiratory and circulatory treatment. There are at present less than 200 completed randomized controlled trials dealing with acute TBI management, mostly smaller ($N < 100$) single-centre studies. Thus, research in management for acute severe brain injury has resulted in little translatable evidence (Bragge et al. 2016). Mortality and morbidity is reduced when the patient with TBI is in a specialized neurointensive care environment (Elf et al. 2002; Varelas et al. 2004; Varelas et al. 2006).

51.3.4.2 Maintenance of MAP and CPP

Cerebral autoregulation in the TBI patient is impaired, and hypotension occurring during the first 6 h after injury has the highest prediction for poor discharge GOS (Hardcastle and Benzon 2014). In addition, many mechanically ventilated patients show signs of hypovolaemia. In the NICU, vasopressor administration is often utilized concurrently with fluid resuscitation in brain-injured patients to avoid even short episodes of low CPP, making estimation of fluid balance even more difficult. A study on optimal CPP using the concept of cerebrovascular pressure reactivity-based individual CPP found that driving CPP in excess of optimal CPP did not yield improvements in $PbrO_2$ and should be avoided and that CPP below optimal CPP might result in secondary ischaemia (Jaeger et al. 2010). In adults, CPP should be kept >60 mmHg, while CPP in children is age dependent (Allen et al. 2014).

51.3.4.3 Which Fluid and When to Transfuse?

Crystalloids are used as the main volume expander in TBI where maintaining a normal concentration of plasma sodium is important in avoiding worsening of cerebral oedema around contusions and controlling ICP. Preservation of normal potassium and chloride ions are also issues in TBI patients. Crystalloids are associated with general tissue oedema including the brain, and saline is associated with hyperchloraemic acidosis, if infused in large amounts. Albumin was associated with higher mortality rates than resuscitation with saline in acute trauma patients with TBI after the SAFE-TBI post hoc study in 2007 (SAFE Study Investigators, Australian and New Zealand Intensive Care Society Clinical Trials Group, Australian Red Cross Blood Service, George Institute for International Health, et al. 2007), and clinical practices of intravenous fluid resuscitation have changed since then (Hammond et al. 2017). Hypertonic saline is a very efficient agent for treatment of ICH and is often used in the NICU in the medical treatment of ICH but is not recommended in a general trauma population.

There are no specific guidelines on fluid therapy in TBI (see chapter on fluid haemodynamics in patients with severe TBI) and only few RCTs on this subject, one of which reported lower mortality in patients receiving fresh frozen plasma compared with placebo (Bragge et al. 2016).

51.3.4.4 Transfusion

Current evidence supports restrictive over liberal red blood cell transfusion practices in critically ill patients. Blood products have potential adverse effects, and there has been an absence of benefit from liberal transfusion strategies (Kramer and Zygun 2009; Figaji et al. 2009; Lelubre et al. 2016; Holst and Perner 2011; Boutin et al. 2016). The association between transfusion and higher mortality seems to be stronger in patients who are transfused at higher haemoglobin levels (Boutin et al. 2016). Further data on RBC transfusion and haemoglobin levels in patients with TBI are required. Presently it is prudent to limit transfusion since haemoglobin threshold is not known neither in adults nor in children.

51.3.4.5 Vasopressors

The choice of vasopressor is guided by the clinical characteristics of the patient and the goals of therapy (Muzevich and Voils 2009; Hylands et al. 2017). In general vasopressors are not recommended in early trauma resuscitation, but in victims with TBI where mortality is doubled by hypotension, they may be beneficial (Hylands et al. 2017). Aggressive vasopressor therapy maintaining a CPP greater than 70 mmHg has been associated with increased incidence of ARDS. With emerging evidence of harm associated with aggressive fluid resuscitation, the alternatives to vasopressor treatment in the NICU are limited. The ideal agent remains unknown. Human data are limited to norepinephrine, dopamine, and phenylephrine, and based on the cerebrovascular effects, norepinephrine and phenylephrine are the preferred agents (Hylands et al. 2017). One RCT of vasopressin vs. catecholamines for CPP control in TBI is ongoing (Hylands et al. 2017; Van Haren et al. 2013). Interestingly, administration of beta-blockers early after TBI has been associated with improved survival in a large retrospective analysis (Ley et al. 2018).

51.3.4.6 Arterial Oxygen Partial Pressure (PaO_2)

Arterial hypoxemia leads to cerebral arteriolar vasodilation (Kontos et al. 1978), increases CBF in healthy humans (Kety and Schmidt 1948), and may increase ICP in patients with TBI. Most studies showing a detrimental effect of hypoxia (usually defined as a PaO_2 <60 mmHg) on outcome after TBI have addressed the prehospital setting (Chesnut et al. 1993); in contrast, the effects of hypoxia after admission to hospital or ICU are less clear. A recent retrospective study from Australia and New Zealand of 24,148 mechanically ventilated ICU patients with TBI, in whom the overall in-hospital mortality was 17.2%, reported that hypoxia as defined by a worst arterial PaO_2 <60 mmHg (8 kPa) within the first 24 h was detected in 4.9% of patients and was associated with an adjusted OR for in-hospital mortality of 1.15 (95% CI 0.96 to 1.38), compared to normoxia defined as PaO_2 60–299 mmHg. Hyperoxia, defined as a worst PaO_2 >299 mmHg, was detected in 12.9% and was associated with an OR of 0.97 (95% CI 0.86–1.11). When patients were divided into 17 subgroups according to PaO_2 in 10 mmHg increments using a PaO_2 of 100–109 mmHg as the reference, only a PaO_2 <40 mmHg (5.3 kPa) was significantly associated with increased mortality at an OR of 1.52 (95% CI 1.03–2.25) (O'Briain et al. 2018). Gómez et al. reported an adjusted OR of verified or suspected hypoxia for a poor neurological outcome (measured by the Glasgow Outcome Scale) after 1 year of 1.87 (1.42–2.46); however, no information was given regarding the definition of hypoxia or whether it was observed before or during admission to hospital (Gómez et al. 2018).

Hyperoxia, either during normobaria or hyperbaria, has been suggested to improve outcome after TBI. In 2012, a Cochrane systematic review and meta-analysis reported that hyperbaric oxygen therapy was associated with a reduction in ICP, as well as a reduced risk of an unfavourable outcome 1 month after injury (relative risk (RR) for unfavourable outcome with hyperbaric oxygen therapy 0.74, 95% CI 0.61 to 0.88, $P = 0.001$) and of dying (RR 0.69, 95% CI 0.54 to 0.88, $P = 0.003$) (Bennett et al. 2012), albeit based on low-quality studies. Subsequently, one small randomized study of low quality reported an improved functional outcome at 6 months in mechanically ventilated TBI patients treated during the first 6 h with an inspired oxygen fraction (FiO_2) of 80% compared to those ventilated with an FiO_2 of 50% (Taher et al. 2016). Another randomized trial reported that 60 min of hyperbaric oxygen at 1.5 atmospheres absolute (ATA) followed by 3 h of normobaric hyperoxia (FiO_2 100%), administered for 3 h, resulted in a 26% absolute reduction in 6-month mortality and a 36% absolute increase in favourable outcome, compared to standard care (Rockswold et al. 2013). However, the current evidence base is currently too weak to justify a recommendation for or against hyperoxia in TBI patients.

In the future, the use of systemic oxygenation targets to avoid secondary brain injury will probably be replaced or supplemented by brain tissue oxygen tension-targeted therapy (Okonkwo et al. 2017). Current guidelines recommend avoidance of PaO_2 <60 mmHg (8.0 kPa) and the maintenance of normoxia. In the case of concomitant severe ARDS, this recommendation should be balanced against the ARDSNet target of a PaO_2 down to 55 mmHg (7.3 kPa). In the case of severe TBI and less severe ARDS, it may be prudent to aim for a slightly higher PaO_2, whereas a patient with mild TBI and severe ARDS may benefit from a lower oxygen target. Monitoring brain tissue oxygen tension may further aid in defining the correct oxygen target in these challenging patients.

51.3.4.7 Intubate: When and How

Following severe brain injury, impaired consciousness and brainstem reflexes induce hypoventilation and lead to aspiration. Therefore, the majority of patients with severe TBI are intubated and mechanically ventilated even though most patients do not have a primary respiratory indication for intubation. Usually intubation takes place in the emergency situation to protect the airway and to control $PaCO_2$. There are several airway considerations and challenges specific to the neurocritically ill patient:

TBI patients with a GCS of <9 should be intubated to secure the airway. Besides the risk of collapse of the upper airway as well as aspiration of gastric contents and impaired cough reflexes, those with injury to the lower pons or medulla or those with elevated ICP especially in the posterior fossa may have an unstable ventilatory drive. For intubation, manual inline stabilization should be used if spinal trauma is suspected. Chin lift and jaw thrust manoeuvers can be safely performed without hyperextending the neck (which is associated with a risk of cervical cord injury) to relieve airway obstruction. In the case of facial trauma, nasopharyngeal airways (as well as nasogastric tubes) are contraindicated. During the process of intubation, patients are at risk of both hypotension and hypoxia. Thus, with induction of anaesthesia and loss of sympathetic tone, a drop in CPP can occur, leading to ischaemia and herniation, if ICP is elevated; conversely, hypertension due to insufficient anaesthesia or analgesia may also increase ICP. Most strong analgesics, intravenous anaesthetics (except ketamine), and neuromuscular blocker drugs are cerebral vasoconstrictors, which will lead to reduced cerebral oxygen metabolism and blood flow and thus to a decreased ICP in most TBI patients.

All trauma patients are at risk of aspiration due to a full stomach. Thus, so-called rapid sequence induction is usually preferred for intubation. Suxamethonium, a fast-acting neuromuscular relaxant, has been reported to increase ICP, but is not contraindicated in patients with a difficult airway. Barbiturates, propofol, and etomidate can be used; however, even a single dose of etomidate may precipitate hypocortisolism and adrenal insufficiency. Propofol is not recommended for long-term sedation in children, but can be used for induction. Ketamine is often used in the acute setting and has been associated with increase in ICP; however, recent studies have reported that ketamine is safe both for induction and sedation in patients with increased ICP and even may confer neuroprotective effects (Oddo et al. 2016; Wazen et al. 2013).

Airway incidents do occur in the NICU (as they do in the general ICU) and pose the same challenges, except that TBI patients are at a high risk of cerebral ischaemia even after short hypoxic episodes.

After intubation, sedatives and analgesics are used for control of pain, anxiety, agitation, and patient-ventilator synchrony. In the brain-injured patient, sedation and analgesia have additional indications, as they lower the cerebral metabolic rate of oxygen consumption and thus may reduce ICP. Sedation is also used to suppress seizures and reduce pain and agitation that may cause arterial hypertension and associated ICH. Overall, sedation and analgesia may protect the brain (Oddo et al. 2016). However, at the same time, the wish to perform serial neurological examinations renders long-acting sedatives and neuromuscular blockers generally undesirable.

Advantages of intubation and sedation	Disadvantages of intubation and sedation
Protects the airway, protects against aspiration, and makes it possible to control PaO_2 and $PaCO_2$	Induction and sedation make serial examinations of consciousness difficult
TBI patients will likely require additional invasive procedures with sedation/anaesthesia (monitor placement, craniotomy)	Sedation may lower MAP and make fluid challenges and vasopressors necessary
Facilitation of transport between units including radiology	General side effects (gastrointestinal motility lowered)

51.3.4.8 Which Neurological Patients Are at Risk of an Airway Catastrophe?

Not every patient with abnormal airway protection needs intubation. In the acute phase of severe TBI, airway protection is usually indicated and may be life-saving, but later, the concept "an adequately protected airway" is more controversial. Normal airway function involves opening of the larynx, vocal folds, and cords during in- and expiration and closure when the airflow stops; coordinated oropharyngeal sensory and muscle activity to move secretion, fluids, and food; a tight lower oesophageal sphincter and low gastric pH; and a robust sensory response to fluid and food at the glottis and lower airways, as well as intact cough pathways. Finally, adequate respiratory muscle strength and tidal volumes are required to generate a strong cough. A clinically unstable patient with impaired airway maintenance requires intubation, but a clinically stable patient with impaired airway maintenance can often be managed without an endotracheal tube by feeding through a tube (often enteral) and by attentive nursing and respiratory care. GCS is routinely used but was not developed for neurologic evaluation in the late phase of TBI and does not address the primary issues related to airway protection. Gag reflex is also routinely assessed, but the gag reflex does not correlate well with laryngeal closure airway protection and may be absent in healthy subjects.

Aspiration leads to fever, pneumonia, ARDS, and systemic inflammation, all of which are associated with worse neurologic outcomes and increased mortality. Intubation and sedation may be required for different acute purposes but must be balanced against the need for an adequate neurological examination and avoidance of the complications of intubation and MV, when possible.

51.3.4.9 Assessment of the Airway and Prediction of a Difficult Airway

An airway evaluation should be performed in every patient prior to intubation. In the unconscious patient, the airway is more difficult to evaluate. A difficult airway algorithm should be adopted.

51.3.4.10 How to Set the Ventilator

After brain injury, a systemic inflammatory state develops, with inflammatory cells also migrating to airways and alveolar spaces. In addition, the TBI patients frequently suffer from lung complications (aspiration, pulmonary contusion related to chest trauma, etc.), and patients are at risk of developing ARDS (Definition Task Force et al. 2012; Rincon et al. 2012). In the presence of an inflammatory state, an injurious ventilatory strategy may significantly add to worsening lung damage. Mechanical ventilation in this situation presents significant challenges, because guidelines recommending strategies in ARDS come into conflicts with what is now considered best practice in TBI (Della Torre et al. 2017). ARDS strategies may include lung-protective mechanical ventilation (LPMV), which is based on low tidal volumes and positive end-expiratory pressures (PEEP) to recruit collapsed alveolar parenchyma. This reduces the sheer forces and the risk of alveolar rupture and the release of inflammatory mediators that occur with repeated opening and closing of collapsed alveoli (Definition Task Force et al. 2012; Finfer et al. 2019). Recruitment manoeuvers, permissive hypercapnia, and prone position are also part of advanced ARDS treatment. The tight interaction between respiratory and cerebral dynamics clearly represents a potential risk for iatrogenic secondary brain damage, when ARDS ventilation recommendations are used; on the other hand, without sufficient arterial oxygenation, even an optimal CPP will not be sufficient to avoid brain damage. As mentioned above, the ARDSNet target of PaO_2 (7.3 kPa) seems too low to be safely applied to patients with TBI. Hypercapnia is associated with cerebral vasodilatation and increase in ICP. Hypercapnia, which is usually accepted in LPMV, can be dangerous in TBI patients. Conversely, hypocapnia and consequent cerebral vasoconstriction decrease ICP. Therefore, in TBI patients, the standard of care is to ventilate to low normocapnia (4.5–5 kPa), but this may be a challenge in ARDS patients.

High TV ventilation in patients with TBI has been associated with development of ARDS. Even though lung-protective ventilation has gained widespread use, many TBI patients are still ventilated with high tidal volumes (Asehnoune et al. 2017; Asehnoune et al. 2018). Brain-injured patient with healthy lungs or only moderately impaired lung function should be ventilated with

LPMV (tidal volume 6–7 mL/kg) (Bruni et al. 2017). When TBI and ARDS coexist, a balance needs to be found between lung protection and CO_2 control. There are no absolute contraindications to the use of protective ventilation in TBI, and the $PaCO_2$ should be set according to ICP and, preferably, brain parenchymal oxygen electrodes.

Presently, choice of ventilator rescue therapies in severe lung injury is best decided on a case-to-case basis.

51.3.4.11 PEEP

A high PEEP can improve pulmonary gas exchange and respiratory mechanics by opening collapsed alveoli and keeping them open, reducing ventilation/perfusion mismatch. However, PEEP also has the potential to impair return of venous flow from the cerebral veins to the heart, decrease mean arterial pressure, and thus increase ICP and decrease CPP. For many years, it was considered prudent to use low or no PEEP in mechanically ventilated patients with brain injury. Recent investigations have challenged the potential harmful effect of PEEP in TBI patients with ARDS and found that in normovolaemic patients, PEEP can be safely applied and may even benefit cerebral brain tissue oxygenation providing that patients were normovolaemic (Della Torre et al. 2017; Asehnoune et al. 2017; Nemer et al. 2015). Others have found a substantial difference in the effect of PEEP on ICP in ARDS depending on whether PEEP caused alveolar hyperinflation or alveolar recruitment. With recruitment, a fall in $PaCO_2$ may occur with a subsequent reduction in ICP, but with hyperinflation (i.e., "over-recruitment"), the effect may be opposite. Similarly, recruitment manoeuvers may cause a significant elevation in ICP in patients with impaired autoregulation, but in TBI patients with ARDS, recruitment may improve oxygenation.

51.3.4.12 Hyperventilation

During acute hyperventilation, increased arteriolar resistance reduces CBF and cerebral blood volume and ultimately decreases ICP. Therapeutic hyperventilation has been widely used to decrease ICP and was an integrated part of the treatment until 10 years ago (Curry et al. 2008). However, the effects are transient, and the risks must be carefully considered before treatment, as diminished CBF may lead to cerebral ischaemia and tissue hypoxia. Therapeutic hyperventilation (at $PaCO_2$ <3.3 kPa) has been debated as a mean to control posttraumatic intracranial hypertension (ICH), but is detrimental to neurologic outcome and should be avoided especially during the acute phase of TBI, i.e. the first 24 h, where CBF is low (Muizelaar et al. 1991).

Prolonged prophylactic hyperventilation is thus not recommended as first-line therapy to reduce ICP, but may be used briefly in emergencies, when other interventions fail, and as a bridge to more definite treatment.

51.3.4.13 Weaning

While it may be life-saving, mechanical ventilation is also associated with life threatening complications and side effects and should be discontinued as soon as possible. Weaning is initiated when the patient is clinically stable, that is, there is no intracranial hypertension, hypoxemia, or hypotension. Most brain-injured patients are able to breathe spontaneously. Weaning is considered successful when the patient can sustain spontaneous breathing unassisted or with minimal support. Weaning delay and failure both increase the risk of complications and may prolong the NICU stay (Bruni et al. 2017; McCredie et al. 2017). When weaning is successful, extubation may be considered.

51.3.4.14 Extubation

Criteria for extubation in the general ICU patient include being awake and able to protect the airway, breathing spontaneously with a PaO_2/FiO_2 >200 mmHg (>27 kPa), FiO_2 <40%, a PEEP <5 cm H_2O, and only low levels of ventilator support (Girard et al. 2017).

Many TBI patients require minimal ventilator support, but little evidence is available to guide their extubation. The risk of extubation failure is higher than in the general ICU population and has been correlated with development of pneumonia and increased mortality, while delayed extubation increases the risk of ventilator-associated pneumonia. GCS has been inconsistently reported as a factor associated with extubation success, but has never been validated in intubated patients; thus, other tools to evaluate arousal are required (Peñuelas et al. 2015; Godet et al. 2017). A multicentre observational study did not support the use of GCS to help predict which TBI patient will fail extubation. Instead, airway protection assessments, such as the presence of cough, should be used as part of the decision process. Younger age and negative fluid balance also predicted extubation success. Neither delayed extubation nor tracheostomy was associated with improved outcome (McCredie et al. 2017).

Based on these considerations, we suggest the following criteria for extubating patients after severe TBI:

- The intracranial pathology has stabilized (e.g. ICP is below 15 mmHg without sedation, and no more than brief and rapidly reversible ICP increases occur during stimulation).
- Coughing occurs during tracheal suctioning and is considered sufficient to mobilize the patient's secretions from the trachea to the pharynx; in a patient with a normal pre-trauma lung function, the PaO_2 >10 kPa, $PaCO_2$ <6.0 kPa, and pH >7.30 with the patient breathing on pressure support ≤10 cm H_2O, FiO_2 of ≤40%, and PEEP ≤5 cm H_2O (other limits may be defined for those with pre-existing pulmonary disease).
- On these settings, the patient's tidal volume is ≥5 mL/kg, and the respiratory rate is ≤30 breaths/min.
- No or minimal circulatory support (e.g. noradrenaline infusion ≤0.05 μg/kg/min) is required.
- The patient is fasting.

If these criteria are met, a trial of extubation can be carried out. In contrast, if one or more of the points are not fulfilled, selected patients may undergo extubation, e.g. if they can follow commands, whereas others may require tracheostomy followed by general weaning of the respiratory support. Reintubation should always be considered possible for patients who fail an extubation trial (e.g. the patient's airway should not be classified as excessively difficult, and doctors who are skilled at airway management and the necessary devices and drugs should be immediately available).

51.3.4.15 Tracheostomy

In general, tracheostomy is associated with reduced time on mechanical ventilation and length of stay in the ICU. However, rates of ventilator-associated pneumonia are not decreased with tracheostomy.

Performing a tracheostomy carries the risk of occult hypoxic or hypotensive periods, which may aggravate secondary brain injury. In patients with severe TBI, early tracheostomy (<7 days) has been associated with increases in ICP and with both increased and reduced in-hospital mortalities (Baron et al. 2016; Stocchetti et al. 2000; Kocaeli et al. 2008; Lu et al. 2018). However, early tracheostomy in patients with a reasonable chance of survival may result in better overall clinical outcome (Rizk et al. 2011).

In conclusion, patients with severe TBI and a need for prolonged mechanical ventilation may benefit from early tracheostomy. However, the procedure may increase ICP and should not be performed before the intracranial pathology has stabilized.

51.3.4.16 Discharge from the NICU

Discharge from the NICU to a neurosurgical ward or a rehabilitation facility can take place when the patient is stable with respect to vital organ functions, in particular the cardiorespiratory and renal systems. Thus, the patient should be able to defend his/her own airway and maintain an acceptable oxygen saturation without advanced respiratory care; hypoxaemia and hypotension should be considered pathological until proven otherwise, as should a low urine output. Those with the highest risk of dying or readmission to intensive care should be discharged to an intermediate care unit (if available), rather than to the general ward, provided that further advanced care is indicated. A discharge protocol which is developed with knowledge of local options and contains threshold values for discharge may improve care (Nates et al. 2016).

51.3.5 Paediatric Aspects

Paediatric normal values for cerebral and systemic haemodynamics differ from those of adults. Furthermore, in children normal intracranial pressure (ICP) and blood pressure differ for different age groups, with potentially important implications for ICP and cerebral perfusion pressure (CPP) thresholds (Allen et al. 2014). The current evidence is based on observational studies reporting that (1) a sustained increase in ICP was associated with lower survival; (2) a higher CPP was associated with a higher chance of survival; (3) the threshold ICP above which survival was reduced was located at 20 mmHg for most studies; and the threshold CPP associated with increased survival was located somewhere between 40 and 50 mmHg (Allen et al. 2014; Kotchanek et al. 2012). These studies included both pro- and retrospective observations, and some observations were done in clinical settings that applied targets for both CPP and ICP. Thus, any relationship between these variables and outcome may have been due to confounding by indication (i.e. the lowest CPP may have been observed in the most severely ill patients, simply because it was harder to increase CPP in these patients, not because CPP in itself defined survival) and self-fulfilling prophecies (i.e. the treating physicians may have given up treatment of those patients with the lowest CPP values, because they expected them to be predictive of a poor outcome). Nevertheless, a level III recommendation is given to consider treating ICP if it exceeds 20 mmHg, and to aim for a CPP between 40 and 50 mmHg, in the low range for infants and in the high range for older children (Kotchanek et al. 2012).

References

Allen BB, Chiu Y-L, Gerber LM, Ghajar J, Greenfield JP. Age-specific cerebral perfusion pressure thresholds and survival in children and adolescents with severe traumatic brain injury*. Pediatr Crit Care Med. 2014;15(1):62–70. http://www.ncbi.nlm.nih.gov/pubmed/24196011.

Asehnoune K, Mrozek S, Perrigault PF, Seguin P, Dahyot-Fizelier C, Lasocki S, et al. A multi-faceted strategy to reduce ventilation-associated mortality in brain-injured patients. The BI-VILI project: a nationwide quality improvement project. Intensive Care Med. 2017;43(7):957–70. https://doi.org/10.1007/s00134-017-4764-6.

Asehnoune K, Roquilly A, Cinotti R. Respiratory management in patients with severe brain injury. J Crit Care. 2018;22(1):76. https://doi.org/10.1186/s13054-018-1994-0.

Baron DM, Hochrieser H, Metnitz PGH, Mauritz W. Tracheostomy is associated with decreased hospital mortality after moderate or severe isolated traumatic brain injury. Wien Klin Wochenschr. 2016;128(11–12):397–403.

Bendjelid, Karim RJ. Fluid responsiveness in mechanically ventilated patients : a review of indices used in intensive care. Intensive Care Med. 2003;29:352–60.

Bennett MH, Trytko B, Jonker B. Hyperbaric oxygen therapy for the adjunctive treatment of traumatic brain injury. Cochrane Database Syst Rev. 2012;12:CD004609. https://doi.org/10.1002/14651858.CD004609.pub3.

Boutin A, Chassé M, Shemilt M, Lauzier F, Moore L, Zarychanski R, et al. Red blood cell transfusion in patients with traumatic brain injury: a systematic review and meta-analysis. Transfus Med Rev. 2016;30(1):15–24. http://www.ncbi.nlm.nih.gov/pubmed/26409622.

Bragge P, Synnot A, Maas AI, Menon DK, Cooper DJ, Rosenfeld JV, et al. A state-of-the-science overview of randomized controlled trials evaluating acute management of moderate-to-severe traumatic brain injury. J Neurotrauma. 2016;33(16):1461–78. https://doi.org/10.1089/neu.2015.4233.

Brazinova A, Rehorcikova V, Taylor MS, Buckova V, Majdan M, Psota M, et al. Epidemiology of traumatic brain injury in europe: a living systematic review. J Neurotrauma. 2016; https://doi.org/10.1089/neu.2015.4126.

Bruni A, Garofalo E, Pelaia C, Longhini F, Navalesi P. Mechanical ventilation in brain injured patients: seeing the forest for the trees. J Thorac Dis. 2017;9(10):3483–7.

Carney N, Totten AM, O'Reilly C, Ullman JS, Hawryluk GWJJ, Bell MJ, et al. Guidelines for the management of severe traumatic brain injury, fourth edition. Neurosurgery. 2017;80(1):6–15.

Chesnut RM, Marshall LF, Klauber MR, Blunt BA, Baldwin N, Eisenberg HM, et al. The role of secondary brain injury in determining outcome from severe head injury. J Trauma. 1993;34(2):216–22. http://www.ncbi.nlm.nih.gov/pubmed/8459458. Accessed 22 Oct 2018.

Cole R. Does central venous pressure predict fluid responsiveness? Chest. 2008;134(6):1351–2. http://linkinghub.elsevier.com/retrieve/pii/S0012369208601634.

Coles JP, Fryer TD, Coleman MR, Smielewski P, Gupta AK, Minhas PS, et al. Hyperventilation following head injury: effect on ischemic burden and cerebral oxidative metabolism. Crit Care Med. 2007;35(2):568–78.

Davies SW, Leonard KL, Falls RK, Mageau RP, Efird JT, Hollowell JP, et al. Lung protective ventilation (ARDSNet) versus airway pressure release ventilation. J Trauma Acute Care Surg. 2015;78(2):240–51. http://www.ncbi.nlm.nih.gov/pubmed/25757107.

Definition Task Force ARDS, Ranieri VM, Rubenfeld GD, Thompson BT, Ferguson ND, Caldwell E, et al. Acute respiratory distress syndrome: the Berlin Definition. JAMA. 2012;307(23):2526–33. http://www.ncbi.nlm.nih.gov/pubmed/22797452.

Della Torre V, Badenes R, Corradi F, Racca F, Lavinio A, Matta B, et al. Acute respiratory distress syndrome in traumatic brain injury: how do we manage it? J Thorac Dis. 2017;9(12):5368–81.

Dunham CM, Cutrona AF, Gruber BS, Calderon JE, Ransom KJ, Flowers LL. Early tracheostomy in severe traumatic brain injury: evidence for decreased mechanical ventilation and increased hospital mortality. Int J Burn Trauma. 2014;4:14–24. www.IJBT.org.

Elf K, Nilsson P, Enblad P. Outcome after traumatic brain injury improved by an organized secondary insult program and standardized neurointensive care. Crit Care Med. 2002;30(9):2129–34.

Eskesen TG, Wetterslev M, Perner A. Systematic review including re-analyses of 1148 individual data sets of central venous pressure as a predictor of fluid responsiveness. Intensive Care Med. 2016;42(3):324–32.

Esnault P, Nguyen C, Bordes J, D'Aranda E, Montcriol A, Contargyris C, et al. Early-onset ventilator-associated pneumonia in patients with severe traumatic brain injury: incidence, risk factors, and consequences in cerebral oxygenation and outcome. Neurocrit Care. 2017;27(2):187–98. https://doi.org/10.1007/s12028-017-0397-4.

Eun M, Seo W. Monitoring of end-tidal CO2: benefits to critically ill neurological patients. 2011;50–5.

Figaji AA, Zwane E, Kogels M, Fieggen AG, Argent AC, Le Roux PD, et al. The effect of blood transfusion on brain oxygenation in children with severe traumatic brain injury*. Pediatr Crit Care Med. 2009;1. https://insights.ovid.com/crossref?an=00130478-900000000-99663.

Finfer SR, Vincent J-L, Slutsky AS, Ranieri VM. Critical care medicine ventilator-induced lung injury. N Engl J Med. 2019;369:2126–62. https://doi.org/10.1056/NEJMra1208707.

Girard TD, Alhazzani W, Kress JP, Ouellette DR, Schmidt GA, Truwit JD, et al. An Official American Thoracic Society/American College of Chest Physicians Clinical Practice Guideline: liberation from mechanical ventilation in critically ill adults. rehabilitation protocols, ventilator liberation protocols, and cuff leak tests. Am J Respir Crit Care Med. 2017;195(1):120–33. http://www.ncbi.nlm.nih.gov/pubmed/27762595.

Godet T, Chabanne R, Marin J, Kauffmann S, Futier E, Pereira B, et al. Extubation failure in brain-injured patients. Anesthesiology. 2017;126(1):104–14.

Godoy DA, Seifi A, Garza D, Lubillo-Montenegro S, Murillo-Cabezas F. Hyperventilation therapy for control of posttraumatic intracranial hypertension. Front Neurol. 2017;8(JUL):1–13.

Gómez PA, Castaño Leon AM, Lora D, Cepeda S, Lagares A. Final outcome trends in severe traumatic brain injury: a 25-year analysis of single center data. Acta Neurochir (Wien). 2018. https://doi.org/10.1007/s00701-018-3705-7.

Gottlieb M, Hunter B. Utility of central venous pressure as a predictor of fluid responsiveness. Ann Emerg Med. 2016;68(1):114–6. https://doi.org/10.1016/j.annemergmed.2016.02.009.

Grände P-O. Critical evaluation of the lund concept for treatment of severe traumatic head injury, 25 years after its introduction. Front Neurol. 2017;8(July). http://journal.frontiersin.org/article/10.3389/fneur.2017.00315/full.

Hadian M, Kim HK, Severyn DA, Pinsky MR. Cross-comparison of cardiac output trending accuracy of LiDCO, PiCCO, FloTrac and pulmonary artery catheters. Crit Care. 2010;14(6):R212.

Hammond NE, Taylor C, Finfer S, Machado FR, An Y, Billot L, et al. Patterns of intravenous fluid resuscitation use in adult intensive care patients between 2007 and 2014: an international cross-sectional study. 2017. https://doi.org/10.1371/journal.pone.0176292.

Hardcastle N, Benzon HAVM. Update on the 2012 guidelines for the management of pediatric traumatic brain injury- information for the anesthesiologist. Pediatr Anaesth. 2014;24(7):703–10.

Holst LB, Perner A. Der er kun sparsom evidens for blodtransfusion til ikkeblødende kritisk syge patienter. Transfusion. 2011:1632–4.

Hylands M, Toma A, Beaudoin N, Frenette AJ, D'Aragon F, Belley-Côté É, et al. Early vasopressor use following traumatic injury: a systematic review. BMJ Open. 2017;7(11):e017559.

Jaeger M, Dengl M, Meixensberger J, Schuhmann MU. Effects of cerebrovascular pressure reactivity-guided optimization of cerebral perfusion pressure on brain tissue oxygenation after traumatic brain injury. Crit Care Med. 2010;38(5):1343–7.

Juul N, Morris GF, Marshall SB, Marshall LF. Intracranial hypertension and cerebral perfusion pressure: influence on neurological deterioration and outcome in severe head injury. J Neurosurg. 2000;92(1):1–6. https://doi.org/10.3171/jns.2000.92.1.0001.

Kalsotra A, Zhao J, Anakk S, Dash PK, Strobel HW. Brain trauma leads to enhanced lung inflammation and injury: Evidence for role of P4504Fs in resolution. J Cereb Blood Flow Metab. 2018;27(5):963–74. www.jcbfm.com.

Kety SS, Schmidt CF. The effects of altered arterial tensions of carbon dioxide and oxygen on cerebral blood flow and cerebral oxygen consumption of normal young men. J Clin Invest. 1948;27(4):484–92. https://www.ncbi.nlm.nih.gov/pmc/articles/PMC439519/pdf/jcinvest00391-0096.pdf.

Kocaeli H, Korfali E, Taşkapilioğlu Ö, Özcan T. Analysis of intracranial pressure changes during early versus late percutaneous tracheostomy in a neuro-intensive care unit. Acta Neurochir. 2008;150(12):1263–7.

Kontos HA, Wei EP, Raper AJ, Rosenblum WI, Navari RM, Patterson JL. Role of tissue hypoxia in local regulation of cerebral microcirculation. Am J Physiol. 1978;234(5):H582–91. https://doi.org/10.1152/ajpheart.1978.234.5.H582.

Kotchanek PMPM, Carney N, Adelson PD, Ashwal S, Bell MJ, Bratton S, et al. Guidelines for the acute medical management of severe traumatic brain injury in infants, children, and adolescents-second edition. Pediatr Crit Care Med. 2012;13:S1–2. http://www.ncbi.nlm.nih.gov/pubmed/22217782.

Kramer AH, Zygun DA. Anemia and red blood cell transfusion in neurocritical care. Crit Care. 2009;13(3).

Lazaridis C. Advanced hemodynamic monitoring: principles and practice in neurocritical care. Neurocrit Care. 2012;

Lelubre C, Bouzat P, Crippa IA, Taccone FS. Anemia management after acute brain injury. Crit Care. 2016;20(1):1–11. https://doi.org/10.1186/s13054-016-1321-6.

Ley EJ, Leonard SD, Barmparas G, Dhillon NK, Inaba K, Salim A, et al. Beta blockers in critically ill patients with traumatic brain injury: results from a multicenter, prospective, observational American Association for the Surgery of Trauma study. J Trauma Acute Care Surg. 2018;84(2):234–44. http://insights.ovid.com/crossref?an=01586154-201802000-00002.

Lu Q, Xie Y, Qi X, Li X, Yang S, Wang Y. Is early tracheostomy better for severe traumatic brain injury? A meta-analysis. World Neurosurg. 2018;112:e324–30.

McCredie VA, Ferguson ND, Pinto RL, Adhikari NKJ, Fowler RA, Chapman MG, et al. Airway management strategies for brain-injured patients meeting standard criteria to consider extubation: a prospective cohort study. Ann Am Thorac Soc. 2017;14(1):85–93.

McNett MM, Bader MK, Livesay S, Yeager S, Moran C, Barnes A, et al. A national trial on differences in cerebral perfusion pressure values by measurement location. Neurocrit Care. 2018;28(2):221–8.

Michard F, Teboul JL. Predicting fluid responsiveness in ICU patients: a critical analysis of the evidence. Chest. 2002;121(6):2000–8. http://www.ncbi.nlm.nih.gov/pubmed/12065368.

Muizelaar JP, Marmarou A, Ward JD, Kontos HA, Choi SC, Becker DP, et al. Adverse effects of prolonged hyperventilation in patients with severe head injury: a randomized clinical trial. J Neurosurg. 1991;75(5):731–9. http://www.ncbi.nlm.nih.gov/pubmed/1919695.

Muzevich KM, Voils SA. Role of vasopressor administration in patients with acute neurologic injury. Neurocrit Care. 2009;11(1):112–9. http://www.ncbi.nlm.nih.gov/pubmed/19387871.

Nates JL, Nunnally M, Kleinpell R, Blosser S, Goldner J, Birriel B, et al. ICU admission, discharge, and triage guidelines: a framework to enhance clinical operations, development of institutional policies, and further research. Crit Care Med. 2016;44(8):1553–602. http://www.ncbi.nlm.nih.gov/pubmed/27428118.

Nemer SN, Caldeira JB, Santos RG, Guimarães BL, Garcia JM, Prado D, et al. Effects of positive end-expiratory pressure on brain tissue oxygen pressure of severe traumatic brain injury patients with acute respiratory distress syndrome: a pilot study. J Crit Care. 2015;30(6):1263–6. https://doi.org/10.1016/j.jcrc.2015.07.019.

Nordström C H. Assessment of critical thresholds for cerebral perfusion pressure by performing bedside monitoring of cerebral energy metabolism. Neurosurg Focus. 2003;15(6):E5. http://ovidsp.ovid.com/ovidweb.cgi?T=JS&PAGE=reference&D=emed6&NEWS=N&AN=15305841%5Cnhttp://ovidsp.ovid.com/ovidweb.cgi?T=JS&PAGE=reference&D=med4&NEWS=N&AN=15305841.

O'Briain D, Nickson C, Pilcher DV, Udy AA. Early hyperoxia in patients with traumatic brain injury admitted to intensive care in Australia and New Zealand: a retrospective multicenter cohort study. Neurocrit Care. 2018;8:443–51.

Oddo M, Crippa IA, Mehta S, Menon D, Payen J-F, Taccone FS, et al. Optimizing sedation in patients with acute brain injury. Crit Care. 2016;20(1):128. https://doi.org/10.1186/s13054-016-1294-5.

Okonkwo DO, Shutter LA, Moore C, Temkin NR, Puccio AM, Madden CJ, et al. Brain oxygen optimization in severe traumatic brain injury phase-II: A Phase II randomized trial. Crit Care Med. 2017;45(11):1907–14. Available from: http://www.ncbi.nlm.nih.gov/pubmed/29028696.

Peñuelas Ó, Thille AW, Esteban A. Discontinuation of ventilatory support: new solutions to old dilemmas. Curr Opin Crit Care. 2015;21:74–81. http://content.wkhealth.com/linkback/openurl?sid=WKPTLP:landingpage&an=00075198-201502000-00012.

Powner DJ, Miller ER, Levine RL. CVP and PAoP measurements are discordant during fluid therapy after traumatic brain injury. J Intensive Care Med. 2005;20(1):28–33.

Prathep S, Sharma D, Hallman M, Joffe A, Krishnamoorthy V, Mackensen GB, et al. Preliminary report on cardiac dysfunction after isolated traumatic brain injury. Crit Care Med. 2014;42(1):142–7. http://www.ncbi.nlm.nih.gov/pubmed/23963125.

Rangel-Castilla L, Lara LR, Gopinath S, Swank PR, Valadka A, Robertson C. Cerebral hemodynamic effects of acute hyperoxia and hyperventilation after severe traumatic brain injury. J Neurotrauma. 2010;27(10):1853–63. https://doi.org/10.1089/neu.2010.1339.

Reilly PM, Sing RF, Giberson FA, Anderson HL, Rotondo MF, Tinkoff GH, et al. Hypercarbia during tracheostomy: a comparison of percutaneous endoscopic, percutaneous Doppler, and standard surgical tracheostomy. Intensive Care Med. 1997;23(8):859–64. http://www.ncbi.nlm.nih.gov/pubmed/9310803.

Rincon F, Ghosh S, Dey S, Maltenfort M, Vibbert M, Urtecho J, et al. Impact of acute lung injury and acute respiratory distress syndrome after traumatic brain injury in the United States. Neurosurgery. 2012;71(4):795–803.

Rivers EP, Ander DS, Powell D. Central venous oxygen saturation monitoring in the critically ill patient. Curr Opin Crit Care. 2001;7(3):204–11. http://www.ncbi.nlm.nih.gov/pubmed/11436529.

Rizk EB, Patel AS, Stetter CM, Chinchilli VM, Cockroft KM. Impact of tracheostomy timing on outcome after severe head injury. Neurocrit Care. 2011;15(3):481–9. http://www.ncbi.nlm.nih.gov/pubmed/21786043.

Rockswold SB, Rockswold GL, Zaun DA, Liu J. A prospective, randomized Phase II clinical trial to evaluate the effect of combined hyperbaric and normobaric hyperoxia on cerebral metabolism, intracranial pressure, oxygen toxicity, and clinical outcome in severe traumatic brain injury. J Neurosurg. 2013;118(6):1317–28. https://doi.org/10.3171/2013.2.JNS121468.

SAFE Study Investigators, Australian and New Zealand Intensive Care Society Clinical Trials Group, Australian Red Cross Blood Service, George Institute for International Health, Myburgh J, Cooper DJ, et al. Saline or albumin for fluid resuscitation in patients with traumatic brain injury. N Engl J Med. 2007;357(9):874–84. https://doi.org/10.1056/NEJMoa067514.

Stocchetti N, Parma A, Songa V, Colombo A, Lamperti M, Tognini L. Early translaryngeal tracheostomy in patients with severe brain damage. Intensive Care Med. 2000;26(8):1101–7. http://www.ncbi.nlm.nih.gov/pubmed/11030167.

Taher A, Pilehvari Z, Poorolajal J, Aghajanloo M. Effects of normobaric hyperoxia in traumatic brain injury: a randomized controlled clinical trial. Trauma Mon. 2016;21(1):e26772. https://www.ncbi.nlm.nih.gov/pmc/articles/PMC4869427/pdf/traumamon-21-01-26772.pdf.

Van Haren RM, Thorson CM, Ogilvie MP, Valle EJ, Guarch GA, Jouria JA, et al. Vasopressin for cerebral perfusion pressure management in patients with severe traumatic brain injury: preliminary results of a randomized controlled trial. J Trauma Acute Care Surg. 2013;75(6):1024–30; discussion 1030. http://www.ncbi.nlm.nih.gov/pubmed/24256677.

Varelas PN, Conti MM, Spanaki MV, Potts E, Bradford D, Sunstrom C, et al. The impact of a neurointensivist-led team on a semiclosed neurosciences intensive care unit. Crit Care Med. 2004;32(11):2191–8. http://www.ncbi.nlm.nih.gov/pubmed/15640630.

Varelas PN, Eastwood D, Yun HJ, Spanaki MV, Hacein Bey L, Kessaris C, et al. Impact of a neurointensivist on outcomes in patients with head trauma treated in a neurosciences intensive care unit. J Neurosurg. 2006;104(5):713–9. https://doi.org/10.3171/jns.2006.104.5.713.

Wazen RM, Kuroda S, Nishio C, Sellin K, Brunski JB, Nanci A. The emerging use of ketamine for anesthesia and sedation in traumatic brain injuries. CNS Neurosci Ther. 2013;19(6):390–5.

52 Renal Aspects

Jens Aage Kølsen-Petersen

Recommendations

Level I

There are insufficient data to support a Level I recommendation for this topic.

Level II

There are insufficient data to support a Level II recommendation for this topic.

Level III

Urinary output, changes in plasma concentrations of creatinine, creatinine clearance, and changes in acid-base status and electrolytes may be used as surrogate parameters for kidney function. At steady state, estimated glomerular filtration rate (eGFR) based on plasma creatinine, age, gender, and race is preferred, while the gold standard, measured GFR using, e.g. plasma clearance of 51 CrEDTA, is expensive and time-consuming.

J. A. Kølsen-Petersen (✉)
Department of Anaesthesia, Aarhus University Hospital, Aarhus, Denmark
e-mail: jenspete@rm.dk

52.1 Overview

The glomerular filtration rate (GFR) is widely accepted as the single best estimate of the overall kidney function in health and disease (Kellum et al. 2012). In critically ill patients, renal function can be monitored by regular measurements of urinary output and plasma concentrations of creatinine taking into account that P-creatinine will not raise until time has elapsed after the renal injury, while urinary output can be measured at once under appropriate fluid supply.

The GFR can be calculated as

$$\text{Creatinine clearance} = \frac{U_{\text{Creatinine}} \times V_{\text{urine}}}{P_{\text{creatinine}}}$$

$U_{\text{Creatinine}}$ and $P_{\text{creatinine}}$ is the concentration of creatinine in urine and plasma, respectively, and V_{urine} is the volume of urine. It must be considered that GFR is overestimated with this method because of tubular secretion of creatinine. At low levels of GFR, this overestimation can be as high as 100%.

Alternatively, GFR can be estimated (eGFR) based on plasma creatinine and certain patient variables such as age, gender, and race (e.g. CKD-EPI (Chronic Kidney Disease Epidemiology), abbreviated (Modification of Diet in Renal Disease) formulas).

© Springer Nature Switzerland AG 2020
T. Sundstrøm et al. (eds.), *Management of Severe Traumatic Brain Injury*,
https://doi.org/10.1007/978-3-030-39383-0_52

Tips, Tricks, and Pitfalls

- Monitor urinary output hourly if rapid changes in kidney function are expected.
- Monitor plasma concentrations of creatinine and urea daily together with acid-base status and electrolytes. If renal function deteriorates, add estimated GFR or GFR calculated from 2 or 24-h urine samples.
- Creatinine [μmol L^{-1}]/urea [mmol L^{-1}] ratio below 10 indicates prerenal cause (hypovolaemia) (Baum et al. 1975).

52.2 Background

Acute kidney injury is a common complication that adversely affects outcome in critically ill trauma patients (Bagshaw et al. 2008). The kidneys regulate intravascular volume, osmolality, and acid-base and electrolyte balance and excrete the end products of metabolism and drugs. Most of these functions depend on the kidney's ability to filtrate sodium and water. The glomerular filtration rate (GFR) is thus widely accepted as the best marker for the overall kidney function (Kellum et al. 2012). The GFR can be measured directly by clearance of a substance that is filtered, but neither reabsorbed nor secreted, e.g. inulin or 51 CrEDTA (Johnson 2005), which is however expensive and time-consuming. The clearance of creatinine, a product of muscle metabolism, closely approximates the GFR (Baum et al. 1975). Creatinine is excreted at a relatively constant speed depending on the muscle mass. It is filtered in the glomeruli and to a minor extent (7–10%) secreted by the tubules in the normal kidney. When kidney function declines and GFR decreases, the creatinine secretion can be even greater than the filtered load, leading to an overestimation of the GFR (Bellomo et al. 2004). For clinical purposes, however, it is important to determine whether renal function is stable or getting worse or better. This can usually be determined by measuring plasma creatinine alone (Kellum et al. 2012). Plasma urea and urine output are non-specific markers of renal function (Bellomo et al. 2004). Urea is formed in the liver as a major end product of the metabolism of the nitrogen-containing substances. It is filtered in the glomerulus but undergoes extensive tubular reabsorption depending on the urine flow (Baum et al. 1975). Apart from the kidney function, the plasma urea concentration depends on the clinical situation, e.g. degree of catabolism, gastrointestinal bleeding, infection, administration of steroids, dietary protein, liver function, and hydration. Urine output may be normal or high despite severe renal failure (nonoliguric). The combination of urine output, plasma creatinine, and creatinine clearance provides the basis for the RIFLE classification of acute renal failure (Bellomo et al. 2004).

Estimated GFR (eGFR) calculated from equations that take into account plasma creatinine and certain patient variables (age, gender, race, and weight) has been shown to be clinically useful for evaluating kidney function in a broad range of clinical settings but has not been sufficiently validated in non-steady-state situations with acute changes in renal function (Johnson 2011). An automated calculator using the best available equation, the Chronic Kidney Disease Epidemiology Collaboration formula (Johnson 2011), can be assessed on the Internet ckdepi.org/equations/gfr-calculator/.

52.3 Specific Paediatric Concerns

The principles outlined above also apply for children. However, the reference values for the glomerular filtration rate and plasma creatinine change as the child grows. GFR is often reported relative to body surface area, i.e. GFR per 1.73 m^2.

The GFR is 15–30% of normal adult values at birth, reaches 50% on the fifth to tenth day, and gradually attains adult values in the second year of life. The normal plasma creatinine increases as the muscle mass increases and reaches adult values in puberty (Schwartz et al. 1976). The plasma concentration of urea is normally 3–6 mmol/L throughout childhood and increases in the same situations as mentioned above.

References

Bagshaw SM, et al. A multi-center evaluation of early acute kidney injury in critically ill trauma patients. Ren Fail. 2008;30:581–9.

Baum N, et al. Blood urea nitrogen and serum creatinine. Physiology and interpretations. Urology. 1975;5:583–8.

Bellomo R, et al. Acute renal failure—definition, outcome measures, animal models, fluid therapy and information technology needs: the Second International Consensus Conference of the Acute Dialysis Quality Initiative (ADQI) Group. Crit Care. 2004;8:R204–12.

Johnson D. The CARI guidelines. Evaluation of renal function. Nephrology(Carlton). 2005;10(Suppl 4):S133–76.

Johnson D. Estimated glomerular filtration rate: which equation is best and how should it be used. Nephrology. 2011;16:483–5.

Kellum JA, Lameire N, Aspelin P, Barsoum RS, Burdmann EA, Goldstein SL, Herzog CA, Joannidis M, Kribben A, Levey AS, MacLeod AM, Mehta RL, Murray PT, Naicker S, Opal SM, Schaefer F, Schetz M, Uchino S. Kidney disease: improving global outcomes (KDIGO) acute kidney injury work group. KDIGO clinical practice guideline for acute kidney injury. Kidney Int Suppl. 2012;2:1–138.

Schwartz GJ, et al. A simple estimate of glomerular filtration rate in children derived from body length and plasma creatinine. Pediatrics. 1976;58:259–63.

53 Neuroendocrine Aspects

Marianne Klose and Ulla Feldt-Rasmussen

Recommendations

Level I

There are insufficient data to support a Level I recommendation for this topic.

Level II

Routine testing for pituitary insufficiency in the acute phase is not recommended, whereas immediate treatment of hypoadrenalism is advised upon clinical suspicion.

Level III

Testing for pituitary insufficiency is recommended upon clinical suspicion after moderate/severe TBI.

Testing for pituitary insufficiency is not recommended in all TBI patients.

If pituitary insufficiency is discovered and treated within the first year after TBI, it is recommended to retest the patient after 1 year or more.

M. Klose (✉) · U. Feldt-Rasmussen
Department of Medical Endocrinology, Copenhagen University Hospital, Copenhagen, Denmark
e-mail: Marianne.christina.klose.01@regionh.dk, klose@rh.dk; ulla.feldt.rasmussen@regionh.dk, ufeldt@rh.dk

53.1 Overview

Severe TBI may impact the hypothalamic-pituitary-peripheral hormone system during the acute phase, but may also lead to long-term consequences in terms of persistent posttraumatic hypopituitarism. Many factors have been shown to influence the normal adaptive hypothalamo-pituitary response to acute critical illness and its treatments including mechanisms affecting, e.g. metabolism, hormone binding, and production. In TBI, there is an additional risk of structural damage causing direct interruption of the normal hypothalamic-pituitary function, with the risk of persistent damage. In the acute phase after TBI, it is therefore particularly difficult to distinguish the two components.

Anterior pituitary hormone alterations are frequently encountered in the acute phase after TBI. However, the diagnosis entails plenty of problems, and the clinical relevance and therapeutic implications of such endocrine changes are still debated. Assessment of the growth hormone, thyroid, and gonadal axes is not recommended in the acute setting, as there is currently no evidence to support a clinical benefit from hormonal replacement in the critically ill. Untreated adrenal insufficiency can on the other hand be life-threatening. The diagnosis of adrenal insufficiency is mainly clinical, as biochemical assessment is difficult in the acute setting, and immediate treatment should be instituted on

© Springer Nature Switzerland AG 2020
T. Sundstrøm et al. (eds.), *Management of Severe Traumatic Brain Injury*,
https://doi.org/10.1007/978-3-030-39383-0_53

clinical suspicion. If possible, a baseline plasma cortisol should be taken prior to treatment, as very low concentrations highly support the diagnosis, whereas normal concentrations do not rule out hypoadrenalism. In these cases, the subsequent treatment response should guide further treatment and follow-up.

The temporal relationship between TBI and hypopituitarism is poorly understood. Longitudinal studies examining TBI patients at variable time points from the acute phase to years after the trauma have reported transient, permanent, and de novo deficiencies all through the time span (Agha et al. 2005; Kleindienst et al. 2009; Klose et al. 2007b; Tanriverdi et al. 2006). Part of this variation may be ascribed to diagnostic difficulties, including those caused by the stress of severe illness, but may also in some cases be related to medication effects.

Tips, Tricks, and Pitfalls

- TBI patients may develop hypopituitarism.
- Involvement of a specialized medical endocrinologist is mandatory for proper choice of hypothalamic-pituitary tests as well as their interpretation.
- Treatment of hypoadrenalism with replacement dosages of hydrocortisone is recommended upon clinical suspicion. Important diagnostic clues are haemodynamic instability despite adequate fluid resuscitation.
- Neither normal plasma sodium nor cortisol excludes presence of severe life-threatening hypoadrenalism.
- Patients with high ICP and basal skull fractures and those with persistent hypogonadal symptoms are at greater risk for hypothalamo-pituitary damage. Diabetes insipidus is a strong indicator for hypothalamo-pituitary damage.
- Long-term treatment of pituitary hormone deficits should follow the general guidelines for treatments of these deficiencies whatever the cause.

Over the last decades, long-term anterior pituitary hormone deficiency has been reported with a prevalence of 15–83% in selected cohorts, suggesting that long-term posttraumatic hypopituitarism might be a more common complication in TBI than previously believed (Table 53.1). Although some studies have failed to show such high frequencies (van der Eerden et al. 2010), this has raised concerns whether undiagnosed and thus untreated hypopituitarism may contribute to the mortality and severe morbidity seen in TBI. The magnitude of this contribution remains

Table 53.1 Symptoms and clinical findings in patients with hypopituitarism

Hormone	Peripheral hormone	Symptoms and clinical findings
GH	IGF-1 (direct effects of GH in muscle and adipose tissue)	Fatigue, muscle weakness, depression, decreased muscle mass/increased fat mass, decreased exercise capacity, hyperlipidaemia, insulin resistance, osteoporosis, growth retardation[a]
FSH/LH	Testosterone, oestradiol	Oligo-/amenorrhoea, decreased libido, infertility, erectile dysfunction, decreased pubic hair, thinning of hair, depression, fatigue, muscle weakness, osteoporosis
TSH	Thyroxine	Fatigue, weakness, dry skin, constipation, bradycardia, cold intolerance, weight gain, thinning of hair, depression, hyperlipidaemia, oligo-/amenorrhoea
ACTH	Cortisol	Fatigue, muscle weakness, nausea/vomiting, anorexia, diarrhoea, weight loss, hypotension, hypoglycaemia, oligo-/amenorrhoea, pale skin
ADH	–	Polyuria, nocturia, thirst

GH growth hormone, *FSH* follicle stimulating hormone, *LH* luteinizing hormone, *TSH* thyroid stimulating hormone, *ACTH* adrenocorticotropic hormone

[a]GH deficiency developed in childhood

to be defined, and although some outcome studies have indicated clinical significance of posttraumatic hypopituitarism with important impacts on health-related quality of life and lipid status (Kelly et al. 2006; Klose et al. 2007c), the findings have not been consistent (Pavlovic et al. 2010). Nevertheless, expert panels have proposed recommendations for hormone assessment of pituitary insufficiency and consequent appropriate replacement after moderate/severe TBI (Ghigo et al. 2005; Ho 2007; Tritos et al. 2015). Unfortunately, the area lacks valid clinical, biochemical, or other predictors, and it has not yet been clarified which part of the TBI population should be tested (Klose and Feldt-Rasmussen 2008). Although some patients have profound hormonal deficiencies and do benefit from treatment, most patients seem to have subtle deficits. Data are still awaited to document the effect of hormone replacement therapy in such patients, and until data are available, one should be cautious to introduce uncritical routine anterior pituitary testing and replacement therapy. Meanwhile, more pragmatic recommendations must be given, e.g. pituitary evaluation should be considered at any stage when clinically indicated in a patient who has suffered TBI (Table 53.1). Certain categories of patients may be at a greater risk, including those with increased ICP and diffuse axonal injury, those with basal skull fractures, as well as those with hypogonadal symptoms (Cuesta et al. 2016), and should be considered at higher priority for pituitary assessment.

53.2 Background

53.2.1 Anterior Pituitary Hormone Deficiency Following

53.2.1.1 TBI: Aetiology

The aetiology of posttraumatic hypopituitarism remains incompletely understood, but current evidence indicates the role of both primary mechanical injury and secondary injury from hypotension, hypoxia, anaemia, and brain swelling causing restriction of flow in the hypophyseal portal vessels. Support of this pathophysiologic concept comes from autopsy studies from fatally head-injured patients in which up to one third sustained anterior pituitary gland necrosis (Ceballos 1966; Crompton 1971; Kornblum and Fisher 1969). It is however unclear whether data from fatal cases can be generalized to explain long-term hypopituitarism in TBI survivors. Two recent MR studies may support the hypothesis. An observational case-control study including 41 patients with non-lethal head trauma demonstrated acute changes in terms of pituitary enlargement, pituitary haemorrhages, infarctions, signal abnormalities, and/or partial stalk transection in about 30% of adult TBI patients (Maiya et al. 2007). Secondly, other observational data have suggested that patients with long-term post-TBI hypopituitarism have a higher frequency of loss of pituitary volume or empty sella, abnormal pituitary gland signal heterogeneity, perfusion deficits, and/or lack of posterior pituitary signal as compared to TBI patients with normal pituitary function (Schneider et al. 2007). Likewise, Bavisetty et al. (2008) reported the degree of injury as defined by acute CT to be the strongest predictor for long-term deficiencies; Klose et al. (2007a) reported that a normal CT excluded development of long-term deficiencies, whereas indirect indicators of severe trauma including increased ICP were predictive of long-term deficiency in their cohort of 104 patients; and Schneider et al. found other indicators of more severe TBI, such as diffuse axonal injury and basal skull fractures, to be predictive (Schneider et al. 2008). Most studies, however, failed to show a relationship between injury-related factors and the development of long-term hypopituitarism (Klose and Feldt-Rasmussen 2008), and the role of acute CT was recently contradicted by Kleindienst et al. (2009) who did not find any relationship between acute or late CT findings and development of hypopituitarism (Table 53.2).

Furthermore, the effects of transient stress from critical illness and medication are mechanisms to be considered in the acute phase. Adrenal cortisol synthesis can be impaired by the anaesthetic agent etomidate and the antifungal agent ketoconazole; exogenous corticosteroid therapy may suppress the HPA axis and induce

Table 53.2 Recent publications on the prevalence of long-term posttraumatic anterior pituitary dysfunction

Authors	*n*	GCS <13	Hypopituitarism Total (%)	Multiple hypopituitarism	GH deficiency[a]	ACTH deficiency	LH/FSH deficiency	TSH deficiency	Predictors
Kelly et al. (2000)	22	–	36	23	18	5	23	5	Diffuse brain swelling, GCS
Lieberman et al. (2001)	70	–	69	18	15	46	1	22	None
Agha et al. (2004)	102	100	29	6	11 (8)	13	12	1	None
Bondanelli et al. (2004)	50	86	54	12	28 (20)	0	14	10	GCS score
Popovic et al. (2004)	67	100	34	10	15 (8)	7	9	4	None
Aimaretti et al. (2005)	70	45	23	10	20	7	11	6	None
Leal-Cerro et al. (2005)	170[b]	100	25	16	6	6	17	6	None
Schneider et al. (2006)	70	78	36	4	10	9	20	3	None
Tanriverdi et al. (2006)	52	40	51	10	33	19	8	6	None
Herrmann et al. (2006)	76	100	24	7	8	2	17	2	None
Klose et al. (2007a)	104	58	15	6	15	5	2	2	Increased ICP, low GCS
Wachter et al. (2009)	53	24	25	2	2	4	1	6	None
Kleindienst et al. (2009)	23	78	83	30	39	0	48	0	Low GH first week
van der Eerden et al. (2010)	107	28	<1	0	0	<1	0	0	ND
Krahulik et al. (2010)	87	-	21	0	14	0	6	0	GCS
Kokshoorn et al. (2011)	112	43%	5	4	3	2	1	0	BMI
Ulfarsson et al. (2013)	51	100%	28	6	22	0	4	2	None

Prodam et al. (2013)	54	100%	28	7	22	12	17	16	–
Silva et al. (2015)	160	31%	31	–	15	10	12	8	Intracranial bleed, MVA
Cuesta et al. (2016)	137[c]	100%	34	–	7	15	16	1	Hypogonadal symptoms
	112[d]	100	33	–	14	21	19	5	
Hannon et al. (2013)	32	100	31	3	19	19	3	–	Acute setting p-cortisol<300nmol/L,

ACTH adrenocorticotropic hormone, *FSH* follicle stimulating hormone, *GCS* Glasgow Coma Scale score, *GH* growth hormone, *ICP* intracranial pressure, *LH* luteinizing hormone, *MVA* motor vehicle accidents, *ND* not done, *TSH* thyroid stimulating hormone

[a]Given as severe GHD (partial GHD)

[b]Only 99 patients were tested

[c]Referred with non-specific symptoms

[d]Referred with symptoms of hypopituitarism

adrenal atrophy that may persist months after cessation, and hepatic metabolism of cortisol may be enhanced by drugs such as phenytoin.

53.2.2 Acute-Phase Anterior Pituitary Hormone Deficiency

Presence of hypothalamic-anterior-pituitary-peripheral hormone alterations is a very common phenomenon in the acute phase after TBI and may resemble the biochemical picture of central hypogonadism or hypothyroidism (Van den Berghe et al. 1998), whereas secretion of stress hormones, such as prolactin, growth hormone (GH), adrenocorticotrophin (ACTH), cortisol (Annane et al. 2000; Beishuizen et al. 2001; Hamrahian et al. 2004), and vasopressin (AVP) (Jochberger et al. 2006), is increased. The degree of such alterations is typically related to disease severity and associated with higher morbidity and mortality (Barton et al. 1987; De Groot 2006; Span et al. 1992). The changes are not disease specific, but a hallmark in acute and critical illness as such and appear to be part of important adaptive mechanisms regulating the inflammatory response, caused by cytokine activation among other factors. Acute illness per se can also result in variable changes of metabolism in all the hormone-binding proteins, and a number of drugs used for life support in intensive care units affect the binding of the hormones to their binding proteins. The interpretation of biochemical findings thus entails plenty of problems, independent on whether total or free hormone measurements are used; currently there are no reliable diagnostic cut-offs for anterior pituitary hormone deficiency in critically ill patients.

The hypothalamic-pituitary-adrenal (HPA) axis deserves special interest, as untreated hypoadrenalism may have a major impact on the patient's outcome. During critical illness, profound and variable changes occur in the HPA axis, including HPA activation (Annane et al. 2000; Hamrahian et al. 2004; Vanhorebeek et al. 2006), decreased cortisol-binding globulin (CBG) the first week after admission (Beishuizen et al. 2001; Hamrahian et al. 2004) leading to increased circulating free cortisol, and suppressed cortisol breakdown (Boonen et al. 2013). All these changes complicate assessment, as the usual biochemical definitions of hypoadrenalism cannot be used (Annane et al. 2017; Cooper and Stewart 2003). Therefore, the threshold that best describes the patients at need for acute or chronic glucocorticoid replacement is still to be defined.

A number of studies have assessed the acute neuroendocrine changes following TBI, in order to investigate the correlation to trauma severity, metabolic derangement, and variables that may predict outcome (Cernak et al. 1999; Cohan et al. 2005; Della et al. 1998; Feibel et al. 1983; Hackl et al. 1991). The clinical implications of these findings however remain unclear. Four longitudinal studies have been designed to evaluate the relation between acute and long-term pituitary hormone status after TBI. Agha et al. (2005) found secondary gonadotropin, growth hormone (GH), corticotrophin (ACTH), and thyrotropin (TSH) deficiency in 80%, 18%, 16%, and 2%, respectively, of 56 patients with moderate or severe TBI. At 1-year follow-up, hormonal abnormalities had recovered in most patients, whereas others had developed de novo deficiencies, and although persistent GH and ACTH deficiency was associated with more severe acute-phase growth hormone and cortisol hyposecretion, the authors were unable to identify biochemical predictors of persistent hypopituitarism. Similar findings were described by others (Tanriverdi et al. 2006; Klose et al. 2007b; Kleindienst et al. 2009). The existing data rely on rather small cohorts only allowing for case description, and therefore clear conclusions and recommendations on this issue are difficult.

Currently, no evidence exists to suggest introduction of routine anterior pituitary hormone screening in critical illness, due to both the aforementioned diagnostic difficulties and lack of evidence of the beneficial effects from hormonal substitution. Treatment with pharmacological doses of GH has been shown to increase morbidity and mortality (Takala et al. 1999), whether or not administration of thyroid hormone is beneficial or harmful remains controversial (De Groot 2006; Stathatos et al. 2001), and no conclusive clinical benefit has been demonstrated for androgen treatment in prolonged critical illness (Angele et al. 1998).

Although the threshold that best describes the patients at need for glucocorticoid replacement in the acute setting remains to be defined, this complication must be considered as potentially lethal. As a rule, baseline plasma cortisol of less than 100 nmol/L indicates adrenal insufficiency, whereas normal or slightly elevated concentrations do not exclude the diagnosis. Important diagnostic clues are haemodynamic instability despite adequate fluid resuscitation, hyponatraemia, and in rare cases hypoglycaemia. Treatment of hypoadrenalism with stress dosages of hydrocortisone is recommended upon clinical suspicion.

Although only based on case reports, the clinical data justify an increased attention towards the potential presence of secondary hypoadrenalism occurring from the acute phase in TBI patients. In order to illustrate the potential pitfall in diagnosing the causes of hyponatraemia in TBI patients, Agha et al. (2007) reported data from three patients with severe TBI, who were initially misdiagnosed as SIADH. In two cases, hypoadrenalism was suspected due to the combination of hyponatraemia, hypoglycaemia, and hypotension and in the third case because plasma sodium did not correct with fluid restriction. All three patients had extremely low baseline cortisol of 33–110 nmol/L and undetectable ACTH levels. The condition ameliorated in all of them upon glucocorticoid replacement. Patients may however present with far more subtle signs and symptoms.

53.2.3 Long-Term Anterior Pituitary Hormone Deficiency

Anterior pituitary hormone deficiency following TBI has traditionally been considered very rare and mainly reported as single cases or case series. With the increased focus on this potential complication over the last decades, long-term anterior pituitary hormone deficiency was reported with a prevalence of 15–83% in selected cohorts (Table 53.2). The diversity in the reported prevalence is likely to be explained by different study populations, study designs, and diagnostic procedures used. The high prevalence has recently lead expert panels to include TBI in endocrine guidelines regarding whom and when to test for hypopituitarism, and several screening programmes have been proposed (Behan et al. 2008; Fleseriu et al. 2016; Ghigo et al. 2005;). Screening was challenged by the study by van der Eerden et al. (2010) including an emergency department-based cohort. Partial hypocortisolism was reported in 1 out of 107 patients, indicating that routine pituitary screening in unselected patients after TBI is unlikely to be cost-effective. Current recommendations are directed towards patients with moderate and severe TBI, and there are data to suggest that persisting hypogonadal symptoms are more predictive of hypopituitarism than non-specific symptoms in screening for pituitary dysfunction (Cuesta et al. 2016).

Very few data exist on the possible clinical implication of anterior pituitary hormone deficiency in TBI patients, and again data are conflicting. Kelly et al. (2006) described higher rates of at least one marker of depression and reduced health-related quality of life (HRQoL) in GH-deficient patients. Klose et al. (2007c) found that posttraumatic hypopituitarism was an independent predictor of the classical phenotypic features of hypopituitarism, including an unfavourable lipid and body composition profile, as well as worsened HRQoL. Bondanelli et al. (2007) found that peak GH was an independent predictor of poorer outcome as measured by rehabilitation scales evaluating cognition, disability, and functional dependency, whereas Pavlovic et al. (2010) found no correlation between neuropsychological variables and stimulated peak GH or insulin-like growth factor I (IGF-I) levels.

The impact of hypopituitarism on QoL, fatigue, sleep changes, and hypogonadal symptoms was recently challenged in a large national TBI cohort (Klose et al. 2015) as symptoms in that study were more heavily explained by concurrent comorbidities and their treatments, including treatment with opioids and antidepressants.

The negative effects of glucocorticoid, thyroid, and gonadal hormone deficiencies are well recognized, as is the beneficial effect from appropriate replacement therapy. These deficiencies and their treatment, however, have more distinct clinical features than GH deficiency, which is the most frequently reported deficiency in TBI patients. GH deficiency is associated with impaired linear growth and attainment of normal body composition in children, but in adults, the features are less specific with reduced lean body mass, decreased exercise capacity, reduced bone mineral density, unfavourable changes in the lipid profile, and decreased QoL. There are only few available data on treatment effect in TBI patients with anterior pituitary hormone deficiency. To evaluate the effect of human GH replacement therapy as documented in the German Pfizer International Metabolic (KIMS) database, clinical and other outcome variables were compared at baseline and after 1 year of hGH replacement in 84 TBI patients and 84 patients with deficiency due to a non-functioning pituitary adenoma (NFPA) (Kreitschmann-Andermahr et al. 2008). At 1-year follow-up, IGF-I SDS levels had increased to the normal range and QoL, as measured by the QoL Assessment of Growth Hormone Deficiency (AGHDA) questionnaire, improved significantly in TBI as in NFPA patients, thus suggesting that TBI patients with GH deficiency benefit from hGH replacement in terms of improved QoL in a similar fashion as do NFPA patients. Additional data suggest that cognitive impairments might be partially reversible with appropriate GH replacement (Maric et al. 2010); however, the underlying mechanisms (such as an obvious potential effect from increased conversion of T_4 to T_3 by GH) were not investigated. This reversal might be relevant, as thyroid hormone has a solidly documented effect on cognition.

53.3 Specific Paediatric Concerns

Paediatric survivors of severe TBI may develop pituitary dysfunction, but as in adults, studies have failed to identify risk factors for development of hypopituitarism. The reported prevalence ranges from 5 to 57%. GH and ACTH deficiency are the most common, followed by gonadotropins and thyroid-stimulating hormone. Given the critical role of anterior pituitary hormones in the regulation of growth, pubertal, and neurocognitive development in childhood, early detection of hormone abnormalities following TBI is important. At this level it is recommended that, as in adults, treatment of long-term posttraumatic hypopituitarism should follow the general guidelines for treatments of the present deficiencies, whatever the cause (Acerini and Tasker 2007; Tritos et al. 2015; Casano-Sancho 2017).

References

Acerini CL, Tasker RC. Traumatic brain injury induced hypothalamic-pituitary dysfunction: a paediatric perspective. Pituitary. 2007;10:373–80.

Agha A, Rogers B, Sherlock M, O'Kelly P, Tormey W, Phillips J, Thompson CJ. Anterior pituitary dysfunction in survivors of traumatic brain injury. J Clin Endocrinol Metab. 2004;89:4929–36.

Agha A, Phillips J, O'Kelly P, Tormey W, Thompson CJ. The natural history of post-traumatic hypopituitarism: implications for assessment and treatment. Am J Med. 2005;118:1416.

Agha A, Walker D, Perry L, Drake WM, Chew SL, Jenkins PJ, Grossman AB, Monson JP. Unmasking of central hypothyroidism following growth hormone replacement in adult hypopituitary patients. Clin Endocrinol (Oxf). 2007;66:72–7.

Aimaretti G, Ambrosio MR, Di Somma C, Gasperi M, Cannavo S, Scaroni C, Fusco A, Del Monte P, De Menis E, Faustini-Fustini M, Grimaldi F, Logoluso F, Razzore P, Rovere S, Benvenga S, Uberti EC, De Marinis L, Lombardi G, Mantero F, Martino E, Giordano G, Ghigo E. Residual pituitary function after brain injury-induced hypopituitarism: a prospective 12-month study. J Clin Endocrinol Metab. 2005;90(11):6085–92.

Angele MK, Ayala A, Cioffi WG, Bland KI, Chaudry IH. Testosterone: the culprit for producing splenocyte immune depression after trauma hemorrhage. Am J Physiol. 1998;274:C1530–6.

Annane D, Sebille V, Troche G, Raphael JC, Gajdos P, Bellissant E. A 3-level prognostic classification in septic shock based on cortisol levels and cortisol response to corticotropin. JAMA. 2000;283:1038–45.

Annane D, Pastores SM, Rochwerg B, Arlt W, Balk RA, Beishuizen A, Briegel J, Carcillo J, Christ-Crain M, Cooper MS, Marik PE, Umberto Meduri G, Olsen KM, Rodgers S, Russell JA, Van den Berghe G. Guidelines for the diagnosis and management of critical illness-related corticosteroid insufficiency (CIRCI) in critically ill patients (Part I): Society of Critical Care Medicine (SCCM) and European Society of Intensive Care Medicine (ESICM) 2017. Intensive Care Med. 2017;43:1751–63.

Barton RN, Stoner HB, Watson SM. Relationships among plasma cortisol, adrenocorticotrophin, and severity of injury in recently injured patients. J Trauma. 1987;27:384–92.

Bavisetty S, Bavisetty S, McArthur DL, Dusick JR, Wang C, Cohan P, Boscardin WJ, Swerdloff R, Levin H, Chang DJ, Muizelaar JP, Kelly DF. Chronic hypopituitarism after traumatic brain injury: risk assessment and relationship to outcome. Neurosurgery. 2008;62:1080–93.

Behan LA, Phillips J, Thompson CJ, Agha A. Neuroendocrine disorders after traumatic brain injury. J Neurol Neurosurg Psychiatry. 2008;79:753–9.

Beishuizen A, Thijs LG, Vermes I. Patterns of corticosteroid-binding globulin and the free cortisol index during septic shock and multitrauma. Intensive Care Med. 2001;27:1584–91.

Bondanelli M, De Marinis L, Ambrosio MR, Monesi M, Valle D, Zatelli MC, Fusco A, Bianchi A, Farneti M, Degli ECI. Occurrence of pituitary dysfunction following traumatic brain injury. J Neurotrauma. 2004;21:685–96.

Bondanelli M, Ambrosio MR, Cavazzini L, Bertocchi A, Zatelli MC, Carli A, Valle D, Basaglia N, Uberti EC. Anterior pituitary function may predict functional and cognitive outcome in patients with traumatic brain injury undergoing rehabilitation. J Neurotrauma. 2007;24:1687–97.

Boonen E, Vervenne H, Meersseman P, Andrew R, Mortier L, Declercq PE, Vanwijngaerden YM, Spriet I, Wouters PJ, Vander PS, Langouche L, Vanhorebeek I, Walker BR, Van den Berghe G. Reduced cortisol metabolism during critical illness. N Engl J Med. 2013;368:1477–88.

Casano-Sancho P. Pituitary dysfunction after traumatic brain injury: are there definitive data in children? Arch Dis Child. 2017;102:572–7.

Ceballos R. Pituitary changes in head trauma (analysis of 102 consecutive cases of head injury). Ala J Med Sci. 1966;3:185–98.

Cernak I, Savic VJ, Lazarov A, Joksimovic M, Markovic S. Neuroendocrine responses following graded traumatic brain injury in male adults. Brain Inj. 1999;13:1005–15.

Cohan P, Wang C, McArthur DL, Cook SW, Dusick JR, Armin B, Swerdloff R, Vespa P, Muizelaar JP, Cryer HG, Christenson PD, Kelly DF. Acute secondary adrenal insufficiency after traumatic brain injury: a prospective study. Crit Care Med. 2005;33:2358–66.

Cooper MS, Stewart PM. Corticosteroid insufficiency in acutely ill patients. N Engl J Med. 2003;348:727–34.

Crompton MR. Hypothalamic lesions following closed head injury. Brain. 1971;94:165–72.

Cuesta M, Hannon MJ, Crowley RK, Behan LA, Tormey W, Rawluk D, et al. Symptoms of gonadal dysfunction are more predictive of hypopituitarism than nonspecific symptoms in screening for pituitary dysfunction following moderate or severe traumatic brain injury. Clin Endocrinol. 2016;84:92–8.

De Groot LJ. Non-thyroidal illness syndrome is a manifestation of hypothalamic-pituitary dysfunction, and in view of current evidence, should be treated with appropriate replacement therapies. Crit Care Clin. 2006;22:57–86, vi.

Della CF, Mancini A, Valle D, Gallizzi F, Carducci P, Mignani V, De ML. Provocative hypothalamo-pituitary axis tests in severe head injury: correlations with severity and prognosis. Crit Care Med. 1998;26:1419–26.

Feibel J, Kelly M, Lee L, Woolf P. Loss of adrenocortical suppression after acute brain injury: role of increased intracranial pressure and brain stem function. J Clin Endocrinol Metab. 1983;57:1245–50.

Fleseriu M, Hashim I, Karavitaki N, Melmed S, Murad M, Salvatori R, Samuels M. Hormonal replacement in hypopituitarism in adults: an Endocrine Society clinical practice guideline. J Clin Endocrinol Metab. 2016;101:3888–921.

Ghigo E, Masel B, Aimaretti G, Leon-Carrion J, Casanueva FF, Dominguez-Morales MR, Elovic E, Perrone K, Stalla G, Thompson C, Urban R. Consensus guidelines on screening for hypopituitarism following traumatic brain injury. Brain Inj. 2005;19: 711–24.

Hackl JM, Gottardis M, Wieser C, Rumpl E, Stadler C, Schwarz S, Monkayo R. Endocrine abnormalities in severe traumatic brain injury—a cue to prognosis in severe craniocerebral trauma? Intensive Care Med. 1991;17:25–9.

Hamrahian AH, Oseni TS, Arafah BM. Measurements of serum free cortisol in critically ill patients. N Engl J Med. 2004;350:1629–38.

Hannon MJ, Crowley RK, Behan LA, O'Sullivan EP, O'Brien MM, Sherlock M, Rawluk D, O'Dwyer R, Tormey W, Thompson CJ. Acute glucocorticoid deficiency and diabetes insipidus are common after acute traumatic brain injury and predict mortality. J Clin Endocrinol Metab. 2013;98:3229–37.

Herrmann BL, Rehder J, Kahlke S, Wiedemayer H, Doerfler A, Ischebeck W, Laumer R, Forsting M, Stolke D, Mann K. Hypopituitarism following severe traumatic brain injury. Exp Clin Endocrinol Diabetes. 2006;114:316–21.

Ho KK. Consensus guidelines for the diagnosis and treatment of adults with GH deficiency II: a statement of the GH Research Society in association with the European Society for Pediatric Endocrinology, Lawson Wilkins Society, European Society of Endocrinology, Japan Endocrine Society, and Endocrine Society of Australia. Eur J Endocrinol. 2007;157:695–700.

Jochberger S, Morgenthaler NG, Mayr VD, Luckner G, Wenzel V, Ulmer H, Schwarz S, Hasibeder WR, Friesenecker BE, Dunser MW. Copeptin and arginine vasopressin concentrations in critically ill patients. J Clin Endocrinol Metab. 2006;91:4381–6.

Kelly DF, Gonzalo IT, Cohan P, Berman N, Swerdloff R, Wang C. Hypopituitarism following traumatic brain injury and aneurysmal subarachnoid hemorrhage: a preliminary report. J Neurosurg. 2000;93:743–52.

Kelly DF, McArthur DL, Levin H, Swimmer S, Dusick JR, Cohan P, Wang C, Swerdloff R. Neurobehavioral and quality of life changes associated with growth hormone insufficiency after complicated mild, moderate, or severe traumatic brain injury. J Neurotrauma. 2006;23:928–42.

Kleindienst A, Brabant G, Bock C, Maser-Gluth C, Buchfelder M. Neuroendocrine function following traumatic brain injury and subsequent intensive care treatment: a prospective longitudinal evaluation. J Neurotrauma. 2009;26:1435–46.

Klose M, Feldt-Rasmussen U. Does the type and severity of brain injury predict hypothalamo-pituitary dysfunction? Does post-traumatic hypopituitarism predict worse outcome? Pituitary. 2008;11:255–61.

Klose M, Juul A, Poulsgaard L, Kosteljanetz M, Brennum J, Feldt-Rasmussen U. Prevalence and predictive factors of post-traumatic hypopituitarism. Clin Endocrinol (Oxf). 2007a;67:193–201.

Klose M, Juul A, Struck J, Morgenthaler NG, Kosteljanetz M, Feldt-Rasmussen U. Acute and long-term pituitary insufficiency in traumatic brain injury: a prospective single-centre study. Clin Endocrinol (Oxf). 2007b;67:598–606.

Klose M, Watt T, Brennum J, Feldt-Rasmussen U. Posttraumatic hypopituitarism is associated with an unfavorable body composition and lipid profile, and decreased quality of life 12 months after injury. J Clin Endocrinol Metab. 2007c;92:3861–8.

Klose M, Stochholm K, Janukonyte J, Christensen LL, Cohen A, Wagner A, et al. Patient reported outcome in posttraumatic pituitary deficiency: results from The Danish National Study on Posttraumatic Hypopituitarism. Eur J Endocrinol. 2015;172:753–62.

Kokshoorn NE, Smit JW, Nieuwlaat WA, Tiemensma J, Bisschop PH, Groote Veldman R, Roelfsema F, Franken AA, Wassenaar MJ, Biermasz NR, Romijn JA, Pereira AM. Low prevalence of hypopituitarism after traumatic brain injury: a multicenter study. Eur J Endocrinol. 2011;165:225–31.

Kornblum RN, Fisher RS. Pituitary lesions in craniocerebral injuries. Arch Pathol. 1969;88:242–8.

Krahulik D, Zapletalova J, Frysak Z, Vaverka M. Dysfunction of hypothalamic-hypophyseal axis after traumatic brain injury in adults. J Neurosurg. 2010;113(3):581–4.

Kreitschmann-Andermahr I, Poll EM, Reineke A, Gilsbach JM, Brabant G, Buchfelder M, Fassbender W, Faust M, Kann PH, Wallaschofski H. Growth hormone deficient patients after traumatic brain injury–baseline characteristics and benefits after growth hormone replacement—an analysis of the German KIMS database. Growth Horm IGF Res. 2008;18:472–8.

Leal-Cerro A, Flores JM, Rincon M, Murillo F, Pujol M, Garcia-Pesquera F, Dieguez C, Casanueva FF. Prevalence of hypopituitarism and growth hormone deficiency in adults long-term after severe traumatic brain injury. Clin Endocrinol (Oxf). 2005;62:525–32.

Lieberman SA, Oberoi AL, Gilkison CR, Masel BE, Urban RJ. Prevalence of neuroendocrine dysfunction in patients recovering from traumatic brain injury. J Clin Endocrinol Metab. 2001;86:2752–6.

Maiya B, Newcombe V, Nortje J, Bradley P, Bernard F, Chatfield D, Outtrim J, Hutchinson P, Matta B, Antoun N, Menon D. Magnetic resonance imaging changes in the pituitary gland following acute traumatic brain injury. Intensive Care Med. 2007;34(3): 468–75.

Maric NP, Doknic M, Pavlovic D, Pekic S, Stojanovic M, Jasovic-Gasic M, Popovic V. Psychiatric and neuropsychological changes in growth hormone-deficient patients after traumatic brain injury in response to growth hormone therapy. J Endocrinol Invest. 2010;33:770–5.

Pavlovic D, Pekic S, Stojanovic M, Zivkovic V, Djurovic B, Jovanovic V, Miljic N, Medic- Stojanoska M, Doknic M, Miljic D, Djurovic M, Casanueva F, Popovic V. Chronic cognitive sequelae after traumatic brain injury are not related to growth hormone deficiency in adults. Eur J Neurol. 2010;17:696–702.

Popovic V, Pekic S, Pavlovic D, Maric N, Jasovic-Gasic M, Djurovic B, Medic SM, Zivkovic V, Stojanovic M, Doknic M, Milic N, Djurovic M, Dieguez C, Casanueva FF. Hypopituitarism as a consequence of traumatic brain injury (TBI) and its possible relation with cognitive disabilities and mental distress. J Endocrinol Invest. 2004;27:1048–54.

Prodam F, Gasco V, Caputo M, Zavattaro M, Pagano L, Marzullo P, Belcastro S, Busti A, Perino C, Grottoli S, Ghigo E, Aimaretti G. Metabolic alterations in patients who develop traumatic brain injury (TBI)-induced hypopituitarism. Growth Horm IGF Res. 2013;23:109–13.

Schneider HJ, Schneider M, Saller B, Petersenn S, Uhr M, Husemann B, von Rosen F, Stalla GK. Prevalence of anterior pituitary insufficiency 3 and 12 months after traumatic brain injury. Eur J Endocrinol. 2006;154:259–65.

Schneider HJ, Samann PG, Schneider M, Croce CG, Corneli G, Sievers C, Ghigo E, Stalla GK, Aimaretti G. Pituitary imaging abnormalities in patients with and without hypopituitarism after traumatic brain injury. J Endocrinol Invest. 2007;30:RC9–RC12.

Schneider M, Schneider HJ, Yassouridis A, Saller B, von Rosen F, Stalla GK. Predictors of anterior pituitary insufficiency after traumatic brain injury. Clin Endocrinol (Oxf). 2008;68:206–12.

Silva P, Bhatnagar S, Herman S, Zafonte R, Klibanski A, Miller K, Tritos N. Predictors of hypopituitarism in patients with traumatic brain injury. J Neurotrauma. 2015;32:1789–95.

Span LF, Hermus AR, Bartelink AK, Hoitsma AJ, Gimbrere JS, Smals AG, Kloppenborg PW. Adrenocortical function: an indicator of severity of disease and survival in chronic critically ill patients. Intensive Care Med. 1992;18:93–6.

Stathatos N, Levetan C, Burman KD, Wartofsky L. The controversy of the treatment of critically ill patients with thyroid hormone. Best Pract Res Clin Endocrinol Metab. 2001;15:465–78.

Takala J, Ruokonen E, Webster NR, Nielsen MS, Zandstra DF, Vundelinckx G, Hinds CJ. Increased mortality associated with growth hormone treatment in critically ill adults. N Engl J Med. 1999;341:785–92.

Tanriverdi F, Senyurek H, Unluhizarci K, Selcuklu A, Casanueva FF, Kelestimur F. High risk of hypopituitarism after traumatic brain injury: a prospective investigation of anterior pituitary function in the acute phase and 12 months after trauma. J Clin Endocrinol Metab. 2006;91:2105–11.

Tritos NA, Yuen KC, Kelly DF, AACE Neuroendocrine and Pituitary Scientific Committee. American Association of Clinical Endocrinologists and American College of Endocrinology disease state clinical review: a neuroendocrine approach to patients with traumatic brain injury. Endocr Pract. 2015;21:823–31.

Ulfarsson T, Gudnason GA, Rosén T, Blomstrand C, Sunnerhagen KS, Lundgren-Nilsson A, Nilsson M. Pituitary function and functional outcome in adults after severe traumatic brain injury: the long-term perspective. J Neurotrauma. 2013;30:271–80.

Van den Berghe G, de Zegher F, Bouillon R. Clinical review 95: acute and prolonged critical illness as different neuroendocrine paradigms. J Clin Endocrinol Metab. 1998;83:1827–34.

van der Eerden AW, Twickler MT, Sweep FC, Beems T, Hendricks HT, Hermus AR, Vos PE. Should anterior pituitary function be tested during follow-up of all patients presenting at the emergency department because of traumatic brain injury? Eur J Endocrinol. 2010;162:19–28.

Vanhorebeek I, Peeters RP, Vander PS, Jans I, Wouters PJ, Skogstrand K, Hansen TK, Bouillon R, Van den Berghe G. Cortisol response to critical illness: effect of intensive insulin therapy. J Clin Endocrinol Metab. 2006;91:3803–13.

Wachter D, Gundling K, Oertel MF, Stracke H, Boker DK. Pituitary insufficiency after traumatic brain injury. J Clin Neurosci. 2009;16:202–8.

Part VIII

Treatment in Neurointensive Care

Per-Olof Grände and Johan Undén

54 Guidelines for Treatment of Patients with Severe Traumatic Brain Injury

Per-Olof Grände and Niels Juul

Recommendations

Level I

There are insufficient data to support a Level I recommendation of a single treatment algorithm and a specific guideline for TBI patients.

Level II

There is no Level II evidence supporting the hypothesis that one of the described guidelines is superior to another.

Level III

There is Level III evidence supporting that care of patients should be performed in a specialized neurointensive care unit. There is Level III evidence from two smaller randomized studies giving support for the Lund therapy and one study giving support for the US guidelines.

54.1 Overview of Guidelines

54.1.1 Comparing Guidelines for the Adult

P.-O. Grände (✉)
Department of Anaesthesia and Intensive Care, Lund University and Lund University Hospital, Lund, Sweden
e-mail: per-olof.grande@med.lu.se

N. Juul
Department of Anaesthesia, Aarhus University Hospital, Aarhus, Denmark
e-mail: d245364@dadlnet.dk

© Springer Nature Switzerland AG 2020
T. Sundstrøm et al. (eds.), *Management of Severe Traumatic Brain Injury*, https://doi.org/10.1007/978-3-030-39383-0_54

	US guideline, 2016, updated version from 2007	European guidelines (EBIC)	Addenbrooke guidelines	Rosner protocol	Lund concept
CPP, blood pressure	CPP 60–70 mmHg	CPP > 60–70 mmHg MAP > 90 mmHg	CPP > 70 mmHg	CPP >70 mmHg	Optimal CPP 60–70 mmHg and min 50 mmHg in selected cases if normovolaemia. Blood pressure-reducing therapy is a recommended option
Ventilation	Volume-controlled normoventilation. Moderate hyperventilation at raised ICP	Volume-controlled hyperventilation to 4.0–4.5 kPa in OBS. May be intensified at high ICP	Volume-controlled hyperventilation at a raised ICP to 3.5–4.0 kPa in OBS if SjO2 > 55%	Hyperventilation accepted	Volume-controlled normoventilation
Oxygenation	PaO_2 > 8 kPa	PaO_2 12–13 kPa	Not specified	Not specified	PaO_2 12–13 kPa
Analgesics, sedatives	Not specified Barbiturate and propofol at high ICP	Yes. Not specified	Propofol, midazolam, fentanyl	Not specified	Deep sedation (midazolam, fentanyl,α_2 agonist). No wake-up tests Propofol in the weaning phase
ICP monitoring	If abnormal CT scan and unconscious	If considered desirable	All patients with severe TBI	All patients with severe TBI	All patients with severe TBI
ICP treatment initiated	ICP > 22 mmHg	ICP > 20–25 mmHg	ICP > 20–25 mmHg	Not specified	Early, independent of ICP
High-dose barbiturates	To control a high ICP if haemodynamically stable	To control a refractory high ICP	Burst suppression pattern to control a refractory high ICP	Not used	Not used. Low dose (1–3 mg/kg/h) for at most 2 days can be used at refractory significantly raised ICP
Hyperosmolar therapy	Mannitol to control a raised ICP, 0.25–1 g/kg Hypertonic saline is an option	Mannitol to control a raised ICP, S-Osm < 315 mosm	Mannitol to control a raised ICP, S-Osm < 320 mosm	Mannitol to control a raised ICP if CPP < 70 mmHg	Not used except to prevent acute brain stem herniation and to offer space during brain operation
CSF drainage	Not specified	Can be used	An option	Can be used to control CPP	Via ventricular drain from a relatively high drainage level to prevent ventricular collapse. CT control of ventricular size
Fluids/fluid balance, erythrocyte transfusion	Normovolaemia Fluids not specified	Normovolaemia. Fluids not specified. Hb > 110 g/L recommended	Normovolaemia. Fluids and optimal Hb values not discussed	Normovolaemia to moderate hypervolaemia Hct 30–35%	Normovolaemia with albumin 20% to be given slowly (s-alb 33–38 g/L) and erythrocytes (leucocyte-depleted blood) to Hb > 110 g/L (Hct 33%) Crystalloids 1–1.5 L/day

Vasopressors/ inotropy	Can be used to maintain CPP	Recommended to maintain CPP	Recommended to maintain CPP	Recommended to maintain a high CPP	If used, in lowest possible doses
Nutrition	Enteral or parenteral nutrition, full supply after 1 week	Early enteral feeding	Early enteral feeding	Not specified	Mainly enteral feeding. Full replacement (15–20 kcal/kg/d) from day 2
Antiseizure prophylaxis	Not recommended, but may be used in patients with high risk of seizure	Not recommended	Can be used	Not discussed	Not used
Surgical therapy		Evacuation of epidural/ subdural haematomas. Craniectomy in exceptional in exceptional cases			Evacuation of haematomas. Decompressive craniectomy when indicated to prevent brainstem herniation
Temp control	Active cooling is not recommended	Not discussed	Active cooling to 33 °C if CPP <70 mmHg and ICP > 25 mmHg	Not discussed	Normothermia. High fever treated pharmacologically. No active cooling

Comparison between various guidelines for treatment of severe isolated TBI in adults in terms of the latest updated version of US guidelines from 2016 (The Brain Trauma Foundation; The American Association of Neurological Surgeons; Congress of Neurological Surgeons 2016), the European Brain Injury Consortium's (EPIC) guidelines (Maas et al. 1997), the Addenbrooke guidelines from Cambridge (Menon 1999), the Rosner protocol (Rosner et al. 1995) and the Lund concept (Grände 2006, 2017)

54.1.2 The Brain Trauma Foundation Guidelines (US Guidelines) and the Lund Concept for Treatment of the Paediatric Population

There are two paediatric guidelines available. The Brain Trauma Foundation Guidelines from 2010, the principles later also published by Bell and Kochanek (2013), here called US guideline, and the Lund concept (Grände 2006, 2017). The US guidelines are mainly based on a meta-analytic approach, while the Lund concept has more of a physiological base.

54.1.2.1 Blood Pressure, CPP and Oxygenation

US guidelines: CPP = 40–65 mmHg. Min SBP 70 mmHg + $(2 \times \text{age})^2$, up to 1 year. Min systolic blood pressure (SBP) 90 mmHg + $(2 \times \text{age})^2$ above 1 year. $PaO_2 > 8$ kPa.

Lund concept: CPP > 38–50 mmHg depending on age from newborn up to 18 years of age. These values provide a normovolaemic condition. SBP not discussed. PaO_2 12–13 kPa.

54.1.2.2 Initiation of ICP Treatment

US guidelines: At an ICP > 20–22 mmHg.

Lund concept: Early independent of ICP to counteract an increase in ICP.

54.1.2.3 Use of Hyperventilation

US guidelines: No prophylactic hyperventilation. Mild hyperventilation 4.0–4.5 kPa at a raised ICP. More aggressive hyperventilation (OBS < 4.0 kPa) may be considered at resistant intracranial hypertension.

Lund concept: Normoventilation, preferably volume controlled.

54.1.2.4 CSF Drainage

US guidelines: An option at a refractory intracranial hypertension.

Lund concept: Intermittently with caution at a high ICP with drainage from a relatively high drainage level via ventricular drainage. CT control to detect and prevent ventricular collapse.

54.1.2.5 Hyperosmolar Therapy

US guidelines: Options for mannitol 0.25–1 g/kg to serum osmol <320 mosm/L and for hypertonic saline to serum osmol <360 mosm/L.

Lund concept: Not recommended. Exceptionally it can be used to prevent acute brainstem herniation, e.g. under transportation, and to offer space during brain operation.

54.1.2.6 Fluid/Fluid Balance and Erythrocyte Therapy

US guidelines: Normovolaemia. Type of fluids and how to verify normovolaemia is not specified.

Lund concept: Normovolaemia. Moderate crystalloid infusions combined with albumin 20% as the main plasma volume expander resulting in an albumin concentration of 32–38 g/L. The albumin infusion should be given slowly. Erythrocyte transfusion (leucocyte-depleted blood) to maintain a haemoglobin concentration of above 110 g/L.

54.1.2.7 Vasopressors

US guidelines: Vasopressors can be used to increase CPP and SPB.

Lund concept: Vasopressors should be used in lowest possible dose.

54.1.2.8 Sedation, Analgesics and Musculorelaxation

US guidelines: Sedation, analgesics and muscle relaxation not specified and left to the treating physician. No propofol.

Lund concept: Midazolam and fentanyl in doses adapted to the age and individually preventing stress and pain. No neuromuscular blockade and no propofol.

54.1.2.9 High-Dose Barbiturates

US guidelines: Can be used at a refractory high ICP.

Lund concept: Not recommended, but lower doses <2–3 mg/kg/h for at most 2 days can be used at a refractory raised ICP.

54.1.2.10 Steroids

US guidelines: Not used.

Lund concept: Not used. One moderate bolus dose of methylprednisolone can be accepted to reduce a life-threatening high fever.

54.1.2.11 Temperature Control

US guidelines: Active cooling to subnormal temperature may be used as brain protection. Hyperthermia should be avoided.

Lund concept: Active cooling should not be used. High fever treated pharmacologically.

54.1.2.12 Antiseizure Prophylaxis

US guidelines: May be used in patients with a high risk of seizure.

Lund concept: Not used.

54.1.2.13 Surgical

US guidelines: Decompressive craniectomy an option to control a refractory high ICP. Surgical evacuation of haematomas and contusions not discussed.

Lund concept: Evacuation of large haematomas and surgical available contusions. Decompressive craniectomy as a last measure to counteract a refractory high ICP.

Tips, Tricks and Pitfalls

- All guidelines for treatment of severe head injury should be looked upon with humbleness, and there must be an individual evaluation of the treatment to choose.

54.2 Background

54.2.1 Guidelines for the Adult

Various guidelines have been presented during the last 25 years for treatment of an isolated severe traumatic brain injury in the adult, of which the most important are presented in the table above. The Rosner protocol (Rosner et al. 1995) and the Lund concept (Asgeirsson et al. 1994) were presented in 1992–1995. The US guideline was presented in its first version in 1996 (Bullock et al. 1996). Other guidelines are the European guideline presented in 1997 (Maas et al. 1997) and the Addenbrooke guideline from Cambridge, England, presented in 1999 (Menon 1999). Elucidatory versions of the Lund concept have been published (Grände 2006, 2017) as well as several updated versions of the US guideline, the latest in 2007 and 2016 (The Brain Trauma Foundation; The American Association of Neurological Surgeons; Congress of Neurological Surgeons 2007, 2016). In addition, national guidelines such as the Danish (Welling et al. 2010) have been published. All guidelines except the Lund concept can be characterized as cerebral perfusion pressure (CPP)-targeted guidelines and show similarities with the US guidelines and are mainly based on meta-analytic surveys. The Lund concept instead is based on basal physiological principles for brain volume and perfusion control and can be characterized as an intracranial pressure (ICP) and perfusion-targeted therapy. While most traditional guidelines including US guidelines are based only on clinical studies, the Lund concept also finds support from experimental studies. None of the published guidelines have been tested in larger randomized controlled studies, but numerous investigations, some with historical controls, have been published both for the Lund concept and more conventional guidelines (Grände 2006; Gerber et al. 2013). Modified versions of the Lund therapy have been compared with more conventional treatments in two smaller randomized studies, showing better outcome with the Lund therapy (Liu et al. 2010; Dizdarevic et al. 2012). Also recent studies with the US guideline have shown good outcome results (Gerber et al. 2013). By now we cannot tell, however, that a specific guideline is better than another.

All guidelines recommend continuous measurement of arterial pressure and ICP as well as the use of artificial ventilation. No guideline recommends treatment with steroids, except that the Lund concept accepts one bolus dose of Solu-Medrol (0.25–0.5 g to the adult) to reduce a life-threatening critically raised body temperature (>39.5 °C). Active cooling is an option in some conventional guidelines, but not in the Lund concept (see Chap. 58). Normal potassium and sodium concentrations are generally recommended. A shift in the treatment paradigm has emerged recently in many "non-Lund centres" by accepting a lower CPP, indicating that the guidelines have approached the Lund concept in some respects, even though the means to reach the goal are different (see Sect. 55.2 for details). Sedation should be sufficient to ameliorate the stress response. Wake-up tests are controversial, but still used in some centres.

There is a general recommendation that patients with severe head injury as soon as possible should be transferred to a neurosurgical unit. The patient should be intubated and receive intensive care treatment as recommended in the guidelines. There are some differences, though, regarding the intensive care treatment, as can be seen from the different guidelines in the table above. One difference is that US guidelines recommend that ICP treatment should not start before ICP is above 20–22 mmHg, while the Lund concept recommends that it should start as soon as possible after arrival to the neurointensive care unit independent of ICP. Focus should be to prevent hypovolaemia, avoidance of hypoxia, avoidance of hyper- or hypoglycaemia and avoidance of hyper- and hypoventilation. Enteral feeding is the goal. The intensive care should endeavour to ensure normality in most areas of the field, such as important physiological parameters.

54.3 Guidelines for the Paediatric Population

Little substantial research has been performed for the paediatric population, defined as <18 years of age. The paediatric brain injury remains poorly investigated. Treatment of children and adolescents therefore is mainly based on deductions from guidelines developed for adults. Important differences from the adult are lower blood pressure and lower peripheral resistance in the whole body, including the brain. This means that perfusion of various organs and the brain is maintained at blood and CPP pressures lower than those recommended for the adult. Like for the adult, enteral feeding is to be preferred. The need of energy/kg is much higher for children than for the adult. Specific recommendations for children and adolescents according to US guidelines are presented by the The Brain Trauma Foundation, Pediatric Guidelines (2010) and Bell and Kochanek (2013) and for the Lund concept (Wahlström et al. 2005; Grände 2006), while the other guidelines do not specifically address the paediatric population. As for the adult, the US paediatric guidelines are based on meta-analytic surveys of clinical studies and are a CPP-targeted therapy, and the Lund therapy is based on physiological principles for brain volume and brain perfusion regulation and is more of an ICP and perfusion-targeted therapy. The Lund concept also considers results from experimental studies.

References

Asgeirsson B, Grände PO, Nordström CH. A new therapy of post-trauma brain oedema based on haemodynamic principles for brain volume regulation. Intensive Care Med. 1994;20(4):260–7.

Bell MJ, Kochanek PM. Pediatric traumatic brain injury in 2012. The year with new guidelines and common data elements. Crit Care Clin. 2013;29(2):223–38.

Bullock R, Chesnut RM, Clifton G, Ghajar J, Marion DW, Narayan RK, Newell DW, Pitts LH, Rosner MJ, Wilberger JW. Guidelines for the management of severe head injury. Brain Trauma Foundation. Eur J Emerg Med. 1996;3(2):109–27.

Dizdarevic K, Hamdan A, Omerhodzic I, Kominlija-Smajic E. Modified Lund concept versus cerebral perfusion pressure-targeted therapy: a randomised controlled study in patients with secondary brain ischemia. Clin Neurol Neurosurg. 2012;114(2):142–8. https://doi.org/10.1016/j.clineuro.2011.10.005.

Gerber LM, Chiu YL, Carney N, Härtl R, Ghajar J. Marked reduction in mortality in patients with severe traumatic brain injury. J Neurosurg. 2013;119:1583–90.

Grände PO. The "Lund concept" for the treatment of severe head trauma—physiological principles and clinical application. Intensive Care Med. 2006;32(10):1475–84.

Grände PO. Critical evaluation of the Lund concept for treatment of severe traumatic head injury, 25 years after its introduction. Front Neurol. 2017;8:315. https://doi.org/10.3389/fneur.2017.00315.

Liu CW, Zheng YK, Lu J, Yu WH, Wang B, Hu W, Zhu KY, Zhu Y, Hu WH, Wang JR, Ma JP. Application of Lund concept in treating brain edema after severe head injury. Zhongguo Wei Zhong Bing Ji Jiu Yi Xue. 2010;22(10):610–3.

Maas AI, Dearden M, Teasdale GM, Braakman R, Chadon F, Iannotti F, Karimi A, Lapierre F, Stochetti

N, Unterberg A. EBIC-guidelines for management of severe head injury in adults. European Brain Injury Consortium. Acta Neurochir (Wien). 1997;139(4):286–94.

Menon DK. Cerebral protection in severe brain injury: physiological determinants of outcome and their optimisation. Br Med Bull. 1999;55(1):226–58.

Rosner MJ, Rosner SD, Johnson AH. Cerebral perfusion pressure: management protocol and clinical results. J Neurosurg. 1995;83(6):949–62.

The Brain Trauma Foundation; Pediatric Guidelines. 2010. https://www.braintrauma.org/coma-guidelines.

The Brain Trauma Foundation; The American Association of Neurological Surgeons; Congress of Neurological Surgeons. Guidelines for the management of severe traumatic brain injury. J Neurotrauma 24 Suppl. 2007;1:S1–106.

The Brain Trauma Foundation; The American Association of Neurological Surgeons; Congress of Neurological Surgeons. Guidelines for management of severe traumatic brain injury 4th edition. J Neurosurg. 2016;354(6314):893–6.

Wahlström MR, Olivecrona M, Koskinen LO, Rydenhag B, Naredi S. Severe traumatic brain injury in pediatric patients: treatment and outcome using an intracranial pressure targeted therapy—the Lund concept. Intensive Care Med. 2005;31(6):832–9.

Welling KI, Eskesen V, Romner B, the Danish Neurotrauma Committee. Neurointensive care of severe traumatic brain injury. Ugeskr Laeger. 2010;172:2091–4. (Danish).

The Lund Therapy: A Physiological Approach

55

Per-Olof Grände and Peter Reinstrup

Recommendations

Level I

There have been no level I studies performed to evaluate the Lund guidelines relative to any alternative guidelines.

Level II

There are no level II randomized studies that support any specific TBI guideline.

Level III

There have been several level III studies including two smaller randomized studies giving some support for the Lund therapy.

P.-O. Grände (✉)
Department of Anaesthesia and Intensive Care, Lund University and Lund University Hospital, Lund, Sweden
e-mail: per-olof.grande@med.lu.se

P. Reinstrup
Department of Anaesthesia and Intensive Care, Lund University and Lund University Hospital, Lund, Sweden

Department of Intensive and Perioperative Care, Skånes University Hospital, Lund, Sweden
e-mail: peter.reinstrup@med.lu.se

55.1 Overview of the Lund Guidelines

1. A vasogenic brain oedema is a consequence of an unbalance of the hydrostatic and the colloid osmotic pressure in the Starling fluid equilibrium, providing a disrupted blood brain barrier (BBB). The intracranial pressure will however increase more than an increase in hydrostatic capillary pressure or decrease in colloid osmotic pressure, as the brain is enclosed in the rigid cranium. Details of this mechanism have been described previously (see Grände 2017). Vasogenic brain oedema may be confined by counteracting a raised hydrostatic capillary pressure, which can be accomplished by antihypertensive treatment (see (2) below). It may also be confined by avoiding low colloid osmotic pressures (see (3) below). A CPP of 60–65 mmHg should be aimed at in most cases for the adult, but somewhat lower values may be necessary to reduce a significantly raised ICP. The ICP-reducing therapy should be started early after arrival to the intensive care, and normovolaemia is assured independent of prevailing ICP.
2. An ICP measuring device should be installed. Zero baseline for ICP should be set in the ear level (midlevel of the brain). Brain oedema can be reduced by normalization of the normally raised arterial blood pressure (providing normovolaemia) by antihypertensive

© Springer Nature Switzerland AG 2020
T. Sundstrøm et al. (eds.), *Management of Severe Traumatic Brain Injury*,
https://doi.org/10.1007/978-3-030-39383-0_55

therapy in terms of β_1 antagonist (e.g. metoprolol 1 mg/mL, 1–2 mL/h i.v., or 50 mg × 1–2 per os for an adult) and α_2 agonist (clonidine diluted to 15 μg/mL, 0.5–1 mL/h i.v., or 150 μg × 1–2 per os for an adult or dexmedetomidine 0.2–1.0 μg/kg/h i.v.). If blood pressure is still too high, use also angiotensin II antagonist (e.g. losartan 50 mg × 1–2 per os for an adult). If necessary, head elevation (max 15–20°) can be used to reduce cerebral perfusion pressure (CPP). In children and adolescents, the doses should be adapted to their age. An arterial blood pressure resulting in too low CPP (CPP below 55 mmHg in adults and below 40 mmHg in small children) may be an indication of a concealed hypovolaemia to be treated with extra fluid substitution before the start of the antihypertensive treatment (see (4) below and Chap. 63). If CPP is still too low, the antihypertensive treatment should be reduced. If there is a need of vasoconstrictors to maintain an adequate CPP, use lowest possible dose. It is important that baseline levels for ICP and blood pressure are the same to get correct CPP values.

3. Normalization of the plasma oncotic pressure with a colloid solution with the purpose to reduce brain oedema by improving transcapillary absorption and to improve perfusion of the brain. Preferably use 20% albumin solutions up to a plasma albumin concentration of 32–36 g/L.
4. A blood volume expanding therapy aimed at preservation of normovolaemia by infusion of albumin (preferably 20% solutions) to normal albumin concentrations (32–36 g/L) and by maintenance of a haemoglobin concentration above 110 g/L (always leucocyte-depleted blood). A crystalloid (normal saline 1.0–1.5 L/day for an adult and correspondingly lower volumes for children) can be given to obtain an adequate general fluid balance and urine production. The blood pressure response from additional volumes of blood and albumin or passive leg elevation will show if a low blood pressure can be explained by hypovolaemia. The volaemic state can also be checked with pulse pressure variations (PPV) (PPV > 10% may indicate hypovolaemia). The need for vasopressors is small when following this therapy and should be avoided. If still used to obtain an adequate blood pressure, it should be used in lowest possible doses. Diuretics can be used (not mannitol).
5. Anti-stress therapy in terms of midazolam 5 mg/mL (0–3 mL/h for an adult) and fentanyl 0.05 mg/mL (0–3 mL/h for the adult). The hypotensive drugs α_2 agonist and ß$_1$ antagonist (see under (1) above) also act as sedatives and reduce catecholamine concentration in plasma. Catecholamine concentration in plasma is also kept low by avoiding noradrenalin and by not using active cooling. Wake-up tests should not be used until start of the weaning procedure, and do not extubate until ICP has stabilized at a relatively normal level.
6. If there are problems with persistent high ICP (above 25 mmHg), the following measures can be taken: (1) surgical removal of available haematomas and contusions, (2) start of thiopental (pentothal, 50 mg/mL) initiated by treatment with a bolus dose of 1–3 mL followed by a continuous infusion of 1–3 mg/kg/h for the adult for at most 2 days (be aware of the risk with respiratory insufficiency with a more long-term use of this drug), or (3) decompressive craniectomy. Osmotherapy to reduce ICP has side effects in terms of renal and electrolyte disturbances and adverse rebound effects at its discontinuation and should be used only for acute prevention of brainstem herniation or to give space during brain surgery. Drainage of CSF—see under (9) below. The therapy may be guided by data from a microdialysis catheter placed in the penumbra zone.
7. Use low-energy nutrition (15–20 kcal/kg/day from days 2–3 for an adult, but relatively more energy for children). An energy supply of 1200–1400 kcal/day to the adult is enough to cover the basal metabolism under sedation and ventilatory support. If possible, use mainly enteral nutrition (high doses of parenteral fat nutrition may cause fever). Avoid over-nutrition. Keep blood glucose in the range of 6–10 mmol/L, and electrolytes should be normal. If there are difficulties to

achieve enough energy supply with enteral nutrition, add glucose (5–10%) with electrolytes i.v. As a last measure, low doses of parenteral nutrition of fat and amino acids can be added.

8. Mechanical ventilation (preferably volume-controlled), keeping a normal PaO_2 and a normal $PaCO_2$. A temporary moderate hyperventilation can be accepted for a short time period to prevent an acute brainstem herniation. PEEP (6–9 cm H_20) is mandatory to prevent atelectasis. Inhalation of a $ß_2$ agonist may help to clean the lung, but the doses should be reduced if there is a blood pressure fall and increase in ICP by a general $ß_2$-induced vasodilation.
9. Drainage of CSF can be performed via a ventricular catheter (not by lumbar puncture) and should be performed from a relatively high ICP pressure level to reduce the risk of ventricular collapse and brainstem herniation. A CT scan can show if the drainage causes a tendency of ventricular collapse.

Tips, Tricks, and Pitfalls

- Use the therapy within the framework of the guidelines.
- Start the therapy early after arrival to the intensive care unit to counteract the development of brain oedema and an increase in ICP prophylactically.
- A not too low haemoglobin concentration helps to avoid hypovolaemia and optimize oxygenation of the penumbra zone (only leucocyte-depleted blood should be used).
- Osmotherapy should be avoided due to the risk of a rebound effect and adverse renal effects and electrolyte disturbances. It can still be used to prevent acute brainstem herniation, e.g. during transportation, and to allow space during brain surgery.
- Decompressive craniectomy can be used to reduce ICP and prevent brainstem herniation.
- Normality of most physiological parameters is worth aiming at.
- Peep is mandatory to counteract atelectasis.

55.2 Background

While most traditional guidelines for treatment of severe head injury, including the US guidelines, are based on a meta-analytic approach, the Lund concept is in its main parts based on basal haemodynamic physiological principles for control of brain volume and brain perfusion. The Lund concept therefore is presented separately in this chapter. The physiological principles of the Lund concept have later on found support in clinical and experimental studies, including clinical outcome studies involving adults and children. Recent updates of the US guidelines have moved closer to the Lund concept (The Brain Trauma Foundation. The American Association of Neurological Surgeons; Congress of Neurological Surgeons 2007, 2016). The Lund concept has not been changed since its introduction, except that the venous vasoconstrictor dihydroergotamine was deleted from the concept after a few years due to the potential side effects always inherent in vasoconstrictors (Grände 2017).

The Lund concept combines two main goals, namely, halting or treating the development of a vasogenic brain oedema (the "ICP goal") and a simultaneously intensified support of the perfusion of the penumbra zone (the "perfusion goal"). The purpose of the therapy is to improve outcome by preventing brainstem herniation and by reducing cell death in the vulnerable penumbra zone. A microdialysis study has shown that these goals are reached with the Lund concept in spite of the use of antihypertensive treatment (Ståhl et al. 2001a). Most likely, this can be explained by improved perfusion and oxygenation, especially of the penumbra zone. This effect may be referred to the avoidance of hypovolaemia with albumin and blood transfusions, the avoidance of norepinephrine, the avoidance of active cooling, and the avoidance of wake-up tests (Skoglund et al. 2012).

The Lund therapy strives towards normalization of essential haemodynamic and biochemical parameters. For an overview of its theoretical background and therapeutic guidelines, see Grände (2006), Koskinen et al. (2014), and Grände (2017). The Lund therapy is applicable to all ages. Outcome studies with the Lund therapy have so far been promising (Eker et al. 1998; Wahlström et al. 2005; Koskinen et al. 2014). No level I and II studies have been performed regarding either the components of the traditional guidelines such as the US guideline and the European guideline in their original versions (Bullock et al. 1996; Maas et al. 1997) or in their updated versions (The Brain Trauma Foundation. The American Association of Neurological Surgeons; Congress of Neurological Surgeons 2007, 2016) or regarding the Lund concept (Grände 2006, 2017; Koskinen et al. 2014). Two smaller randomized studies comparing outcome with a modified version of the Lund concept with that of using conventional treatments, showed a lower mortality rate with the Lund concept (Liu et al. 2010; Dizdarevic et al. 2012). Also US guidelines have found support in a recent study (Gerber et al. 2013).

The "ICP goal" of the therapy is mainly based on the hypothesis that an imbalance between the transcapillary hydrostatic and the oncotic pressures creating filtration will result in a vasogenic brain oedema, provided the blood-brain barrier (BBB) is passively permeable to small solutes. Such a situation can exist in meningitis and after a head trauma. In head trauma patients, the BBB may be disrupted, especially around cerebral contusions. According to this hypothesis, the brain oedema can be counteracted or prevented by reducing a raised hydrostatic capillary pressure, as obtained by the antihypertensive treatment and avoidance of vasopressors, and normalization of a lowered plasma oncotic pressure. As the brain is enclosed in a rigid cranium, the change in ICP by alteration in the vasogenic brain oedema is much larger than the change in hydrostatic capillary pressure initiating the oedema (Grände 2017). It can be calculated that the change in ICP at most can be 5–6 times larger than the initial change in the hydrostatic capillary pressure.

The "perfusion goal" is aimed at maintaining better perfusion and oxygenation of the penumbra zone. This can be obtained by a low plasma concentration of catecholamines, by preventing hypovolaemia (counteracting baroreceptor reflex activation), if possible by avoiding the use of vasoconstrictors, by avoiding stress, by not using active cooling, and by avoiding low haemoglobin concentrations and hyperventilation (the patient should be normocapnic) and by not using wake-up tests. A more normal haemoglobin concentration will help to give a better oxygenation of the injured parts of the brain and to preserve a normovolaemic state. The cytotoxic brain oedema may also be reduced by a better perfusion and oxygenation. Preservation of normovolaemia is essential to maintain perfusion by reducing activation of the baroreceptor reflex, resulting in less peripheral vasoconstriction and lower catecholamine concentration in plasma.

Normal ICP stays in the range of 8–11 mmHg, which is higher than the venous pressure outside the dura of 0–3 mmHg. This pressure difference will increase, subsequent to an increase in ICP. The pressure fall between the subdural venous pressure and the extradural venous pressure (sometimes called the waterfall phenomenon) will create a subdural passive venous collapse, the resistance of which is directly related to the pressure fall. This means that a change in extradural venous pressure (e.g. a venous pressure increase by PEEP or a venous pressure decrease by head elevation) will not be transferred from the venous side into the brain, as the brain is protected by the variable subdural venous collapse. By this passive mechanism, the brain will not be influenced by venous pressure variations, and PEEP will not increase ICP from the venous side and can be used safely. Moderate PEEP (6–9 cm H_2O) is therefore an important component in the Lund concept to prevent development of atelectasis. Details of this physiological mechanism have been published previously (see Koskinen et al. 2014; Grände 2017). Consequently, head elevation will not decrease

ICP from the venous side, but head elevation will still decrease ICP due to the simultaneous reduction in arterial pressure.

Our present knowledge regarding the risk of hyperventilation has been discussed in more detail in a special chapter of this book (Chap. 60). Hyperventilation is not a component of the Lund concept.

In contrast to several other studies (e.g. Tomita et al. 1994; Dubois et al. 2006; Chen et al. 2014), the randomized SAFE-TBI study (The SAFE study investigators 2007) showed worse outcome with albumin in TBI patient. The SAFE-TBI study, however, has been strongly criticized and has not changed the recommendations in the Lund concept that isotonic albumin can be used (Grände 2008, 2017). The use of albumin and critical aspects of the SAFE-TBI study have been discussed in the fluid chapter in this book (Chap. 63). To give albumin as plasma volume expander is also justified due to the relatively small volumes of albumin needed to maintain normovolaemia when following the principles of the Lund therapy (Koskinen et al. 2014). See the chapter on fluid therapy.

Vasopressors such as noradrenalin may compromise circulation of the penumbra zone (Brassard et al. 2009) and should therefore be avoided or used in lowest possible doses. It has also been shown that noradrenaline may trigger ARDS (Contant et al. 2001). Low-dose prostacyclin is an option to improve microcirculation and oxygenation of the penumbra zone (Grände et al. 2000; Grände 2017).

Enteral nutrition is to be preferred, and overnutrition should be avoided, especially when using parenteral nutrition. Blood glucose should be kept between 6 and 10 mmol/L, in agreement with the NICE-SUGAR study (Finfer et al. 2015). Especially lower glucose concentrations than 6 mmol/L in the blood should be avoided, as microdialysis studies have shown that the glucose concentrations in the penumbra zone normally are much lower (sometimes even approaching zero) than in less injured tissues, which most likely cannot be fully compensated by a lower metabolism (Grände et al. 2000; Ståhl et al. 2001b).

A CT scan should be performed soon after arrival at the hospital. To counteract the development of an increase in ICP, the therapy should start early. If possible, extensive intracerebral bleedings and available contusions should be surgically evacuated. The Lund therapy is applicable to all ages if doses and physiological parameters are adapted to the patient's age (Eker et al. 1998; Naredi et al. 1998; Wahlström et al. 2005). The Lund therapy is not dependent on the actual autoregulatory capacity, and the benefit of evaluating autoregulatory capacity is small.

55.3 Specific Paediatric Concerns

The principles of the Lund concept are applicable to all ages if doses of nutrition, pharmacological substances, and fluids are adapted to the age. While a lowest CPP of 55 mmHg occasionally can be accepted in the adult, providing an optimal fluid therapy maintaining normovolaemia, relatively lower values can be accepted in adolescents and children and CPP down to 38–40 mmHg in the smallest children, but always providing an optimal fluid therapy.

References

Brassard P, Seifert T, Secher NH. Is cerebral oxygenation negatively affected by infusion of norepinephrine in healthy subjects? Br J Anaetsth. 2009;102:800–5.

Bullock R, Chesnut RM, Clifton G, Ghajar J, Marion DW, Narayan RK, Newell DW, Pitts LH, Rosner MJ, Wilberger JW. Guidelines for the management of severe head injury. Brain Trauma Foundation. Eur J Emerg Med. 1996;3(2):109–27.

Chen D, Bao L, Lu S, Xu F. Serum albumin and prealbumin predict the poor outcome of traumatic brain injury. PLoS One. 2014;9(3):1–7.

Contant CF, Valadka AB, Gopinath SP, Hannay HJ, Robertsson CS. Adult respiratory distress syndrome: a complication of induced hypertension after severe head injury. J Neurosurg. 2001;95:560–8.

Dizdarevic K, Hamdan A, Omerhodzic I, Kominlija-Smajic E. Modified Lund concept versus cerebral perfusion pressure-targeted therapy: a randomised controlled study in patients with secondary brain ischemia. Clin Neurol Neurosurg. 2012;114(2):142–8. https://doi.org/10.1016/j.clineuro.2011.10.005.

Dubois MJ, Orellana-Jimenez C, Melot C, De Backer D, Berre J, Leeman M, Brimioulle S, Appoloni O, Creteur J, Vincent JL. Albumin administration improves organ function in critically ill hypoalbuminemic patients: a prospective, randomized, controlled, pilot study. Crit Care Med. 2006;34:2536–40.

Eker C, Asgeirsson B, Grände PO, Schalen W, Nordström CH. Improved outcome after severe head injury with a new therapy based on principles for brain volume regulation and preserved microcirculation. Crit Care Med. 1998;26(11):1881–6.

Finfer S, Chittock D, Li Y, Foster D, Dhingra V, Bellomo R, Cook D, Dodek P, Hebert P, Henderson W, Heyland D, Higgins A, McArthur C, Mitchell I, Myburgh J, Robinson B, Ronco J. Intensive versus conventional glucose control in critically ill patients with traumatic brain injury: long-term follow up of a subgroup of patients from the NICE-SUGAR study. Intensive Care Med. 2015;41:1037–47. https://doi.org/10.1007/s00134-015-3757-6.

Gerber LM, Chiu YL, Carney N, Härtl R, Ghajar J. Marked reduction in mortality in patients with severe traumatic brain injury. J Neurosurg. 2013;119:1583–90.

Grände PO. The "Lund concept" for the treatment of severe head trauma—physiological principles and clinical application. Intensive Care Med. 2006;32(10):1475–84.

Grände PO. Time out for albumin or a valuable therapeutic component in severe head injury? Acta Anaesthesiol Scand. 2008;52:738–41.

Grände PO. Critical evaluation of the Lund concept for treatment of severe traumatic head injury, 25 Years after Its Introduction. Front Neurol. 2017;4(8):315. https://doi.org/10.3389/fneur.2017.00315. Review.

Grände PO, Möller AD, Nordström CH, Ungerstedt U. Low-dose prostacyclin in treatment of severe brain trauma evaluated with microdialysis and jugular bulb oxygen measurements. Acta Anaesthesiol Scand. 2000;44(7):886–94.

Koskinen LO, Olivecrona M, Grände PO. Severe traumatic brain injury management and clinical outcome using the Lund concept. Neuroscience. 2014;26(283):245–55. https://doi.org/10.1016/j.neuroscience.2014.06.039. Review.

Liu CW, Zheng YK, Lu J, Yu WH, Wang B, Hu W, Zhu KY, Zhu Y, Hu WH, Wang JR, Ma JP. Application of Lund concept in treating brain edema after severe head injury. Zhongguo Wei Zhong Bing Ji Jiu Yi Xue. 2010;22(10):610–3.

Maas AI, Dearden M, Teasdale GM, Braakman R, Chadon F, Iannotti F, Karimi A, Lapierre F, Stochetti N, Unterberg A. EBIC-guidelines for management of severe head injury in adults. European Brain Injury Consortium. Acta Neurochir (Wien). 1997;139(4):286–94.

Naredi S, Eden E, Zäll S, Stephensen H, Rydenhag B. A standardized neurosurgical neurointensive therapy directed toward vasogenic edema after severe traumatic brain injury: clinical results. Intensive Care Med. 1998;24(5):446–51.

Skoglund K, Enblad P, Hillered L, Marklund N. The neurological wake-up test increases stress hormone levels in patients with severe traumatic brain injury. Crit Care Med. 2012;40(1):216–422. https://doi.org/10.1097/CCM.0b013e31822d7dbd.

Ståhl N, Ungerstedt U, Nordström CH. Brain energy metabolism during controlled reduction of cerebral perfusion pressure in severe head injuries. Intensive Care Med. 2001a;27(7):1215–23.

Ståhl N, Mellergård P, Hallström A, Ungerstedt U, Nordström CH. Intracerebral microdialysis and bedside biochemical analysis in patients with fatal traumatic brain lesions. Acta Anaesthesiol Scand. 2001b;45(8):977–85.

The Brain Trauma Foundation. The American Association of Neurological Surgeons; Congress of Neurological Surgeons. Guidelines for the management of severe traumatic brain injury 3rd edition. J Neurotrauma. 2007;24(Suppl 1):S1–106.

The Brain Trauma Foundation. The American Association of Neurological Surgeons; Congress of Neurological Surgeons. Guidelines for management of severe traumatic brain injury 4th edition. J Neurosurg. 2016;354(6314):893–6.

The SAFE Study Investigators. Saline or albumin for fluid resuscitation in patients with traumatic brain injury. N Engl J Med. 2007;357:874–84.

Tomita H, Ito U, Tone O, Masaoka H, Tominaga B. High colloid oncotic therapy for contusional brain edema. Acta Neurochir Suppl (Wien). 1994;60:547–9.

Wahlström MR, Olivecrona M, Koskinen LO, Rydenhag B, Naredi S. Severe traumatic brain injury in pediatric patients: treatment and outcome using an intracranial pressure targeted therapy—the Lund concept. Intensive Care Med. 2005;31(6):832–9.

56 Pharmacological Neuroprotection

Niklas Marklund

56.1 Neuroprotection in TBI

Recommendations

Level I

There is no Level 1 evidence suggesting that any pharmacological treatment option can improve the outcome of TBI patients. Corticosteroids, magnesium sulfate, erythropoietin, cannabinoids, and progesterone are without demonstrated efficacy for TBI patients and should not be routinely used. Hypothermia decreases ICP although an improved outcome of patients with severe TBI has not been demonstrated.

Level II

There are studies at a Level II evidence with suggested benefits. None of these pharmacological treatments have as of yet been supported at a Level I and cannot be recommended.

Level III

Numerous studies at a Level III evidence exist. These studies are currently not sufficient to recommend or suggest a pharmacological compound to be administered to TBI patients. Thus a Level III recommendation for this topic cannot be provided.

56.2 Overview

A major problem in the management of severe traumatic brain injury (TBI) is that clinical outcome has not been markedly improved over the last decades (Rosenfeld et al. 2012). To date, >1000 studies with a huge variety of exploratory targets for the treatment of TBI are registered at www.clinicaltrials.gov, and important pharmacological treatment targets are also continuously being explored in the experimental TBI setting. A key concept in the management of TBI is that not all cell death occurs at the time of primary injury; instead a cascade of molecular and neurochemical secondary events occur during the initial hours and days with a complex temporal profile. Ultimately, this secondary injury cascade markedly exacerbates the primary injury as outlined in Chap. 6 of this book. As shown in numerous experimental TBI studies, there should be a possibility to attenuate the secondary injury cascades by pharmacological means. This possibility for improving TBI outcome has been explored over several decades, and many drugs with promising preclinical documentation have reached the clinical trial stage (see Maas et al. (2010)), most of which are regarded as neuroprotective.

N. Marklund (✉)
Department of Clinical Sciences Lund, Neurosurgery, Lund University, Skåne University Hospital, Lund, Sweden
e-mail: niklas.marklund@med.lu.se

© Springer Nature Switzerland AG 2020
T. Sundstrøm et al. (eds.), *Management of Severe Traumatic Brain Injury*,
https://doi.org/10.1007/978-3-030-39383-0_56

Neuroprotection in TBI can be defined as "interventions aimed at improving the patient's outcome, and preserving and restoring the integrity, function, and connectivity of the brain cells not irremediably damaged by the initial injury" (Zoerle et al. 2017). With few exceptions, most TBI trials to date have been rather small, only rarely enrolling more than 1000 patients. In their comprehensive overview published in 2016, Bragge and co-workers evaluated multicenter randomized control trials (RCTs) and found 47 completed pharmacological RCTs and 8 ongoing. None of these pharmacological treatments showed a robust clinical benefit, and the vast majority targeted early neuroprotective mechanisms (Bragge et al. 2016). The use of fluid management, hypertonic saline, mannitol, and various sedative compounds is covered in other chapters of this book, and in the following paragraphs, outlining key pharmacological compounds as well as hypothermia, evaluated in several clinical trials for severe TBI.

56.2.1 Early Mechanisms

Rapid intracellular influx of calcium is an immediate event in severe TBI (see Chap. 6). Based on the notion that excess calcium influx is detrimental, the calcium antagonist nimodipine was evaluated in the Head Injury Trials (HITs) (see Vergouwen et al. (2006)). A potential benefit in patients with traumatic subarachnoid hemorrhage was suggested and was explored in the HIT3 and HIT4 studies. In the larger HIT4 trial, a significantly *impaired* outcome in nimodipine-treated patients was observed, and nimodipine cannot be recommended for any subtype of severe TBI. Other immediate events of key pathophysiological importance are glutamate release leading to excitotoxicity and increased formation of reactive oxygen species (ROS), factors consistently identified as important targets in animal models of TBI (Marklund 2016; Marklund and Hillered 2011). Based on the observations that extracellular concentrations of glutamate and aspartate increase early after TBI, their *N*-methyl-D-Aspartate (NMDA) receptors were targeted in several large placebo-controlled trials evaluating compounds such as aptiganel, SNX-111, D-CPP-ene, selfotel, and eliprodil. Invariably, they all failed or even impaired outcome despite successful evaluation in preclinical models. To date, NMDA receptor antagonists should not be used for neuroprotection in severe TBI. A positive role for NMDA receptor *agonists* was suggested in animal models of TBI, finding that they could influence outcome by modifying post-injury plasticity (Shohami and Biegon 2014).

Another early event in severe TBI is calcium- and glutamate-induced mitochondrial dysfunction that may be prolonged. An important event is the opening of the mitochondrial permeability transition pore (mPTP), resulting in a reduced capacity for ATP production as well as the release of apoptosis-inducing factors and generation of ROS (Karlsson et al. 2019). Mitochondrial dysfunction may lead to ongoing tissue atrophy (Xu et al. 2010) and is suggested by microdialysis monitoring (Stovell et al. 2018; Lakshmanan et al. 2010). Ciclosporin (CsA) is a commonly used drug for immunosuppression and was also found neuroprotective due to, e.g., inhibition of the calcium-mediated mPTP activation and attenuation of ROS formation. Across numerous TBI models and time windows, CsA treatment has consistently resulted in neuroprotection with improved histological and/or behavioral outcome. In the clinical trial stage, it was found safe with promising, although not significant treatment results (Mazzeo et al. 2009; Brophy et al. 2013). Microdialysis has also been used in combination with whole blood and CSF sampling to determine the optimal dosing of CsA (Brophy et al. 2013). To date, the available human data is insufficient to recommend its use in severe TBI. The open-label phase II Copenhagen Head Injury Ciclosporin study, evaluating two dosing regimens, is currently ongoing for severe TBI. In a first feasibility study, ciclosporin was found safe, it passed the blood-brain barrier and showed signs of favorable changes in the levels of the biomarkers GFAP, NF-L, Tau, and UCH-L1 (Karlsson et al. 2019).

Thus, mitochondrial dysfunction and glutamate excitotoxicity pave the way for increased oxidative

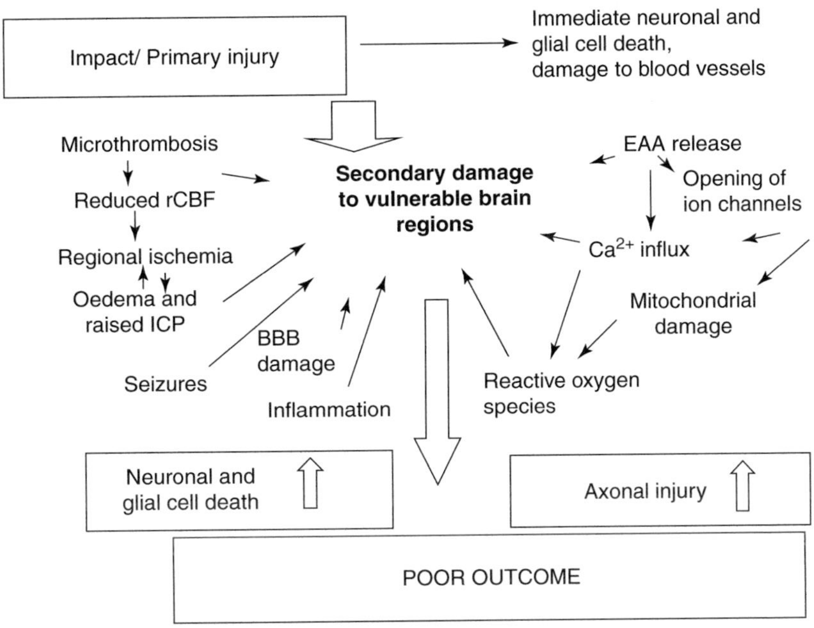

Fig. 56.1 Key events following severe TBI. The secondary injury process provides numerous pharmacological treatment targets that have been successfully evaluated in the experimental TBI setting, while all being unsuccesful in the clinical trial setting. *rCBF* regional cerebral blood flow; *EAA* excitatory amino acids; *BBB* blood-brain barrier

stress post-TBI (O'Connell and Littleton-Kearney 2013). Following the formation of highly reactive, oxygen-based radicals, ROS-induced lipid peroxidation that includes oxidative damage to cellular and organelle membranes ensues. Although the extremely short-acting and reactive radical hydroxyl ion (OH-) is highly toxic to virtually every structure in the cell, others such as the superoxide anion ($O2^-$) and the nitrogen-based radicals (reactive nitrogen species (RNS)), nitric oxide (NO), and peroxynitrite ($ONOO^-$) have been evaluated as pharmacological targets in TBI (Frati et al. 2017). However, both the superoxide radical scavenger polyethylene glycol-conjugated superoxide dismutase (PEG-SOD) and the 21-aminosteroid lipid peroxidation inhibitor tirilazad failed to improve survival or functional outcome in large phase III trials for TBI. Since increased formation of $O2^-$, NO, and $ONOO^-$ influences cerebral blood flow, they remain interesting targets for TBI, although at this point there is no evidence for, or sufficiently tested, a ROS scavening drug being ready for clinical use.

Finally, both the endocannabinoid dexanabinol and magnesium sulfate had unusually solid preclinical documentation showing efficacy in numerous animal models using prolonged time windows. Disappointingly, both compounds failed to demonstrate clinical efficacy, and there were clear suggestions, at least in the high-dose group, that magnesium sulfate *impaired* the outcome of severe TBI patients (Temkin et al. 2007; Maas et al. 2006). Some of the pharmacological targets are outlined in Fig. 56.1.

56.2.2 Steroids

Clinical trials initiated in the late 1970s and early 1980s began evaluating the corticosteroid dexamethasone, and it was found to be ineffective in improving outcome in cohorts of severely brain-injured patients. The multicenter randomized MRC CRASH trial, enrolling more than 10,000 patients, was by far the largest TBI trial (until the recently published CRASH-3 trial), and it evaluated methylprednisolone for patients with severe TBI. The results showed a significant *increase* in death and severe disability (Roberts et al. 2004). It should be remembered that in this trial excessive doses of corticosteroids were administered. In an early study evaluating 396 severe TBI patients, the synthetic corticosteroid triamcinolone was administered within 4 h after trauma and the outcome was improved by treatment in patients with a focal lesion and a GCS score of <8 (Grumme et al. 1995). Currently, there is some renewed interest in a lower-dose corticosteroid approach for selected TBI patients such as those with cortical contusions. There are significant adverse effects, however, emphasizing that corticosteroids should not routinely be administered to TBI patients.

56.2.3 Hormone Treatment

The most widely studied sex hormone progesterone repeatedly showed neuroprotective effects in several animal TBI models, attenuating cerebral edema and neuronal death and improving behavioral outcome. Many, but not all preclinical studies were performed on the bifrontal contusion model. An early clinical study found an improved 3- and 6-month outcome when progesterone was administered to patients within 8 h following severe TBI (Xiao et al. 2008; Skolnick et al. 2014). Thus, two phase III randomized trials were initiated (the ProTECT and SYNAPSE trials), of which the ProTECT trial used a very early <4-hour administration time window. Both the ProTECT and SYNAPSE trials were negative on the primary outcome measures, and even though a recent meta-analysis, evaluating eight RCTs, found an improved outcome at 3 although not at 6 months post-injury (Pan et al. 2019), to date, progesterone cannot be recommended as a routine treatment for severe TBI.

Pituitary deficiency is a common finding in survivors of severe TBI (Tritos et al. 2015; Marina et al. 2015) and may influence clinical outcome. Thus, this is an important factor in the clinical management of severe TBI. This does not imply, however, that early routine supplementation of hormones early post-injury for neuroprotection is warranted.

56.2.4 Hypothermia

Increased body and brain temperature is a well-known secondary injury insult in TBI since it increases brain metabolism and exacerbates neuronal injury. Hypothermia may effectively attenuate the inflammatory response, glutamate release, and ROS production and positively influence neuronal metabolism. In animal models of TBI, it consistently improved histological outcome (Dietrich and Bramlett 2017). This archetypical neuroprotectant has been applied in several clinical trials aiming at a temperature of 32–36.5 °C using various methods of cooling (cooling blankets, gastric lavage, selective head cooling, intravascular methods, etc.). A recent Cochrane assessment (Lewis et al. 2017), updated from an earlier 2009 review, evaluated 37 eligible trials including a total of 3110 randomized participants in both the adult and pediatric age groups. It was concluded that there are no high-quality evidence showing that hypothermia is beneficial in the treatment of severe TBI. The recent POLAR study (Cooper et al. 2018) evaluated early hypothermia (33–35 °C) for a minimum of 72 h up to 7 days post-injury compared to normothermia. A total of 500 patients were included. Even though hypothermia was initiated rapidly (at a median of 1.8 h post-injury) and rewarming was slow, neurological outcomes were not improved by 6 months. However, there were no changes in the rates of pneumonia and intracerebral hemorrhages. The Eurotherm study (Andrews et al. 2018) enrolled 387 patients from 47 centers in 18 countries. This trial used hypothermia titrated to ICP control, where core temperature was initially reduced to 35 °C followed by incremental decreases to a lower limit of 32 °C if needed to maintain ICP at <20 mmHg. Here, the titrated hypothermia approach successfully reduces ICP although mortality was higher and functional outcome worse than in patients treated with normothermia. This study builds on many other findings that hypothermia reduced ICP and it is currently used in many stepwise ICP management protocols.

The reasons for the limited success by hypothermia treatment are likely multifactorial. However, the treatment is risky and should be used with caution and only by experienced physicians since adverse effects include arrhythmias, coagulopathies, sepsis, and, in particular, pneumonia. To avoid the risks associated with systemic hypothermia, selective brain cooling was attempted in a small single-center trial in China, showing reduced ICP and beneficial outcomes at 1 and 2 years post-injury (Qiu et al. 2006), results that await additional, multicenter studies.

In the pediatric population, similar findings of unaltered or even impaired outcome have been found (Bragge et al. 2016; Hutchison et al. 2008). Together, these reports suggest that hypothermia cannot currently be recommended for routine use for TBI, although coming studies may help defining if subsets of TBI patients may benefit from hypothermia, and the most effective hypothermia protocol.

56.2.5 Neuroinflammation

There is robust clinical and experimental evidence showing a rapid and complex inflammatory response post-TBI. A very rapid upregulation at 1 h post-injury of cytokine and chemokine mRNA, followed by their corresponding proteins, has been found in the experimental TBI setting. Immune cells are also found invading the injured brain tissue, initially neutrophils at ca 24 h post-injury and later T cells and macrophages at 3–5 days post-injury (Clausen et al. 2019). Locally, there is also a very early activation of resident microglial cells that may then persist for years post-injury. Cellular membrane disruption caused by the mechanical impact as well as secondary injury factors may result in the release of damage-associated molecular patterns (DAMPs) that can trigger and amplify neuroinflammation (Simon et al. 2017).

Neuroinflammation should be recognized as an interaction between central and peripheral components that are influenced by age, gender, type of TBI and its severity, and other factors. Inflammation is often referred to as a double-edged sword possessing both beneficial and detrimental functions. The removal of injury debris may be one such positive action of the inflammatory mediators. However, chronic neuroinflammation is associated with an ongoing white matter atrophy (Johnson et al. 2013; Ramlackhansingh et al. 2011) and may be associated with impaired regeneration, posing a logical pharmacological treatment target. Although there are many potential treatment targets in this complex system, ever-increasing interest is generated for the action of interleukin (IL)-1β and its receptor. IL-1β is a key pro-inflammatory mediator, and when neutralized in experimental TBI, improved histological and behavioral outcome is consistently found.

Using a novel microdialysis approach in a single-center, phase II randomized control study of recombinant human IL1ra (rhIL1ra, anakinra) in severe TBI, the drug was found safe, to penetrate the extracellular fluid of the brain and to modify the inflammatory response as evident by comparison of the concentrations of 41 cytokines and chemokines. This proof-of-concept study provided evidence that an anti-inflammatory drug may alter the local inflammatory response and suggest an important role for microdialysis in pharmacological studies on TBI (Helmy et al. 2014). In a follow-up study, the IL1ra compound shifted the chemokine profile from an M2 microglia phenotype to an M1, highlighting that the microglial response may be modified by a study drug (Helmy et al. 2016).

Glucocorticoids may be considered anti-inflammatory compounds, and did not improve outcome in severe TBI, although the excessive doses used do not provide arguments either for or against inflammation as a treatment target in TBI. The optimal neuroinflammatory targets have not yet been defined, nor in what TBI subtype neuroinflammation may be most efficacious. Furthermore, the complex temporal response of neuroinflammation makes timing of treatment a challenge. However, neuroinflammation remains a promising target for pharmacological treatment and neuroprotection in severe TBI. To date, there are no specific drugs that can be recommended for administration to severe TBI patients.

56.2.6 Others

56.2.6.1 Erythropoietin (EPO)

EPO is a glycoprotein first used to treat patients with anemia. It has numerous other functions and is considered a neuroprotective drug with roles in apoptosis, radical oxygen species defense, inflammation, and angiogenesis. In experimental TBI, it is neuroprotective and improves functional outcome in animal models (Peng et al. 2014). The large interest in EPO for the treatment of clinical TBI was mainly based on robust preclinical evidence (Liu et al. 2017). In general trauma patients, thromboembolic events were increased by the treatment although early mortality was reduced. More recently, the Erythropoietin in Traumatic Brain Injury (EPO-TBI) was published (Nichol et al. 2015). It was a double-blind, placebo-controlled trial in >600 patients with moderate or severe TBI. EPO did neither improve neurological outcome nor result in an increased number of patients with deep venous thrombosis. In a follow-up post hoc analysis, it was suggested that a reduction in mortality did occur with EPO although only in those patients receiving one to two doses of the compound, not three (Gantner et al. 2018). At present, EPO cannot be recommended to severe TBI patients outside of clinical trials.

56.2.6.2 Beta-Blockers

Severe TBI elicits a severe stress reduction with increased pulse rate and, often, increased blood pressure. Stress reduction using, e.g., clonidine and beta-blockers, is part of the Lund concept for the treatment of severe TBI covered elsewhere in this book. Whether beta-blockers such as propranolol and others have neuroprotective mechanisms of action remains a topic of debate. Emerging observational studies find improved outcome and reduced mortality in those patients provided beta-blockers during neurocritical care. For instance, in an observational study of >2200 patients in 15 North American trauma centers, 50% of TBI patients received beta-blockers, most on day 1 post-injury. Administration of beta-blockers resulted in lower mortality, and propranolol was superior to the other compounds (Ley et al. 2018). In a smaller observational study, the use of beta-blockers shortened hospital stay and markedly improved clinical outcome in severe TBI patients (Ahl et al. 2017). Although these trials showed much promise in the treatment of severe TBI, beta-blockers have not been carefully evaluated in a randomized, systematic fashion, and their use for the purpose of neuroprotection cannot be recommended. Furthermore, there are studies finding increased infection rates and prolonged stay in intensive care unit with their use (Chen et al. 2017), suggesting caution and that better evidence is needed prior to beta-blockers being generally recommended to severe TBI patients.

56.2.6.3 Tranexamic Acid

Coagulation disorders are covered elsewhere in this book. However, rapid correction of coagulation abnormalities may be the best option to achieve neuroprotection. In this chapter, only tranexamic acid (TXA) is discussed. In >20,000 adult trauma patients enrolled in the CRASH-2 study, early <3 h post-injury administration of THX reduced the mortality due to bleeding (Roberts et al. 2013). Early intracranial bleeding is common in severe TBI and associated with increased risk of death and disability, and increased fibrinolysis may worsen the injury progression. The rationale for using TXA is that it inhibits the enzymatic breakdown of fibrinogen and fibrin and may thus prevent hemorrhage, albeit at the price of an increased risk of thromboembolic complications. In the CRASH-3 study, 12,737 TBI patients (9,202 patients treated within 3 hours post-injury) were administered THX or placebo where the primary outcome was death due to TBI within 28 days of injury for patients treated within 3 h of injury. Secondary outcome measures included, e.g., vascular occlusive events, neurosurgical blood loss, days in intensive care, and adverse events (Roberts et al. 2018). The results of the CRASH-3 study showed that there was a small but significant reduction in head-injury related deaths (mortality was 12.5% in the TXA group versus 14.0% in the placebo group), implying and important role for fibrinolysis inhibitors in severe TBI (CRASH-3 trial collaborators 2019).

Tips, Tricks, and Pitfalls

- If you see edema surrounding a traumatic hematoma and consider using corticosteroids, evaluate the available evidence—which will make you refrain from using it. To date, these drugs have not been shown to benefit TBI patients; instead high-dose treatment was shown to impair the outcome of TBI patients in large clinical trials. Still, the interest for using a lower and more refined corticosteroid dose remains in selected centers, particularly in patients with intracerebral contusions.

- Hypothermia reduces ICP when applied to patients with severe TBI and is used as a late step in several ICP-lowering protocols worldwide. The value of hypothermia for neuroprotection in severe TBI is at best limited, and the reader should be aware of the studies finding *impaired* clinical outcome. Thus, routine use of systematic hypothermia for severe TBI cannot be recommended which is supported by the two recent Eurotherm and POLAR RCTs. In pediatric cases, hypothermia has not resulted in improved outcome, and several studies show impaired outcome by the treatment suggesting caution to induce hypothermia in children. The optimal cooling and rewarming strategies, as well as the time window of efficacy, have not been defined.
- Recent RCTs evaluating erythropoietin or progesterone did not show a clinical benefit over control treatment.
- Attenuation of coagulation disorders, although not strictly neuroprotection, may be a pharmacological way of attenuating lesion progression in TBI.
- Large observational studies find that administration of beta-blockers for blood pressure reduction and/or stress relief is associated with reduced mortality and improved outcome. However, they have not as of yet been administered in a randomized fashion, and their role remains debatable.
- Mitochondrial dysfunction may be a key to the energy metabolic disturbance observed post-TBI and be related to the slow recovery experienced by many patients.
- Neuroinflammation remains a promising target for neuroprotection in severe TBI, although the precise treatment targets, timing, and compounds have not been established.
- Is pharmacological neuroprotection dead for severe TBI? Well, not really but clearly suffering. The limitation of providing a drug in sufficient concentrations to the injured brain early enough post-injury will remain a challenge. Likely, to target delayed and/or persistent mechanisms such as mitochondrial dysfunction, axonal injury and neuroinflammation, may have a higher chance for success. Furthermore, the attempt to improve outcome by using a pharmacological compound targeting a single disease mechanism—the "silver bullet"—is likely futile.
- The strict avoidance, detection, and treatment of avoidable factors (seizures, fever, hypotension, hypoxemia, hyper- and hypoglycemia, low CPP, high ICP, etc.) probably remain the best available therapy at the moment to provide neuroprotection for patients suffering from severe TBI.

56.3 Background

In severe TBI, it is well-established that neuronal and glial cells as well as blood vessels may be disrupted at time of impact and that the ensuing hemorrhage and tissue laceration result in exacerbated injury to the brain tissue. One key component of the injury cascade is a massive disturbance of the cellular ion homeostasis initiated by the marked release of the excitatory amino acid neurotransmitters glutamate and aspartate, in turn resulting in an activation of glutamate receptors leading to excitotoxicity (for overview, see Marklund and Hillered (2011) and Chap. 6 in this volume). As a consequence of the glutamate release, cellular influx of Na^+ and Ca^{2+} and efflux of K^+ ensue and lead to traumatic depolarization. The rapid influx of calcium leads to mitochondrial damage, axonal injury, an increase in free radical production, and activation of calcium-dependent destructive proteases such as caspases and calpains resulting in cytoskeletal damage. The mitochondrial dysfunction post-TBI (Hiebert et al. 2015) occurs at the time of increased energy demand due to activation of energy-consuming ion transport systems and cell repair enzymes. A high demand for glucose also occurs at time of reduced regional cerebral blood flow, and this uncoupling of blood flow and cerebral metabolism negatively influences the injured brain (Marklund et al. 2002; Chen et al. 2004). Injured mitochondria are also a potential source for increased production of reactive oxygen/nitrogen species (ROS/RNS), and in combination with a decreased anti-oxidant defense that also occurs following TBI, induces damage to cellular membranes and organelles by lipid peroxidation, protein oxidation, and nucleotide breakdown (Hall 2015).

For obvious reasons, neuronal cell death has attracted the majority of attention in TBI research, although the presence of delayed traumatic axonal injury is increasingly recognized following TBI (Tsitsopoulos et al. 2017).

Inflammation may be a double-edged sword following TBI. Although some inflammatory pathways may be important for regenerative responses and repair, numerous experimental studies suggest that other parts of the immune response is exacerbating the primary injury. The acute inflammatory response following TBI includes breakdown of the blood-brain barrier (BBB) with edema formation, infiltration of peripheral immune cells with production of ROS, activation of resident microglia and astrocytes, and intrathecal release of cytokines (Corps et al. 2015).

In this chapter, I reviewed the key clinical evidence for neuroprotection in patients with severe TBI. Promising preclinical trials have failed when attempting to translate findings from animal models into the clinical setting. Importantly, injury mechanisms, genetic background, gender, age, type and severity of injury, metabolic state of the brain, and other conditions (e.g., other diseases, medication, and coagulation abnormalities) associated with TBI may clearly influence the brain injury and are insufficiently evaluated in preclinical models. Also, much detailed pathophysiological knowledge from experimental TBI has not been confirmed in the injured human brain, and the brain penetration of putative neuroprotective compounds is frequently unknown. Finally, careful selection of patients in terms of injury type and severity based on detailed neuroradiology, age, and additional injuries combined with improved secondary outcome measures is likely crucial in the future development of neuroprotective compounds for human TBI.

The pharmacological and hypothermia TBI trials presented here have all frequently been criticized in terms of study design, route of administration, time window, and patient selection (e.g., see Bragge et al. (2016); Marklund and Hillered (2011)). In particular, it should be emphasized that TBI is not *one* disease; instead the different subtypes of TBI may require markedly different treatments. It is inevitable that the vast clinical heterogeneity creates difficulties when aiming to design a clinical trial (Saatman et al. 2008). Presumably, many previous trials included patients in too good or too severe condition to enable detection of a treatment effect. Also, preclinical studies use rodent TBI models reaching at most a moderate level of injury, and time windows for drug administration beyond the first post-injury hours are rather scarce in the experimental setting. Lack of early mechanistic endpoints and the insensitivity of the more global outcome measures are specific problems in clinical TBI research. Important lessons for future trials include improved patient classifications, knowledge of brain penetration of the study drug and mechanism of its actions, and more carefully defined and detailed clinical outcome measures. The difficulty of achieving high enough concentrations of the drug early enough post-injury is another important obstacle in the pharmacology of TBI. Perhaps may other administration protocols, using for instance intranasal administration (Gucnnoun et al. 2019), be evaluated in future RCTs. More sophisticated RCT design, large multicenter RCTs in priority areas, increased focus on preclinical research, and alternatives to RCTs, such as comparative effectiveness research and precision medicine, are needed to fully

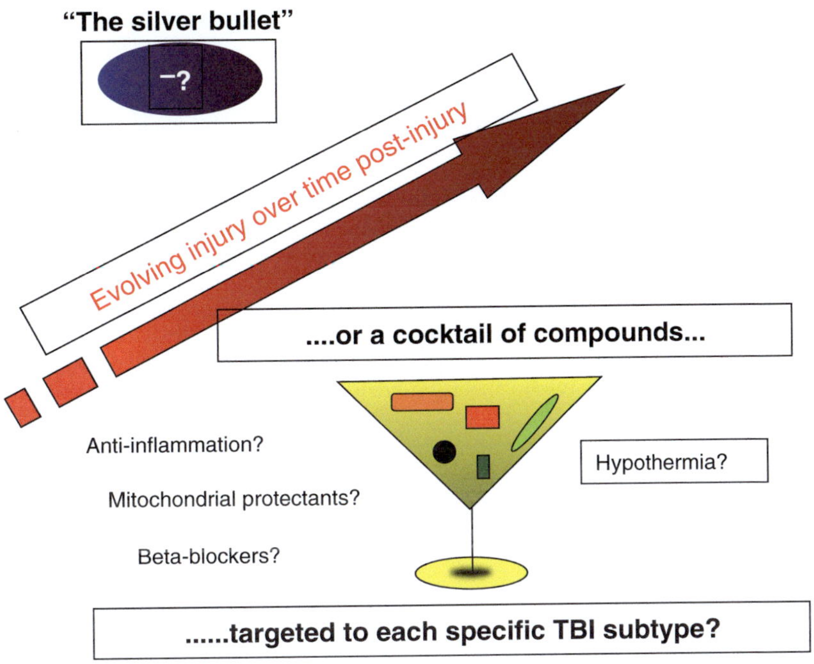

Fig. 56.2 The future pharmacological treatment of TBI may need to include a combination of drugs instead of attempting to use the "silver bullet." Modified from Pitkänen et al. 2005

implement acute TBI research for the benefit of severe TBI patients.

56.4 Summary

Currently, despite a relatively large number of phase III randomized clinical trials, there is no neuroprotective compound with proven clinical benefit available for TBI patients. Whether or not these failures are caused by inadequate trial design, poor brain penetration and/or efficacy of the compound, patient heterogeneity, insufficient preclinical documentation, or insensitive outcome measures, among many other plausible reasons, remains a matter of debate. Furthermore, there is seldom consensus among centers on general neurointensive care management protocols, which further increase patient heterogeneity. It is obvious that numerous mistakes have been made in the past when attempting to translate preclinical information into the complex human situation. The search for the "silver bullet" (Fig. 56.2)—a compound targeting a single neuroprotective mechanism showing efficacy in all subtypes of TBI and in all TBI severities—is not likely to be succesful. The future pharmacological management of TBI patients will probably include both neuroprotective drugs and compounds enhancing regeneration. Until such pharmacological treatments are developed, clinicians should aim for further improvement in the monitoring and neurointensive care management to improve the outcome of severe TBI patients.

References

Ahl R, Thelin EP, Sjolin G, Bellander BM, Riddez L, Talving P, et al. Beta-Blocker after severe traumatic brain injury is associated with better long-term functional outcome: a matched case control study. Eur J Trauma Emerg Surg. 2017;43(6):783–9.

Andrews PJ, Sinclair HL, Rodriguez A, Harris B, Rhodes J, Watson H, et al. Therapeutic hypothermia to reduce intracranial pressure after traumatic brain injury: the Eurotherm3235 RCT. Health Technol Assess. 2018;22(45):1–134.

Bragge P, Synnot A, Maas AI, Menon DK, Cooper DJ, Rosenfeld JV, et al. A state-of-the-science overview of randomized controlled trials evaluating acute management of moderate-to-severe traumatic brain injury. J Neurotrauma. 2016;33(16):1461–78.

Brophy GM, Mazzeo AT, Brar S, Alves OL, Bunnell K, Gilman C, et al. Exposure of cyclosporin A in whole blood, cerebral spinal fluid, and brain extracellular fluid dialysate in adults with traumatic brain injury. J Neurotrauma. 2013;30(17):1484–9.

Chen SF, Richards HK, Smielewski P, Johnstrom P, Salvador R, Pickard JD, et al. Relationship between flow-metabolism uncoupling and evolving axonal injury after experimental traumatic brain injury. J Cereb Blood Flow Metab. 2004;24(9):1025–36.

Chen Z, Tang L, Xu X, Wei X, Wen L, Xie Q. Therapeutic effect of beta-blocker in patients with traumatic brain injury: a systematic review and meta-analysis. J Crit Care. 2017;41:240–6.

Clausen F, Marklund N, Hillered L. Acute inflammatory biomarker responses to diffuse traumatic brain injury in the rat monitored by a novel microdialysis technique. J Neurotrauma. 2019;36(2):201–11.

Cooper DJ, Nichol AD, Bailey M, Bernard S, Cameron PA, Pili-Floury S, et al. Effect of early sustained prophylactic hypothermia on neurologic outcomes among patients with severe traumatic brain injury: the POLAR randomized clinical trial. JAMA. 2018;320(21):2211–20.

Corps KN, Roth TL, McGavern DB. Inflammation and neuroprotection in traumatic brain injury. JAMA Neurol. 2015;72(3):355–62.

CRASH-3 trial collaborators. Effects of tranexamic acid on death, disability, vascular occlusive events and other morbidities in patients with acute traumatic brain injury (CRASH-3): a randomised, placebo-controlled trial. Lancet. 2019;394(10210):1713–23. https://doi.org/10.1016/S0140-6736(19)32233-0. Epub 2019 Oct 14.

Dietrich WD, Bramlett HM. Therapeutic hypothermia and targeted temperature management for traumatic brain injury: experimental and clinical experience. Brain Circ. 2017;3(4):186–98.

Frati A, Cerretani D, Fiaschi AI, Frati P, Gatto V, La Russa R, et al. Diffuse axonal injury and oxidative stress: a comprehensive review. Int J Mol Sci. 2017;18(12):E2600.

Gantner DC, Bailey M, Presneill J, French CJ, Nichol A, Little L, et al. Erythropoietin to reduce mortality in traumatic brain injury: a post-hoc dose-effect analysis. Ann Surg. 2018;267(3):585–9.

Grumme T, Baethmann A, Kolodziejczyk D, Krimmer J, Fischer M, von Eisenhart Rothe B, et al. Treatment of patients with severe head injury by triamcinolone: a prospective, controlled multicenter clinical trial of 396 cases. Res Exp Med (Berl). 1995;195(4):217–29.

Guennoun R, Frechou M, Gaignard P, Liere P, Slama A, Schumacher M, et al. Intranasal administration of progesterone: a potential efficient route of delivery for cerebroprotection after acute brain injuries. Neuropharmacology. 2019;145(Pt B):283–91.

Hall ED. The contributing role of lipid peroxidation and protein oxidation in the course of CNS injury neurodegeneration and neuroprotection: an overview. In: Kobeissy FH, editor. Brain neurotrauma: molecular, neuropsychological, and rehabilitation aspects. Frontiers in neuroengineering. Boca Raton: CRC Press/Taylor & Francis; 2015.

Helmy A, Guilfoyle MR, Carpenter KL, Pickard JD, Menon DK, Hutchinson PJ. Recombinant human interleukin-1 receptor antagonist in severe traumatic brain injury: a phase II randomized control trial. J Cereb Blood Flow Metab. 2014;34(5):845–51.

Helmy A, Guilfoyle MR, Carpenter KLH, Pickard JD, Menon DK, Hutchinson PJ. Recombinant human interleukin-1 receptor antagonist promotes M1 microglia biased cytokines and chemokines following human traumatic brain injury. J Cereb Blood Flow Metab. 2016;36(8):1434–48.

Hiebert JB, Shen Q, Thimmesch AR, Pierce JD. Traumatic brain injury and mitochondrial dysfunction. Am J Med Sci. 2015;350(2):132–8.

Hutchison JS, Ward RE, Lacroix J, Hebert PC, Barnes MA, Bohn DJ, et al. Hypothermia therapy after traumatic brain injury in children. N Engl J Med. 2008;358(23):2447–56.

Johnson VE, Stewart JE, Begbie FD, Trojanowski JQ, Smith DH, Stewart W. Inflammation and white matter degeneration persist for years after a single traumatic brain injury. Brain. 2013;136(Pt 1):28–42.

Karlsson M, Pukenas B, Chawla S, Ehinger JK, Plyler R, Stolow M, et al. Neuroprotective effects of cyclosporine in a porcine pre-clinical trial of focal traumatic brain injury. J Neurotrauma. 2019;36(1):14–24.

Lakshmanan R, Loo JA, Drake T, Leblanc J, Ytterberg AJ, McArthur DL, et al. Metabolic crisis after traumatic brain injury is associated with a novel microdialysis proteome. Neurocrit Care. 2010;12(3):324–36.

Lewis SR, Evans DJ, Butler AR, Schofield-Robinson OJ, Alderson P. Hypothermia for traumatic brain injury. Cochrane Database Syst Rev. 2017;9:CD001048.

Ley EJ, Leonard SD, Barmparas G, Dhillon NK, Inaba K, Salim A, et al. Beta blockers in critically ill patients with traumatic brain injury: results from a multicenter, prospective, observational American Association for the Surgery of Trauma study. J Trauma Acute Care Surg. 2018;84(2):234–44.

Liu WC, Wen L, Xie T, Wang H, Gong JB, Yang XF. Therapeutic effect of erythropoietin in patients with traumatic brain injury: a meta-analysis of randomized controlled trials. J Neurosurg. 2017;127(1):8–15.

Maas AI, Murray G, Henney H 3rd, Kassem N, Legrand V, Mangelus M, et al. Efficacy and safety of dexanabinol in severe traumatic brain injury: results of a phase III randomised, placebo-controlled, clinical trial. Lancet Neurol. 2006;5(1):38–45.

Maas AI, Roozenbeek B, Manley GT. Clinical trials in traumatic brain injury: past experience and current developments. Neurotherapeutics. 2010;7(1):115–26.

Marina D, Klose M, Nordenbo A, Liebach A, Feldt-Rasmussen U. Early endocrine alterations reflect prolonged stress and relate to 1-year functional outcome in patients with severe brain injury. Eur J Endocrinol. 2015;172(6):813–22.

Marklund N. Rodent models of traumatic brain injury: methods and challenges. Methods Mol Biol. 2016;1462:29–46.

Marklund N, Hillered L. Animal modelling of traumatic brain injury in preclinical drug development: where do we go from here? Br J Pharmacol. 2011;164(4):1207–29.

Marklund N, Sihver S, Langstrom B, Bergstrom M, Hillered L. Effect of traumatic brain injury and nitrone radical scavengers on relative changes in regional cerebral blood flow and glucose uptake in rats. J Neurotrauma. 2002;19(10):1139–53.

Mazzeo AT, Brophy GM, Gilman CB, Alves OL, Robles JR, Hayes RL, et al. Safety and tolerability of cyclosporin a in severe traumatic brain injury patients: results from a prospective randomized trial. J Neurotrauma. 2009;26(12):2195–206.

Nichol A, French C, Little L, Haddad S, Presneill J, Arabi Y, et al. Erythropoietin in traumatic brain injury (EPO-TBI): a double-blind randomised controlled trial. Lancet. 2015;386(10012):2499–506.

O'Connell KM, Littleton-Kearney MT. The role of free radicals in traumatic brain injury. Biol Res Nurs. 2013;15(3):253–63.

Pan ZY, Zhao YH, Huang WH, Xiao ZZ, Li ZQ. Effect of progesterone administration on the prognosis of patients with severe traumatic brain injury: a meta-analysis of randomized clinical trials. Drug Des Devel Ther. 2019;13:265–73.

Peng W, Xing Z, Yang J, Wang Y, Wang W, Huang W. The efficacy of erythropoietin in treating experimental traumatic brain injury: a systematic review of controlled trials in animal models. J Neurosurg. 2014;121(3):653–64.

Pitkänen A, Marklund N, Morales, McIntosh TK. Mechanisms of neuronal death and neuroprotective strategies after traumatic brain injury. Drug Discov Today Dis Mech. 2005;2(4):408–18.

Qiu W, Shen H, Zhang Y, Wang W, Liu W, Jiang Q, et al. Noninvasive selective brain cooling by head and neck cooling is protective in severe traumatic brain injury. J Clin Neurosci. 2006;13(10):995–1000.

Ramlackhansingh AF, Brooks DJ, Greenwood RJ, Bose SK, Turkheimer FE, Kinnunen KM, et al. Inflammation after trauma: microglial activation and traumatic brain injury. Ann Neurol. 2011;70(3):374–83.

Roberts I, Yates D, Sandercock P, Farrell B, Wasserberg J, Lomas G, et al. Effect of intravenous corticosteroids on death within 14 days in 10,008 adults with clinically significant head injury (MRC CRASH trial): randomised placebo-controlled trial. Lancet. 2004;364(9442):1321–8.

Roberts I, Shakur H, Coats T, Hunt B, Balogun E, Barnetson L, et al. The CRASH-2 trial: a randomised controlled trial and economic evaluation of the effects of tranexamic acid on death, vascular occlusive events and transfusion requirement in bleeding trauma patients. Health Technol Assess. 2013;17(10):1–79.

Roberts I, Belli A, Brenner A, Chaudhri R, Fawole B, Harris T, et al. Tranexamic acid for significant traumatic brain injury (The CRASH-3 trial): statistical analysis plan for an international, randomised, double-blind, placebo-controlled trial. Wellcome Open Res. 2018;3:86.

Rosenfeld JV, Maas AI, Bragge P, Morganti-Kossmann MC, Manley GT, Gruen RL. Early management of severe traumatic brain injury. Lancet. 2012;380(9847):1088–98.

Saatman KE, Duhaime AC, Bullock R, Maas AI, Valadka A, Manley GT, et al. Classification of traumatic brain injury for targeted therapies. J Neurotrauma. 2008;25(7):719–38.

Shohami E, Biegon A. Novel approach to the role of NMDA receptors in traumatic brain injury. CNS Neurol Disord Drug Targets. 2014;13(4):567–73.

Simon DW, McGeachy MJ, Bayir H, Clark RS, Loane DJ, Kochanek PM. The far-reaching scope of neuroinflammation after traumatic brain injury. Nat Rev Neurol. 2017;13(3):171–91.

Skolnick BE, Maas AI, Narayan RK, van der Hoop RG, MacAllister T, Ward JD, et al. A clinical trial of progesterone for severe traumatic brain injury. N Engl J Med. 2014;371(26):2467–76.

Stovell MG, Mada MO, Helmy A, Carpenter TA, Thelin EP, Yan JL, et al. The effect of succinate on brain NADH/NAD(+) redox state and high energy phosphate metabolism in acute traumatic brain injury. Sci Rep. 2018;8(1):11140.

Temkin NR, Anderson GD, Winn HR, Ellenbogen RG, Britz GW, Schuster J, et al. Magnesium sulfate for neuroprotection after traumatic brain injury: a randomised controlled trial. Lancet Neurol. 2007;6(1):29–38.

Tritos NA, Yuen KC, Kelly DF, Neuroendocrine A, Pituitary Scientific C. American Association of Clinical Endocrinologists and American College of Endocrinology Disease State Clinical Review: a neuroendocrine approach to patients with traumatic brain injury. Endocr Pract. 2015;21(7):823–31.

Tsitsopoulos PP, Abu Hamdeh S, Marklund N. Current opportunities for clinical monitoring of axonal pathology in traumatic brain injury. Front Neurol. 2017;8:599.

Vergouwen MD, Vermeulen M, Roos YB. Effect of nimodipine on outcome in patients with traumatic subarachnoid haemorrhage: a systematic review. Lancet Neurol. 2006;5(12):1029–32.

Xiao G, Wei J, Yan W, Wang W, Lu Z. Improved outcomes from the administration of progesterone for patients with acute severe traumatic brain injury: a randomized controlled trial. Crit Care. 2008;12(2):R61.

Xu Y, McArthur DL, Alger JR, Etchepare M, Hovda DA, Glenn TC, et al. Early nonischemic oxidative metabolic dysfunction leads to chronic brain atrophy in traumatic brain injury. J Cereb Blood Flow Metab. 2010;30(4):883–94.

Zoerle T, Carbonara M, Zanier ER, Ortolano F, Bertani G, Magnoni S, et al. Rethinking neuroprotection in severe traumatic brain injury: toward bedside neuroprotection. Front Neurol. 2017;8:354.

Subacute Surgery in Neurointensive Care

57

Terje Sundstrøm, Eirik Helseth, and Knut Gustav Wester

Recommendations

Level I

Decompressive craniectomy can reduce intracranial pressure (ICP) and mortality in severe traumatic brain injury (TBI) with or without surgical lesions, but it does not improve the rate of patients surviving with a favourable outcome.

Level II

There are insufficient data to support a Level II recommendation for this topic.

Level III

Decompressive craniectomy is an option to treat neurologic deterioration, herniation or intracranial hypertension refractory to medical management in children.

Decompressive craniectomies should be large and include duraplasty.

Post-operative complications can be avoided by meticulous surgical technique and adequate choice of procedure.

57.1 Overview

The possibility of hydrocephalus, brain oedema or a new or recurrent intracranial haematoma must be investigated by repeated computed tomography (CT) scans in case of neurological deterioration or intractable intracranial hypertension in a head-injured patient. Subacute surgery (secondary surgical intervention) should then be considered.

The relevant surgical procedures and their respective indications are described in Part V in this book on acute surgical treatment; these principles also apply to subacute surgery. Drainage of cerebrospinal fluid is moreover discussed in the following section. In general, the monitoring and treatment strategies described elsewhere in Parts VII and VIII should be consulted for detailed information on timing, thresholds and complementary interventions.

T. Sundstrøm (✉)
Department of Neurosurgery, Haukeland University Hospital, Bergen, Norway

Department of Clinical Medicine, University of Bergen, Bergen, Norway
e-mail: tjsu@helse-bergen.no, kgwe@helse-bergen.no

E. Helseth
Institute of Clinical Medicine, University of Oslo, Oslo, Norway

Department of Neurosurgery, Oslo University Hospital, Oslo, Norway
e-mail: ehelseth@ous-hf.no

K. G. Wester
Department of Clinical Medicine, University of Bergen, Bergen, Norway
e-mail: Knut.Wester@uib.no

© Springer Nature Switzerland AG 2020
T. Sundstrøm et al. (eds.), *Management of Severe Traumatic Brain Injury*,
https://doi.org/10.1007/978-3-030-39383-0_57

Tips, Tricks and Pitfalls

- Continuously re-evaluate the level of treatment according to new developments.
- 'Do not treat the patient with a new CT scan'.
- Always look at the patient and think about possible technical malfunctions and the reliability of the monitoring equipment.
- When doubt exists and consciousness is depressed, intracranial pressure should always be monitored, and significant mass lesions should be removed.
- The first 48 h are most critical in a surgical perspective, but intracranial haematomas can occur at any point in time during neurointensive care.
- *Prophylactic* craniectomy is an unwarranted procedure.
- Decompressive craniectomy for refractory high intracranial pressure (ICP) may save lives, but many will have a very poor functional outcome.

57.2 Background

Two major randomized trials have investigated the use of decompressive craniectomy in adults (Cooper et al. 2011; Hutchinson et al. 2016). Decompressive craniectomy has also been studied in two smaller randomized trials, one in adults (Qiu et al. 2009) and one in children (Taylor et al. 2001). There is still uncertainty related to the effectiveness and safety of decompressive craniectomy, but it may be a valid option in selected patients (Sahuquillo and Arikan 2006; Ardissino et al. 2019). For details, please refer to Chap. 26 on decompressive craniectomy.

The randomized controlled Decra study, published in 2011, concluded with an increased risk of a poor outcome for patients with refractory high intracranial pressure (ICP) undergoing bifronto-temporoparietal craniectomy as compared to those receiving conservative medical treatment (Cooper et al. 2011). The craniectomy was performed early (within 72 h) in patients with a moderately increased intracranial pressure (20 mmHg) for a short period of time (15 min) and with diffuse brain injuries without mass lesions. Twenty-three percent of the patients assigned to conservative treatment nevertheless underwent a late craniectomy as a life-saving intervention, and these patients were included in the final analyses demonstrating a poorer outcome with craniectomy. This aggressive approach in a subgroup of patients does not really bring clarification to the major problems. Early prophylactic craniectomy most likely does not have any other effect than preventing a later craniectomy if the ICP cannot be controlled.

The randomized controlled Rescue-ICP study, published in 2016, showed that decompressive craniectomy in patients with traumatic brain injury and refractory high ICP resulted in lower mortality and higher rates of vegetative state and severe disability than in patients receiving medical care (Hutchinson et al. 2016). The rates of moderate disability and good recovery were similar in the two groups. The type of decompressive craniectomy (bifrontal or unilateral) was decided upon by the surgeon.

The ongoing Rescue-ASDH trial (http://www.rescueasdh.org) is a multicentre, pragmatic parallel-group randomized trial of decompressive craniectomy versus craniotomy for adult patients undergoing evacuation of acute subdural haematoma. This study will probably help to define the value of craniectomy in patients with acute subdural haematoma.

In 2016, the Brain Trauma Foundation published the fourth edition of the guidelines for the management of severe traumatic brain injury (https://www.braintrauma.org). In this update, they included recommendations for decompressive craniectomy. The authors stated that these are living guidelines and that new studies, such as the pending results of the Rescue-ICP trial (Hutchinson et al. 2016), would be incorporated as soon as they become available. However, these recommendations have not been updated as of February 2020.

Intracranial haematomas or contusions diagnosed by the initial CT scan can evolve with enlargement of bleeding and/or perifocal oedema, thereby requiring surgery at a later stage. A recent systematic review and meta-analysis of mild TBI patients with brain injuries identified by CT scan, estimated the risk of clinical deterioration to be 11.7% and neurosurgical intervention to be 3.5% (Marincowitz et al. 2018).

Delayed intracranial haemorrhage after blunt head trauma in patients with an initial, normal CT scan is very rare. In a recent study, the authors found an incidence of 0.3% of delayed intracranial haemorrhage in older patients (55 years or older), irrespective of anticoagulant or antiplatelet use (Chenoweth et al. 2018). This finding clearly indicates that routine observation and serial cranial CT scans may not be warranted in these patients.

Carotid dissection and cerebral vasospasms are other conditions to be aware of. Both conditions can cause neurological deterioration in a subacute manner. Carotid dissection is often associated with neck trauma (e.g. seat belt injury) and may be followed by development of a hemiparesis without corresponding findings on initial CT scans. Traumatic arterial spasms are not that uncommon and have a similar time course to that seen with aneurysmal subarachnoid haemorrhage. The clinical significance of vasospasms in traumatic brain injury is still uncertain (Armin et al. 2008).

New or recurrent haematomas are not infrequent after acute surgery for head injuries (Seifman et al. 2011). The vasculature can be injured, and clotting mechanisms can be compromised. Rebleeding at the operative site requiring reoperation has been reported in up to 7% of patients undergoing craniotomy and evacuation of traumatic intracranial haematomas (Bullock et al. 1990). The use of correct surgical techniques and adequate choice of procedures are therefore essential to avoid post-operative complications (see Part V on acute surgical treatment).

57.3 Specific Paediatric Concerns

One small prospective, randomized study has investigated the use of early bitemporal craniectomy without duraplasty in children (Taylor et al. 2001). The children had a median age of 120.9 months. Thirteen children were randomized to craniectomy and 14 children to conservative management; the median GCS scores were 6 and 5, respectively. Notably, children with GCS scores higher than 8 were included in this study. The craniectomy was performed at a median of 19.2 h (range 7.3–29.3 h) after the accident. Children who had sustained intracranial hypertension during the first day after admission (ICP 20–24 mmHg for 30 min, 25–29 mmHg for 10 min, 30 mmHg or more for 1 min) or had evidence of herniation (unilaterally dilated pupil or bradycardia) were eligible for randomization. A trend was shown towards greater improvement in intracranial pressure, less time required in the intensive care unit and improved clinical outcome by adding decompressive craniectomy to conventional medical treatment. Based on this study, a Cochrane review concluded that decompressive craniectomy might be justified in patients below the age of 18 years when full medical treatment is unable to control the intracranial pressure (Sahuquillo and Arikan 2006).

In a systematic review, Ardissino et al. reported a possible benefit of decompressive craniectomy in paediatric patients with TBI for reducing high ICP (>25 mmHg) refractory to medical treatment. The authors also noted that this is supported by low-quality evidence only and that there are substantial uncertainties about the implications for long-term neurological outcome (Ardissino et al. 2019).

The third edition of the Brain Trauma Foundation guidelines for the acute management of paediatric severe traumatic brain injury was published in 2019 (Kochanek et al. 2019). Based on 16 Class III treatment series, they provided a level III recommendation stating that decompressive craniectomy is suggested to treat neurological deterioration, herniation or intracranial hypertension refractory to medical management.

References

Ardissino M, Tang A, Muttoni E, Tsang K. Decompressive craniectomy in paediatric traumatic brain injury: a systematic review of current evidence. Childs Nerv Syst. 2019;35:209–16.

Armin SS, Colohan AR, Zhang JH. Vasospasm in traumatic brain injury. Acta Neurochir Suppl. 2008;104:421–5.

Bullock R, Hanemann CO, Murray L, Teasdale GM. Recurrent hematomas following craniotomy for traumatic intracranial mass. J Neurosurg. 1990;72:9–14.

Chenoweth JA, Gaona SD, Faul M, Holmes JF, Nishijima DK, Sacramento County Prehospital Research Consortium. Incidence of delayed intracranial hemorrhage in older patients after blunt head trauma. JAMA Surg. 2018;153:570–5.

Cooper DJ, Rosenfeld JV, Murray L, Arabi YM, Davies AR, D'Urso P, Kossmann T, Ponsford J, Seppelt I, Reilly P, Wolfe R, DECRA Trial Investigators, Australian and New Zealand Intensive Care Society Clinical Trials Group. Decompressive craniectomy in diffuse traumatic brain injury. N Engl J Med. 2011;364:1493–502.

Hutchinson PJ, Kolias AG, Timofeev IS, Corteen EA, Czosnyka M, Timothy J, Anderson I, Bulters DO, Belli A, Eynon CA, Wadley J, Mendelow AD, Mitchell PM, Wilson MH, Critchley G, Sahuquillo J, Unterberg A, Servadei F, Teasdale GM, Pickard JD, Menon DK, Murray GD, Kirkpatrick PJ, RESCUEicp Trial Collaborators. Trial of decompressive craniectomy for traumatic intracranial hypertension. N Engl J Med. 2016;375:1119–30.

Kochanek PM, Tasker RC, Carney N, Totten AM, Adelson PD, Selden NR, Davis-O'Reilly C, Hart EL, Bell MJ, Bratton SL, Grant GA, Kissoon N, Reuter-Rice KE, Vavilala MS, Wainwright MS, Marincowitz C, Lecky FE, Townend W, Borakati A. Guidelines for the management of pediatric severe traumatic brain injury, third edition: update of the Brain Trauma Foundation guidelines. Pediatr Crit Care Med. 2019;20(3S Suppl 1):S1–S82.

Marincowitz C, Lecky FE, Townend W, Borakati A, Fabbri A, Sheldon TA. The risk of deterioration in GCS 13-15 patients with traumatic brain injury identified by computed tomography imaging: a systematic review and meta-analysis. J Neurotrauma. 2018;35:703–18.

Qiu W, Guo C, Shen H, Chen K, Wen L, Huang H, Ding M, Sun L, Jiang Q, Wang W. Effects of unilateral decompressive craniectomy on patients with unilateral acute post-traumaticbrain swelling after severe traumatic brain injury. Crit Care. 2009;13(6):R185. https://doi.org/10.1186/cc8178.

Sahuquillo J, Arikan F. Decompressive craniectomy for the treatment of refractory high intracranial pressure in traumatic brain injury. Cochrane Database Syst Rev. 2006;1:CD003983. https://doi.org/10.1002/14651858.CD003983.pub2.

Seifman MA, Lewis PM, Rosenfeld JV, Hwang PY. Postoperative intracranial haemorrhage: a review. Neurosurg Rev. 2011;34(4):393–407.

Taylor A, Butt W, Rosenfeld J, Shann F, Ditchfield M, Lewis E, Klug G, Wallace D, Henning R, Tibballs J. A randomized trial of very early decompressive craniectomy in children with traumatic brain injury and sustained intracranial hypertension. Childs Nerv Syst. 2001;17:154–62.

58 Management of Extracranial Injuries

Nikolaj Preus Hatting and Rico Frederik Schou

Recommendations

Level I

There is insufficient data to support a Level 1 recommendation.

Level II

Major extracranial injury is a prognostic factor for mortality in TBI patients.

Level III

In the initial phase, only damage control surgery (DCS) is recommended.

The trauma team should decide and agree upon the timing of the procedures.

ICP monitoring is recommended during extracranial surgery (DCS).

Stabilization in a neuro-ICU is recommended only in isolated TBI; a dedicated trauma ICU is recommended in multitraumatized patients.

Physiological parameters should be maintained within near-normal values. Of special concern is hypotension, where systolic blood pressure above 90 mmHg is advised if concomitant uncontrollable internal bleeding is present.

58.1 Overview

The patient with multitrauma injuries (in addition to traumatic brain injury (TBI)) is at increased risk of adverse events and secondary cerebral insults. After the initial assessment and primary survey (see other chapters), the trauma team is often presented with multiple injuries that require immediate treatment, preferably at the same time.

Therefore, it is important for the trauma team to consent upon an approach for managing the injuries in a prioritized order.

In the initial phase, only the most life-threatening extracranial injuries should be treated. Damage control surgery (DCS), where control of only hemorrhage and contamination is managed, is recommended. It is focused surgery without any unnecessary or time-consuming procedures. DCS is always followed by a "second look" hours or days after the initial DCS. In the meantime, the patient should be admitted to the ICU for further stabilization.

N. P. Hatting
Department of Neuroanesthesiology and Neurointensive Care, Odense University Hospital, Odense, Denmark
e-mail: Nikolaj.Preus.Hatting@rsyd.dk

R. F. Schou (✉)
Department of Neuroanesthesia and Neurocritical Care, Odense University Hospital, Odense, Denmark
e-mail: Rico.Frederik.Schou@rsyd.dk

© Springer Nature Switzerland AG 2020
T. Sundstrøm et al. (eds.), *Management of Severe Traumatic Brain Injury*,
https://doi.org/10.1007/978-3-030-39383-0_58

If DCS is necessary, it is recommended to monitor ICP perioperatively in addition to the standard monitoring setup for anesthesia. It is recommended to seek advice from a specialist in neuroanesthesiology or to invite for joint venture and combine the knowledge of the trauma anesthesiologist and the neuroanesthesiologist.

The timing for extracranial surgery should be considered carefully and weighed against the severity of the TBI; non-vital surgery should be postponed until the patient is stable and beyond the acute phase (1–3 days).

Tips, Tricks, and Pitfalls

- Team decision regarding timing of surgery.
- Establish ICP monitoring in patients undergoing extracranial surgery, especially if GCS <9.
- Seek advice from a neuroanesthesiologist and/or neurosurgeon regarding the level of neuromonitoring, what values to aim for and management of potential adverse events in the perioperative period.
- Choose and titrate anesthetic drugs and opioids according to the level and extent of cumulative injuries.
- Hypovolemia due to bleeding is a major cause for hypotension in the multitrauma patient.
- Beware of coagulopathy and hypotension.

58.2 Background

As for the patient with isolated TBI, the primary concern is to prevent secondary damage and injury from occurring. The multitrauma patient has an increased mortality rate and an even greater risk of adverse events; special care must be undertaken to prevent and counter these complications (McMahon et al. 1999; Lingsma et al. 2013). Pitfalls to avoid are hypotension, hypoxia, fluctuations in $PaCO_2$, hypo-/hyperglycemia, hypo-/hyperthermia, coagulopathy, and raised ICP (Watanabe et al. 2018; van Leeuwen et al. 2012).

The trauma team should agree on a course of action that will prioritize the management of the primary brain injury in relation to extracranial injuries, also in accordance with the general principles for maintaining oxygen supply and adequate perfusion to vital organs.

The team should decide the timing of procedures; intracranial and/or extracranial: resuscitative DCS in the trauma bay area, management of intrahospital transportation to operating theatre, or stabilization in ICU area before and in between surgery.

If the patient is suffering from TBI, bilateral lung contusion, multiple fractures, acid/base disorder, and/or coagulopathy, it is indeed relevant to consider DCS if the magnitude of extracranial injuries, for example, includes large vessel damage, tamponade, pelvic or large bone fractures with concurrent hemorrhage, or intraabdominal organ damage needing resection (Rotondo et al. 1993; Taeger et al. 2005; Keel et al. 2005; DASAIM 2011).

The anesthesiologist in care of the patient should confer with the neurosurgeon and the neuroanesthesiologist regarding the level of neuromonitoring. Patients presenting with GCS <8 should not go through extracranial surgery without ICP monitoring. In patients with a GCS 9–13, ICP monitoring should be considered. Patients with GCS 14–15 should possibly only have ICP monitoring established in the prospect of long-lasting or very extensive extracranial surgery (Farahvar et al. 2012; DASAIM 2011).

In the absence of ICP monitoring, ensuring a MAP >80 mmHg is likely to ensure a CPP >50 mmHg. Intraoperative hypotension has been reported to occur in 60% of TBI patients undergoing surgery for associated orthopedic surgery (Algarra, Lele et al. 2016).

It is recommended to achieve and maintain a systolic blood pressure above 90 mmHg (Brain 2007). When extracranial hemorrhage control is achieved, target a systolic blood pressure 110–

120 mmHg as comparative to isolated TBI (Berry et al. 2012; Brenner et al. 2012).

To ensure adequate circulation and perfusion, normovolemia should be achieved using warm, non-glucose-containing isotonic crystalloid solutions. Hypertonic saline solutions increase intravascular volume and decrease cerebral volume and hence ICP (Algarra, Deepak et al. 2016). The target value of s-Na^+ should be 140–150 mmol/L as hypernatremia (>150 mmol/L) is correlated with increased early mortality (Verdantam et al. 2017).

Albumin is currently not recommended in any guidelines (SAFE Study 2004). Starches and other colloids should be avoided. Vasopressors should be either phenylephrine or norepinephrine (Sookplung et al. 2011). Anemia is associated with increased mortality and poor outcome in TBI (Hare et al. 2008). However, many cerebro-protective mechanisms become effective with anemia, and no studies have yet demonstrated improvement in brain tissue oxygenation with blood transfusion. Optimal hemoglobin level in TBI patients is unclear, but there is no benefit of liberal transfusion strategy (Hgb > 6.2 mmol/L) (Salim et al. 2008). Management of ongoing hemorrhage should follow international guidelines.

There are no guidelines for management of coagulopathy in TBI, though it is present in approximately one third of TBI patients and leads to increased mortality and poor outcome (Talving et al. 2009; Watanabe et al. 2018). The CRASH-2 trial demonstrated that tranexamic acid was associated with a reduction in mortality.

Hyper- and hypoglycemia after TBI are associated with increased morbidity and mortality (Jeremitsky et al. 2005). The current evidence suggests a target glucose range of 5–8 mmol/L (Sharma and Vavilala 2012).

In the period of stabilization, the patient with isolated TBI will benefit from being admitted to neuro-ICU area. If the patient is multitraumatized with concomitant extracranial injuries, a dedicated trauma ICU is recommended over neuro-ICU as this lowers mortality rate (Lombardo et al. 2017)

58.3 Specific Pediatric Concerns

Knowing the pitfalls regarding the compensatory mechanisms in infants and smaller children, it is possible to anticipate and intervene at the earliest possible time.

The recommendation regarding pediatric trauma patients follows the adult protocol, taking into account the difference in reference values and the potential need for expertise in extracranial pediatric surgery and anesthesia (Auner et al. 2014).

References

Algarra NN, Lele AV, Prathep S, et al. Intraoperative secondary insults during orthopedic surgery in traumatic brain injury. J Neurosurg Anesthesiol. 2016;29(3):228–35.

Algarra NN, Deepak S. Perioperative management of traumatic brain injury. Curr Anesthesiol Rep. 2016;6:193–201.

Auner B, et al. Pediatric multiple trauma. Chirurg. 2014;85(5):451–61.

Berry C, Ley EJ, Bukur M, Malinoski D, Margulies DR, Mirocha J, et al. Redefining hypotension in traumatic brain injury. Injury. 2012;43(11):1833–7.

Brain TF. Guidelines for the management of severe traumatic brain injury. J Neurotrauma. 2007;24(suppl 1):S1–106.

Brenner M, Stein DM, Hu PF, Aarabi B, Sheth K, Scalea TM. Traditional systolic blood pressure targets underestimate hypotension-induced secondary brain injury. J Trauma Acute Care Surg. 2012;72(5):1135–9.

DASAIM Neuroanesthesia Group. Recommendation for anesthetic management of patients with TBI and need for extracranial surgery. Danish Society for Anesthesiology and Intensive Care Medicine, DASAIM, Recommendation, Nov. 2011; 2011.

Sharma D, Vavilala MS. Perioperative management of adult traumatic brain injury. Anesthesiol Clin. 2012;30(2):333–46.

Farahvar A, et al. Increased mortality in patients with severe traumatic brain injury treated without intracranial pressure monitoring. J Neurosurg. 2012;117(4):729–34.

Hare GM, Tsui AK, McLaren AT, Ragoonanan TE, Yu J, Mazer CD. Anemia and cerebral outcome: many questions, fewer answers. Anesth Analg. 2008;107:1356–70.

Jeremitsky E, Omert LA, Dunham CM, Wilberger J, Rodriguez A. The impact of hyperglycemia on patients with severe brain injury. J Trauma. 2005;58:47–50.

Keel M, et al. Damage control in severely injured patients. Eur J Trauma. 2005;31:212–21.

Lingsma H, et al. Prognosis in moderate and severe traumatic brain injury: external validation of the IMPACT models and the role of extracranial injuries. J Trauma Acute Care Surg. 2013;74(2):639–46.

Lombardo S, et al. Neuro, trauma, or med/surg intensive care unit: Does it matter where multiple injuries patients with traumatic brain injury are admitted? Secondary analysis of the American Association for the Surgery of Trauma Multi-Institutional Trials Committee decompressive craniectomy study. J Trauma Acute Care Surg. 2017;82(3):489–96.

McMahon CG, et al. Unexpected contribution of moderate traumatic brain injury to death after major trauma. J Trauma. 1999;47(5):891–5.

Rotondo MF, et al. Damage control: an approach for improved survival in exsanguinating penetrating abdominal injury. J Trauma. 1993;35(3):375–83.

Myburgh J, et al. Saline or albumin for fluid resuscitation in patients with traumatic brain injury (SAFE-Study). N Engl J Med. 2004;350:2247–56.

Salim A, Hadjizacharia P, DuBose J, Brown C, Inaba K, Chan L, et al. Role of anemia in traumatic brain injury. J Am Coll Surg. 2008;207:398–406.

Sookplung P, Siriussawakul A, Malakouti A, et al. Vasopressor use and effect on blood pressure after severe adult traumatic brain injury. Neurocrit Care. 2011;15:46–54.

Taeger G, et al. Damage control orthopedics in patients with multiple injuries is effective, time saving and safe. J Trauma. 2005;59(2):409–16; discussion 417.

Talving P, Benfield R, Hadjizacharia P, Inaba K, Chan LS, Demetriades D. Coagulopathy in severe traumatic brain injury: a prospective study. J Trauma. 2009;66:55–61.

van Leeuwen N, et al. Prognostic value of major extracranial injury in traumatic brain injury: an individual patient data meta-analysis in 39,274 patients. Neurosurgery. 2012;70(4):811–8.

Verdantam A, et al. Morbidity and mortality associated with hypernatremia in patients with severe traumatic brain injury. Neurosurg Focus. 2017;43(5):E2.

Watanabe T, et al. Outcomes after traumatic brain injury with concomitant severe extracranial injuries. Neurol Med Chir (Tokyo). 2018;58(9):393–9.

CSF Drainage

59

Lars-Owe D. Koskinen

Recommendations

Level I

There are insufficient data to support a Level I recommendation for this topic.

Level II

There are insufficient data to support a Level II recommendation for this topic.

Level III

Continuous or intermittent CSF drainage is recommended in situations with increased ICP (>20 mmHg) when other measures have failed, such as surgical removal of space-occupying haematomas and contusions and optimization of ventilation and sedation.

59.1 Overview

In an early retrospective study of 39 patients, intermittent or continuous CSF drainage was applied, and it was concluded that early drainage was of little use in influencing ICP while later CSF removal had a more pronounced effect (Papo et al. 1981). In a prospective study of 31 patients, it was shown that various volumes of CSF intermittent drainage significantly decreased the ICP with a few mmHg, but in only six subjects the decrease was more than 3 mmHg and lasted for more than 10 min (Kerr et al. 2000). In a second prospective study from the same group, dose responses of 1, 2 and 3 ml of CSF drainage in 58 severe traumatic brain injury (sTBI) patients with ICP exceeding 20 mmHg were reported (Kerr et al. 2001). The ICP decreased by 2.4, 3.4 and 4.5 mmHg, respectively, immediately after drainage. Ten minutes post-drainage, there was still an effect of the drainage, but approaching the pre-drainage levels. A small transient improvement in cerebral perfusion pressure (CPP) was observed after drainage but no concomitant effect on cerebral blood flow or regional cerebral oxygenation. In a retrospective study of 23 sTBI patients with ICP over 25 mmHg, CSF drainage decreased the ICP by 5.7 mmHg studied 4 min after opening of the drain (Akbik et al. 2017). The CPP was increased by 4.1 mmHg and brain tissue oxygenation by 1.15 mmHg. A prospective study of 24 subjects, with sustained elevated ICP after other ICP decreasing measures, showed that in about 50% of the cases, the ICP was brought under control after continuous drainage (Timofeev et al. 2008). The effect of continuous CSF drainage was studied in an observational

L.-O. D. Koskinen (✉)
Department of Clinical Science-Neurosciences/Neurosurgery, Umeå University and Umeå University Hospital, Umeå, Sweden
e-mail: lars-owe.koskinen@umu.se

© Springer Nature Switzerland AG 2020
T. Sundstrøm et al. (eds.), *Management of Severe Traumatic Brain Injury*,
https://doi.org/10.1007/978-3-030-39383-0_59

retrospective study of 20 sTBI patients 24 h before and after drainage (Lescot et al. 2012). The mean ICP decreased from about 18 mmHg to about 11 mmHg. The need for osmotherapy was diminished during the drainage. However, the threshold for drainage was 20 mmHg, which was not reached before drainage. A retrospective study on prospective collected data using a matched control design in sTBI showed that the mean ICP in the continuous drainage group was 5.66 mmHg lower than in the closed intermittent drainage group (Nwachuku et al. 2014). The ICP burden was also reduced in the continuous drainage group as compared to the closed. However, the clinical outcome at 6 months was unaffected. In a prospective study of 45 patients with sTBI and 55 patients with subarachnoid haemorrhage (SAH) presenting refractory ICP elevation, a combination of ventriculostomy and lumbar drainage was shown to reduce the ICP but not to affect outcome (Tuettenberg et al. 2009). In that study, 12% of the patients were presented with cerebral herniation, and 6% died due to herniation. Some studies have shown an improved outcome after using CSF drainage (Timofeev et al. 2008; Ghajar et al. 1993).

Unfortunately, many of the publications do not consider whether other simultaneous measures such as hyperventilation, osmotherapy and level of sedation interact with the ICP decreasing effect of CSF drainage. Further, the effect on ICP is often studied and reported for a limited time period, making it difficult to draw any solid conclusions.

The decrease in ICP after CSF drainage cannot be expected to be long-lasting and may not be effective in all subjects as the loss of CSF by time will be replaced by brain oedema. It is discussed whether removal of constitutes of the CSF might have a negative effect on cerebral function and repair. In cases with very narrow ventricles, freehand ventriculostomy can be difficult. The method maybe complicated by CSF leakage and infections.

Tips, Tricks and Pitfalls

- CSF drainage can be used when other measures have failed.
- An intermittent drainage is often preferred over continuous.
- The drainage should be against a pressure of 15–20 mmHg or higher in order to avoid slit ventricles.
- If the drain stops functioning, this can be due to blood, debris, mechanical tubing problems, stopcocks or empty ventricles. Empty ventricles are a serious complication to CSF drainage due to increased risk of brainstem herniation.
- Some drainage systems are sensitive to wrong position of the drainage reservoir resulting in non-functioning airing valves.
- If empty ventricles, close the drain for 20 min and check the function again.
- Beware of a dislocation of the ventricular catheter and the relative high risk of infection.
- Be aware of the increased risk of cerebral herniation during drainage, especially with lumbar drainage.

59.2 Background

High ICP is generally considered as one of the main factors influencing the final clinical outcome after TBI (Miller et al. 1977; Narayan et al. 1982; Eisenberg et al. 1988; Jiang et al. 2002; Schreiber et al. 2002; Olivecrona et al. 2010; Marmarou et al. 1991). It has also been reported that those who respond to a given ICP-reducing therapy have a reduced risk of mortality (Farahvar et al. 2011). Several causes of raised ICP can be identified including haematomas, contusions, oedema, disturbance in CSF outflow and resorption. The rationale for removing CSF is based on the Monro-Kellie doctrine (Monro 1783; Kelly 1824), giving space for diffuse cerebral oedema, for example. CSF drainage is thus applied in patients with or without signs of acute hydrocephalus. Lundberg (1960) presented some evidence that CSF drainage decreases elevated ICP. It is well understood that drainage of CSF can be effective in reducing ICP in the emergency situation. It is also commonly pointed out in textbooks and publications that CSF drainage is an effective treatment of elevated ICP, but the scientific evidence is spare.

59.3 Specific Paediatric Concerns

The age of the paediatric patient must be considered in deciding the optimal and critical ICP level (Jones et al. 2003). Furthermore, the lower CSF volume in children must be taken into account when deciding the volume to be drained. In 22 paediatric patients, the ICP decreased after CSF drainage (Shapiro and Marmarou 1982). A study reporting on the use of a combination of CSF drainage by ventriculostomy and lumbar drainage in 16 patients showed that ICP was unaffected in two patients who died; in the remaining 14 patients, an abrupt and lasting decrease in ICP was observed (Levy et al. 1995). Continuous drainage of CSF appears more effective in reducing the ICP than intermittent drainage (Shore et al. 2004). In a multicentre study of 41 paediatric patients, it was shown that the mean ICP was significantly higher (43 ± 26 mmHg, $n = 3$) in the deceased group as compared to the survivors (13 ± 4 mmHg, $n = 38$) (Wahlström et al. 2005).

References

Akbik OS, Krasberg M, Nemoto EM, Yonas H. Effect of cerebrospinal fluid drainage on brain tissue oxygenation in traumatic brain injury. J Neurotrauma. 2017;34:3153–7.

Eisenberg HM, Frankowski RF, Contant CF, Marshall LF, Walker MD. High-dose barbiturate control of elevated intracranial pressure in patients with severe head injury. J Neurosurg. 1988;69:15–23. [Clinical Trial Randomized Controlled Trial Research Support, U.S. Gov't, P.H.S.].

Farahvar A, Gerber LM, Chiu YL, Hartl R, Carney N, Ghajar J. Response to intracranial hypertension treatment as a predictor of death in patients with severe traumatic brain injury. J Neurosurg. 2011;114:1471–8.

Ghajar JBG, Hariri RJ, Patterson RH. Improved outcome from traumatic coma using only ventricular cerebrospinal fluid drainage for intracranial pressure control. Adv Neurosurg. 1993;21:5.

Jiang JY, Gao GY, Li WP, Yu MK, Zhu C. Early indicators of prognosis in 846 cases of severe traumatic brain injury. J Neurotrauma. 2002;19:869–74.

Jones PA, Andrews PJ, Easton VJ, Minns RA. Traumatic brain injury in childhood: intensive care time series data and outcome. Br J Neurosurg. 2003;17:29–39. [Research Support, Non-U.S. Gov't].

Kelly G. Appearances observed in the dissection of two individuals; death from cold and congestion of the brain. Trans Med Chir Sci Edinb. 1824;1:85.

Kerr EM, Marion D, Sereika MS, Weber BB, Orndoff AP, Henker R, et al. The effect of cerebrospinal fluid drainage on cerebral perfusion in traumatic brain injured adults. J Neurosurg Anesthesiol. 2000;12:324–33. [Research Support, Non-U.S. Gov't Research Support, U.S. Gov't, P.H.S.].

Kerr EM, Weber BB, Sereika SM, Wilberger J, Marion DW. Dose response to cerebrospinal fluid drainage on cerebral perfusion in traumatic brain-injured adults. Neurosurg Focus. 2001;11:1–7.

Lescot T, Boroli F, Reina V, Chauvet D, Boch A-L, Puybasset L. Effect of continuous cerebrospinal fluid drainage on therapeutic intensity in severe traumatic brain injury. Neurochirurgie. 2012;58:235–40.

Levy DI, Rekate HL, Cherny WB, Manwaring K, Moss SD, Baldwin HZ. Controlled lumbar drainage in pediatric head injury. J Neurosurg. 1995;83:453–60. [Case Reports].

Lundberg N. Continuous recording and control of ventricular fluid pressure in neurosurgical practice. Acta Psychiatr Scand Suppl. 1960;36:1–193.

Marmarou A, Anderson RL, Ward JD, Choi SC, Young HF, Eisenberg HM, et al. Impact of ICP instability and hypotension on outcome in patients with severe head trauma. J Neurosurg. 1991;75:59–66.

Miller JD, Becker DP, Ward JD, Sullivan HG, Adams WE, Rosner MJ. Significance of intracranial hypertension in severe head injury. J Neurosurg. 1977;47:503–16. [Research Support, U.S. Gov't, P.H.S.].

Monro A. Observations on the structure and function of the nervous system. Edinburgh: Creech & Johnson; 1783.

Narayan RK, Kishore PR, Becker DP, Ward JD, Enas GG, Greenberg RP, et al. Intracranial pressure: to monitor or not to monitor? A review of our experience with severe head injury. J Neurosurg. 1982;56:650–9. [Research Support, U.S. Gov't, P.H.S.].

Nwachuku EL, Puccio AM, Fetzick A, Scruggs B, Chang Y-F, Shutter LA, et al. Intermittent versus continuous cerebrospinal fluid drainage management in adult severe traumatic brain injury: Assessment of intracranial pressure burden. Neurocrit Care. 2014;20:49–53.

Olivecrona M, Wildemyr Z, Koskinen LO. The apolipoprotein E epsilon4 allele and outcome in severe traumatic brain injury treated by an intracranial pressure-targeted therapy. J Neurosurg. 2010;112:1113–9. [Randomized Controlled Trial Research Support, Non-U.S. Gov't].

Papo I, Caruselli G, Luongo A. CSF withdrawal for the treatment of intracranial hypertension in acute head injuries. Acta Neurochir. 1981;56:191–9.

Schreiber MA, Aoki N, Scott BG, Beck JR. Determinants of mortality in patients with severe blunt head injury. Arch Surg. 2002;137:285–90.

Shapiro K, Marmarou A. Clinical applications of the pressure-volume index in treatment of pediatric head injuries. J Neurosurg. 1982;56:819–25. [Research Support, U.S. Gov't, P.H.S.].

Shore PM, Thomas NJ, Clark RS, Adelson PD, Wisniewski SR, Janesko KL, et al. Continuous versus intermittent cerebrospinal fluid drainage after severe traumatic brain injury in children: effect on biochemical markers. J Neurotrauma. 2004;21:1113–22. [Comparative Study (Multicenter Study Research Support, Non--U.S. Gov't Research Support, U.S. Gov't, P.H.S.].

Timofeev I, Dahyot-Fizelier C, Keong N, Nortje J, Al-Rawi PG, Czosnyka M, et al. Ventriculostomy for control of raised ICP in acute traumatic brain injury. Acta Neurochir Suppl. 2008;102:99–104. [Clinical Trial Research Support, Non-U.S. Gov't].

Tuettenberg J, Czabanka M, Horn P, Woitzik J, Barth M, Thome C, et al. Clinical evaluation of the safety and efficacy of lumbar cerebrospinal fluid drainage for the treatment of refractory increased intracranial pressure. J Neurosurg. 2009;110:1200–8.

Wahlström MR, Olivecrona M, Koskinen LO, Rydenhag B, Naredi S. Severe traumatic brain injury in pediatric patients: treatment and outcome using an intracranial pressure targeted therapy – the Lund concept. Intensive Care Med. 2005;31:832–9. [Multicenter Study Research Support, Non-U.S. Gov't].

60 Hyperventilation

Niels Juul

Recommendations

Level I

There are insufficient data to support a Level I recommendation for this topic.

Level II

Prophylactic hyperventilation should be avoided.

Level III

Hyperventilation is recommended as a temporising measure for the reduction of ICP.

Hyperventilation should be avoided during the first 24 h after injury when CBF often is critically reduced. If hyperventilation is still used, it is recommended to monitor brain oxygen delivery by SjO_2 or $PtiO_2$ measurements or other means of continuous brain oxygen monitoring.

60.1 Overview

Aggressive hyperventilation (arterial $PaCO_2 \leq 3.3$ kPa) has been a cornerstone in the management of severe traumatic brain injury (TBI) for more than 20 years because it can cause a rapid reduction in ICP. Brain swelling and elevated ICP develop in 40% of patients with severe TBI (Miller et al. 1977), and high or uncontrolled ICP is one of the most common causes of death and neurologic disability after TBI (Becker et al. 1977). Therefore, the assumption has been made that hyperventilation benefits all patients with severe TBI. In a 1995 survey, Ghajar et al. found that hyperventilation was being used by 83% of US trauma centres (Ghajar et al. 1995). This number has declined over the years, but as recent as 2008, the BrainIT group made a survey in European centres showing that early prophylactic hyperventilation was used in more than 50% of cases (Neumann et al. 2008). However, hyperventilation reduces ICP by causing cerebral vasoconstriction and a subsequent reduction in CBF and cerebral blood volume and not by reducing brain oedema (Raichle and Plum 1972). Research conducted over the past 20 years clearly demonstrate that CBF during the first day after injury is less than half that of normal individuals (Bouma et al. 1992; Muizelaar et al. 1989; Robertson et al. 1988) and that there is a risk of causing or worsening cerebral ischaemia with aggressive hyperventilation, especially in the already ischaemic penumbra zone. Histologic evidence of cerebral ischaemia has been found in most victims of severe TBI who died (Graham and Adams 1971; Ross et al. 1993). A randomised study found significantly poorer outcomes at 3 and

N. Juul (✉)
Department of Anaesthesia, Aarhus University Hospital, Aarhus, Denmark
e-mail: d245364@dadlnet.dk

© Springer Nature Switzerland AG 2020
T. Sundstrøm et al. (eds.), *Management of Severe Traumatic Brain Injury*,
https://doi.org/10.1007/978-3-030-39383-0_60

6 months when prophylactic hyperventilation was used, as compared to when it was not (Muizelaar et al. 1991). Thus, limiting the use of hyperventilation following severe TBI may help to improve neurologic recovery following injury or at least avoid iatrogenic cerebral ischaemia.

Tips, Tricks and Pitfalls

- If the ICP is stable and below 20 mmHg, keep the $PaCO_2$ above 4.5 kPa.
- If the patient is monitored with $ETCO_2$ and the pulmonary condition is stable, compare $ETCO_2$ with $PaCO_2$ on a regular basis (once or twice a day). This will diminish the need for arterial blood gas monitoring since the difference between $PaCO_2$ and $ETCO_2$ will, for all good measures, be approximately the same if the pulmonary condition is stable.
- If the ventilator is on pressure control and you want to decrease $PaCO_2$, increase the frequency of ventilations rather than the tidal volume because this will not alter the difference between $ETCO_2$ and $PaCO_2$.
- If the ventilator is on volume control and you increase the minute volume, keep an eye on the tidal volume to decrease the risk of overextension of the lungs.
- It is easier to keep adequate ventilation volume if the ventilator setting is on volume control.

60.2 Background

60.2.1 CBF Following TBI

Three studies provide Class III evidence that CBF can be dangerously low soon after severe TBI (Bouma et al. 1992; Marion et al. 1991; Sioutos et al. 1995). Two CBF measurements were performed with xenon-CT/CBF method during the first 5 days following severe TBI in a total of 67 patients. CBF measurements were obtained during the first 24 h after injury in one study, and they were less than 18 mL/100 g/min in 31.4% of patients (Bouma et al. 1992). In the second study, the mean CBF during the first few hours after injury was 27 mL/100 g/min (Marion et al. 1991). The third study measured CBF with a thermodiffusion blood flow probe, again during the first 5 days post-injury, in 37 severe TBI patients (Sioutos et al. 1995). Twelve patients had a global CBF less than 18 mL/100 g/min up to 48 h post-injury.

60.2.2 $PaCO_2$/CBF Reactivity and Cerebral Oxygen Utilisation

Three Class III studies provide the evidence base for this topic (Imberti et al. 2002; Oertel et al. 2002 and Sheinberg et al. 1992). Results associating hyperventilation with SjO_2 and $PtiO_2$ values in a total of 102 patients are equivocal. One study showed no consistent positive or negative change in SjO_2 or $PtiO_2$ values (Imberti et al. 2002). A second study associated hyperventilation with a reduction of $PaCO_2$ and subsequent decrease in SjO_2 from 73% to 67%, but the SjO_2 values never dropped below 55% (Oertel et al. 2002). The third study reported hyperventilation to be the second most common identifiable cause of jugular venous oxygen desaturation in a sample of 33 patients (Sheinberg et al. 1992). Studies on regional CBF showed significant variation in reduction in CBF following TBI. Two studies indicated lowest flows in brain tissue surrounding contusions or underlying subdural haematomas and in patients with severe diffuse injuries (Marion et al. 1991; Salvant and Muizelaar 1993). Similarly, a third study found that CO_2 vasoreactivity was most abnormal in contusions and subdural haematomas (McLaughlin and Marion 1996). Considering that CO_2 vasoreactivity could range from almost absent to three times normal in these patients, there could be a dangerous reduction in CBF during hyperventilation, especially in areas surrounding contusions or underlying subdural clots. Only one of these three studies (Marion et al. 1991) had adequate design and sample to be included as evidence. Two studies associated hyperventilation-induced reduction in CBF with a significant increase in oxygen extraction fraction, but they did not find a significant relationship between hyperventilation and change in the $CMRO_2$ (Diringer et al. 2002; Hutchinson et al. 2002).

60.2.3 Effect of Hyperventilation on Outcome

One Class III study involving 890 patients intubated prehospitally showed adverse outcome for both hypo- and hypercapnic patients; intubated patients arriving at the trauma centre with an $PaCO_2$ between 4.0 and 6.5 kPa had a better survival than those who had been hypo- or hyperventilated, after adjustment for confounding factors (adjusted OR 2.17) (Davis et al. 2006).

One Class II RCT of 113 patients used a stratified, randomised design to compare outcomes of severe TBI patients provided normal ventilation ($PaCO_2$ 4.66 ± 0.25 kPa; $n = 41$; control group), hyperventilation ($PaCO_2$ 3.33 + 0.25 kPa; $n = 36$) or hyperventilation with tromethamine ($n = 36$) (Muizelaar et al. 1991). One benefit of hyperventilation is the minimisation of cerebrospinal fluid (CSF) acidosis. However, the effect on CSF pH may not be sustained due to a loss of HCO^{-3} buffer. Tromethamine (THAM) buffer treatment was introduced to test the hypothesis that it could reverse the effects of the loss of buffer. Patients were stratified based on the motor component of the Glasgow Coma Scale (GCS) score (1–3 vs 4–5). The Glasgow Outcome Scale (GOS) score was used to assess patient outcomes at 3, 6 and 12 months. For patients with a motor GCS of 4–5, the 3- and 6-month GOS scores were significantly lower in the hyperventilated patients than in the control or THAM groups. However, the effect was not sustained at 12 months. The recommendation today is that hyperventilation should be avoided.

60.3 Specific Paediatric Concerns

There are no specific paediatric concerns; children should be treated in accordance with the adult guidelines.

References

Becker DP, Miller JD, Ward JD, Greenberg RP, Young HF, Sakalas R. The outcome from severe head injury with early diagnosis and intensive management. J Neurosurg. 1977;47:491–502.

Bouma GJ, Muizelaar JP, Stringer WA, Choi SC, Fatouros P, Young HF. Ultra-early evaluation of regional cerebral blood flow in severely head-injured patients using xenon-enhanced computerized tomography. J Neurosurg. 1992;77:360–8.

Davis DP, Idris AH, Sise MJ, Kennedy F, Eastman AB, Velky T, Vilke GM, Hoyt DB. Early ventilation and outcome in patients with moderate to severe traumatic brain injury. Crit Care Med. 2006;34:1202–8.

Diringer MN, Videen TO, Yundt K, Zazulia AR, Aiyagari V, Dacey RG Jr, Grubb RL, Powers WJ. Regional cerebrovascular and metabolic effects of hyperventilation after severe traumatic brain injury. J Neurosurg. 2002;96:103–8.

Ghajar J, Hariri RJ, Narayan RK, Iacono LA, Firlik K, Patterson RH. Survey of critical care management of comatose, head-injured patients in the United States. Crit Care Med. 1995;23:560–7.

Graham DI, Adams JH. Ischaemic brain damage in fatal head injuries. Lancet. 1971;1:265–6.

Hutchinson PJ, Gupta AK, Fryer TF, al-Rawi PG, Chatfield DA, Coles JP, OConnell MT, Kett-White R, Minhas PS, Aigbirhio FI, Clark JC, Kirkpatrick PJ, Menon DK, Pickard JD. Correlation between cerebral blood flow, substrate delivery, and metabolism in head injury: a combined microdialysis and triple oxygen positron emission tomography study. J Cereb Blood Flow Metab. 2002;22:735–45.

Imberti R, Bellinzona G, Langer M. Cerebral tissue PO_2 and $SjvO_2$ changes during moderate hyperventilation in patients with severe traumatic brain injury. J Neurosurg. 2002;96:97–102.

Marion DW, Darby J, Yonas H. Acute regional cerebral blood flow changes caused by severe head injuries. J Neurosurg. 1991;74:407–14.

McLaughlin MR, Marion DW. Cerebral blood flow and vasoresponsivity within and around cerebral contusions. J Neurosurg. 1996;85:871–6.

Miller JD, Becker DP, Ward JD, Sullivan HG, Adams WE, Rosner MJ. Significance of intracranial hypertension in severe head injury. J Neurosurg. 1977;47:503–10.

Muizelaar JP, Marmarou A, DeSalles AA, Ward JD, Zimmerman RS, Li Z, Choi SC, Young HF. Cerebral blood flow and metabolism in severely head-injured children. Part 1: relationship with GCS score, outcome, ICP, and PVI. J Neurosurg. 1989;71:63–71.

Muizelaar JP, Marmarou A, Ward JD, Kontos HA, Choi SC, Becker DP, Gruermer H, Young HF. Adverse effects of prolonged hyperventilation in patients with severe head injury: a randomized clinical trial. J Neurosurg. 1991;75:731–9.

Neumann JO, Chambers IR, Citerio G, Enblad P, Gregson BA, Howells T, Mattern J, Nilsson P, Piper I, Ragauskas A, Dahuquillo J, Yau YH, Kiening K, BrainT Group. The use of hyperventilation therapy after traumatic brain injury in Europe: an analysis of the BrainIT Group. Intensive Care Med. 2008;34:1676–82.

Oertel M, Kelly DF, Lee JH, McArthur DL, Glenn TC, Vespa P, Boscardin WJ, Hovda DA, Martin NA. Efficacy of hyperventilation, blood pressure elevation, and metabolic suppression therapy in controlling intracranial pressure after head injury. J Neurosurg. 2002;97:1045–53.

Raichle ME, Plum F. Hyperventilation and cerebral blood flow. Stroke. 1972;3:566–75.

Robertson CS, Clifton GL, Grossman RG, Ou CN, Goodman JC, Borum P, Bejot S, Barrodale P. Alterations in cerebral availability of metabolic substrates after severe head injury. J Trauma. 1988;28:1523–32.

Ross DT, Graham DI, Adams JH. Selective loss of neurons from the thalamic reticular nucleus following severe human head injury. J Neurotrauma. 1993;10:151–65.

Salvant JB Jr, Muizelaar JP. Changes in cerebral blood flow and metabolism related to the presence of subdural hematoma. Neurosurgery. 1993;33:387–93.

Sheinberg M, Kanter MJ, Robertson CS, Contant CF, Narayan RK, Grossman RG. Continuous monitoring of jugular venous oxygen saturation in head-injured patients. J Neurosurg. 1992;76:212–7.

Sioutos PJ, Orozco JA, Carter LP, Weinand ME, Hamilton AJ, Williams FC. Continuous regional cerebral cortical blood flow monitoring in head-injured patients. Neurosurgery. 1995;36:943–9.

Osmotherapy

61

Jens Aage Kølsen-Petersen

Recommendations

Level I

There are insufficient data to support a Level I recommendation on this topic.

Level II

Reduction in intracranial pressure (ICP) has been consistently demonstrated with both mannitol and hypertonic saline.

Mannitol is effective for control of raised intracranial pressure (ICP) at doses of 0.25–1 g/kg body weight. Mannitol should be avoided with arterial systolic blood pressure <90 mmHg.

Hypertonic saline (HTS) can be infused intravenously as a bolus or continuous infusion in concentrations of 1.6–7.5%.

Level III

The choice of mannitol or hypertonic saline as a first-line hyperosmolar agent should be left to the treating physician. The plasma sodium, renal condition and intravascular volume status of the patient should be included in the decision. Electrolytes should be monitored, and plasma sodium maintained below 155 mmol/L. Restrict mannitol use prior to ICP monitoring to patients with signs of transtentorial herniation or progressive neurological deterioration not attributable to extracranial causes.

61.1 Overview

Reducing the volume of the intracranial content, decreasing ICP and increasing cerebral perfusion pressure (CPP) by drawing water out of the brain into the vascular compartment along an osmotic gradient is a cornerstone in the medical treatment of elevated ICP (Carney et al. 2017; Gu et al. 2018). Solutions of mannitol and hypertonic saline are effective to reduce ICP and are used frequently in clinical practice (White et al. 2006; Bhardwaj 2007; Carney et al. 2017; Mangat 2018; Gu et al. 2018). Both solutions exert an early effect on ICP due to optimisation of rheological properties of the blood resulting in decreased blood viscosity and haematocrit, increasing cerebral blood flow (CBF) and oxygen delivery, resulting in reflex autoregulatory vasoconstriction of cerebral arterioles that reduces CBV and ICP. This is followed by an osmotic shrinkage of brain cells that peaks after 15–30 min (Ziai et al. 2007).

In the absence of definitive evidence regarding administration regimens related to different kinds of brain injury and side effects such as osmotic

J. A. Kølsen-Petersen (✉)
Department of Anaesthesia, Aarhus University Hospital, Aarhus, Denmark
e-mail: jenspete@rm.dk

© Springer Nature Switzerland AG 2020
T. Sundstrøm et al. (eds.), *Management of Severe Traumatic Brain Injury*,
https://doi.org/10.1007/978-3-030-39383-0_61

diuresis, kidney failure and rebound cerebral oedema, the clinician must weigh the value of long-standing clinical acceptance and safety (mannitol) against a newer, potentially more effective therapy with a limited clinical record (hypertonic saline).

Tips, Tricks and Pitfalls

- When osmotherapy is required for intracranial hypertension, administer a bolus of 20% mannitol 0.25–1.0 g/kg or 1–2 mL/kg, 3–5.6% NaCl over 10–20 min. Alternatively, use a continuous IV infusion of 3–5.6% NaCl 1–2 mL/kg/h.
- Use hypertonic saline for patients who are hypotensive with sinus tachycardia due to prerenal dehydration because mannitol induces osmotic diuresis, which may worsen hypotension.
- Maintain Na between 145 and 155 mmol/L.
- Monitor sodium and potassium every 4 h. Allow Na to normalise gradually after ICP has been stabilised.

61.2 Background

The effect of circulating osmotic agents on the brain was first described by Weed and McKibben using intravenous infusion of 30% NaCl solutions in doses from 2.2 mL/kg to 8.8 mL/kg in cats (Weed and Mckippen 1919). Later, hyperosmolar solutions of urea, glycerol and sorbitol were used in the treatment of elevated ICP (Knapp 2005). These agents were largely replaced by mannitol in the 1960s (Knapp 2005). Within the last two decades, concentrated saline solutions have received renewed attention (Gu et al. 2018). In this chapter, only mannitol and hypertonic saline will be discussed, since they are the main substances used in current clinical practice (Ragland and Lee 2016; Carney et al. 2017).

61.2.1 Mannitol

61.2.1.1 Mechanism of Action

The exact mechanism behind the ICP-lowering effect of mannitol in the injured brain is still controversial. It is generally proposed to be biphasic with an immediate effect on blood rheology followed by an osmotic effect on brain water (Diringer and Zazulia 2004; Knapp 2005; Ogden et al. 2005; Carney et al. 2017). Infusion immediately lowers ICP because of cerebral autoregulatory vasoconstriction in response to (1) increased cerebral perfusion pressure and oxygenation due to osmotically induced plasma volume expansion and increased cardiac output (Rosner and Coley 1987; White et al. 2006) and/or (2) increased microcirculation due to shrinkage of erythrocytes and endothelial cells and decreased haematocrit and blood viscosity (Burke et al. 1981; Ogden et al. 2005). After 15–30 min, an osmotic gradient is established over the blood–brain barrier (BBB) that draws water from the brain into the intravascular space (Paczynski 1997; Diringer and Zazulia 2004; Bratton et al. 2007). The water efflux depends on (1) the osmotic gradient created, (2) the osmotic reflection coefficient of the membrane for that solute (ranging from 0 to 1, where 1 is impermeable) and (3) the hydraulic conductivity of the membrane (Diringer and Zazulia 2004). Mannitol has a reflection coefficient of 0.9 over the intact blood–brain barrier.

Infusion of mannitol to normal rabbits and monkeys in clinical doses (Diringer and Zazulia 2004) and to brain-injured rats in supra-clinical doses (Todd et al. 2006) reduces brain water by approximately 2%. The rather modest decrease in brain water may explain why the initial ICP seems to be important for the ICP-lowering effect of mannitol since the intracranial compliance curve is steeper at a higher pressure. In a recent meta-analysis of 18 clinical studies, it was found that the ICP decrease was significantly greater when initial ICP was higher than 30 mmHg compared to when it was lower. The dose of mannitol seemed to be of less importance (Sorani and Manley 2008).

A longer-lasting effect on ICP, though never satisfactorily documented, has been attributed to accelerated absorption of cerebrospinal fluid brought about by the plasma hyperosmolarity (Paczynski 1997; White et al. 2006).

61.2.1.2 Dose and Pharmacokinetics

The Brain Trauma Foundation recommends a dose of mannitol for control of elevated ICP after traumatic brain injury of 0.25–1.0 g/kg body weight (Carney et al. 2017), whereas other authors recommend 1–1.5 g/kg (Ragland and Lee 2016). The peak ICP-lowering effect is seen 15–30 min after infusion and lasts about 60 min (Sorani and Manley 2008), although a duration of 6 h or more has been reported (Bratton et al. 2007).

There are insufficient data to support a standard treatment (Carney et al. 2017; Oddo et al. 2018). Intermittent boluses may be as good as continuous infusion. Mannitol is not metabolised in mammalian tissues and is excreted unchanged in the urine with an elimination half-life of 0.5–2.5 h (Paczynski 1997). In the presence of intact renal function, accumulation within tissues is unlikely to occur (Paczynski 1997).

61.2.1.3 Side Effects

Infusion of mannitol may cause hypotension that challenges the cerebral perfusion through two different mechanisms. Firstly, rapid infusions may cause a decrease in systemic vascular resistance and hypotension, especially in the hypovolaemic patient (Paczynski 1997; Ragland and Lee 2016). However, it is rarely a clinical problem during infusions of 0.5–1.5 g/kg over 15–30 min (Paczynski 1997). Secondly, mannitol is a strong osmotic diuretic that may cause a diuresis five times the infused volume (Paczynski 1997). Hence, a reduction in intravascular volume often accompanies infusion, rendering the patient at risk for hypovolaemia (Knapp 2005). Consequently, appropriate fluid replacement is important, e.g. with 0.9% sodium chloride. A Foley catheter is recommended.

Mannitol is excreted unchanged in the urine. A serum osmolality >320 mOsm/L has been associated with acute tubular necrosis and renal failure (Knapp 2005). However, the data supporting this are limited and come from studies with hypovolaemic patients (Diringer and Zazulia 2004; Knapp 2005).

Infusion of hyperosmolar solutions leads to plasma dilution and acute hyponatraemia followed by osmotic diuresis with a loss of 'free water' that results in hypernatraemia (Paczynski 1997). Potassium, phosphate and magnesium are lost in urine, putting the patient at risk for electrolyte disturbances (Paczynski 1997). Hyperkalaemia has been reported after infusion of mannitol in clinical doses (Hassan et al. 2007), even complicated with ventricular tachycardia (Seto et al. 2000). Measuring electrolytes and serum osmolality every 2–6 h has been proposed (Knapp 2005).

Continuous or repeated administration of mannitol may lead to osmotic equilibration between the intra- and extracellular compartments through the accumulation of intracellular osmolytes in the brain and risk of rebound cerebral oedema when the hyperosmolar infusion is stopped (Diringer and Zazulia 2004). Furthermore, mannitol may cross even the intact BBB (reflection coefficient 0.9) and especially the injured BBB and may cause water movement back into the brain (Diringer and Zazulia 2004). There may be a risk of midline shift in the presence of a unilateral lesion (Diringer and Zazulia 2004). However, mannitol is not metabolically trapped in the brain, and by time it would exit the way it entered, down its concentration gradient (Diringer and Zazulia 2004). The matter of rebound cerebral oedema after mannitol administration is controversial (Paczynski 1997; Diringer and Zazulia 2004).

61.2.1.4 Clinical Studies

In spite of the reduction in ICP and its clinical use for more than 60 years, the beneficial effect of mannitol on outcome is still debated (Grape and Ravussin 2012; Grände and Romner 2012). In a recent Cochrane review on mannitol for traumatic brain injury (Wakai et al. 2013), only four randomised controlled clinical studies were found (Schwartz et al. 1984; Smith et al. 1986; Sayre et al. 1996; Vialet et al. 2003). The authors of the Cochrane review concluded that there is insufficient reliable evidence to make recommendations on the use of mannitol in the management of patients with traumatic brain injury (Wakai et al. 2013). The latest guideline from the Brain Trauma Foundation restates that mannitol is effective for control of raised intracranial pressure and that the use of mannitol prior to ICP monitoring should be restricted to patients with signs of transtentorial herniation or progressive neurological deterioration not attributable to extracranial causes (Carney et al. 2017).

Although mannitol is a time-honoured means of treating intracranial hypertension, hypertonic saline is emerging as an alternative. Hypertonic saline (HTS) is efficacious in the treatment of cerebral oedema and elevations in ICP even in cases refractory to mannitol (Ogden et al. 2005; White et al. 2006; Bhardwaj 2007; Tyagi et al. 2007; Ziai et al. 2007; Ragland and Lee 2016; Mangat 2018; Gu et al. 2018).

61.2.2 Hypertonic Saline

61.2.2.1 Mechanism of Action

The principal ICP-lowering effect of hypertonic saline (HTS) infusion is possibly due to osmotic mobilisation of water from the brain to the intravascular space (Ogden et al. 2005; Bratton et al. 2007; Tyagi et al. 2007). Sodium chloride has a reflection coefficient of 1.0 over the intact blood–brain barrier, making it, theoretically, more efficient than mannitol with a reflection coefficient of 0.9 (Bhardwaj 2007; Himmelseher 2007). It appears from animal studies that the integrity of the BBB is important for the effect of hypertonic saline (White et al. 2006). Thus, hypertonic crystalloid infusions (3% to 6.5%) primarily dehydrated the uninjured parts of the brain, while the water content in the injured parts was unaffected by fluid tonicity (Wisner et al. 1990; Shackford et al. 1992). Similar results come from MRI scans of a patient with traumatic brain injury after infusion of 18% HTS (Saltarini et al. 2002).

Infusion of hypertonic saline has several other consequences that may benefit the brain. Plasma volume increases due to almost instantaneous mobilisation of water from the intracellular compartment of mainly erythrocytes and endothelial cells into the vascular fluid spaces along the osmotic gradient (Tølløfsrud et al. 1998). The mean arterial pressure (MAP) and hence the CPP are better preserved or even augmented compared to mannitol (Berger et al. 1994; Qureshi et al. 1999). A typical dose in trauma of 250 ml 7.5% NaCl expands plasma volume by about two to three times the infused volume (Vassar and Holcroft 1992; Kramer 2003; Järvelä et al. 2003).

In addition to increased preload, HTS infusion decreases both right (Kien et al. 1991) and left ventricular afterload through hyperosmotic-induced arteriolar vasodilation (Read et al. 1960; Gazitùa et al. 1971; Goertz et al. 1995). Despite reports of short-lived hyperosmotic-induced impairment of cardiac contractility (Gazitùa et al. 1971), overall cardiac performance increases because of augmented preload and decreased afterload (Goertz et al. 1995). In a porcine model of haemorrhagic shock and brain injury, HTS resuscitation was found to decrease ICP and increase cerebral perfusion pressure, pial arteriolar diameter, cerebral blood flow and cerebral oxygen delivery compared to resuscitation with Ringer's lactate (Schmoker et al. 1991; Shackford et al. 1994).

In addition to these salutary effects, HTS infusion improves the microcirculation through shrinkage of erythrocytes and ischaemic swollen endothelial cells (Mazzoni et al. 1989; Mazzoni et al. 1990; Corso et al. 1998). Thus, enhanced microcirculation was demonstrated in animal visceral organs after resuscitation from haemorrhagic (Maningas 1987; Kreimeier et al. 1988; Kreimeier et al. 1990; Behrman et al. 1991; Bauer et al. 1993; Vollmar et al. 1994; Corso et al. 1998) and endotoxic (Oi et al. 2000) shock compared to infusion of Ringer's lactate (Pascual et al. 2003). Reduction in endothelial–leukocyte interaction decreases capillary plugging by activated sticking leukocytes, which further augments nutritional flow (Nolte et al. 1992; Bauer et al. 1993; Vollmar et al. 1994; Härtl et al. 1997; Pascual et al. 2002). Recovery of the microcirculation may explain why both the resting membrane potential and cell volume changed towards pre-shock values after infusion of hypertonic saline compared to isotonic saline with equal amounts of Na and Cl in bled rats (Nakayama et al. 1985), and it may also explain why oxygen consumption (VO_2) returned to above baseline after resuscitation with HTS in haemorrhaged larger animals (Kramer et al. 1986; Kreimeier et al. 1990).

Finally, recent studies found hypertonicity to affect immune responses in animals and in human blood cell cultures. It was shown that hypertonicity attenuated neutrophil cytotoxicity (Hampton et al. 1994; Rosengren et al. 1994; Rizoli et al. 1998; Ciesla et al. 2000; Pascual et al. 2002) and at the same time upregulated immunologic protection furnished by lymphocytes (Junger et al. 1997; Loomis et al. 2001; Loomis et al. 2003). The few clinical studies, conducted to date, specifically addressing the immune effect of hypertonic saline infusion, showed little, if any, effect on markers of immune function, and large clinical trials did not convincingly demonstrate benefit in terms of morbidity or mortality (Kolsen-Petersen 2004). Whether the observed immunomodulatory properties of hypertonic saline infusion translate into a clinically significant effect is thus still an open question.

61.2.2.2 Dose and Pharmacokinetics

There is no evidence, yet, to support one concentration of sodium chloride or administration protocol over another for the control of elevated ICP (Tyagi et al. 2007; Carney et al. 2017; Mangat 2018; Gu et al. 2018). HTS as both bolus and continuous infusions lowers ICP (Tyagi et al. 2007). Concentrations between 1.6% and 7.5% have been used successfully (Himmelseher 2007; Tyagi et al. 2007; Gu et al. 2018). Many studies used 200–300 mL of 3% NaCl since it is equiosmolar with a 'standard' 20% mannitol regimen (White et al. 2006). The goal is ICP control with a sodium level between 145 and 155 mmol/L either through continuous infusion of 3% HTS solution 1–2 mL/kg/h (Bhardwaj 2007) or through repeated doses of 250 ml (White et al. 2006). Studies with hypotensive trauma patients including those with brain injury often use 250 mL 7.5% NaCl with or without added colloid (Wade et al. 1997a; Wade et al. 1997b; Cooper et al. 2004; Bulger et al. 2010) based on animal experiments (Dubick et al. 1995).

The pharmacokinetics were studied in healthy men after infusion of 7.5% NaCl 5 mL/kg over 30 min (Drobin and Hahn 2002). Plasma volume was increased by approximately 25% at the end of infusion and decreased over the next 240 min with a half-life about 60 min. The efficacy of ICP reduction and the exact duration of the ICP-lowering effect are difficult to predict in general. Most studies show that ICP remains decreased 1–2 h after infusion (Himmelseher 2007).

61.2.2.3 Side Effects

Infusion of hypertonic saline increases the plasma concentrations of sodium and chloride. The increase in Cl induces a hyperchloraemic acidosis (Kolsen-Petersen et al. 2005) that is unlikely to be clinically relevant, except in the most severe cases (Gunnerson et al. 2006). The increase in Na depends on the dose, concentration and speed of administration of the HTS solution (Kolsen-Petersen 2004). In trauma patients, Na generally reached 150–155 mM measured 30–60 min after infusion of 250 mL NaCl 7.5% with or without colloids over 1–5 min (Maningas et al. 1989; Vassar et al. 1991; Mattox et al. 1991; Younes et al. 1992; Vassar et al. 1993a; Vassar et al. 1993b). Plasma Na exceeded 155 mM in one tenth of trauma patients receiving a 250 mL bolus of HSD (Mattox et al. 1991; Younes et al. 1992). Sodium levels below 160 mEq/L are generally well tolerated without worsened outcome in the neurologic intensive care unit (Aiyagari et al. 2006). Thus, as long as plasma sodium is kept in the recommended range (145–155 mmol/L), the hypernatraemia possibly benefits ICP and is unlikely to adversely affect outcome (White et al. 2006; Bhardwaj 2007; Himmelseher 2007).

A rapid increase in plasma Na in patients with chronic hyponatraemia carries the risk of central pontine myelinolysis. Consequently, pre-existing chronic hyponatraemia should be excluded before administration of hypertonic saline, especially in malnourished and alcoholics (Bratton et al.

2007). No human studies with HTS have demonstrated central pontine myelinolysis (Tyagi et al. 2007). Even a mean peak sodium concentration of 171 mmol/L after continuous infusion of 3% NaCl in a paediatric intensive care unit caused no signs on myelinolysis on MRI or post-mortem (Khanna et al. 2000; Peterson et al. 2000).

Highly concentrated sodium chloride infusions, albeit effective in reducing ICP, may impair the BBB and lead to increased water accumulation in the injured brain (Himmelseher 2007). Thus, infusion of 40 ml of 20% NaCl over 20 min 1–5 days after traumatic brain injury decreased the volume of the non-contused hemisphere, whereas it increased the volume of the contused hemisphere based on quantitative assessments of CT scans (Lescot et al. 2006). The exact clinical relevance of this observation remains to be determined (Himmelseher 2007). As with mannitol, continuous osmotherapy with HTS may lead to accumulation of intracellular osmolytes and rebound oedema when serum sodium returns towards normal (Ogden et al. 2005; White et al. 2006).

Potassium has been reported by some authors to decrease because of dilution and urinary loss in exchange for sodium (Qureshi and Suarez 2000; Kolsen-Petersen et al. 2005). In other studies, however, a transient increase was found of about 0.5 mM after infusion of 7.5% NaCl 4 mL/kg (Kolsen-Petersen et al. 2005).

In a single study of resuscitation of burn patients, HTS was associated with a fourfold increase in acute renal failure compared with a historical control group receiving Ringer's lactate (Huang et al. 1995). However, no correlation was found between serum sodium and biochemical markers of kidney function in retrospective chart studies in kids with traumatic brain injury (Peterson et al. 2000) or adults with elevated ICP (Froelich et al. 2009) treated with continuous 3% HTS infusion. Nevertheless, patients with Na >155 mmol/L had a higher risk of developing blood urea nitrogen >8.9 mmol/L or creatinine >132.6 μmol/L (Froelich et al. 2009).

Dilution of normal human plasma with hypertonic saline significantly increased prothrombin (PT) and activated partial thromboplastin times (APTT) and decreased platelet aggregation when 10% or more of the plasma was replaced by 7.5% HTS, raising concerns of potential coagulopathy after HTS infusion (Reed et al. 1991). In a later experiments on euvolaemic and haemorrhaged swine, no coagulopathy was found after infusion of 4 mL/kg 7.5% NaCl with 6% dextran (Dubick et al. 1993). None of the clinical trials involving patients with active haemorrhage from penetrating or other non-tamponaded blunt injuries produced evidence that these solutions increase blood loss or mortality (Vassar and Holcroft 1992).

61.2.2.4 Clinical Studies

HTS solutions have been studied for resuscitation of patients with traumatic brain injury. Subgroup analysis in randomised prospective clinical trials with hypotensive trauma patients showed that infusion of 250 mL 7.5% NaCl with 6% dextran 70 (HSD) in addition to standard of care increased survival to discharge compared to Ringer's lactate alone (Vassar et al. 1991) and that the effect was caused by HSD (Vassar et al. 1993a). Subsequent analysis of individual patient data from trials comparing HSD with isotonic crystalloid solution included 223 hypotensive trauma patients with head injury and concluded that patients treated with HSD solutions are twice as likely to survive until discharge (Wade et al. 1997b). However, two prospective randomised double-blinded trials of prehospital infusion of hypertonic saline in trauma patients with GCS <9 found no significant difference in mortality or neurologic outcome compared to Ringer's lactate (Cooper et al. 2004) and normal saline (Bulger et al. 2010). It can be argued, though, that the ICP-lowering effect of a single dose of HTS is temporary and further doses or infusion may be needed in order to show benefit.

Control of ICP in the intensive care unit by repeated doses or infusion of HTS has been investigated in several small, mainly observational or retrospective studies in both children and adults with traumatic brain injury (White et al. 2006; Bhardwaj 2007; Gu et al. 2018). From these studies, it appears that HTS solutions are efficacious in ameliorating cerebral oedema and reducing ICP after brain injury and surgery. However, definitive human trials using hard endpoints are lacking (White et al. 2006; Bhardwaj 2007; Carney et al. 2017).

61.2.3 Sugar or Salt?

Mannitol and HTS for treatment of elevated ICP have been compared in small clinical studies using equiosmolar regimens (White et al. 2006; Li et al. 2015; Gu et al. 2018). Based on these human trials, it appears that HTS may be more effective than mannitol in reducing ICP and has a longer duration of action (White et al. 2006; Ziai et al. 2007; Mangat et al. 2015; Carney et al. 2017). HTS may even reduce ICP refractory to mannitol administration (Ziai et al. 2007; Mangat 2018). Whether this affects mortality is, as yet, unknown.

The two regimens are compared in Table 61.1.

61.3 Specific Paediatric Concerns

In a recent guideline from the Brain Trauma Foundation, regarding acute medical management of severe traumatic brain injury in infants, children and adolescents, it was concluded that there is Class II evidence supporting the use of 3% hypertonic saline, 6.5–10 mL/kg for the acute treatment of intracranial hypertension in severe paediatric TBI, and Class III evidence supporting its use as a continuous infusion, 0.1–1.0 mL/kg/h during the intensive care unit course (Kochanek et al. 2012). There is insufficient evidence to support or refute the use of mannitol, concentrations of hypertonic saline higher that 3% or other hyperosmolar agents for the treatment of severe paediatric TBI (Kochanek et al. 2012). This calls for further investigations in children aimed at identifying the best hyperosmolar agent and the optimal treatment regimen and evaluating the long-term neurology outcome.

Table 61.1 Comparison of mannitol and hypertonic saline

	Mannitol	Hypertonic saline
Dose	Bolus 0.25–1.0 g/kg = 1.25–5 mL/kg 20% mannitol	Bolus 1–2 ml/kg 3–5.6% NaCl or infusion 1–2 ml/kg/t 3–5.6% NaCl. Target [Na^+] 145–155 mmol/L
Effectiveness	Reflection coefficient 0.9. Effect may decrease with repeated administration	Reflection coefficient 1.0. Potentially greater and more prolonged effect. May work when mannitol refractory
Effect on mortality	Unknown	Unknown
Rheologic effect	Yes	Yes
Diuretic effect	Osmotic diuresis up to five times infused volume	Diuresis up to twice infused volume via decreased ANP
Haemodynamic effect	Diuresis may compromise intravascular volume causing hypovolaemia and hypotension	Augments intravascular volume, maintains MAP, CVP and CO Increased microcirculation
Other effects	Antioxidant via free-radical scavenging	Restores resting membrane potential and cell volume Immunomodulatory
Maximum serum osmolality	320 mOsm/L	360 mOsm/L
Potential for rebound oedema	Yes	Yes
Half-life	2–4 h	Unknown
Known and potential adverse effects	Hypotension, rebound elevation in ICP, hypokalaemia, haemolysis, renal failure	Rebound elevation in ICP, hypo- and hyperkalaemia, congestive heart failure, haemolysis, coagulopathy, central pontine myelinolysis

ANP atrial natriuretic peptide; *MAP* mean arterial pressure; *CVP* central venous pressure; *CO* cardiac output
Adapted after Ziai et al. (2007) and Knapp (2005)

References

Aiyagari V, Deibert E, Diringer MN. Hypernatremia in the neurologic intensive care unit: how high is too high? J Crit Care. 2006;21:163–72.

Bauer M, Marzi I, Ziegenfuss T, Seeck G, Bühren V, Larsen R. Comparative effects of crystalloid and small volume hypertonic hyperoncotic fluid resuscitation on hepatic microcirculation after hemorrhagic shock. Circ Shock. 1993;40:187–93.

Behrman SW, Fabian TC, Kudsk KA, Proctor KG. Microcirculatory flow changes after initial resuscitation of hemorrhagic shock with 7.5% hypertonic saline/6% dextran 70. J Trauma. 1991;31:589–98; discussion 599–596.

Berger S, Schürer L, Härtl R, Deisböck T, Dautermann C, Murr R, Messmer K, Baethmann A. 7.2% NaCl/10% dextran 60 versus 20% mannitol for treatment of intracranial hypertension. Acta Neurochir Suppl (Wien). 1994;60:494–8.

Bhardwaj A. Osmotherapy in neurocritical care. Curr Neurol Neurosci Rep. 2007;7:513–21.

Bratton SL, Chestnut RM, Ghajar J, McConnell Hammond FF, Harris OA, Hartl R, Manley GT, Nemecek A, Newell DW, Rosenthal G, Schouten J, Shutter L, Timmons SD, Ullman JS, Videtta W, Wilberger JE, Wright DW. Guidelines for the management of severe traumatic brain injury II Hyperosmolar therapy. J Neurotrauma. 2007;24(Suppl 1):S14–20.

Bulger EM, May S, Brasel KJ, Schreiber M, Kerby JD, Tisherman SA, Newgard C, Slutsky A, Coimbra R, Emerson S, Minei JP, Bardarson B, Kudenchuk P, Baker A, Christenson J, Idris A, Davis D, Fabian TC, Aufderheide TP, Callaway C, Williams C, Banek J, Vaillancourt C, van Heest R, Sopko G, Hata JS, Hoyt DB, ROC Investigators. Out-of-hospital hypertonic resuscitation following severe traumatic brain injury: a randomized controlled trial. JAMA. 2010;304(13):1455–64. https://doi.org/10.1001/jama2010.1405.

Burke AM, Quest DO, Chien S, Cerri C. The effects of mannitol on blood viscosity. J Neurosurg. 1981;55:550–3.

Carney N, Totten AM, O'Reilly C, Ullman JS, Hawryluk GW, Bell MJ, Bratton SL, Chesnut R, Harris OA, Kissoon N, et al. Guidelines for the management of severe traumatic brain injury, fourth edition. Neurosurgery. 2017;80(1):6–15.

Ciesla DJ, Moore EE, Zallen G, Biffl WL, Silliman CC. Hypertonic saline attenuation of polymorphonuclear neutrophil cytotoxicity: timing is everything. J Trauma. 2000;48:388–95.

Cooper DJ, Myles PS, FT MD, Murray LJ, Laidlaw J, Cooper G, Tremayne AB, Bernard SS, Ponsford J, HTS Study Investigators. Prehospital hypertonic saline resuscitation of patients with hypotension and severe traumatic brain injury: a randomized controlled trial. JAMA. 2004;291:1350–7.

Corso CO, Okamoto S, Leiderer R, Messmer K. Resuscitation with hypertonic saline dextran reduces endothelial cell swelling and improves hepatic microvascular perfusion and function after hemorrhagic shock. J Surg Res. 1998;80:210–20.

Diringer MN, Zazulia AR. Osmotic therapy: fact and fiction. Neurocrit Care. 2004;1:219–33.

Drobin D, Hahn RG. Kinetics of isotonic and hypertonic plasma volume expanders. Anesthesiology. 2002;96:1371–80.

Dubick MA, Kilani AF, Summary JJ, Greene JY, Wade CE. Further evaluation of the effects of 7.5% sodium chloride/6% Dextran-70 (HSD) administration on coagulation and platelet aggregation in hemorrhaged and euvolemic swine. Circ Shock. 1993;40:200–5.

Dubick MA, Davis JM, Myers T, Wade CE, Kramer GC. Dose response effects of hypertonic saline and dextran on cardiovascular responses and plasma volume expansion in sheep. Shock. 1995;3:137–44.

Froelich M, Ni Q, Wess C, Ougorets I, Härtl R. Continuous hypertonic saline therapy and the occurrence of complications in neurocritically ill patients. Crit Care Med. 2009;37:1433–41.

Gazitùa S, Scott JB, Swindall B, Haddy FJ. Resistance responses to local changes in plasma osmolality in three vascular beds. Am J Phys. 1971;220:384–91.

Goertz AW, Mehl T, Lindner KH, Rockemann MG, Schirmer U, Schwilk B, Georgieff M. Effect of 7.2% hypertonic saline/6% hetastarch on left ventricular contractility in anesthetized humans. Anesthesiology. 1995;82:1389–95.

Grände PO, Romner B. Osmotherapy in brain edema: a questionable therapy. J Neurosurg Anesthesiol. 2012;24(4):407–12.

Grape S, Ravussin P. PRO: Osmotherapy for the treatment of acute intracranial hypertension. J Neurosurg Anesthesiol. 2012;24(4):402–6.

Gu J, Huang H, Huang Y, Sun H, Xu H. Hypertonic Saline or mannitol for treating elevated intracranial pressure in traumatic brain injury: a meta-analysis of randomised controlled trials. Neurosurg Rev. 2018. https://doi.org/10.1007/s10143-018-0991-8.

Gunnerson KJ, Saul M, He S, Kellum JA. Lactate versus nonlactate metabolic acidosis: a retrospective outcome evaluation of critically ill patients. Crit Care. 2006;10:R22.

Hampton MB, Chambers ST, Vissers MC, Winterbourn CC. Bacterial killing by neutrophils in hypertonic environments. J Infect Dis. 1994;169:839–46.

Härtl R, Medary MB, Ruge M, Arfors KE, Ghahremani F, Ghajar J. Hypertonic/hyperoncotic saline attenuates microcirculatory disturbances after traumatic brain injury. J Trauma. 1997;42:S41–7.

Hassan ZU, Kruer JJ, Fuhrman TM. Electrolyte changes during craniotomy caused by administration of hypertonic mannitol. J Clin Anesth. 2007;19:307–9.

Himmelseher S. Hypertonic saline solutions for treatment of intracranial hypertension. Curr Opin Anaesthesiol. 2007;20:414–26.

Huang PP, Stucky FS, Dimick AR, Treat RC, Bessey PQ, Rue LW. Hypertonic sodium resuscitation is associated with renal failure and death. Ann Surg. 1995;221:543–54; discussion 554–557.

Järvelä K, Koskinen M, Kööbi T. Effects of hypertonic saline (7.5%) on extracellular fluid volumes in healthy volunteers. Anaesthesia. 2003;58:878–81.

Junger WG, Coimbra R, Liu FC, Herdon-Remelius C, Junger W, Junger H, Loomis W, Hoyt DB, Altman A. Hypertonic saline resuscitation: a tool to modulate immune function in trauma patients? Shock. 1997;8:235–41.

Khanna S, Davis D, Peterson B, Fisher B, Tung H, O'Quigley J, Deutsch R. Use of hypertonic saline in the treatment of severe refractory posttraumatic intracranial hypertension in pediatric traumatic brain injury. Crit Care Med. 2000;28:1144–51.

Kien ND, Kramer GC, White DA. Acute hypotension caused by rapid hypertonic saline infusion in anesthetized dogs. Anesth Analg. 1991;73:597–602.

Knapp JM. Hyperosmolar therapy in the treatment of severe head injury in children: mannitol and hypertonic saline. AACN Clin Issues. 2005;16:199–211.

Kochanek PM, et al. Guidelines for the acute medical management of severe traumatic brain injury in infants, children, and adolescents-second edition. Pediatr Crit Care Med. 2012;13(1 Suppl):S1–82.

Kolsen-Petersen JA. Immune effect of hypertonic saline: fact or fiction? Acta Anaesthesiol Scand. 2004;48:667–78.

Kolsen-Petersen JA, Nielsen JO, Tonnesen E. Acid base and electrolyte changes after hypertonic saline (7.5%) infusion: a randomized controlled clinical trial. Scand J Clin Lab Invest. 2005;65:13–22.

Kramer GC. Hypertonic resuscitation: physiologic mechanisms and recommendations for trauma care. J Trauma. 2003;54:S89–99.

Kramer GC, Perron PR, Lindsey DC, Ho HS, Gunther RA, Boyle WA, Holcroft JW. Small-volume resuscitation with hypertonic saline dextran solution. Surgery. 1986;100:239–47.

Kreimeier U, Brückner UB, Messmer K. Improvement of nutritional blood flow using hypertonic-hyperoncotic solutions for primary treatment of hemorrhagic hypotension. Eur Surg Res. 1988;20:277–9.

Kreimeier U, Brueckner UB, Schmidt J, Messmer K. Instantaneous restoration of regional organ blood flow after severe hemorrhage: effect of small-volume resuscitation with hypertonic-hyperoncotic solutions. J Surg Res. 1990;49:493–503.

Lescot T, Degos V, Zouaoui A, Preteux F, Coriat P, Puybasset L. Opposed effects of hypertonic saline on contusions and noncontused brain tissue in patients with severe traumatic brain injury. Crit Care Med. 2006;34(12):3029–33.

Li M, Chen T, Chen SD, Cai J, Hu YH. Comparison of equimolar doses of mannitol and hypertonic saline for the treatment of elevated intracranial pressure after traumatic brain injury. a systematic review and meta-analysis. Medicine (Baltimore). 2015;94(17):e668. https://doi.org/10.1097/MD.0000000000000668.

Loomis WH, Namiki S, Hoyt DB, Junger WG. Hypertonicity rescues T cells from suppression by trauma-induced anti- inflammatory mediators. Am J Physiol Cell Physiol. 2001;281:C840–8.

Loomis WH, Namiki S, Ostrom RS, Insel PA, Junger WG. Hypertonic stress increases T cell interleukin-2 expression through a mechanism that involves ATP release, P2 receptor, and p38 MAPK activation. J Biol Chem. 2003;278:4590–6.

Mangat HS. Hypertonic saline infusion for treating intracranial hypertension after severe traumatic brain injury. Crit Care. 2018;22:37. https://doi.org/10.1186/s13054-018-1963-7.

Mangat HS, Chiu YL, Gerber LM, Alimi M, Ghajar J, Hartl R. Hypertonic saline reduces cumulative and daily intracranial pressure burdens after severe traumatic brain injury. J Neurosurg. 2015;122(1):202–10. https://doi.org/10.3171/2014.10.JNS132545.

Maningas PA. Resuscitation with 7.5% NaCl in 6% dextran-70 during hemorrhagic shock in swine: effects on organ blood flow. Crit Care Med. 1987;15:1121–6.

Maningas PA, Mattox KL, Pepe PE, Jones RL, Feliciano DV, Burch JM. Hypertonic saline-dextran solutions for the prehospital management of traumatic hypotension. Am J Surg. 1989;157:528–33; discussion 533–534.

Mattox KL, Maningas PA, Moore EE, Mateer JR, Marx JA, Aprahamian C, Burch JM, Pepe PE. Prehospital hypertonic saline/dextran infusion for post- traumatic hypotension. The U.S.A. Multicenter Trial. Ann Surg. 1991;213:482–91.

Mazzoni MC, et al. Lumenal narrowing and endothelial cell swelling in skeletal muscle capillaries during hemorrhagic shock. Circ Shock. 1989;29:27–39.

Mazzoni MC, Borgström P, Intaglietta M, Arfors KE. Capillary narrowing in hemorrhagic shock is rectified by hyperosmotic saline-dextran reinfusion. Circ Shock. 1990;31:407–18.

Nakayama S, Kramer GC, Carlsen RC, Holcroft JW. Infusion of very hypertonic saline to bled rats: membrane potentials and fluid shifts. J Surg Res. 1985;38:180–6.

Nolte D, Bayer M, Lehr HA, Becker M, Krombach F, Kreimeier U, Messmer K. Attenuation of postischemic microvascular disturbances in striated muscle by hyperosmolar saline dextran. Am J Phys. 1992;263:H1411–6.

Oddo M, Poole D, Helbok R, Meyfroidt G, Stocchetti N, Bouzat P, Cecconi M, Geeraerts T, Martin-Loeches I, Quintard H, Taccone FS, Geocadin RG, Hemphill C, Ichai C, Menon D, Payen JF, Perner A, Smith M, Suarez J, Videtta W, Zanier ER, Citerio G. Fluid therapy in neurointensive care patients: ESICM consensus and clinical practice recommendations. Intensive Care Med. 2018;44(4):449–63. https://doi.org/10.1007/s00134-018-5086-z.

Ogden AT, Mayer SA, Connolly ESJ. Hyperosmolar agents in neurosurgical practice: the evolving role of hypertonic saline. Neurosurgery. 2005;57:207–15.

Oi Y, Aneman A, Svensson M, Ewert S, Dahlqvist M, Haljamäe H. Hypertonic saline-dextran improves intestinal perfusion and survival in porcine endotoxin shock. Crit Care Med. 2000;28:2843–50.

Paczynski RP. Osmotherapy. Basic concepts and controversies. Crit Care Clin. 1997;13:105–29.

Pascual JL, Ferri LE, Seely AJ, Campisi G, Chaudhury P, Giannias B, Evans DC, Razek T, Michel RP, Christou NV. Hypertonic saline resuscitation of hemorrhagic shock diminishes neutrophil rolling and adherence to endothelium and reduces in vivo vascular leakage. Ann Surg. 2002;236:634–42.

Pascual JL, Khwaja KA, Chaudhury P, Christou NV. Hypertonic saline and the microcirculation. J Trauma. 2003;54:S133–40.

Peterson B, Khanna S, Fisher B, Marshall L. Prolonged hypernatremia controls elevated intracranial pressure in head- injured pediatric patients. Crit Care Med. 2000;28:1136–43.

Qureshi AI, Suarez JI. Use of hypertonic saline solutions in treatment of cerebral edema and intracranial hypertension. Crit Care Med. 2000;28:3301–13.

Qureshi AI, Wilson DA, Traystman RJ. Treatment of elevated intracranial pressure in experimental intracerebral hemorrhage: comparison between mannitol and hypertonic saline. Neurosurgery. 1999;44:1055–63.

Ragland J, Lee K. Critical care management and monitoring of intracranial pressure. J Neurocrit Care. 2016;9(2):105–12. https://doi.org/10.18700/jnc.160101.

Read RC, Johnson JA, Vick JA, Meyer MW. Vascular effects of hypertonic solutions. Circ Res. 1960;8:538–48.

Reed RL 2nd, Johnston TD, Chen Y, Fischer RP. Hypertonic saline alters plasma clotting times and platelet aggregation. J Trauma. 1991;31:8–14.

Rizoli SB, Kapus A, Fan J, Li YH, Marshall JC, Rotstein OD. Immunomodulatory effects of hypertonic resuscitation on the development of lung inflammation following hemorrhagic shock. J Immunol. 1998;161:6288–96.

Rosengren S, Henson PM, Worthen GS. Migration-associated volume changes in neutrophils facilitate the migratory process in vitro. Am J Phys. 1994;267:C1623–32.

Rosner MJ, Coley I. Cerebral perfusion pressure: a hemodynamic mechanism of mannitol and the postmannitol hemogram. Neurosurgery. 1987;21:147–56.

Saltarini M, Massarutti D, Baldassarre M, Nardi G, De Colle C, Fabris G. Determination of cerebral water content by magnetic resonance imaging after small volume infusion of 18% hypertonic saline solution in a patient with refractory intracranial hypertension. Eur J Emerg Med. 2002;9:262–5.

Sayre MR, Daily SW, Stern SA, Storer DL, van Loveren HR, Hurst JM. Out-of-hospital administration of mannitol to head-injured patients does not change systolic blood pressure. Acad Emerg Med. 1996;3:840–8.

Schmoker JD, Zhuang J, Shackford SR. Hypertonic fluid resuscitation improves cerebral oxygen delivery and reduces intracranial pressure after hemorrhagic shock. J Trauma. 1991;31:1607–13.

Schwartz ML, Tator CH, Rowed DW, Reid SR, Meguro K, Andrews DF. The University of Toronto head injury treatment study: a prospective, randomized comparison of pentobarbital and mannitol. Can J Neurol Sci. 1984;11:434–40.

Seto A, Murakami M, Fukuyama H, Niijima K, Aoyama K, Takenaka I, Kadoya T. Ventricular tachycardia caused by hyperkalemia after administration of hypertonic mannitol. Anesthesiology. 2000;93:1359–136.

Shackford SR, Zhuang J, Schmoker J. Intravenous fluid tonicity: effect on intracranial pressure, cerebral blood flow, and cerebral oxygen delivery in focal brain injury. J Neurosurg. 1992;76:91–8.

Shackford SR, Schmoker JD, Zhuang J. The effect of hypertonic resuscitation on pial arteriolar tone after brain injury and shock. J Trauma. 1994;37:899–908.

Smith HP, Kelly DL Jr, McWhorter JM, Armstrong D, Johnson R, Transou C, Howard G. Comparison of mannitol regimens in patients with severe head injury undergoing intracranial monitoring. J Neurosurg. 1986;65:820–4.

Sorani MD, Manley GT. Dose-response relationship of mannitol and intracranial pressure: a metaanalysis. J Neurosurg. 2008;108:80–7.

Todd MM, Cutkomp J, Brian JE. Influence of mannitol and furosemide, alone and in combination, on brain water content after fluid percussion injury. Anesthesiology. 2006;105:1176–81.

Tølløfsrud S, Tønnessen T, Skraastad O, Noddeland H. Hypertonic saline and dextran in normovolaemic and hypovolaemic healthy volunteers increases interstitial and intravascular fluid volumes. Acta Anaesthesiol Scand. 1998;42:145–53.

Tyagi R, Donaldson K, Loftus CM, Jallo J. Hypertonic saline: a clinical review. Neurosurg Rev. 2007;30:277–89.

Vassar MJ, Holcroft JW. Use of hypertonic-hyperoncotic fluids for resuscitation of trauma patients. J Int Care Med. 1992;7:189–98.

Vassar MJ, Perry CA, Gannaway WL, Holcroft JW. 7.5% sodium chloride/dextran for resuscitation of trauma patients undergoing helicopter transport. Arch Surg. 1991;126:1065–72.

Vassar MJ, Fischer RP, O'Brien PE, Bachulis BL, Chambers JA, Hoyt DB, Holcroft JW. A multicenter trial for resuscitation of injured patients with 7.5% sodium chloride. The effect of added dextran 70. The Multicenter Group for the Study of Hypertonic Saline in Trauma Patients. Arch Surg. 1993a;128:1003–11.

Vassar MJ, Perry CA, Holcroft JW. Prehospital resuscitation of hypotensive trauma patients with 7.5% NaCl versus 7.5% NaCl with added dextran: a controlled trial. J Trauma. 1993b;34:622–32; discussion 632–633.

Vialet R, Albanèse J, Thomachot L, Antonini F, Bourgouin A, Alliez B, Martin C. Isovolume hypertonic solutes (sodium chloride or mannitol) in the treatment of refractory posttraumatic intracranial hypertension: 2 mL/kg 7.5% saline is more effective than 2 mL/kg 20% mannitol. Crit Care Med. 2003;31:1683–7.

Vollmar B, Lang G, Menger MD, Messmer K. Hypertonic hydroxyethyl starch restores hepatic microvascular perfusion in hemorrhagic shock. Am J Phys. 1994;266:H1927–34.

Wade CE, Kramer GC, Grady JJ, Fabian TC, Younes RN. Efficacy of hypertonic saline dextran (HSD) in patients with traumatic hypotension: meta-analysis of individual patient data. Acta Anaesthesiol Scand Suppl. 1997a;110:77–9.

Wade CE, Grady JJ, Kramer GC, Younes RN, Gehlsen K, Holcroft JW. Individual patient cohort analysis of the efficacy of hypertonic saline/dextran in patients with traumatic brain injury and hypotension. J Trauma. 1997b;42:S61–5.

Wakai A, McCabe A, Roberts I, Schierhout G. Mannitol for acute traumatic brain injury. Cochrane Database Syst Rev. 2013;8:CD001049.

Weed lH, Mckippen PS. Experimental alteration of brain bulk. Am J Phys. 1919;48(4):531–58.

White H, Cook D, Venkatesh B. The use of hypertonic saline for treating intracranial hypertension after traumatic brain injury. Anaesth Analg. 2006;102:1836–46.

Wisner DH, Schuster L, Quinn C. Hypertonic saline resuscitation of head injury: effects on cerebral water content. J Trauma. 1990;30:75–8.

Younes RN, Aun F, Accioly CQ, Casale LP, Szajnbok I, Birolini D. Hypertonic solutions in the treatment of hypovolemic shock: a prospective, randomized study in patients admitted to the emergency room. Surgery. 1992;111:380–5.

Ziai WC, Toung TJ, Bhardwaj A. Hypertonic saline: first-line therapy for cerebral edema? J Neurol Sci. 2007;261:157–66.

Barbiturates for ICP Management 62

Mads Rasmussen

Recommendations

Level I

There are insufficient data to support a Level I recommendation for this topic.

Level II

Prophylactic administration of barbiturates to induce burst suppression EEG is not recommended. Barbiturate administration can be used to control elevated ICP refractory to maximum standard medical and surgical treatment. Haemodynamic stability is essential before and during barbiturate therapy.

Level III

No barbiturate regimen has been shown to be superior to another. We still lack any study showing improved outcome with barbiturate therapy.

M. Rasmussen (✉)
Department of Anaesthesia and Intensive Care, Section of Neuroanaesthesia, Aarhus University Hospital, Aarhus, Denmark
e-mail: mads.rasmussen@vest.rm.dk

62.1 Overview

The ICP-lowering and cerebral protective effects of barbiturates are believed to be due to the coupling of cerebral blood flow to regional cerebral metabolic demand. By suppression of cerebral metabolic demand, barbiturates reduce cerebral metabolism inducing vasoconstriction and thereby lower cerebral blood flow and cerebral blood volume and thus ICP. Other effects of barbiturates include alterations in vascular tone and resistance and inhibition of excitotoxicity (Shapro 1985).

During the last six decades, barbiturates have been used to manage high ICP (Horsley 1937). Currently, high dosages of barbiturates are used in patients with severe head injury and high ICP refractory to standard medical and surgical treatment. This practice is recommended by the Brain Trauma Foundation Guidelines because this is the only second-level measure for which there is Level II evidence to reduce intracranial pressure (Brain Trauma Foundation Guidelines 2016; Carney et al. 2017).

A systematic review conducted by the Cochrane Injuries Group concluded that there is no evidence that barbiturate therapy in patients with severe head injury improves outcome in spite of the ICP-reducing effect. Barbiturate therapy results in a fall in blood pressure in one of four patients. This hypotensive effect may offset any ICP-lowering effect on cerebral perfusion pressure (Roberts and Sydenham 2009).

© Springer Nature Switzerland AG 2020
T. Sundstrøm et al. (eds.), *Management of Severe Traumatic Brain Injury*,
https://doi.org/10.1007/978-3-030-39383-0_62

A number of different therapeutic regimens using thiopental have been applied. No documentation has been presented, however, that one regimen is superior to another. I suggest the following protocol:

Use a loading dose of 10 mg/kg over 30 min followed by infusion of 5 mg/kg/h for 3 h and a subsequent infusion of 1–3 mg/kg/h thereafter. If the effect is absent after the initial 30 min, it is unlikely that barbiturate therapy will work and you should discontinue further thiopentone infusion. The need for barbiturate therapy can be re-evaluated. An electroencephalographic monitoring may be used to evaluate the existence of a burst suppression pattern, which implies near-maximal reduction in cerebral metabolism.

Tips, Tricks and Pitfalls

- Initiate barbiturate therapy only in haemodynamically stable patients.
- Patients may receive vasopressors to counteract severe hypotension.
- Use barbiturate therapy in patients with ICP greater than 20 mmHg refractory to other standard treatments with appropriate sedation (propofol/midazolam), mannitol, hypertonic saline, ventricular drainage and moderate hyperventilation (3.6–4.5 kPa).

∗Use lowest possible doses.

62.2 Background

62.2.1 Effect of Barbiturate Therapy on Intracranial Pressure

Two studies have examined the effect of barbiturate administration on intracranial pressure. Eisenberg et al. randomly assigned 73 patients with severe head injury with GCS of 4–8 and intractable ICP to either pentobarbital or no pentobarbital (Eisenberg et al. 1988). The results indicated a 2:1 benefit for those treated with pentobarbital with regard to ICP control. A smaller proportion of the patients in the barbiturate group had uncontrolled ICP (68% versus 83%). The relative risk for uncontrolled ICP was 0.81 (95% CI 0.62–1.06). Ward et al. (1985) allocated 53 patients with severe head injury to receive either pentobarbital or no pentobarbital (Ward et al. 1985). Similar to the Eisenberg study, mean ICP was lower in the barbiturate-treated patients. There was no difference in 1-year mortality. Hypotension (systolic blood pressure < 80 mmHg) occurred in 54% of the patients in the pentobarbital group and in 7% of the patients in the control group.

62.2.2 Barbiturate Therapy Versus Mannitol: Effect on Intracranial Pressure

Schwartz et al. compared prophylactic pentobarbital and mannitol for ICP control in 59 patients with severe head injury. Pentobarbital was less effective than mannitol for control of elevated ICP, and there was no difference in mortality between the two drugs (RR = 1.21; 95% CI 0.75–1.94) (Schwartz et al. 1984).

62.2.3 Pentobarbital Versus Thiopental for ICP Control

Pérez-Bárcena et al. randomised 44 patients suffering from severe head injury to either pentobarbital or thiopental. Inclusion criteria were GCS <8 after resuscitation or neurological deterioration during the first week after trauma and with an ICP >20 mmHg refractory to first tier measures as defined by the Brain Trauma Foundation.

Fewer patients had uncontrollable ICP with thiopental. There was no significant difference with regard to neurological outcome. Incidence of hypotension was equal in the two groups (Pérez-Bárcena et al. 2008).

62.2.4 Systematic Review of Barbiturate Randomised Controlled Trials

In 1999 and 2009, the Cochrane Injuries Group completed a systematic review of barbiturates for acute traumatic brain injury. They included data from six trials. The pooled risk ratio for death (barbiturate versus no barbiturate) was 1.09 (95% CI 0.81–1.47). Two randomised studies examined the effect of barbiturates on ICP. In one study, the results indicated that ICP was better controlled with barbiturate treatment. In another study, however, there was no effect on ICP with prophylactic barbiturate treatment. Barbiturate therapy is associated with increased incidence of hypotension (RR = 1.80; 95% CI 1.19–2.70) (Roberts and Sydenham 2009), depressed cardiac output and respiratory depression including adult respiratory distress syndrome (ARDS) (Ellens et al. 2015).

62.3 Specific Paediatric Concerns

The 2012 Guidelines (Kochanet et al. 2012) recommend barbiturate therapy in haemodynamically stable patients when maximal medical and surgical therapy has failed to control ICP. Concerns regarding barbiturates include reductions in blood pressure and cardiac output and increased intrapulmonary shunt, while a specific concern in children is the wide variability in drug clearance. When barbiturate therapy is used, continuous arterial blood pressure monitoring and cardiovascular support to maintain adequate CPP are suggested. The suggested therapeutic regime mentioned in the overview section may be used as a guide with careful consideration of age and weight (Adelson et al. 2003).

References

Adelson PD, Bratton SL, Carney NA, Chesnut RM, du Coudray HE, Goldstein B, Kochanek PM, Miller HC, Partington MD, Selden NR, Warden CR, Wright DW, American Association for Surgery of Trauma, Child Neurology Society, International Society for Pediatric Neurosurgery, International Trauma Anesthesia and Critical Care Society, Society of Critical Care Medicine, World Federation of Pediatric Intensive and Critical Care Societies. Guidelines for the management of severe traumatic head injury in infants, children and adolescents. Chapter 13. The use of barbiturates in the control of intracranial hypertension in severe pediatric brain injury. Pediatr Crit Care Med. 2003;4(3 suppl):S49–52.

Carney N, Totten AM, O'Reilly C, Ullman JS, Hawryluk GW, Bell MJ, Bratton SL, Chesnut R, Harris OA, Kissoon N, Rubiano AM, Shutter L, Tasker RC, Vavilala MS, Wilberger J, Wright DW, Ghajar J. Guidelines for the management of severe traumatic brain injury, fourth edition. Neurosurgery. 2017;80(1):6–15. https://doi.org/10.1227/NEU.0000000000001432. PubMed PMID: 27654000.

Eisenberg HM, Frankowski RF, Contant CF, Marshall LF, Walker MD. High-dose barbiturate control of elevated intracranial pressure in patients with severe head injury. J Neurosurg. 1988;69:15–23.

Ellens NR, Figuera BE, Clarc JC. The use of barbiturate-induced coma during cerebrovascular neurosurgical procedures. A review of the literature. Brain Circ. 2015;1:140–5.

Horsley JS. The intracranial pressure during barbital narcosis. Lancet. 1937;1:141–3.

Kochanek PM, Carney N, Adelson PD, Ashwal S, Bell MJ, Bratton S, Carson S, Chesnut RM, Ghajar J, Goldstein B, Grant GA, Kissoon N, Peterson K, Selden NR, Tasker RC, Tong KA, Vavilala MS, Wainwright MS, Warden CR, American Academy of Pediatrics-Section on Neurological Surgery; American Association of Neurological Surgeons/Congress of Neurological Surgeons; Child Neurology Society; European Society of Pediatric and Neonatal Intensive Care; Neurocritical Care Society; Pediatric Neurocritical Care Research Group; Society of Critical Care Medicine; Paediatric Intensive Care Society UK; Society for Neuroscience in Anesthesiology and Critical Care; World Federation of Pediatric Intensive and Critical CareSocieties. Guidelines for the acute medical management of severe traumatic brain injury in infants, children, and adolescents – second edition. Pediatr Crit Care Med. 2012;13(Suppl 1):S1–82.

Pérez-Bárcena J, Llompart-Pou JA, Homar J, Abadal JM, Raurich JM, Frontera G, Brell M, Ibáñez J, Ibáñez J. Pentobarbital versus thiopental in the treatment of refractory intracranial hypertension in patients with traumatic brain injury: a randomized controlled trial. Crit Care. 2008;12(4):R112.

Roberts I, Sydenham E. Barbiturates for acute traumatic brain injury. Cochrane Database Syst Rev. 2009;(4):CD 000033. https://doi.org/10.1002/14651858.

Schwartz ML, Tator CH, Rowed DW, Reid SR, Meguro K, Andrews DF. The University of Toronto head injury treatment study: a prospective, randomized comparison of pentobarbital and mannitol. Can J Neurol Sci. 1984;11:434–40.

Shapro HM. Barbiturates in brain ischemia. Br J Anaesth. 1985;57:82–95.

Ward JD, Becker DP, Miller JD, Choi SC, Marmarou A, Wood C, Newlon PG, Keenan R. Failure of prophylactic barbiturate coma in the treatment of severe head injury. J Neurosurg. 1985;62:383–8.

Management of Fluids and Electrolytes

63

Per-Olof Grände and Niels Juul

Recommendations

Level I

There are insufficient data to support a Level I recommendation for a specific fluid therapy in traumatic brain injury (TBI) patients.

Level II

There has been one Level II study (the SAFE-TBI study) supporting the use of normal saline rather than 4% hypotonic albumin in TBI patients.

Level III

There have been several Level III studies supporting the use of albumin in TBI patients.

There are insufficient data to support the use of synthetic colloids in severe TBI.

P.-O. Grände (✉)
Department of Anaesthesia and Intensive Care, Lund University and Lund University Hospital, Lund, Sweden
e-mail: per-olof.grande@med.lu.se

N. Juul
Department of Anaesthesia, Aarhus University Hospital, Aarhus, Denmark
e-mail: d245364@dadlnet.dk

63.1 Overview

The infusion of plasma volume expanders is essential after a TBI to counteract hypovolaemia. Hypovolaemia increases the risk of compromised circulation in the most injured part of the brain. A recent experimental study on the cat showed that significant hypovolaemia develops rather quickly after a traumatic head injury (Bentzer and Grände 2017).

The support for saline or other *crystalloid* solutions as the main plasma volume expanders in TBI patients is supported by the results of the SAFE-TBI study (The SAFE Study Investigators 2007). This fluid regimen is cheaper than other fluid regimens using albumin or synthetic colloids.

A crystalloid solution is distributed throughout the whole extracellular space of the body, which means that only 20–25% of the volume infused will stay intravascularly and the rest will be relatively quickly distributed to the interstitial space of the body. The maintenance of normovolaemia with saline or other crystalloids therefore means the need for large volumes, resulting in interstitial oedema with potential side effects in terms of increased lung water, greater diffusion distances and an increased risk of compartment syndrome. What may be more important in TBI patients is that distribution of crystalloids will occur also to the brain interstitium, provided the blood–brain barrier (BBB) is disrupted and becomes permeable for small solutes. There is apparently a risk

© Springer Nature Switzerland AG 2020
T. Sundstrøm et al. (eds.), *Management of Severe Traumatic Brain Injury*,
https://doi.org/10.1007/978-3-030-39383-0_63

that the use of crystalloids will trigger the development of tissue oedema not only in organs away from the brain but also in the brain itself in TBI patients (Grände 2006; Jungner et al. 2010).

Albumin has a molecular weight of 69 kDa and is the most essential natural plasma protein. In contrast to synthetic colloids, all the molecules are of the same size, are negatively charged and are not degraded to smaller molecules. As will be discussed below, the fact that albumin is not degraded may be an advantage by exerting a more sustained plasma volume expansion, but it may also be a disadvantage if albumin accumulates in the interstitium. Allergic reactions with albumin are rare. The protein concentration in plasma is reduced after a TBI, reflecting increased leakage of plasma proteins to the interstitium—being beyond the recirculation capacity of the lymphatic system (Bentzer and Grände 2017; Haskell et al. 1997). According to the two-pore theory for transvascular fluid exchange (Rippe and Haraldsson 1994), plasma proteins are transferred to the interstitium through the relatively few large pores at the end of the capillary network and in venules, following the fluid stream mainly through convection. The hydrostatic pressure is the dominating force in the large pores, as the transcapillary oncotic absorbing force is significantly reduced across these pores. This means that even in the normal state, there is a continuous leakage of plasma and plasma proteins from the intravascular space to the extravascular space through these pores, but the capacity of the recirculating lymphatic system is large enough to prevent hypovolaemia and tissue oedema. The loss of plasma fluid is dependent on the number of large pores and on the magnitude of the force of the hydrostatic pressure. This means that there is a risk that the more albumin infused to compensate for hypovolaemia, the more leakage of plasma fluid there will be. Thus, the use of albumin as plasma volume expander should include measures that reduce the transcapillary leakage to volumes below the capacity of the lymphatic system. According to physiological principles of transcapillary fluid exchange as described by the two-pore theory, leakage of plasma fluid to the interstitium can be reduced by maintaining the hydrostatic capillary pressure low. This can be accomplished by avoiding high arterial pressures and avoidance of vasopressors such as noradrenaline (Dubniks et al. 2007; Nygren et al. 2010). The leakage can also be reduced using low infusion rates (Bark and Grände 2014) and higher concentrations of the albumin solution. Physiotherapy may also reduce the need for albumin by stimulating the lymphatic drainage system. As discussed below, the need for albumin infusions may also be reduced by avoidance of low haemoglobin concentrations.

By increasing the plasma oncotic pressure, albumin may induce absorption of fluid from the brain, provided BBB is permeable to small solutes (Tomita et al. 1994; Grände 2006; Jungner et al. 2010). This regime may be questioned if the BBB is disrupted to a large extent, resulting in leakage of albumin to the brain. However, considering the low protein concentration in cerebrospinal fluid of 2–3 g/L at most after a severe head injury, most likely reflecting approximately the same concentrations in the brain interstitium, these concentrations are very low compared to the normal plasma protein concentration of approximately 60 g/L. Protein leakage cannot therefore have any significant influence on the transcapillary oncotic absorbing force in the brain. The plasma oncotic effect may help to maintain ICP at an adequate level or to reduce a raised ICP. There are insufficient data to give support for the use of synthetic colloids to severe TBI patients.

63.1.1 Erythrocyte Transfusion

No studies have been performed to date that can be used for guidance in the treatment with erythrocyte transfusion in patients with severe TBI. One study from Canada (Hébert et al. 1999) could not show any beneficial effects of erythrocyte transfusion in a general intensive care material, but no TBI patients were included and leukocyte-depleted blood was not used. A more recent study, on the other hand, showed that higher haemoglobin concentrations are associated with improved outcome after subarachnoid haemorrhage (Naidech et al. 2007), and another study showed improved oxygenation of red blood cell transfusion regardless of baseline haemoglobin concentration (Zygun et al. 2009). Due to the uncertainty regarding optimal haemoglobin concentration, very low haemoglobin concentrations down to 70 g/L (4.3 mmol/L) have been accepted in many neurointensive care units, while other units aim at a haemoglobin concentrations above 110 g/L, as also recommended in the Lund concept (see Chap. 58).

Low haemoglobin concentrations mean larger plasma volume to maintain normovolaemia. This means a greater need for plasma volume expanders to reach normovolaemia from a hypovolaemic state, which also means more transcapillary leakage of plasma and more tissue oedema according to the two-pore theory. It has also been shown in the dog that plasma leakage to the interstitium is higher with a low haemoglobin concentration than with a more normal one (Valeri et al. 1986). These considerations indicate that haemoglobin concentration is of importance in the fluid therapy of TBI patients, and a relatively normal haemoglobin level may be optimal. Normalisation of a low haemoglobin value also improves oxygenation of the injured brain (Smith et al. 2005; Dhar et al. 2009). This may be of special importance for outcome in TBI patients as the hypoxic penumbra zone is the critical area of a traumatised brain to be saved.

As transplantation from another human being, blood transfusion does have side effects. Especially, it has proinflammatory effects when using non-leukocyte-depleted blood and when using blood stored for longer periods of time. Side effects of erythrocyte transfusion can be reduced by using leukocyte-depleted blood and fresher blood products (Bilgin et al. 2011). It is still not verified, however, to what extent the blood volume expanding effect and oxygenation effect of blood transfusion in TBI patients override any potentially adverse effects.

63.1.2 How to Confirm the Status of the Volumetric State

A relatively normal protein and haemoglobin concentration may help to maintain an adequate intravascular volume. The use of Swan-Ganz catheters, PiCCO catheters and other advanced vascular monitoring devices is rarely indicated in the treatment of TBI patients. The arterial blood pressure response on a bolus dose of a plasma volume expander or erythrocytes, the arterial blood pressure response following leg tilting and the PPV index of the arterial curve may be tools by which to evaluate the volumetric state of the patient.

63.1.3 Guidance on Fluid Treatment With Crystalloids and Albumin

The use of crystalloids as the dominating plasma volume expander means that relatively large volumes must be infused to maintain normovolaemia, and there is often a need for vasopressors to keep an adequate cerebral perfusion pressure. Be aware of the fact that this fluid therapy means general tissue oedema, including the lung and the injured brain with a disrupted BBB and that there is a potential risk of hyperchloraemic acidosis when using large volumes of saline.

In spite of the SAFE-TBI study, there is still support for the use of albumin up to relatively normal albumin concentrations (33–37 g/L), if used adequately. Even though 20% albumin is to be preferred, also lower concentrations can be used. Avoid over-transfusion with albumin. In addition, a crystalloid solution should be used (e.g. 1–1.5 L/day for an adult) to maintain an adequate fluid balance and urine production.

The need for albumin as a plasma volume expander can be restricted by (1) giving albumin at a low infusion rate (e.g. 100 mL of 20% albumin over 4 h), (2) avoiding high arterial pressures by avoiding vasopressors and using antihypertensive treatment at supranormal blood pressures and (3) avoiding low haemoglobin concentration (>110 g/L) (leukocyte-depleted blood should be used).

63.1.4 Electrolytes

As with other patients in the intensive care setting, preservation of normal concentrations of electrolytes such as sodium, potassium and chloride ions is important in patients with a severe head injury. The infusion of potassium should be adapted to maintain its concentration within normal limits of 3.6–4.4 mmol/L. It is especially emphasised that low concentrations of sodium may have severe adverse effects in head-injured patients, as hyponatraemia can be associated with the development of brain oedema. Hypotonic solutions (both for albumin and crystalloid solutions) therefore must be avoided. If not adequately treated, hyponatraemia is quite common in these patients. Note the risk with adverse hyperchloraemic acidosis with large volumes of crystalloids resulting in high values of chloride ions. Treatment with osmotherapy in terms of hypertonic saline or mannitol may cause pronounced adverse hypernatremia. Hyponatremia, hypocalcaemia, hypophosphataemia, hypokalaemia and hypomagnesaemia may appear in head trauma patients, and these electrolytes should be determined regularly and if necessary be adequately supplemented.

Hyponatraemia after a head injury can be classified by the cerebral salt-wasting syndrome (CSWS) and the syndrome of inappropriate antidiuretic hormone secretion (SIADH). In CSWS, there is an elevation of brain natriuretic peptide (BNP) levels, which results in reduction in the efficacy of aldosterone and hence reduction in the ability to reabsorb sodium in the kidneys. This results in excretion of salt in the urine. The SIADH is more common in neurological patients and results from an excessive secretion of antidiuretic hormone; water is retained with risk of hypervolaemia and reduced plasma sodium and should be treated with sodium substitution in combination with diuretics. CSWS is a more rare cause of hyponatraemia, but it may be diagnosed as hyponatraemia in combination with excessive production of slightly hypertonic urine. It should be treated with sodium substitution in combination with fluid substitution in volumes related to the amount of urine production. If the polyuria is extensive, the patient may be treated with low doses of ADH analogue. Adrenal gland failure may occur early after a traumatic brain injury and can be diagnosed from analysis of pituitary and adrenal hormones. If it results in severe hypoglycaemia, hypotension and hyponatraemia, treatment with adrenocorticotropin hormones can be considered.

63.1.5 Vasopressors

Previously, all traditional guidelines recommended the use of vasopressors to maintain a CPP of above 70 mmHg, and both inotropic support and vasoconstrictors such as phenylephrine and noradrenaline were used. By the change in the recommendations of CPP from a minimal value of 70 mmHg down to 50–60 mmHg in the update of the US guidelines from 2007 (The Brain Trauma Foundation 2007) and to 60–70 mmHg in the latest update from 2016 (The Brain Trauma Foundation 2016), the need for vasopressors has been reduced, if these guidelines are followed.

The use of lowest possible dose of vasopressors is recommended with the Lund therapy. Still, CPP stays in the range of 60–70 mmHg in most patients using this guideline in spite of the use of antihypertensive therapy. Most likely this is due to a more strict treatment of hypovolaemia by albumin infusions towards a relatively normal albumin concentration in plasma and by giving erythrocyte transfusion at low haemoglobin concentrations. According to the principles behind the Lund therapy, the use of lowest possible dose of vasopressors may reduce the increase in ICP, reduces the need for plasma volume expanders and results in a less compromised microcirculation and better oxygenation of hypoxic areas of the brain and in the rest of the body (see Chap. 55).

Tips, Tricks and Pitfalls

If using a crystalloid (always isotonic solutions) as the main plasma volume expander, be aware of the following:

- Relatively large volumes are needed to maintain normovolaemia.
- Crystalloids are associated with general tissue oedema, including the injured brain.
- Saline is associated with hyperchloraemic acidosis.

If using albumin (always isotonic solutions) as plasma volume expander, the need of albumin and the risk of hypovolemia may be reduced by:

- Using high-concentration solutions.
- Using low infusion rates.
- Avoiding high blood pressures and vasopressors.
- Avoiding low haemoglobin concentrations.
- Frequent physiotherapy to activate the lymphatic recirculation system.

63.2 Background

As in other trauma patients, the TBI patient suffers from a general increase in microvascular permeability, resulting in an increase in transcapillary leakage of plasma fluid to the interstitium (Bentzer and Grände 2017). This leakage results in hypovolaemia if the transcapillary escape rate (TER) (normally 5–8% of total plasma volume per hour) is increased above the capacity of the lymphatic recirculation system (Haskell et al. 1997). If not adequately treated, most patients with severe TBI suffer from hypovolaemia, resulting in activation of the baroreceptor reflex with increased sympathetic discharge and catecholamine release. Avoidance of hypovolaemia is essential in patients with severe TBI for maintenance of perfusion and oxygenation of the injured brain, especially the most injured parts of the brain (Rise et al. 1998). This means that there is a need for transfusion with blood volume expanders to restore blood volume to a normovolaemic condition.

In principle, we lack generally accepted clinical studies that could be used for guidance on fluid treatment in these patients. Saline and albumin are the most common plasma volume expanders used in clinical practice today for TBI patients. The only randomised study regarding fluid therapy in severe TBI patients published so far (The SAFE Study Investigators 2007) showed better outcome with normal saline than with 4% hypotonic albumin, while other smaller studies have all indicated beneficial effects with albumin (Tomita et al. 1994; Dubois et al. 2006; Bernard et al. 2008; Rodling Wahlström et al. 2009; Jungner et al. 2010). A large recent study also showed that low serum albumin and prealbumin predict a significantly worse outcome of traumatic brain injury (Chen et al. 2014). The SAFE-TBI study has resulted in more frequent use of normal saline and other crystalloids and much less frequent use of albumin during the last few years in many neurointensive care units all over the world.

Traditional guidelines such as the American Guidelines or the European Brain Injury Consortium guidelines—in their original or updated versions for treatment of TBI—do not suggest any strategies for fluid management (Bullock et al. 1996; Maas et al. 1997; Stocchetti et al. 2001; The Brain Trauma Foundation 2007; 2016). Thus, no consensus about the type of fluid substitution, which volumes and infusion rates to use, or which concentration of albumin solution to use for an optimal fluid treatment, has been developed. We also lack studies and recommendations about the optimal haemoglobin concentration in patients with severe TBI, an issue of importance not only regarding oxygenation of the brain, but also regarding maintaining of an adequate blood volume, as erythrocytes comprise a large proportion of the blood volume. This is of added importance at a time where restraints, due to the risk of transfusion with contaminated blood, give rise to strict local criteria for blood transfusion. The two main plasma volume-expanding alternatives used today, crystalloids and albumin, in combination with their most important physiological features have been described above.

The unexpected results from the SAFE-TBI study may indicate that normal saline is a better choice than 4% albumin as plasma volume expander in TBI patients. The SAFE-TBI study has been criticised, however, for several reasons (Drummond et al. 2011; Van Aken et al. 2012). It was a subgroup study of 350 patients selected from a much larger study with 7000 general intensive care patients not designed to identify how human albumin affects outcome in patients with TBI. The SAFE-TBI study has been criticised because of this and the fact that subgroup analyses are always doubtful from a statistical point of view, especially if the groups differ at baseline. This was also the case in the SAFE-TBI study regarding baseline ICP and number of older patients, both differences negative for the albumin group. More important, however, was that they used a hypotonic human albumin solution of 250 mosm/kg compared with normal plasma osmolarity of 290 mosm/kg. Hypotonic solutions are contraindicated in TBI patients due to the risk of brain oedema development. Van Aker and co-workers (Van Aken et al. 2012) even declared that the albumin compound was not the deleterious factor in the SAFE-TBI study, but that it just confirmed that hypotonic solutions are deleterious in TBI patients. Considering the critic raised and the unexpected results of the SAFE-TBI study, it is reasonable to conclude that this study alone cannot be used to question the use of albumin in severely injured TBI patients. It was also concluded in a recent review that evidence from trials, no matter how impressive, should be interpreted with caution when only one trial is available (Ioannidis 2005). This statement is applicable to the SAFE-TBI study.

The fact that norepinephrine was used in high doses in the SAFE-TBI study to reach a CPP of above 70 mmHg may have been negative for outcome in the albumin group. It has been documented both experimentally and in patients that norepinephrine induces a significant loss of plasma proteins to the interstitium (Dubniks et al. 2007; Nygren et al. 2010). Increased loss of plasma by norepinephrine can be explained according to the two-pore theory for transcapillary exchange by an increase in hydrostatic capillary pressure and convection (Rippe and Haraldsson 1994). Especially for the albumin group, this may have resulted in extracranial complications in terms of general tissue oedema and ARDS (Contant et al. 2001; Grände 2008) and hypovolaemia. Thus, even though the SAFE-TBI study has been the only randomised study to be published so far regarding fluid therapy in TBI patients and to formally fulfil the demand for a Level II study, after critical evaluation, the results cannot be used for a general recommendation of avoiding albumin and using only normal saline or other crystalloids as plasma volume expander.

With the lack of recommendations in conventional guidelines on how to treat patients with severe TBI regarding plasma volume substitution, this chapter has described the two main alternatives used in clinical practice today: (1) a fluid regime using mainly crystalloids as recommended by the SAFE-TBI study and (2) an alternative regimen based on physiological and pathophysiological principles for transcapillary fluid exchange using albumin as colloid combined with crystalloids. In principle, the latter regimen agrees with that suggested in the Lund concept for treatment of severe TBI patients (Grände 2006, 2017), which is described in another chapter of this book (Chap. 55). This regimen recommends 1–1.5 L of an isotonic crystalloid combined with albumin 20% up to 33 g/L and normovolaemia. Synthetic colloids such as HES solutions and gelatin have previously been given as plasma volume expanders in TBI patients in Europe, but no human trials have been published giving support on TBI patients. A recent study also showed in a general intensive care material that HES solutions may cause renal insufficiency. Gelatin consists of small molecules and behaves more or less like a crystalloid. Synthetic fluids therefore should not be used in head-injured patients.

References

Bark BP, Grände PO. Infusion rate and plasma volume expansion of dextran and albumin in the septic guinea pig. Acta Anaesthesiol Scand. 2014;58:44–51. https://doi.org/10.1111/aas.12228.

Bentzer P, Grände PO. Isolated brain trauma in cats triggers rapid onset of hypovolemia. Neurocrit Care. 2017;26:450–6. https://doi.org/10.1007/s12028-016-0348-5.

Bernard F, Al-Tamimi YZ, Chatfield D, Lynch AG, Matta BF, Menon DK. Serum albumin level as a predictor of outcome in traumatic brain injury: potential for treatment. J Trauma. 2008;64(4):872–5.

Bilgin YM, van Watering LMG, Brand A. Clinical effects of leucoreduction of blood transfusions. Neth J Med. 2011;69:441–5.

Bullock R, Chesnut RM, Clifton G, Ghajar J, Marion DW, Narayan RK, Newell DW, Pitts LH, Rosner MJ, Wiberger JW. Guidelines for the management of severe head injury. Brain Trauma Foundation. Eur J Emerg Med. 1996;3(2):109–27.

Chen D, Bao L, Lu S, Xu F. Serum albumin and prealbumin predict the poor outcome of traumatic brain injury. PLoS One. 2014;9(3):1–7.

Contant CF, Valadka AB, Gopinath SP, Hannay HJ, Robertson CS. Adult respiratory distress syndrome: a complication of induced hypertension after severe head injury. J Neurosurg. 2001;95(4):560–8. https://doi.org/10.3171/jns.2001.95.4.0560.

Dhar R, Zazulia AR, Videen TO, Zipfel GJ, Derdeyn CP, Diringer MN. Red blood cell transfusion increases cerebral oxygen delivery in anemic patients with subarachnoid hemorrhage. Stroke. 2009;40(9):3039–44.

Drummond JC, Patel P, Lemkull B. Proscribing the use of albumin in the head-injured patient is not warranted. Anesth Analg. 2011;113:426–7. https://doi.org/10.1213/ANE.0b013e31821ed699.

Dubniks M, Persson J, Grände PO. Effect of blood pressure on plasma volume loss in the rat under increased permeability. Intensive Care Med. 2007;33(12):2192–8.

Dubois MJ, Orellana-Jimenez C, Melot C, De Backer D, Berre J, Leeman M, Brimioulle S, Appoloni O, Creteur J, Vincent JL. Albumin administration improves organ function in critically ill hypoalbuminemic patients: a prospective, randomized, controlled, pilot study. Crit Care Med. 2006;34:2536–40.

Grände PO. The "Lund Concept" for the treatment of severe head trauma – physiological principles and clinical application. Intensive Care Med. 2006;32(10):1475–84.

Grände PO. Time out for albumin or a valuable therapeutic component in severe head injury? Acta Anaesthesiol Scand. 2008;52(6):738–41.

Grände PO. Critical evaluation of the Lund concept for treatment of severe traumatic head injury, 25 years after its introduction. Front Neurol. 2017. https://doi.org/10.3389/fneur.2017.00315.

Haskell A, Nadel ER, Stachenfeld NS, Nagashima K, Mack GW. Transcapillary escape rate of albumin in humans during exercise-induced hypervolemia. J Appl Physiol. 1997;83(2):407–13.

Hébert PC, Wells G, Blajchman MA, Marshal J, Martin C, Pagliarello G, Tweeddale M, Schweitzer I, Yetisir E. A multicenter, randomized, controlled clinical trial of transfusion requirements in critical care. Transfusion Requirements in Critical Care Investigators, Canadian Critical Care Trials Group. N Engl J Med. 1999;340(6):409–17.

Ioannidis JP. Contradicted and initially stronger effects in highly cited clinical research. JAMA. 2005;294:218–28. https://doi.org/10.1001/jama.294.2.218.

Jungner M, Grände PO, Mattiasson G, Bentzer P. Effects on brain edema of crystalloid and albumin fluid resuscitation after brain trauma and hemorrhage in the rat. Anesthesiology. 2010;112(5):1194–203.

Maas AI, Dearden M, Teasdale GM, Braakman R, Chadon F, Iannotti F, Karimi A, Lapierre F, Stochetti N, Unterberg A. EBIC-guidelines for management of severe head injury in adults. European Brain Injury Consortium. Acta Neurochir. 1997;139(4):286–94.

Naidech AM, Jovanovic B, Wartenberg KE, Parra A, Ostapkovich N, Cinnolly ES, Mayer SA, Commichau C. Higher hemoglobin is associated with improved outcome after subarachnoid hemorrhage. Crit Care Med. 2007;35(10):2383–9.

Nygren A, Redfors B, Thorén A, Ricksten SE. Norepinephrine causes a pressure-dependent plasma volume decrease in clinical vasodilatory shock. Acta Anaesthesiol Scand. 2010;54(7):814–20.

Rippe B, Haraldsson B. Transport of macromolecules across microvascular walls: the two-pore theory. Physiol Rev. 1994;74(1):163–219.

Rise IR, Risöe C, Kirkeby O. Cerebrovascular effects of high intracranial pressure after moderate hemorrhage. J Neurosurg Anesthesiol. 1998;10(4):224–30.

Rodling Wahlström M, Olivecrona M, Nyström F, Koskinen LO, Naredi S. Fluid therapy and the use of albumin in the treatment of severe traumatic brain injury. Acta Anaesthesiol Scand. 2009;53(1):18–25.

Smith M, Stiefel MF, Magge S, Frangos S, Bloom S, Gracias V, Le Roux PD. Packed red blood cell transfusion increases local cerebral oxygenation. Crit Care Med. 2005;33(5):1104–8.

Stocchetti N, Penny KI, Dearden M, Braakman R, Cohadon F, Iannotti F, Lapierre F, Karimi A, Maas A, Murray GD, Ohman J, Persson L, Servadei F, Teasdale GM, Trojanowski T, Unterberg A, European

Brain Injury Consortium. Intensive care management of head-injured patients in Europe: a survey from the European brain injury consortium. Intensive Care Med. 2001;27(2):400–6.

The Brain Trauma Foundation. The American Association of Neurological Surgeons; Congress of Neurological Surgeons. Guidelines for the management of severe traumatic brain injury 3rd edition. J Neurotrauma. 2007;24(Suppl 1):S1–106.

The Brain Trauma Foundation. The American Association of Neurological Surgeons; Congress of Neurological Surgeons. Guidelines for management of severe traumatic brain injury 4th edition. J Neurosurg. 2016;354(6314):893–6.

The SAFE Study Investigators. Saline or albumin for fluid resuscitation in patients with traumatic brain injury. N Engl J Med. 2007;357:874–84.

Tomita H, Ito U, Tone O, Masaoka H, Tominaga B. High colloid oncotic therapy for contusional brain edema. Acta Neurochir Suppl (Wien). 1994;60:547–9.

Valeri CR, Donahue K, Feingold HM, Cassidy GP, Altschule MD. Increase in plasma volume after the transfusion of washed erythrocytes. Surg Gynecol Obstet. 1986;162(1):30–6.

Van Aken HK, Kampmeier TG, Ertmer C, Westphal M. Fluid resuscitation in patients with traumatic brain injury: what is a SAFE approach? Curr Opin Anaesthesiol. 2012;25:563–5. https://doi.org/10.1097/ACO.0b013e3283572274.

Zygun DA, Nortje J, Hutchinson PJ, Timofeev I, Menon DK, Gupta AK. The effect of red blood cell transfusion on cerebral oxygenation and metabolism after severe traumatic brain injury. Crit Care Med. 2009;37:1074–8.

64 Sedation: Including Pain Treatment and Withdrawal Symptoms

Geir Olav Dahle

Recommendations

Level I

There are insufficient data to support a Level I recommendation for sedation and analgesia.

Level II

Prophylactic use of barbiturates to the level of burst suppression on EEG is not recommended. Barbiturate administration to control elevated ICP can be used, but careful control of hemodynamic stability and pulmonary side effects is essential during barbiturate therapy. Propofol can be used for the control of ICP, but high-dose propofol can be associated with significant morbidity.

Level III

When barbiturates and propofol are used, normovolemia must be maintained in order to avoid hypotension. To minimize the risk for the propofol infusion syndrome, the maximum dose of propofol administered should be below 4 mg/kg/h, and caution must be taken when propofol infusion exceeds 48 h, especially in children.

Tips, Tricks, and Pitfalls

- A strategy to reduce the incidence of withdrawal symptoms is to gradually reduce drug doses.
- In trauma emergency situations, ketamine is probably safe to use.

64.1 Overview

Several different sedative and analgesic agents have been used for sedation and analgesia in severe TBI (Table 64.1). Treatment of pain and avoidance of stress and agitation with the help of sedatives and analgesics could theoretically help to keep ICP within acceptable levels. Sedation and analgesia may thus be beneficial. However, sedation with long-acting sedative drugs makes it difficult to perform repeated neurological exams (wake-up tests). All sedative agents have adverse hemodynamic effects. The scientific evidence for the effect of sedation and analgesia in patients with severe TBI has been lacking. In the last two guideline editions from the Brain Trauma Foundation from 2007 and 2017, a chapter on "Anesthetics, Analgesics, and Sedatives" has been added, but they contain relatively few recommendations based on high quality evidence (Carney et al. 2017).

G. O. Dahle (✉)
Department of Anaesthesia and Intensive Care, Haukeland University Hospital, Bergen, Norway
e-mail: geir.olav.dahle@helse-bergen.no

© Springer Nature Switzerland AG 2020
T. Sundstrøm et al. (eds.), *Management of Severe Traumatic Brain Injury*,
https://doi.org/10.1007/978-3-030-39383-0_64

Table 64.1 Effects of commonly employed anesthetics/analgesics in patients with severe traumatic brain injury

Anesthetic/analgesic agent	Cerebral metabolism	ICP	Adverse effects	Comments
Propofol	⇓	⇔ (⇓)	Hypotension propofol infusion syndrome	Maintain normovolemia <4 mg/kg/h
Midazolam	⇓	⇔		Long duration
Barbiturates	⇓	⇓	Hypotension	Maintain normovolemia Monitor with EEG
Ketamine	⇔	⇔		Hemodynamic stability Limited data available in severe TBI
Dexmedetomidine		⇔ (⇓)	Hypotension Bradycardia	Limited data available in severe TBI Maintains arousal
Opioids	⇔	⇔ (⇑)	Hypotension	Maintain normovolemia Continuous infusion

64.2 Background

Administration of sedatives and analgesics is necessary for stress reduction in the treatment of severe TBI. The scientific evidence regarding which drugs to use is scarce, and all available drugs used have their pros and cons. Specific concern should be taken when using propofol for longer periods of time and in high doses, due to the propofol infusion syndrome (PRIS).

64.2.1 Propofol

Propofol is extensively used for sedation in critically ill patients, including patients with severe TBI. The drug has a rapid onset and short duration, which makes it possible to examine a patient neurologically short after termination of infusion (wake-up tests). In experimental studies, propofol has been shown to reduce cerebral metabolism, and in clinical studies, it has maintained or decreased ICP. Propofol can cause hypotension, and careful titration is therefore needed in hemodynamically unstable or hypovolemic patients (Carney et al. 2017; Flower and Hellings 2012; Oddo et al. 2016).

Although propofol has been administered safely in millions of patients during the last three decades, some patients, both children and adults, develop the propofol infusion syndrome. This syndrome includes adverse effects with myocardial failure, lactic acidosis, hyperkalemia, rhabdomyolysis, lipemia, and acute renal failure and is often fatal in reported cases. In a recent structured review of experimental studies and 153 case reports, TBI was associated with increased risk for development of PRIS together with high and prolonged duration of propofol treatment and development of fever (Krajcova et al. 2015). To avoid PRIS, a maximum infusion rate of 4 mg/kg/h in patients with severe TBI is recommended. Caution is also warranted when propofol infusion exceeds 48 h. If lactic acidosis develops or the need for inotropic support increases, in the absence of obvious reasons, propofol should be discontinued (Carney et al. 2017; Oddo et al. 2016; Otterspoor et al. 2008).

64.2.2 Midazolam

Midazolam is commonly used for sedation in neurosurgical intensive care units. The drug has minimal cardiovascular effects, at least in the normovolemic patient. Since midazolam has a high volume of distribution, it will accumulate continuous infusion for a prolonged period of time. This results in substantially prolonged sedation and subsequent difficult assessment of patients after termination of infusion. Midazolam reduces cerebral metabolism and blood flow, but in a more variable fashion compared to propofol. This may be because it is more difficult to achieve burst suppression with benzodiazepines. Even though some studies indicate more ICP reduction with propofol, meta-analyses still have not shown different outcome nor intracerebral pressure control between management with midazolam and propofol sedation in patients with TBI. More sufficiently powered studies are still needed (Gu et al. 2014; Oddo et al. 2016; DJ Roberts et al. 2011).

64.2.3 Barbiturates

Historically, barbiturates have been used as sedative agents in TBI. However, because of more severe side effect than alternative sedative agents, barbiturates are nowadays reserved for anesthesia induction, for treatment of refractory elevated ICP, and for treatment of status epilepticus. Current guidelines from the Brain Trauma Foundation restrict the recommendation of high-dose barbiturates to the treatment of elevated ICP refractory to other treatment, including appropriate sedation with other drugs (Carney et al. 2017). Barbiturates are believed to decrease ICP by the coupling of decreased cerebral metabolic demands to reduced cerebral blood flow, thus reducing cerebral blood volume and intracranial pressure. In a systematic review updated in 2012, the Cochrane Injuries Group concluded that there is no evidence supporting improved outcome with barbiturate therapy in patients with severe TBI based on data from six trials (Roberts and Sydenham 2012). The lack of effect could be due to hypotensive effects induced by the barbiturates, especially in hypovolemic patients, abolishing the positive effect which lowered ICP could have on the cerebral perfusion pressure. When barbiturates are used, caution must therefore be taken to maintain normovolemia in order to avoid hypotension. High-dose barbiturates may also trigger the development of ARDS (Ellens et al. 2015). Barbiturate therapy should preferably be monitored by continuous electroencephalography in order to titrate the lowest possible dose (Carney et al. 2017; Flower and Hellings 2012).

64.2.4 Ketamine

Ketamine is a short-acting N-methyl-D-aspartate (NMDA) receptor antagonist with rapid onset of action associated with better hemodynamic stability than other sedatives. Traditionally, ketamine was withheld in patients with TBI as early studies indicated it being associated with an increase in ICP. However, ketamine is becoming more accepted for use in TBI after more recent studies have not managed to confirm this association in children nor adults (Zeiler et al. 2014). Lately, ketamine also has received increased attention, as it may exhibit neuroprotective properties with greater restriction of cortical spreading depolarization compared to other sedatives, including midazolam and propofol during TBI, subarachnoid hemorrhage, and malignant stroke (Hertle et al. 2012).

64.2.5 α_2-Agonists

Dexmedetomidine is an α_2-agonist commonly used as a sedative in intensive care units. It produces a unique sedation that maintains arousal despite deep level of sedation. Dexmedetomidine causes minimal respiratory depression, has opioid-sparing effects, and may reduce delirium. Lately, the drug has been proposed for sedation in TBI patients. Studies have shown comparable effects to propofol with regard to sedation (Erdman et al. 2014; Humble et al. 2016). However, it has also been associated with hypotension, which may have negative consequences for cerebral perfusion in TBI (Pajoumand et al. 2016). Today, there is not enough evidence to recommend the use of dexmedetomidine for the sedation of TBI patients.

Alpha$_2$-agonists may also be used in combination with sedatives and analgesics for stress reduction in severe TBI. This therapeutic approach is used in the "Lund concept," where clonidine is used for two purposes: reduction of systolic blood pressure and reduction of stress response. Dexmedetomidine may however be a better choice than clonidine, as it is more selective and thus less prone to α_1-mediated vasoconstriction (Grände 2017).

64.2.6 Analgesics

The most commonly used analgesics in patients with severe TBI have been opioid agonists. Morphine is the most extensively used, but fentanyl, sufentanil, alfentanil, and remifentanil are also used. The choice of opioid agonist often relies on the clinical situation. If steady sedation with control of ICP and minimal reaction to stimuli is needed, a moderate to long-lasting opioid agonist, i.e. morphine, may be appropriate. Otherwise, the need of early neurological assessment may require a shorter-acting opioid agonist, i.e. remifentanil (Flower and Hellings 2012; Karabinis et al. 2004; Oddo et al. 2016).

Studies have shown an increase in ICP and a decrease in MAP after bolus doses of opioid agonists. The underlying mechanism of opioid effects on ICP is not evaluated in detail. Opioids may induce histamine release, leading to a decrease in cerebral vascular resistance and a fall in systemic blood pressure. Elevation of ICP by opioid agonists could also be caused by a compensatory autoregulatory cerebral vasodilation following a decrease in MAP. To avoid a reduction in MAP and in order to use opioid agonists safely, patients with a severe TBI should always be kept normovolemic, and it may be better to administer analgesics in continuous infusion instead of giving bolus injections (Albanese et al. 1999; Flower and Hellings 2012; Roberts et al. 2011).

64.2.7 Withdrawal

Opioid and benzodiazepine administration for a longer period of time (>5–7 days) increases the risk of abstinence symptoms after termination of the drugs. The risk of withdrawal abstinence increases with abrupt termination or rapid tapering. Prevention and management of withdrawal symptoms are important in that it can aggravate patient distress. One strategy to reduce the incidence of withdrawal symptoms has been weaning the drugs slowly over several days. Also, utilization of α_2-agonists (clonidine, dexmedetomidine) for avoidance of withdrawal symptoms is used. Evidence is somewhat limited but growing. Consensus regarding the best strategy to avoid drug withdrawal symptoms in critically ill patients is lacking (Awissi et al. 2013; Barr et al. 2013; Devlin et al. 2010).

64.3 Specific Pediatric Concerns

Children seem to be overrepresented among the reported cases of propofol infusion syndrome. This could be due to their lower glycogen stores and higher dependency on fat metabolism (Kam and Cardone 2007; Krajcova et al. 2015; Otterspoor et al. 2008). Administration of benzodiazepines and/or opioids for sedation in critically ill children may induce withdrawal symptoms after termination of the drugs. To reduce the incidence of withdrawal symptoms, the total doses of benzodiazepines and/or opioids administered should be kept as low as possible to control ICP. A daily tapering rate of 10–20% has been recommended in several studies; however, this strategy did not result in total absence of withdrawal symptoms (Ista et al. 2007). The European Society of Paediatric and Neonatal Intensive Care recommends the use of standardized iatrogenic withdrawal syndrome assessment instruments (i.e., WAT-1 or SOS) during tapering of sedation with opioids or benzodiazepines (Harris et al. 2016).

References

Albanese J, et al. Sufentanil, fentanyl, and alfentanil in head trauma patients: a study on cerebral hemodynamics. Crit Care Med. 1999;27(2):407–11.

Awissi DK, et al. Alcohol, nicotine, and iatrogenic withdrawals in the ICU. Crit Care Med. 2013;41(9 Suppl 1):S57–68.

Barr J, et al. Clinical practice guidelines for the management of pain, agitation, and delirium in adult patients in the intensive care unit. Crit Care Med. 2013;41(1):263–306.

Carney N, et al. Guidelines for the management of severe traumatic brain injury, fourth edition. Neurosurgery. 2017;80(1):6–15.

Devlin JW, et al. Adverse drug events associated with the use of analgesics, sedatives, and antipsychotics in the intensive care unit. Crit Care Med. 2010;38(6 Suppl):S231–43.

Ellens NR, Figuera BE, Clarc JC. The use of barbiturate-induced coma during cerebrovascular neurosurgical procedures A review of the literature. Brain Circ. 2015;1:140–5.

Erdman MJ, et al. A comparison of severe hemodynamic disturbances between dexmedetomidine and propofol for sedation in neurocritical care patients. Crit Care Med. 2014;42(7):1696–702.

Flower O, Hellings S. Sedation in traumatic brain injury. Emerg Med Int. 2012;2012:637171.

Grände PO. Critical evaluation of the lund concept for treatment of severe traumatic head injury, 25 years after its introduction. Front Neurol. 2017;8:315.

Gu JW, et al. Comparison of the safety and efficacy of propofol with midazolam for sedation of patients with severe traumatic brain injury: a meta-analysis. J Crit Care. 2014;29(2):287–90.

Harris J, et al. Clinical recommendations for pain, sedation, withdrawal and delirium assessment in critically ill infants and children: an ESPNIC position statement for healthcare professionals. Intensive Care Med. 2016;42(6):972–86.

Hertle DN, et al. Effect of analgesics and sedatives on the occurrence of spreading depolarizations accompanying acute brain injury. Brain. 2012;135(Pt 8):2390–8.

Humble SS, et al. ICU sedation with dexmedetomidine after severe traumatic brain injury. Brain Inj. 2016;30(10):1266–70.

Ista E, et al. Withdrawal symptoms in children after long-term administration of sedatives and/or analgesics: a literature review. "Assessment remains troublesome". Intensive Care Med. 2007;33(8):1396–406.

Kam PC, Cardone D. Propofol infusion syndrome. Anaesthesia. 2007;62(7):690–701.

Karabinis A, et al. Safety and efficacy of analgesia-based sedation with remifentanil versus standard hypnotic-based regimens in intensive care unit patients with brain injuries: a randomised, controlled trial [ISRCTN50308308]. Crit Care. 2004;8(4):R268–80.

Krajcova A, et al. Propofol infusion syndrome: a structured review of experimental studies and 153 published case reports. Crit Care. 2015;19:398.

Oddo M, et al. Optimizing sedation in patients with acute brain injury. Crit Care. 2016;20(1):128.

Otterspoor LC, et al. Update on the propofol infusion syndrome in ICU management of patients with head injury. Curr Opin Anaesthesiol. 2008;21(5):544–51.

Pajoumand M, et al. Dexmedetomidine as an adjunct for sedation in patients with traumatic brain injury. J Trauma Acute Care Surg. 2016;81(2):345–51.

Roberts I, Sydenham E. Barbiturates for acute traumatic brain injury. Cochrane Database Syst Rev. 2012;12:Cd000033.

Roberts DJ, et al. Sedation for critically ill adults with severe traumatic brain injury: a systematic review of randomized controlled trials. Crit Care Med. 2011;39(12):2743–51.

Zeiler FA, et al. The ketamine effect on ICP in traumatic brain injury. Neurocrit Care. 2014;21(1):163–73.

65 Nutrition

Anne Berit Guttormsen, Bram Johan de Hoog, and Jennie Witte Hernæs

Recommendations

Level I

Additional parenteral nutrition (PN) should be avoided in patients who tolerate enteral nutrition (EN) to target energy intake.

There are insufficient data to support Level I recommendation for when to start artificial nutrition, the preferable route of feeding (enteral (EN) or parenteral (PN)), the energy and protein requirements and the level of blood sugar in patients with severe traumatic brain injury (TBI).

Level II

There is Level II evidence supporting that starting tailored nutrition early improves outcome in intensive care patients. Both hypocaloric nutrition and hypercaloric nutrition seem harmful.

Level III

Evaluation of nutritional status, i.e. body weight, height, weight loss and food intake, the last week before admission is recommended. Continuous infusion of insulin is feasible to control blood sugar in the intensive care setting. Both hypoglycaemia and hyperglycaemia are deleterious in patients with TBI. The suggested target range for blood sugar is 6–9 mmol/L.

65.1 Overview

Individual nutritional support is an important component in patient care and might contribute to better outcome and optimal rehabilitation (Singer et al. 2011; Carney et al. 2017). Hyperglycaemia is associated with worse outcome, and serum glucose of 6–9 mmol/L seems optimal (Béchir et al. 2010; Meierhans et al. 2010; Kansagara et al. 2011).

In the acute phase, nutrition is the third priority after stabilisation of vital functions (ventilation, haemodynamics) and intracranial pressure. Enteral nutrition (EN) is preferred and should be initiated within 24–48 h after the injury. EN should be supplied through a soft tube through the mouth (only if the patient is

A. B. Guttormsen (✉)
Department of Anaesthesia and Intensive Care, Haukeland University Hospital, Bergen, Norway

Department of Clinical Medicine, University of Bergen, Bergen, Norway
e-mail: anne.guttormsen@helse-bergen.no

B. J. de Hoog
Department of Anaesthesia and Intensive Care, Haukeland University Hospital, Bergen, Norway
e-mail: bram.johan.de.hoog@helse-bergen.no

J. W. Hernæs
Eating Disorders Unit, Skaraborgs Hospital, Skövde, Sweden
e-mail: Jennie.witte.hernaes@vgregion.se

© Springer Nature Switzerland AG 2020
T. Sundstrøm et al. (eds.), *Management of Severe Traumatic Brain Injury*, https://doi.org/10.1007/978-3-030-39383-0_65

on a ventilator) or nasal cavity to the stomach. In the rehabilitation phase, percutaneous enteral gastrostomy (PEG) may be the preferable route. The technique is debatable and has complications (Kurien et al. 2010). If less than 1500 kcal (1500 mL) is administered, EN needs to be supplemented with vitamins and micronutrients to cover basal requirements. To increase energy intake, a concentrated EN formula may be used, i.e. 1.5–2 kcal/mL. In a recent publication performed in Australian and New Zealand intensive care units, higher energy intake given as an energy dense solution did not affect survival in a general ICU population (Chapman et al. 2018). EN containing fibre may be used to normalise bowel function, especially in the rehabilitation phase. There are possible interactions between continuous EN and peroral medications. Be aware that concomitant administration of EN might diminish or delay absorption of phenytoin (Cook et al. 2008).

Table 65.1 Nutrition guideline

TBI patients that cannot eat should start artificial nutrition
If there are no contraindications for EN, insert a gastric feeding tube and start EN within 24–48 h
Measure (indirect calorimetry) or estimate EE (25–50 kcal/kg/24 h, dependent on days after injury). Repeat at regular intervals, preferably every week in unstable patients
Use a feeding protocol to increase and monitor EN
If EE cannot be measured, increase EN to 70% of target in the first week. PN may be added if energy target is not reached after 5–7 days
Use small bowel feeding when gastric retention prevents full EN
Assess protein requirement and loss once to twice weekly in intensive care until nitrogen balance is achieved
Stable patients who can feed themselves should be assessed regularly for malnutrition with a screening tool (Kondrup et al. 2003)
Fortify ordinary food and give ONS, EN or PN if needed. Measure body weight at least once a week

ONS oral nutritional supplements in the form of liquid sip feeds, bars, puddings and powders, *EN* enteral nutrition, *PN* parenteral nutrition

Parenteral nutrition (PN) might be added if nutritional needs are not gained within 3–7 days (Singer et al. 2018). However, the EPaNIC study (Casaer et al. 2011), comparing early (24–48 h) and late (8 days) PN in critically ill patients, has questioned early initiation of PN if EN fails. Several studies point out that about 80% of targeted energy should be provided in the ICU setting (Singer et al. 2011). In the intensive care phase, most TBI patients have a multi-lumen central venous catheter. One of the lumens should be dedicated to i.v. nutrition if PN is needed. PN with lower osmolality can be supplied via a peripheral line for a shorter period of time, i.e. 2–3 days. The line should be inspected at least once a day and changed on clinical indication rather than routinely (Webster et al. 2015). PN is most conveniently administered from three-chamber bags comprising glucose, fat and amino acids. These solutions contain 1 kcal/mL solution; the content of glucose, fat and amino acids differs between manufacturers. Bags for peripheral administration contain <1 kcal/mL, i.e. administered volume must be higher to reach energy target.

Energy supply should be tailored. Stress metabolism is unpredictable, and therefore energy demand is best measured with indirect calorimetry (Cook et al. 2008; Rattanachaiwong and Singer 2018). Although recommended, few departments use indirect calorimetry because the equipment is expensive and the technique is cumbersome. If the ventilator has volumetric measurement of end-tidal CO_2, this measure can be used to estimate energy expenditure (Stapel et al. 2015). Overfeeding is harmful (Griffiths 2007; Turner 2010; Casaer et al. 2011) due to increased metabolism, excessive CO_2 and heat production and a risk that body temperature will increase. These metabolic changes might increase ICP (dilatation of brain arteries), especially in patients that are not on a ventilator.

The following basal needs can be used when calculating energy and nutrient requirements, but individual adaptations must be considered.

Catabolic state (early)	25 kcal/kg/24 h
Anabolic state (late)	30–50 kcal/kg/24 h[a]
Glucose requirements	
Glucose	2–3 g/kg/24 h
Lipid requirements	
Lipid	0.5–2 g/kg/24 h
Protein requirements	
Protein (nitrogen)	1–1.5 g/kg/24 t (~0.16–0.24 g N/kg/24 h)
Electrolyte requirements	
Sodium	1–1.4 mmol/kg/24 h (might be considerably higher in salt-wasting conditions)
Potassium	0.7–0.9 mmol/kg/24 h
Phosphate	0.15–0.30 mmol/kg/24 h
Magnesium	0.04 mmol/kg/24 h
Calcium	0.11 mmol/kg/24 h

[a]The highest energy supply during rehabilitation. In the rehabilitation phase body weight should guide energy supply

65.1.1 Fluid Requirements

The supplement of fluid is an integrated part of nutritional support. The basal requirement of fluid is approximately 30 mL/kg/24 h, and the administered volume has to be adjusted according to the clinical situation.

Tips, Tricks and Pitfalls

- *Ordinary food and oral nutritional supplements*
  - If the patient is able to drink and/or eat, he/she should be encouraged to do so. Measure food intake.
- *Enteral nutrition*
  - Start EN with 20 mL/h of a standard solution (1.0 kcal/mL). Increase with 10–20 mL every 8 h while monitoring gastric retention. Modest increase in delivery may prevent diarrhoea.
  - In patients with gastric retention, a motility agent can be added like erythromycin (200 mg × 2–3/day) over a period of maximal 3 days.
  - In case of gastrointestinal paresis due to opioids, use peripherally functioning antagonists: naloxone 3–6 mg × 3 orally or parenteral methylnaltrexone.
  - In failed enteral nutrition, also treat constipation.
  - If motility agents do not solve gastric retention, the feeding tube can be positioned in the small bowel.
  - If need for EN for more than 2–4 weeks, PEG might be the preferred route.
- *Parenteral nutrition*
  - During administration of PN, a central venous access is preferable.
  - Daily requirements should be administered by three-chamber bags. Trace elements and micronutrients (water-soluble and fat-soluble vitamins) must be added.
- *Amount of energy*
  - In the rehabilitation phase, body weight should be measured one to two times a week.
  - Stable body weight, or slowly increased body weight, hints that energy supply is sufficient. Be aware that oedema will also increase body weight.

65.2 Background

After TBI, dysphagia are common, leading to malnutrition, dehydration and aspiration pneumonia. TBI induces a hypermetabolic response mediated by cytokines, other inflammatory mediators, hormones (norepinephrine, epinephrine, ACTH and cortisol, growth hormone, prolactin and vasopressin) and endorphins (Cook et al. 2008).

Concomitant production of glucose coupled with insulin resistance leads to hyperglycaemia.

Due to a hypermetabolic response, resting energy expenditure (REE) might be increased compared with estimates done according to the Harris-Benedict formula (Frankenfield et al. 2007). There is an inverse relationship between Glasgow Coma Scale score and REE. Energy requirement is difficult to predict because many factors influence metabolism. Muscle relaxants, mechanical ventilation, opioids and sedation all reduce REE. Agitation, seizures, increased body temperature and catecholamines increase metabolism.

EN is preferred if tolerated (Lochs et al. 2006; Singer et al. 2018). However, failed enteral feeding because of high gastric residual volume is a common problem in critically ill patients (Fraser and Bryant 2010). Prokinetic drugs can enhance gastric motility. Metoclopramide 10 mg q 3–4/day is used in general intensive care patients, but may not be effective in TBI patients. Erythromycin is a motilin agonist. Its use as prokinetic to achieve nutritional goals may be equivalent to small bowel feeding in the short term (Boivin and Levy 2001). There are resistance issues with erythromycin, and it is not efficient with prolonged use (Nguyen et al. 2007). Combining both agents has better results with prolonged feeding (Fraser and Bryant 2010). There are no studies on the effect of methylnaltrexone on opioid-induced constipation in TBI patients. Small bowel feeding is recommended if gastric feeding is still unsuccessful despite motility agents. It may also reduce the incidence of ventilator-associated pneumonia in patients at risk (Heyland et al. 2003).

PN is indicated in heavily sedated patients (barbiturate coma) due to gastric retention and GI paralyses, or if EN does not reach nutritional requirements. Close monitoring of electrolytes (sodium, potassium and phosphate), acid-base balance, blood glucose, liver status and triglycerides are important during the critical care phase of injury.

In TBI patients, standard equations for estimating energy demand, such as Harris-Benedict, Mifflin-St-Jeor and Ireton-Jones (Frankenfield et al. 2007), are inaccurate, and indirect calorimetry should be used if available. Patients with severe TBI can lose 10–15% of lean body mass in one week if nutritional intervention is not started. Tailored energy intake probably improves outcome (Singer et al. 2011).

During intensive care, patients with TBI might have problems with fluid and electrolyte (primarily sodium) balance. It is therefore mandatory to closely monitor fluid balance, serum sodium and excretion of sodium in the urine to avoid hyponatraemia and hypovolaemia. Stress metabolism induces a catabolic state with gluconeogenesis and breakdown of skeletal muscle. Loss of nitrogen and muscle is high (>20 gN/24 h or >600 g of muscle tissue/24 h). Restoration of nitrogen balance is often not achieved until 2–3 weeks after injury. Protein requirements are a matter of debate in critically ill patients (Wolfe et al. 1983; Larsson et al. 1990; Ishibashi et al. 1998; Seron Arbeloa et al. 1999). There is scarce evidence supporting that amino acid infusion of more than 1.5 g/kg/day leads to a better nitrogen balance. It may instead lead to augmented urea production. Correcting nitrogen balance will not reverse the catabolic state (Clifton et al. 1986; Streat and Hill 1987; Young et al. 1987) but will lead to a positive nitrogen balance earlier (Twyman et al. 1985). Supplementation of amino acids is necessary to maintain protein syntheses. It is possible to calculate nitrogen balance in patients with normal renal function. To do so, 24-h urine is collected to measure urea excretion. Nitrogen supply = (protein intake (g))/6.25, and nitrogen loss = urine urea (mmol) times 0.028 + 4 g (correcting for non-urinary loss) (Sobotka 2004).

Studies on cerebral glucose level using microdialysis suggest that a blood glucose level between 6 and 9 mmol/L results in optimal cerebral glucose concentration in TBI patients. Insulin therapy started at blood glucose levels above 7 mmol/L had positive effect on cerebral metabolism (Béchir et al. 2010; Meierhans et al. 2010). Kansagara and collaborators (Kansagara et al. 2011) have performed a systematic review summarising available data from 1950 to 2010. They conclude that tight blood glucose control often causes hypoglycemia and that there is no consistent evidence that tight blood glucose control is better than a less strict glycemic control. Still, evidence is conflicting (Bilotta and Rosa 2012; Shi et al. 2016). ESPEN guidelines advocate a serum glucose level below 10 mmol/L (Singer et al. 2018). During intensive care, blood glucose is controlled with continuous infusion of insulin.

In TBI patients, serum zinc concentration declines due to sequestration in the liver and increased secretion in the urine. Zinc is a cofactor for substrate metabolism and is important for immune and NMDA receptor function (Cook et al. 2008). One study indicates that zinc supplementation in the immediate period after head injury is favourable, as the study group had improved neurologic recovery. Further, serum prealbumin concentrations were significantly higher in the zinc-supplemented group 3 weeks after injury, which might indicate better nutritional status (Young et al. 1996). Decreased food intake or insufficient nutritional support aggravates malnutrition and effects outcome. Despite this, it is important not to feed too much energy, eventually causing obesity, which has negative effects for the daily care of the patient. Support with artificial nutrition should decrease in line with increase in oral food intake, always making sure energy demands are met.

65.3 Specific Paediatric Concerns

There are not enough data to support a level I recommendation for how to perform nutritional support in paediatric patients with TBI. Energy and protein requirements per kg are increased, and guidelines (Carney et al. 2017; Malakouti et al. 2012) recommend supplementation of 130–160% of measured or calculated basal energy expenditure. There are few studies on the optimal route or timing of nutrition. However, one study found that hyperglycemia was an independent predictor for death and poor cerebral outcome in children (Cochran et al. 2003).

References

Béchir M, Meierhans R, Brandi G, Sommerfeld J, Fasshauer M, Cottini SR, Stocker R, Stover JF. Insulin differentially influences brain glucose and lactate in traumatic brain injured patients. Minerva Anestesiol. 2010;76:896–904.

Bilotta F, Rosa G. Optimal glycemic control in neurocritical care patients. Crit Care. 2012;16(5):163. https://doi.org/10.1186/cc11521.

Boivin MA, Levy H. Gastric feeding with erythromycin is equivalent to transpyloric feeding in the critically ill. Crit Care Med. 2001;29:1916–9.

Carney N, Totten AM, O'Reilly C, Ullman JS, Hawryluk GW, Bell MJ, Bratton SL, Chesnut R, Harris OA, Kissoon N, Rubiano AM, Shutter L, Tasker RC, Vavilala MS, Wilberger J, Wright DW, Ghajar J. Guidelines for the management of severe traumatic brain injury, fourth edition. Neurosurgery. 2017;1(80):6–15.

Casaer MP, Mesotten D, Hermans G, Wouters PJ, Schetz M, Meyfroidt G, Van Cromphaut S, Ingels C, Meersseman P, Muller J, Vlasselaers D, Debaveye Y, Desmet L, Dubois J, Van Assche A, Vanderheyden S, Wilmer A, Van den Berghe GN. Early versus late parenteral nutrition in critically ill adults. N Engl J Med. 2011;365(6):506–17.

Chapman M, Peake SL, Bellomo R, Davies A, Deane A, Horowitz M, Hurford S, Lange K, Little L, Mackle D, O'Connor S, Presneill J, Ridley E, Williams P, Young P, TARGET Investigators, for the ANZICS Clinical Trials Group. Energy-dense versus routine enteral nutrition in the critically ill. N Engl J Med. 2018;379(19):1823–34. https://doi.org/10.1056/NEJMoa1811687.

Clifton GL, Robertson CS, Choi SC. Assessment of nutritional requirements of head-injured patients. J Neurosurg. 1986;64:895–0.

Cochran A, Scaife ER, Hansen KW, Downey EC. Hyperglycemia and outcomes from pediatric traumatic brain injury. J Trauma. 2003;55:1035–8.

Cook AM, Peppard A, Magnuson B. Nutrition considerations in traumatic brain injury. Nutr Clin Pract. 2008;23:608–20.

Frankenfield D, Hise M, Malone A, Russell M, Gradwell E, Compher C. Prediction of resting metabolic rate in critically ill adult patients: results of a systematic review of the evidence. J Am Diet Assoc. 2007;107:1552–61.

Fraser RJ, Bryant L. Current and future therapeutic prokinetic therapy to improve enteral feed intolerance in the ICU patient. Nutr Clin Pract. 2010;25:26–31.

Griffiths RD. Too much of a good thing: the curse of overfeeding. Crit Care. 2007;11:176.

Heyland DK, Dhaliwal R, Drover JW, Gramlich L, Dodek P. Canadian clinical practice guidelines for nutrition support in mechanically ventilated, critically ill adult patients. JPEN J Parenter Enteral Nutr. 2003;27:355–73.

Ishibashi N, Plank LD, Sando K, Hill GL. Optimal protein requirements during the first 2 weeks after the onset of critical illness. Crit Care Med. 1998;26:1529–35.

Kansagara D, Fu R, Freeman M, Wolf F, Helfand M. Intensive insulin therapy in hospitalized patients: a systematic review. Ann Intern Med. 2011;154:268–82.

Kondrup J, Rasmussen HH, Hamberg O, Stanga Z. Nutritional risk screening (NRS2002): a new method based on analyses of controlled clinical trials. Clin Nutr. 2003;22:321–36.

Kurien M, McAlindon ME, Westaby D, Sanders DS. Percutaneous endoscopic gastrostomy (PEG) feeding. BMJ. 2010;340:c2414.

Larsson J, Lennmarken C, Martensson J, Sandstedt S, Vinnars E. Nitrogen requirements in severely injured patients. Br J Surg. 1990;77:413–6.

Lochs H, Allison SP, Meier R, Pirlich M, Kondrup J, Schneider S, van den Berghe G, Pichard C. Introductory to the ESPEN guidelines on enteral nutrition: terminology, definitions and general topics. Clin Nutr. 2006;25:180–6.

Malakouti A, Sookplung P, Siriussawakul A, Philip S, Bailey N, Brown M, Farver K, Zimmerman JJ, Bell MJ, Vavilala MS. Nutrition support and deficiencies in children with severe traumatic brain injury. Pediatr Crit Care Med. 2012;13(1):e18–24. https://doi.org/10.1097/PCC.0b013e31820aba1f.

Meierhans R, Bechir M, Ludwig S, Sommerfeld J, Brandi G, Haberthur C, Stocker R, Stover JF. Brain metabolism is significantly impaired at blood glucose below 6 mM and brain glucose below 1 mM in patients with severe traumatic brain injury. Crit Care. 2010;14:R13.

Nguyen NQ, Chapman MJ, Fraser RJ, Bryant LK, Holloway RH. Erythromycin is more effective than metoclopramide in the treatment of feed intoler- ance in critical illness. Crit Care Med. 2007;35:483–9.

Rattanachaiwong S, Singer P. Should we calculate or measure energy expenditure? Practical aspects in the ICU. Nutrition. 2018;55-56:71–5. https://doi.org/10.1016/j.nut.2018.05.001.

Sobotka L. Basics in clinical nutrition. Prague: Publishing House Galen; 2004.

Seron Arbeloa C, Avellanas Chavala M, Homs Gimeno C, Larraz Vileta A, Laplaza Marin J, Foncillas P. Evaluation of a high protein diet in critical care patients. Nutr Hosp. 1999;14:203–9.

Shi J, Dong B, Mao Y, Guan W, Cao J, Zhu R, Wang S. Traumatic brain injury and hyperglycemia, a potentially modifiable risk factor. Oncotarget. 2016;7(43):71052–61. https://doi.org/10.18632/oncotarget.11958. Review.

Singer P, Anbar R, Cohen J, Shapiro H, Shalita-Chesner M, Lev S, Grozovski E, Theilla M, Frishman S, Madar Z. The tight calorie control study (TICACOS): a prospective, randomized, controlled pilot study of nutritional support in critically ill patients. Intensive Care Med. 2011;37:601–9.

Singer P, Blaser AR, Berger MM, Alhazzani W, Calder PC, Casaer MP, Hiesmayr M, Mayer K, Montejo JC, Pichard C, Preiser JC, van Zanten ARH, Oczkowski S, Szczeklik W, Bischoff SC. ESPEN guideline on clinical nutrition in the intensive care unit. Clin Nutr. 2018;29. S0261-5614(18)32432-4. https://doi.org/10.1016/j.clnu.08.037.

Stapel SN, de Grooth HJ, Alimohamad H, Elbers PW, Girbes AR, Weijs PJ, Oudemans-van Straaten HM. Ventilator-derived carbon dioxide production to assess energy expenditure in critically ill patients: proof of concept. Crit Care. 2015;19:370. https://doi.org/10.1186/s13054-015-1087-2.

Streat SJ, Hill GL. Nutritional support in the man- agement of critically ill patients in surgical intensive care. World J Surg. 1987;11:194–201.

Turner P. Providing optimal nutritional support on the intensive care unit: key challenges and practical solutions. Proc Nutr Soc. 2010;69:574–81.

Twyman D, Young AB, Ott L, Norton JA, Bivins BA. High protein enteral feedings: a means of achieving positive nitrogen balance in head injured patients. JPEN J Parenter Enteral Nutr. 1985;9:679–84.

Webster J, Osborne S, Rickard CM, New K. Clinically-indicated replacement versus routine replacement of peripheral venous catheters. Cochrane Database Syst Rev. 2015;(8):CD007798. https://doi.org/10.1002/14651858.CD007798.pub4.

Wolfe RR, Goodenough RD, Burke JF, Wolfe MH. Response of protein and urea kinetics in burn patients to different levels of protein intake. Ann Surg. 1983;197:163–71.

Young B, Ott L, Twyman D, Norton J, Rapp R, Tibbs P, Haack D, Brivins B, Dempsey R. The effect of nutritional support on outcome from severe head injury. J Neurosurg. 1987;67:668–76.

Young B, Ott L, Kasarskis E, Rapp R, Moles K, Dempsey RJ, Tibbs PA, Kryscio R, McClain C. Zinc supplementation is associated with improved neurologic recovery rate and visceral protein levels of patients with severe closed head injury. J Neurotrauma. 1996;13:25–34.

Management of CNS-Related Infection

66

Christian A. Helland, Steinar Skrede, and Jens Kjølseth Møller

Recommendations

Level I

There are insufficient data to support Level I recommendations for this topic.

Level II

Use of antimicrobial-impregnated CSF drains is recommended.

Periprocedural antibiotic prophylaxis is recommended.

Level III

Prophylactic catheter exchange, irrigation of catheters or prolonged prophylactic antibiotic therapy for patients with an EVD is *not* recommended.

C. A. Helland (✉)
Department of Neurosurgery, Haukeland University Hospital, Bergen, Norway
e-mail: chhe@helse-bergen.no

S. Skrede
Department of Medicine, Section of Infectious Diseases, Haukeland University Hospital, Bergen, Bergen, Norway
e-mail: sskr@helse-bergen.no

J. K. Møller
Department of Clinical Microbiology, Vejle Hospital, Vejile, Denmark
e-mail: jkm@dadlnet.dk

© Springer Nature Switzerland AG 2020
T. Sundstrøm et al. (eds.), *Management of Severe Traumatic Brain Injury*,
https://doi.org/10.1007/978-3-030-39383-0_66

Strict adherence to a sterile protocol for insertion and maintenance of a closed system is advised. The EVD should be removed on a timely fashion.

Parenteral antibiotic treatment should be guided by the results of CSF gram stain and microbiological culture.

In patients with clinical signs of post-operative meningitis or VRI (ventriculostomy-related infections), systemic administration of vancomycin combined with either ceftriaxone or meropenem as empirical therapy is recommended for coverage of gram-positive microbes, including coagulase-negative staphylococci (CoNS), *Staphylococcus aureus* and gram-negative bacilli, taking local bacteria and susceptibility patterns into account.

Meropenem i.v. is recommended as empirical therapy in the event of a gram-negative isolate.

Subsequent antimicrobial treatment should be adjusted to bacterial culture and susceptibility results.

66.1 Overview

Central nervous system (CNS) infection is a serious complication to head trauma or to invasive procedures, most commonly implantation of an external ventricular drain (EVD). The etiological agents associated with these infections (e.g. resistant gram-negative bacilli and staphylococci) are different to those found in community-acquired meningitis, and the pathogenic mechanisms are different. Furthermore, the diagnosis may be difficult to establish as both clinical presentation and CSF abnormalities related to trauma and surgery in these patients confound the usual diagnostics.

This chapter focuses on management of drain-related infections, as these require highly specialised handling. Furthermore, it also focuses on the evaluation, diagnosis and management of CNS infection in the traumatic brain injury (TBI) patient.

If possible, the drain should be removed - or exchanged.

In the following, EVD-related infections are defined by the presence of clinical symptoms of CNS infection such as new fever, nuchal rigidity, decreased mental status and neurological deterioration. Supporting the clinical diagnosis are laboratory parameters indicating a deterioration of the biochemical profile of the CSF and/or a positive gram stain/culture from CSF.

Progressively advancing CSF pleocytosis, declining CSF glucose and increasing CSF protein define deterioration of the CSF biochemical profile.

An operational algorithm for the management of ventriculostomy-related infections (VRIs) is shown in Fig. 66.1.

Risk factors for external CSF drain-related infections are prophylactic catheter exchange, unnecessary manipulation of catheters, neurosurgical procedures, cranial fractures, haemorrhagic CSF and CSF leaks. The use of antimicrobial-impregnated catheters shows promise in preventing CSF infections; however, further studies are required. Antibiotic therapy should not be instituted in patients with external CSF drains prophylactically, as such use of systemic antibiotics selects for more resistant pathogens leading to increased mortality in neurosurgical infection.

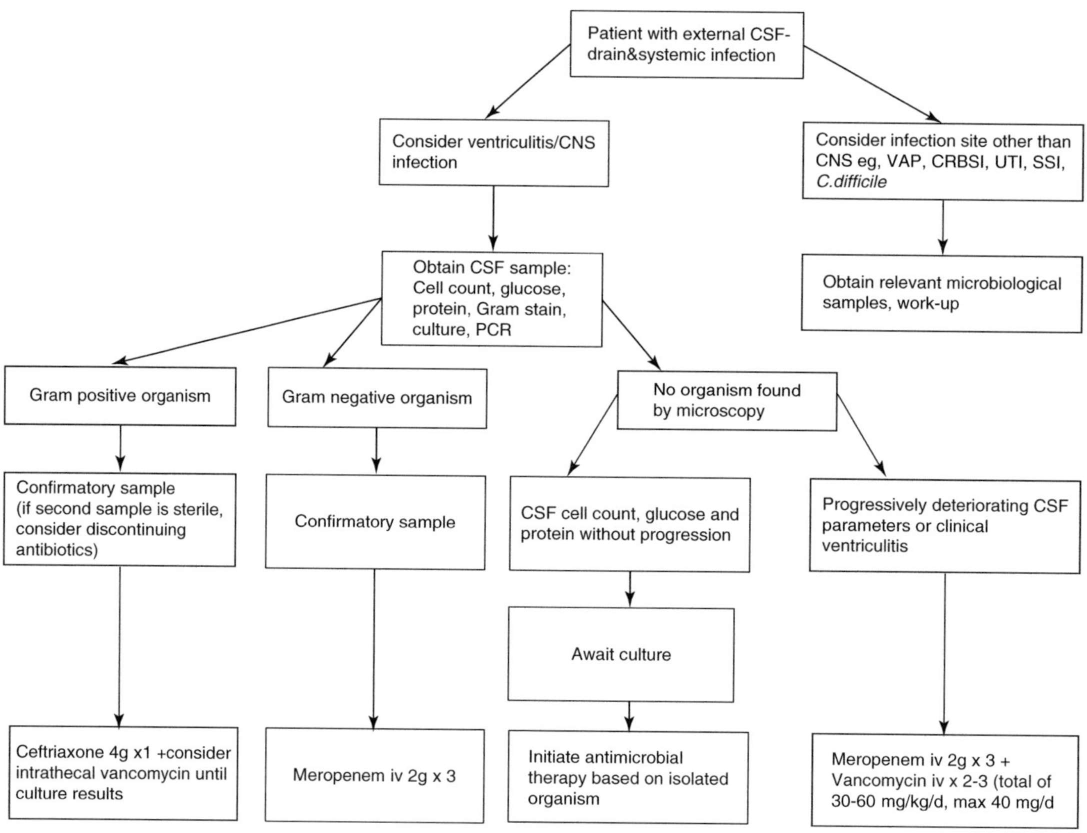

Fig. 66.1 Operational algorithm/flow chart for management of VRIs. *VAP* ventilator associated pneumonia; *CRBSI* catheter-related blood stream infection; *UTI* urinary tract infection; *SSI* surgical site infection

Tips, Tricks and Pitfalls

- Obtain microbiological samples before initiating antimicrobial therapy:
  - CSF for gram stain, culture, nonculture diagnostic laboratory (PCR), cell count, glucose and protein
  - Blood cultures × 2 (from central venous catheter and peripheral blood)
  - Sputum for culture/PCR
  - Swabs/aspirates from possible surgical site infection (SSI)
  - Urine for culture
  - Faeces for *Clostridium difficile* (if patient has diarrhoea)
- Consider other origins of infection: ventilator-associated pneumonia (VAP), catheter-related bloodstream infection (CRBSI), urinary tract infection (UTI), *Clostridium difficile* enterocolitis, sinusitis and surgical site infection (SSI).
- Duration of treatment is individualised and adjusted to microbial aetiology. It may range from 10 to 14 days for confirmation of gram-positive microbes. The treatment in gram-negative infections is given for 14 (up to 21) days.
- In ventriculostomy-related infection (VRI), we recommend intrathecal therapy (primarily vancomycin or gentamicin) sparingly used, but to be considered in situations where intravenous antibiotic therapy failed when the primary EVD has been removed or if the causal microbe displays susceptibility limited to antibiotics with poor CSF penetration.
- If institutional CSF infection rate is >10%, an investigation of the institutional procedures for the insertion and care of the EVD should be initiated

66.2 Background

CNS infection in the TBI patient is primarily caused by the breach of barriers due to trauma or by neurosurgical interventions such as the placement of CSF drains.

This chapter focuses mainly on the management of drain-related CNS infections, as these require highly specialised knowledge. This chapter also suggests a general empirical treatment strategy for CNS infections in the TBI patient.

66.2.1 Diagnosis

The interpretation of studies on infections related to external ventricular drains (EVDs) has been impeded by the lack of a universally agreed upon definition of ventriculostomy-related infection (VRI), which has made a comparison of results exceedingly difficult.

Previously, VRI has been defined by a positive cerebrospinal fluid (CSF) culture drawn from an EVD or lumbar puncture (LP) (Mayhall et al. 1984) without taking the CSF biochemical profile or the clinical status of the patient into consideration. This definition has led to an overestimate of the true incidence, as the possibility of contamination or colonisation was not taken into account. Efforts to establish more stringent diagnostic criteria for VRI have been partly hindered by the fact that both clinical symptoms and laboratory findings can be relatively non-specific. The traditional symptoms of CNS infection—nuchal rigidity, fever, decreased level of consciousness and neurological deterioration—can be difficult to ascertain in the brain trauma patient with decreased level of consciousness. Furthermore, the less pathogenic organisms that are commonly isolated in VRI, such as coagulase-negative staphylococci, generally cause mild symptoms. Moreover, the aseptic CNS inflammation caused by the presence of a foreign body, e.g. an EVD, can create a similar CSF profile as seen in CNS infection with pleocytosis, decreased CSF glucose and increased CSF protein.

Lozier et al. have proposed new diagnostic criteria for VRI where the abnormal CSF profile is not defined in absolute terms, but rather viewed as a change of the biochemical profile of the patient compared to previous examination results. By these criteria, *ventriculitis* is defined by the presence of clinical symptoms of CNS infection such as fever, nuchal rigidity, decreased mental status and neurological deterioration in conjunction with progressively advancing CSF pleocytosis, declining CSF glucose, increasing CSF protein and a positive gram stain/culture.

VRI is defined by the same laboratory findings, but no clinical symptoms other than fever. A suspected VRI is defined by abnormal CSF profile, lack of clinical symptoms other than fever and the absence of a positive gram stain/culture. In a patient with an expected CSF profile and no other symptoms of infection than fever, the finding of a positive gram stain/culture is considered a contaminant. If isolated in repeat culture from the same patient with no changes in CSF profile or clinical status, it is deemed colonisation of the catheter (Lozier et al. 2002).

The Centers for Disease Control and Prevention´s National Healthcare Safety Network definition of nosocomial ventriculitis or meningitis includes at least one of the following criteria (CDC/NHSN 2017):

- Organism cultured from CSF
- At least two of the following symptoms with no other recognised cause in patients aged >1 year: fever >38 °C or headache, meningeal signs or cranial nerve signs, or at least two of the following symptoms with no other recognised cause in patients aged ≤1 year: fever >38 °C or hypothermia <36 °C, apnoea, bradycardia, irritability and at least one of the following:
  - Increased white cells, elevated protein and decreased glucose in CSF
  - Organisms seen on gram stain of CSF
  - Organisms cultured from blood
  - Positive nonculture diagnostic laboratory test from CSF, blood or urine
  - Diagnostic single-antibody titre (immunoglobulin M) or fourfold increase in paired sera (immunoglobulin G) for organism.

However, a nonculture diagnostic laboratory test or antibody titres for specific organisms are not often used in patients with healthcare-associated ventriculitis or meningitis.

In conjunction with this, VRI is defined as the presence of clinical symptoms of CNS infection such as new fever, nuchal rigidity, decreased mental status and neurological deterioration. Supporting the clinical diagnosis are laboratory parameters indicating a deterioration of the biochemical profile of the CSF (advancing CSF pleocytosis, declining CSF glucose and increasing CSF protein) and/or a positive gram stain/culture from CSF.

66.2.2 Epidemiology

In patients with EVD, the reported frequency of infection is ranging from 0% to more than 20% (Tunkel et al. 2017). The overall pooled incidence of EVD-related CSF infection in a large meta-analysis was 11.4 per 1000 catheter days (Ramanan et al. 2015).

The true incidence of VRI remains elusive due to the varying definitions of drain-related CNS infection. Ventriculostomy-related infections have a reported low mortality from 0 to 2.8%, but they are associated with increased morbidity (Bota et al. 2005; Flibotte et al. 2004; Holloway et al. 1996). The majority of reports show a preponderance of gram-positive cocci—mainly coagulase-negative staphylococci and *Staphylococcus aureus*—consistent with skin flora comprising up to 75–85% of isolates. Gram-negative bacilli are also commonly isolated and normally comprise up to 15–20%. Fungi, although occasionally found, are still a rare cause of VRI. The mortality of VRI appears to depend on the causative agent, as studies with a large proportion of gram-negative infections report a far higher mortality rate of up to 58% (Ramanan et al. 2015; Buckwold et al. 1977; Lu et al. 1999; Lyke et al. 2001; Mombelli et al. 1983). Gram-negative CNS infections have been associated with the prophylactic use of antibiotics covering the gram-positive spectrum, thus selecting for gram-negative organisms, multi-resistant bacteria and fungi (Lyke et al. 2001; Alleyne et al. 2000; Aucoin et al. 1986; Korinek et al. 2006; May et al. 2006; Poon et al. 1998; Stoikes et al. 2008). Furthermore, a long hospital stay in head trauma patients also predispose for gram-negative CNS infection (Buckwold et al. 1977; Mombelli et al. 1983; Berk and McCabe 1980).

66.2.3 Risk Factors

A number of risk factors for VRI of relevance to head trauma patients have been identified. Several reports show that haemorrhagic CSF increases the risk of VRI (Mayhall et al. 1984; Holloway et al. 1996; Aucoin et al. 1986; Sundbärg et al. 1988). Cranial fractures, both basilar cranial fractures and depressed cranial fractures, have also been demonstrated to have a statistically significant association with VRIs (Mayhall et al. 1984; Holloway et al. 1996; Aucoin et al. 1986). Likewise, neurosurgical procedures such as craniotomy have been reported to increase the incidence of VRIs (Mayhall et al. 1984; Holloway et al. 1996; Sundbärg et al. 1988). Interestingly, it has also been shown that concomitant systemic infection increases the risk of VRI. It is not always by the same organism causing the systemic infection, leading to the speculation that this could be due to relative immunosuppression caused by the systemic infection (Bota et al. 2005; Holloway et al. 1996; Clark et al. 1989).

Regarding risk factors pertaining to the catheter, maintenance of a closed drainage system has been hypothesised to be essential to prevent infection. In line with this theory, irrigation of the EVD has been demonstrated to significantly increase the risk of CNS infection (Mayhall et al. 1984; Aucoin et al. 1986). Recently, Korinek et al. reported that the implementation of a rigid protocol for insertion and care for the EVD, with strict adherence to sterile technique and maintenance of a closed system, resulted in a significant reduction in drain-related infections from 12.2 to 5.7%. Protocol violations such as catheter manipulations and inappropriate CSF sampling were major risk factors for infection in this study, as the score for protocol violation was four times higher in the infected group than in non-infected patients (Korinek et al. 2005). Another major risk factor for infection identified in this study was CSF leakage around the EVD in concurrence with other reports (Holloway et al. 1996; Lyke et al. 2001; Sundbärg et al. 1988; Bogdahn et al. 1992; Rebuck et al. 2000; Schade et al. 2005). These studies emphasise the importance of maintenance of a closed system and adherence to strict procedures in the insertion and management of the EVD in order to prevent infection.

There is controversy in the literature concerning the significance of the duration of catheterisation as pertaining to the risk of infection. A number of studies have found duration of drainage to be a risk factor for VRI with variable data regarding when the infection rate starts increasing. Several of these reports suggest that more than 5 days of catheterisation is a risk factor for VRI (Mayhall et al. 1984; Holloway et al. 1996; Aucoin et al. 1986; Clark et al. 1989; Paramore and Turner 1994), and one report by Holloway et al. notes a decline in infection after day 10 (Holloway et al. 1996). However, other reports demonstrate increasing infection rates up to day 6, after which infection rates decline (Paramore and Turner 1994; Kanter et al. 1985). Conversely, numerous studies show no relationship between duration of EVD and infection (Sundbärg et al. 1988; Korinek et al. 2005; Pfisterer et al. 2003; Smith and Alksne 1976; Winfield et al. 1993). Duration of treatment as a risk factor for VRI is not supported from the findings in a recent meta-analysis (Ramanan et al. 2015). As the incidence and mechanism of infection depends on the local practice regarding sterile technique and maintenance of a closed system in the management of external ventricular drains, we believe that a unifying conclusion pertaining to duration of catheterisation as a risk factor may not be possible to draw.

66.2.4 Prevention

In order to prevent ventriculostomy-related infections, various interventions such as prophylactic catheter exchange, tunnelling of external ventricular drains, prophylactic antibiotics and impregnated catheters have been investigated. The results of these interventions will be reviewed in this section.

Based on the assumption that duration of catheterisation is a risk factor for VRI, prophylactic catheter exchange has been proposed as a means to decrease EVD-related infections (Mayhall et al. 1984). However, prophylactic catheter exchange does not reduce the likelihood of VRI (Holloway et al. 1996). On the contrary, some studies suggest a higher CSF infection rate with routine revision of EVDs as opposed to no change (Arabi et al. 2005; Wong et al. 2002). In line with these observations, several studies have reported a correlation between multiple catheters and VRI (Sundbärg et al. 1988; Clark et al. 1989; Rebuck et al. 2000; Arabi et al. 2005; Lo et al. 2007). This correlation, however, has been disputed by others, who report no such association (Mayhall et al. 1984; Holloway et al. 1996; Lyke et al. 2001; Alleyne et al. 2000). Based on these reports, a single external ventricular drain can be used as long as clinically indicated, unless a change is necessary because of CSF infection or catheter malfunction. We do not recommend prophylactic change of catheters.

The use of an extended tunnelling technique for EVDs has been proposed to reduce infection rates and was initially reported to result in a zero rate of infection (Friedman and Vries 1980). However, subsequent studies reported drain-related infections despite tunnelling of catheters, but reported lower rates of infection than untunnelled catheters (Khanna et al. 1995; Kim et al. 1995; Leung et al. 2007). Tunnelling of EVDs has become common practice amongst neurosurgeons and shown to reduce infection rates in the context of central venous catheters (CVCs) (Mermel 2000).

Another common practice in order to prevent drain-related infection is the administration of prophylactic antimicrobial therapy, either periprocedural or for the duration of the drainage period. A recent meta-analyses reported a reduction of infection rate by approximately 50% in patients (Sheppard et al. 2018). This number is in accordance with the figures reported for systemic periprocedural antimicrobial prophylaxis for VP-shunts (Haines and Walters 1994; Langley et al. 1993; Ratilal et al. 2006). Although no RCTs have been conducted, the use of periprocedural antibiotics for the insertion of EVDs is recommended (Tunkel et al. 2017).

There are several studies on the effect of giving systemic antibiotics before the drainage period. One randomised prospective study demonstrated significant reduction in CSF infection in patients receiving prophylactic antibiotics before the drainage period compared to those who did not receive antibiotics. This reduction, however, was at the expense of more resistant pathogens such as MRSA and *Candida* species and a higher mortality rate in the prolonged antimicrobial arm (Poon et al. 1998). Other studies have shown no effect on infection rates by the administration of prophylactic antibiotics (Mayhall et al. 1984; Alleyne et al. 2000; Aucoin et al. 1986; May et al. 2006; Stoikes et al. 2008; Rebuck et al. 2000; Rosner and Becker 1976), but a shift towards multi-drug-resistant organisms, fungi and gram-negative microbes was likewise observed among patients receiving continuous antibiotic treatment (Aucoin et al. 1986; May et al. 2006; Stoikes et al. 2008). The shift towards more resistant pathogens can lead to higher mortality rates and significant morbidity in the infected group (Lyke et al. 2001).

This is in striking contrast to reported low mortality rates (0–2.8%) in patient groups where no prophylactic antibiotics were given (Bota et al. 2005; Flibotte et al. 2004; Holloway et al. 1996; Schade et al. 2005). On the basis of these reports and the availability of an efficacious alternative (antimicrobial-impregnated EVD catheters, see below), the administration of prolonged prophylactic antibiotics is *not* supported, as there is insufficient evidence supporting a reduction in infection incidence. More importantly, several studies using prophylactic antibiotics demonstrate increased mortality and morbidity due to a selection for more resistant microorganisms.

Antimicrobial-impregnated catheters are commonly used in clinical practice, both in CSF shunts and in EVD. They are impregnated with either minocycline or clindamycin, combined with rifampicin.

Their ability to significantly reduce the risk of infection is well documented for CSF shunts (Govender et al. 2003; Thomas et al. 2012; Parker et al. 2011; Parker et al. 2015). Similar results have been reported for antimicrobial-impregnated EVDs (Zabramski et al. 2003; Tamburrini et al. 2008). Although other studies do not report a significant difference in favour of anti-microbial EVDs (Wong et al. 2008), meta-analyses and pooled analysis from systematic reviews demonstrate a significant reduction of VRI in favour of antimicrobial impregnated EVD (Thomas et al. 2012; Sonabend et al. 2011; Cui et al. 2015).

Although there were no reports of induction of bacterial resistance in these studies (Zabramski et al. 2003; Tamburrini et al. 2008; Wong et al. 2008), the concern has been expressed from in vitro studies demonstrating induced resistance in staphylococci exposed minocycline-rifampicin catheters (Sampath et al. 2001; Tambe et al. 2001). However, the increased rifampicin resistance of staphylococci in vivo by these catheters has still not been found in other clinical trials (Turnbull et al. 2018). Another cause for concern is reports demonstrating significant increase in *Candida* colonisation when using minocycline-rifampicin-coated CVCs (Sampath et al. 2001; Leon et al. 2004).

Catheters impregnated with silver nanoparticles have also been studied for use in external drainage. In CVCs, the efficacy of silver-coated catheters has still not been demonstrated, but the results in external drains seem to be encouraging. In vitro studies have demonstrated their antibacterial effect and indicated that silver toxicity is not a problem (Galiano et al. 2008; Roe et al. 2008). Previous studies reported reduction in positive CSF cultures in patients with silver-impregnated catheters (Lackner et al. 2008; Fichtner et al. 2010). In the 'SILVER trial', silver-impregnated catheters significantly reduced the risk of VRI (Keong et al. 2012), which was further supported in a meta-analysis (Cui et al. 2015).

Silver resistance has previously been described in burn units due to use of silver as an antiseptic, and there is concern that the use of silver-coated catheters will select for antibiotic resistance as studies suggest that silver resistance can confer cross-resistance to multiple antibiotics (McHugh et al. 1975; Pirnay et al. 2003).

Based on the documented efficacy, we recommend the use of antimicrobial-impregnated catheters in preventing VRI. There is no conclusive evidence for the preference of antimicrobial or silver-impregnated for the prevention of VRI.

Overall, the implementation of a strict protocol for insertion and care for the catheter with emphasis on sterile technique and avoidance of unnecessary catheter manipulation still remains the best way to prevent drain-related CNS infection.

66.2.5 Treatment

The principles for empirical treatment of patients with nosocomial meningitis are generally equal to those for treatment of acute bacterial meningitis (van de Beek et al. 2016). The antimicrobial agent(s) must penetrate the CNS, attain adequate concentration and have bactericidal activity against the infecting microbe.

With clinical symptoms of CNS infection in conjunction with CSF findings as described above, antimicrobial therapy should be initiated after appropriate cultures. When possible, antimicrobial therapy should be tailored to the specific microorganism and its in vitro susceptibility. Preferably, treatment should be monitored by infectious specialist or by staff in units experienced in selecting antibiotic therapy and in clinical treatment.

CSF device infections usually appear early and are therefore most often, but not exclusively, caused by skin flora. The most important pathogens associated with VRI are coagulase-negative staphylococci and *Staphylococcus aureus* as well as gram-negative bacilli (van de Beek et al. 2010).

Empirical therapy with intravenous vancomycin plus third-generation of cephalosporin is warranted (van de Beek et al. 2010). Targeted therapy should be given whenever possible. In cases with coagulase-negative staphylococci that are methicillin susceptible, oxacillin is the first choice. In susceptible cases with unfavourable response, oral rifampicin can be an additional antimicrobial therapy. Vancomycin is the drug of choice in methicillin-resistant CoNS. In this situation, doses must be high with concentrations >15–20 μg/mL. *Staphylococcus aureus* are most commonly methicillin sensitive and should be treated as for CoNS as described above. Other possible gram-positive microbes are *Propionibacterium acnes*, which should be treated with benzylpenicillin in monotherapy. The empirical choice to treat a presumptive gram-negative pathogen should be determined on basis of the local antimicrobial susceptibility pattern of these pathogens.

Meropenem is the recommended empirical choice or, if contraindicated, alternative agents are either aztreonam or a fluoroquinolone that offer gram-negative covering.

Once a pathogen is identified and susceptibility patterns are available, treatment will be customised accordingly for optimal management (Tunkel et al. 2017; van de Beek et al. 2010).

In many VRI cases, the meningeal inflammation is milder, and this can hamper the distribution of systemically administered antimicrobials to CNS. Other factors adding to the difficulty in eradicating the microbiological agents causing VRI or nosocomial meningitis/ventriculitis are troublesome pattern of susceptibility (e.g. multidrug-resistant gram-negative bacilli).

Intraventricular antimicrobial therapy should be considered for patients with healthcare-associated ventriculitis and meningitis, in which the infection responds poorly to systemic antimicrobial therapy or where the microbe is resistant to relevant antibiotics and susceptible to agents that do not pass the blood brain barrier well (Tunkel et al. 2017).

Intrathecal administration bypasses the blood-CSF barrier. Therefore, it has the advantage (at least theoretically) to achieve high CSF concentrations without high systemic blood concentrations and hence lower systemic toxicities (Tunkel et al. 2017; Wen et al. 1992; Ng et al. 2014). However, it remains to confirm the efficacy and safety of this route of administration, as it has not been demonstrated in controlled trials. However, the experience reported with intraventricular or intrathecal administration of several antimicrobials (e.g. vancomycin, gentamycin, polymyxin B, amikacin, colistin) suggests no severe or irreversible toxicity (van de Beek et al. 2010; Ng et al. 2014; Ziai and Lewin 2009). Nonetheless, penicillins and cephalosporins should not be administered by the intrathecal route because of their neurotoxicity (Wen et al. 1992).

Recommended doses of selected antimicrobial agents administered by the intraventricular route are summarised in Table 66.1 (Tunkel et al. 2017).

Antimicrobial agents administered intrathecally should be preservative-free.

When administered through a ventricular drain, the drain should be clamped for 15–60 min to allow for equilibration of agent in the CSF before opening the drain (Cook et al. 2009).

Intraventricularly administered gentamicin is not recommended in neonates (McCracken et al. 1980).

With regard to the duration of antimicrobial therapy in healthcare-associated meningitis and ventriculitis, it should be adjusted to microbiological aetiology. In general, gram-positive microbes can be treated for a shorter time than gram-nega-

Table 66.1 Recommended dosage of antimicrobial agents administered by the intraventricular route

Antimicrobial agent	Daily intraventricular dose
Amikacin	5–50 mg[a]
Amphotericin B deoxycholate	0.01–0.5 mg in 2 mL of 5% dextrose in water
Colistin (formulated as colistimethate sodium)	10 mg
Daptomycin	2–5 mg[b]
Gentamicin	1–8 mg[c,d,e]
Polymyxin B	5 mg
Quinupristin/dalfopristin	2–5 mg
Tobramycin	5–20 mg
Vancomycin	5–20 mg[d,e,f]

[a]The usual intraventricular dose is 30 mg daily

[b]One study used 10 mg every day for 2 days and more than 10 mg every 48 h. Another study used 5 mg or 10 mg every 72 h. Data are based on isolated case reports

[c]Dose is 4–8 mg in adults

[d]Dosage recommendations in adults based on ventricle size/volume are as follows: (1) Slit ventricles: 5 mg vancomycin and 2 mg gentamicin. (2) Normal size: 10 mg vancomycin and 3 mg gentamicin. (3) Enlarged ventricles: 15–20 mg vancomycin and 4–5 mg gentamicin

[e]Recommendations for frequency of administration based on external ventricular drain output over 24 h are as follows: (1) <50 mL/24 h: every third day. (2) 50–100 mL/24 h: every second day. (3) 100–150 mL/24 h: every day. (4) 150–200 mL/24 h: increase the dosage by 5 mg of vancomycin and 1 mg of gentamicin and give once daily. (5) 200–250 mL/24 h: increase the dosage by 10 mg of vancomycin and 2 mg of gentamicin and give once daily

[f]Most studies used a 10-mg or a 20-mg dose

tive cases. In most, but not all, CoNS (*coagulase-negative staphylococci*) and *Propionibacterium acnes* infections, it is recommended that treatment to be suspended after 10 to 14 days; the shorter duration restricted to cases with few symptoms and minimal CSF changes. The same is valid for *Staphylococcus aureus* infections. In gram-negative bacillary infections, 10–14 days may be sufficient, but some experts advocate treatment duration of up to 21 days. In such cases, treatment effect should be monitored by culture. In situations where cultures are repeatedly growth positive, treatment should extend to 10–14 days following the last day of culture positivity.

66.3 Specific Paediatric Concerns

Intraventricularly administered gentamicin is not recommended in neonates.

References

Alleyne CH Jr, Hassan M, Zabramski JM. The efficacy and cost of prophylactic and perioprocedural antibiotics in patients with external ventricular drains. Neurosurgery. 2000;47(5):1124–7; discussion 7-9.

Arabi Y, Memish ZA, Balkhy HH, Francis C, Ferayan A, Al Shimemeri A, et al. Ventriculostomy-associated infections: incidence and risk factors. Am J Infect Control. 2005;33(3):137–43.

Aucoin PJ, Kotilainen HR, Gantz NM, Davidson R, Kellogg P, Stone B. Intracranial pressure monitors. Epidemiologic study of risk factors and infections. Am J Med. 1986;80(3):369–76.

Berk SL, McCabe WR. Meningitis caused by gram-negative bacilli. Ann Intern Med. 1980;93(2):253–60.

Bogdahn U, Lau W, Hassel W, Gunreben G, Mertens HG, Brawanski A. Continuous-pressure controlled, external ventricular drainage for treatment of acute hydrocephalus-evaluation of risk factors. Neurosurgery. 1992;31(5):898–903; discussion -4.

Bota DP, Lefranc F, Vilallobos HR, Brimioulle S, Vincent J. Ventriculostomy-related infections in critically ill patients: a 6-year experience. J Neurosurg. 2005;103(3):468–72.

Buckwold FJ, Hand R, Hansebout RR. Hospital-acquired bacterial meningitis in neurosurgical patients. J Neurosurg. 1977;46(4):494–500.

CDC/NHSN. Surveillance definitions for specific types of infections. 2017. https://www.cdc.gov/nhsn/PDFs/pscManual/17pscNosInfDef_current.pdf.

Clark WC, Muhlbauer MS, Lowrey R, Hartman M, Ray MW, Watridge CB. Complications of intracranial pressure monitoring in trauma patients. Neurosurgery. 1989;25(1):20–4.

Cook AM, Mieure KD, Owen RD, Pesaturo AB, Hatton J. Intracerebroventricular administration of drugs. Pharmacotherapy. 2009;29(7):832–45.

Cui Z, Wang B, Zhong Z, Sun Y, Sun Q, Yang G, et al. Impact of antibiotic- and silver-impregnated external ventricular drains on the risk of infections: a systematic review and meta-analysis. Am J Infect Control. 2015;43(7):e23–32.

Fichtner J, Guresir E, Seifert V, Raabe A. Efficacy of silver-bearing external ventricular drainage catheters: a retrospective analysis. J Neurosurg. 2010;112(4):840–6.

Flibotte JJ, Lee KE, Koroshetz WJ, Rosand J, McDonald CT. Continuous antibiotic prophylaxis and cerebral spinal fluid infection in patients with intracranial pressure monitors. Neurocrit Care. 2004;1(1):61–8.

Friedman WA, Vries JK. Percutaneous tunnel ventriculostomy. Summary of 100 procedures. J Neurosurg. 1980;53(5):662–5.

Galiano K, Pleifer C, Engelhardt K, Brossner G, Lackner P, Huck C, et al. Silver segregation and bacterial growth of intraventricular catheters impregnated with silver nanoparticles in cerebrospinal fluid drainages. Neurol Res. 2008;30(3):285–7.

Govender ST, Nathoo N, van Dellen JR. Evaluation of an antibiotic-impregnated shunt system for the treatment of hydrocephalus. J Neurosurg. 2003;99(5):831–9.

Haines SJ, Walters BC. Antibiotic prophylaxis for cerebrospinal fluid shunts: a metanalysis. Neurosurgery. 1994;34(1):87–92.

Holloway KL, Barnes T, Choi S, Bullock R, Marshall LF, Eisenberg HM, et al. Ventriculostomy infections: the effect of monitoring duration and catheter exchange in 584 patients. J Neurosurg. 1996;85(3):419–24.

Kanter RK, Weiner LB, Patti AM, Robson LK. Infectious complications and duration of intracranial pressure monitoring. Crit Care Med. 1985;13(10):837–9.

Keong NC, Bulters DO, Richards HK, Farrington M, Sparrow OC, Pickard JD, et al. The SILVER (Silver Impregnated Line Versus EVD Randomized trial): a double-blind, prospective, randomized, controlled trial of an intervention to reduce the rate of external ventricular drain infection. Neurosurgery. 2012;71(2):394–403; discussion-4.

Khanna RK, Rosenblum ML, Rock JP, Malik GM. Prolonged external ventricular drainage with percutaneous long-tunnel ventriculostomies. J Neurosurg. 1995;83(5):791–4.

Kim DK, Uttley D, Bell BA, Marsh HT, Moore AJ. Comparison of rates of infection of two methods of emergency ventricular drainage. J Neurol Neurosurg Psychiatry. 1995;58(4):444–6.

Korinek AM, Reina M, Boch AL, Rivera AO, De Bels D, Puybasset L. Prevention of external ventricular drain-related ventriculitis. Acta Neurochir. 2005;147(1):39–45; discussion-6.

Korinek AM, Baugnon T, Golmard JL, van Effenterre R, Coriat P, Puybasset L. Risk factors for adult nosocomial meningitis after craniotomy role of antibiotic prophylaxis. Neurosurgery. 2006;59(1):126–33.

Lackner P, Beer R, Broessner G, Helbok R, Galiano K, Pleifer C, et al. Efficacy of silver nanoparticles-impregnated external ventricular drain catheters in patients with acute occlusive hydrocephalus. Neurocrit Care. 2008;8(3):360–5.

Langley JM, LeBlanc JC, Drake J, Milner R. Efficacy of antimicrobial prophylaxis in placement of cerebrospinal fluid shunts: meta-analysis. Clin Infect Dis. 1993;17(1):98–103.

Leon C, Ruiz-Santana S, Rello J, de la Torre MV, Valles J, Alvarez-Lerma F, et al. Benefits of minocycline and rifampin-impregnated central venous catheters. A prospective, randomized, double-blind, controlled, multicenter trial. Intensive Care Med. 2004;30(10):1891–9.

Leung GK, Ng KB, Taw BB, Fan YW. Extended subcutaneous tunnelling technique for external ventricular drainage. Br J Neurosurg. 2007;21(4):359–64.

Lo CH, Spelman D, Bailey M, Cooper DJ, Rosenfeld JV, Brecknell JE. External ventricular drain infections are independent of drain duration: an argument against elective revision. J Neurosurg. 2007;106(3):378–83.

Lozier AP, Sciacca RR, Romagnoli MF, Connolly ES Jr. Ventriculostomy-related infections: a critical review of the literature. Neurosurgery. 2002;51(1):170–81; discussion 81-2.

Lu CH, Chang WN, Chuang YC, Chang HW. Gram-negative bacillary meningitis in adult post-neurosurgical patients. Surg Neurol. 1999;52(5):438–43; discussion 43-4.

Lyke KE, Obasanjo OO, Williams MA, O'Brien M, Chotani R, Perl TM. Ventriculitis complicating use of intraventricular catheters in adult neurosurgical patients. Clin Infect Dis. 2001;33(12):2028–33.

May AK, Fleming SB, Carpenter RO, Diaz JJ, Guillamondegui OD, Deppen SA, et al. Influence of broad-spectrum antibiotic prophylaxis on intracranial pressure monitor infections and subsequent infectious complications in head-injured patients. Surg Infect (Larchmt). 2006;7(5):409–17.

Mayhall CG, Archer NH, Lamb VA, Spadora AC, Baggett JW, Ward JD, et al. Ventriculostomy-related infections. A prospective epidemiologic study. N Engl J Med. 1984;310(9):553–9.

McCracken GH Jr, Mize SG, Threlkeld N. Intraventricular gentamicin therapy in gram-negative bacillary meningitis of infancy. Report of the Second Neonatal Meningitis Cooperative Study Group. Lancet. 1980;1(8172):787–91.

McHugh GL, Moellering RC, Hopkins CC, Swartz MN. Salmonella typhimurium resistant to silver nitrate, chloramphenicol, and ampicillin. Lancet. 1975;1(7901):235–40.

Mermel LA. Prevention of intravascular catheter-related infections. Ann Intern Med. 2000;132(5):391–402.

Mombelli G, Klastersky J, Coppens L, Daneau D, Nubourgh Y. Gram-negative bacillary meningitis in neurosurgical patients. J Neurosurg. 1983;59(4):634–41.

Ng K, Mabasa VH, Chow I, Ensom MH. Systematic review of efficacy, pharmacokinetics, and administration of intraventricular vancomycin in adults. Neurocrit Care. 2014;20(1):158–71.

Paramore CG, Turner DA. Relative risks of ventriculostomy infection and morbidity. Acta Neurochir. 1994;127(1-2):79–84.

Parker SL, Anderson WN, Lilienfeld S, Megerian JT, McGirt MJ. Cerebrospinal shunt infection in patients receiving antibiotic-impregnated versus standard shunts. J Neurosurg Pediatr. 2011;8(3):259–65.

Parker SL, McGirt MJ, Murphy JA, Megerian JT, Stout M, Engelhart L. Comparative effectiveness of antibiotic-impregnated shunt catheters in the treatment of adult and pediatric hydrocephalus: analysis of 12,589 consecutive cases from 287 US hospital systems. J Neurosurg. 2015;122(2):443–8.

Pfisterer W, Muhlbauer M, Czech T, Reinprecht A. Early diagnosis of external ventricular drainage infection: results of a prospective study. J Neurol Neurosurg Psychiatry. 2003;74(7):929–32.

Pirnay JP, De Vos D, Cochez C, Bilocq F, Pirson J, Struelens M, et al. Molecular epidemiology of Pseudomonas aeruginosa colonization in a burn unit: persistence of a multidrug-resistant clone and a silver sulfadiazine-resistant clone. J Clin Microbiol. 2003;41(3):1192–202.

Poon WS, Ng S, Wai S. CSF antibiotic prophylaxis for neurosurgical patients with ventriculostomy: a randomised study. Acta Neurochir Suppl. 1998;71:146–8.

Ramanan M, Lipman J, Shorr A, Shankar A. A meta-analysis of ventriculostomy-associated cerebrospinal fluid infections. BMC Infect Dis. 2015;15:3.

Ratilal B, Costa J, Sampaio C. Antibiotic prophylaxis for surgical introduction of intracranial ventricular shunts. Cochrane Database Syst Rev. 2006;(3):CD005365.

Rebuck JA, Murry KR, Rhoney DH, Michael DB, Coplin WM. Infection related to intracranial pressure monitors in adults: analysis of risk factors and antibiotic prophylaxis. J Neurol Neurosurg Psychiatry. 2000;69(3):381–4.

Roe D, Karandikar B, Bonn-Savage N, Gibbins B, Roullet JB. Antimicrobial surface functionalization of plastic catheters by silver nanoparticles. J Antimicrob Chemother. 2008;61(4):869–76.

Rosner MJ, Becker DP. ICP monitoring: complications and associated factors. Clin Neurosurg. 1976;23:494–519.

Sampath LA, Tambe SM, Modak SM. In vitro and in vivo efficacy of catheters impregnated with antiseptics or antibiotics: evaluation of the risk of bacterial resistance to the antimicrobials in the catheters. Infect Control Hosp Epidemiol. 2001;22(10):640–6.

Schade RP, Schinkel J, Visser LG, Van Dijk JM, Voormolen JH, Kuijper EJ. Bacterial meningitis caused by the use of ventricular or lumbar cerebrospinal fluid catheters. J Neurosurg. 2005;102(2):229–34.

Sheppard JP, Ong V, Lagman C, Udawatta M, Duong C, Nguyen T, et al. Systemic antimicrobial prophylaxis and antimicrobial-coated external ventricular drain catheters for preventing ventriculostomy-related infections: a meta-analysis of 5242 cases. Neurosurgery. 2018;86(1):19–29.

Smith RW, Alksne JF. Infections complicating the use of external ventriculostomy. J Neurosurg. 1976;44(5):567–70.

Sonabend AM, Korenfeld Y, Crisman C, Badjatia N, Mayer SA, Connolly ES Jr. Prevention of ventriculostomy-related infections with prophylactic antibiotics and antibiotic-coated external ventricular drains: a systematic review. Neurosurgery. 2011;68(4):996–1005.

Stoikes NF, Magnotti LJ, Hodges TM, Weinberg JA, Schroeppel TJ, Savage SA, et al. Impact of intracranial pressure monitor prophylaxis on central nervous system infections and bacterial multi-drug resistance. Surg Infect (Larchmt). 2008;9(5):503–8.

Sundbärg G, Nordström CH, Söderstrom S. Complications due to prolonged ventricular fluid pressure recording. Br J Neurosurg. 1988;2(4):485–95.

Tambe SM, Sampath L, Modak SM. In vitro evaluation of the risk of developing bacterial resistance to antiseptics and antibiotics used in medical devices. J Antimicrob Chemother. 2001;47(5):589–98.

Tamburrini G, Massimi L, Caldarelli M, Di Rocco C. Antibiotic impregnated external ventricular drainage and third ventriculostomy in the management of hydrocephalus associated with posterior cranial fossa tumours. Acta Neurochir. 2008;150(10):1049–55; discussion 55-6.

Thomas R, Lee S, Patole S, Rao S. Antibiotic-impregnated catheters for the prevention of CSF shunt infections: a systematic review and meta-analysis. Br J Neurosurg. 2012;26(2):175–84.

Tunkel AR, Hasbun R, Bhimraj A, Byers K, Kaplan SL, Michael Scheld W, et al. 2017 Infectious Diseases Society of America's Clinical Practice Guidelines for healthcare-associated ventriculitis and meningitis. Clin Infect Dis. 2017;64:e34–65.

Turnbull IR, Buckman SA, Horn CB, Bochicchio GV, Mazuski JE. Antibiotic-impregnated central venous catheters do not change antibiotic resistance patterns. Surg Infect (Larchmt). 2018;19(1):40–7.

van de Beek D, Drake JM, Tunkel AR. Nosocomial bacterial meningitis. N Engl J Med. 2010;362(2):146–54.

van de Beek D, Cabellos C, Dzupova O, Esposito S, Klein M, Kloek AT, et al. ESCMID guideline: diagnosis and treatment of acute bacterial meningitis. Clin Microbiol Infect. 2016;22(Suppl 3):S37–62.

Wen DY, Bottini AG, Hall WA, Haines SJ. Infections in neurologic surgery. The intraventricular use of antibiotics. Neurosurg Clin N Am. 1992;3(2):343–54.

Winfield JA, Rosenthal P, Kanter RK, Casella G. Duration of intracranial pressure monitoring does not predict daily risk of infectious complications. Neurosurgery. 1993;33(3):424–30; discussion 30-1.

Wong GK, Poon WS, Wai S, Yu LM, Lyon D, Lam JM. Failure of regular external ventricular drain exchange to reduce cerebrospinal fluid infection: result of a randomised controlled trial. J Neurol Neurosurg Psychiatry. 2002;73(6):759–61.

Wong GK, Poon WS, Ng SC, Ip M. The impact of ventricular catheter impregnated with antimicrobial agents on infections in patients with ventricular catheter: interim report. Acta Neurochir Suppl. 2008;102:53–5.

Zabramski JM, Whiting D, Darouiche RO, Horner TG, Olson J, Robertson C, et al. Efficacy of antimicrobial-impregnated external ventricular drain catheters: a prospective, randomized, controlled trial. J Neurosurg. 2003;98(4):725–30.

Ziai WC, Lewin JJ 3rd. Improving the role of intraventricular antimicrobial agents in the management of meningitis. Curr Opin Neurol. 2009;22(3):277–82.

67 Management of Extracranial Infections

Jan-Erik Berdal

Recommendations

Level I

There are no Level I recommendations.

Level II

There are a number of Level II recommendations for the majority of infection issues discussed in this chapter.

Level III

There are a large number of recently published major guidelines and their supporting literature giving support for the recommendations given in this chapter.

67.1 Overview

Infections acquired in the intensive care unit (ICU) are a major cause of morbidity and excess mortality. In the Extended Prevalence of Infection in Intensive Care (EPIC II) study, a prospective, point-prevalence study across 1265 ICUs in 75 countries, 51% of patients were considered infected, and 71% were receiving antibiotics (Vincent et al. 2009). The lungs were the most common focus of infections, followed by abdominal and bloodstream infections (BSI), and mortality rates in infected patients were twice those of non-infected (33.1% vs 14.8%). Distinguishing between community-acquired, hospital-acquired, and ICU-acquired infections was not attempted in EPIC II, but data from surveillance studies of ICU-acquired infections show a similar pattern and infection burden. The European Centre for Disease Prevention and Control (ECDC) 2018 report on ICU health care-associated infections (HAI) noted that 8.4% of patients staying in an ICU for more than 2 days presented with at least one ICU-acquired health care-associated infection, 6% pneumonias, 4% bloodstream infections (BSI), and 2% with urinary tract infections (UTIs). Close to all of the episodes of pneumonia and UTI were associated with intubation or indwelling catheters, respectively, and almost half of BSI episodes were catheter related (European Centre for Disease Prevention and Control 2018). Data on nosocomial infections in specific neuro-intensive care units are sparse, but show a similar spectrum and infection density with HAP, VAP, UTIs, and BSI dominating. Post-craniotomy and external drain-related infections constitute a smaller share, with variations

J.-E. Berdal (✉)
Infectious Diseases Department, Akershus University Hospital, Nordbyhagen, Norway

University of Oslo, Oslo, Norway
e-mail: jan.erik.berdal@ahus.no

© Springer Nature Switzerland AG 2020
T. Sundstrøm et al. (eds.), *Management of Severe Traumatic Brain Injury*,
https://doi.org/10.1007/978-3-030-39383-0_67

in frequency depending on the case mix and length of stay in the units (Dettenkofer et al. 1999; Laborde et al. 1993).

Traumatic brain injury patients may be at particular risk for pneumonia. In a study from a large traumatic head injury database, pneumonia occurred in 41% of patients, developing at intermediary and late stages, 5–11 days after injury, and having a significant negative effect on overall outcome (Jürgen et al. 1992). Brain injury has been shown to induce immunosuppression in both animal and humans. It is thought to be the result of dysregulated brain-immune interactions, which may last for weeks and contribute to the infection proneness in brain injury patients of diverse etiologies (Busl 2018). The diagnosis of infection after brain injury is complicated by the high frequency of fever, being a manifestation of both infection and the brain injury per se. Fever was in one study reported in 87% of patients in the first week, correlated to severity of injury (Stocchetti et al. 2002).

A high exposure to antibiotics and long hospital stays put the neuro-intensive care unit patients at risk for *Clostridium difficile* infections (CDIs). CDI illness may range from mild self-limiting diarrhea to fulminant and life-threatening colitis. From 2003 onward, the emergence and spread of more virulent strains (BI/NAP1/027) associated with fluoroquinolone use have led to large outbreaks with more severe disease. After treatment in the intensive care unit, patients with reduced consciousness and neurologic deficits continue to be at risk for nosocomial infections, in particular HAP due to the increased risk of micro and macro aspirations. In the following sections, the prevention and management of the aforementioned infections will be discussed. External drain-related infections and suggestions for general empiric therapy for CNS infections in the TBI patients are discussed separately in Chap. 66.

Tips, Tricks, and Pitfalls

- Nosocomial infections are common in neuro-intensive care units, and pneumonia is by far the most common infection in brain injury patients peaking 5–7 days post-injury.
- Brain injury-induced immunosuppression, a result of dysregulated brain-immune interactions, contributes to the infection proneness in brain injury patients of diverse etiologies.
- Antibiotic treatment should be guided by microbial sampling results, and empiric treatment should be informed by regularly updated local hospital and ICU antibiograms.
- Treatment lengths are being shortened to one week for most ventilator-associated pneumonia (VAP), UTIs, and BSIs except *S. aureus* infections, aimed at reducing the growing concerns of antibiotic resistance pressure and risk of *C. difficile* infections.

67.2 Hospital- and Ventilator-Acquired Pneumonia

67.2.1 Prevention

Hospital-acquired pneumonia (HAP) is by far the most common nosocomial infection in general and neuro-intensive care units (Busl 2018; Vincent et al. 2009). It is defined as pneumonia occurring 48 h after hospital admittance. Ventilator-associated pneumonia (VAP) is a subgroup of HAP and defined as pneumonia occurring 48 h after intubation. The category health care-associated pneumonia (HCAP) has been abandoned, realizing that risk of pneumonia with antibiotic-resistant organisms is more dependent on local resistance patterns and recent antibiotic treatment than on residence in a health-care facility (Kalil et al. 2016). Further discussion will focus on VAP, as it is of particular concern in ICUs.

The risk of VAP is a function of (1) the length of invasive mechanical ventilation because cumulative risk increases with time, (2) the accumulation and leakage of oropharyngeal and gastric fluids from above the endotracheal tube cuff, and (3) the microbial composition of these fluids, all potentially modifiable. Preventive strategies have therefore focused on preventing intubation choosing noninvasive ventilation whenever possible, and when unavoidable, using weaning and sedation protocols to keep ventilation time as short as possible (Blackwood et al. 2011). Because intubation as such poses an increased risk for VAP, a balance must be struck between too early extubation that may necessitate re-intubation and shortening of ventilation time. A strategy to reduce aspiration of gastric fluids has focused on positioning, keeping the patient in a semi-recumbent (45°) rather than supine position. This has however proven hard to achieve in real-life outside studies, because patients inevitably slide down the bed. Raising the bed to at least 30° is a recommended compromise (Hellyer et al. 2016). Reduction of leakage into the lungs can be achieved by keeping and regularly checking for correct cuff pressure and, increasingly, in patients expected to need more than very short mechanical ventilation, by utilizing endotracheal tubes with a designated suction catheter draining the otherwise inaccessible fluid pool above the cuff but underneath the vocal cords. In different meta-analyses, this strategy has been shown to both reduce length of ventilation and ICU stay and VAP and is recommended in VAP prevention bundle (Hellyer et al. 2016). Decontamination of oral secretions with chlorhexidine has been shown to decrease VAP incidence, however without reduction in mortality. In a recent meta-analysis, there was a signal of increased mortality (Price et al. 2014), and chlorhexidine mouthwash is no longer recommended in VAP prevention bundles. Selective oral decontamination (SOD) and selective digestive decontamination (SDD) with oral administration of broad-spectrum non-absorbable antibiotics have been found to reduce VAP incidence, but studies have mostly been conducted in settings with a low prevalence of resistant microbes (de Smet et al. 2009). Together with increasing concerns of antibiotic usage-driven resistance development, a modest effect on mortality with a high number needed to treat (NTT), and lack of data from countries with higher prevalence of resistance, SOD and SDD have not been widely adopted for the prevention of VAP.

67.2.2 Diagnosis

New lung infiltrate, new onset of fever, purulent sputum, leukocytosis, and decline in oxygenation are the classic clinical criteria for diagnosis. There is insufficient data to support routine use of invasive airways sampling with quantitative cultures thresholds (10^4 colony forming units/mL for BAL) used as a trigger to withhold or stop antibiotics. Clinical criteria alone may however overestimate the incidence of VAP, and antibiotic discontinuation in patients with suspected VAP whose invasive quantitative culture results are below the diagnostic threshold for VAP may decrease unnecessary antibiotic use and reduce antibiotic-related adverse events. There is no evidence that this strategy worsens outcomes (Kalil et al. 2016). Noninvasive or invasive microbial (when performed) sampling should always be used to guide and adjust antibiotic therapy. Although only a minority of VAP episodes are accompanied with bacteremia, blood cultures should be performed as part of diagnostic workup, not the least to confirm or exclude other infectious complications. Biomarkers such as CRP and PCT should *not* be used to overrule a clinical decision to initiate therapy, but can be useful in the re-evaluation of the diagnosis and stopping or shortening of antibiotic therapy.

67.2.3 Antibiotic Treatment

Empiric antibiotic treatment for VAP should consist of antibiotics with activity against both *S. aureus* and *Pseudomonas*, such as piperacillin/tazobactam and carbapenems, with de-escalation to narrower antibiotics when possible according to culture results (Kalil et al. 2016). An alternative carbapenem-sparing "escalation" strategy is preferable if local antibiograms show a low occurrence of *Pseudomonas* and extended-spectrum beta-lactamase (ESBL)-producing microbes. In an escalation strategy, empiric therapy is commenced with a third-generation cephalosporin and escalated to a carbapenem only if necessitated by culture results *and* poor response to therapy, as cultures do not necessarily discriminate between infections and colonization, leading to many false positives and antibiotic overtreatment. The need for coverage for MRSA or multi-drug-resistant organisms is highly dependent on local resistance patterns. Major guidelines emphasize the need to establish local resistance surveillance preferably both at hospital and ICU levels and regularly communicate antibiogram results to clinicians.

A recent Cochrane analysis did not find evidence for improved outcomes with antibiotic combination therapy (Arthur et al. 2016). Unless necessitated by high local resistance patterns risking under-coverage with monotherapy, combination therapy is neither recommended for empiric nor directed therapy for hard-to-treat organisms such as *Pseudomonas*. A fixed short-course treatment length of 7 days was not inferior to 10–14 days in recent meta-analyses of six RCTs (Pugh et al. 2015) and is now recommended length of treatment (Kalil et al. 2016). Longer courses may reduce relapse rates in VAP due to *Pseudomonas* and other non-fermenting microbes, but the supporting evidence is weak. In "possible" but low probability VAP, stopping antibiotics after 3 days may be possible (Pugh et al. 2015).

67.3 Intravascular Catheter-Related Infections (CRBSI)

Indwelling catheters are a leading cause of bloodstream and health care-associated infections in general, with ICU and chronically ill cancer patients at particular risk. Catheter-related blood stream infections (CRBSI) are associated with increased morbidity and mortality, but tend to be overdiagnosed, leading to unnecessary catheter removals (Raad et al. 2007). The clinical diagnosis is challenging. Fevers and chills in ICU patients are nonspecific, and though catheter insertion site inflammation has a high specificity, the sensitivity for CRBSI is very poor (Safdar and Maki 2002). Probable CRBSI can be diagnosed with positive peripheral blood culture when there is no other apparent source of the bloodstream infection, and findings of *S. aureus*, coagulase-negative staphylococci, and *Candida* species should increase suspicion (Kiehn and Armstrong 1990). A definite diagnosis requires finding the same microorganism from the catheter tip if removed or that blood culture drawn from the catheter becomes positive ≥2 h *before* simultaneously drawn blood culture from a peripheral vein (Rijnders et al. 2001). Unless patients are hemodynamically unstable or otherwise appearing severely ill, catheters need not be removed in suspected CRBSI, but results of blood cultures can be awaited before management decisions. In general, short-term catheters (<14 days) should be removed. Long-term catheters can be managed with catheter retention and antibiotic lock solutions depending on the organism. Isolation of *S. aureus*, gram-negatives, enterococci, and *Candida* generally requires catheter removal if feasible, whereas coagulase-negative staphylococci can be treated with a short 7–10-day antibiotic course or with catheter removal without antibiotic therapy if not longer needed. For more details on the multiple variables determining management, more comprehensive guidelines should be consulted (Mermel et al. 2009).

S. aureus bacteremia carries a risk of metastatic spread by bloodstream seeding, in particular with bacteremia persisting >72 h in spite of therapy. Blood cultures should thus be repeated daily until negative and deep-seated infectious complications, foremost endocarditis and skeletal infections, should be sought when appropriate. If ruled out, a 14-day antibiotic course is sufficient for uncomplicated *S. aureus* bacteremia, but the jury is still out on the safety of even shorter durations. Vancomycin is the preferred empiric antibiotic when MRSA is prevalent and also the safest empiric option for coagulase-negative staphylococci, but beta-lactam antibiotics such as cloxacillin are more potent and preferred for susceptible staphylococci. The need for empiric gram-negative coverage must be decided on a case-by-case basis depending on the host factors and severity of presentation.

67.4 Urinary Tract Infections

Despite figuring prominently on the list of nosocomial infections, notably in the aforementioned EPIC II study (Vincent et al. 2009), the true magnitude of ICU-acquired UTIs is hard to discern. Clinical UTI diagnosis is challenging in the ICU, with a near-universal use of urinary catheters and the resulting unreliability of clinical symptoms of dysuria, pollakisuria, and urinary retention in their presence. Inability of communicating symptoms in sedated and ventilated patients adds to diagnostic uncertainty (Shuman and Chenoweth 2010). The placement of a catheter leads to universal bacterial colonization within few days of insertion, and dipstick tests for leukocytes and protein frequently become positive in the presence of a catheter. The diagnosis thus becomes one of exclusion when no other source of infection can be found. In the ICU patient, this is further complicated by the difficulty of differentiating infectious from noninfectious causes of inflammation, with both being able to cause fever, elevated inflammatory markers, and hemodynamic instability. A more confident diagnosis can be made with a close temporal relation between the placement of the catheter and a presumed infectious episode, the rare UTI episodes which are blood culture positive, or when a CT scan reveals pyelonephritis or obstructions. The most important preventive measures are avoidance of catheterization whenever possible and limiting the duration when catheterization is unavoidable (Lo et al. 2008).

Asymptomatic bacteriuria should not be treated with antibiotics. When UTIs are treated in catheterized patients, the catheter should be replaced if it has been in place for more than 7–14 days, as the formation of a biofilm may impair clearance of infection. There is increasing evidence to support a shorter antibiotic duration of 7 days, also in bacteremic UTIs, at least in patients who are rapidly stabilized (van Nieuwkoop et al. 2017; Yahav et al. 2018). As in the case of VAP, local resistance data should guide antibiotic therapy.

Enterobacteriaceae are by far the most important organisms, and third-generation cephalosporins or penicillins with increased gram-negative spectrum are reasonable options, with the need for added initial coverage for *Pseudomonas* or ESBL-producing microbes with a carbapenem depending on the severity of presentation, host factors, and local antibiograms. Because patients who are at increased risk of developing organ failures and renal failure in particular congregate in the ICU, aminoglycosides, otherwise excellent antibiotics for UTIs, are less attractive.

67.5 *Clostridium difficile* Infections

CDI is a major cause of health care-associated infections (HAI) and the most common cause of antibiotic associated diarrhea, accounting for 10–25% of cases and nearly all cases of pseudomembranous colitis (Bartlett 1994). *C. difficile* is acquired by the fecal-oral route from asymptomatic carriers or patients, via transiently colonized hands of health personnel, or via contaminated surfaces and equipment. Antibiotic disruption of the gut flora promotes transition from colonization to symptomatic disease, and both length of treatment and exposure to multiple antibiotics increase the risk. Certain antibiotics, notably quinolones, have been linked to the spread of more virulent strains like the hypervirulent ribotype 027. However, in clinical practice, any antibiotic can cause CDI and must therefore be prescribed with CDI risk in mind. Broad-spectrum antibiotics are nevertheless recognized to pose the greater risk, and antibiotic stewardship with feedback on appropriate use of narrow-spectrum antibiotics has been shown to significantly reduce CDI incidence (Fowler et al. 2007). Nonmodifiable risk factors are high age, general debility, and serious underlying disease. Chemotherapy and neutropenia also promote CDIs (Guh and Kutty 2018). The entry point for the clinical diagnosis is diarrhea, defined as ≥3 loose stools in 24 h. Diarrhea can be profuse in colitis but may be absent in seriously ill patients with paralytic ileus and toxic megacolon. Fever, abdominal pain, and leukocyte count >15 × 10^9 cells/L are markers of severe disease, and values >25 × 10^9 cells/L with lactate level ≥5 mmol/L are indicators of need for early surgery. Tests detect either the presence of *C. difficile* in stool (GHD), toxins in stool (toxin EIA), or genes for toxin production (NAATS). Different test combinations are in clinical use, but when testing is restricted to appropriate patients, NAATS alone, or after screening for GHD, is recommended. Repeat testing does not increase sensitivity. If CDI is strongly suspected despite a negative test, sigmoidoscopy may be diagnostic. Tests remain positive long after clinical cure and retesting as treatment control is not indicated. Treatment recommendations have recently been updated by the Infectious Diseases Society of America (IDSA) (McDonald et al. 2018). Ongoing antibiotic therapy should be discontinued if not jeopardizing recovery from other infections and may suffice in mild disease. Vancomycin (125 mg × 4 p.o) or fidaxomicin (200 mg × 2 p.o) for 10 days is recommended over metronidazole, also in non-severe disease. In fulminant cases, and if ileus is present, i.v. metronidazole 500 mg × 3 should be added. In the latter, rectal instillation of vancomycin (500 mg × 4) may also be administered. Recurrences are common, and fecal microbiota transplant (FMT) is highly efficacious and should be considered after more than two recurrences. A novel monoclonal toxin-binding antibody (bezlotoxumab) has recently been approved to reduce risk of recurrences in high-risk patients, and a severely ill neurointensive care unit patient would arguably fit that category. Bezlotoxumab must be given together with conventional CDI therapy as it does not interrupt ongoing infection.

67.6 Specific Pediatric Concerns

With few exceptions (fluoroquinolones, tetracyclines) where age limitations for usage in children are given, most antibiotics can safely be administered respecting weight-based dosage recommendations. There are very limited data for FMT in children.

References

Arthur LE, Kizor RS, Selim AG, van Driel ML, Seoane L. Antibiotics for ventilator-associated pneumonia. Cochrane Database Syst Rev. 2016;10:CD004267. https://doi.org/10.1002/14651858.CD004267.pu.

Bartlett JG. Clostridium difficile: history of its role as an enteric pathogen and the current state of knowledge about the organism. Clin Infect Dis. 1994;18:S265–72. https://doi.org/10.1093/clinids/18.Supplement_4.S265.

Blackwood B, Alderdice F, Burns K, Cardwell C, Lavery G, O'Halloran P. Use of weaning protocols for reducing duration of mechanical ventilation in critically ill adult patients: Cochrane systematic review and meta-analysis. BMJ. 2011;342:c7237. https://doi.org/10.1136/bmj.c7237.

Busl KM. Nosocomial infections in the neurointensive care unit. Neurosurg Clin N Am. 2018;29:299–314. https://doi.org/10.1016/j.nec.2017.11.008.

de Smet AMGA, Kluytmans JAJW, Cooper BS, Mascini EM, Benus RFJ, van der Werf TS, et al. Decontamination of the digestive tract and oropharynx in ICU patients. N Engl J Med. 2009;360:20–31. https://doi.org/10.1056/NEJMoa0800394.

Dettenkofer M, Ebner W, Hans F-J, Forster D, Babikir R, Zentner J, et al. Nosocomial infections in a neurosurgery intensive care unit. Acta Neurochir (Wien). 1999;141:1303–8. https://doi.org/10.1007/s007010050434.

European Centre for Disease Prevention and Control. Healthcare-associated infections acquired in intensive care units. In: ECDC, editor. Annual epidemiological report for 2016 ECDC, Stockholm. 2018.

Fowler S, Webber A, Cooper BS, Phimister A, Price K, Carter Y, et al. Successful use of feedback to improve antibiotic prescribing and reduce Clostridium difficile infection: a controlled interrupted time series. J Antimicrob Chemother. 2007;59:990–5. https://doi.org/10.1093/jac/dkm014.

Guh AY, Kutty PK. Clostridioides difficile infection. Ann Intern Med. 2018;169:ITC49–64. https://doi.org/10.7326/AITC201810020.

Hellyer TP, Ewan V, Wilson P, Simpson AJ. The Intensive Care Society recommended bundle of interventions for the prevention of ventilator-associated pneumonia. J Intensive Care Soc. 2016;17:238–43. https://doi.org/10.1177/1751143716644461.

Jürgen P, Randall MC, Lawrence FM, Marjan van B-C, Melville RK, Barbara AB, et al. Extracranial complications of severe head injury. J Neurosurg. 1992;77:901–7. https://doi.org/10.3171/jns.1992.77.6.0901.

Kalil AC, Metersky ML, Klompas M, Muscedere J, Sweeney DA, Palmer LB, et al. Management of adults with hospital-acquired and ventilator-associated Pneumonia: 2016 Clinical Practice Guidelines by the Infectious Diseases Society of America and the American Thoracic Society. Clin Infect Dis. 2016;63:e61–e111. https://doi.org/10.1093/cid/ciw353.

Kiehn TE, Armstrong D. Changes in the spectrum of organisms causing bacteremia and fungemia in immunocompromised patients due to venous access devices. Eur J Clin Microbiol Infect Dis. 1990;9:869–72. https://doi.org/10.1007/bf01967501.

Laborde G, Grosskopf U, Schmieder K, Harders A, Klimek L, Hardenack M, Gilsbach JM. Nosocomial infections in a neurosurgical intensive care unit. Der Anaesthesist. 1993;42:724–31.

Lo E, Nicolle L, Classen D, Arias KM, Podgorny K, Anderson DJ, et al. Strategies to prevent catheter-associated urinary tract infections in acute care hospitals. Infect Control Hosp Epidemiol. 2008;29:S41–50. https://doi.org/10.1086/591066.

McDonald LC, Gerding DN, Johnson S, Bakken JS, Carroll KC, Coffin SE, et al. Clinical practice guidelines for Clostridium difficile infection in adults and children: 2017 update by the Infectious Diseases Society of America (IDSA) and Society for Healthcare Epidemiology of America (SHEA). Clin Infect Dis. 2018;66:e1–e48. https://doi.org/10.1093/cid/cix1085.

Mermel LA, Allon M, Bouza E, Craven DE, Flynn P, O'Grady NP, et al. Clinical practice guidelines for the diagnosis and management of intravascular catheter-related infection: 2009 update by the Infectious Diseases Society of America. Clin Infect Dis. 2009;49:1–45. https://doi.org/10.1086/599376.

Price R, MacLennan G, Glen J. Selective digestive or oropharyngeal decontamination and topical oropharyngeal chlorhexidine for prevention of death in general intensive care: systematic review and network meta-analysis. BMJ. 2014;348:g2197. https://doi.org/10.1136/bmj.g2197.

Pugh R, Grant C, Cooke RPD, Dempsey G. Short-course versus prolonged-course antibiotic therapy for hospital-acquired pneumonia in critically ill adults. Cochrane Database Syst Rev. 2015;8:CD007577. https://doi.org/10.1002/14651858.CD007577.pub3.

Raad I, Hanna H, Maki D. Intravascular catheter-related infections: advances in diagnosis, prevention, and management. Lancet Infect Dis. 2007;7:645–57. https://doi.org/10.1016/S1473-3099(07)70235-9.

Rijnders BJA, Verwaest C, Peetermans WE, Wilmer A, Vandecasteele S, Van Eldere J, Van Wijngaerden E. Difference in time to positivity of hub-blood versus nonhub-blood cultures is not useful for the diagnosis of catheter-related bloodstream infection in critically ill patients. Crit Care Med. 2001;29:1399–403.

Safdar N, Maki DG. Inflammation at the insertion site is not predictive of catheter-related bloodstream infection with short-term, noncuffed central venous catheters*. Crit Care Med. 2002;30:2632–5.

Shuman EK, Chenoweth CE. Recognition and prevention of healthcare-associated urinary tract infections in the intensive care unit. Crit Care Med. 2010;38:S373–9. https://doi.org/10.1097/CCM.0b013e3181e6ce8f.

Stocchetti N, Rossi S, Zanier E, Colombo A, Beretta L, Citerio G. Pyrexia in head-injured patients admitted to intensive care. Intensive Care Med. 2002;28:1555–62. https://doi.org/10.1007/s00134-002-1513-1.

van Nieuwkoop C, van der Starre WE, Stalenhoef JE, van Aartrijk AM, van der Reijden TJK, Vollaard AM, et al. Treatment duration of febrile urinary tract infection: a pragmatic randomized, double-blind, placebo-controlled non-inferiority trial in men and women. BMC Med. 2017;15:70. https://doi.org/10.1186/s12916-017-0835-3.

Vincent J, Rello J, Marshall J, Silva E, Anzueto A, Martin CD, et al. International study of the prevalence and outcomes of infection in intensive care units. JAMA. 2009;302:2323–9. https://doi.org/10.1001/jama.2009.1754.

Yahav D, Turjeman A, Babitch T, Koppel F, Bitterman R, Neuberger A, et al. Seven versus 14 antibiotic days for the treatment of Gram-negative bacteraemia: non-inferiority randomized controlled trial. (Abstract O1120). Paper presented at the European Congress of Clinical Microbiology and Infectious Diseases, Madrid, April 21–24. 2018.

Temperature Management

68

Per-Olof Grände and Peter Reinstrup

Recommendations

Level I

Active cooling to subnormal temperature in traumatic brain injury (TBI) patients does not improve outcome.

Level II

There is support for the avoidance of high fever, but no support for active cooling.

Level III

Level III studies support the use of active cooling in TBI patients, a conclusion not supported from Level I or II studies. Paracetamol can be used to reduce fever in TBI patients.

68.1 Overview

Body temperature can be measured at different sites where rectal temperature is the classical standard position for body core measurement. Other sites have been vagina, bladder, ear, oral and oesophagus. Measurement of brain temperature with a temperature probe inserted in the brain (positioned in the parenchyma or in a ventricle) has shown that brain temperature is only slightly higher (≈ 0.3 °C) than body core temperature in spite of the much higher metabolism of the brain (Mellergård and Nordström 1991). The high blood flow to the brain will counteract a difference between body core temperature and brain temperature. Normal rectal temperature is 36.7 ± 0.7 °C.

Based on experimental and clinical studies, there is a general view that high fever is detrimental to TBI patients (Thompson et al. 2003). An important goal in the treatment of these patients has therefore been to prevent or reduce fever. So far, we lack evidence-based consensus regarding how to reduce temperature in TBI patients. Fever can be reduced pharmacologically by affecting the hypothalamic thermostat or by active cooling of the patient. During the last 15 years, it has also been suggested that active cooling to subnormal temperatures (32–34 °C) should be beneficial due to its well-known neuroprotective effect, as demonstrated in animal studies after brain ischaemia and also in humans after near drowning in cold water and after active cooling following heart resuscitation (Polderman 2008; Grände et al. 2009; Sandestig et al. 2014). There was no improved outcome, however, in a recent randomised heart resuscitation hypothermia study

P.-O. Grände (✉) · P. Reinstrup
Department of Anaesthesia and Intensive Care, Lund University and Lund University Hospital, Lund, Sweden
e-mail: per-olof.grande@med.lu.se; peter.reinstrup@med.lu.se

© Springer Nature Switzerland AG 2020
T. Sundstrøm et al. (eds.), *Management of Severe Traumatic Brain Injury*,
https://doi.org/10.1007/978-3-030-39383-0_68

in the group treated with active cooling down to 33 °C compared to a temperature of 36 °C (Nielsen et al. 2013). The fact that hypothermia decreases an increased intracranial pressure has also been taken as an indication for beneficial effect of hypothermia in head trauma patients (Polderman 2008; Andrews et al. 2015).

The mechanisms behind the suggested hypothermia-induced neuroprotection are not clarified, but the reduced neuronal metabolism, reduced inflammatory response, reduction in toxic substances such as glutamate and a scavenging effect are discussed to be involved. It was therefore believed that active cooling should be beneficial in TBI patients. In this chapter, we give recommendations on how and when temperature should be reduced and the goal temperature in TBI patients, based on the results of the most recent studies and current knowledge in this field. It is concluded that active cooling is associated with side effects and that we lack support for its use in TBI patients, and it can therefore not be recommended (see below).

Tips, Tricks and Pitfalls

- Avoid active cooling in TBI patients.
- Too high body temperature can be reduced by affecting the thermostat pharmacologically with paracetamol (1 g × 2–4 p.o.). A persistent life-threatening high fever above 39 °C can be reduced with one bolus dose of metylprednisolone (Solu-Medrol) (0.25–0.5 g i.v.).
- Normothermia is the optimal temperature.

68.2 Background

68.2.1 Active Cooling of the TBI Patient

There have been many studies on TBI patients that have analysed the effect of active cooling to normal and subnormal temperatures on outcome. Cooling of the whole body (systemic cooling) has been used in most studies so far.

Local cooling of the brain has been discussed to reduce complications of systemic cooling, such as pulmonary complications and coagulation disturbances. Selective brain cooling can be obtained by a cooling cap or by intranasal cooling with circulating cold water via a tubing/balloon system inserted into the nose. Local cooling, especially with an intranasal cooling technique, so far has had difficulty in reducing brain temperature, and additional technical development is necessary before it can be recommended (Springborg et al. 2013).

In spite of the fact that reduction of fever by active cooling to a normal temperature or lower has been used in clinical practice in TBI patients for decades, there have been no randomised or larger studies confirming any beneficial effect of this therapeutic measure on outcome. Several smaller studies have suggested that there is improved outcome with active cooling (Marion et al. 1997; Adelson et al. 2005), but, as mentioned, the best trials on children and adults could not confirm such an effect (Clifton et al. 2001, 2011; Hutchison et al. 2008). The well-known hypothermia-induced reduction in ICP most likely is an effect of hypothermia-induced vasoconstriction with a simultaneous decrease in cerebral blood flow and blood volume. The ICP effect of hypothermia to 33–35 °C on outcome in TBI patients starting with an ICP above 20 mmHg was recently analysed in a large multicentre European randomised study (Andrews et al. 2015). As expected, they found that ICP decreased with hypothermia, but there was no improvement in outcome, and the study was interrupted in advance due to signs of adverse effects.

A comprehensive analysis of the best studies supported the view that active cooling to subnormal temperatures has no beneficial effect on outcome in TBI patients; instead, these studies indicated that active cooling even worsens outcome. This conclusion was supported by a recent Cochrane analysis (Sydenham et al. 2009). Thus, we still lack any support for the view that treatment of a severe head injury with or without fever and with or without a raised ICP by active cooling to normal or subnormal temperature is beneficial. Thus, at this stage, active cooling systemically or locally cannot be recommended as a general therapy or a therapy to reduce temperature or ICP in TBI patients.

There are some specific characteristics that may explain why the well-established neuroprotective effect of active cooling does not improve outcome in TBI patients (Grände et al. 2009; Sandestig et al. 2014). Active systemic or local cooling always means a difference between the body or brain temperature and the temperature stipulated by the hypothalamic thermostat. This difference creates a pronounced metabolic stress with the purpose of restoring body temperature to the level before cooling, resulting in an increase in plasma catecholamines. Muscle shivering is a visible component of this stress response, but the increase in stress and catecholamine release most likely is present without shivering. There is a great risk that the increased catecholamine concentration after active cooling will further reduce the already compromised circulation of the penumbra zone. There is also a risk that ventilatory adjustment to the hypothermia-induced lower metabolism is not performed, leading to a condition corresponding to hyperventilation, resulting in worse perfusion of the penumbra zone. Hypothermia also means a lower blood pressure, resulting in more frequent use of vasopressors, which may not only reduce perfusion of the penumbra zone, but also increase the risk of development of ARDS (Robertson et al. 1999) and loss of plasma volume to the interstitium (Dubniks et al. 2007; Nygren et al. 2010). Finally, reduction of the body temperature to subnormal values may induce coagulation disturbances and increase the volumes of contusional bleedings (Rundgren and Engström 2008).

68.2.2 Pharmacological Reduction of Fever

From a physiological point of view, fever should be treated by adjusting the hypothalamic thermostat. Several types of new temperature-reducing substances have been tested experimentally, but so far none of these substances can be used clinically due to severe side effects. This means that at the moment, paracetamol and steroids are the only temperature-reducing substances affecting the hypothalamic thermostat available in clinical practice. Paracetamol can be used to reduce fever, but it reduces temperature by only about 0.5 °C in acceptable doses. In higher doses, it has side effects in terms of inhibition of the endogenous production of prostacyclin, and it has toxic effects on the liver.

Steroids (e.g. methylprednisolone) effectively reduce fever by affecting the hypothalamic temperature centre. A randomised study on TBI patients (the CRASH study), including both moderately injured and more severely injured patients (GCS <14), analysed the effect of routine use methylprednisolone (Edwards et al. 2005). It showed worse outcome in TBI patients given steroids. Note that steroids were given in a very high dose of more than 20 g for 2 days in that study and were used independently of fever or not and independently of the severity of the head injury. The results of the CRASH study support the conclusion that corticosteroids in high doses should not be used in the treatment of moderate and severe head injury and especially not for several days. This does not mean, however, that the fever-reducing effect of just one bolus dose of methylprednisolone at the relatively low dose of 0.25–0.5 g to an adult with a severe TBI cannot be used to reduce a life-threatening high fever. Such a dose may significantly reduce fever for up to 2 days, and the beneficial fever-reducing effect most likely overrides the potential adverse effects shown by the 20–30 times larger doses in the CRASH study and the well-known adverse effect of a very high fever. A subsequent increase in blood glucose can be controlled by insulin.

68.3 Specific Paediatric Concerns

The highest-quality randomised trials performed for the adult and the paediatric population have not shown any beneficial effects of active cooling following TBI (Clifton et al. 2001, 2011). The best paediatric study performed so far (Hutchison et al. 2008) strongly indicated that hypothermia even worsens outcome. This means that according to our present knowledge, active hypothermia should not be used in the paediatric population.

References

Adelson PD, Ragheb J, Kanev P, Brockmeyer D, Beers SR, Brown SD, Cassidy LD, Chang Y, Levin H. Phase II clinical trial of moderate hypothermia after severe traumatic brain injury in children. Neurosurgery. 2005;56(4):740–54.

Andrews PJ, Sinclair HL, Rodriguez A, Harris BA, Battison CG, Rhodes JK, Murray GD, Eurotherm3235 Trial Collaborators. Hypothermia for intracranial hypertension after traumatic brain injury. N Engl J Med. 2015;373(25):2403–12. https://doi.org/10.1056/NEJMoa1507581.

Clifton GL, Miller ER, Choi SC, Levin HS, McCauley S, Smith KR Jr, Muizelaar JP, Wagner FC Jr, Marion DW, Luerssen TG, Chesnut RM, Schwartz M. Lack of effect of induction of hypothermia after acute brain injury. N Engl J Med. 2001;344(8):556–63.

Clifton GL, Valadka A, Zygun D, Coffey CS, Drever P, Fourwinds S, Janis LS, Wilde E, Taylor P, Harshman K, Conley A, Puccio A, Levin HS, McCauley SR, Bucholz RD, Smith KR, Schmidt JH, Scott JN, Yonas H, Okonkwo DO. Very early hypothermia induction in patients with severe brain injury (the National Acute Brain Injury Study: Hypothermia II): a randomised trial. Lancet Neurol. 2011;10(2):131–9.

Dubniks M, Persson J, Grände PO. Effect of blood pressure on plasma volume loss in the rat under increased permeability. Intensive Care Med. 2007;33(12):2192–8.

Edwards P, Arango M, Balica L, Cottingham R, El-Sayed H, Farrell B, Fernandes J, Gogichaisvili T, Golden N, Hartzenberg B, Husain M, Ulloa MI, Jerbi Z, Khamis H, Komolafe E, Laloë V, Lomas G, Ludwig S, Mazairac G, Muñoz Sanchéz Mde L, Nasi L, Olldashi F, Plunkett P, Roberts I, Sandercock P, Shakur H, Soler C, Stocker R, Svoboda P, Trenkler S, Venkataramana NK, Wasserberg J, Yates D, Yutthakasemsunt S, CRASH trial collaborators. Final results of MRC CRASH, a randomised placebo-controlled trial of intravenous corticosteroid in adults with head injury-outcomes at 6 months. Lancet. 2005;365(9475):1957–9.

Grände PO, Reinstrup P, Romner B. Active cooling in traumatic brain-injured patients: a questionable therapy? Acta Anaesthesiol Scand. 2009;53(10):1233–8.

Hutchison JS, Ward RE, Lacroix J, Hébert PC, Barnes MA, Bohn DJ, Dirks PB, Doucette S, Fergusson D, Gottesman R, Joffe AR, Kirpalani HM, Meyer PG, Morris KP, Moher D, Singh RN, Skippen PW, Hypothermia Pediatric Head Injury Trial Investigators and the Canadian Critical Care Trials Group. Hypothermia therapy after traumatic brain injury in children. N Engl J Med. 2008;358(23):2447–56.

Marion DW, Penrod LE, Kelsey SF, Obrist WD, Kochanek PM, Palmer AM, Wisniewski SR, DeKosky ST. Treatment of traumatic brain injury with moderate hypothermia. N Engl J Med. 1997;336(8):540–6.

Mellergård P, Nordström CH. Intracerebral temperature in neurosurgical patients. Neurosurgery. 1991;28(5):709–13.

Nielsen N, Wetterslev J, Cronberg T, Erlinge D, Gasche Y, Hassager C, Horn J, Hovdenes J, Kjaergaard J, Kuiper M, Pellis T, Stammet P, Wanscher M, Wise MP, Åneman A, Al-Subaie N, Boesgaard S, Bro-Jeppesen J, Brunetti I, Bugge JF, Hingston CD, Juffermans NP, Koopmans M, Køber L, Langørgen J, Lilja G, Møller JE, Rundgren M, Rylander C, Smid O, Werer C, Winkel P, Friberg H, TTM Trial Investigators. Targeted temperature management at 33°C versus 36°C after cardiac arrest. N Engl J Med. 2013;369(23):2197–206. https://doi.org/10.1056/NEJMoa1310519.

Nygren A, Redfors B, Thorén A, Ricksten SE. Norepinephrine causes a pressure-dependent plasma volume decrease in clinical vasodilatory shock. Acta Anaesthesiol Scand. 2010;54:814–20.

Polderman KH. Induced hypothermia and fever control for prevention and treatment of neurological injuries. Lancet. 2008;7(371):1955–69.

Robertson CS, Valadka AB, Hannay HJ, Contant CF, Gopinath SP, Cormio M, Uzura M, Grossman RG. Prevention of secondary ischemic insults after severe head injury. Crit Care Med. 1999;27(10):2086–95.

Rundgren M, Engström M. A thromboelastometric evaluation of the effects of hypothermia on the coagulation system. Anesth Analg. 2008;107(5):1465–8.

Sandestig A, Romner B, Grände PO. Therapeutic hypothermia in children and adults with severe traumatic brain injury. A review. Ther Hypothermia Temp Manag. 2014;4:10–20. https://doi.org/10.1089/ther.2013.0024.

Springborg JB, Springborg KK, Romner B. First clinical experience with intranasal cooling for hyperthermia in brain-injured patients. Neurocrit Care. 2013;18:400–5.

Sydenham E, Roberts I, Alderson P. Hypothermia for traumatic head injury. Cochrane Database Syst Rev. 2009;2:CD001048.

Thompson HJ, Tkacs NC, Saatman KE, Raghupathi R, McIntosh TK. Hyperthermia following traumatic brain injury: a critical evaluation. Neurobiol Dis. 2003;12(3):163–73.

Seizures

69

Elisabeth Ronne-Engström and Jon Axel Forsse

Recommendations

Level I

There are insufficient data to support a Level I recommendation regarding either treatment for early posttraumatic seizures (PTS) or anti-seizure prophylaxis after head trauma.

Level II

Early posttraumatic seizures should be treated. Anticonvulsants may be used to decrease the incidence of early PTS (within 7 days of injury).

Level III

When seizures occur, it is important to re-evaluate the clinical situation with respect to intracranial lesions requiring surgical intervention. Prophylactic anti-seizure therapy may be considered as a treatment option to prevent early PTS in young paediatric patients and infants at high risk for seizures following head injury.

E. Ronne-Engström (✉)
Department of Neuroscience, Neurosurgery, Uppsala University, Uppsala, Sweden
e-mail: elisabeth.ronne.engstrom@akademiska.se

J. A. Forsse
Department of Neurosurgery, Odense University Hospital, Odense, Denmark
e-mail: jon.axel.forsse@rsyd.dk

69.1 Overview

There are no randomised, controlled, double-blind studies regarding treatment of early seizures after TBI, but observational studies support that seizures should be treated as soon as they occur. The basic idea of neurointensive care of TBI is to identify and treat conditions that compromise the brain's supply and use of oxygen and glucose. Seizure activity in the acute phase impairs this in a number of ways and can therefore worsen the brain injury. Neuronal firing causes a massive release of the potentially neurotoxic transmitter glutamate (GLU). In order to clear the synaptic space from GLU, there is an efficient glial uptake; however, it is highly energy dependent. Seizures increase energy demand, which can cause an energy failure in the brain developing into manifest ischaemia. Seizure activity can also cause significant changes in cerebral blood flow, with both increases and decreases observed.

It is debated whether anticonvulsant prophylaxis after head trauma should be used or not. The Brain Trauma Foundation states in its latest review that an adequate treatment with phenytoin or levetiracetam reduces the incidence of early seizures, but that evidence of effect on outcome is lacking (Carney et al. 2017). A major confounding factor is that earlier studies based their conclusions only on clinically observable seizures. The Brain Trauma Foundation states that further studies are needed and that such studies should

© Springer Nature Switzerland AG 2020
T. Sundstrøm et al. (eds.), *Management of Severe Traumatic Brain Injury*,
https://doi.org/10.1007/978-3-030-39383-0_69

use continuous EEG (cEEG) monitoring to identify seizures. Once seizures occur, they could either be a result of the original trauma or an indication that new intracranial lesions have developed. Treatment of repeated seizures and status epilepticus is a matter for qualified neurointensive care, multimodality monitoring and a team approach including neurosurgeons, neurologists, neurophysiologists and neurointensivists.

69.1.1 Background

Seizures occurring after traumatic brain injury (TBI) are usually described as either early (within first week after trauma) or late (thereafter). These are two qualitatively different phenomena, probably to some extent with separate pathophysiological mechanisms. The true incidence of early seizures is presently discussed. Based on clinical observations, the incidence was estimated to ~10%. However, continuous EEG monitoring shows that early seizures are more common and are seen in up to 50% of TBI patients who are admitted to neurointensive care. Early seizures are more often seen in younger children and the elderly and in those with subdural/epidural haematomas (alone or in combination with brain contusions) (Bennett et al. 2017; Arndt et al. 2016; Vespa et al. 1999; Ronne-Engstrom and Winkler 2006).

Late seizures manifest as posttraumatic epilepsy and develop in approximately 5% of TBI. Posttraumatic epilepsy accounts for 20% of symptomatic epilepsy in the population (Lowenstein 2009) and is more common after penetrating injury, severe closed injury, focal lesions and age >65 (Pohlmann-Eden and Bruckmeir 1997; Annegers and Coan 2000).

Early seizures are also believed to be a risk factor for posttraumatic epilepsy, and there seems to be a time window for therapeutic intervention before the traumatic brain scar matures into a chronic epileptic region.

There are two main indications for monitoring and treatment of seizures after head trauma: to avoid worsening of traumatic brain injuries in the acute phase and to avoid fatal status epilepticus.

69.1.2 The Relation of Seizures to the Acute Brain Injury

There are several mechanisms by which seizure activity in the acute phase can exacerbate the brain trauma. Neuronal firing causes a massive release of the potentially neurotoxic transmitter glutamate (GLU). Extracellular GLU release during seizure activity has been demonstrated with intracerebral microdialysis in patients with chronic epilepsy (During and Spencer 1993; Ronne-Engstrom et al. 1992) and in TBI patients (Vespa et al. 1998). Another problem is that the postsynaptic glial uptake of GLU is highly energy dependent (Magistretti and Pellerin 1999). Seizure activity can thus cause a significant increase in the energy demand. In the acute phase after trauma, with an already strained brain metabolism, an increased energy demand can result in manifest ischaemia due to energy failure with demands higher than availability (Samuelsson et al. 2007). Seizure activity can also cause significant changes in cerebral blood flow (CBF). This has been demonstrated with several techniques, e.g. cortical blood flow measurements using laser Doppler fibre attached to subdural strip electrodes (Ronne-Engstrom et al. 1993). Increased as well as decreased CBF was detected during seizures, and both these situations are potentially harmful. Increased CBF can increase ICP by vasodilatation, and a decreased CBF can worsen an energy failure situation. The blood flow changes are probably coupled with dynamic changes in metabolic demands. Vespa showed that patients with TBI and repetitive nonconvulsive seizures had both higher mean ICP and higher lactate/pyruvate ratio measured with intracerebral microdialysis, marking perturbed energy metabolism (Vespa et al. 2007).

69.2 NICU Management

69.2.1 Seizure Monitoring

The general idea with NICU monitoring is to identify and treat conditions that compromise the oxygen and glucose supply to the brain or increase metabolic demands, e.g. fever and epileptic seizures. As EEG patterns depend on the integrity of the brain structures as well as on the cerebral blood flow and metabolism, continuous EEG is theoretically an ideal monitoring modality. EEG is in fact so far the only available method for online real-time monitoring of the brain's functions. There are still problems with the technique, such as the availability of EEG reading on a 24-h basis. However, since EEG today is done digitally, computerised treatment of the EEG signal can facilitate the EEG reading. An example of this is the use of the trends of the EEG's total power (Vespa 2005). High values can indicate seizure activity, and when this is found, raw EEG during this time period is studied. Another advantage of digital EEG is that it allows for web-based reading.

69.2.2 Prophylaxis

It is debated whether anticonvulsant prophylaxis should be used or not. A major confounding factor when reading the literature is that early studies base their conclusions only on clinically observable seizures. The Brain Trauma Foundation has in their guidelines for treatment of TBI also reviewed the scientific basis for anti-seizure prophylaxis (Carney et al. 2017). Their conclusion is that there is evidence that an adequate treatment with phenytoin reduces the incidence of early seizures, but not that of posttraumatic epilepsy. Valproate may have a comparable effect but may also be associated with a higher mortality. They also state that more studies are needed on the effect on outcome by reducing early seizures and that such studies should use continuous EEG monitoring to identify seizures. Using drugs with anticonvulsant properties, e.g. midazolam, in sedating intubated patients could be an alternative to anti-seizure prophylaxis. No seizures were monitored in a study were most of the patients were sedated with thiopental and midazolam (Olivecrona et al. 2009).

69.2.3 Treatment of Seizures

When seizures occur, it is important to re-evaluate the clinical situation to see if something has changed. This could be the development of a brain contusion, subdural haematoma or a cortical venous thrombosis. One should also keep in mind the possibility of withdrawal symptoms for alcohol/drug addicts with TBI. Early posttraumatic seizures should be treated as soon as they occur, which is easier if the unit has a protocolled treatment. The suggested treatments below are from the Uppsala University Hospital treatment program for seizures in neurointensive care. *Single seizures* could be treated with diazepam 10 mg i.v. or lorazepam 2–4 mg i.v. Secondary prophylaxis with phenytoin or levetiracetam should be considered.

In case of *repeated seizures*, treatment as well as prophylaxis should be started. It is preferred that continuous EEG monitoring is used to ensure that the patient becomes seizure-free from the treatment. Respiration and cardiovascular functions should also be monitored, and the threshold for intubation and mechanical ventilation should be low. The choice of pharmacological substances should be based on local guidelines for sedation of intubated patients. Propofol infusion is often used. A bolus dose of 1–3 mg/kg is given, followed by 1–5 mg/kg/h. Treatment should not extend 48 h. Midazolam infusion is also efficient. Midazolam is administered with a bolus of 0.2 mg/kg i.v. followed by 0.1–0.5 mg/kg/h. To this is added phenytoin infusion, 15–20 mg FE/kg, followed by intermittent doses of 250 mg FE/kg × 3. It is important that adequate serum concentrations are achieved and daily checks are advised. Levetiracetam can be used at this stage as an alternative to phenytoin and may have a preferable adverse event profile (initial dose 500 mg × 2 daily, oral or i.v. with loading dose 30–70 mg/kg max 3 g considered safe).

If seizures still are present, lorazepam, levetiracetam, lamotrigine, carbamazepine or valproate can be added. Anticonvulsant drugs have many side effects including interaction with other drugs, skin reactions, deranged liver function and haematologic disturbances, such as clotting disturbances, which can be especially serious for TBI patients.

Status epilepticus that does not resolve with the treatment above can be treated with thiopental infusion. Bolus dose is 100–250 mg and is followed by 50 mg every 2–3 min until EEG is low voltage without seizure activity or burst suppression. This is followed by an infusion of 3–5 mg/kg/h. There should be at least a period of 12–24 h free from seizures before the treatment stops. The patient with thiopental treatment must be on mechanical ventilation with a strict control on electrolytes, temperature and vital organ functions.

69.3 Specific Paediatric Concerns

There are only a few studies in the literature regarding children and early posttraumatic seizures. In one study, 7% had immediate seizures (Emanuelson and Uvebrant 2009). This contrasts to a study showing that as much as 68% of children with moderate and severe TBI developed early posttraumatic seizures. The two groups probably represent different severities of TBI (Liesemer et al. 2011). In a large retrospective cohort study from 2017, Bennet et al. concluded that posttraumatic seizures were diagnosed in 25.2% of children with severe TBI (Bennett et al. 2017).

The Brain Trauma Foundation guidelines state that prophylactic use of anti-seizure therapy is not recommended for children with severe traumatic brain injury (TBI) for preventing *late* posttraumatic seizures (Level II) (Kochanek et al. 2012). However, it may be considered a treatment option in young paediatric patients and infants at high risk, for the prevention of *early* seizures (Level III).

Treatment of seizures and status epilepticus in children should follow similar strategies as in adults. However, the doses and choices of drugs should be carefully considered after the individual circumstances. For example, propofol is only recommended for starting sedation of children >1 month of age and should not be used for continuous sedation >24 h (Kaye et al. 2017). Continuous EEG monitoring can be very valuable in paediatric patients.

Tips, Tricks, and Pitfalls

- When seizures occur, exclude development of new intracranial lesions needing surgical intervention.
- Remember possible withdrawal symptoms for alcohol/drug addicts with TBI.
- *Treatment of single seizures*:
  - Intravenous diazepam 10 mg or lorazepam 2–4 mg.
  - Consider prophylaxis with phenytoin.
- *Treatment of repeated seizures*:
  - Start continuous treatment as well as prophylaxis.
  - Monitor vital functions and EEG.
  - Low threshold for intubation and artificial ventilation to enable more intense treatment.
  - Propofol infusion is commonly used. A bolus dose of 1–3 mg/kg is followed by infusion of 1.0–7.5 mg/kg/h until seizure activity is relieved. Midazolam can also be used, combined with propofol or as monotherapy, and starts with a bolus of 0.2 mg/kg i.v. followed by infusion of 0.1–0.5 mg/kg/h.
  - Phenytoin is added as prophylaxis with 15–20 mg FE/kg i.v. followed by 250 FE × 3. It is important that adequate serum concentrations are achieved, and daily checks are advised. Levetiracetam is considered a sufficient alternative to phenytoin.
  - If seizures persist, lorazepam, levetiracetam, lamotrigine, carbamazepine or valproate can be added.
- *Treatment of status epilepticus if not resolved with the treatment above*:
  - Thiopental infusion. Bolus dose is 100–250 mg and is followed by 50 mg every 2–3 min until EEG is low voltage without seizure activity or burst suppression. This is followed by an infusion of 3–5 mg/kg/h. There should be 12–24 h free from seizures before the treatment stops. Note: the patient must be on mechanical ventilation with strict control of electrolytes, temperature and vital organ functions.

References

Annegers JF, Coan SP. The risks of epilepsy after traumatic brain injury. Seizure. 2000;9(7):453–7.

Arndt DH, Goodkin HP, Giza CC. Early posttraumatic seizures in the pediatric population. J Child Neurol. 2016;31(1):46–56.

Bennett KS, DeWitt PE, Harlaar N, Bennett TD. Seizures in children with severe traumatic brain injury. Pediatr Crit Care Med. 2017;18(1):54–63.

Carney N, Totten AM, O'Reilly C, Ullman JS, Hawryluk GWJ, Bell MJ, Bratton SL, Chesnut R, Harris OA, Kissoon N, Rubiano AM, Shutter L, Tasker RC, Vavilala MS, Wilberger J, Wright DW, Ghajar J. Guidelines for the management of severe traumatic brain injury, fourth edition. Neurosurgery. 2017;80(1):6–15.

During MJ, Spencer DD. Extracellular hippocampal glutamate and spontaneous seizure in the conscious human brain. Lancet. 1993;341(8861):1607–10.

Emanuelson I, Uvebrant P. Occurrence of epilepsy during the first 10 years after traumatic brain injury acquired in childhood up to the age of 18 years in the south western Swedish population-based series. Brain Inj. 2009;23(7):612–6.

Kaye AD, Fox CJ, Padnos IW, Ehrhardt KP, Diaz JH, Cornett EM, Chandler D, Sen S, Patil S. Pharmacologic considerations of anesthetic agents in pediatric patients: a comprehensive review. Anesthesiol Clin. 2017;35:e73–94.

Kochanek PM, Carney N, Adelson PD, Ashwal S, Bell MJ, Bratton S, Carson S, Chesnut RM, Ghajar J, Goldstein B, et al. Guidelines for the acute medical management of severe traumatic brain injury in infants, children, and adolescents, second edition. Pediatr Crit Care Med. 2012;13(1):1–82.

Liesemer K, et al. Early post-traumatic seizures in moderate to severe pediatric traumatic brain injury: rates, risk factors, and clinical features. J Neurotrauma. 2011;28(5):755–62.

Lowenstein DH. Epilepsy after head injury: an overview. Epilepsia. 2009;50(Suppl 2):4–9.

Magistretti PJ, Pellerin L. Astrocytes couple synaptic activity to glucose utilization in the brain. News Physiol Sci. 1999;14:177–82.

Olivecrona M, et al. Absence of electroencephalographic seizure activity in patients treated for head injury with an intracranial pressure-targeted therapy. J Neurosurg. 2009;110(2):300–5.

Pohlmann-Eden B, Bruckmeir J. Predictors and dynamics of posttraumatic epilepsy. Acta Neurol Scand. 1997;95(5):257–62.

Ronne-Engstrom E, Winkler T. Continuous EEG monitoring in patients with traumatic brain injury reveals a high incidence of epileptiform activity. Acta Neurol Scand. 2006;114(1):47–53.

Ronne-Engstrom E, et al. Intracerebral microdialysis of extracellular amino acids in the human epileptic focus. J Cereb Blood Flow Metab. 1992;12(5):873–6.

Ronne-Engstrom E, Carlson H, Blom S, Flink R, Gazelius B, Spännare B, Hillered L. Monitoring of cortical blood flow in human epileptic foci using laser doppler flowmetry. J Epilepsy. 1993;6:145–51.

Samuelsson C, et al. Cerebral glutamine and glutamate levels in relation to compromised energy metabolism: a microdialysis study in subarachnoid hemorrhage patients. J Cereb Blood Flow Metab. 2007;27(7):1309–17.

Vespa P. Continuous EEG monitoring for the detection of seizures in traumatic brain injury, infarction, and intracerebral hemorrhage: "to detect and protect". J Clin Neurophysiol. 2005;22(2):99–106.

Vespa P, et al. Increase in extracellular glutamate caused by reduced cerebral perfusion pressure and seizures after human traumatic brain injury: a microdialysis study. J Neurosurg. 1998;89(6):971–82.

Vespa PM, et al. Increased incidence and impact of nonconvulsive and convulsive seizures after traumatic brain injury as detected by continuous electroencephalographic monitoring. J Neurosurg. 1999;91(5):750–60.

Vespa PM, et al. Nonconvulsive electrographic seizures after traumatic brain injury result in a delayed, prolonged increase in intracranial pressure and metabolic crisis. Crit Care Med. 2007;35(12):2830–6.

70 Paroxysmal Sympathetic Hyperactivity

Christina Rosenlund

Recommendations

Level I

Hypermetabolism and nitrogen loss follow acute severe cerebral injury, and high protein diet is vital.

Level II

Weight loss following dystonia is causing problems in rehabilitation settings.

It is a recommendation that full nutritional replacement be instituted by day 7 post-injury.

About 15–20% nitrogen calories in nutritional replacement reduce nitrogen loss.

Level III

If there are clinical signs of paroxysmal sympathetic hyperactivity and other explanations for the symptoms are ruled out, it is recommended to try treatment with intrathecal baclofen.

If there is no response to treatment with a lumbar dosage of 200 g baclofen, further testing is without purpose.

C. Rosenlund (✉)
Department of Neurosurgery, Odense University Hospital, Odense, Denmark

70.1 Overview

Paroxysmal sympathetic hyperactivity is defined by dystonia (paroxystic increase in muscle tone) and at least one of the following symptoms below:

1. Hyperthermia
2. Arterial hypertension
3. Tachypnoea
4. Tachycardia
5. Sweating
6. Hypersalivation/increase in bronchial secretion

Paroxysmal sympathetic hyperactivity can cause systemic disorders, contractures (joints) and excessive weight loss because of a massive loss of muscle protein. If there are clinical signs of paroxysmal sympathetic hyperactivity and other explanations for the symptoms are ruled out, it is recommended to try treatment with intrathecal baclofen. The differential diagnoses for these symptoms are as follows:

- New cerebral lesions Hydrocephalus
- Shunt infection Shunt dysfunction Systemic infection Cardiac disorder

When the decision to treat is made, a test dose of baclofen is given to test the response to treatment.

© Springer Nature Switzerland AG 2020
T. Sundstrøm et al. (eds.), *Management of Severe Traumatic Brain Injury*,
https://doi.org/10.1007/978-3-030-39383-0_70

The test dose is given through a lumbar puncture; 2 ml CSF is sent to microbiological examination. Give only one dose of baclofen per day.

	Day 1	Day 2	Day 3
Dosage adults			
(Baclofen)	100 g	200 g	
Dosage children			
<10 kg	25 g	35 g	50 g
10–30 kg	35 g	50 g	75 g
>30 kg	50 g	75 g	100 g

If there is an effect on the symptoms (reduction or disappearance of symptoms) following administration of 100 g, consider placing a spinal catheter and an external pump. If there is no response to treatment with 200 g, further testing is without purpose. This is also the recommendation following the third test dosage when treating children (Rosenlund 2017).

Placement of a spinal catheter for continuous infusion with baclofen through an external pump (Rosenlund 2017):

1. Pre-puncture antibiotics (dicloxacillin 1 g i.v. or cefuroxime 1.5 g i.v.).
2. Use a thin epidural/spinal catheter.
3. Sterile cover after thorough cleansing.
4. The catheter is placed in the subarachnoid space via puncture at level L3/L4.
5. The catheter is lead approximately 10 cm in cranial direction.
6. Catheter loop at access point. Sterile drape afterwards.
7. The catheter is fastened with a patch along the back and fixated at the level of the clavicle.
8. A catheter filter is mounted.
9. An injection pump is mounted.

Initial dosage is 5–10 g/h, which gives a daily dose of 120–240 g. Treatment dosages of up to 800 g/day can be necessary to have maximal effect on the condition, in a few cases even more than that. With a concentration in the injection pump of 50 g baclofen/ml, the infusion is programmed to run at a speed of 0.1–0.2 ml/h.

Dosage baclofen (50 g/ml):

g/h	5	10	15	20	25	30
ml/h (à 10 g/ml)	0.1	0.2	0.3	0.4	0.5	0.6
g/24 h	120	240	360	480	600	720

The dosage can be increased with 10–15% every 6 h until maximal effect is reached (disappearance of symptoms) while observing for effect and/or side effects. The spinal catheter can be used for 3–6 days. The patient must be observed for signs of infection, and daily measurement of CRP and leukocytes is necessary. Sometimes the paroxysmal sympathetic hyperactivity has disappeared completely within a few days of treatment with baclofen (<1 week). If this is not the case and the treatment cannot be discontinued, the patient needs to get a subcutaneous pump implanted. Side effects of the treatment are rare and are in that case related to an overdose (Ertzgaard et al. 2017; Rosenlund 2017):

- Urine retention Muscle hypotonia Excessive salivation
- Confusion, vertigo and somnolence Nausea, vomiting
- Depression of respiration (very seldom) Coma
- Convulsions
- Interaction: antihypertensives and tricyclic antidepressants (Ertzgaard et al. 2017)

Tips, Tricks and Pitfalls

- If the patient has an external drain from the ventricular system, you can use this to administrate baclofen. NB. The dosage of baclofen is of the dosage given through a lumbar puncture, i.e. test dosage is 15 g instead of 100 g baclofen.
- It is possible to give bolus baclofen through the spinal catheter instead of administering continuous baclofen. The maximal dosage is 200 g (adults), and the bolus interval must be at least 6 h.
- Paroxysmal sympathetic hyperactivity has previously been called autonomic dysfunction.

70.2 Background

70.2.1 Dystonia

The stretch and bend reflexes are under normal circumstances regulated from the superior centres in the brainstem and the brain through-neurons, which are balancing the stimulating and inhibitory impulses. Damage to the brain or spinal cord can cause a downregulation of the threshold for synaptic excitation at the level of the segmental anterior horn cell, which causes an abnormal increase in reflex activity. This is the definition of spasticity, clinically seen as resistance of the muscle to stretch until a point of sudden collapse (clasp-knife effect). Dystonia is a variant of spasticity and are clinically characterised as abnormal, involuntary and often painful contractions of muscles with both agonistic and antagonistic functions, resulting in a persisting contracture, for example, torticollis and talipes equinus (club foot) (Baguley et al. 2014; Hilz et al. 2018; Hughes and Rabinstein 2014; Laxe et al. 2013).

70.2.2 Paroxysmal Sympathetic Hyperactivity

A review of 349 paroxysmal sympathetic hyperactivity case reports published before 2010 found that about 80% of cases followed TBI, 10% followed anoxic brain injury, 5% followed stroke and the remaining 5% occurred in association with hydrocephalus, tumours, hypoglycaemia, infections or unspecified cases. Prevalence is reported from various countries in a range from 8% to 33%. In one study, the prevalence was affected by the time of assessment, with 24% of the patients meeting the criteria for paroxysmal sympathetic hyperactivity 7 days after injury, decreasing to 8% after 2 weeks. The overall clinical impression is that paroxystic sympathetic hyperactivity is an independent risk factor for poorer neurological outcomes in patients who had a brain injury (Meyfroidt et al. 2017)

Current theories regarding the pathophysiology propose that combinations of diffuse or focal injuries disconnect one or more cerebral centres from caudal excitatory centres. Disconnection is thought to cause spinal circuit excitation; paroxysm then resolves in response to recovery of the inhibitory drivers. The periaqueductal grey matter has been described as a central inhibitory driver that implicates midbrain lesions in the functional or structural disconnections that underlie the more severe end of the paroxysmal sympathetic hyperactivity spectrum. The combination of this theory also supports the fact that some patients with paroxysmal sympathetic hyperactivity has a short period of the symptoms while others have the syndrome for months and even years, suggesting that those with more rapid recovery of the supraspinal inhibition has less brainstem involvement. Available data suggest that allodynic hyper-responsiveness in paroxystic sympathetic hyperactivity develops as a consequence of impaired control by higher cortical centres, resulting in sympathetic storms. Maladaptive spinal cord plasticity is also possible, with subclinical allodynic or sympathetic over-responsiveness persisting for at least 5 years after injury (Meyfroidt et al. 2017).

Paroxysmal sympathetic hyperactivity typically appears following diffuse and severe cerebral lesions, such as diffuse axonal injury, hypoxia and severe CNS infection, and is characterised by tachycardia, tachypnoea, arterial hypertension, sweating, hypersalivation, hypersecretion and dystonia. Paroxysmal sympathetic hyperactivity ('paroxystic autonomic instability disorder', 'dysautonomia', 'autonomic dysfunction') is paroxysmal in nature and can be provoked by minor sensory stimuli (light touch or a sound). The condition is often clinically visible in the period of coma remission, when the patient is out of, or reduced in, sedation from days to a few weeks after the cerebral damage (Meyfroidt et al. 2017; Baguley et al. 2014; Rosenlund 2017). Paroxysmal sympathetic hyperactivity can result in systemic dysfunction, contractures and a severe weight loss because of loss of muscle protein (Caldwell et al. 2013). The initiating time for neurorehabilitation is delayed because of a prolonged stay in the intensive care unit. The condition can be fatal and can alternatively persist for weeks, months or even years if left untreated, resulting in painful contractures and problems regarding rehabilitation and care. If the condition is not treated with intrathecal baclofen, it is often chosen to sedate the patient in order to get control over the symptoms. Sedation is not a treatment as such, and the patients are still suffering from paroxysmal sympathetic hyperactivity. Prolonged sedation increases the risk of complications such as bacteraemia, ventilation-associated pneumonia (VAP), secondary complications to immobility/inactivity and those related to drugs (accumulation, tolerance, withdrawal symptoms, circulatory problems) (Baguley et al. 2014). Baclofen treatment has been shown to eliminate the autonomic symptoms and dystonia in several studies (Hinson et al. 2017; Hilz et al. 2018; Kim et al. 2018; Letzkus et al. 2016; Mathew et al. 2016; Samuel et al. 2016). There are no reported complications to the treatment except for a few with catheter-related infections or ruptures and the risk of withdrawal symptoms if treatment is too abruptly stopped. In some cases, it is sufficient to treat only for a few days (3–4) in the acute phase, which means that the patient does not need further treatment. Intrathecal baclofen treatment is used in Denmark in the neurointensive care units and is given to patients suffering from paroxysmal sympathetic hyperactivity following a severe cerebral injury hence diffuse axonal injury (DAI), stroke (e.g. malignant arteria cerebri media infarction), anoxic damage, CNS infection, sequelae from subarachnoid haemorrhage or CNS tumours (Rosenlund 2017).

70.2.3 Weight Loss

It is well documented (Brain Trauma Foundation et al. 2007) that hypermetabolism and excessive nitrogen loss follow acute severe cerebral injury. Thus, it is found that a resting patient, in coma and with an isolated TBI, has an energy expenditure of 140% of expected metabolic rate (variability 120–250%). The same patient in relaxation (pancuronium bromide or barbiturate) has an energy use of 100–120% of the expected metabolic rate. This finding suggests that most of the excessive use of energy is related to muscle tone. Less than 10% of the expended calories are from protein resources under normal circumstances (healthy, average men). In a patient with an acute severe cerebral injury, who receives a total coverage of expended energy through the diet including 10 g of nitrogen/day, the catabolism of protein reaches as high as 30% of the energy sources used; this results in a loss of nitrogen of 14–25 g/day. It has been shown that the earliest normalisation of the nitrogen balance begins in the third week posttraumatically and often later than that. It is also shown that there is a tendency for the nitrogen loss to increase in the beginning of the posttraumatic phase with a peak in the second week. Most of the parenteral and enteral dietary products for hypermetabolic conditions have a maximal content of protein of 20%. Excessive weight loss is still the result because the nitrogen balance will be negative despite the reduced nitrogen loss (Brain Trauma Foundation et al. 2007). Weight loss is a huge problem in patients suffering from paroxysmal sympathetic hyperactivity (Baguley et al. 2014).

70.2.4 Baclofen

Baclofen (4-amino-3-(4-chlorophenyl)-gamma-aminobutyric acid) is a well-known and well-tested product, which has been used as treatment for spinal spasticity for the last 40 years and for dystonia for the latest years as well, also when the dystonia is a part of a paroxysmal sympathetic hyperactivity (Leland Albright 1996; Sidenius 2010; Kock-Jensen 2007). Baclofen has an agonistic impact on the GABA-B receptors, which binds to and stimulates the pre-synaptic GABA-B receptors in the brainstem and spinal cord. Baclofen inhibits the mono- and poly-synaptic reflexes and GABA metabolism hence spasticity. When administered intrathecally, the dosage needed to treat is much lower compared with orally administered baclofen, especially because of the poor passage of orally administered baclofen across the blood-brain barrier (Sidenius 2010; Meythaler et al. 1999).

70.3 Specific Paediatric Concerns

Children are treated as adults except regarding the dosage (see Sect. 65.1). There are no randomised studies to document the effect of intrathecal treatment with baclofen on paroxystic sympathetic hyperactivity. There is on the other hand a convincing amount of cases that show the effectiveness of the treatment (Meyfroidt et al.

2017). Baclofen itself is a well-known pharmacologic compound with no side effects when administered intrathecally. Paroxysmal sympathetic hyperactivity is a potentially fatal condition and at least a condition that complicates and lowers the outcome significantly for the patients.

References

Baguley IJ, Perkes IE, Fernandez-Ortega JF, Rabinstein AA, Dolce G, Hendricks HT, Consensus Working Group. Paroxysmal sympathetic hyperactivity after acquired brain injury: consensus on conceptual definition, nomenclature, and diagnostic criteria. J Neurotrauma. 2014;31(17):1515–20. https://doi.org/10.1089/neu.2013.3301. Epub 2014 Jul 28

Brain Trauma Foundation; American Association of Neurological Surgeons; Congress of Neurological Surgeons; Joint Section on Neurotrauma and Critical Care, AANS/CNS, Bratton SL, Chestnut RM, Ghajar J, FF MCH, Harris OA, Hartl R, Manley GT, Nemecek A, Newell DW, Rosenthal G, Schouten J, Shutter L, Timmons SD, Ullman JS, Videtta W, Wilberger JE, Wright DW. Guidelines for the management of severe traumatic brain injury. XII. Nutrition. J Neurotrauma. 2007;2007(24 Suppl 1):S77–82. No abstract available. Erratum in: J Neurotrauma. 2008 Mar;25(3):276–8

Caldwell SB, Smith D, Wilson FC. Impact of paroxysmal sympathetic hyperactivity on nutrition management after brain injury: a case series. Brain Inj. 2013;28(3):370–3. https://doi.org/10.3109/02699052.2013.865265. Epub 2013 Dec 30

Ertzgaard P, Campo C, Calabrese A. Efficacy and safety of oral baclofen in the management of spasticity: a rationale for Intrathecal Baclofen. J Rehabil Med. 2017;49(3):193–203.

Hilz MJ, Liu M, Roy S, Wang R. Autonomic dysfunction in the neurological intensive care unit. Clin Auton Res. 2018;29:301–11. https://doi.org/10.1007/s10286-018-0545-8.

Hinson HE, Schreiber MA, Laurie AL, Baguley IJ, Bourdette D, Ling GSF. Early fever as a predictor of paroxysmal sympathetic hyperactivity in traumatic brain injury. J Head Trauma Rehabil. 2017;32(5):E50–4. https://doi.org/10.1097/HTR.0000000000000271.

Hughes JD, Rabinstein AA. Early diagnosis of paroxysmal sympathetic hyperactivity in the ICU. Neurocrit Care. 2014;20(3):454–9. https://doi.org/10.1007/s12028-013-9877-3.

Kim HS, Kim NY, Kim YW. Successful Intrathecal Baclofen therapy for intractable paroxysmal sympathetic hyperactivity in patient with Pontine Hemorrhage: a case report. Clin Neuropharmacol. 2018;41(4):138–41. https://doi.org/10.1097/WNF.0000000000000289.

Kock-Jensen C. Intrathekal baclofen through bolus/external pump. Hammel: Regionshospitalet Hammel Neurocenter; 2007. Instruks. Local Publication 1–8.

Laxe S, Terré R, León D, Bernabeu M. How does dysautonomia influence the outcome of traumatic brain injured patients admitted in a neurorehabilitation unit? Brain Inj. 2013;27(12):1383–7. https://doi.org/10.3109/02699052.2013.823648. Epub 2013 Oct 8

Leland Albright A. Topical review: baclofen in the treatment of cerebral palsy. J Child Neurol. 1996;11(2):77–83.

Letzkus L, Keim-Malpass J, Kennedy C. Paroxysmal sympathetic hyperactivity: autonomic instability and muscle over-activity following severe brain injury. Brain Inj. 2016;30(10):1181–5. https://doi.org/10.1080/02699052.2016.1184757. Epub 2016 Jul 7

Mathew MJ, Deepika A, Shukla D, Devi BI, Ramesh VJ. Paroxysmal sympathetic hyperactivity in severe traumatic brain injury. Acta Neurochir (Wien). 2016;158(11):2047–52. Epub 2016 Aug 31

Meyfroidt G, Baguley IJ, Menon DK. Paroxysmal sympathetic hyperactivity: the storm after acute brain injury. Lancet Neurol. 2017;16(9):721–9. https://doi.org/10.1016/S1474-4422(17)30259-4.

Meythaler JM, Guin-Renfroe S, Grabb P, Hadley MN. Long-term continuously infused intrathecal baclofen for spastic-dystonic hypertonia in traumatic brain injury: 1-year experience. Arch Phys Med Rehabil. 1999;80(1):13–9.

Rosenlund C. Autonomic dysfunction—diagnostics and treatment. Guideline. Odense University Hospital. Infonet, Dok-ID 315661. Local publication. 2017.

Samuel S, Allison TA, Lee K, Choi HA. Pharmacologic management of paroxysmal sympathetic hyperactivity after brain injury. J Neurosci Nurs. 2016;48(2):82–9. https://doi.org/10.1097/JNN.0000000000000207.

Sidenius P. Medicin.dk. Spasticitet. Infomatum a/s. 34. udgave, 1.oplag 2010;327.

71 Prophylaxis Against Venous Thromboembolism (VTE) in Patients with Traumatic Brain Injury (TBI)

Ulf Schott and Morten Zebitz Steiness

Recommendations

Level I

No evidence level I in guiding thromboprophylaxis in TBI exists and stresses the need for adequately powered prospective randomized trials to guide clinical management in different types and severities of TBI.

Level II

There are reliable data supporting mechanical thromboprophylaxis of the lower extremities should start as early as possible and be continued until full mobilization. Several guidelines also recommend this.

Level III

Pharmacological prophylaxis with a low molecular weight heparin (LMWH) should be used in combination with mechanical prophylaxis, when there is no expansion or risk for expansion of hematomas, evaluated by coagulation assays and repetitive CT scans. This area is a typical gray zone area, and there is a high variance when LMWH actually is started due to concerns of hematoma progression. Cava filters should be considered in complex cases.

71.1 Overview

Patients with severe traumatic brain injury (TBI) are at significant risk of developing venous thromboembolic complications. Patients with intracerebral hemorrhages generally have an altered coagulation profile and often have excessive coagulation after the bleeding has stopped. While in neurointensive care, these patients are often unconscious or sedated and lie still for long periods, potentially causing blood stasis in the deep veins (Kaufman et al. 1983). Intracerebral hemorrhages are an indirect evidence of injured endothelial cells in the brain; some TBI patients have damaged endothelium in other parts of the body as well. The injured areas cause inflammation, increasing the concentration of acute phase reactants, making the blood even more hypercoagulative. All these factors are included in Virchow's triad, a theory that explains the pathogenesis of venous thrombosis. Venous thromboembolism (VTE) is estimated to occur in 20% of patients with TBI, so guidelines recommend

U. Schott
Department of Anaesthesia and Intensive Care, Institution of Clinical Sciences, Lund University, Lund, Sweden
e-mail: ulf.schott@skane.se

M. Z. Steiness (✉)
Spine Section, Department of Neurosurgery, Aalborg University Hospital, Aalborg, Denmark
e-mail: mzs@rn.dk

© Springer Nature Switzerland AG 2020
T. Sundstrøm et al. (eds.), *Management of Severe Traumatic Brain Injury*,
https://doi.org/10.1007/978-3-030-39383-0_71

the use of mechanical and pharmacologic thromboprophylaxis (Kaufman et al. 1983; Knudson et al. 2004; Haddad and Arabi 2012). The more severe pulmonary embolism (PE) was estimated to occur in 0.38% of patients with severe TBI (Page et al. 2004). Advanced age, excess weight, and the severity of the TBI all increase the risk of VTE.

There are no specific pediatric concerns, except that children are less prone to thrombotic complications than adults. After start of puberty, children have the same risk as adults.

A number of studies have demonstrated the efficacy and safety of mechanical prophylaxis with either graduated compression stockings or intermittent pneumatic compression. The relative risk of venous thrombosis has been reduced to >50% (Skillman et al. 1978; Turpie et al. 1989) without any changes in mean arterial pressure, intracranial pressure (ICP), or central venous pressure as documented by Davidson et al. (1993). There is a general consensus that thromboprophylaxis of the lower extremities should start as early as possible and be continued until full mobilization, which is also highlighted in guidelines from the Neurocritical Care Society and the Society of Critical Care Medicine (Nyquist et al. 2016).

Among *elective* neurosurgical patients, there is level I evidence regarding pharmacological prophylaxis (Agnelli et al. 1998), but these data cannot automatically be transferred to TBI patients. Studies among patients with TBI suggest that LMWH is efficacious in reducing the risk of VTE. However, data also show a trend toward an increased risk of intracranial bleeding. LMWH seems to be favorable on survival and VTE frequencies as compared to unfractionated heparin (Benjamin et al. 2017).

There is no clear evidence indicating when it is safe to initiate LMWH treatment. Case studies suggest that LMWH prophylaxis should not be initiated before a 24-h control computed tomography (CT) scan has been performed, demonstrating no progression in existing hematomas or new intracranial bleedings (Black et al. 1986; Gerlach et al. 2003; Kleindienst et al. 2003; Norwood et al. 2002). Later studies suggest starting LMWH between 24 and 72 hours (h) after the trauma while monitoring the patient's progress with consecutive CTs to avoid initiating LMWH in patients with an expanding intracerebral hemorrhage (ICH) (Haddad and Arabi 2012; Minshall et al. 2011; Dudley et al. 2010).

The risks and benefits of LMWH were evaluated by Dudley et al. in a retrospective study of 287 TBI patients. In this study, patients received LMWH treatment between 48 and 72 h post-trauma after two CTs showing no sign of hemorrhage expansion. There was a low incidence of VTE (7.3%), and only one patient (0.4%) had a symptomatic expansion of a pre-existing ICH (Dudley et al. 2010). No difference in VTE frequencies was seen between two types of LMWH—enoxaparin and dalteparin.

A large observational cohort study of 2468 TBI patients compared early (<72 h) and late (>72 h) initiation of LMWH. The patients who received early prophylaxis had lower incidences of both deep venous thrombosis (DVT) and PE without any increased risk of neurosurgical intervention or death (Byrne et al. 2016). Two other studies have corroborated these results (Koehler et al. 2011; Jamjoom and Jamjoom 2013).

A small randomized, double-blinded pilot study found that patients with minor TBIs who received LMWH after a stable CT within 24 h post trauma (34 patients) had ICH progression rates similar to the placebo group (28 patients) (Phelan et al. 2012). Norwood et al. (2002) found similar results in a prospective, single-cohort observational study including 150 patients. Kurtoglu et al. found no significant differences in mortality or the incidence of DVT or pulmonary embolism (PE) in a small prospective, randomized, controlled trial on brain and spinal trauma patients who were treated with either intermittent graded pneumatic compression devices (60 patients) or LMWH (60 patients). LMWH was administrated after a stable control CT within 24 h post trauma. There was only one exacerbation of an epidural hematoma in each group (Kurtoglu et al. 2004). In a recent systematic review of 21 studies, Margolick et al. concluded that pharmacological prophylaxis started 24–48 h post trauma was safe in "low"-hemorrhagic-risk TBIs with no expansion upon repeated CT scans (Margolick et al. 2018).

The largest prospective study comes from Australia (Skrifvars et al. 2017), but is actually a post hoc analysis of the erythropoietin in traumatic brain injury (EPO-TBI) trial that included twice-weekly lower limb ultrasound screening. VTE was defined as an ultrasound-proven proximal DVT or a clinically detected PE. Of 603 patients, 119 (19.7%) developed VTE, mostly comprising DVT (102 patients, 16.9%) with a smaller number of PE events (24 patients, 4.0%) even if mechanical and pharmacological prophylaxis were adopted in most cases.

However, a national UK survey among 62 neurosurgeons indicated a wide variation when LMWHs were actually started in different types of TBIs, with median LMWH initiation from 1 to 7 days after trauma (Jamjoom et al. 2016). ICP monitoring with or without intraventricular drainage of hemorrhagic cerebrospinal fluid (CSF) may also affect when LMWH treatment is started, sometimes first after catheter withdrawal. A recent retrospective study of 155 patients, however, indicated that both standard heparin and LMWH were safe to administer while using active invasive monitoring devices (Dengler et al. 2016). A concern is at withdrawal, when to optimally stop and when to readminister LMWH.

In complex multitrauma patients who survived to ICU admission, prescreened for high VTE risk, TBI did not further increase the risk for VTE, especially in patients receiving pharmacological and mechanical thromboprophylaxis (Valle et al. 2014). Byrne et al. found LMWH to be superior to heparin in preventing PE in patients after major trauma. Their propensity-matched analysis included 153,474 patients. The matched results were 1.4% PE in patients receiving LMWH and 2.4% PE in the group that received heparin (Byrne et al. 2017).

Minshall et al. compared the safety and efficacy of heparin with the LMWH enoxaparin and found that patients who received LMWH after TBI had fewer complications. However, patients receiving heparin had more severe TBIs, suggesting that heparin was favored by the physicians treating those patients, perhaps due to better monitoring capabilities, a shorter half-life, and the option of better reversal with protamine (Minshall et al. 2011). Dengler et al. retrospectively evaluated heparin and LMWH in TBI patients and found no difference in DVT or hemorrhage expansion using intracranial pressure monitoring devices. In that study, heparin was not reserved for the more severe TBI cases (Dengler et al. 2016).

In addition to the risks discussed above, brain trauma patients can also develop an early acute coagulopathy of trauma shock (aCoTS) (Johansson et al. 2011) or a later disseminated intravascular coagulation (DIC). DIC usually occurs 6–72 hours' post trauma (Mukhopadhyay et al. 2013). Both aCoTS and DIC are strong predictors of a poor outcome after TBI.

Coagulation monitoring in trauma has evolved to involve tests like thromboelastography (TEG®/ROTEM®) and thrombin generation (TGA) to better reflect hypo- or hypercoagulation than standard laboratory coagulation tests (Johansson et al. 2011; Miao et al. 2017). A recent trauma study reported that although TGA parameters indicated hypercoagulable states, they did not identify patients with DVT or PE (Voils et al. 2016). Hincker et al. identified a preoperative hypercoagulable ROTEM® both with thromboplastin reagent InTEM and tissue factor reagent ExTEM activated profiles (clot formation time (CFT), alpha angle (AA), and maximal clot formation (MCF)) in 10 out of 333 noncardiac surgery patients who developed postoperative DVTs even after LMWH or heparin thromboprophylaxis. There was no indication of this hypercoagulation in the activated partial thromboplastin time (aPTT), protrombin time (PT), or platelet count analyses (Hincker et al. 2014). In TBI patients and other trauma patients, alcohol can induce a hypocoagulable thromboelastographic profile in the initial trauma setting, possibly explaining the DVT-reducing effect of alcohol (Cook et al. 2015).

There are several types of LMWHs. They all inhibit the common coagulation pathway by indirectly inhibiting factor Xa (fXa) and directly inhibiting factor IIa (fIIa) to varying extents as described by each type's anti-fXa/anti-fIIa ratio. The current gold standard for monitoring

LMWH treatment measures the anti-fXa activity in a patient's plasma. However, this method neglects its anti-fIIa effect. TGA reflects the LMWH inhibition of both fXa and fIIa, potentially providing a better analysis that describes the full effect of the LMWH (Thomas et al. 2015). Usually thromboprophylactic doses of LMWH do not need laboratory monitoring other than platelet count to detect heparin-induced thrombocytopenia.

Also, the LMWH enoxaparin is primarily eliminated through the kidneys, making renal insufficiency an important factor for potential accumulation and thereby increased bleeding risk. Body weight (BW) is also known to affect the enoxaparin dose response (Costantini et al. 2013), with low BW posing a risk of overdose and high BW leading to potentially insufficient thromboprophylaxis under the standard dose regimes. Individual differences in bleeding risk and dose response to LMWH further complicate this issue. LMWHs are generally administered by a subcutaneous injection once a day and exhibit peak and trough effects during treatment. The LMWH anti-fIIa effect can be reversed with protamine more or less depending on the specific type of LMWH's anti-fXa/anti-fIIa ratio (Thomas et al. 2015).

Finally, recent guidelines from Neurocritical Care Society (NCS) and Society of Critical Care Medicine (SCCM) recommend to start LMWH in patients with stable hematomas and no ongoing coagulopathy within 48 h after hospital admission together with mechanical devices (Nyquist et al. 2016). This strategy is also recommended by the updated TBI guidelines from the UK Brain Trauma Foundation (Carney et al. 2017). They consider that the benefits outweigh the risks—the survey referred to above indicates however that these guidelines are not followed (Jamjoom et al. 2016). A concern is the severity of the TBI and the risk for a progressive hemorrhagic injury (PHI). A risk score to predict PHI has been suggested and might increase the safety of LMWH administration after TBI (Yuan et al. 2012). The systematic review by Shen et al. (2015) concludes that LMWH thromboprophylaxis appears to be safe among TBI patients with stabilized hemorrhagic patterns. Still, there are many issues remaining to optimize its efficiency and safety (Shen et al. 2015; Carney et al. 2017). Vena cava filters are also an option in many trauma centers, especially in multitrauma patients with lower limb, pelvic, and spinal fractures together with TBI (Jeremitsky et al. 2013).

Tips, Tricks, and Pitfalls

- Today we have no optimal laboratory technique to monitor various anticoagulants or thromboprophylactic drugs.
- There is a thin balance between aggravating TBI haemorrage with too early pharmacologic thromboprophylaxis and increasing risk for thromboembolism by delaying it.
- Clinical judgement and evaluation from repetitive CT scans during the first 2–5 (or longer) days is the mainstay.
- Calf compression and then starting with low dose LMWH thromboprophylaxis after 2–4 days if the TBI induced haemorrhage seems to be stabilised is recommended by most guidelines.
- High alert to stop LMWH if haemorrhage is expanded – protamin can revert some of its effect depending on the anti-Xa/anti-Iia ratio of the specific LMWH.
- LMWH should be stopped 12 h before manipulation or withdrawal of intracerebral pressure monitoring/ventricular drainage catheters.
- Simultaneous DIC, thrombocytopenia should be resolved/treated before considering LMWH.

References

Agnelli G, Piovella F, Buoncristiani P, et al. Enoxaparin plus compression stocking compared with compression stocking alone in the prevention of venous thromboembolism after elective neurosurgery. N Engl J Med. 1998;339:80–5.

Benjamin E, Recinos G, Aiolfi A, et al. Pharmacological thromboembolic prophylaxis in traumatic brain injuries: low molecular weight heparin is superior to unfractionated heparin. Ann Surg. 2017;266:463–9.

Black PM, Baker MF, Snook CP. Experience with external pneumatic calf compression in neurology and neurosurgery. Neurosurgery. 1986;18:440–4.

Byrne J, Mason S, Gomez D, et al. Timing of pharmacologic venous thromboembolism prophylaxis in severe traumatic brain injury: a propensity-matched cohort study. J Am Coll Surg. 2016;223:621–31.

Byrne J, Geerts W, Mason S, et al. Effectiveness of low-molecular-weight heparin versus unfractionated heparin to prevent pulmonary embolism following major trauma. J Trauma Acute Care Surg. 2017;82:252–62.

Carney N, Totten AM, O'Reilly C, et al. Guidelines for the management of severe traumatic brain injury, fourth edition. Neurosurgery. 2017;80:6–15.

Cook M, Louis S, McCully S, et al. Positive blood alcohol is associated with reduced DVT in trauma. Injury. 2015;46:131–5.

Costantini T, Min E, Box K, et al. Dose adjusting enoxaparin is necessary to achieve adequate venous thromboembolism prophylaxis in trauma patients. J Trauma Acute Care Surg. 2013;74:128–35.

Davidson JE, Williams DC, Hoffman MS. Effect of intermittent pneumatic leg compression on intracranial pressure in brain-injured patients. Crit Care Med. 1993;21:224–7.

Dengler B, Mendez-Gomez P, Chavez A, et al. Safety of chemical DVT prophylaxis in severe traumatic brain injury with invasive monitoring devices. Neurocrit Care. 2016;25:215–23.

Dudley R, Aziz I, Bonnici A, et al. Early venous thromboembolic event prophylaxis in traumatic brain injury with low-molecular-weight heparin: risks and benefits. J Neurotrauma. 2010;27:2165–72.

Gerlach R, Scheuer T, Beck J, et al. Risk of postoperative hemorrhage intracranial surgery after early nadroparin administration: results of a prospective study. Neurosurgery. 2003;53:1028–34.

Haddad S, Arabi Y. Critical care management of severe traumatic brain injury in adults. Scand J Trauma Resusc Emerg Med. 2012;20:12.

Hincker A, Feit J, Sladen R, et al. Rotational thromboelastometry predicts thromboembolic complications after major non-cardiac surgery. Crit Care. 2014;18:549.

Jamjoom A, Jamjoom A. Safety and efficacy of early pharmacological thromboprophylaxis in traumatic brain injury: systematic review and meta-analysis. J Neurotrauma. 2013;30:503–11.

Jamjoom AA, Chari A, Salijevska J, et al. A national survey of thromboprophylaxis in traumatic brain injury in the United Kingdom. Br J Neurosurg. 2016;30:240–5.

Jeremitsky E, St Germain N, Kao AH, et al. Risk of pulmonary embolism in trauma patients: not all created equal. Surgery. 2013;154:810–4.

Johansson P, Sørensen A, Perner A, et al. Disseminated intravascular coagulation or acute coagulopathy of trauma shock early after trauma? An observational study. Crit Care. 2011;15:272.

Kaufman H, Satterwhite T, McConnell B, et al. Deep vein thrombosis and pulmonary embolism in head injured patients. Angiology. 1983;34:627–38.

Kleindienst A, Harvey HB, Mater E, et al. Early antithrombotic prophylaxis with low molecular weight heparin in neurosurgery. Acta Neurochir. 2003;145:1085–90.

Knudson MM, Ikossi DG, Khaw L, et al. Thromboembolism after trauma: an analysis of 1602 episodes from the American College of Surgeons National Trauma Data Bank. Ann Surg. 2004;240:490–6.

Koehler D, Shipman J, Davidson M, et al. Is early venous thromboembolism prophylaxis safe in trauma patients with intracranial hemorrhage. J Trauma. 2011;70:324–9.

Kurtoglu M, Yanar H, Bilsel Y, et al. Venous thromboembolism prophylaxis after head and spinal trauma: intermittent pneumatic compression devices versus low molecular weight heparin. World J Surg. 2004;28:807–11.

Margolick J, Dandurand C, Duncan K, et al. A systematic review of the risks and benefits of venous thromboembolism prophylaxis in traumatic brain injury. Can J Neurol Sci. 2018;45:432–44.

Miao W, Zhao K, Deng W, Teng J. Coagulation factor hyperfunction after subarachnoid hemorrhage induces deep venous thrombosis. World Neurosurg. 2017;110:46–50.

Minshall C, Eriksson E, Leon S, et al. Safety and efficacy of heparin or enoxaparin prophylaxis in blunt trauma patients with a head abbreviated injury severity score >2. J Trauma Injury. 2011;71:396–400.

Mukhopadhyay A, Chhabra G, Sharma S, et al. Coagulopathy as prognostic marker in acute traumatic brain injury. J Emerg Trauma Shock. 2013;6:180–5.

Norwood SH, McAuley CE, Berne JD, et al. Prospective evaluation of the safety of enoxaparin prophylaxis for venous thromboembolism in patients with intracranial hemorrhagic injuries. Arch Surg. 2002;137:696–701.

Nyquist P, Bautista C, Jichici D, et al. Prophylaxis of venous thrombosis in neurocritical care patients: an evidence-based guideline: a statement for healthcare professionals from the Neurocritical Care Society. Neurocrit Care. 2016;24:47–60.

Page RB, Spott MA, Krishnamurthy S, et al. Head injury and pulmonary embolism: a retrospective report based on the Pennsylvania Trauma Outcomes study. Neurosurgery. 2004;54:143–8.

Phelan H, Wolf S, Norwood S, et al. A randomized, double-blinded, placebo-controlled pilot trial of anticoagulation in low-risk traumatic brain injury. J Trauma Acute Care Surg. 2012;73:1434–41.

Shen X, Dutcher SK, Palmer J, et al. A systematic review of the benefits and risks of anticoagulation following traumatic brain injury. J Head Trauma Rehabil. 2015;30:29–37.

Skillman JJ, Collins RE, Coe NP, et al. Prevention of deep vein thrombosis in neurosurgical patients: a controlled, randomized trial of external pneumatic compression boots. Surgery. 1978;83:354–8.

Skrifvars MB, Bailey M, Presneill J, et al. EPO-TBI investigators and the ANZICS Clinical Trials Group. Venous thromboembolic events in critically ill traumatic brain injury patients. Intensive Care Med. 2017;43:419–28.

Thomas O, Lybeck E, Strandberg K, et al. Monitoring low molecular weight heparins at therapeutic levels: dose-responses of, and correlations and differences between aPTT, anti-factor Xa and thrombin generation assays. PLoS One. 2015;10(1):e0116835.

Turpie AG, Hirsh J, Gent M, et al. Prevention of deep vein thrombosis in potential neurosurgical patients. A randomized trial comparing graduated compression stockings alone or graduated compression stockings plus intermittent compression with control. Arch Intern Med. 1989;149:679–81.

Valle EJ, Van Haren RM, Allen CJ, et al. Does traumatic brain injury increase the risk for venous thromboembolism in polytrauma patients? J Trauma Acute Care Surg. 2014;77:243–25.

Voils S, Lemon S, Jordan J, et al. Early thrombin formation capacity in trauma patients and association with venous thromboembolism. Thromb Res. 2016;147:13–5.

Yuan F, Ding J, Chen H, et al. Predicting progressive hemorrhagic injury after traumatic brain injury: derivation and validation of a risk score based on admission characteristics. J Neurotrauma. 2012;29:2137–42.

Coagulopathy (Bleeding Tendency)

72

Bo-Michael Bellander, Alexander Fletcher-Sandersjöö, and Martin Engström

Recommendations

Tranexamic acid should be administered within 3 hours to patients with multitrauma that includes head injury (CRASH-2 collaborators, 2011), and considered for patients with isolated TBI as well (The CRASH-3 collaborators 2019).

Level I

The addition of TBI to hemorrhagic shock is associated with worsened coagulopathy and increased mortality (Galvagno et al. 2017).

Tranexamic acid administered within 3 hours after trauma improves outcome in patients suffering from major multitrauma (CRASH 2, 2011).

Tranexamic acid administered within 3 hours after trauma reduces head injury-related death in patients suffering from isolated TBI (CRASH 3, 2019).

Level II

Normalization of INR is associated with improved mortality in patients with acute traumatic coagulopathy and isolated TBI.

Level III

Routine clinical practice includes early and repeated monitoring of coagulation, using a traditional laboratory determination including prothrombin time (PT), activated partial thromboplastin time (APTT) platelet counts, and fibrinogen and/or a viscoelastic method.

Despite weak scientific evidence, platelet transfusion is recommended to maintain a platelet count above 50×10^9/L and, in case of ongoing bleeding, above 100×10^9/L.

Tips, Tricks, and Pitfalls

- Ensure access to early and repeated monitoring of coagulation status and platelet function.
- Multitrauma and isolated TBI patients behave differently.
- Ensure that a protocol is established for massive transfusion practice and treatment of patients with anticoagulants and antiplatelet agents.
- Thromboembolic prophylaxis should be instituted early in patients with TBI.

B.-M. Bellander (✉)
Department of Clinical Neuroscience, Karolinska Institutet, Stockholm, Sweden

Department of Neurosurgery, Karolinska University Hospital, Stockholm, Sweden
e-mail: bo-michael.bellander@sll.se

A. Fletcher-Sandersjöö
Department of Neurosurgery, Karolinska University Hospital, Solna, Sweden

M. Engström
Department of Health Care, Region Halland, Halmstad, Sweden
e-mail: Martin.Engstrom@regionhalland.se

© Springer Nature Switzerland AG 2020

T. Sundstrøm et al. (eds.), *Management of Severe Traumatic Brain Injury*,
https://doi.org/10.1007/978-3-030-39383-0_72

72.1 Introduction: TBI and Bleeding

Approximately 30–50% of patients suffering from cerebral contusions present hemorrhagic progression on the second CT scan after admission to the hospital (Beaumont and Gennarelli 2006; Juratli et al. 2014; Alahmadi et al. 2010; Narayan et al. 2008a). Hematoma progression after TBI has also been shown for epidural hematomas (EDH) (Zangbar et al. 2016), traumatic subarachnoid hemorrhage (trSAH) (Chieregato et al. 2005), and acute subdural hematomas (acSDH) (Oertel et al. 2002; Asan 2018). In fact, progressive intracranial bleeding is among the leading causes of preventable death following TBI (McCully and Schreiber 2013; Wafaisade et al. 2010; Talving et al. 2009). Acute traumatic coagulopathy (ATC) is common following traumatic brain injury (TBI) (Kumar 2013). It has been shown to increase the risk for hemorrhagic progression (Stein et al. 1992) and is an independent predictor of complications (Stein et al. 2002) and poor outcome, following TBI (Juratli et al. 2014; Murray et al. 2007; Selladurai et al. 1997; Harhangi et al. 2008). In addition to ATC, patients suffering from TBI are getting older (Roozenbeek et al. 2013). Thus, the amount of TBI patients on anticoagulant and antiplatelet drugs (Siracuse et al. 2010) has increased with an associated increased risk for hemorrhagic progression.

Hemorrhagic progress occurs even when conventional coagulation measurements are normal (Allard et al. 2009). This has led to the adoption of complementary tests, for example, analysis methods to measure platelet function (Nekludov et al. 2007a). Still the development of new biomarkers and laboratory tests are needed to support future preventive measures and targeted therapies.

Posttraumatic bleeding, due to torn arteries and/or veins, that can be surgically controlled, differs from coagulopathic bleeding with its inability to form clots at the capillary bed and subsequent diffuse bleeding and is not covered in this chapter.

In contrast to increased bleeding, thromboembolic complications also follow TBI. More extensive thromboembolic complications occur in 6–13% of patients after TBI (Narayan et al. 2008a, b). In a study analyzing the presence of secondary peaks of the biomarker S100B, nearly 30% of patients with TBI developed intracerebral thromboembolic complications (Thelin et al. 2014). Thus, it is important to monitor the temporal changes between hemorrhagic diathesis and thromboembolism in patients suffering from TBI.

72.2 Who Is Going to Bleed?

Considering the adverse effects associated with hemorrhage progression following TBI, identifying patients prone to bleeding is crucial. Risk factors for hemorrhagic progression following isolated TBI have been identified in the literature and thoroughly presented in a recent review (Maegele et al. 2017) (Table 72.1). In general, increased risk is associated with old age, more severe injury, and shock (Alahmadi et al. 2010; Chieregato et al. 2005; Oertel et al. 2002; Wafaisade et al. 2010; Talving et al. 2009; Maegele et al. 2017; Epstein et al. 2015; Chang et al. 2006), and laboratory findings may further strengthen the predicted risk (Juratli et al. 2014; Maegele et al. 2017; Karri et al. 2017; Lustenberger et al. 2010).

It is important to note that the definition of ATC varies between different publications (Epstein et al. 2014). The international normalized ratio, INR, $\geq$1.3 appears to be one of the most prevalent definitions, although it only measures "the extrinsic pathway" of the coagulation cascade. By adding APT time also, the intrinsic pathway of the coagulation pathway will be covered. If the patient exhibits a pathological level of INR, APT (Activated Partial Thromboplastin) time, or platelet count, the risk for hemorrhagic progression increases up to 85% (Stein et al. 1992).

The development of platelet dysfunction that develops following TBI despite the absence of ongoing antiplatelet medication leads to a subsequent increased risk for hemorrhage.

Hyperfibrinolytic activity (Cotton et al. 2012) and a high FDP/fibrinogen ratio (Lee

Table 72.1 Risk factors for progressive hemorrhage

Clinical risk factors	Laboratory risk factors
Age ≥50 years and 75 years	B-glucose >8 mmol/L
Male sex (Oertel et al. 2002)	Base deficit >6 mmol/L
GCS ≤8 before intubation	Hb <124 g/L
Worsened GCS between CT 1 and 2 (Chang et al. 2006)	Tissue plasminogen activators (tPA) ↑
Pathological pupil reaction	D-Dimer ↑
CT findings showing	Thrombocytopenia (<100?)
– trSAH	
– acSDH (Chang et al. 2006)	
– Edema	
– Midline shift	
– Initial size of ICH (Chang et al. 2006)	
– Effacement of basal cisterns (Chang et al. 2006)	
ISS ≥16	Thrombocyte dysfunction
SAP ≤90 mmHg	Fibrinogen ↓
Shock index (=HR/SAP) ≥1	FDP (Fibrin Degradation Product)/ fibrinogen ratio ↑
Iv fluids <2 L prehospital	INR ≥1.3
Time from trauma and first CT scan (Oertel et al. 2002)	APT time (Oertel et al. 2002)
Two of the following: age >50, SI ≥1, and abnormal pupil reaction	

et al. 2018) are correlated to outcome. Depletion of plasma levels of fibrinogen is an independent predictor for massive transfusion in the multi-trauma patient (Nakamura et al. 2017) and is an important parameter to follow closely (See Table 72.1).

72.3 Why Do They Bleed?

Approximately half of patients with traumatic intracerebral contusions show hemorrhagic progress within the first 24 h (Narayan et al. 2008a). A primary CT scan performed early after injury may of course increase the risk for hemorrhagic progression on the follow-up CT scan (Oertel et al. 2002), but is this not the only explanation. This bleeding tendency appears to be due to several different factors, including consumption coagulopathy, inhibition of coagulation, fibrinolysis, platelet dysfunction (Laroche et al. 2012), and injuries to the neurovascular unit (Simard et al. 2012). Below, we present the most studied mechanisms behind coagulopathy in patients with TBI.

72.3.1 Consumption Coagulopathy

Consumption of coagulation factors and iatrogenic hemodilution from fluid therapy following general trauma may severely impair the ability to hemostasis after severe bleeding following multitrauma (Armand and Hess 2003). Tissue hypoperfusion, defined as arterial blood gas (ABG) base deficit (BD) >6 mmol/L, in combination with the TBI is necessary to create coagulopathy (Brohi et al. 2007; Cohen et al. 2007). Hypoperfusion has been suggested to initiate coagulopathy by activating protein C (Cohen et al. 2007), probably with a subsequent inhibition of coagulation factors Va and VIIIa (Rittirsch et al. 2008).

72.3.2 Drug-Induced Coagulopathy

72.3.2.1 Anticoagulants

Warfarin induces an anticoagulant effect by blocking the vitamin K cycle. Vitamin K is necessary to complete the synthesis of coagulation factors II, VII, IX, and X in the liver. Ongoing warfarin treatment increases the risk for intracranial bleeding (Alrajhi et al. 2015; Smits et al. 2007) and mortality (Siracuse et al. 2010; Franko et al. 2006; Batchelor and Grayson 2012). The risk for a positive CT scan for TBI patients on warfarin is approximately 5% in minimal TBI (GCS 15) and 22% in mild TBI (GCS 14–15) (Alrajhi et al. 2015). The risk for delayed hemorrhage 6–24 h after a negative first CT scan is approximately 1% in these patients (Chauny et al. 2016). Even non-anticoagulated patients often present an increased INR at admission following TBI. Mortality decreases substantially, from 65–69% to 20–25%, if INR is normalized following TBI (Epstein et al. 2016). Warfarin can be reversed using prothrombin complex concentrate (PCC), aiming at a reduction of INR to <1.3 (Epstein et al. 2015). To the best of our knowledge, there are no studies that have assessed early prophylactic treatment with PCC or FFP in patients taking warfarin and suffering from minimal or mild TBI to prevent hemorrhage. According to present recommendations at the Karolinska University Hospital, intracranial bleeding in patients taking warfarin should be reversed with prothrombin complex concentrate (PCC), which has a direct effect and a half-life of 6–8 h, and vitamin K, which has its maximum effect after 6–12 h.

New oral anticoagulants (NOAC), such as the reversible direct thrombin inhibitor dabigatran and the factor X inhibitors rivaroxaban, apixaban, and edoxaban, seem to result in lower mortality following TBI when compared to warfarin (Maung et al. 2016). Initially, there were no available reversal agents for NOACs until idarucizumab was introduced for dabigatran. Recently, a reversal agent for rivaroxaban and apixaban, named Andexanet alfa (Connolly et al. 2019), has been approved by the FDA and is on inquiry in the EU (Burnett et al. 2017). An updated expert consensus decision pathway on management of bleeding in patients on oral anticoagulant was published by the American College of Cardiology (Tomaselli et al. 2017). The use of anticoagulants is included in the Scandinavian guidelines as a risk factor for the development of intracranial hemorrhage (Unden et al. 2013). According to present recommendations at the Karolinska University Hospital, patients on NOAC who suffer from minor TBI (GCS 15) with normal CT scans should still be admitted for observation and their anticoagulation temporarily paused. Patients with mild to severe TBI, or with intracranial hemorrhage on their CT scan, should be administered a reversal agent (if possible) and have the plasma concentration of the NOAC measured. For dabigatran, the half-life of the reversal agent is shorter than that for the anticoagulant; thus a new dose might be necessary 8–12 h later. For patients where no reversal agent exists, four units of factor PCC 20–30 U/kg BW should be administered. PCC has been shown to be beneficial in 26 of 31 patients suffering from bleeding during factor X inhibition (Allison et al. 2018) and is recommended by the European Heart Rhythm Association (Steffel et al. 2018).

72.3.2.2 Platelet Inhibitors

Platelet inhibitors are more common in the elderly and also increase the risk of bleeding complications (Serebruany et al. 2004). Acetylsalicylic acid irreversibly acetylates platelet cyclooxygenase by blocking thromboxane (Multiplate ASPI), thereby inhibiting the formation of prostaglandin. Clopidogrel, prasugrel, and ticagrelor block the ADP P2Y12 receptor (Multiplate ADP). In patients on platelet inhibitors who suffer from mild TBI (GCS 13–15), approximately 9–13 % have an intracranial hemorrhage on their initial CT scan (Vedin et al. 2019; Moustafa et al. 2018; Uccella et al. 2018). Of note, patients on aspirin had the highest hematoma rate, 35%, compared to patients on clopidogrel, warfarin, dabigatran, rivaroxaban, or apixaban in a blended TBI cohort of 1847 patients (Kobayashi et al. 2017).

In TBI patients on platelet inhibitors, aspirin, clopidogrel, or both, a platelet count of less than 135×10^9/L has been predictive of both radiographic and clinical deterioration (Joseph et al. 2014). Inhibiting this by platelet transfusion has limited effect as the platelet inhibitors will have the same effect on the transfused platelets as on the patient's own platelets as long as there is a significant circulating concentration of the agent (Makris et al. 2013). When assessing the timing of platelet transfusions in patients on platelet inhibitors with traumatic intracranial hemorrhage, a 9.5% progression in hemorrhage size was found. When adding the presence of subdural hematoma and lower admission Glasgow coma score, predictors of hemorrhage progression, to a logistic regression analysis, there remained no significant difference in minutes to platelet transfusion (Pandya et al. 2018). A slight increased mortality for TBI patients on antiplatelet medication has also been presented in a meta-analysis (Batchelor and Grayson 2013), but the literature is limited concerning this issue (Beynon et al. 2012), and the increased mortality has also been suggested to be associated with the severity of pre-existing conditions rather than the antiplatelet medications itself (Sumiyoshi et al. 2017).

72.3.3 Thrombocytopenia and Platelet Dysfunction

Thrombocytopenia is associated with progressive bleeding (Engström et al. 2005; Carrick et al. 2005) and affects outcome negatively (Juratli et al. 2014). In 310 patients with blunt severe TBI, a platelet count of $<100 \times 10^9$/L has been associated with a ninefold adjusted risk of death, and a platelet count of $<175 \times 10^9$/L has been identified as a significant predictor of hemorrhagic progression (Schnuriger et al. 2010).

In addition to platelet inhibitors, platelet dysfunction can be initiated by the trauma per se and plays a role in bleeding progression (Wohlauer et al. 2012). A normal platelet count does not tell us anything about platelet function, and coagulation disturbances may occur even when standard parameters for coagulation are normal (Allard et al. 2009). Platelet dysfunction can be revealed using multiple electrode aggregometry (MEA; e.g. Multiplate®, thromboelastography with platelet mapping (TEG-PM), etc.), which can detect platelet responsiveness. By using MEA the receptor function on the platelets can be assessed and used to evaluate clotting performance following TBI, even in patients without known antiplatelet therapies.

The ASPI-test reagent consists of arachidonic acid which is the substrate for the enzyme cyclooxygenase in the platelets. Cyclooxygenase converts arachidonic acid to thromboxane A2 which is a potent platelet activator. When cyclooxygenase is blocked, the formation of thromboxane A2 is inhibited and no or little platelet activation can occur. This test is primarily sensitive to acetylsalicylic acid (ASA) and nonsteroid anti-inflammatory drugs (NSAID).

The Multiplate's adenosine diphosphate (ADP) test reagent consists of ADP which activates platelets via the ADP receptor. The test is sensitive to drugs such as clopidogrel, prasugrel, and ticagrelor. These drugs have a mechanism of action through the P2Y12 receptor, which is believed to be most important for ADP. The test is insensitive to ASA and NSAIDs.

The thrombin receptor activating peptide (TRAP) test reagent consists of a thrombin receptor activating peptide (TRAP-6) which is a platelet activator that stimulates platelet aggregation via the thrombin receptors. The test reacts to drugs that are GpIIb/IIIa antagonists. The TRAP reaction is inhibited by abciximab (ReoPro) and tirofiban (Aggrastat) with little or no inhibition of ASA or clopidogrel.

Early platelet dysfunction, assessed by using TEG-PM, is prevalent after severe TBI and correlates with mortality (Davis et al. 2013; Kutcher et al. 2012). Patients not on antiplatelet treatment suffering from TBI and presenting a low responsiveness to arachidonic acid (AA), using TEG-PM, at admittance to the hospital were likely to develop bleeding complications later (Nekludov et al. 2007a). Similar findings have been shown concerning the ADP-receptor response after TBI compared to uninjured controls (Castellino et al. 2014). Thus, analyzing the thrombocyte function might increase the chance to identify potential progressive bleeders after TBI (Gozal et al. 2017).

In a retrospective analysis of 178 TBI patients, treated at a NICU, MEA analysis showed that ASPI levels were low after TBI and increased in a time-dependent fashion. Patients on cyclooxygenase (COX) inhibitors demonstrated lower ASPI levels than non-treated patients. Platelet transfusion increased the ASPI levels. In univariate analysis, the initial ASPI and TRAP values were significant predictors of outcome, but not of lesion progression. The findings were though not confirmed in multivariable analysis (Lindblad et al. 2018) which might be explained by the retrospective nature of the study and by the plethora of different treatments the patients were exposed to.

72.3.4 Fibrinolysis

Primary fibrinolysis is an important part of acute coagulopathy after trauma (Kashuk et al. 2010). Approximately 2–10% of patients admitted due to general trauma suffer from severe hyperfibrinolysis, defined as lysis index >3% after 30 min (LI30) in rotation thromboelastometry (ROTEM) analysis, which has been correlated to progressive bleeding (Karri et al. 2017), increased injury severity, increased number of transfusions, longer ventilator treatment, longer in-hospital stay, and higher mortality (Cotton et al. 2012; Cardenas et al. 2014).

Physiological fibrinolysis following general trauma is defined as LI30 0.8–3% using ROTEM. Fibrinolysis shutdown (Moore et al. 2016) has been proposed as another pathological event after general trauma. While hyperfibrinolysis is defined as LI30 >3% in ROTEM analysis, fibrinolysis shutdown is defined as LI30 <0.8%. It mainly affects males of older age with lower number of thrombocytes. Both hyperfibrinolysis and fibrinolysis shutdown have been shown to correlate to mortality (Moore et al. 2016). A relationship between fibrinolysis in multitrauma patients with severe TBI and subsequent progressive hemorrhage has been shown (Karri et al. 2017). Patients suffering from isolated TBI that develops disseminated intravascular coagulation (DIC) in combination with hyperfibrinolysis show a significant higher mortality compared to patients with DIC without hyperfibrinolysis (58.9% and 10.7%, respectively) (Wada et al. 2017).

72.3.5 Injury to the Neurovascular Unit: Microvascular Failure

The hemorrhagic progression of contusions may continue for hours or even days after admission to hospital, thoroughly reviewed by Kurland and co-workers (Kurland et al. 2012) who stressed the hypothesis that the progression is not only the result from coagulopathy but also involves a delayed, progressive microvascular failure initiated by the impact. Even if coagulopathy after TBI presents a risk for poor outcome, Kurland and co-workers state that the literature does not support a simple causative relationship between coagulopathy and progressive delayed hemorrhage (Kurland et al. 2012).

Microvessels may be fractured immediately at impact, but also hours or days later. The zones affected by a traumatic contusion can be defined as the contusion, penumbra and para-penumbra. The contusion itself is where tissue and microvessels are disrupted with an immediate hemorrhage at impact. Outside the contusion lies the penumbra, were the energy does not shear microvessels immediately, but instead activates molecular processes initiating events that will lead to microvascular disruption and delayed progressive hemorrhage (Simard et al. 2009). Outside the penumbra lies the para-penumbra, where the transmitted energy at impact is not enough to create delayed vascular impairment, but may initiate other pathophysiological events such as apoptosis (Patel et al. 2010). The SURF-receptor blocker glibenclamide has been suggested as a possible treatment targeting the penumbra zone and has been shown to significantly lower the expansion of cerebral contusions on CT scans (Khalili et al. 2017). Glibenclamide inhibits the sulfonylurea receptor 1 (Sur1)-regulated NC(Ca-ATP) channel which is upregulated in cells of the neurovascular unit after traumatic brain injury. The channel has been connected to edema formation and delayed secondary hemorrhage (Simard et al. 2012).

Other mechanisms may include complement activation where the terminal membrane attack complex has been shown to attack neurons in the border zone after TBI (Bellander et al. 2001) but also lead to disintegration of the blood-brain barrier (Stahel et al. 2001).

72.3.6 General Trauma Versus Isolated TBI

It has been suggested that the mechanism of trauma-induced coagulopathy and platelet dysfunction following isolated TBI differs from general (extracranial) trauma. In isolated TBI, there is less blood loss and thus less shock. Moreover, the brain parenchyma contains more tissue factor (TF) than other organs (Mackman 2009), and the disintegrated blood-brain barrier may allow for interactions between circulating plasma proteins and the brain parenchyma after TBI (Chang et al. 2016). Patients with penetrating TBI also appear to be more coagulopathic than patients with blunt TBI (Folkerson et al. 2018).

In general trauma, bleeding-induced shock, generation of thrombin-thrombomodulin complex (which inhibits both thrombin-catalyzed fibrin formation and factor V activation), and activation of coagulant and fibrinolytic pathways have been recognized as conditions explaining early acute coagulopathy (Rossaint et al. 2016), further exacerbated by hemodilution due to resuscitation (Chang et al. 2016), consumption of coagulation factors, hypothermia, hypoperfusion-induced metabolic acidosis, and inflammation (Floccard et al. 2012).

A post hoc analysis from the Pragmatic, Randomized Optimal Platelet and Plasma Ratios (PROPPR) trial (Holcomb et al. 2015) found that patients with TBI in combination with hemorrhagic shock showed higher serum lactate, higher activated prothrombin times, and lower platelet counts compared to patients with isolated TBI. Mortality 30 days after injury was higher in the group of isolated TBI and in the group with TBI and hemorrhagic shock, compared to the group with only hemorrhagic shock and the group of patients without TBI and hemorrhagic shock. An adjusted odds of death were 8–11 times higher in the groups with TBI (Galvagno et al. 2017).

TBI alone has been shown to induce profound platelet dysfunction (Castellino et al. 2014). The increased number of circulating microparticles, exclusive for TBI (Nekludov et al. 2014), has been associated with outcome (Morel et al. 2008). Microparticles (MP) are small particles emanating from different cell types, including activated platelets and endothelial cells, as well as astrocytes. They carry the same receptors on the cell surface as the parent cells, and they can promote a physiological response, such as initiating neuroinflammation and activating coagulation, by expressing various types of proinflammatory or procoagulative markers. Circulating MP is part of the biological response after TBI.

In TBI, brain-derived microparticles have been shown to act as disseminating factors leading to consumption coagulopathy in mice (Tian et al. 2015).

Platelet-derived microparticles exposing p-selectin, and endothelial microparticles exposing tissue factor, have presented a significantly increased transcranial gradient (cerebrovenous > arterial) in patients suffering from severe TBI. This indicates that the microparticles generated in the injured brain lead to a similar systemic coagulative response as seen in multitrauma (Nekludov et al. 2014).

The presence of MP from platelets, endothelial cells, and astrocytes released after trauma can be analyzed using flow cytometry (Nekludov et al. 2017). They reflect pathological changes in the damaged brain, but also function as a link between the coagulation and complement system.

Thus, it is important to monitor the temporal course of this complicated chain of events, to support the physician's decision-making concerning future therapeutical interventions.

72.4 Preventive Measures and Therapy

Considering the detrimental effects associated with coagulopathy and TBI, treatment of coagulopathy should start as early as possible (Rossaint et al. 2016). Correction of INR, medically or spontaneously, decreases mortality significantly, from 65–70% down to 20–25% (Epstein et al. 2016). The use of plasma and platelets concentrates, as well as different recombinant coagulation factors and hemostatic drugs like tranexamic acid and desmopressin, is part of the neurosurgeon's armament, but the subsequent effects on outcome are debatable. The reasons for this might be patient heterogeneity and inexact outcome measures, which are general problems in performed randomized clinical trials concerning TBI (Bullock et al. 2002). Thus, there are today no specific guidelines for the treatment of coagulopathy following isolated TBI and why treatments generally are following those for general trauma, including massive transfusion protocols and the use of viscoelastic assays.

72.5 Protocol for Massive Transfusion

Blood Sampling

- Blood type grouping and base test
- APTT, PK (INR), TPK, and fibrinogen
- Arterial blood gas analysis (Hb, pH, Ca^{2+})
- Viscoelastic analysis, e.g., thromboelastography (TEG) or thromboelastometry (ROTEM)

modified from Karolinska Trauma Center

1. Transfuse erythrocyte concentrate, plasma, and platelet concentrate as 4:4:1.
2. Fibrinogen concentrate 2–4 g i.v.
3. Tranexamic acid 2 g i.v.
4. Calcium glubionate 10 mL i.v. until serum level of free Ca^{2+} >1 mmol.
5. Treat acidosis (ABG repeatedly) and hypothermia.
6. Monitor coagulation using thromboelastometry (ROTEM®).
7. If need of transfusion exceeds one erythrocyte concentrate/10 kg BW and hour despite abovementioned measures and adequate surgical measures, consider recombinant FVIIa (NovoSeven®). Prior to administration of FVIIa, try fibrinogen 4 g + tranexamic acid 2 g + 2 units of platelet concentrates.

Transfusion Targets

- Hb ≥100 g/L
- Fibrinogen >2 g/L
- APT time: normal
- Free Ca^{2+} >1 mmol/L
- TPK >100 × 10^9
- PK(INR) <1.3
- APT time: normalization
- Body temp >36.5 °C
- pH >7.2

72.5.1 Ongoing Cerebral Bleeding

If hemorrhagic diathesis is recognized, it is important to promptly correct potential hypothermia and acidosis. In a multitrauma situation with severe bleeding, the protocol for massive transfusion should be followed.

72.5.2 Local Procoagulants

During surgery there are different local procoagulant products that can be used.

Collagen-based agents, such as Avitene, which is an active absorbable collagen hemostat, that accelerate clot formation.

Gelatin-based agents**,** e.g., Floseal, which is a tissue glue consisting of gelatin and thrombin. The gelatin granules swell to produce a tamponade effect, and when the blood meets the thrombin, the high concentrations of human thrombin convert fibrinogen into fibrin monomers, accelerating clot formation, and a strong clot is formed.

Another gelatin-based resorbable hemostatic is Spongostan, which may be dipped into tranexamic acid to prevent local fibrinolysis.

Cellulose-based agents, e.g., Surgicel, which is a hemostatic agent made of an oxidized cellulose polymer to control postsurgical bleeding.

Fibrin and synthetic glue, e.g., Tisseel, which is a two-component tissue glue consisting of fibrinogen, fibronectin, factor XIII, bovine aprotinin and plasminogen, human thrombin, and calcium chloride dihydrate. The fibrin adhesion system initiates the final phase of physiological blood coagulation and is possible to administer as spray.

Another example is TachoSil, which consists of a matrix including human fibrinogen and thrombin that can be used to cover the bleeding site

72.5.3 Coagulation Factors

Prothrombin complex concentrate (PCC) is made up of blood clotting factors II, IX, and X, and some versions also contain factor VII. The risk for associated thromboembolic complications is (though not well studied) why the European Trauma Bleeding Guidelines presently recommend PCC primarily for emergency reversal of vitamin K antagonists and in patients where bleeding is evident due to a delayed initiation of coagulation, assessed using viscoelastic monitoring (Rossaint et al. 2016). The use of recombinant coagulation factor VII is only recommended if the traumatic coagulopathy persists despite all other attempts to control bleeding (Rossaint et al. 2016).

72.5.3.1 Fresh Frozen Plasma (FFP) and Cryoprecipitate

Infusion of FFP in patients with severe head injury does not always appear to improve outcome (Anglin et al. 2013; Etemadrezaie et al. 2007), despite for a subgroup of patients suffering from multifocal intracranial hemorrhage if the plasma is administered early, within 4 h after trauma, (Chang et al. 2017) or in combination with red blood cells and platelets (Chang et al. 2017). FFP is recommended to maintain INR and APTT <1.5 times normal control, and FFP or fibrinogen concentrate in combination with red blood cell transfusion is recommended when massive hemorrhage is expected (Rossaint et al. 2016).

72.5.4 Platelet Transfusion

Platelet transfusion is questioned due to its short half-life and risk for transfusion complications leading to a worse outcome when transfused (Spiess 2010). The American Association of Blood Banks (AABB) performed a major review concerning platelet transfusion and was not able to give any recommendation regarding platelet transfusion for patients receiving antiplatelet therapy who suffer from an intracranial hemorrhage. There are weak recommendations based on low-quality evidence that platelet transfusion may benefit patients having elective central venous catheter placement with a platelet count less than 20×10^9 cells/L and for patients having elective diagnostic lumbar puncture with a platelet count less than 50×10^9 cells/L (Kaufman et al. 2015). Kumar performed a review on 11 papers including 1.300 patients suffering from intracranial hemorrhage, concerning prophylactic platelet transfusion and found that the overall results did not indicate any significant difference in mortality between transfused and not transfused patients (Kumar et al. 2015).

Platelet transfusion has been shown to correct low TBI-induced platelet MEA values (Lindblad et al. 2018; Nekludov and Bellander 2008; Naidech et al. 2012).

Massive transfusion with high platelet ratio (platelets:RBC ≥1:2) was associated with improved survival in massively transfused trauma patients (Brasel et al. 2011), while platelet transfusion to patients suffering from moderate thrombocytopenia, defined as platelet count 50–107 × 10^9/L, did not affect outcome (Anglin et al. 2013).

Despite a weak scientific evidence, platelet transfusion is recommended to maintain a platelet count above 50 × 10^9/L and, in case of ongoing bleeding, above 100 × 10^9/L (Rossaint et al. 2016).

72.5.5 Fibrinogen

Fibrinogen is the final component in the coagulation cascade. In addition to its role in the coagulation system, fibrinogen also is a pleiotropic protein with essential roles in inflammation and tissue repair (Davalos and Akassoglou 2012). It is not detectable in normal brain tissue, but when BBB disintegrates, fibrinogen enters the CNS and acts as a primary astrocyte activation signal, with a subsequent deposition of inhibitory proteoglycans inducing glial scar formation (Schachtrup et al. 2010).

In multitrauma, plasma fibrinogen reaches critical low levels at an early stage and is the primary coagulation factor deficiency during major bleeding (Chambers et al. 2011). It is associated with increased blood loss and transfusion requirements in trauma (Rourke et al. 2012). In a retrospective analysis of 1266 multitrauma patients, a high FDP/fibrinogen ratio on arrival was shown as a predictor of 28-day mortality (Lee et al. 2018). Its role in bleeding control is pivotal, and it appears reasonable to maintain plasma fibrinogen as early as possible. Even though fibrinogen in patients with isolated TBI is significantly higher than in trauma patients without TBI (Yuan et al. 2016), it should not be overlooked. Administration of fibrinogen concentrate effectively treats early and critical fibrinogen depletion (Schochl et al. 2014) and is recommended when there is significant bleeding with viscoelastic signs of fibrinogen dysfunction or plasma level of fibrinogen is less than 1.5–2.0 g/L (Rossaint et al. 2016).

72.5.6 Antifibrinolytic Treatment

Prospective randomized clinical trials using the antifibrinolytic agent tranexamic acid (TXA) have shown improved outcome following general trauma (The CRASH-2 collaborators, 2011; Cole et al. 2015; Morrison et al. 2012) even though contradictory findings have been reported (Valle et al. 2014; Harvin et al. 2015). Still, the European Trauma Bleeding Guidelines recommend prehospital use of TXA on patients suffering from major multitrauma (grade 1B) within 3 h after trauma (Rossaint et al. 2016; Jokar et al. 2017).

The CRASH-3 randomized trial found that early (<3 h) administration of TXA was associated with a non-significant reduction of head injury-related mortality in patients with isolated TBI (The CRASH- 3 collaborators, 2019). However, there was a significant reduction in head injury-related mortality when TXA was administered within 3 h to patients with mild-to-moderate TBI. Thus, time and severity seemed to be key parameters underlying these findings, with early administration decrease the extent of the bleeding before the hemorrhagic volume may become dangerous, and late administration could be inadequate once a significant hemorrhage has accumulated. There has also been some debate regarding the use of "head injury-related mortality" as the primary outcome variable, as oppose to "all-cause mortality" which was used in CRASH 2 study. Based on this trial, many argue that there is enough evidence to support early TXA in moderate-to-mild TBI, while it is too scarce to support its use in severe TBI.

72.5.7 Desmopressin

In a retrospective meta-analysis including 596 patients with platelet dysfunction during cardiac surgery, administration of desmopressin reduced red cell transfusions, blood loss, and risk of reoperation due to bleeding (Desborough et al. 2017a). However, in a recent Cochrane report of randomized control trials including a total of 3874 patients receiving desmopressin during surgery, the authors concluded that the reduction in volume of red cells transfused and total blood loss was small and clinically unimportant (Desborough et al. 2017b). The administration of platelets and desmopressin to patients suffering blunt TBI is not associated with a decreased risk for early radiographic hemorrhage progression (Kim et al. 2015) and is only recommended for patients treated with platelet inhibiting drugs or with von Willebrand disease (Rossaint et al. 2016).

72.6 Who Will Develop Thromboembolic Complications?

72.6.1 Hypercoagulability

Approximately 54% of patients not subjected to prophylaxis against thromboembolism develop deep vein thrombosis (Geerts et al. 1994). More extensive thromboembolic complications occur after TBI in 6–13% of patients with TBI (Narayan et al. 2008a, b). However, microthrombosis can be detected in most patients who have died as a result of TBI (Stein et al. 2004). The number of microthrombi, or "shock bodies," appears to increase during the first 8–9 days after TBI (Huber et al. 1993; Lafuente and Cervos-Navarro 1999). Furthermore, nearly 40% of patients suffering from TBI presents secondary peaks in the serum levels of the biomarker S100B during their NICU stay. The majority of these secondary peaks corresponds to CT- or MRI-verified ischemia or cerebral infarcts within the first 3 weeks after admission (Thelin et al. 2014). The cause of this is unclear, but hypercoagulability may be one explanation, and if so, these findings indicate that thromboembolic complications following TBI might be even more common than previously known. The brain is a rich source of tissue factor (Keimowitz and Annis 1973) which may stimulate the development of intravascular coagulation in the brain. TBI patients show increasing changes in thromboelastography indicating an increasing hypercoagulability over the days after the initial TBI (Massaro et al. 2015). A maladaptive protein C response to trauma and hypoperfusion has been suggested to cause an immediate coagulopathy followed by a chronic susceptibility to thromboembolic events (Lustenberger et al. 2010; Laroche et al. 2012). The complement activation elicited by the TBI (Bellander et al. 2001) interferes with the coagulation system on several levels (Ekdahl et al. 2016) and may contribute to the coagulopathy after TBI (Nekludov et al. 2007b).

72.6.2 Inflammation

Interaction between the complement, coagulation, and kallikrein/kinin systems is well described (Ekdahl et al. 2016). The complement system, which is a phylogenetically old part of our innate immune system, is activated by the TBI (Bellander et al. 1996, 2001). The anaphylactic toxin C5a, which is formed during complement activation, is one of the most potent inflammatory mediators capable of stimulating chemotaxis of inflammatory cells to the lesion area. The finally assembled terminal membrane complex C5b-9 (membrane attack complex; MAC) has cytolytic capability which, attach to neurons in the peripheral zone of cerebral contusions, creating pores in the cell membrane, and allowing water and solutes to enter the cell with a subsequent cytolysis. Affected cells respond by synthesizing complement inhibitors, such as clusterin, which prevent the assembly of C5b-9, thereby losing its cytolytic effect.

Both the coagulation system and the complement system are made up of complex serine proteases that are activated following TBI and interact at several levels (Foley and Conway 2016). The complement system's C5b-9 attacks, in addition to neurons in the peripheral zone of cerebral contusions (Bellander et al. 2001), also endothelial cells (Tedesco et al. 1997; Ikeda et al. 1997) and platelets (Peerschke et al. 2006; Sims 1991), affecting the blood-brain barrier (Stahel et al. 2001) as well as thrombocyte function (Lood et al. 2012; Mehta et al. 2008). Platelet aggregation and release of serotonin is significantly increased if complement is present (Polley and Nachman 1978). Complement activation can thus be an explanation for changes in platelet reactivity after TBI.

72.7 Specific Pediatric Concerns

Massive bleeding is less common after pediatric trauma.

Age-related changes in the coagulation system occur during the first months after birth.

The reference intervals for prothrombin time, activated partial thromboplastin time APTT, and fibrinogen are similar to adults, while many other assays may differ (Christiaans et al. 2014).

72.8 Conclusions

Post-traumatic coagulopathy and hypercoagulopathy are important players in the development of secondary injuries after traumatic brain injury. The intricate interaction between the different biochemical cascades and the temporal course is important to identify and understand. We need to be able to define what targeted treatments should be instituted to each individual patient and at what time point to minimize these devastating effects and improve patient outcome.

References

Alahmadi H, Vachhrajani S, Cusimano MD. The natural history of brain contusion: an analysis of radiological and clinical progression. J Neurosurg. 2010;112:1139–45.

Allard CB, Scarpelini S, Rhind SG, Baker AJ, Shek PN, Tien H, Fernando M, Tremblay L, Morrison LJ, Pinto R, Rizoli SB. Abnormal coagulation tests are associated with progression of traumatic intracranial hemorrhage. J Trauma. 2009;67:959–67.

Allison TA, Lin PJ, Gass JA, Chong K, Prater SJ, Escobar MA, Hartman HD. Evaluation of the use of low-dose 4-factor prothrombin complex concentrate in the reversal of direct oral anticoagulants in bleeding patients. J Intensive Care Med. 2018:885066618800657.

Alrajhi KN, Perry JJ, Forster AJ. Intracranial bleeds after minor and minimal head injury in patients on warfarin. J Emerg Med. 2015;48:137–42.

Anglin CO, Spence JS, Warner MA, Paliotta C, Harper C, Moore C, Sarode R, Madden C, Diaz-Arrastia R. Effects of platelet and plasma transfusion on outcome in traumatic brain injury patients with moderate bleeding diatheses. J Neurosurg. 2013;118:676–86.

Armand R, Hess JR. Treating coagulopathy in trauma patients. Transfus Med Rev. 2003;17:223–31.

Asan Z. Growth potential of subdural hematomas under clinical observation: which subdural hematomas tend to grow and why they do. World Neurosurg. 2018;113:e598–603.

Batchelor JS, Grayson A. A meta-analysis to determine the effect of anticoagulation on mortality in patients with blunt head trauma. Br J Neurosurg. 2012;26:525–30.

Batchelor JS, Grayson A. A meta-analysis to determine the effect of preinjury antiplatelet agents on mortality in patients with blunt head trauma. Br J Neurosurg. 2013;27:12–8.

Beaumont A, Gennarelli T. CT prediction of contusion evolution after closed head injury: the role of pericontusional edema. Acta Neurochir Suppl. 2006;96:30–2.

Bellander BM, von Holst H, Fredman P, Svensson M. Activation of the complement cascade and increase of clusterin in the brain following a cortical contusion in the adult rat. J Neurosurg. 1996;85:468–75.

Bellander BM, Singhrao SK, Ohlsson M, Mattsson P, Svensson M. Complement activation in the human brain after traumatic head injury. J Neurotrauma. 2001;18:1295–311.

Beynon C, Hertle DN, Unterberg AW, Sakowitz OW. Clinical review: traumatic brain injury in patients receiving antiplatelet medication. Crit Care. 2012;16:228.

Brasel KJ, Vercruysse G, Spinella PC, Wade CE, Blackbourne LH, Borgman MA, Zarzabal LA, Du F, Perkins JG, Maegele M, Schreiber M, Hess JR, Jastrow KM 3rd, Gonzalez EA, Holcomb JB, Kozar R, Trauma Outcomes G, Brasel KJ, Vercruysse G, MacLeod J, Dutton RP, Duchesne JC, McSwain NE, Muskat P, Johannigamn J, Cryer HM, Cryer HM, Pittet JF, Knudson P, De Moya MA, Tieu B, Brundage S, Napolitano LM, Brunsvold M, Sihler KC, Beilman G, Peitzman AB, Zenait MS, Sperry J, Alarcon L, Croce MA, Minei JP, Stewart RM, Cohn SM, Mickalek JE, Bulger EM, Cotton BA, Nunez TC, Ivatury R, Meredith JW, Miller P, Pomper GJ, Marin B. The association of blood component use ratios with the survival of massively transfused trauma patients with and without severe brain injury. J Trauma. 2011;71:S343–52.

Brohi K, Cohen MJ, Ganter MT, Matthay MA, Mackersie RC, Pittet JF. Acute traumatic coagulopathy: initiated by hypoperfusion: modulated through the protein C pathway? Ann Surg. 2007;245:812–8.

Bullock MR, Merchant RE, Choi SC, Gilman CB, Kreutzer JS, Marmarou A, Teasdale GM. Outcome measures for clinical trials in neurotrauma. Neurosurg Focus. 2002;13(1):ECP1.

Burnett A, Siegal D, Crowther M. Specific antidotes for bleeding associated with direct oral anticoagulants. BMJ. 2017;357:j2216.

Cardenas JC, Matijevic N, Baer LA, Holcomb JB, Cotton BA, Wade CE. Elevated tissue plasminogen activator and reduced plasminogen activator inhibitor promote hyperfibrinolysis in trauma patients. Shock. 2014;41:514–21.

Carrick MM, Tyroch AH, Youens CA, Handley T. Subsequent development of thrombocytopenia and coagulopathy in moderate and severe head injury: support for serial laboratory examination. J Trauma. 2005;58:725–9; discussion 729–30.

Castellino FJ, Chapman MP, Donahue DL, Thomas S, Moore EE, Wohlauer MV, Fritz B, Yount R, Ploplis V, Davis P, Evans E, Walsh M. Traumatic brain injury causes platelet adenosine diphosphate and arachidonic acid receptor inhibition independent of hemorrhagic shock in humans and rats. J Trauma Acute Care Surg. 2014;76:1169–76.

Chambers LA, Chow SJ, Shaffer LE. Frequency and characteristics of coagulopathy in trauma patients treated with a low- or high-plasma-content massive transfusion protocol. Am J Clin Pathol. 2011;136:364–70.

Chang EF, Meeker M, Holland MC. Acute traumatic intraparenchymal hemorrhage: risk factors for progression in the early post-injury period. Neurosurgery. 2006;58:647–56; discussion 647–56.

Chang R, Cardenas JC, Wade CE, Holcomb JB. Advances in the understanding of trauma-induced coagulopathy. Blood. 2016;128:1043–9.

Chang R, Folkerson LE, Sloan D, Tomasek JS, Kitagawa RS, Choi HA, Wade CE, Holcomb JB. Early plasma transfusion is associated with improved survival after isolated traumatic brain injury in patients with multifocal intracranial hemorrhage. Surgery. 2017;161:538–45.

Chauny JM, Marquis M, Bernard F, Williamson D, Albert M, Laroche M, Daoust R. Risk of delayed intracranial hemorrhage in anticoagulated patients with mild traumatic brain injury: systematic review and meta-analysis. J Emerg Med. 2016;51:519–28.

Chieregato A, Fainardi E, Morselli-Labate AM, Antonelli V, Compagnone C, Targa L, Kraus J, Servadei F. Factors associated with neurological outcome and lesion progression in traumatic subarachnoid hemorrhage patients. Neurosurgery. 2005;56:671–80; discussion 671–80.

Christiaans SC, Duhachek-Stapelman AL, Russell RT, Lisco SJ, Kerby JD, Pittet JF. Coagulopathy after severe pediatric trauma. Shock. 2014;41:476–90.

Cohen MJ, Brohi K, Ganter MT, Manley GT, Mackersie RC, Pittet JF. Early coagulopathy after traumatic brain injury: the role of hypoperfusion and the protein C pathway. J Trauma. 2007;63:1254–61; discussion 1261–2.

Cole E, Davenport R, Willett K, Brohi K. Tranexamic acid use in severely injured civilian patients and the effects on outcomes: a prospective cohort study. Ann Surg. 2015;261:390–4.

Connolly SJ, Crowther M, Eikelboom JW, Gibson CM, Curnutte JT, Lawrence JH, Yue P, Bronson MD, Lu G, Conley PB, Verhamme P, Schmidt J, Middeldorp

S, Cohen AT, Beyer-Westendorf J, Albaladejo P, Lopez-Sendon J, Demchuk AM, Pallin DJ, Concha M, Goodman S, Leeds J, Souza S, Siegal DM, Zotova E, Meeks B, Ahmad S, Nakamya J, Milling TJ Jr, A.-. Investigators. Full study report of andexanet Alfa for bleeding associated with factor Xa inhibitors. N Engl J Med. 2019;380(14):1326–35.

Cotton BA, Harvin JA, Kostousouv V, Minei KM, Radwan ZA, Schochl H, Wade CE, Holcomb JB, Matijevic N. Hyperfibrinolysis at admission is an uncommon but highly lethal event associated with shock and prehospital fluid administration. J Trauma Acute Care Surg. 2012;73:365–70; discussion 370.

Davalos D, Akassoglou K. Fibrinogen as a key regulator of inflammation in disease. Semin Immunopathol. 2012;34:43–62.

Davis PK, Musunuru H, Walsh M, Cassady R, Yount R, Losiniecki A, Moore EE, Wohlauer MV, Howard J, Ploplis VA, Castellino FJ, Thomas SG. Platelet dysfunction is an early marker for traumatic brain injury-induced coagulopathy. Neurocrit Care. 2013;18:201–8.

Desborough MJ, Oakland KA, Landoni G, Crivellari M, Doree C, Estcourt LJ, Stanworth SJ. Desmopressin for treatment of platelet dysfunction and reversal of antiplatelet agents: a systematic review and meta-analysis of randomized controlled trials. J Thromb Haemost. 2017a;15:263–72.

Desborough MJ, Oakland K, Brierley C, Bennett S, Doree C, Trivella M, Hopewell S, Stanworth SJ, Estcourt LJ. Desmopressin use for minimising perioperative blood transfusion. Cochrane Database Syst Rev. 2017b;7:CD001884.

Ekdahl KN, Teramura Y, Hamad OA, Asif S, Duehrkop C, Fromell K, Gustafson E, Hong J, Kozarcanin H, Magnusson PU, Huber-Lang M, Garred P, Nilsson B. Dangerous liaisons: complement, coagulation, and kallikrein/kinin cross-talk act as a linchpin in the events leading to thromboinflammation. Immunol Rev. 2016;274:245–69.

Engström M, Romner B, Schalen W, Reinstrup P. Thrombocytopenia predicts progressive hemorrhage after head trauma. J Neurotrauma. 2005;22:291–6.

Epstein DS, Mitra B, O'Reilly G, Rosenfeld JV, Cameron PA. Acute traumatic coagulopathy in the setting of isolated traumatic brain injury: a systematic review and meta-analysis. Injury. 2014;45:819–24.

Epstein DS, et al. Acute traumatic coagulopathy in the setting of isolated traumatic brain injury: definition, incidence and outcomes. Br J Neurosurg. 2015;29(1): 118–122.

Epstein DS, Mitra B, Cameron PA, Fitzgerald M, Rosenfeld JV. Normalization of coagulopathy is associated with improved outcome after isolated traumatic brain injury. J Clin Neurosci. 2016;29:64–9.

Etemadrezaie H, Baharvahdat H, Shariati Z, Lari SM, Shakeri MT, B G. The effect of fresh frozen plasma in severe closed head injury. Clin Neurol Neurosurg. 2007;109:166–71.

Floccard B, Rugeri L, Faure A, Saint Denis M, Boyle EM, Peguet O, Levrat A, Guillaume C, Marcotte G, Vulliez A, Hautin E, David JS, Negrier C, Allaouchiche B. Early coagulopathy in trauma patients: an on-scene and hospital admission study. Injury. 2012;43:26–32.

Foley JH, Conway EM. Cross talk pathways between coagulation and inflammation. Circ Res. 2016;118:1392–408.

Folkerson LE, Sloan D, Davis E, Kitagawa RS, Cotton BA, Holcomb JB, Tomasek JS, Wade CE. Coagulopathy as a predictor of mortality after penetrating traumatic brain injury. Am J Emerg Med. 2018;36:38–42.

Franko J, Kish KJ, O'Connell BG, Subramanian S, Yuschak JV. Advanced age and preinjury warfarin anticoagulation increase the risk of mortality after head trauma. J Trauma. 2006;61:107–10.

Galvagno SM Jr, Fox EE, Appana SN, Baraniuk S, Bosarge PL, Bulger EM, Callcut RA, Cotton BA, Goodman M, Inaba K, O'Keeffe T, Schreiber MA, Wade CE, Scalea TM, Holcomb JB, Stein DM, P.S. Group. Outcomes after concomitant traumatic brain injury and hemorrhagic shock: a secondary analysis from the pragmatic, randomized optimal platelets and plasma ratios trial. J Trauma Acute care Surg. 2017;83:668–74.

Geerts WH, Code KI, Jay RM, Chen E, Szalai JP. A prospective study of venous thromboembolism after major trauma. N Engl J Med. 1994;331:1601–6.

Gozal YM, Carroll CP, Krueger BM, Khoury J, Andaluz NO. Point-of-care testing in the acute management of traumatic brain injury: identifying the coagulopathic patient. Surg Neurol Int. 2017;8:48.

Harhangi BS, Kompanje EJ, Leebeek FW, Maas AI. Coagulation disorders after traumatic brain injury. Acta Neurochir (Wien). 2008;150(2):165–75; discussion 175. Epub 2008 Jan 2.

Harvin JA, Peirce CA, Mims MM, Hudson JA, Podbielski JM, Wade CE, Holcomb JB, Cotton BA. The impact of tranexamic acid on mortality in injured patients with hyperfibrinolysis. J Trauma Acute Care Surg. 2015;78:905–9; discussion 909–11.

Holcomb JB, Tilley BC, Baraniuk S, Fox EE, Wade CE, Podbielski JM, del Junco DJ, Brasel KJ, Bulger EM, Callcut RA, Cohen MJ, Cotton BA, Fabian TC, Inaba K, Kerby JD, Muskat P, O'Keeffe T, Rizoli S, Robinson BR, Scalea TM, Schreiber MA, Stein DM, Weinberg JA, Callum JL, Hess JR, Matijevic N, Miller CN, Pittet JF, Hoyt DB, Pearson GD, Leroux B, van Belle G, P.S. Group. Transfusion of plasma, platelets, and red blood cells in a 1:1:1 vs a 1:1:2 ratio and mortality in patients with severe trauma: the PROPPR randomized clinical trial. JAMA. 2015;313:471–82.

Huber A, Dorn A, Witzmann A, Cervos-Navarro J. Microthrombi formation after severe head trauma. Int J Leg Med. 1993;106:152–5.

Ikeda K, Nagasawa K, Horiuchi T, Tsuru T, Nishizaka H, Niho Y. C5a induces tissue factor activity on endothelial cells. Thromb Haemost. 1997;77:394–8.

Jokar A, Ahmadi K, Salehi T, Sharif-Alhoseini M, Rahimi-Movaghar V. The effect of tranexamic acid in traumatic brain injury: a randomized controlled trial. Chin J Traumatol. 2017;20:49–51.

Joseph B, Pandit V, Meyer D, Butvidas L, Kulvatunyou N, Khalil M, Tang A, Zangbar B, O'Keeffe T, Gries L, Friese RS, Rhee P. The significance of platelet count in traumatic brain injury patients on antiplatelet therapy. J Trauma Acute Care Surg. 2014;77(3):417–21.

Juratli TA, Zang B, Litz RJ, Sitoci KH, Aschenbrenner U, Gottschlich B, Daubner D, Schackert G, Sobottka SB. Early hemorrhagic progression of traumatic brain contusions: frequency, correlation with coagulation disorders, and patient outcome: a prospective study. J Neurotrauma. 2014;31:1521–7.

Karri J, Cardenas JC, Matijevic N, Wang YW, Choi S, Zhu L, Cotton BA, Kitagawa R, Holcomb JB, Wade CE. Early fibrinolysis associated with hemorrhagic progression following traumatic brain injury. Shock. 2017;48:644–50.

Kashuk JL, Moore EE, Sawyer M, Wohlauer M, Pezold M, Barnett C, Biffl WL, Burlew CC, Johnson JL, Sauaia A. Primary fibrinolysis is integral in the pathogenesis of the acute coagulopathy of trauma. Ann Surg. 2010;252:434–42; discussion 443–4.

Kaufman RM, Djulbegovic B, Gernsheimer T, Kleinman S, Tinmouth AT, Capocelli KE, Cipolle MD, Cohn CS, Fung MK, Grossman BJ, Mintz PD, O'Malley BA, Sesok-Pizzini DA, Shander A, Stack GE, Webert KE, Weinstein R, Welch BG, Whitman GJ, Wong EC, Tobian AA, Aabb. Platelet transfusion: a clinical practice guideline from the AABB. Ann Intern Med. 2015;162:205–13.

Keimowitz RM, Annis BL. Disseminated intravascular coagulation associated with massive brain injury. J Neurosurg. 1973;39:178–80.

Khalili H, Derakhshan N, Niakan A, Ghaffarpasand F, Salehi M, Eshraghian H, Shakibafard A, Zahabi B. Effects of oral glibenclamide on brain contusion volume and functional outcome of patients with moderate and severe traumatic brain injuries: a randomized double-blind placebo-controlled clinical trial. World Neurosurg. 2017;101:130–6.

Kim DY, O'Leary M, Nguyen A, Kaji A, Bricker S, Neville A, Bongard F, Putnam B, Plurad D. The effect of platelet and desmopressin administration on early radiographic progression of traumatic intracranial hemorrhage. J Neurotrauma. 2015;32:1815–21.

Kobayashi L, Barmparas G, Bosarge P, Brown CV, Bukur M, Carrick MM, Catalano RD, Holly-Nicolas J, Inaba K, Kaminski S, Klein AL, Kopelman T, Ley EJ, Martinez EM, Moore FO, Murry J, Nirula R, Paul D, Quick J, Rivera O, Schreiber M, Coimbra R, AMPOSoTPoNOAS Group. Novel oral anticoagulants and trauma: the results of a prospective American Association for the Surgery of Trauma Multi-Institutional Trial. J Trauma Acute Care Surg. 2017;82:827–35.

Kumar MA. Coagulopathy associated with traumatic brain injury. Curr Neurol Neurosci Rep. 2013;13:391.

Kumar A, Mhaskar R, Grossman BJ, Kaufman RM, Tobian AA, Kleinman S, Gernsheimer T, Tinmouth AT, Djulbegovic B, Panel APTG. Platelet transfusion: a systematic review of the clinical evidence. Transfusion. 2015;55:1116–27; quiz 1115.

Kurland D, Hong C, Aarabi B, Gerzanich V, Simard JM. Hemorrhagic progression of a contusion after traumatic brain injury: a review. J Neurotrauma. 2012;29:19–31.

Kutcher ME, Redick BJ, McCreery RC, Crane IM, Greenberg MD, Cachola LM, Nelson MF, Cohen MJ. Characterization of platelet dysfunction after trauma. J Trauma Acute Care Surg. 2012;73:13–9.

Lafuente JV, Cervos-Navarro J. Craniocerebral trauma induces hemorheological disturbances. J Neurotrauma. 1999;16:425–30.

Laroche M, Kutcher ME, Huang MC, Cohen MJ, Manley GT. Coagulopathy after traumatic brain injury. Neurosurgery. 2012;70:1334–45.

Lee DH, Lee BK, Noh SM, Cho YS. High fibrin/fibrinogen degradation product to fibrinogen ratio is associated with 28-day mortality and massive transfusion in severe trauma. Eur J Trauma Emerg Surg. 2018;44:291–8.

Lindblad C, Thelin EP, Nekludov M, Frostell A, Nelson DW, Svensson M, Bellander BM. Assessment of platelet function in traumatic brain injury—a retrospective observational study in the neuro-critical care setting. Front Neurol. 2018;9:15.

Lood C, Eriksson S, Gullstrand B, Jonsen A, Sturfelt G, Truedsson L, Bengtsson AA. Increased C1q, C4 and C3 deposition on platelets in patients with systemic lupus erythematosus—a possible link to venous thrombosis? Lupus. 2012;21:1423–32.

Lustenberger T, Talving P, Kobayashi L, Barmparas G, Inaba K, Lam L, Branco BC, Demetriades D. Early coagulopathy after isolated severe traumatic brain injury: relationship with hypoperfusion challenged. J Trauma. 2010;69:1410–4.

Mackman N. The role of tissue factor and factor VIIa in hemostasis. Anesth Analg. 2009;108:1447–52.

Maegele M, Schochl H, Menovsky T, Marechal H, Marklund N, Buki A, Stanworth S. Coagulopathy and haemorrhagic progression in traumatic brain injury: advances in mechanisms, diagnosis, and management. Lancet Neurol. 2017;16:630–47.

Makris M, Van Veen JJ, Tait CR, Mumford AD, Laffan M, British Committee for Standards in Haematology. Guideline on the management of bleeding in patients on antithrombotic agents. Br J Haematol. 2013;160:35–46.

Massaro AM, Doerfler S, Nawalinski K, Michel B, Driscoll N, Ju C, Patel H, Quattrone F, Frangos S, Maloney-Wilensky E, Sean Grady M, Stein SC, Kasner SE, Kumar MA. Thromboelastography defines late hypercoagulability after TBI: a pilot study. Neurocrit Care. 2015;22:45–51.

Maung AA, Bhattacharya B, Schuster KM, Davis KA. Trauma patients on new oral anticoagulation agents have lower mortality than those on warfarin. J Trauma Acute Care Surg. 2016;81:652–7.

McCully SP, Schreiber MA. Traumatic brain injury and its effect on coagulopathy. Semin Thromb Hemost. 2013;39:896–901.

Mehta N, Uchino K, Fakhran S, Sattar MA, Branstetter BFt, Au K, Navratil JS, Paul B, Lee M, Gallagher KM, Manzi S, Ahearn JM, Kao AH. Platelet C4d is associated with acute ischemic stroke and stroke severity. Stroke. 2008;39:3236–41.

Moore HB, Moore EE, Liras IN, Gonzalez E, Harvin JA, Holcomb JB, Sauaia A, Cotton BA. Acute fibrinolysis shutdown after injury occurs frequently and increases mortality: a multicenter evaluation of 2,540 severely injured patients. J Am Coll Surg. 2016;222:347–55.

Morel N, Morel O, Petit L, Hugel B, Cochard JF, Freyssinet JM, Sztark F, Dabadie P. Generation of procoagulant microparticles in cerebrospinal fluid and peripheral blood after traumatic brain injury. J Trauma. 2008;64:698–704.

Morrison JJ, Dubose JJ, Rasmussen TE, Midwinter MJ. Military Application of Tranexamic Acid in Trauma Emergency Resuscitation (MATTERs) Study. Arch Surg. 2012;147:113–9.

Moustafa F, Roubin J, Pereira B, Barres A, Saint-Denis J, Perrier C, Mondet M, Dutheil F, Schmidt J. Predictive factors of intracranial bleeding in head trauma patients receiving antiplatelet therapy admitted to an emergency department. Scand J Trauma Resusc Emerg Med. 2018;26:50.

Murray GD, Butcher I, McHugh GS, Lu J, Mushkudiani NA, Maas AI, Marmarou A, Steyerberg EW. Multivariable prognostic analysis in traumatic brain injury: results from the IMPACT study. J Neurotrauma. 2007;24:329–37.

Naidech AM, Liebling SM, Rosenberg NF, Lindholm PF, Bernstein RA, Batjer HH, Alberts MJ, Kwaan HC. Early platelet transfusion improves platelet activity and may improve outcomes after intracerebral hemorrhage. Neurocrit Care. 2012;16:82–7.

Nakamura Y, Ishikura H, Kushimoto S, Kiyomi F, Kato H, Sasaki J, Ogura H, Matsuoka T, Uejima T, Morimura N, Hayakawa M, Hagiwara A, Takeda M, Kaneko N, Saitoh D, Kudo D, Maekawa K, Kanemura T, Shibusawa T, Hagihara Y, Furugori S, Shiraishi A, Murata K, Mayama G, Yaguchi A, Kim S, Takasu O, Nishiyama K. Fibrinogen level on admission is a predictor for massive transfusion in patients with severe blunt trauma: analyses of a retrospective multicentre observational study. Injury. 2017;48:674–9.

Narayan RK, Maas AI, Servadei F, Skolnick BE, Tillinger MN, Marshall LF, G. Traumatic Intracerebral Hemorrhage Study. Progression of traumatic intracerebral hemorrhage: a prospective observational study. J Neurotrauma. 2008a;25:629–39.

Narayan RK, Maas AI, Marshall LF, Servadei F, Skolnick BE, Tillinger MN, r.T.I.S. Group. Recombinant factor VIIA in traumatic intracerebral hemorrhage: results of a dose-escalation clinical trial. Neurosurgery. 2008b;62:776–86.

Nekludov M, Bellander BM. Efficacy of platelet concentrates in patients with brain trauma and bleeding diathesis. In: 26th Annual National-Neurotrauma-Society Symposium, Journal of Neurotrauma, Orlando, FL, USA, 2008. p. 887.

Nekludov M, Bellander BM, Blombäck M, Wallen HN. Platelet dysfunction in patients with severe traumatic brain injury. J Neurotrauma. 2007a;24(11):1699–706.

Nekludov M, Antovic J, Bredbacka S, Blombäck M. Coagulation abnormalities associated with severe isolated traumatic brain injury: cerebral arterio-venous differences in coagulation and inflammatory markers. J Neurotrauma. 2007b;24:174–80.

Nekludov M, Mobarrez F, Gryth D, Bellander BM, Wallen H. Formation of microparticles in the injured brain of patients with severe isolated traumatic brain injury. J Neurotrauma. 2014;31:1927–33.

Nekludov M, Bellander BM, Gryth D, Wallen H, Mobarrez F. Brain-derived microparticles in patients with severe isolated TBI. Brain Injury. 2017;31:1856–62.

Oertel M, Kelly DF, McArthur D, Boscardin WJ, Glenn TC, Lee JH, Gravori T, Obukhov D, McBride DQ, Martin NA. Progressive hemorrhage after head trauma: predictors and consequences of the evolving injury. J Neurosurg. 2002;96:109–16.

Pandya U, Malik A, Messina M, Albeiruti AR, Spalding C. Reversal of antiplatelet therapy in traumatic intracranial hemorrhage: does timing matter? J Clin Neurosci. 2018;50:88–92.

Patel AD, Gerzanich V, Geng Z, Simard JM. Glibenclamide reduces hippocampal injury and preserves rapid spatial learning in a model of traumatic brain injury. J Neuropathol Exp Neurol. 2010;69: 1177–90.

Peerschke EI, Yin W, Grigg SE, Ghebrehiwet B. Blood platelets activate the classical pathway of human complement. J Thromb Haemost. 2006;4:2035–42.

Polley MJ, Nachman R. The human complement system in thrombin-mediated platelet function. J Exp Med. 1978;147:1713–26.

Rittirsch D, Flierl MA, Ward PA. Harmful molecular mechanisms in sepsis. Nat Rev Immunol. 2008;8:776–87.

Roozenbeek B, Maas AI, Menon DK. Changing patterns in the epidemiology of traumatic brain injury. Nat Rev Neurol. 2013;9:231–6.

Rossaint R, Bouillon B, Cerny V, Coats TJ, Duranteau J, Fernandez-Mondejar E, Filipescu D, Hunt BJ, Komadina R, Nardi G, Neugebauer EA, Ozier Y, Riddez L, Schultz A, Vincent JL, Spahn DR. The European guideline on management of major bleeding and coagulopathy following trauma: fourth edition. Crit Care. 2016;20:100.

Rourke C, Curry N, Khan S, Taylor R, Raza I, Davenport R, Stanworth S, Brohi K. Fibrinogen levels during trauma hemorrhage, response to replacement therapy, and association with patient outcomes. J Thromb Haemost. 2012;10:1342–51.

Schachtrup C, Ryu JK, Helmrick MJ, Vagena E, Galanakis DK, Degen JL, Margolis RU, Akassoglou K. Fibrinogen triggers astrocyte scar formation by promoting the availability of active TGF-beta after vascular damage. J Neurosci. 2010;30:5843–54.

Schnuriger B, Inaba K, Abdelsayed GA, Lustenberger T, Eberle BM, Barmparas G, Talving P, Demetriades D. The impact of platelets on the progression

of traumatic intracranial hemorrhage. J Trauma. 2010;68:881–5.
Schochl H, Schlimp CJ, Maegele M. Tranexamic acid, fibrinogen concentrate, and prothrombin complex concentrate: data to support prehospital use? Shock. 2014;41(Suppl 1):44–6.
Selladurai BM, Vickneswaran M, Duraisamy S, Atan M. Coagulopathy in acute head injury—a study of its role as a prognostic indicator. Br J Neurosurg. 1997;11:398–404.
Serebruany VL, Malinin AI, Eisert RM, Sane DC. Risk of bleeding complications with antiplatelet agents: meta-analysis of 338,191 patients enrolled in 50 randomized controlled trials. Am J Hematol. 2004;75:40–7.
Simard JM, Kilbourne M, Tsymbalyuk O, Tosun C, Caridi J, Ivanova S, Keledjian K, Bochicchio G, Gerzanich V. Key role of sulfonylurea receptor 1 in progressive secondary hemorrhage after brain contusion. J Neurotrauma. 2009;26:2257–67.
Simard JM, Woo SK, Schwartzbauer GT, Gerzanich V. Sulfonylurea receptor 1 in central nervous system injury: a focused review. J Cereb Blood Flow Metab. 2012;32:1699–717.
Sims W. The response of human platelets to activated components of the complement system. Immunol Today. 1991;12:338–41.
Siracuse JJ, Robich MP, Gautam S, Kasper EM, Moorman DW, Hauser CJ. Antiplatelet agents, warfarin, and epidemic intracranial hemorrhage. Surgery. 2010;148:724–9; discussion 729–30.
Smits M, Dippel DW, Steyerberg EW, de Haan GG, Dekker HM, Vos PE, Kool DR, Nederkoorn PJ, Hofman PA, Twijnstra A, Tanghe HL, Hunink MG. Predicting intracranial traumatic findings on computed tomography in patients with minor head injury: the CHIP prediction rule. Ann Intern Med. 2007;146:397–405.
Spiess BD. Platelet transfusions: the science behind safety, risks and appropriate applications. Best Pract Res Clin Anaesthesiol. 2010;24:65–83.
Stahel PF, Morganti-Kossmann C, Perez D, Redaelli C, Gloor B, Trentz O, Kossmann T. Intrathecal levels of complement-derivied soluble membrane attack complex (sC5b-9) correlate with blood-brain barrier dysfunction in patients with traumatic brain injury. J Neurotrauma. 2001;18:773–81.
Steffel J, Verhamme P, Potpara TS, Albaladejo P, Antz M, Desteghe L, Haeusler KG, Oldgren J, Reinecke H, Roldan-Schilling V, Rowell N, Sinnaeve P, Collins R, Camm AJ, Heidbuchel H, The E.S.C.S.D. Group. European Heart Rhythm Association Practical Guide on the use of non-vitamin K antagonist oral anticoagulants in patients with atrial fibrillation. Eur Heart J. 2018;39(16):1330–93.
Stein SC, Young GS, Talucci RC, Greenbaum BH, Ross SE. Delayed brain injury after head trauma: significance of coagulopathy. Neurosurgery. 1992;30:160–5.
Stein SC, Chen XH, Sinson GP, Smith DH. Intravascular coagulation: a major secondary insult in nonfatal traumatic brain injury. J Neurosurg. 2002;97:1373–7.
Stein SC, Graham DI, Chen XH, Smith DH. Association between intravascular microthrombosis and cerebral ischemia in traumatic brain injury. Neurosurgery. 2004;54:687–91; discussion 691.
Sumiyoshi K, Hayakawa T, Yatsushige H, Shigeta K, Momose T, Enomoto M, Sato S, Takasato Y. Outcome of traumatic brain injury in patients on antiplatelet agents: a retrospective 20-year observational study in a single neurosurgery unit. Brain Injury. 2017;31:1445–54.
Talving P, Benfield R, Hadjizacharia P, Inaba K, Chan LS, Demetriades D. Coagulopathy in severe traumatic brain injury: a prospective study. J Trauma. 2009;66:55–61; discussion 61–2.
Tedesco F, Pausa M, Nardon E, Introna M, Mantovani A, Dobrina A. The cytolytically inactive terminal complement complex activates endothelial cells to express adhesion molecules and tissue factor procoagulant activity. J Exp Med. 1997;185:1619–27.
The Crash-2 collaborators, The importance of early treatment with tranexamic acid in bleeding trauma patients: an exploratory analysis of the CRASH-2 randomised controlled trial." Lancet. 2011;377(9771): 1096-1101, 1101 e1091–1092.
The CRASH-3 trial collaborators: "Effects of tranexamic acid on death, disability, vascular occlusive events and other morbidities in patients with acute traumatic brain injury (CRASH-3): a randomised, placebo-controlled trial." Lancet. 2019. https://doi.org/10.1016/S0140-6736(19)32233-0.
Thelin EP, Nelson DW, Bellander BM. Secondary peaks of S100B in serum relate to subsequent radiological pathology in traumatic brain injury. Neurocrit Care. 2014;20:217–29.
Tian Y, Salsbery B, Wang M, Yuan H, Yang J, Zhao Z, Wu X, Zhang Y, Konkle BA, Thiagarajan P, Li M, Zhang J, Dong JF. Brain-derived microparticles induce systemic coagulation in a murine model of traumatic brain injury. Blood. 2015;125(13):2151–9.
Tomaselli GF, Mahaffey KW, Cuker A, Dobesh PP, Doherty JU, Eikelboom JW, Florido R, Hucker W, Mehran R, Messe SR, Pollack CV Jr, Rodriguez F, Sarode R, Siegal D, Wiggins BS. 2017 ACC Expert Consensus Decision Pathway on Management of Bleeding in Patients on Oral Anticoagulants: a report of the American College of Cardiology Task Force on Expert Consensus Decision Pathways. J Am Coll Cardiol. 2017;70:3042–67.
Uccella L, Zoia C, Bongetta D, Gaetani P, Martig F, Candrian C, Rosso R. Are antiplatelet and anticoagulants drugs a risk factor for bleeding in mild traumatic brain injury? World Neurosurg. 2018;110:e339–45.
Unden J, Ingebrigtsen T, Romner B, Scandinavian Neurotrauma C. Scandinavian guidelines for initial management of minimal, mild and moderate head injuries in adults: an evidence and consensus-based update. BMC Med. 2013;11:50.
Valle EJ, Allen CJ, Van Haren RM, Jouria JM, Li H, Livingstone AS, Namias N, Schulman CI, Proctor

KG. Do all trauma patients benefit from tranexamic acid? J Trauma Acute Care Surg. 2014;76:1373–8.

Vedin T, Svensson S, Edelhamre M, Karlsson M, Bergenheim M, Larsson PA. Management of mild traumatic brain injury-trauma energy level and medical history as possible predictors for intracranial hemorrhage. Eur J Trauma Emerg Surg. 2019;45(5):901–7.

Wada T, Gando S, Maekaw K, Katabami K, Sageshima H, Hayakawa M, Sawamura A. Disseminated intravascular coagulation with increased fibrinolysis during the early phase of isolated traumatic brain injury. Crit Care. 2017;21:219.

Wafaisade A, Lefering R, Tjardes T, Wutzler S, Simanski C, Paffrath T, Fischer P, Bouillon B, Maegele M, Trauma Registry of D.G.U. Acute coagulopathy in isolated blunt traumatic brain injury. Neurocritical Care. 2010;12(2):211–9.

Wohlauer MV, Moore EE, Thomas S, Sauaia A, Evans E, Harr J, Silliman CC, Ploplis V, Castellino FJ, Walsh M. Early platelet dysfunction: an unrecognized role in the acute coagulopathy of trauma. J Am Coll Surg. 2012;214:739–46.

Yuan Q, Sun YR, Wu X, Yu J, Li ZQ, Du ZY, Wu XH, Zhou LF, Hu J. Coagulopathy in traumatic brain injury and its correlation with progressive hemorrhagic injury: a systematic review and meta-analysis. J Neurotrauma. 2016;33:1279–91.

Zangbar B, Serack B, Rhee P, Joseph B, Pandit V, Friese RS, Haider AA, Tang AL. Outcomes in trauma patients with isolated epidural hemorrhage: a single-institution retrospective cohort study. Am Surg. 2016;82:1209–14.

Corticosteroids

73

Jens Jakob Riis

Recommendations

Level I

Administration of high-dose corticosteroids in brain trauma patients is harmful with significant side effects and should not be used.

Level II

Data are insufficient to support Level II recommendations on this topic.

Level III

Data are insufficient to support Level III recommendations on this topic.

73.1 Overview

Because no studies have shown benefit in using steroids in brain trauma, the use of corticosteroids has for long been controversial and therefore been questioned. The randomised CRASH study showed that mortality was increased in patients receiving very high doses of steroids. No consensus exists, however, regarding the benefits or adverse effect in using low to moderate doses of corticosteroids in brain trauma patients.

The previously recommended high-dose methylprednisolone to patients with trauma-induced spinal transection has now been abandoned for some years in many Nordic trauma centres because of the following:

1. Lack of evidence for beneficial effect
2. Harmful effect on brain trauma patients with spinal cord injuries
3. Significant side effects such as hyperglycaemia, gastric ulcers/bleeding, increased risk of infection, psychosis and impaired wound healing

Cerebral oedema caused by head trauma can be seen as an isolated phenomenon or can be seen after removal of an acute subdural haematoma. In brain trauma, the cerebral oedema is a mixture of vasogenic and cytotoxic oedema (Papadopoulos et al. 2004). Today, it has not been proven that corticosteroids to brain trauma patients have the same beneficial effect as it has in patients with brain tumours and meningitis. Administration of corticosteroids in order to decrease traumatically induced oedema, e.g. around cerebral contusions, has not been widespread due to lack of evidence. Serious side effects in brain injured patients are probably another explanation.

The purpose of using corticosteroids in brain trauma patients has been targeting the oedema

J. J. Riis (✉)
Department of Neurosurgery, Aalborg University Hospital, Aalborg, Denmark
e-mail: j.riis@rn.dk

© Springer Nature Switzerland AG 2020
T. Sundstrøm et al. (eds.), *Management of Severe Traumatic Brain Injury*,
https://doi.org/10.1007/978-3-030-39383-0_73

surrounding, e.g. contusions and the general cerebral oedema and inflammation arising after the insult (Dearden et al. 1986; Giannotti et al. 1984; Kamano 2000; Rabinstein 2006).

As shown by Audibert et al. (2009) and Ginsbury and Busto (2003), hyperpyrexia is negatively influencing prognosis in traumatic brain injury. A moderate single dose of corticosteroid has also been used in head trauma patients with very high fever (Grände 2006).

Tips, Tricks and Pitfalls

- Avoid using corticosteroids in brain trauma patients, especially in high doses.

73.2 Background

A systematic review in *British Medical Journal* by Alderson and Roberts (1997) suggested that the mortality in brain trauma patients was reduced with approx. 1–2% if given corticosteroids. Two thousand patients were included in this study that encouraged the use of corticosteroids.

Corticosteroids to patients with brain tumours with peritumoural oedema is a well-established routine, and the effect is significant, e.g. on hemiparesis. The tumour-induced oedema is thought to be secondary to disrupted BBB, and the mechanism of action by corticosteroids is supposed to be decreasing the permeability of tight junctions and stabilising the damaged BBB (Raslan and Bhardwaj 2007; Sinha et al. 2004).

The randomised CRASH study (Roberts et al. 2004) has become a cornerstone regarding the use of corticosteroids in brain trauma. It was supposed to include 2000 patients, but the inclusion was terminated prematurely because an interim analysis showed that 21% of patients given corticosteroids were dead within 2 weeks compared to 18% in the group given placebo. The patients received either a bolus dose of 2 g of methylprednisolone within 8 h after the head injury, and afterwards 0.4 g/h for the next 48 h, or an infusion of placebo. The study included both moderately injured patients and more severely injured patients—all included patients had a GCS of 14 or less. Ten thousand and eight patients had been included when the study was closed. The relative risk (RR) for death for all causes was 1.18 (95% CI; 1.09–1.27; $p = 0.001$). There was no increase in complications (infections, gastric bleedings, etc.) in the groups allocated to corticosteroids, which is contrary to the findings in the Cochrane review mentioned earlier (Alderson and Roberts 2005). The reason for the increased mortality has never been elucidated, but the irrelevantly very high doses of methylprednisolone used may have affected outcome negatively (Roberts et al. 2004).

Because of that, corticoids are no longer given routinely to brain trauma patients. Since the last edition of this book, no new scientific evidence has emerged that contradicts this practice, although some authors have emphasised that low-dose corticosteroids may be used under specific circumstances (Grände 2006; Giannotti et al. 1984; Kamano 2000). In a recent study (Huijben et al. 2018), corticosteroids were used very infrequently and for targeting vasopressor-resistant hypotension and sepsis.

The above-mentioned Cochrane review (Alderson and Roberts 2005) states that "the largest trial with about 80% of all randomised participants found a significant increase in the risk ratio of death with steroids of 1.15 (95% CI 1.07–1.24) and a relative risk of severe disability of 1.05 (95%; CI 0.99–1.07).

The risk of GI bleeding, hyperglycaemia and infection was also increased. This is of special concern because hyperglycaemia is hazardous in patients with cerebral contusions. The importance of keeping blood sugar within normal range in patients with brain trauma has been emphasised in many trials (Jeremitsky et al. 2005; Laird and Miller 2004; Rovlias and Kotsou 2000; Salim et al. 2009; Yag et al. 1989).

So far, the use of corticosteroids has also been directed against the inflammatory response after head injury, but the exact role of inflammatory mediators in brain trauma is not fully elucidated and the use of corticosteroids in this setting is not justified.

Overall, there is no evidence that administration of (high-dose) corticosteroids in traumatic brain injury has any beneficial effect on survival or long-term outcome; actually Level 1 evidence states that administration of very-high-dose corticosteroids to brain trauma patients is harmful and increase mortality without any obvious benefit for the patients (Roberts et al. 2004).

73.3 Specific Paediatric Concerns

High-dose corticosteroids in paediatric patients with brain trauma should *not* be used.

References

Alderson P, Roberts I. Corticosteroids in acute traumatic brain injury: systematic review of randomised controlled trials. Br Med J. 1997;314:1855–9.

Alderson P, Roberts IG. Corticosteroids for acute traumatic brain injury. Cochrane Database Syst Rev. 2005;1:CD000196. https://doi.org/10.1002/14651858.CD000196.pub.2.

Audibert G, Baumann A, et al. Deleterious role of hyperthermia in neurocritical care. Ann Fr Anesth Reanim. 2009;28(4):345–51.

Dearden NM, Gibson JS, et al. Effect of high-dose dexamethasone on outcome from severe head injury. J Neurosurg. 1986;64:81–8.

Giannotti SL, Weiss MH, et al. High dose glucocorticosteroids in the management of severe head injury. Neurosurgery. 1984;15:497–501.

Ginsbury MD, Busto R. Combating hyperthermia in acute stroke: a significant clinical concern. Stroke. 2003;34(1):5–6.

Grände PO. The "Lund concept" for the treatment of severe head trauma– physiological principles and clinical applications. Intensive Care Med. 2006;32:1475–84.

Huijben JA, et al. Variation in general supportive and preventive intensive care management of traumatic brain injury: a survey in 66 neurotrauma centers participating in the Collaborative European NeuroTrauma Effectiveness Research in Traumatic Brain injury (CNETER-TBI) study. Crit Care. 2018;22(1):90.

Jeremitsky E, Omert LA, et al. The impact of hyperglycaemia on patients with severe head injury. J Trauma. 2005;58:47–50.

Kamano S. Are steroids really ineffective for severely head injured patients? Neurosurg Focus. 2000;8(1):Article 7.

Laird AM, Miller PR. Relationship of early hyperglycaemia to mortality in trauma patients. J Trauma. 2004;56(5):1058–60.

Papadopoulos MC, Saadoun S, et al. Molecular mechanisms of brain tumour edema. Neuroscience. 2004;129:1011–20.

Rabinstein AA. Treatment of brain edema. Neurologist. 2006;12:59–73.

Raslan A, Bhardwaj A. Medical management of cerebral edema. Neurosurg Focus. 2007;22(5):E12: 1–E12:9.

Roberts I, Yates D, et al. Effect of intravenous corticosteroids on death within 14 days in 10008 adults with clinically significant head injury (MRS CRASH-trial). Lancet. 2004;364:1321–8.

Rovlias A, Kotsou S. The influence of hyperglycaemia on neurological outcome in patients with severe head injury. Neurosurgery. 2000;46:335–43.

Salim A, Hadjizachoria A, et al. Persistent hyperglycaemia in severe traumatic brain injury; an independent predictor of outcome. Am Surg. 2009;75(1):25.

Sinha S, Bastin ME, et al. Effect of dexamethasone on peritumoural oedematous brain: a DT-MRI study. J Neurol Neurosurg Psychiatry. 2004;75:1632–5.

Yag B, Ott L, et al. Relationship between admission hyperglycaemia and neurologic outcome of severely brain injured patients. Ann Surg. 1989;210(4):466–72.

Management of Acute Psychiatric Problems

74

Arne Einar Vaaler

Recommendations

Level I

There are insufficient data to support a Level 1 recommendation for this topic.

Level II

There are insufficient data to support a Level 2 recommendation for this topic.

Level III

Patients with recent TBI are in acute life crises often complicated by substance abuse, polypharmacy, challenging behavior, and multiple psychiatric and somatic conditions. Single clinical factors or combinations may induce or increase symptoms and disruptive behavior. Clinical decisions have to be made in spite of limited control of possible risk factors. Benzodiazepines and mood-stabilizing antiepileptics are safe and effective options in numerous clinical situations. Antipsychotics should be used with caution.

Tips, Tricks, and Pitfalls

- Target the agitation in the emergency situation.
- Benzodiazepines are always effective and safe with the exceptions of ongoing alcohol intoxication or severe respiratory problems.
- Mood-stabilizing antiepileptics (e.g., valproate or carbamazepine) are effective as add-on in numerous situations.
- Antipsychotics are used worldwide. However, they have side effects that may increase the agitation.
- Patients with TBI are especially more prone to side effects from antipsychotics.
- If an antipsychotic is used, choose low-dose second-generation (quetiapine, olanzapine).
- Treat abstinence from opiates and nicotine.
- Some patients are extremely agitated due to a combination of causes. Sometimes general anesthesia with barbiturates, propofol, or medical GHB is wise.

A. E. Vaaler (✉)
Department of Mental Health, Norwegian University of Science and Technology (NTNU), Trondheim, Norway
e-mail: arne.einar.vaaler@stolav.no, arne.e.vaaler@ntnu.no

© Springer Nature Switzerland AG 2020
T. Sundstrøm et al. (eds.), *Management of Severe Traumatic Brain Injury*,
https://doi.org/10.1007/978-3-030-39383-0_74

74.1 Background

There is a lack of scientific evidence, handbooks, and guidelines in the pharmacological, emergency treatment of patients with neuropsychiatric disorders following a traumatic brain injury (TBI) (Plantier et al. 2016). The patients have not received sufficient attention in RCTs.

In psychiatric emergency services, a similar lack of scientific evidence is compensated for by "expert consensus guidelines" (Allen et al. 2005) with principles of treatment based on "first do no harm." The guidelines indicate alternatives for psychoactive medications having both positive effects in numerous clinical situations and minimal potential to increase the acute, clinical challenges (Allen et al. 2005; Garriga et al. 2016). The present overview is based on these principles adapted to the emergency patients with acute TBI. The prime focus is on the treatment in intensive care the first days after the trauma and not on the long-term psychopharmacological treatment and rehabilitation. A guideline for the long-term pharmacological treatment of neuropsychiatric disorders after TBI has recently been published (Plantier et al. 2016).

When patients wake up in the intensive care after any TBI, the psychiatric symptoms, function, and behavior are consequences of both the recent injury, and the medical history and behaviors often years prior to the event. The challenges in treatment and care are comparable to the multitude of problems presenting to psychiatric acute and emergency services. The patients are in acute life crises complicated by substance abuse, polypharmacy, challenging behavior, and multiple psychiatric and somatic conditions (Zealberg and Brady 1999). Single clinical factors or combinations may induce or increase symptoms and disruptive behavior. The clinicians may face complex and dynamic situations with limited knowledge of the background, lack of cooperation from the patient, and possibilities of fast deterioration with increasing behavioral problems. Clinical decisions have to be made in spite of limited control of possible risk factors. Immediate interventions or lack of such may both have adverse effects, and even reasonable treatment options may leave the patient feeling traumatized and angered.

Table 74.1 Ten domains of de-escalation

1. Respect personal space
2. Do not be provocative
3. Establish verbal contact
4. Be concise
5. Identify wants and feelings
6. Listen closely to what the patient is saying
7. Agree or agree to disagree
8. Lay down the law and set clear limits
9. Offer choices and optimism
10. Debrief the patient and staff

From Fiskind. "Calming agitation with words not drugs – 10 commandments for safety." Current Psych 2002; 1(4) Reprinted with permission from Current Psychiatry/ Frontline Medical Communications. *All rights reserved*

74.2 Problematic Behavior

Agitation, a state of extreme arousal, physical restlessness, hypervigilance, or of heightened irritability, can be seen in numerous clinical situations. Agitation predicts imminent violent behavior towards oneself or others (Hankin et al. 2011; McClure et al. 2015). Escalation from anxiety to agitation and violent behavior is unpredictable, and violent behavior often occurs without warning signs (Hankin et al. 2011). The priority in intensive care units is to decrease the agitation in order to prevent further deterioration and aggressive incidents. A therapeutic ward attitude towards the patients based on the principles of de-escalation ("talking down") is reassuring for many (Table 74.1) (Fiskind 2002; Richmond et al. 2012).

74.3 Etiology of Agitated, Problematic Behavior

Agitation may be due to any general medical condition causing brain dysfunction, substance abuse, a primary psychiatric disorder, the recent TBI, or a combination of multiple factors (Table

Table 74.2 Medical and psychiatric conditions that may cause agitation

Agitation from general medical condition
• Head trauma
• Encephalitis, meningitis, or other infection
• Encephalopathy (particularly from liver or renal failure)
• Exposure to environmental toxins
• Metabolic derangement (e.g., hyponatremia, hypocalcemia, hypoglycemia)
• Hypoxia
• Thyroid disease
• Seizure (postictal)
• Toxic levels of medication (e.g., psychiatric or anticonvulsant)
Agitation from intoxication/withdrawal
• Alcohol
• Other drugs (cocaine, ecstasy, ketamine, bath salts, inhalants, methamphetamines)
Agitation from psychiatric disorder
• Psychotic disorder
• Manic and mixed states
• Agitated depression
• Anxiety disorder
• Personality disorder
• Reactive or situational agitation (adaptive disorder)
• Autism spectrum disorder
Undifferentiated agitation
(Presumed to be from a general medical condition until proved otherwise)

From Garriga et al. "Assessment and management of agitation in psychiatry: Expert consensus." The world journal of biological psychiatry 2016; 17
Reprinted with permission from Eduard Vieta (corresponding author) and Siegfried Kasper (chief editor). All rights reserved

74.2) (Garriga et al. 2016; Battaglia 2005). Substance abuse is very frequent prior to TBI. The longer time from the trauma to the clinical evaluation, the higher the probability of abstinence. Complicating conditions like seizures, infections, and hypoxia tend to increase the agitation. Prior long-term use of psychoactive medications like antidepressants (AD), antipsychotics (AP), or benzodiazepines (BNZ) may increase the agitation as an effect of the sudden discontinuation.

Usually the clinician will have some clues about the factors that fuel the agitation. These factors have to be targeted immediately. However, sometimes anti-agitation treatment must be started without knowledge about possible trigger factors for the agitation.

74.4 Comorbid Substance Abuse

Agitation related to substance abuse may be due to acute intoxication, abstinence, and/or long-term sequela causing organic brain dysfunction. It is very frequent in emergency settings. A Norwegian study found traces of multiple substances in nearly 50% of patients admitted to psychiatric inpatient care with 15% showing positive screens for amphetamines (Mordal et al. 2010). Methamphetamine (MA) is the dominating amphetamine. MA abuse induces excessive neurotoxicity, and 40% of the users exhibit global neuropsychological impairment (Panenka et al. 2013). This suggests that a number of patients with recent TBI have neurocognitive dysfunctions also prior to the event.

The most frequent substance is alcohol. Frequently used substances are also cannabinoids, stimulants, new psychoactive substances (NPS), gamma hydroxybutyrate (GHB), and opioids. In intensive care, it is possible only to have a very limited overview of possible compounds. More than a thousand new, different substances have been described only in the last 10 years.

Acute intoxications are usually not in need of specific treatment. In polysubstance abuse, intoxication and abstinence may be present simultaneously. Symptoms and behaviors due to abstinence are usually the acute, therapeutic challenge. Immediate treatment is vital to prevent deterioration into delirious conditions and increased harm. Most somatic disorders, infections, and trauma increase the possibility of development into delirium.

"The expert consensus guidelines" for psychiatric emergency services generally recommend BNZ as first-line treatment of abstinence in most situations with a known substance, all situations with an unknown agent, and in clinical situations with abstinence after use of multiple substances. The exceptions are patients still in acute intoxication from alcohol, or patients with chronic, severe respiratory disorders.

BNZ are standard treatment of abstinence from alcohol in most countries. BNZ are also safe first-line options in abstinence from stimulants, hallucinogens, new psychoactive substances, and GHB.

Substances may have specific effects on cardiac function (hallucinogens, opioids), induce seizures (cocaine), or increase extrapyramidal side effects (EPS) when used together with AP (stimulants) (van Harten et al. 1998; Toce et al. 2018). In addition of being an immediate hazard to the somatic health, these "side-effects" from the substances may increase the agitation and the challenging behavior. AP may induce acute EPS, prolong the QTc, and lower the seizure threshold, thus further enhancing these hazards. Reservation in the use of AP is wise. If an AP should be used in this clinical situation, the indication is add-on to further reduce agitation after other anti-agitation medications have been started. Low-dose second-generation AP should be preferred before a first-generation.

The effects of BNZ can be increased by adding a mood-stabilizing antiepileptic like valproic acid or carbamazepine. These compounds will decrease the agitation, have mood-stabilizing properties, prevent paroxysmal cerebral hyperactivity and seizures, and reduce effects of antipsychotic or antidepressant rebound. The immediate effect of valproic acid can be increased by using loading doses. This means starting with a high dose (20–30 mg/kg/day. i.v./p.o.) and gradually decreasing it after a few days.

Sometimes substance-related conditions induce medical emergencies with extreme agitation, confusion, psychosis, hypertension, and rhabdomyolysis. One example is withdrawal from "around-the-clock" use of GHB and related compounds. Even very high doses of BNZ may not be sufficient indicating the use of barbiturates, propofol, or pharmaceutical GHB (van Noorden et al. 2015).

People living a life dominated by polysubstance abuse, personality disorders, and lack of social structure are at risk of violence both as perpetrators and as victims. These patients pose a special challenge in emergency settings when having a TBI of any kind. However, also these patients usually accept BNZ and valproic acid. Adding a transdermal opioid will be helpful for the frequent opioid abstinence. Almost all of them are smokers making it wise also to add nicotine replacement in some form (Allen et al. 2011).

74.5 Organic Brain Disorders

A number of acute organic brain disorders and dysfunctions are associated with sudden behavioral changes dominated by polymorphous psychiatric symptoms, agitation, and risk of violent behavior. The conditions are often induced by paroxysmal cerebral hyperactivity, including epileptic seizures. After TBI, these conditions may be an effect of the recent trauma, sequela from past trauma, or abstinence from abuse of alcohol, psychoactive drugs, or substances prior to the trauma (Vaaler et al. 2010; Boutros et al. 2015). Immediate medication may be needed before an exact diagnosis can be established. Psychotropic medications lowering the seizure threshold may increase the cerebral hyperactivity. AP should thus be used with caution. The principles of "first do no harm" suggest raising the seizure threshold with BNZ and fast-acting, mood-stabilizing antiepileptics (Allen et al. 2005; Riss et al. 2008). Valproic acid loading is usually safe and effective. BNZ is also an effective alternative both in monotherapy and as an add-on medication.

74.6 Affective Disorders, Depression, and Suicide

Patients suffering from depressive episodes dominated by agitation, panic, and desperation pose a special risk for imminent suicidal acts (McClure et al. 2015; Popovic et al. 2015). When admitted to the emergency department after suicide attempts, AD and especially SSRIs (selective serotonin reuptake inhibitors) and SNRIs (serotonin-norepinephrine reuptake inhibitors) must be discontinued due their potential to increase agitation and suicidal intention. If high-dose AD has been used for more than 1–2 moths, the patient may suffer a discontinuation reaction (AD rebound) which also have anxiety and agitation as core symptoms. In such cases continuing small-dose AD for a few weeks is wise. Valproic acid may be helpful for AD rebound as well as having effects on the affective disorder, mood-stabilizing properties, and effects on the frequent comorbid substance-related disorders.

Even though these patients suffer from depressive episodes, the prime target for treatment is not "the depression" with the class of drugs called AD. The anxiety, panic, desperation, and major sleep problems are all symptoms secondary to the depressive episode. These are the symptoms fueling the agitation and thus the prime targets in the pharmacological treatment. BNZ and mood-stabilizing antiepileptics are the drugs of choice. However, AP in the form of low-dose quetiapine (50–100 mg) or olanzapine (5–10 mg) may be helpful in inducing sleep even though this is off-label use.

74.7 Psychoses

In the emergency setting, psychotic symptoms may be present in a number of conditions like affective disorders and depressions, abstinence from substances and medication, paroxysmal cerebral hyperactivity, delirium, or schizophrenia. The presence of psychosis does not primarily indicate the use of AP. Anxiety secondary to delusions and hallucinations fuels the agitation. Thus, addressing the agitation is the prime priority also when psychotic symptoms are present.

In patients with known psychiatric disorders (schizophrenia, bipolar 1 disorder), there is an increased indication for use of low-dose AP. Second-generation AP are preferred over first-generation. If the patient cannot cooperate with peroral medication, intramuscular olanzapine is an alternative. BNZ has an effect on the agitation as well as an additive antipsychotic effect to the AP (Wilson et al. 2012).

74.8 Delirium

Fluctuating symptoms dominated by a rapid onset, clouding of consciousness, altered level of awareness, and problems with directing, focusing, sustaining, and shifting attention indicate delirium (Stowell et al. 2012). Agitation and psychosis are frequently associated with the condition. Delirium indicates an ongoing medical disorder affecting brain function, or a rapid change in the established environment of the brain. The latter may take part with a sudden withdrawal from a chronically ingested agent like alcohol or medication, or a recent ingestion of a drug like an anticholinergic in an elderly person (Wilson et al. 2012). In medical conditions causing delirium (e.g., hypoxia, electrolyte imbalance, hypoglycemia), a correction of the cause usually also reduces the agitation.

BNZ is the drug of choice in delirious conditions complicated by agitation. In the elderly patient a more cautious use of BNZ may be indicated. Second-generation antipsychotics in low doses are an alternative both in monotherapy and as add-on.

74.9 Catatonia

Patients with symptoms of catatonia are admitted to intensive care due to clinical presentations of stupor (Jaimes-Albornoz and Serra-Mestres 2012). Catatonia may be caused by numerous neurological, medical, pharmacological, and psychiatric conditions. It can also be a syndrome secondary to TBI. The symptoms are highly polymorphous but dominated by motor, affective, autonomous, and behavioral signs. It may present as a retarded-stuporous or an exited variety. Both forms may present in a patient at different times during the same episode of the illness.

Catatonia may develop into a life-threatening form called lethal or malignant catatonia with autonomous symptoms like hyperthermia, tachycardia, hypertension, thromboembolism, diaphoresis, and alternating excitement and stupor. Malignant catatonia may be secondary to a variety of general medical or psychiatric causes, or a complication to antidopaminergic (neuroleptic malignant syndrome) (NMS) (Strawn et al. 2007) or serotonergic compounds (serotonergic syndrome).

BNZ and especially lorazepam are the drug of choice for catatonia. AP should be avoided at least in the acute phase. Electroconvulsive therapy (ECT) may be life-saving for patients unresponsive to lorazepam (Zisselman and Jaffe 2010).

74.10 Agitation from Unknown or Possibly Multiple Factors

If agitation has to be managed immediately in the emergency department, BNZ is the drug of choice as first-line treatment. An antiepileptic mood stabilizer is generally safe as add-on.

74.11 The Different Classes of Drugs in Agitation

74.11.1 First-Generation AP (FGA)

FGA (e.g., haloperidol and zuclopenthixol) inhibit dopaminergic transmission in the brain giving a relatively immediate anti-agitation effect. Due to its long tradition, haloperidol is probably still the most used drug for the purpose worldwide. Parenteral haloperidol has an effect on agitation after 30 min lasting up to 24 h. The side-effects causing behavioral problems are EPS including dystonia, akathisia, and Parkinson-like symptoms. Dystonia and akathisia may be extensive and painful, increasing the discomfort and agitation. All FGA have potentials to induce cardiac arrhythmias, lowering the seizure threshold, and induce symptoms of catatonia including NMS (Battaglia 2005).

74.11.2 Second-Generation AP (SGA)

The SGA or "atypical antipsychotics" (e.g., risperidone and olanzapine) are combined serotonin/dopamine antagonists. The pharmacological profile and thus the side-effect profile are different between the SGA. The SGA generally have comparable effects on agitation as FGA. The advantage of some SGA is the reduced risk of imminent EPS (dystonia and akathisia) (Battaglia 2005; Wilson et al. 2012). This is especially apparent for olanzapine and quetiapine. However, risperidone has a relatively high frequency of EPS, especially in elevated doses.

SGA may also induce cardiac arrhythmias. A special caution is warranted for ziprasidone. SGA also lower the seizure threshold, however, probably not in the same extent as FGA.

There are studies indicating a general caution when using AP after TBI due to a possible increased risk of cognitive side effects, as well as an increased risk of developing NMS (Plantier et al. 2016). AP have been used in this clinical situation for many years. This indicates that AP is effective as an anti-agitation medication. However, in the emergency department after a TBI, AP may give rise to more problems than they solve. If a patient wakes up from anesthesia and suddenly experiences EPS, this will induce immediate anxiety, agitation, and anger. Thus a general rule is to use non-pharmacological approaches or use alternatives to AP in patients with TBI (Plantier et al. 2016).

74.11.3 BNZ

BNZ are safe, well tolerated, and accepted by the patients in most clinical emergency situations (Starcevic 2014). The few exceptions are patients in acute alcohol intoxication or patients with an underlying severe respiratory condition. BNZ are as effective as haloperidol in calming agitation in most clinical situations. Most studies have been conducted with lorazepam. It can be given orally, intramuscularly, or intravenously in increments of 1–2 mg (Battaglia 2005).

74.11.4 Other Groups of Drugs

Fast-acting mood-stabilizing antiepileptics (e.g., valproate, carbamazepine, and oxcarbamazepine) have anti-agitation effects in a number of clinical situations. They can be used in monotherapy or as add-on to BNZ and/or AP.

Transdermal opioids and nicotine replacement have documented effects in the emergency populations.

Clonidine has a documented, rapid effect in suppressing symptoms of opiate abstinence (Toce et al. 2018). Clonidine is also used in akathisia induced by AP and insomnia induced by stimulants. However, data from populations of patients in intensive care is lacking.

References

Allen MH, Currier GW, Carpenter D, Ross RW, Docherty JP, E. Expert Consensus Panel for Behavioral. The expert consensus guideline series. Treatment of behavioral emergencies 2005. J Psychiatr Pract. 2005;11(Suppl 1):5–108; quiz 110–102.

Allen MH, Debanne M, Lazignac C, Adam E, Dickinson LM, Damsa C. Effect of nicotine replacement therapy on agitation in smokers with schizophrenia: a double-blind, randomized, placebo-controlled study. Am J Psychiatry. 2011;168(4):395–9.

Battaglia J. Pharmacological management of acute agitation. Drugs. 2005;65(9):1207–22.

Boutros NN, Bowyer S, Wang J, Urfy MZ, Loeb JA. Epilepsy spectrum disorders: a concept in need of validation or refutation. Med Hypotheses. 2015;85(5):656–63.

Fiskind A. Calming agitation with words not drugs: 10 commandments for safety. Curr Psychiatry. 2002;1(4):32–9.

Garriga M, Pacchiarotti I, Kasper S, Zeller SL, Allen MH, Vazquez G, Baldacara L, San L, McAllister-Williams RH, Fountoulakis KN, Courtet P, Naber D, Chan EW, Fagiolini A, Moller HJ, Grunze H, Llorca PM, Jaffe RL, Yatham LN, Hidalgo-Mazzei D, Passamar M, Messer T, Bernardo M, Vieta E. Assessment and management of agitation in psychiatry: expert consensus. World J Biol Psychiatry. 2016;17(2):86–128.

Hankin CS, Bronstone A, Koran LM. Agitation in the inpatient psychiatric setting: a review of clinical presentation, burden, and treatment. J Psychiatr Pract. 2011;17(3):170–85.

Jaimes-Albornoz W, Serra-Mestres J. Catatonia in the emergency department. Emerg Med J. 2012;29(11):863–7.

McClure JR, Criqui MH, Macera CA, Ji M, Nievergelt CM, Zisook S. Prevalence of suicidal ideation and other suicide warning signs in veterans attending an urgent care psychiatric clinic. Compr Psychiatry. 2015;60:149–55.

Mordal J, Holm B, Morland J, Bramness JG. Recent substance intake among patients admitted to acute psychiatric wards: physician's assessment and on-site urine testing compared with comprehensive laboratory analyses. J Clin Psychopharmacol. 2010;30(4):455–9.

Panenka WJ, Procyshyn RM, Lecomte T, MacEwan GW, Flynn SW, Honer WG, Barr AM. Methamphetamine use: a comprehensive review of molecular, preclinical and clinical findings. Drug Alcohol Depend. 2013;129(3):167–79.

Plantier D, Luaute J, S. group. Drugs for behavior disorders after traumatic brain injury: systematic review and expert consensus leading to French recommendations for good practice. Ann Phys Rehabil Med. 2016;59(1):42–57.

Popovic D, Vieta E, Azorin JM, Angst J, Bowden CL, Mosolov S, Young AH, Perugi G. Suicide attempts in major depressive episode: evidence from the BRIDGE-II-Mix study. Bipolar Disord. 2015;17(7):795–803.

Richmond JS, Berlin JS, Fishkind AB, Holloman GH Jr, Zeller SL, Wilson MP, Rifai MA, Ng AT. Verbal de-escalation of the agitated patient: consensus statement of the American Association for Emergency Psychiatry Project BETA De-escalation Workgroup. West J Emerg Med. 2012;13(1):17–25.

Riss J, Cloyd J, Gates J, Collins S. Benzodiazepines in epilepsy: pharmacology and pharmacokinetics. Acta Neurol Scand. 2008;118(2):69–86.

Starcevic V. The reappraisal of benzodiazepines in the treatment of anxiety and related disorders. Expert Rev Neurother. 2014;14(11):1275–86.

Stowell KR, Florence P, Harman HJ, Glick RL. Psychiatric evaluation of the agitated patient: consensus statement of the American Association for Emergency Psychiatry Project Beta Psychiatric Evaluation Workgroup. West J Emerg Med. 2012;13(1):11–6.

Strawn JR, Keck PE Jr, Caroff SN. Neuroleptic malignant syndrome. Am J Psychiatry. 2007;164(6):870–6.

Toce MS, Chai PR, Burns MM, Boyer EW. Pharmacologic treatment of opioid use disorder: a review of pharmacotherapy, adjuncts, and toxicity. J Med Toxicol. 2018;14(4):306–22.

Vaaler AE, Morken G, Iversen VC, Kondziella D, Linaker OM. Acute Unstable Depressive Syndrome (AUDS) is associated more frequently with epilepsy than major depression. BMC Neurol. 2010;10:67.

van Harten PN, van Trier JC, Horwitz EH, Matroos GE, Hoek HW. Cocaine as a risk factor for neuroleptic-induced acute dystonia. J Clin Psychiatry. 1998;59(3):128–30.

van Noorden MS, Kamal RM, Dijkstra BA, Mauritz R, de Jong CA. A case series of pharmaceutical gamma-hydroxybutyrate in 3 patients with severe benzodiazepine-resistant gamma-hydroxybutyrate withdrawal in the hospital. Psychosomatics. 2015;56(4):404–9.

Wilson MP, Pepper D, Currier GW, Holloman GH Jr, Feifel D. The psychopharmacology of agitation: consensus statement of the American Association for Emergency Psychiatry Project Beta Psychopharmacology Workgroup. West J Emerg Med. 2012;13(1):26–34.

Zealberg JJ, Brady KT. Substance abuse and emergency psychiatry. Psychiatr Clin North Am. 1999;22(4):803–17.

Zisselman MH, Jaffe RL. ECT in the treatment of a patient with catatonia: consent and complications. Am J Psychiatry. 2010;167(2):127–32.

Part IX

Rehabilitation and Follow-Up

Olli Tenovuo

Rehabilitation After Severe TBI

75

Nada Andelic, Solrun Sigurdardottir, and Olli Tenovuo

Tips, Tricks, and Pitfalls

- Prevention of secondary insults due to autonomic dysfunction, upper airway dysfunction/dysphagia, severe endocrine disturbances and detection and treatment of nonconvulsive seizures will improve the final outcome (tertiary prevention).
- It is imperative to develop rehabilitation programs at the neurointensive care that are able to encounter adverse reactions to the primary injury (detect and treat secondary and tertiary injury).
- During the recovery phase after end of sedation, patients often present with severe hypertension, tachycardia, spontaneous hyperventilation, fever and profuse sweating, and excessive amount of salivation. These symptoms are often misdiagnosed and consequently given the wrong treatment. The patient is returned to sedation, artificially ventilated, and given antibiotic treatment. In many cases, these symptoms are due to autonomic dysfunction and they should be treated accordingly.

N. Andelic
Department of Physical Medicine and Rehabilitation, Oslo University Hospital Ullevål, Oslo, Norway

Research Centre for Habilitation and Rehabilitation Models and Services, Faculty of Medicine, Institute of Health and Society, University of Oslo, Oslo, Norway
e-mail: nadand@ous-hf.no

S. Sigurdardottir
Department of Research, Sunnaas Rehabilitation Hospital, Bjørnemyr, Norway
e-mail: solrun.sigurdardottir@sunnaas.no

O. Tenovuo (✉)
Department of Clinical Medicine, Turku Brain Injury Centre, Turku University Hospital, University of Turku, Turku, Finland

75.1 Overview

Rehabilitation for severe TBI should begin as early after injury as possible (Andelic et al. 2012). Growing evidence supports the effectiveness of intensive rehabilitation once the patient is medically stable (Turner-Stokes et al. 2015). Internationally, cognitive rehabilitation is provided in 95% of rehabilitation facilities serving the patients with TBI, including combinations of individual, group, and community-based therapies (Cicerone et al. 2000). A systematic review (Cicerone et al. 2011) suggested that comprehensive holistic neuropsychological rehabilitation is able to improve functional

© Springer Nature Switzerland AG 2020
T. Sundstrøm et al. (eds.), *Management of Severe Traumatic Brain Injury*,
https://doi.org/10.1007/978-3-030-39383-0_75

independence, community integration, and productivity, even years after the injury. A holistic approach is also considered as a treatment standard for patients with behavioral and psychological disorders following acquired brain injuries (Cattelani et al. 2010). Inclusion of family members during the rehabilitation process is important and their needs should be addressed (Norup et al. 2015).

75.2 Definition of Rehabilitation

World Health Organization (WHO) defines rehabilitation as "a set of measures that assist individuals, who experience or are likely to experience disability, to achieve and maintain optimum functioning in interaction with their environments" (World Health Organization 2001). Consequently, rehabilitation reduces the impact of a broad range of health conditions, including neurological diseases and brain injuries. In contrast to other medical specialties, which focus on prevention and treatment of disease, rehabilitation focuses on the improvement in physical and cognitive functioning and independence. During the last decades rehabilitation outcomes have been extended to include not only levels of impairment, but also domains of activity and participation and a quality of life. Severe TBI causes physical and mental impairments, as well as problems in speech, movement, sensation, and self-care. However, behavioral, cognitive, and emotional impairments are often the most important barriers to successful community reintegration and require detailed, coordinated assessment and a comprehensive holistic rehabilitation approach to achieve the best outcomes.

The International Classification of Functioning, Disability, and Health (ICF) provides a framework that can be used for all aspects of rehabilitation. The ICF views health conditions from biological, personal, and social (bio-psycho-social) perspectives and targets body functions and structure, activity and participation, environmental factors, and personal factors (World Health Organization 2001). Using the ICF model is the key in identifying the rehabilitation needs and designing effective rehabilitation interventions for patients with severe TBI (Scarponi et al. 2009). To make the ICF practical for everyday use, the comprehensive and brief ICF Core Sets have been developed in order to describe the functional profile of patients with TBI (see Table 75.1). The comprehensive ICF Core Sets reflect the entire spectrum of typical problems that a patient with TBI may face, and can serve as a checklist to guide the multidisci-

Table 75.1 Brief **ICF Core Sets** for traumatic brain

ICF code	ICF category title
Body functions	
b164	Higher-level cognitive functions
b152	Emotional functions
b130	Energy and drive functions
b760	Control of voluntary movement functions
b144	Memory functions
b280	Sensation of pain
b140	Attention functions
b110	Consciousness functions
Body structures	
s110	Structure of brain
Activities and participation	
d230	Carrying out daily routine
d350	Conversation
d450	Walking
d720	Complex interpersonal interactions
d845	Acquiring, keeping, and terminating a job
d5	Self-care
d920	Recreation and leisure
d760	Family relationships
Environment factors	
e310	Immediate family
e580	Health services, systems, and policies
e115	Products and technology for personal use in daily living
e320	Friends
e570	Social security services, systems, and policies
e120	Products and technology for personal indoor and outdoor mobility and transportation

https://www.icf-research-branch.org/icf-core-sets-projects2/neurological-conditions/development-of-icf-core-sets-for-traumatic-brain-injury-tbi plinary assessment of functioning. The brief ICF Core Sets capture the essence of patient's functioning and disability and is used when a brief assessment is necessary, for example, in single-discipline settings or in primary care.

Neurorehabilitation is usually provided by multidisciplinary teams, which include two or more of the following disciplines working in a coordinated effort: a physiatrist or physician with specialized training in TBI rehabilitation, neuropsychologist, rehabilitation nurse, psychologist, physical therapist, occupational therapist, social worker, speech therapist, psychiatrist, and eventually pharmacologist. The rehabilitation team is working with the patient and his/her family in partnership (person-centered approach). Rehabilitation professionals share a common goal to help individuals with physical and cognitive impairments to function optimally, either by focusing on the impairment itself or the activities affected by the impairment. The working alliance in holistic neuropsychological rehabilitation has been studied in Denmark, indicating that a good working alliance is the basis of successful rehabilitative work (Schonberger et al. 2006).

The available research supports that multidisciplinary neurorehabilitation has a great potential to improve functional recovery after severe TBI, through neuroplasticity and development of compensatory mechanisms (Hylin et al. 2017). Neuroplasticity has been defined as "the ability of the nervous system to respond to intrinsic and extrinsic stimuli by reorganizing its structure, function, and connections" (Cramer et al. 2011). The crucial parameters that can influence the rehabilitation efficiency are timing and intensity of rehabilitative training (Hylin et al. 2017; Konigs et al. 2018). However, the exact time window to introduce rehabilitative training is still unclear. The experimental research suggests that an early onset, but not immediately after the injury, is more beneficial for both structural plasticity and functional recovery (Hylin et al. 2017). In addition, the training intensity may influence both the rate of behavioral changes and neural consequences associated with new learning (Hylin et al. 2017). A Cochrane review (Turner-Stokes et al. 2015) and recently published systematic review and meta-analysis of controlled clinical trials (Konigs et al. 2018) have also suggested that more intensive training, initiated early after the injury, may be the most effective rehabilitation strategy for patients with brain injuries.

75.3 Models of Rehabilitation Services Delivery Following Severe TBI

The continuity and quality of care from early to late phases following TBI should be the main issue involved in the organization of rehabilitation services for patients with TBI. This is a major concern within the rehabilitation field of severe TBI in the Nordic countries (Andelic et al. 2012; Borg et al. 2011; Godbolt et al. 2015; Sorbo et al. 2005). According to Borg et al. (2011), "there is a wealth of data lending support to a clinical management model that integrates neurointensive care and a qualified rehabilitation program and ensures a continuum of care in the early rehabilitation process." This statement is supported by a study of cost-effectiveness of the continuous chain of rehabilitation after severe TBI (Andelic et al. 2014), which indicated that a continuous chain of rehabilitation had lower hospitalization costs and better health outcomes than a broken chain of rehabilitation over a period of 5 years. Growing evidence indicates the effectiveness of early rehabilitation in individuals with severe TBI (Andelic et al. 2012; Sorbo et al. 2005; Engberg et al. 2006). Moreover, medical care has improved greatly for patients with "disorders of consciousness" (Engberg et al. 2006), and this subpopulation has specific rehabilitation needs that should be targeted using neurological, radiological, and neurophysiological assessments (Whyte et al. 2013).

75.4 Acute (Early) Care Rehabilitation

A coordinated rehabilitation already starts during the acute trauma care at ICU after hemodynamic and intracranial pressure (ICP) stabilization of the patient, in the state when he/she is emerging from coma (Konigs et al. 2018). In addition to traditional acute care efforts (i.e., maintaining joint and limb flexibility, bowel and bladder function, skin care, and pulmonary function), rehabilitation focuses on preventing complications and promoting functional recovery through multisensory stimulation. Such interventions are directed at the daily multisensory stimulation, positioning, range of movement exercises, and mobilization (Andelic et al. 2012; Mackay et al. 1992). Early multidisciplinary neurorehabilitation, provided in the trauma center within 2 weeks after injury, increased gains in self-care, mobility, and cognition compared with usual care while also reducing the length of hospital stay (Andelic et al. 2012). Moreover, an early stimulation of visual, auditory, olfactory, tactile, and gustatory modalities, as well as stimulation of sensory modalities using autobiographic stimuli provided by the family members, promotes functional recovery of patients in coma (Abbasi et al. 2009; Moattari et al. 2016).

In the early stage of recovery, extreme agitation is frequently seen during the period of post-traumatic amnesia, with psychotic symptoms incorporated into confusion and inattention (Ponsford et al. 2014a). Neuropsychiatric problems (e.g., psychosis, agitation, aggression, depression, anxiety, and post-traumatic stress disorder) are major barriers for rehabilitation during this phase as well as in the later phases following TBI and should be treated by environmental adaptations in order to keep the patients and caregivers safe. If these efforts are insufficient, pharmacotherapy should be added (Iaccarino et al. 2015).

75.5 Inpatient Post-Acute Rehabilitation

When sufficient medical stability in the acute care has been achieved, more intensive inpatient rehabilitation may be provided at a hospital ward or at a specialized acute or subacute rehabilitation unit. The primary focus is the restoration of lost functional skills. In general, this level of care is for patients who are able to participate and show improvements but are not yet ready to return home after discharge from acute hospital. Comprehensive, inpatient neurorehabilitation aims to reduce impairment; increase physical, cognitive, and psychosocial independence; compensate for disability; and minimize distress of the patient as well as family caregivers. Based on the patient's needs, this may contain physical, cognitive, and behavioral therapies provided by a specialized multidisciplinary team through a goal-oriented rehabilitation plan. There is evidence that more intensive neurorehabilitation in the inpatient rehabilitation facility for at least 20 h per week promotes recovery in global functioning compared to the program at routine intensity (10 h per week) (Zhu et al. 2007). Moreover, intensive multidisciplinary neurorehabilitation with focus on neuropsychological rehabilitation and psychotherapy (>25 h per week) increased the likelihood of better productive status in the long-term perspective (Sarajuuri et al. 2005).

A significant proportion of patients with motor deficits (73%) improve in their physical ability and ambulation during the first 6 months following TBI (Katz et al. 2004). The recovery of motor function after severe TBI is an active process supported by physiotherapy and occupational therapy and aimed at improving strength, endurance, mobility, sitting and standing balance, coordination, walking, as well as independence in daily tasks (i.e., dressing, washing, cooking, and leisure activities). Physical exercises may modulate the motor cortex; for example, it has been reported that the density of the primary motor cortex was increased with more intense exercise, whereas activity of the primary sensory cortex and the prefrontal cortex was not altered with exercise (Brummer et al. 2011). In addition, repetitive task-specific training provided by occupational therapist incorporates motor programming, which is important for accurate timing, speed, coordination, and reconstruction of the whole task (Hubbard et al. 2009). Spasticity can be a particular problem after severe TBI and should be treated in order to avoid muscle contractures and functional limb deficits. A passive stretching, heat and cold, use of orthoses, and positioning are important in order to prevent contractures. A number of studies have demonstrated the efficacy of botulinum toxin in the management of troublesome limb spasticity post-stroke or following TBI (Dong et al. 2017). Communication deficits such as dysarthria and aphasia require assessment and interventions provided by speech therapist in order to improve understanding and expressing written and spoken language and speech clarity. In addition, the speech therapists may assess swallowing difficulties (dysphagia) and provide guidance on how this should be managed safely. Patients with very severe motor, communication, and cognitive deficits may require different assistive devices to reduce disability and promote participation. These may include wheelchairs, mechanical lifts, bracing to maintain positioning, orthoses, walkers and canes, adaptive technologies for communication (from simple pointing boards to more complex preprogrammed artificial voice communicators), and environment controlling devices. Assistive devices should be selected carefully and fitted properly. To minimize a mismatch between the patient's need and the device, a comprehensive assessment of needs and coordination between the patient, rehabilitation team, orthotists, device vendors, and family members, and knowledge of home environment are needed (Iaccarino et al. 2015).

75.6 Outpatient Rehabilitation

Following an inpatient rehabilitation stay, individuals with ongoing disability may need further treatment as an outpatient at variable rehabilitation facilities. Some may receive support from a community-based rehabilitation team/therapist working with the person in his/her home. The main aims are to facilitate continued progress and successful community reintegration (family, social, and work reintegration). In addition to previously mentioned efforts, services may contain vocational rehabilitation, recreational therapy, and psychosocial counseling. First after the discharge from hospital environment, patients and their families may realize the cognitive and behavioral deficits that prevent community integration and alter the family dynamics. Family members have a very important role in helping the patient through the rehabilitation process. The patients who make the best recovery after TBI are those whose families are actively involved in rehabilitation. However, it is important that the family members focus primarily on their role that provides love and affection and not on a "therapist" role.

For many patients, severe TBI becomes a chronic disease, and rehabilitation team members are important sources of support and counseling in the community and vocational reintegration. Cognitive therapy may aim to enhance mental, psychological, and independent functioning; occupational therapy to help patients to manage daily activities and vocational skills; physiotherapy (somatic or relaxation exercises) to regain walking, balance, or physical hobby activities; and speech therapy to help patients to restore speech and communication. As the patient with severe TBI may experience prolonged social isolation due to difficulties to fulfill or resume an accepted social role, the rehabilitation team should also focus on reestablishing of social and recreational activities. Depression and fatigue may frequently influence social participation and should be addressed if needed. Driving can be a difficult issue for patients because it is a highly desired goal. However, relicensing may be considered first 6–12 months after a severe TBI depending on conditions such as cognitive impairment, visual field defects, or seizures that may affect driving safety.

Efforts to evaluate the effectiveness of multidisciplinary rehabilitation in working age adults found evidence that intensive neurorehabilitation in residential settings may improve community integration after severe TBI (Turner-Stokes et al. 2015). In a controlled clinical trial, intensive multidisciplinary outpatient neuropsychological rehabilitation program (5 h per day, 4 days per week) based on the milieu model, with more group-based interventions provided in a therapeutic environment, resulted in greater improvements in community integration, productivity, life satisfaction, and self-efficacy (Cicerone et al. 2008). In a large controlled randomized study of community-based rehabilitation after severe TBI, the interventions were based on individualized goals in collaboration with the patient and the multidisciplinary team, and better outcomes (personal care, community mobility, socializing, employment, psychological well-being) were shown in the treatment group compared to the control group (Powell et al. 2002). Another large study also showed that intensive programs resulted in functional improvements, whereas supported living programs produced stable functioning (Eicher et al. 2012).

The Common Data Element (CDE) recommendations (Hicks et al. 2013) are intended to apply to rehabilitation research conducted within acute hospital, inpatient rehabilitation, and outpatient settings. For adults, the outcome measure recommended as a core recommendation is the Glasgow Outcome Score – Extended (see Table 75.2).

Table 75.2 Core and basic rehabilitation outcome measures based on CDE recommendations for adults with moderate-severe traumatic brain injury (Hicks et al. 2013)

Assessment	Instruments
	Core measure:
	Glasgow Outcome Score—Extended
Neuropsychological functions:	Basic measures:
Memory	Rey Auditory Verbal Learning Test (RAVLT) or California Verbal Learning Test-II (CVLT-II)
Speed of processing	Wechsler Adult Intelligence Scale (WAIS-IV), Processing Speed Index
Attention and mental control	Trail Making Test (TMT)
Psychological status	Brief Symptom Inventory-18 Item (BSI-18)
Quality of life	Satisfaction with Life Scale (SWLS)
Global outcome	Disability Rating Scale (DRS)
Motor and cognitive activity limitations	Functional Independence Measure (FIM): Motor Subscale and Cognition Subscale
Societal participation	Craig Handicap Assessment and Reporting Technique, Short Form (CHART-SF)

75.7 Cognitive Rehabilitation

Cognitive rehabilitation is defined as "a systematic, functionally oriented service of therapeutic activities that is based on the assessment and understanding of the patient's brain-behavioral deficits" (Cicerone et al. 2000). Taking into consideration the frequent cognitive disabilities after severe TBI in, e.g., memory, attention, concentration, and executive functions, neuropsychological assessment is often useful as the first step in cognitive rehabilitation and should be essential part of any rehabilitation program and intervention (Ponsford et al. 2014b). Understanding of the principles and mechanisms of neuroplasticity also holds potential for developing treatments for cognitive deficits after brain injury (Nordvik et al. 2014). The most common sequels of severe TBI are in the areas of cognition, communication, behavioral functioning, and mental health. These deficits vary greatly among individuals with severe TBI and represent a complex system of comorbidities in a single individual. The complexity of disabilities often present challenges in treatment program design and are dependent on many factors beyond those that are used to grade injury severity. Outcomes can thus be very heterogeneous, and clinicians need to rely on the best available evidence to guide clinical practice in TBI. Using the Manual for Cognitive Rehabilitation published by the American Congress of Rehabilitation Medicine (ACRM) can be recommended, but it is not freely available. The set of guidelines by the INCOG group (Bayley et al. 2014) focused on TBI can also be recommended in the clinical practice.

75.8 Cognitive Interventions

Restoration, compensation, and meta-cognition interventions are commonly used approaches in cognitive rehabilitation, used in all phases of recovery and in different settings (e.g., inpatient, outpatient, and community). In the 1970s to 1980s, the restorative approach was impairment-focused with the aim to restore lost function through drill and practice activities, often used in the acute and post-acute phases of recovery. However, restorative interventions are controversial, showing disappointing effect and lack of generalization to real-world tasks. From the 1990s, cognitive rehabilitation started to focus on compensatory strategy training with the aim to lessen the disabling impact of impairment, often with the use of internal and/or external strategies. Compensatory strategies are often used after cognitive recovery has occurred (i.e., 1–2 years post-injury), showing more success (Wilson et al. 2009). Metacognitive strategies are those that foster anticipation and planning, response monitoring, and self-evaluation and can be applied in all phases of cognitive rehabilitation. Rehabilitation programs need to target the level of cognitive dysfunction with certain intensity and should be theoretically based according to principles of cognitive remediation (Sohlberg and Turkstra 2011) as well as promote generalization, incorporating also metacognitive and emotional strategies. Interventions can be applied through technology and compensatory strategies that may allow the individuals with cognitive impairment to more fully participate in their life activities such as work, family life, and society.

Goal Assessment. Setting goals are important in cognitive TBI rehabilitation. It encourages patients to define their own goals and increases their self-awareness as well as engagement to rehabilitation interventions. Identifying goals of treatment allows the rehabilitation to be monitored in a consistent manner. Goals need to be identified by their time frame (short or long term) and rehabilitation setting (inpatient or outpatient). Short-term goals often focus on changes at the level of activity (e.g., ADL) or functioning (e.g., behavioral), while long-term goals are often set at the level of participation (e.g., work). The SMART acronym (specific, measurable, achievable, realistic, and timed) offers a practical means to define goals in a concrete manner (Bovend'Eerdt et al. 2009).

Both the INCOG group guidelines for TBI (Ponsford et al. 2014b; Velikonja et al. 2014) and Cochrane reviews (Cicerone et al. 2000, 2011) have drawn similar conclusions for cognitive interventions for attention, memory, and executive functions:

Attention. For mild-moderate attentional impairment, training with metacognitive strategies applied in everyday life and dual-task training (i.e., each task trained separately and then together) are recommended. For severe attentional impairment, dual-task training and environmental modification is recommended (Cicerone et al. 2011; Ponsford et al. 2014b). However, training on basic tasks of reaction time or focused attention in the acute phase and practice on computerized tasks without intervention by a professional are not recommended.

Memory. For mild-moderate memory impairment, both internal (e.g., visual imagery, repeated practice) and external (i.e., mobile/smartphone, notebook, whiteboard) compensatory devices are recommended. External compensatory devices and errorless learning can benefit persons with severe memory problems, even for those who are many years post-injury (Cicerone et al. 2011; Velikonja et al. 2014).

Executive functions and self-awareness. For patients who are aware of their cognitive deficits, using of metacognitive strategies (e.g., goal setting, goal management training (GMT) (Tornas et al. 2016), problem orientation and problem solving) and their applications in everyday life is recommended (Cicerone et al. 2011; Tate et al. 2014). However, reviews have drawn varying conclusions regarding effective treatment for self-awareness, where the INCOG group supports the use of direct corrective feedback.

75.9 Virtual Reality

Virtual reality (VR) represents a new, 3D synthetic environment created by computer graphics, where the patient interacts with and controls his/her movements within the VR using a joystick or a keyboard. VR allows the development of real-life, context-specific experiences, such as cooking in a virtual kitchen, driving a virtual car, or shopping in a virtual supermarket. In these ecologically valid VR environments, patients can be assessed and trained (cognitive, sensory, motor, and social training) while maintaining experimental control over stimulus measurement and delivery. There is evidence that such training may improve brain plasticity and regenerative processes (Zanier et al. 2018). However, the use of VR in clinical practice is still limited by the accessibility and costs.

75.10 Telerehabilitation

Telerehabilitation involves interventions delivered via telecommunication and the Internet (i.e., video and teleconferencing technologies; mobile phones; telehealth and telemedicine) in order to improve accessibility of healthcare services for patients with disabilities or geographic barriers. There is evidence that telerehabilitation may be equally effective, but not superior to other forms of rehabilitation (Betts et al. 2018). Telerehabilitation may incorporate specific cognitive interventions or educational and training strategies, which may result in positive outcomes (Betts et al. 2018). However, current evidence is limited due to small number of studies, lack of standardized intervention parameters and outcome measures, and larger sample sizes. Further research is needed on resource allocation and costs to guide the decision-makers and clinical practice.

75.11 Future Prospects

There have been increasing efforts at summing up what is the current "scientific knowledge base" within the field of brain injury rehabilitation. Systematic reviews have mostly relied on randomized controlled trials and expert consensus and less on small patient groups reflecting personalized care. Rehabilitation of severe TBI comprises many phases: from emergency and in-hospital acute medical care to admission and post-acute care in a rehabilitation center and to chronic care in the community. It covers the full breadth of medical neuroscience, cognitive neuroscience, pharmacology, brain imaging, and assistive and smart technology. Future challenge is to integrate these areas of expertise to guide TBI rehabilitation into widespread research and clinical practice. The use of smart technologies and new brain imaging has an important future in the rehabilitation of patients with a variety of cognitive difficulties and disabilities. There is also need for international collaboration to establish a research base for practice-based evidence from larger multicenter clinical trials (Bodien et al. 2018; Maas et al. 2017) in order to define the effective service provision and to reach consensus on the best evidence-based practice of TBI rehabilitation.

References

Abbasi M, Mohammadi E, Sheaykh Rezayi A. Effect of a regular family visiting program as an affective, auditory, and tactile stimulation on the consciousness level of comatose patients with a head injury. Japan J Nursing Science. 2009;6:21–6.

Andelic N, Bautz-Holter E, Ronning P, et al. Does an early onset and continuous chain of rehabilitation improve the long-term functional outcome of patients with severe traumatic brain injury? J Neurotrauma. 2012;29:66–74.

Andelic N, Ye J, Tornas S, et al. Cost-effectiveness analysis of an early-initiated, continuous chain of rehabilitation after severe traumatic brain injury. J Neurotrauma. 2014;31:1313–20.

Bayley MT, Tate R, Douglas JM, et al. INCOG guidelines for cognitive rehabilitation following traumatic brain injury: methods and overview. J Head Trauma Rehabil. 2014;29:290–306.

Betts S, Feichter L, Kleinig Z, et al. Telerehabilitation versus standard care for improving cognitive function and quality of life for adults with traumatic brain injury: a systematic review. Internet J Allied Health Sci Pract. 2018;16:article 9.

Bodien YG, McCrea M, Dikmen S, et al. Optimizing outcome assessment in multicenter TBI trials: perspectives from TRACK-TBI and the TBI endpoints development initiative. J Head Trauma Rehabil. 2018;33:147–57.

Borg J, Roe C, Nordenbo A, et al. Trends and challenges in the early rehabilitation of patients with traumatic brain injury: a Scandinavian perspective. Am J Phys Med Rehabil. 2011;90:65–73.

Bovend'Eerdt TJ, Botell RE, Wade DT. Writing SMART rehabilitation goals and achieving goal attainment scaling: a practical guide. Clin Rehabil. 2009;23:352–61.

Brummer V, Schneider S, Struder HK, Askew CD. Primary motor cortex activity is elevated with incremental exercise intensity. Neuroscience. 2011;181:150–62.

Cattelani R, Zettin M, Zoccolotti P. Rehabilitation treatments for adults with behavioral and psychosocial disorders following acquired brain injury: a systematic review. Neuropsy Review. 2010;20:52–85.

Cicerone KD, Dahlberg C, Kalmar K, et al. Evidence-based cognitive rehabilitation: recommendations for clinical practice. Arch Phys Med Rehabil. 2000;81:1596–615.

Cicerone KD, Mott T, Azulay J, et al. A randomized controlled trial of holistic neuropsychologic rehabilitation after traumatic brain injury. Arch Phys Med Rehabil. 2008;89:2239–49.

Cicerone KD, Langenbahn DM, Braden C, et al. Evidence-based cognitive rehabilitation: updated review of the literature from 2003 through 2008. Arch Phys Med Rehabil. 2011;92:519–30.

Cramer SC, Sur M, Dobkin BH, et al. Harnessing neuroplasticity for clinical applications. Brain. 2011;134:1591–609.

Dong Y, Wu T, Hu X, Wang T. Efficacy and safety of botulinum toxin type A for upper limb spasticity after stroke or traumatic brain injury: a systematic review with meta-analysis and trial sequential analysis. Eur J Phys Med Rehab. 2017;53:256–67.

Eicher V, Murphy MP, Murphy TF, Malec JF. Progress assessed with the Mayo-Portland adaptability inventory in 604 participants in 4 types of post-inpatient rehabilitation brain injury programs. Arch Phys Med Rehabil. 2012;93:100–7.

Engberg AW, Liebach A, Nordenbo A. Centralized rehabilitation after severe traumatic brain injury: a population-based study. Acta Neurol Scand. 2006;113:178–84.

Godbolt AK, Stenberg M, Lindgren M, et al. Associations between care pathways and outcome 1 year after severe traumatic brain injury. J Head Trauma Rehabil. 2015;30:E41–51.

Hicks R, Giacino J, Harrison-Felix C, et al. Progress in developing common data elements for traumatic brain injury research: version two-the end of the beginning. J Neurotrauma. 2013;30:1852–61.

Hubbard IJ, Parsons MW, Neilson C, Carey LM. Task-specific training: evidence for and translation to clinical practice. Occup Ther International. 2009;16:175–89.

Hylin MJ, Kerr AL, Holden R. Understanding the mechanisms of recovery and/or compensation following injury. Neural Plast. 2017;2017:7125057.

Iaccarino M, Bhatnagar S, Zafonte R. Rehabilitation after traumatic brain injury. Handb Clin Neurol. 2015;127:411–22.

Katz DI, White DK, Alexander MP, Klein RB. Recovery of ambulation after traumatic brain injury. Arch Phys Med Rehabil. 2004;85:865–9.

Konigs M, Beurskens EA, Snoep L, Scherder EJ, Oosterlaan J. Effects of timing and intensity of neurorehabilitation on functional outcome after traumatic brain injury: a systematic review and meta-analysis. Arch Phys Med Rehabil. 2018;99:1149–59.

Maas AIR, Menon DK, Adelson PD, et al. Traumatic brain injury: integrated approaches to improve prevention, clinical care, and research. Lancet Neurol. 2017;16:987–1048.

Mackay LE, Bernstein BA, Chapman PE, Morgan AS, Milazzo LS. Early intervention in severe head injury: long-term benefits of a formalized program. Arch Phys Med Rehabil. 1992;73:635–41.

Moattari M, Alizadeh Shirazi F, Sharifi N, Zareh N. Effects of a sensory stimulation by nurses and families on level of cognitive function and basic cognitive sensory recovery of comatose patients with severe traumatic brain injury: a randomized control trial. Trauma Mon. 2016;21(4):e23531.

Nordvik JE, Walle KM, Nyberg CK, et al. Bridging the gap between clinical neuroscience and cognitive rehabilitation: the role of cognitive training, models of neuroplasticity and advanced neuroimaging in future brain injury rehabilitation. NeuroRehabilitation. 2014;34:81–5.

Norup A, Perrin PB, Cuberos-Urbano G, et al. Family needs after brain injury: a cross cultural study. NeuroRehabilitation. 2015;36:203–14.

Ponsford J, Janzen S, McIntyre A, et al. INCOG recommendations for management of cognition following traumatic brain injury, part I: posttraumatic amnesia/delirium. J Head Trauma Rehabil. 2014a;29:307–20.

Ponsford J, Bayley M, Wiseman-Hakes C, et al. INCOG recommendations for management of cognition following traumatic brain injury, part II: attention and information processing speed. J Head Trauma Rehabil. 2014b;29:321–37.

Powell J, Heslin J, Greenwood R. Community based rehabilitation after severe traumatic brain injury: a randomised controlled trial. J Neurol Neurosurg Psychiatry. 2002;72:193–202.

Sarajuuri JM, Kaipio ML, Koskinen SK, Niemela MR, Servo AR, Vilkki JS. Outcome of a comprehensive neurorehabilitation program for patients with traumatic brain injury. Arch Phys Med Rehabil. 2005;86:2296–302.

Scarponi F, Sattin D, Leonardi M, Raggi A, Zampolini M. The description of severe traumatic brain injury in light of the ICF classification. Disability Rehab. 2009;31:S134–43.

Schonberger M, Humle F, Teasdale TW. The development of the therapeutic working alliance, patients' awareness and their compliance during the process of brain injury rehabilitation. Brain Inj. 2006;20:445–54.

Sohlberg MM, Turkstra LS. Optimizing cognitive rehabilitation. Effective instructional methods. New York: The Guilford Press; 2011.

Sorbo A, Rydenhag B, Sunnerhagen KS, Blomqvist M, Svensson S, Emanuelson I. Outcome after severe brain damage, what makes the difference? Brain Inj. 2005;19:493–503.

Tate R, Kennedy M, Ponsford J, et al. INCOG recommendations for management of cognition following traumatic brain injury, part III: executive function and self-awareness. J Head Trauma Rehabil. 2014;29:338–52.

Tornas S, Lovstad M, Solbakk AK, et al. Rehabilitation of executive functions in patients with chronic acquired brain injury with goal management training, external cuing, and emotional regulation: a randomized controlled trial. J Int Neuropsychol Soc. 2016;22:436–52.

Turner-Stokes L, Pick A, Nair A, Disler PB, Wade DT. Multi-disciplinary rehabilitation for acquired brain injury in adults of working age. Cochrane Database Syst Rev. 2015;12:CD004170.

Velikonja D, Tate R, Ponsford J, et al. INCOG recommendations for management of cognition following traumatic brain injury, part V: memory. J Head Trauma Rehabil. 2014;29:369–86.

Whyte J, Nordenbo AM, Kalmar K, et al. Medical complications during inpatient rehabilitation among patients with traumatic disorders of consciousness. Arch Phys Med Rehabil. 2013;94:1877–83.

Wilson BA, Gracey F, Evans JJ, Bateman A. Neuropsychological rehabilitation theory, models, therapy and outcome. New York: Cambridge University Press; 2009.

World Health Organization. The international classification of functioning, disability and health-ICF. Geneva: World Health Organization; 2001.

Zanier ER, Zoerle T, Di Lernia D, Riva G. Virtual reality for traumatic brain injury. Front Neurol. 2018;9:345.

Zhu XL, Poon WS, Chan CC, Chan SS. Does intensive rehabilitation improve the functional outcome of patients with traumatic brain injury (TBI)? A randomized controlled trial. Brain Inj. 2007;21:681–90.

Long-Term Follow-Up

76

Olli Tenovuo, Nada Andelic, and Solrun Sigurdardottir

76.1 Overview

The long-term sequels of severe TBI include increased mortality and reduced life expectancy; increased morbidity to many health problems, including neurodegenerative diseases, epilepsy, and psychiatric disorders; poor ability to adjust in changing life situations due to cognitive problems, and psychosocial problems including difficulties in maintaining relationships and alienation (Wilson et al. 2017). Despite a reasonable number of studies describing these lifelong consequences (Masel and DeWitt 2010), there are few studies, which have tried to address how these problems should be managed by the healthcare system (Stocchetti and Zanier 2016).

O. Tenovuo (✉)
Department of Clinical Medicine, Turku Brain Injury Centre, Turku University Hospital, University of Turku, Turku, Finland

N. Andelic
Department of Physical Medicine and Rehabilitation, Oslo University Hospital Ullevål, Oslo, Norway

Research Centre for Habilitation and Rehabilitation Models and Services, Faculty of Medicine, Institute of Health and Society, University of Oslo, Oslo, Norway
e-mail: nadand@ous-hf.no

S. Sigurdardottir
Department of Research, Sunnaas Rehabilitation Hospital, Bjørnemyr, Norway
e-mail: solrun.sigurdardottir@sunnaas.no

A number of studies have addressed the ways to cope with the sequels of TBI (Mueller et al. 2018). While this "try to make it" approach might be the only option in many cultures and health systems, at least in low- and middle-income countries, this does not mean that these patients do not need professional support or that coping is not important. There is full consensus within the healthcare system that other chronic conditions such as hypertension or diabetes require regular medical follow-up in order to prevent later complications and consequences, although the patients finally are themselves responsible for how they take care of themselves (active self-management). In the case of severe TBI, despite knowing the increased risk for many severe medical conditions, regular medical care is rare after the first year post-injury, even though these patients are not able to take care of themselves equally with those having healthy brains and normal cognition.

76.2 Supportive Rehabilitation

Rehabilitation is commonly considered to mean the actions during the acute and subacute period of recovery, aiming at restoring physical, cognitive, and social functioning (see Chap. 20). However, especially in severe TBI, it is common to see impairment in the individual's functioning in all these three levels, as well as restrictions in

© Springer Nature Switzerland AG 2020
T. Sundstrøm et al. (eds.), *Management of Severe Traumatic Brain Injury*,
https://doi.org/10.1007/978-3-030-39383-0_76

participation and reduced quality of life, when the planned rehabilitation has ended. Individuals with severe TBI may live with multiple different disabilities in need of long-lasting, and in some cases permanent, rehabilitation in order to enhance participation and quality of life, to maintain the achieved level of functioning, or to prevent decline, which otherwise would take place, e.g., because of the additive effects of injury and aging.

It is generally accepted that patients with marked spasticity are in need of constant physiotherapy, and occasionally surgical interventions such as tendon lengthening and tenotomies, in order to maintain functioning and prevent, e.g., contractures and pain. Although spasticity is fairly uncommon after a TBI, the need is independent of the etiology of spasticity. A long-lasting and increased spasticity and decreased ambulation are among the main factors associated with development of heterotopic ossification (in the hips, elbows, and shoulders). Physiotherapy is important both as a preventive effort and the mainstay of therapy. In addition, a radiation therapy and surgery can be considered as late interventions in order to prevent new bone growth and to restore motion (Chalidis et al. 2007).

A much more common indication for long-lasting physiotherapy after a TBI is impaired balance, which may stem from many different causes commonly seen after a severe TBI (Perez et al. 2018). Poor balance is a significant risk for new TBIs or other severe injuries, such as femur fractures. From the point of maintaining physical functioning, some patients may have multitrauma and thus increased need for physical well-being; they may also have poor initiation, fatigue, and executive dysfunction that limit their ability to take care of their physical condition. This combination easily leads to a vicious circle, necessitating supportive rehabilitation to prevent it.

Many patients with severe TBI—especially without other major injuries—do have fairly normal physical functioning, but severely impaired cognition (Dikmen et al. 2009). The most frequent sequels of severe TBI—memory problems, poor attention and initiation, impaired communication, executive dysfunction, and fatigue—predispose these patients for many everyday problems in modern society. For example, individuals might struggle with understanding of financial and legal issues, seeking for social welfare, and adopting in new technologies and regulations. In addition, severe TBI is associated with psychosocial deficits and increased risk of developing psychiatric diseases, which may cause emotional distress in family members, friends, and work colleagues. Once a "stable" life situation is reached, this balance is often delicate and easily ruined when the patient faces new challenges, such as divorce, loosing friends, or loosing work (Arango-Lasprilla et al. 2008; Kelley et al. 2014).

Deficits in executive functioning, especially when combined with the often-occurring poor self-awareness, may drive the life of these patients in chaos. In order to prevent these problems, cognitive rehabilitation may be needed not only during the first 1–2 years after the injury, but possibly much longer, at least when big life changes or major stressors occur. The problem is often that the patient—especially if living alone—is unable to seek for help in these situations. Offering every patient with severe TBI a lifelong follow-up is not cost-effective or possible in any healthcare system. Instead, these patients should have a place with sufficient expertise and understanding, where they could get in contact easily and with a low threshold if the achieved balance of life is threatened. Offering preventive measures and low-threshold services is definitely cost saving for the society.

Cognitive supportive rehabilitation can be carried out in many ways, but a common requirement is the provider's understanding of TBI-related, usually invisible problems. Few places have a sufficient supply of neuropsychologists, who are experienced with TBI rehabilitation. Other options are psychologists, psychotherapists, or (semi)professional support persons, who have both knowledge and preferably also experience in the field of TBI rehabilitation. In some cases, when there is a severe problem in self-awareness, the most efficient way of support may be to offer counseling for the proxies.

76.3 Medical Professional Follow-Up

A major problem in many healthcare systems is the lack of coordination and contingency of care for patients with TBI (Maas et al. 2017). Typically, the acute stage is taken care of by neurosurgeons, but after hospital discharge, the follow-up may be at a neurologist, physical medicine specialist, occupational medicine, basic healthcare, or nowhere at all. There is a high risk for these patients to fall in-between, which easily leads to even more complex problems by time. It is not rare that patients will at some point drift to psychiatric care and be considered to suffer from depression and anxiety, personality disorder, panic disorder, substance abuse, or psychosis (Ponsford et al. 2018). While it is common that these kinds of psychiatric disorders develop after a TBI, the underlying cause may remain unrecognized, leading frequently to insufficient or lacking therapeutic responses or even deterioration of the clinical condition.

One of the major challenges in clinical TBI medicine is the endless individuality, and this applies also to chronic stages. Therefore, clinical expertise and experience are crucial if aiming at high-quality follow-up for these patients. Due to the vast number of TBIs, the highest level of care cannot be offered for all patients. In an ideal pathway of care for severe TBI after the initial hospital period, specialized outpatient clinics or rehabilitation units for TBI will treat these patients. These must have access for multidisciplinary assessments, including physician, rehabilitation nurse, neuropsychologist, speech therapist, occupational therapist, physiotherapist, and social worker. This unit should be responsible for the follow-up until the patient's situation has sufficiently stabilized, which includes assessments of vocational rehabilitation, medications needed, and eventual need for long-term rehabilitation. Thereafter, a family doctor or some other doctor from basic healthcare could do long-term follow-up, someone who has the possibility to follow the patient in the long run. A stable therapeutic relationship is especially important for these patients, because they are often unable to tell their problems properly, and may well give an impression of well-being, due to the invisible nature of their problems. The specialized unit should still be easily consulted, if needed.

Over the last decades, the Chronic Care Model (CCM) (Wagner et al. 1996) has been used in the management of patients with chronic illnesses (such as diabetes, chronic cardiovascular disease, and cancer) in order to address chronic needs of the patients and integrate care across specialists and primary care providers. Such a model may probably capture the complexity of TBI care and be applicable to the long-term healthcare management. However, the knowledge-base on the implementation and effectiveness of this model in TBI care is still lacking.

76.4 Social/Psychosocial Support

Depending on the social security and insurance system of the country, patients with TBI easily end up in complex, problematic situations including independence, financial resources, insurance coverage, medical insurance, work, and community participation, which may last for years. Although cases with litigation are more common in milder TBI cases, they may occur also after a severe TBI. The working ability is frequently impaired as a consequence of combined physical and cognitive deficits. However, fatigue and executive problems are the most disabling conditions, which may be difficult to comprehend by authorities or working environment. Patients are sometimes offered a sheltered working environment, whereas the return to previous work positions is fairly rarc.

The chronic stress that these situations may cause and the patient's frequent inability to handle and cope with them may effectively destroy the benefits from rehabilitation and cause deterioration of the patient's clinical condition. Therefore, sufficient social and sometimes legal support may be important in order to avoid exhaustion of the limited cognitive and psychic resources.

Similarly, these patients often end up in problems in their relationships or in establishing new, participating in volunteer activities, or taking care of children and may develop various psychiatric disorders, either by reactive or organic mechanisms. Secondary psychiatric problems combined with the cognitive TBI sequels are a difficult, but common combination and may require long-lasting therapeutic support. As for all care for TBI, sufficient understanding about the nature of TBI and its symptoms is a prerequisite for successful care.

Care for patients with severe TBI in the chronic phase is frequently provided by nonprofessionals and family caregivers, who are in need of information and family interventions to manage this situation (Hart et al. 2018). Many family caregivers experience increasing, multifaceted burden related to the extent and type of care provided, difficulties adapting to the role of a caregiver, and social disintegration, leading to psychological distress and low quality of life. In general, family support services after TBI may depend on the country, region and available local resources. Especially in healthcare systems where the resources are limited, this field can easily become a low priority, despite the fact that it may be appropriate to assume that the patient outcome is influenced by the support provided by the family caregiver (Norup et al. 2015). The major challenge is that the needs of family caregivers are not identified systematically and in a differentiated manner, and they are not addressed by proper interventions. Therefore, it is important to advise family caregivers to seek help and social support when they need it.

76.5 Conclusion

An ultimate goal of treatment and rehabilitation after severe TBI is to give patients a meaningful existence and a life within their expectancies. Despite its importance, the number of studies on long-term treatment/rehabilitation possibilities is still very limited and should be improved. Given the facts that severe TBIs cause persistent, lifelong, multidimensional consequences, the individualized care and tailored rehabilitation to each patient and his/her family is of major importance in the long run.

References

Arango-Lasprilla JC, Ketchum JM, Dezfulian T, Kreutzer JS, O'Neil-Pirozzi TM, Hammond F, Jha A. Predictors of marital stability 2 years following traumatic brain injury. Brain Inj. 2008;22(7–8):565–74. https://doi.org/10.1080/02699050802172004.

Chalidis B, Stengel D, Giannoudis PV. Early excision and late excision of heterotopic ossification after traumatic brain injury are equivalent: a systematic review of the literature. J Neurotrauma. 2007;24(11):1675–86. https://doi.org/10.1089/neu.2007.0342.

Dikmen SS, Corrigan JD, Levin HS, Machamer J, Stiers W, Weisskopf MG. Cognitive outcome following traumatic brain injury. J Head Trauma Rehabil. 2009;24(6):430–8. https://doi.org/10.1097/HTR.0b013e3181c133e9.

Hart T, Driver S, Sander A, Pappadis M, Dams-O'Connor K, Bocage C, et al. Traumatic brain injury education for adult patients and families: a scoping review. Brain Inj. 2018;32(11):1295–306. https://doi.org/10.1080/02699052.2018.1493226.

Kelley E, Sullivan C, Loughlin JK, Hutson L, Dahdah MN, Long MK, et al. Self-awareness and neurobehavioral outcomes, 5 years or more after moderate to severe brain injury. J Head Trauma Rehabil. 2014;29(2):147–52. https://doi.org/10.1097/HTR.0b013e31826db6b9.

Maas AIR, Menon DK, Adelson PD, Andelic N, Bell MJ, Belli A, et al. Traumatic brain injury: integrated approaches to improve prevention, clinical care, and research. Lancet Neurol. 2017;16(12):987–1048. https://doi.org/10.1016/S1474-4422(17)30371-X.

Masel BE, DeWitt DS. Traumatic brain injury: a disease process, not an event. J Neurotrauma. 2010;27(8):1529–40. https://doi.org/10.1089/neu.2010.1358.

Mueller C, Wesenberg S, Nestmann F, Stubbs B, Bebbington P, Raymond V. Interventions to enhance coping after traumatic brain injury: a systematic review. Int J Ther Rehabil. 2018;25(3). https://doi.org/10.12968/ijtr.2018.25.3.107.

Norup A, Perrin PB, Cuberos-Urbano G, Anke A, Andelic N, Doyle ST, et al. Family needs after brain injury: a cross cultural study. NeuroRehabilitation. 2015;36(2):203–14. https://doi.org/10.3233/NRE-151208.

Perez H, Green RE, Mochizuki G. Spectral analysis of centre of pressure identifies altered balance control in individuals with moderate-severe traumatic brain injury. Disabil Rehabil. 2018:1–9. https://doi.org/10.1080/09638288.2018.1501101.

Ponsford J, Alway Y, Gould KR. Epidemiology and natural history of psychiatric disorders after TBI. J Neuropsychiatry Clin Neurosci. 2018;30(4):262–70. https://doi.org/10.1176/appi.neuropsych.18040093.

Stocchetti N, Zanier ER. Chronic impact of traumatic brain injury on outcome and quality of life: a narrative review. Crit Care. 2016;20(1):148. https://doi.org/10.1186/s13054-016-1318-1.

Wagner EH, Austin BT, Von Korff M. Improving outcomes in chronic illness. Manag Care Q. 1996;4(2):12–25.

Wilson L, Stewart W, Dams-O'Connor K, Diaz-Arrastia R, Horton L, Menon DK, Polinder S. The chronic and evolving neurological consequences of traumatic brain injury. Lancet Neurol. 2017;16(10):813–25. https://doi.org/10.1016/S1474-4422(17)30279-X.

Part X

Outcome and Prognosis

Teemu Luoto

General Overview

77

Eirik Vikane and Teemu Luoto

77.1 General Aspects

Traumatic brain injury (TBI) is a leading cause of death and disability and is a critical health and socioeconomic problem worldwide (Hyder et al. 2007; Roozenbeek et al. 2013). TBI results in cognitive, behavioural and physical impairment, which significantly impacts independent living and social skills, interpersonal relationships, social and leisure activities and participation in work or school. However, due to diffuse and variable pathophysiological effects, there is a considerable variability in outcomes between individuals with TBI, even with severe injury (Ponsford 2013). TBI results in different impairments in the physical and mental functions, which not only produces life changes to the patient, but also to the patient's family and others with a relation to the patient (Laxe et al. 2015). To help in providing information regarding the identification of patients' problems and needs as well as planning, implementation and coordination of the rehabilitation process, the WHO International Classification of Functioning, Disability and Health (ICF) has been developed. This comprehensive classification constitutes a wide range of categories that aims to cover all the relevant aspects of functioning after TBI (Laxe et al. 2013). Two versions of the classification are available: (1) comprehensive core set (139 ICF categories) and (2) brief core set (23 ICF categories).

The introduction of the GCS in 1974 and the Glasgow Outcome Scale (GOS) in 1975 have been of great importance to the standardization of injury severity and outcome after TBI (Teasdale and Jennett 1974; Jennett and Bond 1975). Although GCS serves as the cornerstone in the clinical assessment of patients with TBI, it falls short in its prognostic abilities. Whereas GOS (more recently Glasgow Outcome Scale Extended [GOS-E]) gives a good gross characterization of the patient's global TBI outcome, it lacks detail on different outcome domains (e.g. cognitive and social functioning). More recently, the National Institute of Neurological Disorders and Stroke (NINDS) and several co-sponsoring federal agencies developed data standards for clinical TBI research. Out of this effort, Common Data Elements (CDEs) were produced in order to improve research and clinical treatment, increase data quality and promote data sharing in the field of TBI (Hicks et al. 2013; The National Institute of Neurological Disorders and Stroke (NINDS) n.d.). By harmonizing the data elements among different international studies, the comparability

E. Vikane (✉)
Department of Physical Medicine and Rehabilitation, Haukeland University Hospital, Bergen, Norway
e-mail: eirik.vikane@helse-bergen.no

T. Luoto
Department of Neurosurgery, Tampere University Hospital and Tampere University, Tampere, Finland
e-mail: teemu.luoto@pshp.fi

© Springer Nature Switzerland AG 2020
T. Sundstrøm et al. (eds.), *Management of Severe Traumatic Brain Injury*,
https://doi.org/10.1007/978-3-030-39383-0_77

of inter-study findings can be established. The CDEs encompass a variety of prognostic factors as well as different outcome domains. The main multidimensional outcome domains are (1) recovery of consciousness, (2) physical functioning, (3) neuropsychological impairment, (4) global outcome, (5) health-related quality of life, (6) TBI symptoms and (7) psychological status.

77.2 Mortality and Morbidity

The overall TBI mortality has been stable around 25% of the last two decades, and approximately 50% have a favourable outcome after a severe TBI (Lindfors et al. 2018; Murray et al. 2018). The mortality is highest within the first week post-injury. Some studies have observed an improvement in mortality rates among younger patients, whereas the mortality among elderly TBI patients is still high. The mortality increases from 50% at the age of 70 to above 75% at the age of 86 years and older (Murray et al. 2018; El-Menyar et al. 2018). Higher mortality is in particular observed among elderly patients with lower level of consciousness, high-energy trauma, one pupil fixed and dilated and more extensive intracranial pathology (Herou et al. 2015).

Different prognostic calculators for TBI have been developed (Perel et al. 2008; Steyerberg et al. 2008; Gao and Zheng 2015). In these prognostic models (e.g. IMPACT and CRASH), different injury characteristics, clinical parameters and neuroradiological findings are combined to predict outcome in individual patients. The models provide estimates of prognostic probabilities with an inherent degree of uncertainty. Common outcome measures used in these prognostic models are mortality and GOS/GOS-E as a global outcome scale (Maas et al. 2015). The prognostic model risk factors that have the most detrimental effect on TBI outcome are the following: (1) age, (2) GCS motor score, (3) pupillary reactivity and (4) secondary insults (hypotension, hypoxia and hypothermia) (Maas et al. 2015). In the future, outcome models can possibly be improved by integrating biomarker (e.g. blood-based neurotrauma biomarkers, genetic factors) findings into the equation.

Severe TBI is associated with an increased risk of multiple comorbidities acutely or chronically after injury, and the injury may even accelerate cognitive ageing (Wood 2017). These diseases and conditions can complicate recovery and result in an unfavourable outcome. Some of the most common TBI-related comorbidities include (1) somatic problems (e.g. post-traumatic epilepsy, headache and dementia), (2) psychiatric disorders (e.g. depression and post-traumatic stress disorder), (3) neuropsychological sequelae (e.g. cognitive deficits and behavioural changes) and (4) neurosurgical problems (e.g. post-traumatic hydrocephalus and syndrome of the trephined). Additionally, a minority of patients with severe TBI have a very poor recovery and remain in a vegetative or minimally conscious state. The aforementioned aspects of severe TBI recovery and outcome are discussed in detail in the following chapters.

References

El-Menyar A, Consunji R, Abdelrahman H, Latifi R, Wahlen BM, Al-Thani H. Predictors and time-based hospital mortality in patients with isolated and polytrauma brain injuries. World J Surg. 2018;42(5):1346–57.

Gao J, Zheng Z. Development of prognostic models for patients with traumatic brain injury: a systematic review. Int J Clin Exp Med. 2015;8(11):19881–5.

Herou E, Romner B, Tomasevic G. Acute traumatic brain injury: mortality in the elderly. World Neurosurg. 2015;83(6):996–1001.

Hicks R, Giacino J, Harrison-Felix C, Manley G, Valadka A, Wilde EA. Progress in developing common data elements for traumatic brain injury research: version two--the end of the beginning. J Neurotrauma. 2013;30(22):1852–61.

Hyder AA, Wunderlich CA, Puvanachandra P, Gururaj G, Kobusingye OC. The impact of traumatic brain injuries: a global perspective. NeuroRehabilitation. 2007;22(5):341–53.

Jennett B, Bond M. Assessment of outcome after severe brain damage. Lancet. 1975;1(7905):480–4.

Laxe S, Zasler N, Selb M, Tate R, Tormos JM, Bernabeu M. Development of the International Classification of Functioning, Disability and Health core sets for traumatic brain injury: an International consensus process. Brain Inj. 2013;27(4):379–87.

Laxe S, Cieza A, Castano-Monsalve B. Rehabilitation of traumatic brain injury in the light of the ICF. NeuroRehabilitation. 2015;36(1):37–43.

Lindfors M, Vehvilainen J, Siironen J, Kivisaari R, Skrifvars MB, Raj R. Temporal changes in outcome following intensive care unit treatment after traumatic brain injury: a 17-year experience in a large academic neurosurgical centre. Acta Neurochir. 2018;160(11):2107–15.

Maas AI, Lingsma HF, Roozenbeek B. Predicting outcome after traumatic brain injury. Handb Clin Neurol. 2015;128:455–74.

Murray GD, Brennan PM, Teasdale GM. Simplifying the use of prognostic information in traumatic brain injury. Part 2: graphical presentation of probabilities. J Neurosurg. 2018;128(6):1621–34.

Perel P, Arango M, Clayton T, Edwards P, Komolafe E, Poccock S, et al. Predicting outcome after traumatic brain injury: practical prognostic models based on large cohort of international patients. BMJ. 2008;336(7641):425–9.

Ponsford J. Factors contributing to outcome following traumatic brain injury. NeuroRehabilitation. 2013;32(4):803–15.

Roozenbeek B, Maas AI, Menon DK. Changing patterns in the epidemiology of traumatic brain injury. Nat Rev Neurol. 2013;9(4):231–6.

Steyerberg EW, Mushkudiani N, Perel P, Butcher I, Lu J, McHugh GS, et al. Predicting outcome after traumatic brain injury: development and international validation of prognostic scores based on admission characteristics. PLoS Med. 2008;5(8):e165; discussion e.

Teasdale G, Jennett B. Assessment of coma and impaired consciousness. A practical scale. Lancet. 1974;2(7872):81–4.

The National Institute of Neurological Disorders and Stroke (NINDS). https://www.commondataelements.ninds.nih.gov.

Wood RL. Accelerated cognitive aging following severe traumatic brain injury: a review. Brain Inj. 2017;31(10):1270–8.

78 Somatic Consequences

Johan Ljungqvist

Recommendations

Level I

There are insufficient data to support a Level I recommendation for this topic.

Level II

There are insufficient data to support a Level II recommendation for this topic.

Level III

There is no evidence to support the use of antiepileptic drugs to reduce the risk of late-onset seizures after TBI in adults. Hormone deficiency is a common finding after severe TBI and screening should be considered.

Tips, Tricks, and Pitfalls

- Somatic consequences are common after traumatic brain injury (TBI) and require prompt recognition and treatment in order to optimize the neurological outcome for the patient.
- General treatment guidelines are often adequate also for patients with TBI.
- Patients with clinical signs of adrenal insufficiency require immediate treatment, and screening for hormone deficiency should be considered, as this occurs also in the subacute and chronic phase after TBI.

78.1 Background

Traumatic brain injury should not be considered a distinct event, as a sequence of damage occurs to the central nervous system that continues to affect the patient in the subacute and chronic periods after injury. While some sequelae, such as seizures, are more common within the first months after injury, levels of fatigue often increase during the first year after severe TBI.

J. Ljungqvist (✉)
Department of Neurosurgery, Sahlgrenska University Hospital, Gothenburg, Sweden

Institute of Neuroscience and Physiology, Sahlgrenska Academy University of Gothenburg, Gothenburg, Sweden
e-mail: johan.ljungqvist@vgregion.se

© Springer Nature Switzerland AG 2020
T. Sundstrøm et al. (eds.), *Management of Severe Traumatic Brain Injury*,
https://doi.org/10.1007/978-3-030-39383-0_78

78.2 Post-traumatic Seizures

Late seizures are seizures that occur later than 1 week after TBI. Depending on the series, the incidence of late seizures ranges from 1.9 to >30% (Frey 2003). The wide range likely reflects the variability in the populations studied, particularly with respect to injury severity. In a population study by Annegers and colleagues, the standardized incidence ratio for late seizures in patients with severe TBI was 17.0 (95% confidence interval, 12.3–23.6) (Annegers et al. 1998), and in a Finnish study, the incidence was 24.5% (Asikainen et al. 1999). Older age, early seizures, and more severe TBI have been associated with an increased risk of late seizures (DeGrauw et al. 2018). Moreover, injuries that involve depressed skull fractures, dural penetration, and focal tissue destruction are at particular risk. In a series by Englander and colleagues, patients with biparietal contusions had a cumulative probability of late post-traumatic seizures of 66%, and patients with dural penetration along with bone and metal fragments, 62.5% (Englander et al. 2003).

Late seizures often occur within the first year of injury (Annegers et al. 1998; Englander et al. 2003), but the increased risk after TBI may persist for up to 10 or 20 years (Annegers et al. 1998; Frey 2003).

A Cochrane review from 2015 did not find evidence to support the use of antiepileptic drugs to reduce the risk of late seizures or mortality (Thompson et al. 2015). Similarly, a review by Picenna and colleagues found no evidence for the effectiveness of pharmacological treatments in the prevention or treatment of symptomatic seizures in adults with post-traumatic epilepsy; however, they did find limited high-level evidence for the effectiveness of levetiracetam for children with post-traumatic epilepsy (Piccenna et al. 2017). See also Chap. 69.

78.3 Hypopituitarism

Hypopituitarism, or presence of pituitary hormone alterations, is commonly found in the acute phase after TBI (c.f. Chap. 56). However, the relevance and therapeutic implications of these findings are uncertain (Klose and Feldt-Rasmussen 2015; Tolli et al. 2017). The general prevalence of post-traumatic hypopituitarism has been reported to be 27%, growth hormone deficiency being the commonest deficiency (Schneider et al. 2007). For clinicians who see patients in the subacute or chronic phase after TBI, it is important to recognize clinical signs of adrenal insufficiency and to institute immediate treatment (Klose and Feldt-Rasmussen 2015). Patients with overt post-traumatic multiple pituitary hormone deficiencies also require treatment, and screening for hormone deficiency should be considered (Klose and Feldt-Rasmussen 2015; Tolli et al. 2017).

78.4 Paroxysmal Sympathetic Hyperactivity

Paroxysmal sympathetic hyperactivity occurs in about 10% of patients after severe TBI, particularly those with worse outcomes (c.f. Chap. 73) (Hendricks et al. 2010; Fernandez-Ortega et al. 2012). The condition may persist for weeks to months and is characterized by "periodic episodes of increased heart rate and blood pressure, sweating, hyperthermia, and motor posturing, often in response to external stimuli" (Meyfroidt et al. 2017). In the subacute and chronic phases after TBI, it is important to diagnose paroxysmal sympathetic hyperactivity and to optimize treatment. The main goals of treatment, suggested by Meyfroidt and colleagues, are "to avoid the triggers that provoke the paroxysms, to mitigate the excessive sympathetic outflow, and to address the effects of paroxysmal sympathetic hyperactivity on other organ systems through supportive therapy" (Meyfroidt et al. 2017).

78.5 Headache and Pain

Complaints of frequent or continuous headache are common after TBI. The *International Classification of Headache Disorders* 3rd edition (ICHD-3) defines "headache attributed to trauma or injury to the head and/or neck", which encompasses both a new headache that occurs after the trauma and worsening of a pre-existing headache after the trauma (Headache Classification Committee of the International Headache Society (IHS) 2018). Different studies have shown a prevalence of significant headache at 1 year after trauma in 18–33% of patients (Lew et al. 2006; Kamins and Charles 2018). Nordhaug and colleagues found that patients hospitalized after mild head injury had an increased risk of new-onset headache (OR 1.74, 95% CI 1.05–2.87) as well as an increased risk of exacerbation of previously reported headache (OR 1.93, 95% CI 1.24–3.02) compared to a control group (Nordhaug et al. 2018). Other chronic pain syndromes also occur more frequently compared to the general population, particularly in patients with mild TBI (Nampiaparampil 2008). Patients with severe TBI may have difficulties reporting or processing their symptoms because of other cognitive or executive impairments.

Headache and pain are associated with other consequences of TBI such as post-traumatic depression, cognition, and fatigue, but the causality is not known (Kumar et al. 2018). Hoffmann and colleagues found a relationship between pain and community participation at 1 year after injury, but this relationship became insignificant when depression was taken into account, hence demonstrating the complex relationship between different sequelae of TBI (Hoffman et al. 2007).

Management of chronic headache and pain in patients with TBI is difficult because of the complex underlying mechanisms (Kamins and Charles 2018) and the relative paucity of studies on specific post-traumatic headache or pain. However, a majority of studies have reported that patients present with tension-type or migraine-like headaches, and for these symptoms, simple analgesics and nonsteroid inflammatory drugs are commonly used (Lew et al. 2006). Prophylactic therapies and acute migraine-specific treatments may also be given. Overuse of analgesics is not uncommon in patients with chronic headache, including patients after TBI, and this could lead to a paradoxical increase in headache that may become refractory (Lew et al. 2006).

Thorough examination, appreciation of the complex nature of the pathophysiology of the disease, and awareness of coexisting symptoms (such as fatigue and depression) are important factors in the management of post-traumatic headache and pain. Therefore, physical therapy, psychologic evaluation, and cognitive therapy may be more effective than pharmacologic treatment (Kamins and Charles 2018).

78.6 Fatigue and Sleep Disorders

Fatigue is a common sequela of TBI that affects a majority of patients, regardless of injury severity and regardless of time since the injury (Mollayeva et al. 2014; Beaulieu-Bonneau and Ouellet 2017). Cantor and colleagues found that 75% of the sample of individuals with TBI, included in their study, reported significant levels of fatigue as opposed to 40% of those in a non-injured comparison group (Cantor et al. 2008). Lequerica and colleagues followed patients longitudinally and found that less than half of their patients experienced a remission of fatigue over time (Lequerica et al. 2017). Beaulieu-Bonneau and Ouellet also performed a longitudinal study and found a pattern of reduction of fatigue levels in patients with mild TBI, stable fatigue levels in patients with moderate TBI, and increased fatigue levels in patients with severe TBI (Beaulieu-Bonneau and Ouellet 2017). An increase of fatigue over time in patients with severe TBI could possibly be linked to increased levels of awareness and overall activity (Bjorkdahl et al. 2016; Beaulieu-Bonneau and Ouellet 2017). Fatigue is also strongly linked to post-traumatic depression, with fatigue preceding depression (Kumar et al. 2018).

There is no objective measure or generally accepted definition of fatigue after TBI, but the experience of fatigue can be both physical and cognitive. Cantor and colleagues noted that fatigue is "often associated with a felt sense of disproportionate exertion and associated mental or physical exhaustion and inability to perform" (Cantor et al. 2013). The "Mental Fatigue Scale" is a questionnaire for the self-assessment of mental fatigue that describes the condition (Johansson et al. 2009). The scale includes 15 questions in different areas associated with mental fatigue, i.e., fatigue in general, lack of initiative, mental fatigue, mental recovery, concentration difficulties, memory problems, slowness of thinking, sensitivity to stress, increased tendency to become emotional, irritability, sensitivity to light or noise, as well as decreased or increased duration of sleep or diurnal variations (Johansson et al. 2009).

Fatigue is closely linked to other sequelae of TBI, including cognitive deficits, insomnia, anxiety, depression, and pain, and it affects global well-being (Beaulieu-Bonneau and Ouellet 2017). Despite the association between fatigue and sleepiness, sleep does not seem to have a restorative effect on fatigue (Cantor et al. 2013). However, problems with sleep are also common after TBI, and in a meta-analysis by Mathias and Alvaro, 50% of patients suffered from sleep disturbance after TBI, and 25–29% had a diagnosed sleep disorder (insomnia, hypersomnia, apnea) (Mathias and Alvaro 2012). Thus, it is important to recognize and treat these conditions to avoid their potential impact on recovery and outcome.

While there are no structural neuroimaging correlations of fatigue that can be used in routine practice, structural and functional MRI studies have given some clues. Schonberger and colleagues have found a relation between cognitive fatigability and right frontal and temporal brain lesions as well as to the total lesion load (Schonberger et al. 2017). Moreover, the group speculates that the findings "could be the result of decreased functional connectivity of attentional networks that results in accelerated exhaustion during cognitive task performance" (Schonberger et al. 2017). Wylie and colleagues have demonstrated a relationship between fatigue and activation in the caudate nucleus, a structure involved in the control of motor processes and cognitive behavior (Wylie et al. 2017).

There is currently insufficient evidence to recommend or contraindicate any treatments of fatigue after TBI (Cantor et al. 2014). However, several pharmacological studies are underway, and studies of cognitive behavioral therapy have shown promising results in pilot studies (Cantor et al. 2014; Nguyen et al. 2017).

References

Annegers JF, Hauser WA, Coan SP, Rocca WA. A population-based study of seizures after traumatic brain injuries. N Engl J Med. 1998;338(1):20–4.

Asikainen I, Kaste M, Sarna S. Early and late posttraumatic seizures in traumatic brain injury rehabilitation patients: brain injury factors causing late seizures and influence of seizures on long-term outcome. Epilepsia. 1999;40(5):584–9.

Beaulieu-Bonneau S, Ouellet MC. Fatigue in the first year after traumatic brain injury: course, relationship with injury severity, and correlates. Neuropsychol Rehabil. 2017;27(7):983–1001.

Bjorkdahl A, Esbjornsson E, Ljungqvist J, Skoglund T, Sunnerhagen KS. Decline in cognitive function due to diffuse axonal injury does not necessarily imply a corresponding decline in ability to perform activities. Disabil Rehabil. 2016;38(10):1006–15.

Cantor JB, Ashman T, Gordon W, Ginsberg A, Engmann C, Egan M, Spielman L, Dijkers M, Flanagan S. Fatigue after traumatic brain injury and its impact on participation and quality of life. J Head Trauma Rehabil. 2008;23(1):41–51.

Cantor JB, Gordon W, Gumber S. What is post TBI fatigue? NeuroRehabilitation. 2013;32(4):875–83.

Cantor JB, Ashman T, Bushnik T, Cai X, Farrell-Carnahan L, Gumber S, Hart T, Rosenthal J, Dijkers MP. Systematic review of interventions for fatigue after traumatic brain injury: a NIDRR traumatic brain injury model systems study. J Head Trauma Rehabil. 2014;29(6):490–7.

DeGrauw X, Thurman D, Xu L, Kancherla V, DeGrauw T. Epidemiology of traumatic brain injury-associated epilepsy and early use of anti-epilepsy drugs: an analysis of insurance claims data, 2004-2014. Epilepsy Res. 2018;146:41–9.

Englander J, Bushnik T, Duong TT, Cifu DX, Zafonte R, Wright J, Hughes R, Bergman W. Analyzing risk factors for late posttraumatic seizures: a prospective, multicenter investigation. Arch Phys Med Rehabil. 2003;84(3):365–73.

Fernandez-Ortega JF, Prieto-Palomino MA, Garcia-Caballero M, Galeas-Lopez JL, Quesada-Garcia G, Baguley IJ. Paroxysmal sympathetic hyperactivity after traumatic brain injury: clinical and prognostic implications. J Neurotrauma. 2012;29(7):1364–70.

Frey LC. Epidemiology of posttraumatic epilepsy: a critical review. Epilepsia. 2003;44(s10):11–7.

Headache Classification Committee of the International Headache Society (IHS). The International Classification of Headache Disorders, 3rd edition. Cephalalgia. 2018;38(1):1–211.

Hendricks HT, Heeren AH, Vos PE. Dysautonomia after severe traumatic brain injury. Eur J Neurol. 2010;17(9):1172–7.

Hoffman JM, Pagulayan KF, Zawaideh N, Dikmen S, Temkin N, Bell KR. Understanding pain after traumatic brain injury: impact on community participation. Am J Phys Med Rehabil. 2007;86(12):962–9.

Johansson B, Berglund P, Ronnback L. Mental fatigue and impaired information processing after mild and moderate traumatic brain injury. Brain Inj. 2009;23(13–14):1027–40.

Kamins J, Charles A. Posttraumatic headache: basic mechanisms and therapeutic targets. Headache. 2018;58(6):811–26.

Klose M, Feldt-Rasmussen U. Hypopituitarism in traumatic brain injury-a critical note. J Clin Med. 2015;4(7):1480–97.

Kumar RG, Gao S, Juengst SB, Wagner AK, Fabio A. The effects of post-traumatic depression on cognition, pain, fatigue, and headache after moderate-to-severe traumatic brain injury: a thematic review. Brain Inj. 2018;32(4):383–94.

Lequerica AH, Botticello AL, Lengenfelder J, Chiaravalloti N, Bushnik T, Dijkers MP, Hammond FM, Kolakowsky-Hayner SA, Rosenthal J. Factors associated with remission of post-traumatic brain injury fatigue in the years following traumatic brain injury (TBI): a TBI model systems module study. Neuropsychol Rehabil. 2017;27(7):1019–30.

Lew HL, Lin PH, Fuh JL, Wang SJ, Clark DJ, Walker WC. Characteristics and treatment of headache after traumatic brain injury: a focused review. Am J Phys Med Rehabil. 2006;85(7):619–27.

Mathias JL, Alvaro PK. Prevalence of sleep disturbances, disorders, and problems following traumatic brain injury: a meta-analysis. Sleep Med. 2012;13(7):898–905.

Meyfroidt G, Baguley IJ, Menon DK. Paroxysmal sympathetic hyperactivity: the storm after acute brain injury. Lancet Neurol. 2017;16(9):721–9.

Mollayeva T, Kendzerska T, Mollayeva S, Shapiro CM, Colantonio A, Cassidy JD. A systematic review of fatigue in patients with traumatic brain injury: the course, predictors and consequences. Neurosci Biobehav Rev. 2014;47:684–716.

Nampiaparampil DE. Prevalence of chronic pain after traumatic brain injury: a systematic review. JAMA. 2008;300(6):711–9.

Nguyen S, McKay A, Wong D, Rajaratnam SM, Spitz G, Williams G, Mansfield D, Ponsford JL. Cognitive behavior therapy to treat sleep disturbance and fatigue after traumatic brain injury: a pilot randomized controlled trial. Arch Phys Med Rehabil. 2017;98(8):1508–1517.e1502.

Nordhaug LH, Hagen K, Vik A, Stovner LJ, Follestad T, Pedersen T, Gravdahl GB, Linde M. Headache following head injury: a population-based longitudinal cohort study (HUNT). J Headache Pain. 2018;19(1):8.

Piccenna L, Shears G, O'Brien TJ. Management of post-traumatic epilepsy: an evidence review over the last 5 years and future directions. Epilepsia Open. 2017;2(2):123–44.

Schneider HJ, Kreitschmann-Andermahr I, Ghigo E, Stalla GK, Agha A. Hypothalamopituitary dysfunction following traumatic brain injury and aneurysmal subarachnoid hemorrhage: a systematic review. JAMA. 2007;298(12):1429–38.

Schonberger M, Reutens D, Beare R, O'Sullivan R, Rajaratnam SMW, Ponsford J. Brain lesion correlates of fatigue in individuals with traumatic brain injury. Neuropsychol Rehabil. 2017;27(7):1056–70.

Thompson K, Pohlmann-Eden B, Campbell LA, Abel H. Pharmacological treatments for preventing epilepsy following traumatic head injury. Cochrane Database Syst Rev. 2015;(8):CD009900.

Tolli A, Borg J, Bellander BM, Johansson F, Hoybye C. Pituitary function within the first year after traumatic brain injury or subarachnoid haemorrhage. J Endocrinol Invest. 2017;40(2):193–205.

Wylie GR, Dobryakova E, DeLuca J, Chiaravalloti N, Essad K, Genova H. Cognitive fatigue in individuals with traumatic brain injury is associated with caudate activation. Sci Rep. 2017;7(1):8973.

79 Neuropsychiatric Consequences

Salla Koponen

Recommendations

Level I

There are insufficient data to support a Level I recommendation for this topic.

Level II

A subset of individuals with major depressive disorder after TBI probably respond to antidepressive medication.

Level III

Individuals with severe TBI are susceptible to the side effects of psychotropic agents. Agents with significant anticholinergic effects should be avoided. Benzodiazepines are not recommended due to their effects on cognitive function and impulse control.

S. Koponen (✉)
Department of Psychiatry, Hospital District of Helsinki and Uusimaa, Helsinki, Finland
e-mail: salla.koponen@hus.fi

Tips, Tricks, and Pitfalls

- A psychiatric consultation should be considered, when a patient with TBI has disabling psychiatric symptoms. Major depressive disorder, posttraumatic stress disorder, and anxiety disorders are common after TBI.
- All psychotropic agents should be started at a low dose to avoid side effects.

79.1 Overview

Mental disorders and other neurobehavioral changes are commonly seen after traumatic brain injury (TBI). They typically cause significant disability and poorer quality of life. In patients with severe TBI, the decreased health-related quality of life has been associated with depressive symptoms (Grauwmeijer et al. 2018) and posttraumatic stress symptoms (Bosma et al. 2018). Substance use disorders are known to be common prior to severe TBI (Alway et al. 2016a), and substance use often continues causing difficulties in the rehabilitation. To improve the outcome of severe TBI, neuropsychiatric consequences need to be recognized and managed at an early stage. A psychiatric consultation should be considered, when a patient has apparent symptoms of, for example, posttraumatic stress disorder or moder-

© Springer Nature Switzerland AG 2020
T. Sundstrøm et al. (eds.), *Management of Severe Traumatic Brain Injury*,
https://doi.org/10.1007/978-3-030-39383-0_79

ate to severe major depressive disorder. Unfortunately, the evidence-based knowledge of their treatment after TBI is scarce. Patients with severe TBI are particularly susceptible to the side effects of psychotropic agents. For *acute* neuropsychiatric conditions, see Chap. 74.

79.2 Neurobehavioral Changes

In a study with 120 individuals with severe TBI, the most common neuropsychiatric symptoms (assessed with the Neuropsychiatric Inventory, NPI) were apathy (42%), irritability (37%), dysphoric or depressed mood (29%), disinhibition (28%), eating disturbances (27%), and agitation (24%) (Ciurli et al. 2011). The high occurrence of apathy is noteworthy, as apathy often impedes the rehabilitation attempts. In apathy, the diminished motivation can manifest itself in diminished goal-directed behavior, goal-directed cognitive activity, or emotions (Arnould et al. 2016).

Impulsivity is another well-known consequence of TBI. It can be defined as a tendency to experience strong reactions (especially in association with negative affects), a difficulty to think and reflect on the consequences of an act, or a difficulty to remain focused on a task (Arnould et al. 2016). Particularly after severe TBI, impulsive aggressive behavior may also be seen.

A marked personality change has been found in 33% of patients with severe TBI (Diaz et al. 2012). The diagnosis of organic personality disorder can be applied in these cases (F07.0 in ICD-10). The prominent symptoms of organic personality disorder are usually either apathetic features or impulsive and aggressive features.

The assessment of neurobehavioral changes is often complicated by the lack of self-awareness after severe TBI. Information from family members or other caregivers is essential to carry out a reliable assessment.

The evidence-based knowledge of the management of neurobehavioral symptoms is scarce. Chronic impulsive or aggressive behavior is often targeted with pharmacotherapy. However, the data to support this approach is insufficient. Consequently, psychosocial interventions should be considered first (Fisher et al. 2015). In a Cochrane review by Fleminger et al. (2006), the best evidence of effectiveness for agitation or aggression after TBI was found for propranolol and pindolol at high doses, but even this evidence was weak. In clinical practice, beta-blockers are not commonly used due to their cardiovascular effects. SSRIs (selective serotonin reuptake inhibitors) or antiepileptics are usually the first choice to treat severe impulsivity or aggressive behavior after TBI (Arciniegas and Wortzel 2014). Buspirone can also be used. Benzodiazepines should be avoided, as they impair impulse control and cognitive function. Antipsychotics, particularly first-generation (typical) antipsychotics, should also be avoided due to their side effects (e.g. extrapyramidal side effects). All psychotropic medications should be started at a low dose and the dose should be increased slowly. Before starting any psychotropic medication for agitation or aggression, pain and other somatic etiological factors should be excluded. It is meant to be said that pain and other somatic factors can cause agitation or aggression. There are no evidence-based means to manage apathy.

79.3 Mental Disorders

The diagnosis and treatment of the following relatively common mental disorders is important to enable patients to benefit from the rehabilitation of TBI. The diagnostics is often complicated, as the symptoms of many mental disorders, e.g., major depressive disorder, overlap with the symptoms of chronic TBI. The data on the effectiveness of pharmacotherapy and psychotherapeutic interventions in individuals with TBI is insufficient.

79.3.1 Major Depressive Disorder

An increased risk of depression has been found in individuals with TBI (Tsai et al. 2014; Perry et al. 2016). In a study with 559 patients, 53% had major depressive disorder (MDD) during the 12-month follow-up after TBI (Bombardier et al. 2010). Subjects with severe TBI also had an increased risk of depression in all three abovementioned studies. According to some reports, MDD has been more common after mild TBI (26%) than after moderate to severe TBI (15%) (Ouellet et al. 2018). Depression prior to injury is a predictor of the development of MDD after TBI (Bombardier et al. 2010; Cnossen et al. 2017; Ouellet et al. 2018). In clinical practice, particularly patients with a history of MDD should be monitored for depressive symptoms after TBI.

The core symptoms of MDD are depressed mood, marked loss of interest or ability to enjoy activities (anhedonia), and decreased energy. The diagnosis of MDD can be difficult after TBI, as there is an overlap in some symptoms of MDD and TBI. The symptoms seen in both of these conditions are decreased energy, sleep disturbance of any type, diminished ability to concentrate, and irritability. This overlap should be taken into account also when interpreting self-rating scales for depression, such as Beck Depression Inventory (BDI). After severe TBI, the lack of self-awareness can also complicate the diagnosis of depression.

Although the diagnostic criteria of MDD are not fulfilled, TBI patients may have milder depressive symptoms. In this case, the ICD-10 diagnosis of "adjustment disorder with depressed mood" can be used. Patients with this kind of adjustment disorder should be followed, as depressive symptoms may worsen and eventually fulfill the criteria of MDD, causing more disability. Psychosocial treatment for depressive symptoms should be considered at an early stage.

Suicide risk should be monitored especially in individuals whose TBI is a consequence of a suicide attempt or who otherwise have a history of suicidal behavior. TBI is associated with an increased suicide risk (Madsen et al. 2018).

Antidepressive agents are used to treat MDD after TBI, although the evidence to support this is insufficient (Price et al. 2011; Salter et al. 2016; Fann et al. 2017; Kreitzer et al. 2019). SSRIs are usually preferred, but SNRIs (serotonin-norepinephrine reuptake inhibitors) and mirtazapine can also be used. In addition, mirtazapine often has a beneficial effect on sleep, but in some individuals, it causes daytime sleepiness. All psychotropic medications, including antidepressants, should be started at a low dose to avoid side effects. In one study, sertraline (SSRI) appeared to be efficacious in preventing depression after TBI (Jorge et al. 2016). Tricyclic antidepressants are not recommended (in doses needed to treat depression) due to their anticholinergic side effects. Bupropion should be avoided after severe TBI, as it increases the risk of epileptic seizures.

Psychotherapeutic interventions should be considered, although all patients with severe TBI are not able to benefit from these interventions due to impaired cognitive function and lack of self-awareness. There is very limited knowledge of the effectiveness of psychotherapy in patients with TBI (Gertler et al. 2015; Wiart et al. 2016). In clinical practice, primarily cognitive behavioral methods have appeared to be useful after severe TBI.

The risk of bipolar disorder is also increased after TBI (Tsai et al. 2014; Perry et al. 2016). However, milder and more rapid fluctuation in mood, not fulfilling the criteria of mania or hypomania, is remarkably more common after TBI.

79.3.2 Posttraumatic Stress Disorder

Posttraumatic stress disorder (PTSD) can evolve after an exceptionally threatening event, e.g., assault or motor vehicle accident. In addition, some individuals develop a subsyndromal PTSD. In this case, the diagnostic criteria of PTSD are not fulfilled, but anxiety and other posttraumatic symptoms can nevertheless be disabling and should be treated.

PTSD is more common in patients with mild TBI, but it can also develop after severe TBI, even when no conscious memory of the event is present (Bahraini et al. 2014; Alway et al. 2016b). After moderate to severe TBI, PTSD was found in 17% of 85 patients during a 4-year follow-up period (Alway et al. 2016b). The onset of PTSD was typically delayed: it peaked between 6 and 12 months after TBI (Alway et al. 2016b). Thus, the mental state of patients should be followed even after the first few months.

The diagnosis of PTSD is often challenging in patients with TBI. The symptoms of PTSD are diverse, and there is an overlap in symptoms of PTSD and TBI. Sleep disturbance, irritability, and difficulty in concentrating are common symptoms in both conditions (Bahraini et al. 2014). The core symptoms of PTSD are persistent re-experiencing of the traumatic event (e.g., nightmares or flashbacks), avoidance of trauma-related stimuli, and trauma-related arousal and reactivity (e.g., difficulty sleeping, irritability or aggression, difficulty concentrating, or heightened startle reaction). Also, symptoms resembling depression, such as decreased interest in activities and difficulty experiencing positive emotions, can occur in PTSD.

When symptoms of PTSD are suspected, a psychiatric consultation is recommended. A proper treatment plan is needed, as PTSD often has a chronic course. Psychotherapeutic interventions are primary, but pharmacotherapy is often also necessary for severe anxiety and sleep disturbance. Benzodiazepines should be avoided, as they can impair cognitive function and impulse control. In addition, the risk of problematic benzodiazepine use and even dependence is relatively high in PTSD, as anxiety is often persistent. Data on the treatment of PTSD in individuals with TBI is insufficient. Antidepressive agents, primarily SSRIs, are recommended. The use of SNRIs is possible, especially when pain relief is also needed. Mirtazapine can be used to treat insomnia.

79.3.3 Substance Use Disorders

A significant proportion of patients with TBI have a history of substance use. After moderate to severe TBI, preinjury alcohol or drug use disorders were found in 38% of 161 patients (Alway et al. 2016a). The occurrence of alcohol or drug use disorders was lower after TBI, the rate being 9–17% during the 5-year follow-up period (Alway et al. 2016a). In another study with 1-year follow-up, alcohol and drug use declined during the first 4 months after TBI, but after that increased close to the preinjury level (Beaulieu-Bonneau et al. 2018). Patients with mild TBI returned to alcohol use earlier than those with moderate to severe TBI (Beaulieu-Bonneau et al. 2018). In clinical practice, substance use should be brought up, and counselling and access to addiction services should be ensured.

References

Alway Y, Gould KR, Johnston L, McKenzie D, Ponsford J. A prospective examination of Axis I psychiatric disorders in the first 5 years following moderate to severe traumatic brain injury. Psychol Med. 2016a;46(6):1331–41. https://doi.org/10.1017/S0033291715002986.

Alway Y, Gould KR, McKay A, Johnston L, Ponsford J. The evolution of post-traumatic stress disorder following moderate-to-severe traumatic brain injury. J Neurotrauma. 2016b;33(9):825–31. https://doi.org/10.1089/neu.2015.3992.

Arciniegas DB, Wortzel HS. Emotional and behavioral dyscontrol after traumatic brain injury. Psychiatr Clin North Am. 2014;37(1):31–53. https://doi.org/10.1016/j.psc.2013.12.001.

Arnould A, Dromer E, Rochat L, Van der Linden M, Azouvi P. Neurobehavioral and self-awareness changes after traumatic brain injury: towards new multidimensional approaches. Ann Phys Rehabil Med. 2016;59(1):18–22. https://doi.org/10.1016/j.rehab.2015.09.002.

Bahraini NH, Breshears RE, Hernández TD, Schneider AL, Forster JE, Brenner LA. Traumatic brain injury and posttraumatic stress disorder. Psychiatr Clin North Am. 2014;37(1):55–75. https://doi.org/10.1016/j.psc.2013.11.002.

Beaulieu-Bonneau S, St-Onge F, Blackburn M, Banville A, Paradis-Giroux A, Ouellet MC. Alcohol and drug use before and during the first year after traumatic brain injury. J Head Trauma Rehabil. 2018;33(3):E51–60. https://doi.org/10.1097/HTR.0000000000000341.

Bombardier CH, Fann JR, Temkin NR, Esselman PC, Barber J, Dikmen SS. Rates of major depressive disorder and clinical outcomes following traumatic brain injury. JAMA. 2010;303(19):1938–45. https://doi.org/10.1001/jama.2010.599.

Bosma CM, Mansoor N, Haller CS. Association of post-traumatic stress symptom severity with health-related quality of life and self-reported functioning across 12 months after severe traumatic brain injury. Arch Phys Med Rehabil. 2018;99(8):1576–83. https://doi.org/10.1016/j.apmr.2018.02.008.

Ciurli P, Formisano R, Bivona U, Cantagallo A, Angelelli P. Neuropsychiatric disorders in persons with severe traumatic brain injury: prevalence, phenomenology, and relationship with demographic, clinical, and functional features. J Head Trauma

Rehabil. 2011;26(2):116–26. https://doi.org/10.1097/HTR.0b013e3181dedd0e.

Cnossen MC, Scholten AC, Lingsma HF, Synnot A, Haagsma J, Steyerberg PEW, Polinder S. Predictors of major depression and posttraumatic stress disorder following traumatic brain injury: a systematic review and meta-analysis. J Neuropsychiatry Clin Neurosci. 2017;29(3):206–24. https://doi.org/10.1176/appi.neuropsych.16090165.

Diaz AP, Schwarzbold ML, Thais ME, Hohl A, Bertotti MM, Schmoeller R, Nunes JC, Prediger R, Linhares MN, Guarnieri R, Walz R. Psychiatric disorders and health-related quality of life after severe traumatic brain injury: a prospective study. J Neurotrauma. 2012;29(6):1029–37. https://doi.org/10.1089/neu.2011.2089.

Fann JR, Bombardier CH, Temkin N, Esselman P, Warms C, Barber J, Dikmen S. Sertraline for major depression during the year following traumatic brain injury: a randomized controlled trial. J Head Trauma Rehabil. 2017;32(5):332–42. https://doi.org/10.1097/HTR.0000000000000322.

Fisher A, Lennon S, Bellon M, Lawn S. Family involvement in behaviour management following acquired brain injury (ABI) in community settings: a systematic review. Brain Inj. 2015;29(6):661–75. https://doi.org/10.3109/02699052.2015.1004751.

Fleminger S, Greenwood RJ, Oliver D. Pharmacological management for agitation and aggression in people with acquired brain injury. Cochrane Database Syst Rev. 2006;(4):CD003299.

Gertler P, Tate RL, Cameron ID. Non-pharmacological interventions for depression in adults and children with traumatic brain injury. Cochrane Database Syst Rev. 2015;(12):CD009871. https://doi.org/10.1002/14651858.CD009871.pub2.

Grauwmeijer E, Heijenbrok-Kal MH, Peppel LD, Hartjes CJ, Haitsma IK, de Koning I, Ribbers GM. Cognition, health-related quality of life, and depression ten years after moderate to severe traumatic brain injury: a prospective cohort study. J Neurotrauma. 2018;35(13):1543–51. https://doi.org/10.1089/neu.2017.5404.

Jorge RE, Acion L, Burin DI, Robinson RG. Sertraline for preventing mood disorders following traumatic brain injury: a randomized clinical trial. JAMA Psychiat. 2016;73(10):1041–7. https://doi.org/10.1001/jamapsychiatry.2016.2189.

Kreitzer N, Ancona R, McCullumsmith C, Kurowski BG, Foreman B, Ngwenya LB, Adeoye O. The effect of antidepressants on depression after traumatic brain injury: a meta-analysis. J Head Trauma Rehabil. 2019;34:E47–54. https://doi.org/10.1097/HTR.0000000000000439. [Epub ahead of print].

Madsen T, Erlangsen A, Orlovska S, Mofaddy R, Nordentoft M, Benros ME. Association between traumatic brain injury and risk of suicide. JAMA. 2018;320(6):580–8. https://doi.org/10.1001/jama.2018.10211.

Ouellet MC, Beaulieu-Bonneau S, Sirois MJ, Savard J, Turgeon AF, Moore L, Swaine B, Roy J, Giguère M, Laviolette V. Depression in the first year after traumatic brain injury. J Neurotrauma. 2018;35(14):1620–9. https://doi.org/10.1089/neu.2017.5379.

Perry DC, Sturm VE, Peterson MJ, Pieper CF, Bullock T, Boeve BF, Miller BL, Guskiewicz KM, Berger MS, Kramer JH, Welsh-Bohmer KA. Association of traumatic brain injury with subsequent neurological and psychiatric disease: a meta-analysis. J Neurosurg. 2016;124(2):511–26. https://doi.org/10.3171/2015.2.JNS14503.

Price A, Rayner L, Okon-Rocha E, Evans A, Valsraj K, Higginson IJ, Hotopf M. Antidepressants for the treatment of depression in neurological disorders: a systematic review and meta-analysis of randomised controlled trials. J Neurol Neurosurg Psychiatry. 2011;82(8):914–23. https://doi.org/10.1136/jnnp.2010.230862.

Salter KL, McClure JA, Foley NC, Sequeira K, Teasell RW. Pharmacotherapy for depression posttraumatic brain injury: a meta-analysis. J Head Trauma Rehabil. 2016;31(4):E21–32. https://doi.org/10.1097/HTR.0000000000000193.

Tsai MC, Tsai KJ, Wang HK, Sung PS, Wu MH, Hung KW, Lin SH. Mood disorders after traumatic brain injury in adolescents and young adults: a nationwide population-based cohort study. J Pediatr. 2014;164(1):136–141.e1. https://doi.org/10.1016/j.jpeds.2013.08.042.

Wiart L, Luaute J, Stefan A, Plantier D, Hamonet J. Non pharmacological treatments for psychological and behavioural disorders following traumatic brain injury (TBI). A systematic literature review and expert opinion leading to recommendations. Ann Phys Rehabil Med. 2016;59(1):31–41. https://doi.org/10.1016/j.rehab.2015.12.001.

80 Neuropsychological Perspectives

Aniko Bartfai and Eirik Vikane

Recommendations

Level I

There are insufficient data to support a Level I recommendation for this topic.

Level II

Neuropsychological assessment, behavioral treatment, and cognitive rehabilitation after a severe TBI are recommended (American Congress of Rehabilitation Medicine, Brain Injury-Interdisciplinary Special Interest Group, Disorders of Consciousness Task Force, et al. 2010; Bayley et al. 2014; Schrijnemaekers et al. 2014).

Level III

There is limited evidence for pharmacological treatment of behavioral disturbances or other psychiatric symptoms (except major depressive disorders) in the later stage after a TBI (Anghinah et al. 2018; Hammond et al. 2017; Fann et al. 2017).

Tips, Tricks, and Pitfalls

- The principles of proactive intervention should permeate the whole hospital setting (physical environment, treatment philosophy, staff-patient relationship, and staff education) when treating patients with severe TBI.
- In the early stage, it is essential to provide the patients with a relatively quiet, structured environment where external stimulation can easily be regulated.
- When insight is severely impaired, patients might deny suffering an injury. Despite having obvious problems, they still might want to return to their home or work.

A. Bartfai (✉)
Division of Rehabilitation Medicine, Department of Clinical Sciences, Danderyd Hospital, Karolinska Institute, Stockholm, Sweden
e-mail: aniko.bartfai@ki.se

E. Vikane
Department of Physical Medicine and Rehabilitation, Haukeland University Hospital, Bergen, Norway
e-mail: eirik.vikane@helse-bergen.no

© Springer Nature Switzerland AG 2020
T. Sundstrøm et al. (eds.), *Management of Severe Traumatic Brain Injury*,
https://doi.org/10.1007/978-3-030-39383-0_80

80.1 Neuropsychological Perspectives on the Rehabilitation in the Early Stages After Severe Traumatic Brain Injury

In the early stage of recovery after severe TBI, patients, if responsive at all, exhibit changes in arousal, altered responsivity, behavioral disturbances, and psychiatric symptoms. For acute and chronic psychiatric conditions following TBI, see Chaps. 74 and 79, respectively. About a third of patients show impaired awareness, and about the same proportion might show agitated behavior and lack of insight into their injury. An essential early observation to describe these phenomena was Kurt Goldstein's description of "catastrophic anxiety," a state of altered consciousness, perception, and cognition (Goldstein 1952). Today, we know that a considerable proportion of disruptive, challenging behavior is related to problematic communication. Communication-related problems include verbal aggression, profanity, verbal outbursts, shouting, sexually inappropriate language, and sometimes physical aggression as a substitute for defective communication (Ylvisaker et al. 2007). In contrast, patients with negative symptoms, such as apathy, withdrawal, and passivity, are much less noticed and they in fact receive less attention regarding treatment. Behavioral interventions require specialized expertise. Thus, the task of a neuropsychologist in an acute TBI setting is fivefold:

1. Diagnosis (cognitive, emotional)
2. Therapeutic support to the patient
3. Planning and managing behavioral interventions, including teaching the other team members
4. Representing the neuropsychological perspective in teamwork, including supervision and teaching of staff
5. Providing support to the family

The principles of proactive intervention should permeate the whole hospital setting (physical environment, treatment philosophy, staff-patient relationship, and staff education) treating patients with acute severe TBI.

Measurements to characterize injury severity in the acute stage, such as the GCS, Reaction Level Scale (RLS), and Pediatric Trauma Score (PTS), are described in Chap. 7. The Center for Outcome Measurement in Brain Injury, COMBI (http://tbims.org/combi/), is an online resource regarding outcome measurement in brain injury rehabilitation. COMBI is a collaborative project of many brain injury centers in the United States. For each measure, rating forms in English, training information, and data on validity and reliability are provided along with a reference list of studies using the instrument. Some frequently used scales oriented toward characterization of functional cognitive status will be presented here.

For patients with post-traumatic amnesia (PTA), the Galveston Orientation and Amnesia Test (GOAT) was developed to evaluate cognition serially during the subacute stage of recovery (Levin et al. 1979). This practical scale measures orientation to person, place, time, and memory for events preceding and following the injury. The questions are rated with error points subtracted from 100. When the patient scores at least 75 points on the GOAT on 2 consecutive days, the period of PTA is considered ceased.

Disorders of consciousness (DOC) are discussed in detail in the chapter about minimally conscious and vegetative state.

80.1.1 Neuropsychological Assessments in the Early Stages After Moderate or Severe Brain Injury

There are wide variations in the behavioral effects of a brain injury. Treatment and rehabilitation need to be individually tailored for each patient. Neuropsychological evaluation in the early stage after injury aims to provide detailed information on the patient's cognitive status, resources, and limitations. The neuropsychological examination can be carried out while the patient is still in PTA if the patient can cooperate concerning other cognitive dimensions (e.g., concentration, communication, spatial abilities, learning of new information, and executive functions). However, the examination needs to be tailored considering the short attention span, high fatigability, motor, and other limitations. The traditional model of a neuropsychological assessment in an office with an extensive battery of standardized, psychometrically evaluated tests needs to be abandoned. For bedside assessment or early assessment in the ward, simple and flexible methods are needed. Luria's neuropsychological investigation, systematized by Anne-Lise Christensen, was developed with these requirements in mind (Christensen and Luria 1979).

Luria's basic approach, to evaluate systematically cognitive functions, starting with easy tasks and then to increase the complexity, can be utilized by using easier tasks presented in different textbooks. Lezak's neuropsychological assessment is a significant source for these kinds of tests (Lezak et al. 2012). Another book containing useful information is the handbook of Strub and Black providing a simplified explanation of examination procedures on assessment of level of consciousness, language, memory, and attention (Strub and Black 2000). Start with simple, straightforward tasks in each modality. Observe not only *what* the patient can do but also *how* the patient performs. This assessment situation is not aimed at establishing numerical data for performance and cognitive capacity, but as a base for treatment planning. How does the patient deal with the failure during the execution of an earlier easy task? Does the patient try to find other solutions or give up? What are the emotional reactions? It is crucial to guide the patient if the patient is unable to carry out the task. For rehabilitation, it is essential how the patient utilizes the provided cues. What kind of strengths can the patient rely on during the challenging period of recovery and rehabilitation? The examination procedure is based on hypothesis testing, recommended by both Luria and Edith Kaplan within the context of the Boston Process Approach (Christensen and Luria 1979; Casaletto and Heaton 2017; Kaplan 1988). This approach puts high demands on the clinical neuropsychologist. As Walsh puts it, the method requires the clinician to develop a frame of reference made up of two major elements: (1) familiarity with the current body of knowledge of neuropsychological findings and (2) personal experience of a wide range (Walsh 1995).

There are shorter fixed neuropsychological batteries for patients with more cognitive capacity, such as the *Repeatable Battery for the Assessment of Neuropsychological Status, RBANS*, a screening tool following head injury (Randolph et al. 1998). It is a standardized screening instrument for adults. The test provides the following measurements: immediate and delayed memory, visuospatial and constructional ability, attention, and language. It is comprised of 12 subtests that take approximately 30 min to administer. The RBANS is recommended for screening in an acute care setting and tracking recovery by conducting repeated measures.

For isolated syndromes, such as neglect, dysexecutive behavior, and impairment in everyday attention and memory, there are tests, which are more closely related to everyday problems. Occupational therapists can also use these tests. *The Behavioural Assessment of the Dysexecutive Syndrome (BADS*) includes tests for impairment in planning, organization, problem-solving, and attention (Evans et al. 1997). The test measures six cognitive areas: temporal judgment, mental flexibility, problem-solving, planning, strategy formation, and performance monitoring. Furthermore, the Dysexecutive Questionnaire (DEX) can be used to assess problem areas concerning personality, motivation, and behavioral problems. *The Rivermead Behavioural Memory Test* includes 14 subtests assessing aspects of visual, verbal, recall, recognition, and immediate and delayed everyday memory (Wills et al. 2000). Additionally, prospective memory skills and the ability to learn new information can be assessed. *The Behavioral Inattention Test* (BIT) is designed to assess the presence and the extent of visual neglect on a sample of everyday problems faced by patients with visual inattention (Halligan et al. 1990). *The Test of Everyday Attention (TEA)* is designed to measure three aspects of attentional functioning: selective and sustained attention and mental shifting (Robertson et al. 1996).

80.1.2 Behavioral Disturbances

Lack of insight—when insight is severely impaired, patients might deny suffering an injury. Despite having obvious problems, they might want to return to their home or work. There is also a risk for psychotic perceptions, psychotic symptoms, misunderstandings, and paranoid ideation. Patients are often restless and agitated and might try to pull out catheters. When able to walk around, they might wander into the rooms of other patients or leave the ward unit. Sexually disinhibited behavior is particularly challenging both for the staff and family. Other patients might also be at risk.

80.1.3 Management of Challenging Behavior in an Institutional Setting

Applied Behavior Analysis (ABA) is an applied form of behavior therapy to develop procedures of observable changes in behavior. The method has been used to modify behavior in persons with varying cognitive and communication capacities in connection with challenging behavior (Ylvisaker et al. 2007). Initially, the focus was more concentrated on sanctions, negative consequences of undesired behavior, or positive consequences of a behavioral change in the desired direction. Lately, the emphasis has shifted to proactive interventions to structure the environment and communication to minimize frustration and challenging behavior, i.e., method of positive behavior interventions and support (PBIS) (Ylvisaker et al. 2007).

Ylvisaker and his co-workers summarize the active elements of this approach:

1. Specifically planned environmental structuring
2. Proactive adjustment of tasks and expectations
3. Provision of meaningful and well-understood daily routines (possibly including external graphic organizers to ensure orientation to tasks, schedules, and habits)
4. Assurance of adequate amount of choice and control
5. Engagement in personally meaningful activities
6. Exercising with desired people
7. Planned development of positive behavioral momentum before difficult tasks
8. Assurance of errorless learning with proper antecedent supports/prompts
9. Planned guarantee of positive, supportive communication from communication partners
10. Development of positive communication alternatives to negative behavior (Bayley et al. 2014)

Ylvisaker and co-workers conclude that behavioral intervention in general should be considered a practice guideline for behavior problems after TBI affecting both children and adults, both in the acute and post-acute stages of recovery. Individuals with challenging behavior after TBI should be provided with systematically organized behavioral interventions and support, consistent with the available evidence based on individualized functional behavior assessments.

80.1.4 General Considerations for the Rehabilitation Setting

In the early stage, it is essential to provide the patients with a relatively quiet, structured environment where external stimulation can easily be managed. Structuring the environment assists in regaining orientation to place, time, and person. Single rooms or stable partitions from other patients are recommended, along with clear and easy signs on doors to identify who is staying in which room or functionality, such as the bath. A large calendar on the wall showing the current date and dimming lights overnight might assist in regaining orientation to time. A few large photographs of the most important persons in the patient's life provide a connection to the past and identity, mainly if nursing and treatment staff utilizes this information in their daily work and interaction with the patient. A few emotionally relevant objects might also be helpful. However, avoid the clutter of many things around the patient, and store gifts from visitors. For the patient to remember this critical period in life, a simple notebook can be introduced. Family and visitors could be encouraged to document a visit or note events the patient might have been interested in or want to participate in, had he/she been in good health. Generous visiting hours are recommended.

Similar principles should apply for the design of the entire ward. Digital locks to open entrance doors might be an easy way to limit disoriented patients to the ward. The codes are available to everybody, but some cognitive skills are required for their use. The day a patient can apply the code, usually, the patient is also responsible and oriented to behave safely. Noise, clutter, and distracting or dangerous objects need to be avoided and handled by the staff in a safe manner. Clear floor plans and proximity to training areas for physiotherapy and occupational therapy facilitate spatial learning and memory, enabling increased independence.

Limited attention span, poor memory, and cognitive and physical fatigability put strong time constraints on rehabilitation. In the inpatient setting, short, repeated training sessions are recommended. Regular routines for scheduling 30- or 45-min rehabilitation sessions often exceed capacity. On the other hand, with training hours between 9 AM–4 PM, the afternoons and evenings are very long for restless, disoriented patients needing external stimuli for structure. Transdisciplinary teamwork, where occupational therapists and physiotherapists teach and delegate rehabilitation exercises to nurses or nurse's aides, might allow the scheduling of short training sessions. Repetitive sessions also promote learning.

80.1.5 Considerations for Staff Support and Education

In the inpatient rehabilitation phase after severe TBI, nurses and nurse's aides are closest to the patient. They play an essential role and spend the most time with the patient. However, nurses and foremost nurse's aides have significant variations in training concerning TBI. Motor impairments might necessitate assistance in personal care, and the presence of cognitive and communication impairments often require adjustments in the typical care process. Care plans need to be adjusted following the patients difficulties. Difficulties with communication, comprehension, and memory require other strategies like more written information and repeated oral information. Patients and their significant others seek information from nurses regarding unusual behavior, need for care, and expectations for recovery. It is essential that nurses and nurse aides provide correct information (Oyesanya et al. 2017). The staff also needs to be familiar with concepts, such as disinhibition of behavior, emotional dyscontrol, neglect, and different forms of communication problems.

Thus, staff education is essential and currently, given the shortage and significant turnover in hospital staff, a never-ending task. Routine continuing education and team supervision is crucial. At the Clinic of Rehabilitation Medicine, Danderyd University Hospital, Stockholm, Sweden, there is a model for continuing education for the staff on the inpatient ward. An ongoing course, where classes are given once a month, during each academic year. It is organized locally, and clinical staff, physicians and representatives of each profession in the rehabilitation team serve as instructors. A small, practical examination is given at the end of each course.

TBI often places new demands for the patient regarding personal care and skills of daily living. Hemiplegia and impaired motor coordination require new strategies and skills in personal care in a situation where cognitive capacity is limited for new learning. The patient needs to get acquainted with new routines on the ward, learn new names, and learn how to find their way in the ward and in training areas while being confused and having a restricted attention span and inadequate capacity for new learning.

Among the more successful techniques for teaching information for patients with moderate or severe TBI, is the technique of errorless learning. The basic idea is to enable the encoding of new information, learning without error.

To achieve this, patients are given correct information at each learning occasion (Tailby and Haslam 2003). This method is often counterintuitive to hospital staff, who are used to other problem-solving techniques currently applied in the school system. To allow a patient to guess an answer (e.g., "What is my name?") makes the task more difficult. Guessing results in conflicting information and hampers new learning. The proper procedure for the staff is to give the correct answer immediately (e.g. "My name is Daisy."). Research shows that elaborating an answer is helpful (e.g. "Daisy, like the flower."). After several occasions, the clues can be shortened (e.g., "My name is Dai…."), and later even less information is given (e.g., "My name starts with a D." and so on). The advantages of errorless learning have been repeatedly documented for patients with severe memory impairment. The method can be successfully applied for skill learning. Adherence to apply this technique needs a lot of effort from the staff and requires both education concerning the rationale of the method and support during everyday work, as an essential part of staff education.

80.2 Neuropsychological Perspectives on the Long-Term Outcome After Severe Traumatic Brain Injury

80.2.1 General Considerations

In contrast with earlier expectations about the static long-term nature of the disability for a person after a moderate or severe TBI, recent longitudinal studies show that the brain injury initiates fluctuations in the functional status during the whole lifetime (Hart et al. 2018). Moreover, a third of this population declines in function within a 10-year perspective (Corrigan and Hammond 2013). Thus, TBI should be treated as a chronic condition and should be managed as such with appropriate self-management and competent support to prevent deterioration during lifetime (Hart et al. 2018).

Generally, in health care, the focus on management of chronic conditions has shifted to self-management training involving teaching and internalization of personal responsibility. In practical terms, self-management requires problem-solving, decision-making, establishing goals, planning, and cooperating with health-care providers—requiring the very same cognitive and executive functions which are often impaired after TBI. These problems would automatically disqualify brain injury patients from participation in self-management. However, there are considerable variations in the type and level of impairments in higher cognitive functions, and the resources and motivation of an individual patient should be taken into account to a greater extent, than customary in today's praxis. We have recently found that chronic patients after moderate acquired brain injury regarded themselves as personally responsible, even if the action was carried out by another person (Markovic et al. 2018). Thus, increased self-management seems to be a possibility in this patient group, but the method needs significant adjustments (Corrigan and Hammond 2013).

Although the comprehensive health-care systems in the Scandinavian countries extend in to the chronic phase after a TBI, several studies have found that the patient's immediate family, spouses, and parents carry a heavy load in daily life (Manskow et al. 2015; Doser and Norup 2016). Results indicate that not only the severity of the injury is associated with increased caregiver burden, but also unmet needs for the caregiver are important for the experience of burden. Feelings of loneliness, dysexecutive functioning, lack of social network, and depression are other contributing factors that may increase caregiver burden. There are some differences in the reaction pattern between spouses and parents to a TBI patient. Spouses face a significant change in roles for the whole family, while parents might have to slip back into an unexpected and unwanted role of renewed parenting. Studies indicate that over a more extended time range, spouses were more distressed and depressed (Manskow et al. 2015).

Based on clinical observation and examination, pharmacological treatment may be an option in addition to behavioral treatment for behavioral disturbances or other psychiatric symptoms in the later stage after a TBI. The treatment follows the same principles as in the earlier stages described in earlier chapters, with the main principle "start low, go slow." Single studies demonstrate promising results of amantadine on decreasing aggression and to improve functional outcome after a TBI (Hammond et al. 2017; Liepert 2016). Selective serotonin reuptake inhibitors are widely used for major depression after a TBI, but pharmacological studies demonstrate conflicting results on efficacy (Fann et al. 2017). Due to evidence still being limited, there is a need for research on the effectiveness of pharmacological treatment in the later stages after a TBI (Fann et al. 2017).

80.2.2 Behavioral Outcome and Rehabilitation

There is a wide variation in the outcome after moderate to severe brain injury. Generally, factors that influence the outcome after TBI are admission GCS, age, educational level, duration of PTA, and length of stay in the intensive care unit (Ludin and Rashid 2018). Improved neurosurgical procedures and developments in acute care have contributed to a more favorable outcome. Occasionally, patients do recover to a great extent, having only mild cognitive problems, such as decreased mental energy, mental fatigue, and concentration difficulties, but the major part of patients with moderate to severe brain injury do exhibit motor, cognitive, or behavioral symptoms. In the Scandinavian countries, the majority of patients receive rehabilitation during the first year after TBI when recovery is at its fastest. Access to rehabilitation is limited after the early years following a TBI, although studies have shown that patients after moderate and severe TBI (including older patients) can make significant, meaningful improvements beyond the acute phase of recovery (Rosenbaum et al. 2018).

Methods for remediation of impairment in cognitive functions can be grouped in two major categories: (1) the use of compensatory techniques, such as memory books, and (2) cognitive training of specific cognitive areas, such as training of attention or language. In compensatory training the underlying assumption is that the function level of the impaired cognitive domain can be elevated by using different strategies.

A strategy can be internal or external. An example of an internal memory strategy would be creating a categorized list in your mind, for example, before going to the grocery store. Placing the different groceries in different groups according to some principle, like vegetables, dairy products, hygiene products, etc., would make them easier to remember. One external memory strategy would be to write a shopping list at home and take it to the store.

Cognitive training of specific areas, such as working memory, attention, or language, is a hierarchic training based on cognitive theory. The training is goal-oriented and measurable, and goals and subgoals are also organized in a hierarchic order. A successful practice should also contain elements of generalization to everyday situations. The above distinction is frequently used for pedagogical purposes, but in reality, both approaches contain elements from one of the other. Compensatory strategies require the learning of new compensatory method or the use of assistive technology (Bartfai and Boman 2014). Cognitive training, on the other hand, involves the training of strategies for everyday situations (Toglia 1991).

80.2.3 Cognitive Training

Cognitive training is resource-intensive, and 15–20 1-h individual training sessions within a 5–6-week period are required as a minimum. A neuropsychologist, occupational therapist, or speech and language therapist usually performs it. These methods are relatively new and also need an intensive teaching program for the therapists. For TBI, an international group of researchers and clinicians has provided specific instructions (INCOG guidelines) for further clinical praxis implementation (Bayley et al. 2014). One interactive program, Goal Management Training, has demonstrated some promising results to improve emotional regulation skills and executive functions after a TBI (Tornas et al. 2016; Stamenova and Levine 2018). Computer-assisted cognitive training methods have been developed for some functions, such as working memory and language training (Spencer-Smith and Klingberg 2015; Des Roches and Kiran 2017). Bogdanova and colleagues summarize the positive results in their review (Bogdanova et al. 2016). An essential feature of computer-based cognitive training is the need of regular personal coaching.

80.2.4 Assistive Technology for Compensating Cognitive Impairment

The use of assistive technology to compensate cognitive impairment has a long tradition in the Scandinavian countries. Examples are timers for electric stoves, reminders to turn off running water, locks to entrance doors, and similar safety features at home (Boman et al. 2010). Mobile devices can assist persons with moderate to severe cognitive impairments to increase independency outside the home environment (Leopold et al. 2015). Finding a suitable device, teaching the use, and providing the patient with assistive devices are the tasks of the occupational therapist. The rapid technological development has created a lot of products, which could be used for assistive purposes. However, persons with brain injury often have concomitant problems to use these new functionalities and require still extensive training or simplified solutions.

80.2.5 Neuropsychological Assessments in the Late Stages After Moderate to Severe Brain Injury

GCS describes only the patient's initial status after brain injury. Glasgow Outcome Scale (GOS) and its extended version (GOS-E) are the most frequently used outcome measures in TBI research and clinical praxis. These are recommended due to advantages of brevity, modest requirement for assessor training, and high reliability. However, they exhibit a ceiling effect, particularly in the region of mild to moderate cognitive impairment. Current studies recommend the use of additional neuropsychological measures (as described earlier in this chapter). There is also the possibility to use larger, psychometrically more evaluated batteries, such as the Wechsler Adult Intelligence Scales and Wechsler Memory Scales (Lezak et al. 2012). In Sweden, the use of the Wechsler scales is mandatory, as a basis for a decision for publicly supported personal assistance.

80.2.6 Support and Education for Family and Carers

As mentioned earlier, the immediate family, parents, and spouses carry a lifelong burden. Patients with a moderate and severe brain injury might also require additional external support in daily living involving many external carers simultaneously, sometimes in 24/7 shifts. Laws and regulations vary in the Scandinavian countries, but the common denominator is that external carers have widely differing educational backgrounds and knowledge within the field of brain injury and require information and education. Carers also change very frequently. Thus, support and education for significant others is a complicated matter. Some help and education for families and carers is provided during the discharge phase of rehabilitation and also some outpatient settings. The extent of this support is largely depending on the organization of care in the different countries. However, the patients' need for continuity and flexibility in the services delivered is rarely met. Systematic educational programs are rare, although some studies have indicated beneficial effects on outcome. Long-distance communication on the telephone or the Internet should be utilized to a greater extent as proven by a recent Australian study (Lorig et al. 2013).

References

American Congress of Rehabilitation Medicine, Brain Injury-Interdisciplinary Special Interest Group, Disorders of Consciousness Task Force, Seel RT, Sherer M, Whyte J, Katz DI, Giacino JT, et al. Assessment scales for disorders of consciousness: evidence-based recommendations for clinical practice and research. Arch Phys Med Rehabil. 2010;91(12):1795–813.

Anghinah R, Amorim RLO, Paiva WS, Schmidt MT, Ianof JN. Traumatic brain injury pharmacological treatment: recommendations. Arq Neuropsiquiatr. 2018;76(2):100–3.

Bartfai A, Boman I-L. A multiprofessional client-centered guide to implementing assistive technology for clients with cognitive impairments. Technol Disabil. 2014;26(1):11–21.

Bayley MT, Tate R, Douglas JM, Turkstra LS, Ponsford J, Stergiou-Kita M, et al. INCOG guidelines for cognitive rehabilitation following traumatic brain injury: methods and overview. J Head Trauma Rehabil. 2014;29(4):290–306.

Bogdanova Y, Yee MK, Ho VT, Cicerone KD. Computerized cognitive rehabilitation of attention and executive function in acquired brain injury: a systematic review. J Head Trauma Rehabil. 2016;31(6):419–33.

Boman IL, Lindberg Stenvall C, Hemmingsson H, Bartfai A. A training apartment with a set of electronic memory aids for patients with cognitive problems. Scand J Occup Ther. 2010;17(2):140–8.

Casaletto KB, Heaton RK. Neuropsychological assessment: past and future. J Int Neuropsychol Soc. 2017;23(9–10):778–90.

Christensen A-L, Luria AR. Luria's neuropsychological investigation (text). Kopenhagen: Munksgaard; 1979.

Corrigan JD, Hammond FM. Traumatic brain injury as a chronic health condition. Arch Phys Med Rehabil. 2013;94(6):1199–201.

Des Roches CA, Kiran S. Technology-based rehabilitation to improve communication after acquired brain injury. Front Neurosci. 2017;11:382.

Doser K, Norup A. Caregiver burden in Danish family members of patients with severe brain injury: the chronic phase. Brain Inj. 2016;30(3):334–42.

Evans JJ, Chua SE, McKenna PJ, Wilson BA. Assessment of the dysexecutive syndrome in schizophrenia. Psychol Med. 1997;27(3):635–46.

Fann JR, Bombardier CH, Temkin N, Esselman P, Warms C, Barber J, et al. Sertraline for major depression during the year following traumatic brain injury: a randomized controlled trial. J Head Trauma Rehabil. 2017;32(5):332–42.

Goldstein K. The effect of brain damage on the personality. Psychiatry. 1952;15(3):245–60.

Halligan P, Wilson B, Cockburn J. A short screening test for visual neglect in stroke patients. Int Disabil Stud. 1990;12(3):95–9.

Hammond FM, Malec JF, Zafonte RD, Sherer M, Bogner J, Dikmen S, et al. Potential impact of amantadine on aggression in chronic traumatic brain injury. J Head Trauma Rehabil. 2017;32(5):308–18.

Hart T, Driver S, Sander A, Pappadis M, Dams-O'Connor K, Bocage C, et al. Traumatic brain injury education for adult patients and families: a scoping review. Brain Inj. 2018;32(11):1295–306.

Kaplan E. A process approach to neuropsychological assessment. In: Boll T, Bryant BK, editors. Clinical neuropsychology and brain function: research, measurement, and practice. Washington, DC: American Psychological Association; 1988. p. 125–67.

Leopold A, Lourie A, Petras H, Elias E. The use of assistive technology for cognition to support the performance of daily activities for individuals with cognitive disabilities due to traumatic brain injury: the current state of the research. NeuroRehabilitation. 2015;37(3):359–78.

Levin HS, O'Donnell VM, Grossman RG. The Galveston Orientation and Amnesia Test. A practical scale to assess cognition after head injury. J Nerv Ment Dis. 1979;167(11):675–84.

Lezak M, Howieson D, Bigler E, Tranel D. Neuropsychological assessment. 5th ed. New York: Oxford University Press; 2012.

Liepert J. Update on pharmacotherapy for stroke and traumatic brain injury recovery during rehabilitation. Curr Opin Neurol. 2016;29(6):700–5.

Lorig K, Ritter PL, Plant K, Laurent DD, Kelly P, Rowe S. The South Australia health chronic disease self-management Internet trial. Health Educ Behav. 2013;40(1):67–77.

Manskow US, Sigurdardottir S, Roe C, Andelic N, Skandsen T, Damsgard E, et al. Factors affecting caregiver burden 1 year after severe traumatic brain injury: a prospective Nationwide Multicenter Study. J Head Trauma Rehabil. 2015;30(6):411–23.

Markovic G, Bartfai A, Ekholm J, Nilsson C, Schult ML, Lofgren M. Daily management of attention dysfunction two-four years after brain injury and early cognitive rehabilitation with attention process training: a qualitative study. Neuropsychol Rehabil. 2018;27:1–22.

Ludin MS and Rashid AN. Functional outcomes and health-related quality of life after severe traumatic brain injury: a review. Clin Nurs Res. 2018:1054773818792459.

Oyesanya TO, Brown RL, Turkstra LS. Caring for patients with traumatic brain injury: a survey of nurses' perceptions. J Clin Nurs. 2017;26(11–12):1562–74.

Randolph C, Tierney MC, Mohr E, Chase TN. The Repeatable Battery for the Assessment of Neuropsychological Status (RBANS): preliminary clinical validity. J Clin Exp Neuropsychol. 1998;20(3):310–9.

Robertson IH, Ward T, Ridgeway V, Nimmo-Smith I. The structure of normal human attention: the test of everyday attention. J Int Neuropsychol Soc. 1996;2(6):525–34.

Rosenbaum AM, Gordon WA, Joannou A, Berman BA. Functional outcomes following post-acute rehabilitation for moderate-to-severe traumatic brain injury. Brain Inj. 2018;32(7):907–14.

Schrijnemaekers AC, Smeets SM, Ponds RW, van Heugten CM, Rasquin S. Treatment of unawareness of deficits in patients with acquired brain injury: a systematic review. J Head Trauma Rehabil. 2014;29(5):E9–E30.

Spencer-Smith M, Klingberg T. Benefits of a working memory training program for inattention in daily life: a systematic review and meta-analysis. PLoS One. 2015;10(3):e0119522.

Stamenova V, Levine B. Effectiveness of goal management training (R) in improving executive functions: a meta-analysis. Neuropsychol Rehabil. 2018;29(10):1569–99.

Strub R, Black W. The mental status examination in neurology. 4th ed. Philadelphia: F. A. Davis; 2000.

Tailby R, Haslam C. An investigation of errorless learning in memory-impaired patients: improving the technique and clarifying theory. Neuropsychologia. 2003;41(9):1230–40.

Toglia JP. Generalization of treatment: a multicontext approach to cognitive perceptual impairment in adults with brain injury. Am J Occup Ther. 1991;45(6):505–16.

Tornas S, Lovstad M, Solbakk AK, Schanke AK, Stubberud J. Goal management training combined with external cuing as a means to improve emotional regulation, psychological functioning, and quality of life in patients with acquired brain injury: a randomized controlled trial. Arch Phys Med Rehabil. 2016;97(11):1841–52.e3.

Walsh KW. A hypothesis-testing approach to assessment. In: Mapou RL, Spector J, editors. Clinical neuropsychological assessment. Critical issues in neuropsychology. Boston: Springer; 1995.

Wills P, Clare L, Shiel A, Wilson BA. Assessing subtle memory impairments in the everyday memory performance of brain injured people: exploring the potential of the extended Rivermead Behavioural Memory Test. Brain Inj. 2000;14(8):693–704.

Ylvisaker M, Turkstra L, Coehlo C, Yorkston K, Kennedy M, Sohlberg MM, et al. Behavioural interventions for children and adults with behaviour disorders after TBI: a systematic review of the evidence. Brain Inj. 2007;21(8):769–805.

81 Neurosurgical Challenges

Jussi P. Posti

> **Tips, Tricks and Pitfalls**
> - Syndrome of the trephined is often reversed by cranioplasty. Cranioplasty performed within 3 months after decompressive hemicraniectomy may further enhance recovery.
> - In patients treated with decompressive hemicraniectomy, post-traumatic hydrocephalus should be managed with cranioplasty and case-dependently, with or without shunting with adjustable or gravity-controlled devices.
> - Synthetic implants should be preferred in cranioplasty. Autologous bone should not be used in young patients and smokers and in case of a fracture in the bone flap.

81.1 Subacute Phase Complications

Recommendation

Level I

There are insufficient data to support a Level I recommendation for this topic.

Level II

There are insufficient data to support a Level II recommendation for this topic.

Level III

There are insufficient data to support a Level III recommendation for this topic.

Patients with severe traumatic brain injury (TBI) present diverse subacute phase complications that may necessitate neurosurgical attention. The most commonly occurring matters are syndrome of the trephined (SOT), post-traumatic hydrocephalus (PTH) and post-traumatic cerebrospinal fluid (CSF) fistulae. They may already develop during the initial hospital stay following TBI, but not unfrequently, patients are referred to a neurosurgical centre presenting with late-onset post-traumatic hydrocephalus or subtle and long-lasting cerebrospinal fluid (CSF) leakage from the nose or ear.

81.1.1 Syndrome of the Trephined

SOT, "sinking skin flap syndrome" or "paradoxical herniation" (Choi et al. 2011; Joseph and Reilly 2009), is a condition observed in some neurosurgical patients who have undergone decompressive craniectomy (DC), see Chap. 26. The condition is most often described in male

J. P. Posti (✉)
Clinical Neurosciences, Department of Neurosurgery and Turku Brain Injury Centre, Turku University Hospital and University of Turku, Turku, Finland
e-mail: jussi.posti@utu.fi

© Springer Nature Switzerland AG 2020
T. Sundstrøm et al. (eds.), *Management of Severe Traumatic Brain Injury*,
https://doi.org/10.1007/978-3-030-39383-0_81

patients after TBI, manifesting as an unexplained neurological and cognitive decline (Ashayeri et al. 2016). SOT was first described by Grant and Norcross in 1939 as an aggregate symptom comprising headache, dizziness, pain/discomfort at the DC site, apprehension and/or mental depression (Grant and Norcross 1939). The condition was first thought to be psychiatric in nature and caused by the open cranial vault. During the following decades, SOT has been redefined many times. Along with cognitive and motor deficits, delayed dysautonomic syndrome (Romero et al. 2013), levodopa-resistant parkinsonian symptoms (Bijlenga et al. 2007), midbrain syndrome with eye movement disorders (Gottlob et al. 2002), disturbed and altered sensory functions (Joseph and Reilly 2009), orthostatic headaches (Mokri 2010) and impaired speech and language function (Hagan and Bradley 2017) have all been reported to be a part of the syndrome.

Ashayeri et al. reported in a recent systemic review article (Ashayeri et al. 2016) that SOT can be identified as a composition of symptoms including three main components: (1) long-term neurological deficits usually beginning weeks to months after craniectomy, (2) presentation not depending on the location of the lesion and (3) clinical improvement after subsequent cranioplasty (CP). SOT has been associated with a long interval between DC and CP and with larger bone defect size, but the findings show unreliable consistency in relation to symptom onset and clinical improvement (Ashayeri et al. 2016; Jeyaraj 2015; Paredes et al. 2015). It has been proposed that the effect of atmospheric pressure on reduced CSF flow, decreased cerebral perfusion and disturbed glucose metabolism constitute the syndrome (Ashayeri et al. 2016). Figure 81.1 shows a patient case with SOT.

The severity of the symptoms usually fluctuates, and the incidence of the syndrome in patients treated with DC has been reported to vary between 1 and 24% (Honeybul 2010; Sedney et al. 2016). Based on clinical experience, it is likely that the syndrome is underdiagnosed. SOT is important to recognise, because it usually indicates the need for an earlier CP to reverse the debilitating symptoms and improve the eventual outcome (Coelho et al. 2014; Di Stefano et al. 2016; Posti et al. 2018). Ashayeri et al. concluded that the syndrome commonly occurs in male patients at 5.1 ± 10.8 months after DC with defect ranging from 88.3 ± 34.4 cm^2 with improvement within 3.8 ± 3.9 days after CP (Ashayeri et al. 2016).

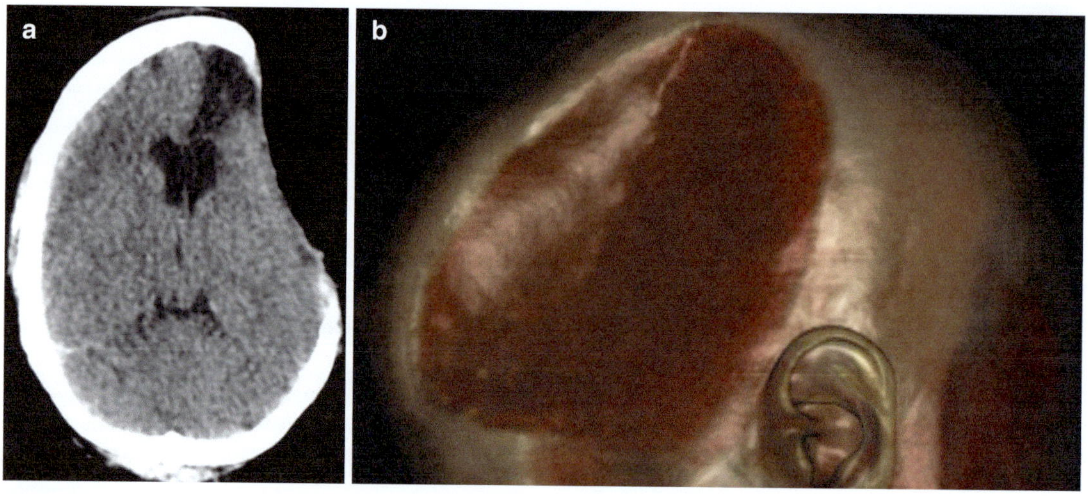

Fig. 81.1 Forty-two-year-old man with a history of primary decompressive craniectomy due to traumatic brain injury before cranioplasty exhibiting typical syndrome of the trephined. The bone flap was left out after evacuation of subdural haematoma. Cognitive deficits and speech impairment were partially reversed after cranioplasty. (**a**) Axial CT scan showing a left-sided sinking flap and chronic phase of frontobasal injury, (**b**) 3D reconstruction of the CT scan

81.1.2 Post-traumatic Hydrocephalus

PTH is an excess accumulation of intraventricular CSF following TBI. Up to half of the patients who have sustained TBI may develop PTH (Kowalski et al. 2018). In patients treated with DC, the incidence of PTH has been reported to be up to 36% (Vedantam et al. 2017). It has been demonstrated that DC after TBI is associated with development of PTH especially in paediatric patients (Fattahian et al. 2018). However, the association of PTH with DC has been challenged (Rahme et al. 2010).

The diagnosis of PTH is based on a combination of clinical characteristics and ventricular enlargement. Neither one alone is satisfactory for diagnosis, because signs and symptoms may be difficult to distinguish from the presentation of the injury per se, and ventricular enlargement may be due to a compensatory widening after loss of brain parenchyma. PTH most commonly occurs in the first few months after injury. Kammersgaard et al. found that 25% of patients were diagnosed within 2 weeks, 50% within 3 weeks and 75% within 8 weeks of rehabilitation (Kammersgaard et al. 2013). Denes and colleagues presented a mean time for CSF diversion of 80 days (range 20–270 days) after TBI in a similar series of patients (Denes et al. 2011). A gradual decline in functional status during the first months of the rehabilitation phase, coupled with a progressive ventricular enlargement shown on repeat computed tomography (CT) scans, is key to the diagnosis of PTH.

The acute presentation of PTH causing elevated intracranial pressure may also include papilloedema, headache, seizures and deteriorating neurological status during the subacute recovery phase of TBI (Denes et al. 2011; Kammersgaard et al. 2013; Li et al. 2008). However, PTH does not necessarily cause elevated ICP and does not associate with gait disturbance, urinary incontinence or dementia observed in normal pressure hydrocephalus (Kammersgaard et al. 2013; Tribl and Oder 2000).

Careful selection of patients benefiting from a ventriculoperitoneal shunt is important, as the procedure is associated with significant complications. It has been reported that earlier CSF diversion is associated with improved recovery in patients with PTH (Kowalski et al. 2018). However, there are no evidence-based guidelines on CSF diversion in patients with PTH. Based on our experience, adjustable or gravitation-regulated devices are the preferred choice for CSF diversion to reduce the risk of overdrainage. There are contradictory reports on the benefit of endoscopic third ventriculostomy in management of PTH (De Bonis et al. 2013; Singh et al. 2008). It has also been suggested to avoid CSF diversion in patients treated with DC, because CP reliably improves CSF dynamics and may reverse verticulomegaly (Ashayeri et al. 2016).

81.1.3 Post-traumatic CSF Fistulae

Traumatic nasal CSF fistulae result from a dural and arachnoidal disruption and are most often found in association with a frontal sinus, sphenoid sinus, ethmoid bone, cribriform plate and sphenoethmoid recess fractures (Banks et al. 2009; Friedman et al. 2001; Prosser et al. 2011) that communicate with the nasal cavity and paranasal sinuses. CSF leakage into middle ear or from the ear typically occurs in association with fractures of petrous part of the temporal bone. In case of a temporal fracture extending from the greater wing of the sphenoid to the sphenoid sinus, rhinorrhoea may also occur (Friedman et al. 2001; Oh et al. 2017).

Leakage of CSF from the nose or ear can result in meningitis or intracranial abscess if left untreated. A traumatic fistula may also be detected by intracranial air on CT, with or without post-traumatic leakage of CSF, and be manifested by intracranial infection after basal skull fracture. Post-traumatic CSF leakage usually begins within 2 days following TBI. The late-onset leakage may be defined as a presentation at least 1 week after TBI (Oh et al. 2017). The incidence of post-traumatic CSF leakage that occurs years after TBI is unknown, but may be higher than is generally recognised. The rate of meningitis associated with persistent CSF leakage is reported to be 7–30%, and the rate increases over time if the leakage continues (Friedman et al. 2001).

Management of CSF leakage is variable and remains somewhat controversial. Conservative management is commonly advocated because 28–85% of traumatic CSF leaks will be spontaneously blocked (Bell et al. 2004; Friedman et al. 2001; Mincy 1966). The mechanism behind the spontaneous block is usually coagulated blood or inflammatory adhesions at the site of the meningeal disruption and associated skull fracture (Friedman et al. 2001). The efficacy of prophylactic antibiotics is controversial and is currently not supported by the latest Cochrane systematic review (Ratilal et al. 2015). Management of CSF leakage usually begins conservatively with bed rest. If the leakage is not resolved within 24 h, an intervention should be considered. The site of leakage should be detected using a thin-slice CT scan. As a first-tier therapy, we advocate the use of lumbar drainage in case of small non-displaced fractures following blunt trauma and in case of late-onset CSF leakage. If the leakage is not resolved with lumbar drainage within days, or if the fracture site suggests a high risk that leakage will continue, surgical treatment should be undertaken.

81.2 Cranioplasty

Recommendations

Level I

There are insufficient data to support a Level I recommendation for this topic.

Level II

There are insufficient data to support a Level II recommendation for this topic.

Level III

There are insufficient data to support a Level III recommendation for this topic.

81.2.1 Introduction

Cranial reconstruction (CP) is a common neurosurgical procedure with a high complication rate with infection being the commonest complication (De Bonis et al. 2012; Piitulainen et al. 2015a). Although CP is considered a routine procedure, it is associated with significant morbidity in some patients: complication rates of 10–40% have been reported, often leading to reoperations, long-term antibiotic treatment, increased need for rehabilitation and poor neurological recovery (Bobinski et al. 2013; Coulter et al. 2014; Halani et al. 2017; Piitulainen et al. 2015b). The number of CPs is increasing due to the utilisation of DC in the neurosurgical emergency setting. During the first decade after the millennium shift, CPs are performed in 20–25 per 1,000,000 inhabitants per year in Europe, the Middle East and Asia (Servadei 2011).

In the procedure, the cranium is repaired by returning the previously removed autologous bone flap or by placing a synthetic implant in the bony defect area. A successful CP will restore the contour of the cranium and cosmesis, protect the brain and restore the physiological ICP, CSF flow and cerebral metabolism (Ashayeri et al. 2016; Coelho et al. 2014; Di Stefano et al. 2016). CP also prevents hemisphere collapses and midline displacements. A recent systematic review suggests that cerebral perfusion is decreased after DC and CP significantly improves cerebral perfusion (Halani et al. 2017).

CP is reported to improve cognitive, language and motor performance and thus the procedure is important for patients who suffer from the sequela of severe TBI and DC (Malcolm et al. 2017; Sakamoto et al. 2006; Shahid et al. 2017; Stiver et al. 2008). Cognitive and neurological deficits occur typically in patients with severe TBI after DC (Ashayeri et al. 2016), and due to the serious nature of the condition, patients with severe TBI are also prone to develop surgical complications after CP. It is generally accepted that CP is advocated for patients treated with DC, because CP improves functional outcome, but there is a lack of consensus about selection of patients for cranial reconstruction (Halani et al. 2017). It has recently been reported in a relatively small cohort that a successful CP predicts favourable functional outcome 1 year after the procedure, and the rate of major complications was not affected by the neurological state of a patient at the time of CP (Posti et al. 2018).

However, some patients appear unfit for CP due to poor recovery, and often there are concerns of causing additional harm with surgery to a patient with unfavourable outcome. Furthermore, selection of materials and timing of CP are a part of the complex clinical decision-making related to the procedure.

81.2.2 Materials

The choice of CP material has received substantial interest as a potential modifiable risk factor (Korhonen et al. 2018; Piitulainen et al. 2015b; Schwarz et al. 2016; Yadla et al. 2011). Despite the common prevalence of the procedure in the neurosurgical practice, there is still no clear consensus regarding the most appropriate material to be used.

The choice of material is usually done at discretion of a surgical team, single surgeon or institution consensus based on the patient clinical characteristics or implant costs. Theoretically, the ideal material for CP should possess many favourable characteristics. It should not conduct heat or trigger inflammatory responses and should also be biocompatible and biologically inert, radiolucent, lightweight, osteoinductive and osteoconductive and mechanically strong. Furthermore, the material should be suitable for custom design to perfectly cover the bony deficit and provide acceptable cosmesis (Zanotti et al. 2016).

Most commonly, cryopreserved autologous bone is utilised in cranial reconstruction, but a variety of synthetic materials has been introduced. In a recent systematic review comprising 2 randomised, 14 prospective and 212 retrospective studies, after autologous bone flap (32%), the most commonly utilised materials were titanium (18%), polymethyl methacrylate (PMMA) (16%), hydroxyapatite (HA) (9%) and polyether ether ketone (PEEK) (2%), while in 23% of the procedures, other synthetic materials were used (van de Vijfeijken et al. 2018).

There is a multitude of prospective and retrospective studies on different CP implant materials. The single-material and single-surgeon series often present results that are strikingly good, but larger cohorts including multiple materials or more than one centre present higher complication rates.

Table 81.1 demonstrates summary properties of autologous bone, HA, titanium, PMMA and PEEK in the context of CP. Glass fibre-reinforced

Table 81.1 Summary of common materials utilised in cranioplasty

	AB	HA	Ti	PMMA	PEEK	FRC–BG
Biocompatibility	Yes	Yes	Yes	Yes	Yes	Yes
Osteointegration/osteoconduction	Yes	Yes	No[a]	No[a]	No[a]	Yes
Durability	Good	Moderate	Good	Good	Good	Good
Aesthetic outcome	Good[b]	Good	Moderate[c]	Good	Good	Good
Infection rate	Moderate	Low	Low	High	Low	Low[d]
Paediatric usage	Yes	Yes	Possibly	No	No	Yes
Radiolucency	Yes	Yes	No	Yes	Yes	Yes
Resterilisation	Possibly	No	Yes	No	No	No
Toxicity	No	No	Possible	Possible	No	No
Literature	Wide	Wide	Wide	Wide[e]	Narrow	Minimal

AB autologous bone, *HA* hydroxyapatite, *Ti* titanium, *PMMA* polymethyl methacrylate, *PEEK* polyether ether ketone, *FRC-BG* glass fibre-reinforced composite–bioactive glass

[a]May exhibit some fibrous tissue ingrowth or bone formation at the implant margins

[b]Aesthetic result may be compromised by bone resorption

[c]Aesthetic result may be compromised by heat and cold conduction properties

[d]Minimal body of literature suggests low infection rate

[e]Literature is mainly outdated

composite–bioactive glass (FRC–BG) implant is a novel option for CP and presented in the table due to author's own research and clinical experience.

81.2.2.1 Autologous Bone

Frozen autologous bone flap is traditionally used for primary reconstruction because it is biocompatible, cheap, viable and readily available and has equivalent strength characteristics to the cranial bone. Additionally, there is no risk of disease transmission (Zanotti et al. 2016). Autologous bone shows osseointegration capacity and is suitable for paediatric CP (Da Silva et al. 2007; Rocque et al. 2013). However, the use of autologous bone may be limited due to bone flap contamination following scalp lacerations or bony fracture. Increased storage costs and international regulations have led to discontinuation of institutional bone banking activity in some European centres.

Recent studies suggest that problems after CP with autologous bone are more frequent than was thought previously, the most common problem being bone flap resorption. The risk factors of resorption are younger age, shunt-dependent hydrocephalus, current smoking and injury-related bone flap fractures (Dünisch et al. 2013; Korhonen et al. 2018). A recent review and meta-analysis suggests that infection rates are similar between autologous bone and synthetic materials in both overall CP population and patients with TBI (Malcolm et al. 2018). Nevertheless, a recent systematic review including a larger set of studies without subanalysis of patients with TBI suggests that infection rates are higher in autologous bone than synthetic materials (van de Vijfeijken et al. 2018). CPs performed with autologous bone are significantly associated with more reoperations mostly due to bone flap resorption (Malcolm et al. 2018). Based on the current knowledge, it can be suggested that an initial synthetic implant should be considered especially in younger patients and in a case of a fragmented bone flap.

81.2.2.2 Polymethyl Methacrylate

Methyl methacrylate was discovered in 1939 and was extensively experimented in the 1940s (Woodhall and Spurling 1945). PMMA is a mouldable acrylic resin with strength similar to the cranial bone tissue, and it has widely been used in craniofacial reconstruction. Acrylic resins do not conduct heat, and they are stable, durable, chemically inert, well tolerated by tissue and easily placed and modified (Shah et al. 2014; Zanotti et al. 2016). In terms of CP, PMMA is the cheapest, most widely used and easiest material to produce (Moreira-Gonzalez et al. 2003; Marchac and Greensmith 2008). Furthermore, PMMA does not interfere in imaging studies, electroencephalography or radiotherapy (Chiarini et al. 2004). PMMA has also raised a special interest in computer-assisted design and 3D printing as a promising implant material (Kim et al. 2012; Morales-gómez et al. 2018). These techniques have decreased the need for intraoperative moulding.

Due to the lack of porosity, PMMA implants cannot be infiltrated by new bone tissue. PMMA interferes with vascularisation and does not have osseointegration capacity and does not interact with the surrounding tissue (Goiato et al. 2009; Zanotti et al. 2016). Focal and systemic inflammatory and allergic responses to PMMA have been described (Goodman et al. 1991; Goon et al. 2008; Khader and Towler 2016; Zanotti et al. 2016). It has been reported that PMMA may be susceptible to higher or similar infection rate that is reported using autologous bone and other synthetic implants (Bobinski et al. 2013; Cho and Gosain 2004; Gosain 2005; Höhne et al. 2018; van de Vijfeijken et al. 2018). Some of the PMMA implants are moulded and cut intraoperatively without polishing. This may result in bacterial adhesion and biofilm deposition, which could contribute to an increased infection rate compared to other synthetic materials (Katsikogianni et al. 2004; van de Vijfeijken et al. 2018). Due to these properties of the material, resterilisation cannot be suggested. In terms of paediatric CP, PMMA implants are not recommended, because the material does not accommodate bone growth of the skull (Goiato et al. 2009; Zanotti et al. 2016). However, Fiaschi and colleagues reported a series of 12 paediatric CPs performed with custom-made PMMA implants with acceptable results with a relatively long follow-up interval (Fiaschi et al. 2016).

81.2.2.3 Polyether Ether Ketone

PEEK is an aromatic semicrystalline polymer that is resistant to high temperatures, displays strength and elastic properties that are similar to cranial bone and is chemically inert (Zanotti et al. 2016). Though being resistant to temperatures even as high 300 °C, the material does not conduct heat (Camarini et al. 2011; Lethaus et al. 2014), and thus, PEEK implants can be sterilised in moist and dry heat (Zanotti et al. 2016). PEEK does not interfere in imaging (Kurtz and Devine 2007). Custom PEEK implants can be shaped by computer-assisted design/computer-assisted manufacture technology to fit the specific size of any given defect (Camarini et al. 2011).

Currently, the literature on usage of PEEK in CP is scarce. Many studies report promising results in utilising PEEK in CP (Punchak et al. 2017; van de Vijfeijken et al. 2018). In a meta-analysis by Punchak et al., the authors report a trend towards lower postoperative complication rates after PEEK CP procedures compared to autologous bone CP procedures. Furthermore, in two studies, among patients undergoing PEEK and titanium mesh CP, lower failure rates of PEEK versus titanium mesh implants have been reported (Punchak et al. 2017; Zhang et al. 2018). PEEK does not possess osteomimetic properties, and thus its utilisation in paediatric CP should be considered with caution, as in the case of PMMA. However, porous polyethylene shows revascularisation and soft tissue ingrowth into pores of the implant margin (Wheeler et al. 2000). At the moment, PEEK implants are expensive (van de Vijfeijken et al. 2018).

81.2.2.4 Hydroxyapatite

Calcium phosphates (tricalcium phosphate and HA) have been used to fill cranial defects throughout the twentieth century (Harris et al. 2014). Calcium phosphates present excellent tissue compatibility and the advantages of being osteoactive and radiolucent with characteristics that mimic bone tissue.

These features promote osteogenesis, which can result in partial or complete bone formation through osteoinduction and osteoconduction (Fricia et al. 2015; Martini et al. 2012; Zanotti et al. 2016). HA is one of the commonest forms of calcium phosphate for clinical use. Traditionally, it has been available as a nonabsorbable ceramic and has been widely studied (Di Rienzo et al. 2012; Zanotti et al. 2016). HA is radiolucent (Goiato et al. 2009). HA cement has been extensively used for CP in adults (van de Vijfeijken et al. 2018), and it has also been used in children during growth stage (Gosain 1997). Due to porous structure of HA, resterilisation is not possible. Reconstruction of large bony defects can be difficult, because significant remodelling can occur as the cement hardens and may even break into fragments (Frassanito et al. 2013), and thus HA is probably most suitable for reconstruction of small defects (Ratnayake et al. 2017). The use of HA cement in combination with tantalum and titanium mesh provides structural support and increased stability of the implant construction (Durham et al. 2003).

The infection rates of HA implants have been reported to be very low in a recent systematic review (van de Vijfeijken et al. 2018). The systematic review included a Finnish study in which HA implants exhibited also a very low infection rate, but the implants were relatively small compared to other materials (Piitulainen et al. 2015b). In a relatively small study cohort, HA implants had a lower infection rate than titanium implants, but at the same time, have a higher postoperative risk for epidural haematoma (Lindner et al. 2017), which may be attributed to the implant design and required surgical technique.

81.2.2.5 Titanium

Titanium, introduced for CP in 1965, is currently the only metal used in CP (Blake et al. 1990; Goldstein et al. 2013). The advantages over other metals include good biocompatibility, resistance to infection, mechanical strength and inexpensiveness (Honeybul et al. 2018). Titanium implants are used in two forms: intraoperatively moulded and preformed (standard plates and custom made) (Joffe et al. 1999). Titanium is biologically inert and is considered a reliable material for CP providing a good long-term clinical outcome (Zanotti et al. 2016).

The disadvantages of titanium are related to the heat and cold conduction properties and suboptimal quality of follow-up imaging due to radiopaqueness (Cabraja et al. 2009; Zanotti et al. 2016). However, titanium is MRI-compatible. Titanium produces less imaging artefacts when combined with ceramics or other metals (Ducic 2002; Khader and Towler 2016). Based on our clinical experience, mesh titanium implants produce less artefacts, but may still interfere with, e.g. tumour resection evaluation on follow-up imaging. Heat and cold conduction may interfere with the aesthetic results of CP with titanium. One of the largest concerns related to utilisation of titanium in CP is its tendency to cause thinning of subcutaneous tissue leading to implant exposure and subsequent removal of the implant (Frodel 2008; Thien et al. 2015). Sun et al. reported that patients showing hypersensitivities to more than three kinds of metal had higher risks of titanium implant exposure, and they suggested that a routine allergy screening should be performed before titanium CP (Sun et al. 2018).

Titanium has been successfully used in adults (Honeybul et al. 2018; Lindner et al. 2017) and adolescents (Williams et al. 2016). However, titanium does not exhibit capacity for growth and may be problematic for applications in paediatric cranioplasty. Titanium exhibits lower infection rate than autologous bone (Honeybul et al. 2017) and intraoperatively moulded PMMA implants (Höhne et al. 2018).

81.2.2.6 Other Materials

Utilisation of polyethylene (PE) in CP was originally reported in 1950 and was considered an advantageous material compared with other available materials for CP of that time (Eben and Dillard 1950). PE is inert and non-resorbable and has low tissue reactivity and high long-term structural stability (Goiato et al. 2009). Later, bone ingrowth into porous PE was reported (Klawitter et al. 1976), and the material was introduced in facial deformity (Frodel and Lee 1998) and cranial reconstruction procedures (Couldwell et al. 1994; Wang et al. 2012). Studies on outcome of CPs utilising PE implants are rare. However, in small case series, successful utilisation of PE implants has been reported in adolescents (Lin et al. 2012) and adults (Kumar et al. 2016).

Recently, a FRC–BG implant has been developed to mimic the properties and structure of the cranial bone (Vallittu 2017). The advantages of FRC–BG implants are strong and lightweight design, and they have low thermal conductivity. The composite material allows computer-assisted design/computer-assisted manufacture technology for custom design. FRC–BG implants have a porous structure, which allows extracellular liquid perfusion and ingrowth of bone with bacteriostatic and osteoinductive properties by bioactive glass (Aitasalo et al. 2014). These properties promote new bone formation (Tuusa et al. 2008). We have recently reported about FRC–BG implant safety, cosmesis and biocompatibility in children (Piitulainen et al. 2015b, 2019) and adults (Piitulainen et al. 2015a; Posti et al. 2015). FRC–BG implants are radiolucent and no toxic adverse events have been detected (Piitulainen et al. 2019; Posti et al. 2015).

81.2.3 Timing

DC leaves a large bony defect in the calvarium exposing the brain to atmosphere pressure resulting in disturbance of physiological brain perfusion (Picard and Zanardi 2013) and cerebrospinal fluid circulation (Fodstad et al. 1984). CP is typically delayed several months after DC to allow the patient to recover from the acute phase of injury and ensure resolution of elevated intracranial pressure. CP is of paramount importance for patients who show capacity for recovery, because the procedure may reverse cognitive, language and motor deficits—in other words, SOT (Ashayeri et al. 2016; Sakamoto et al. 2006; Shahid et al. 2017; Stiver et al. 2008). Consequently, timing of CP has attracted much discussion.

Malcolm et al. conducted a systematic review and meta-analysis on the relation of complications following CP to procedure timing (Malcolm et al.

2016). The analysis comprised 25 articles including 3126 CP procedures of which 1421 were early (within 3 months) and 1795 late (beyond 3 months). The results suggest that early CP is associated with greater odds of hydrocephalus than late CP, but otherwise early CP is as safe as late CP. Subsequently, the same group conducted a systematic review on the effect of timing for CP to augment neurological outcome (Malcolm et al. 2017). The analysis comprised 8 articles including 551 CP procedures of which 248 were early and 303 late. The results demonstrated that CP is associated with improved neurological function and that early CP may further enhance recovery.

The optimal CP timing remains a controversial issue. Both of the reviews include heterogeneous studies with groups of patients with different indications for DC. Most of the patients had undergone DC due to trauma in both datasets. Currently, there are no published clinical trials examining the effect of timing of CP on neurological outcome. Hence, the latter study included only retrospective and observational studies. In the future, large prospective studies are needed to standardise the best timing of performing CP in patients with predefined indications for DC. To achieve viable and clinically relevant results, the DC and CP techniques, implant materials and design, complication types and quantitative neurological outcome assessments need to be rigorously standardised. Based on the current evidence and considering the overall outcome, early CP can be considered preferable while recognising the possible risk of post-CP hydrocephalus.

81.2.4 Complications

Despite CP being a fairly straightforward routine procedure in neurosurgery, it is still associated with a relatively high complication rate, ranging from 10 to 40%, often leading to significant morbidity, delayed rehabilitation and compromised outcome (Bobinski et al. 2013; Coulter et al. 2014; Halani et al. 2017; Posti et al. 2018). Postoperative complications related to CP can be divided to early and late complications (Sahoo et al. 2018).

Early postoperative complications include intracranial postoperative haematoma or CSF collection, skin flap necrosis, wound dehiscence and implant infection. Meticulous perioperative haemostasis should be maintained during CP in order to avoid postoperative haematoma. CSF collection indicates meningeal disruption and is usually a self-limiting condition. The initial DC should be planned so that the skin incision is placed beyond the bone deficit (see Chap. 26). In CP, the initial incision line should always be used to preserve vasculature and prevent flap necrosis and wound dehiscence. Primary implant infections are likely rare, because synthetic implants are sterilised by manufacturers and carefully packed. In the past at our centre, when autologous bone flaps were used, we obtained swab sample before storage. If bacterial growth was detected, the bone flap was discarded.

Late postoperative complications include late infection, exposure of implant and loss of implant fixation. Latent infection or (allergic) reaction to implant material such as titanium (see Sect. 81.2.2.5) may result in late wound dehiscence and implant exposure. Based on our experience, implant exposure necessitates implant removal and antibiotic therapy. Subsequent CP should not be undertaken before contrast-enhanced and diffusion MRI sequences, and blood infection parameters have been totally normalised and wound is perfectly healed. We recommend waiting at least 3–6 months before re-CP. Implant migration may occur because of growth of skull when non-ossifying synthetic implant materials are used. Loss of fixation may also lead to implant migration. In these cases, the original implant may be preserved using refixation in a revision procedure, if the wound has remained intact.

References

Aitasalo KM, Piitulainen JM, Rekola J, Vallittu PK. Craniofacial bone reconstruction with bioactive fiber-reinforced composite implant. Head Neck. 2014;36:722–8.

Ashayeri K, Jackson EM, Huang J, Brem H, Gordon CR. Syndrome of the trephined: a systematic review. Neurosurgery. 2016;79(4):525–34. https://doi.org/10.1227/NEU.0000000000001366.

Banks CA, Palmer JN, Chiu AG, O'Malley BW, Woodworth BA, Kennedy DW. Endoscopic closure of CSF rhinorrhea: 193 cases over 21 years. Otolaryngol Head Neck Surg. 2009;140(6):826–33. https://doi.org/10.1016/j.otohns.2008.12.060.

Bell RB, Dierks EJ, Homer L, Potter BE. Management of cerebrospinal fluid leak associated with craniomaxillofacial trauma. J Oral Maxillofac Surg. 2004;62(6):676–84. https://doi.org/10.1016/j.joms.2003.08.032.

Bijlenga P, Zumofen D, Yilmaz H, Creisson E, De Tribolet N. Orthostatic mesodiencephalic dysfunction after decompressive craniectomy. J Neurol Neurosurg Psychiatry. 2007;78:430–3.

Blake GB, MacFarlane MR, Hinton JW. Titanium in reconstructive surgery of the skull and face. Br J Plast Surg. 1990;43(5):528–35. https://doi.org/10.1016/0007-1226(90)90115-G.

Bobinski L, Koskinen L-O, Lindvall P. Complications following cranioplasty using autologous bone or polymethylmethacrylate--retrospective experience from a single center. Clin Neurol Neurosurg. 2013;115:1788–91.

Cabraja M, Klein M, Lehmann T-N. Long-term results following titanium cranioplasty of large skull defects. Neurosurg Focus. 2009;26:E10.

Camarini ET, Tomeh JK, Dias RR, Da Silva EJ. Reconstruction of frontal bone using specific implant polyether-ether- ketone. J Craniofac Surg. 2011;22(6):2205–7. https://doi.org/10.1097/SCS.0b013e3182326f2c.

Chiarini L, Figurelli S, Pollastri G, Torcia E, Ferrari F, Albanese M, Nocini PF. Cranioplasty using acrylic material: a new technical procedure. J Craniomaxillofac Surg. 2004;32(1):5–9. https://doi.org/10.1016/j.jcms.2003.08.006.

Cho YR, Gosain AK. Biomaterials in craniofacial reconstruction. Clin Plast Surg. 2004;31(3):377–85. https://doi.org/10.1016/j.cps.2004.03.001.

Choi JJ, Cirivello MJ, Neal CJ, Armonda RA. Paradoxical herniation in wartime penetrating brain injury with concomitant skull-base trauma. J Craniofac Surg. 2011;22(6):2163–7. https://doi.org/10.1097/SCS.0b013e3182323fd5.

Coelho F, Maynart Oliveira A, Silva Paiva W, Rios Freire F, Tome Calado V, Luis Amorim R, et al. Comprehensive cognitive and cerebral hemodynamic evaluation after cranioplasty. Neuropsychiatr Dis Treat. 2014;10:695–701. https://doi.org/10.2147/NDT.S52875.

Couldwell WT, Chen TC, Weiss MH, Fukushima T, Dougherty W. Cranioplasty with the Medpor porous polyethylene Flexblock implant. J Neurosurg. 1994;81(3):483–6. https://doi.org/10.3171/jns.1994.81.3.0483.

Coulter I, Pesic Smith J, Cato Addison W, Khan S, Thompson D, Jenkins A, et al. Routine but risky: a multi-centre analysis of the outcomes of cranioplasty in the Northeast of England. Acta Neurochir. 2014;156:1361–8.

Da Silva RV, Bertran CA, Kawachi EY, Camilli JA. Repair of cranial bone defects with calcium phosphate ceramic implant or autogenous bone graft. J Craniofac Surg. 2007; https://doi.org/10.1097/scs.0b013e31802d8ac4.

De Bonis P, Frassanito P, Mangiola A, Nucci CG, Anile C, Pompucci A. Cranial repair: how complicated is filling a "hole"? J Neurotrauma. 2012;29:1071–6.

De Bonis P, Tamburrini G, Mangiola A, Pompucci A, Mattogno PP, Porso M, Anile C. Post-traumatic hydrocephalus is a contraindication for endoscopic third-ventriculostomy: isn't it? Clin Neurol Neurosurg. 2013;115(1):9–12. https://doi.org/10.1016/j.clineuro.2012.08.021.

Denes Z, Barsi P, Szel I, Boros E, Fazekas G. Complication during postacute rehabilitation: patients with posttraumatic hydrocephalus. Int J Rehabil Res. 2011;34(3):222–6. https://doi.org/10.1097/MRR.0b013e328346e87d.

Di Rienzo A, Iacoangeli M, di Somma LGM, Alvaro L, Nocchi N, Scerrati M. Shape modifications of porous hydroxyapatite prostheses to improve rigid implant fixation: experience in 12 cases. Surg Neurol Int. 2012;3:161. https://doi.org/10.4103/2152-7806.105100.

Di Stefano C, Rinaldesi M, Quinquinio C, Ridolfi C, Vallasciani M, Sturiale C, Piperno R. Neuropsychological changes and cranioplasty: a group analysis. Brain Inj. 2016;30:164–71.

Ducic Y. Titanium mesh and hydroxyapatite cement cranioplasty: a report of 20 cases. J Oral Maxillofac Surg. 2002;60(3):272–6. https://doi.org/10.1053/joms.2002.30575.

Dünisch P, Walter J, Sakr Y, Kalff R, Waschke A, Ewald C. Risk factors of aseptic bone resorption: a study after autologous bone flap reinsertion due to decompressive craniotomy. J Neurosurg. 2013;118(5):1141–7. https://doi.org/10.3171/2013.1.JNS12860.

Durham SR, McComb JG, Levy ML, Cohen AR, Menezes AH, Sutton LN. Correction of large (>25 cm2) cranial defects with "reinforced" hydroxyapatite cement: technique and complications. Neurosurgery. 2003;52(4):842–5. https://doi.org/10.1227/01.NEU.0000054220.01290.8E.

Eben A, Dillard PH. The use of pure polyethylene plate for cranioplasty. J Neurosurg. 1950;7(6):492–8. https://doi.org/10.3171/jns.1950.7.6.0492.

Fattahian R, Bagheri S, Sadeghi M. Development of posttraumatic hydrocephalus requiring ventriculoperitoneal shunt after decompressive craniectomy for traumatic brain injury: a systematic review and meta-analysis of retrospective studies. Med Arch. 2018;72(3):214–9. https://doi.org/10.5455/medarh.2018.72.214-219.

Fiaschi P, Pavanello M, Imperato A, Dallolio V, Accogli A, Capra V, et al. Surgical results of cranioplasty with a polymethylmethacrylate customized cranial implant in pediatric patients: a single-center experience. J Neurosurg Pediatr. 2016;17(6):705–10. https://doi.org/10.3171/2015.10.PEDS15489.

Fodstad H, Love JA, Ekstedt J, Friden H, Liliequist B. Effect of cranioplasty on cerebrospinal fluid hydrodynamics in patients with the syndrome of the trephined. Acta Neurochir. 1984;70:21–30.

Frassanito P, De Bonis P, Mattogno PP, Mangiola A, Novello M, Brinchi D, et al. The fate of a macroporous hydroxyapatite cranioplasty four years after implantation: macroscopical and microscopical findings in a case of recurrent atypical meningioma. Clin Neurol Neurosurg. 2013;115(8):1496–8. https://doi.org/10.1016/j.clineuro.2012.11.032.

Fricia M, Passanisi M, Salamanna F, Parrilli A, Giavaresi G, Fini M. Osteointegration in custom-made porous hydroxyapatite cranial implants: from reconstructive surgery to regenerative medicine. World Neurosurg. 2015;84(2):591.e11–6. https://doi.org/10.1016/j.wneu.2015.03.027.

Friedman JA, Ebersold MJ, Quast LM. Post-traumatic cerebrospinal fluid leakage. World J Surg. 2001;25(8):1062–6. https://doi.org/10.1007/s00268-001-0059-7.

Frodel JL. Computer-designed implants for fronto-orbital defect reconstruction. Facial Plast Surg. 2008;24(1):22–34. https://doi.org/10.1055/s-2007-1021459.

Frodel JL, Lee S. The use of high-density polyethylene implants in facial deformities. Arch Otolaryngol Head Neck Surg. 1998;124:1219–23. https://doi.org/10.1001/archotol.124.11.1219.

Goiato MC, Anchieta RB, Pita MS, Dos Santos DM. Reconstruction of skull defects: currently available materials. J Craniofac Surg. 2009;20(5):1512–8. https://doi.org/10.1097/SCS.0b013e3181b09b9a.

Goldstein JA, Paliga JT, Bartlett SP. Cranioplasty: indications and advances. Curr Opin Otolaryngol Head Neck Surg. 2013;21(4):400–9. https://doi.org/10.1097/MOO.0b013e328363003e.

Goodman SB, Fornasier VL, Keil J. Quantitative comparison of the histological effects of particulate polymethylmethacrylate versus polyethylene in the rabbit tibia. Arch Orthop Trauma Surg. 1991;110(3):123–6. https://doi.org/10.1007/BF00395792.

Goon ATJ, Bruze M, Zimerson E, Goh CL, Soo-Quee Koh D, Isaksson M. Screening for acrylate/methacrylate allergy in the baseline series: our experience in Sweden and Singapore. Contact Dermatitis. 2008;59(5):307–13. https://doi.org/10.1111/j.1600-0536.2008.01440.x.

Gosain AK. Hydroxyapatite cement paste cranioplasty for the treatment of temporal hollowing after cranial vault remodeling in a growing child. J Craniofac Surg. 1997;8(6):506–11. https://doi.org/10.1097/00001665-199711000-00017.

Gosain AK. Biomaterials for reconstruction of the cranial vault. Plast Reconstr Surg. 2005;116(2):663–6. https://doi.org/10.1097/01.prs.0000176289.05374.5b.

Gottlob I, Simonsz-Tòth B, Heilbronner R. Midbrain syndrome with eye movement disorder: dramatic improvement after cranioplasty. Strabismus. 2002;10(4):271–7. https://doi.org/10.1076/stra.10.4.271.13830.

Grant F, Norcross N. Repair of cranial defects by cranioplasty. Ann Surg. 1939;110:488–512.

Hagan M, Bradley JP. Syndrome of the trephined: functional improvement after reconstruction of large cranial vault defects. J Craniofac Surg. 2017;28(5):1129–30. https://doi.org/10.1097/SCS.0000000000003747.

Halani SH, Chu JK, Malcolm JG, Rindler RS, Allen JW, Grossberg JA, et al. Effects of cranioplasty on cerebral blood flow following decompressive craniectomy: a systematic review of the literature. Neurosurgery. 2017;81(2):204–16. https://doi.org/10.1093/neuros/nyx054.

Harris DA, Fong AJ, Buchanan EP, Monson L, Khechoyan D, Lam S. History of synthetic materials in alloplastic cranioplasty. Neurosurg Focus. 2014;36:E20.

Höhne J, Werzmirzowsky K, Ott C, Hohenberger C, Hassanin BG, Brawanski A, Schebesch KM. Outcomes of cranioplasty with preformed titanium versus freehand molded polymethylmethacrylate implants. J Neurol Surg A Cent Eur Neurosurg. 2018;79(3):200–5. https://doi.org/10.1055/s-0037-1604362.

Honeybul S. Complications of decompressive craniectomy for head injury. J Clin Neurosci. 2010;17(4):430–5. https://doi.org/10.1016/j.jocn.2009.09.007.

Honeybul S, Morrison DA, Ho KM, Lind CR, Geelhoed E. A randomized controlled trial comparing autologous cranioplasty with custom-made titanium cranioplasty. J Neurosurg. 2017;160(5):885–91. https://doi.org/10.3171/2015.12.JNS152004.

Honeybul S, Morrison DA, Ho KM, Lind CRP, Geelhoed E. A randomised controlled trial comparing autologous cranioplasty with custom-made titanium cranioplasty: long-term follow-up. Acta Neurochir. 2018;160(5):885–91. https://doi.org/10.1007/s00701-018-3514-z.

Jeyaraj P. Importance of early cranioplasty in reversing the "syndrome of the trephine/motor trephine syndrome/sinking skin flap syndrome". J Maxillofac Oral Surg. 2015;14(3):666–73. https://doi.org/10.1007/s12663-014-0673-1.

Joffe J, Harris M, Kahugu F, Nicoll S, Linney A, Richards R. A prospective study of computer-aided design and manufacture of titanium plate for cranioplasty and its clinical outcome. Br J Neurosurg. 1999;13(6):576–80. https://doi.org/10.1080/02688699943088.

Joseph V, Reilly P. Syndrome of the trephined. J Neurosurg. 2009;111:650–2. https://doi.org/10.3171/2009.3.JNS0984.

Kammersgaard LP, Linnemann M, Tibæk M. Hydrocephalus following severe traumatic brain injury in adults. Incidence, timing, and clinical predictors during rehabilitation. NeuroRehabilitation. 2013;33(3):473–80. https://doi.org/10.3233/NRE-130980.

Katsikogianni M, Missirlis YF, Harris L, Douglas J. Concise review of mechanisms of bacterial adhesion to biomaterials and of techniques used in estimating bacteria-material interactions. Eur Cells Mater. 2004;8:37–57. https://doi.org/10.22203/eCM.v008a05.

Khader BA, Towler MR. Materials and techniques used in cranioplasty fixation: a review. Mater Sci Eng C. 2016;66:315–22. https://doi.org/10.1016/j.msec.2016.04.101.

Kim BJ, Hong KS, Park KJ, Park DH, Chung YG, Kang SH. Customized cranioplasty implants using three-dimensional printers and polymethyl-methacrylate casting. J Korean Neurosurg Soc. 2012;52(6):541–6. https://doi.org/10.3340/jkns.2012.52.6.541.

Klawitter JJ, Bagwell JG, Weinstein AM, Sauer BW, Pruitt JR. An evaluation of bone growth into porous high density polyethylene. J Biomed Mater Res. 1976;10(4):595–603. https://doi.org/10.1002/jbm.820100212.

Korhonen TK, Tetri S, Huttunen J, Lindgren A, Piitulainen JM, Serlo W, et al. Predictors of primary autograft cranioplasty survival and resorption after craniectomy. J Neurosurg. 2018;1:1–8. https://doi.org/10.3171/2017.12.jns172013.

Kowalski RG, Weintraub AH, Rubin BA, Gerber DJ, Olsen AJ. Impact of timing of ventriculoperitoneal shunt placement on outcome in posttraumatic hydrocephalus. J Neurosurg. 2018; https://doi.org/10.3171/2017.7.JNS17555.

Kumar NG, Sreenivas M, Gowda S. Cranioplasty of large cranial defects with porous polyethylene implants. J Craniofac Surg. 2016;27(4):e333–5. https://doi.org/10.1097/SCS.0000000000002480.

Kurtz SM, Devine JN. PEEK biomaterials in trauma, orthopedic, and spinal implants. Biomaterials. 2007;28(32):4845–69. https://doi.org/10.1016/j.biomaterials.2007.07.013.

Lethaus B, Bloebaum M, Essers B, ter Laak M, Steiner T, Kessler P. Patient-specific implants compared with stored bone grafts for patients with interval cranioplasty. J Craniofac Surg. 2014;25:206–9.

Li G, Wen L, Zhan RY, Shen F, Yang XF, Fu WM. Cranioplasty for patients developing large cranial defects combined with post-traumatic hydrocephalus after head trauma. Brain Inj. 2008;22(4):333–7. https://doi.org/10.1080/02699050801958353.

Lin AY, Kinsella CR, Rottgers SA, Smith DM, Grunwaldt LJ, Cooper GM, Losee JE. Custom porous polyethylene implants for large-scale pediatric skull reconstruction: early outcomes. J Craniofac Surg. 2012;23(1):67–70. https://doi.org/10.1097/SCS.0b013e318240c876.

Lindner D, Schlothofer-Schumann K, Kern B-C, Marx O, Müns A, Meixensberger J. Cranioplasty using custom-made hydroxyapatite versus titanium: a randomized clinical trial. J Neurosurg. 2017;126(1):175–83. https://doi.org/10.3171/2015.10.JNS151245.

Malcolm JG, Rindler RS, Chu JK, Grossberg JA, Pradilla G, Ahmad FU. Complications following cranioplasty and relationship to timing: a systematic review and meta-analysis. J Clin Neurosci. 2016;33:39–51. https://doi.org/10.1016/j.jocn.2016.04.017.

Malcolm JG, Rindler RS, Chu JK, Chokshi F, Grossberg JA, Pradilla G, Ahmad FU. Early cranioplasty is associated with greater neurological improvement: a systematic review and meta-analysis. Neurosurgery. 2017;82(3):278–88. https://doi.org/10.1093/neuros/nyx182.

Malcolm JG, Mahmooth Z, Rindler RS, Allen JW, Grossberg JA, Pradilla G, Ahmad FU. Autologous cranioplasty is associated with increased reoperation rate: a systematic review and meta-analysis. World Neurosurg. 2018;116:60–8. https://doi.org/10.1016/j.wneu.2018.05.009.

Marchac D, Greensmith A. Long-term experience with methylmethacrylate cranioplasty in craniofacial surgery. J Plast Reconstr Aesthet Surg. 2008;61(7):744–52. https://doi.org/10.1016/j.bjps.2007.10.055.

Martini L, Staffa G, Giavaresi G, Salamanna F, Parrilli A, Serchi E, et al. Long-term results following cranial hydroxyapatite prosthesis implantation in a large skull defect model. Plast Reconstr Surg. 2012;129(4):625e–35e. https://doi.org/10.1097/PRS.0b013e318244220d.

Mincy JE. Posttraumatic cerebrospinal fluid fistula of the frontal fossa. J Trauma. 1966;6(5):618–22. https://doi.org/10.1097/00005373-196609000-00007.

Mokri B. Orthostatic headaches in the syndrome of the trephined: resolution following cranioplasty. Headache. 2010;50(7):1206–11. https://doi.org/10.1111/j.1526-4610.2010.01715.x.

Morales-gómez JA, Garcia-estrada E, Leos-bortoni JE, Delgado-brito M, Flores-huerta LE, La Cruz-arriaga AAD, et al. Cranioplasty with a low-cost customized polymethylmethacrylate implant using a desktop 3D printer. J Neurosurg. 2018;15:1–7. https://doi.org/10.3171/2017.12.JNS172574.

Moreira-Gonzalez A, Jackson IT, Miyawaki T, Barakat K, DiNick V. Clinical outcome in cranioplasty: critical review in long-term follow-up. J Craniofac Surg. 2003;14:144–53.

Oh J-W, Kim S-H, Whang K. Traumatic cerebrospinal fluid leak: diagnosis and management. Korean J Neurotrauma. 2017;13(2):63–7. https://doi.org/10.13004/kjnt.2017.13.2.63.

Paredes I, Castaño-León AM, Munarriz PM, Martínez-Perez R, Cepeda S, Sanz R, et al. Cranioplasty after decompressive craniectomy. A prospective series analyzing complications and clinical improvement. Neurocirugia. 2015;26(3):115–25. https://doi.org/10.1016/j.neucir.2014.10.001.

Picard NA, Zanardi CA. Brain motion in patients with skull defects: B-mode ultrasound observations on respiration-induced movements. Acta Neurochir. 2013;155:2149–57.

Piitulainen JM, Kauko T, Aitasalo KMJ, Vuorinen V, Vallittu PK, Posti JP. Outcomes of cranioplasty with synthetic materials and autologous bone grafts. World Neurosurg. 2015a;83:708–14. https://doi.org/10.1016/j.wneu.2015.01.014.

Piitulainen JM, Posti JP, Aitasalo KMJM, Vuorinen V, Vallittu PKK, Serlo W. Paediatric cranial defect reconstruction using bioactive fibre-reinforced composite implant: early outcomes. Acta Neurochir. 2015b;157:681–7.

Piitulainen JM, Posti JP, Vallittu PK, Aitasalo KM, Serlo W. A large calvarial bone defect in a child: osteointegration of an implant. World Neurosurg. 2019; https://doi.org/10.1016/j.wneu.2019.01.028.

Posti JP, Piitulainen J, Hupa L, Fagerlund S, Frantzén J, Aitasalo KMJ, et al. A glass fiber-reinforced composite - bioactive glass cranioplasty implant: a case study of an early development stage implant removed due to a late infection. J Mech Behav Biomed Mater. 2015;55:191–200.

Posti JP, Yli-Olli M, Heiskanen L, Aitasalo KMJ, Rinne J, Vuorinen V, et al. Cranioplasty after severe traumatic brain injury: effects of trauma and patient recovery on cranioplasty outcome. Front Neurol. 2018;9:223. https://doi.org/10.3389/fneur.2018.00223.

Prosser JD, Vender JR, Solares CA. Traumatic cerebrospinal fluid leaks. Otolaryngol Clin North Am. 2011;44(4):857–73. https://doi.org/10.1016/j.otc.2011.06.007.

Punchak M, Chung LK, Lagman C, Bui TT, Lazareff J, Rezzadeh K, et al. Outcomes following polyetheretherketone (PEEK) cranioplasty: systematic review and meta-analysis. J Clin Neurosci. 2017;41:30–5. https://doi.org/10.1016/j.jocn.2017.03.028.

Rahme R, Weil AG, Sabbagh M, Moumdjian R, Bouthillier A, Bojanowski MW. Decompressive craniectomy is not an independent risk factor for communicating hydrocephalus in patients with increased intracranial pressure. Neurosurgery. 2010;67(3):675–8. https://doi.org/10.1227/01.NEU.0000383142.10103.0B.

Ratilal BO, Costa J, Pappamikail L, Sampaio C. Antibiotic prophylaxis for preventing meningitis in patients with basilar skull fractures. Cochrane Database Syst Rev. 2015;(4):CD004884.

Ratnayake JTB, Mucalo M, Dias GJ. Substituted hydroxyapatites for bone regeneration: a review of current trends. J Biomed Mater Res B Appl Biomater. 2017;105(5):1285–99. https://doi.org/10.1523/JNEUROSCI.4925-04.2005.

Rocque BG, Amancherla K, Lew SM, Lam S. Outcomes of cranioplasty following decompressive craniectomy in the pediatric population. J Neurosurg Pediatr. 2013;12:120–5. https://doi.org/10.3171/2013.4.peds12605.

Romero FR, Zanini MA, Ducati LG, Gabarra RC. Sinking skin flap syndrome with delayed dysautonomic syndrome - an atypical presentation. Int J Surg Case Rep. 2013;4(11):1007–9. https://doi.org/10.1016/j.ijscr.2013.08.013.

Sahoo NK, Tomar K, Thakral A, Rangan NM. Complications of cranioplasty. J Craniofac Surg. 2018;29(5):1344–8. https://doi.org/10.1097/SCS.0000000000004478.

Sakamoto S, Eguchi K, Kiura Y, Arita K, Kurisu K. CT perfusion imaging in the syndrome of the sinking skin flap before and after cranioplasty. Clin Neurol Neurosurg. 2006;108:583–5.

Schwarz F, Dünisch P, Walter J, Sakr Y, Kalff R, Ewald C. Cranioplasty after decompressive craniectomy: is there a rationale for an initial artificial bone-substitute implant? A single-center experience after 631 procedures. J Neurosurg. 2016;124:710–5.

Sedney CL, Dillen W, Julien T. Clinical spectrum and radiographic features of the syndrome of the trephined. J Neurosci Rural Pract. 2016;6(3):438–41. https://doi.org/10.4103/0976-3147.158778.

Servadei F. Clinical value of decompressive craniectomy. N Engl J Med. 2011;364:1558–9. https://doi.org/10.1056/NEJMe1102998.

Shah AM, Jung H, Skirboll S. Materials used in cranioplasty: a history and analysis. Neurosurg Focus. 2014;36(4):E19. https://doi.org/10.3171/2014.2.FOCUS13561.

Shahid A, Mohanty M, Singla N, Mittal B, Gupta S. The effect of cranioplasty following decompressive craniectomy on cerebral blood perfusion, neurological, and cognitive outcome. J Neurosurg. 2017;128:229–35.

Singh I, Haris M, Husain M, Husain N, Rastogi M, Gupta RK. Role of endoscopic third ventriculostomy in patients with communicating hydrocephalus: an evaluation by MR ventriculography. Neurosurg Rev. 2008;31(3):319–25. https://doi.org/10.1007/s10143-008-0137-5.

Stiver S, Wintermark M, Manley G. Reversible monoparesis following decompressive hemicraniectomy for traumatic brain injury. J Neurosurg. 2008;109:245–54.

Sun Y, Hu Y, Yuan Q, Yu J, Wu XX, Du Z, et al. Association between metal hypersensitivity and implant failure in patients who underwent titanium cranioplasty. J Neurosurg. 2018;1:1–7. https://doi.org/10.3171/2018.1.JNS171804.

Thien A, King NKK, Ang BT, Wang E, Ng I. Comparison of polyetheretherketone and titanium cranioplasty after decompressive craniectomy. World Neurosurg. 2015;83(2):176–80. https://doi.org/10.1016/j.wneu.2014.06.003.

Tribl G, Oder W. Outcome after shunt implantation in severe head injury with post-traumatic hydrocephalus. Brain Injury. 2000;14:345–54.

Tuusa SM, Peltola MJ, Tirri T, Puska MA, Roytta M, Aho H, et al. Reconstruction of critical size calvarial bone defects in rabbits with glass-fiber-reinforced composite with bioactive glass granule coating. J Biomed Mat Res B Appl Biomater. 2008;84:510–9.

Vallittu PK. Bioactive glass-containing cranial implants: an overview. J Mater Sci. 2017;52:8772–84. https://doi.org/10.1007/s10853-017-0888-x.

Vedantam A, Yamal J-M, Hwang H, Robertson CS, Gopinath SP. Factors associated with shunt-dependent hydrocephalus after decompressive craniectomy for traumatic brain injury. J Neurosurg. 2017;128(5):1547–52. https://doi.org/10.3171/2017.1.JNS162721.

van de Vijfeijken SECM, Münker TJAG, Spijker R, Karssemakers LHE, Vandertop WP, Becking AG, et al. Autologous bone is inferior to alloplastic cranioplasties: safety of autograft and allograft materials for cranioplasties, a systematic review. World Neurosurg. 2018;117:443–452.e8. https://doi.org/10.1016/j.wneu.2018.05.193.

Wang JC, Wei L, Xu J, Liu JF, Gui L. Clinical outcome of cranioplasty with high-density porous polyethylene. J Craniofac Surg. 2012;23(5):1404–6. https://doi.org/10.1097/SCS.0b013e31825e3aeb.

Wheeler DL, Eschbach EJ, Hoellrich RG, Montfort MJ, Chamberland DL. Assessment of resorbable bioactive material for grafting of critical-size cancellous defects. J Orthop Res. 2000;18(1):140–8. https://doi.org/10.1002/jor.1100180120.

Williams L, Fan K, Bentley R. Titanium cranioplasty in children and adolescents. J Craniomaxillofac Surg. 2016;44(7):789–94. https://doi.org/10.1016/j.jcms.2016.03.010.

Woodhall B, Spurling RG. Tantalum cranioplasty for war wounds of the skull. Ann Surg. 1945;121(5):649–68.

Yadla S, Campbell PG, Chitale R, Maltenfort MG, Jabbour P, Sharan AD. Effect of early surgery, material, and method of flap preservation on cranioplasty infections: a systematic review. Neurosurgery. 2011;68:9; discussion 1130.

Zanotti B, Zingaretti N, Verlicchi A, Robiony M, Alfieri A, Parodi PC. Cranioplasty: review of materials. J Craniofac Surg. 2016;27(8):2061–72. https://doi.org/10.1097/SCS.0000000000003025.

Zhang Q, Yuan Y, Li X, Sun T, Zhou Y, Yu H, Guan J. A large multicenter retrospective research on embedded cranioplasty and covered cranioplasty. World Neurosurg. 2018;112:e645–51. https://doi.org/10.1016/j.wneu.2018.01.114.

82 Minimally Conscious and Vegetative State

Alison K. Godbolt

Recommendations

Level I

Treat with amantadine, unless contraindicated, if assessment confirms a PDOC, commencing treatment 4–16 weeks post injury.

Level II

Repeated assessment including standardized behavioural scales is needed before a diagnosis of a PDOC (VS or MCS) can be confirmed.

Level III

When sufficiently medically stable for discharge from acute care, patients with STBI and likely PDOC should be referred to rehabilitation services with specialized interdisciplinary teams for further assessment, medical management and rehabilitation care.

Assessment of conscious level should be preceded by assessment for and treatment of other conditions that could contribute to impaired behavioural responses.

Evidence for treatments other than amantadine is insufficient to allow a recommendation, despite some promising examples.

The American Academy of Neurology's recommendations in additional areas can be found in their 2018 practice guideline.

Tips, Tricks and Pitfalls

- Rule out other explanations for lack of response before concluding that the patient has a disorder of consciousness: Are they sedated, in pain, suffering from an infection or other complication, or did they just sleep badly?
- Use the Coma Recovery Scale-Revised (CRS-R) repeatedly, in addition to clinical assessment, for increased sensitivity in detecting signs of consciousness.
- Treat with amantadine to promote recovery unless there is a good reason not to.

82.1 Terminology

Severe traumatic brain injury (STBI) is usually followed by some period of coma (i.e. unconsciousness with no eye opening). Patients who survive usually emerge from coma, begin to communicate and gradually regain a greater or

A. K. Godbolt (✉)
University Department of Rehabilitation Medicine, and Department of Clinical Sciences, Karolinska Institute, Danderyd Hospital, Stockholm, Sweden
e-mail: alison.godbolt@sll.se

© Springer Nature Switzerland AG 2020
T. Sundstrøm et al. (eds.), *Management of Severe Traumatic Brain Injury*,
https://doi.org/10.1007/978-3-030-39383-0_82

lesser degree of independence. A small group of patients, however, open their eyes, but show no or extremely limited behavioural signs of consciousness, and are described as having a disorder of consciousness (DOC). Prolonged DOC (PDOC, ≥4 weeks (Royal College of Physicians 2013)) encompasses vegetative state (VS) (Jennett and Plum 1972) and minimally conscious state (MCS) (Giacino et al. 2002). In VS, patients show no behavioural signs of consciousness. In contrast, in MCS, patients show "clearly discernible" but inconsistent signs of consciousness, for example, sustained visual tracking, localization of painful stimuli and/or attempts at communication, without these reaching a functional level. Emergence from MCS is marked by the emergence of functional communication and/or functional object use. The term "vegetative" has unfortunately derogatory connotations, and the alternative term "unresponsive wakefulness syndrome" (UWS) is used by some authors (Laureys et al. 2010).

82.2 Epidemiology

There is a lack of robust data regarding incidence and prevalence of PDOC after STBI, due to multiple factors. Some studies pre-date the definition of MCS in 2002 (prior to which some, but not all, MCS patients would have been classified as in a VS); there is a lack of consensus regarding routines for systematic assessment, a lack of ICD-10 codes to document the occurrence of PDOC and a lack of systematic follow-up. A few prospective studies have attempted epidemiological estimates. Godbolt et al. (2013) used data from a Swedish prospective longitudinal study of STBI (n = 114) in adults aged 18–65 years to estimate the annual rates of post-traumatic disorders of consciousness (PT-DOC) persisting for specified time periods after injury. PT-DOC persisting for at least 3 months occurred in three per million working-age people (ages 18–65) annually. More transient PT-DOC, present 3 weeks after injury, but not at 3 months, occurred in five per million working-age people. Longer lasting PT-DOC, persisting 1 year after injury, had an annual incidence of 1.4 per million working-age people. A Norwegian prospective study of STBI (Andelic et al. 2012) found that only one of 61 patients had a PDOC (defined as Glasgow Outcome Scale Extended score = 2) a year after injury. A systematic review (van Erp et al. 2014) including acquired brain injury of different aetiologies (including STBI) found a reported prevalence of VS/UWS of 0.2–6.1 per 100,000 population. Overall, prognosis is better for patients with PDOC of traumatic aetiology than for other aetiologies.

82.3 Theoretical Model

Work by Schiff and others has provided a model for the underlying pathophysiological substrates for PDOC. The "meso-circuit" model (Schiff 2010) emphasizes the central role of the thalamus and the disturbance of brain networks involved in maintaining impaired consciousness and also suggests mechanisms for the effect of medications known to promote consciousness such as amantadine.

82.4 Diagnosis

Diagnosis of a PDOC is based on a synthesis of the following: exclusion or minimization of other factors that can impact behavioural responses (e.g. sedation from medications, critical illness neuro/myopathy, pituitary disturbance and other medical complications), findings on clinical examination, use of standardized behavioural assessment scales and knowledge of radiological and electroencephalogram (EEG) findings. Patients with STBI are very sensitive to factors such as pain, sleep disturbance, environmental noise and the amount of sensory stimulation of all types, and there is a risk that these factors contribute to the absence of behavioural responses. Optimization of the patient's general condition through careful attention to these aspects is a prerequisite for interpretation of behavioural responses.

Despite growing interest in sophisticated technological methods for identifying consciousness (e.g. with functional magnetic resonance imaging (fMRI) (Monti et al. 2010) or high-density EEG (Cruse et al. 2011)), at the time of writing this chapter, these methods are not established in routine health care. fMRI and high-density EEG have shown preserved consciousness in a small minority of patients who seem to be in VS when assessed with behaviourally based methods, but these methods are insufficiently sensitive and specific to be useful in the clinical care of individual patients. Jox et al.'s 2012 opinion article on ethical aspects of using new diagnostic and treatment methods remains a relevant basis for discussions with patients' relatives.

82.4.1 Standardized Scales

It is now well established that the use of standardized behaviourally based assessment scales adds sensitivity to clinical examination in the detection of signs of awareness (Schnakers et al. 2009). Of the available scales, a 2010 review (Seel et al. 2010) recommended the Coma Recovery Scale-Revised (CRS-R) most highly, despite some limitations. CRS-R is available in several languages, including Swedish, Spanish, Italian, German, French, Dutch and Norwegian. Several other scales had acceptable psychometric properties, and a limited literature suggests that the Sensory Modality Assessment and Rehabilitation Technique (SMART) methodology may have some advantages in terms of sensitivity to very subtle behavioural signs of consciousness (Godbolt et al. 2012). Whichever scale is chosen, assessments should be repeated to avoid missing reproducible but inconsistent signs of consciousness that may be masked by other treatable or transient factors (e.g. lack of sleep, pain).

82.4.2 Confirming Emergence from the Minimally Conscious State (MCS)

Patients are considered to have emerged from MCS if they demonstrate functional communication and/or functional object use. In clinical practice, patients commonly show a fluctuation in ability, and it can be unclear whether conscious responses are sufficiently consistent to be able to confirm emergence from MCS. Functional interactive communication can be demonstrated via correct yes/no responses to 6/6 basic situational questions on two consecutive evaluations, whilst functional object use can be confirmed by generally appropriate use of at least two different objects on two consecutive evaluations (Giacino et al. 2002). Operational difficulties remain, however, for patients who after STBI commonly have severe motor impairments, poor vision or hearing, language deficits and/or confusion. A practical guide to evaluation, taking such difficulties into consideration, is found in the 2013 British National Guidelines on PDOC (electronic annex 1a, via this https://www.rcplondon.ac.uk/guidelines-policy/prolonged-disorders-consciousness-national-clinical-guidelines).

82.5 Prognosis

Prognosis for recovery of consciousness and further improvement thereafter is variable and can be surprisingly good (Katz et al. 2009; Godbolt et al. 2013). Some patients who initially meet the criteria for PDOC go on to regain independence in personal care, and a few even return to work. However, assessment of prognosis for individual patients remains imprecise. For those patients who show no or limited recovery over an extended period, relatively little is known about how best to promote quality of life and what little communicative ability the patient may have. Patients who improve from VS/UWS to MCS in the early months after injury have a better prognosis for recovery of consciousness and function, emphasizing the relevance of discriminating between these conditions.

82.6 Management

Careful attention must initially be given to optimization of the patient's general condition including treatment of complications and may be followed by methods targeting promotion of consciousness more directly, such as pharmacotherapy, rehabilitation therapy, sensory stimulation and neuromodulation. The evidence base, other than for amantadine, is generally weak.

82.6.1 Sensory Stimulation (Box 82.1)

Sensory stimulation has an interesting theoretical basis and has been used in some centres for many years, but like many other complex interventions within neurorehabilitation has a poor evidence base for effect. Recently, theoretical models have been proposed promoting multimodal rather than unimodal sensory stimulation (Abbate et al. 2014), but sufficient research data to guide clinical practice is lacking.

Box 82.1. Sensory Stimulation for PDOC: Examples of Studies

1. Specific methods (unimodal stimulation)
   (a) FAST, Familiar Auditory Sensory Training
   - Pape et al. (2015), RCT, $n = 7$ treatment group, TBI: Greater improvement on one of two behavioural measures of consciousness for treatment group.

   (b) Music therapy
   - Magee and O'Kelly (2015), review: Indirect evidence for positive effects on arousal and attention.

   (c) Other auditory stimulation
   - Cheng et al. (2013), case series, $n = 86$, within-subject comparison. Auditory localization demonstrated more frequently in response to patient's own name than to a bell.
2. Multimodal stimulation
   (a) Auditive, tactile, kinetic, olfactory and/or gustatory stimulation in various combinations.
   - Padilla and Domina (2016), review. Some evidence of effect, but conclusions not fully supported.

   (b) Physiotherapy-based methods incorporating sensory stimulation, for example, the Affolter method, have been used for many years in some countries in Europe and are considered by their users to have worthwhile effects. No published evaluations of effect could be found in the English language literature.

82.6.2 Pharmacotherapy

The first priority should be to review the patient's medications and minimize sedation. If no improvement is observed, drugs aimed at promoting consciousness can be considered.

The strongest evidence of benefit is from treatment with the dopamine agonist and *N*-methyl-D-aspartate (NMDA) receptor antagonist amantadine. A methodologically robust randomized controlled study (Giacino et al. 2012) demonstrated more rapid improvement in patients treated with amantadine compared to placebo, without any difference in unwanted effects between the study arms. The trial design treated patients only for a relatively short time period, for largely logistical research reasons, and there remains a lack of data regarding when or whether to stop treatment for patients who improve on amantadine. A pragmatic approach can be taken with a planned dose reduction and cessation of treatment for a period when the patient's functional level is considered to have stabilized (usually from several months to a few years after injury), with follow-up and reinstatement of treatment if reduction in function occurs. The insomnia medication zolpidem (a sedative, hypnotic drug) has been shown to have useful paradoxical effects, with improved awareness, in a small minority of patients (1 in 15 patients, Whyte and Myers 2009), which was however not confirmed in a larger study (clinically relevant improvement in 0 of 60 patients (Thonnard et al. 2013)).

82.6.3 Neuromodulation (Box 82.2)

Neuromodulation, for example, with transcranial magnetic stimulation or direct current stimulation, is a promising technique which is often combined with some form of traditional therapy, whereby the brain is "primed" for maximal neuroplastic effects from therapy. Research is still at a relatively early stage (Ragazzoni et al. 2017), and it is likely to be some years before evidence-based clinical recommendations can be formulated.

Box 82.2. Neuromodulation for PDOC: A Promising Intervention for the Future

1. tDCS, transcranial direct current stimulation
   - Ragazzoni et al. (2017), review
     - One randomized, controlled, cross-over study ($n = 55$), no clear effect
     - One non-randomized, controlled study ($n = 10$), effect only in MCS
2. rTMS, repetitive transcranial magnetic stimulation
   - Ragazzoni et al. (2017), review
     - Two small controlled studies, case reports, case series. Conflicting results
   - Controlled study did not show effect (Cincotta et al. 2015).
3. Median nerve stimulation
   - Included in multimodal approach in the case series of deFina et al. (2010), inconclusive
4. Deep brain stimulation
   - Vanhoecke and Hariz, review (2017), sceptical, ethical issues, "no clear evidence"
5. Vagal stimulation
   - Single case study showed improvement (Corazzol et al. 2017)
6. Epidural spinal cord stimulation
   - Ragazzoni et al. (2017), review, case studies, uncontrolled case series, inconclusive findings

82.6.4 Maintaining Function and Preventing Complications (Box 82.3)

In recent years, literature has emerged (Whyte et al. 2013; Godbolt et al. 2015) highlighting that medical complications are common in patient with PDOC over an extended period (weeks to months, including the period after discharge from neurosurgical care). As medical complications and/or their consequences can impact the patient's arousal level and ability to interact with the environment, their prevention and continuing management is an important element in promoting function and a necessity before attempting to assess a possible PDOC due to STBI.

Active follow-up by physicians with brain injury expertise (e.g. rehabilitation medicine specialists) is necessary for optimal detection and management of complications such as continuing paroxysmal sympathetic hyperactivity, late detection of hydrocephalus, heterotopic ossification and pituitary dysfunction, amongst others. See earlier chapters in this book for discussion of specific complications. A summary of other factors is given in Box 82.3.

Box 82.3. Treatments Aiming to Maintain Function and Prevent Complications

1. Spasticity management and prevention of contractures
   - Includes some or all of specialized seating (wheelchair to promote an optimal, relaxed sitting position), positioning through 24 h to minimize spasticity, orthotics, passive movements, tip table, pharmacological treatment of spasticity (but note risk of sedation with enteral treatment)
2. Epilepsy management
3. Respiratory management with mobilization of secretions
   - May include positioning, use of positive expiratory pressure (PEP) breathing, assisted coughing

4. Urinary tract management
    - Some patients may have symptoms related to a neurogenic bladder. A few are managed with a suprapubic catheter. Urinary stones and catheter-related problems may occur.
5. Gastrointestinal management
    - Most patients require feeding via gastrostomy tube and require bowel management monitoring and interventions.
    - Mouth hygiene can be a challenge when mouth opening is limited.
6. Prevention of pressure sores
    - Regular turning needed. Air mattresses may however trigger spasticity.
7. Environmental regulation
    - It is generally accepted that excessive sensory stimulation can have negative effects with "overloading" of neural networks, resulting in fatigue and/or further reduced arousal and/or cognitive function. How this aspect is best balanced against the need to avoid understimulation (sensory deprivation), and synthesized with emerging evidence regarding sensory stimulation, remains to be defined.
8. Promoting sleep
9. Pain management
    - Behaviourally based scales can be used to assess pain in patients with PDOC. Management must balance ethical and physiological need to treat pain, with unwanted effects including sedation from pain medication.
10. Minimizing, detecting and treating other medical complications

82.6.5 National Guidelines

Several countries have published national guidelines for the care of patients with PDOC. Of particular interest for the clinician are the American Academy of Neurology guidelines (Giacino et al. 2018) and the British Royal College of Physicians guidelines (2013).

82.6.6 Concluding Remarks

Careful assessment of patients with PDOC is central to medical and rehabilitation management and is also necessary in order to give an adequate basis for consideration of ethical issues. Brain injury competence continues to be necessary after initial neurosurgical care and can be found within several related medical specialties, with some differences in national traditions and work distributions. Specialities include rehabilitation medicine (physiatry in the USA) and neurology. The needs and involvement of relatives of patients with PDOC after STBI should be considered, and dialogue with health-care professionals encouraged.

References

Abbate C, Trimarchi PD, Basile I, Mazzucchi A, Devalle G. Sensory stimulation for patients with disorders of consciousness: from stimulation to rehabilitation. Front Hum Neurosci. 2014;8:616.

Andelic N, Bautz-Holter E, Ronning P, Olafsen K, Sigurdardottir S, Schanke AK, Sveen U, Tornas S, Sandhaug M, Roe C. Does an early onset and continuous chain of rehabilitation improve the long-term functional outcome of patients with severe traumatic brain injury? J Neurotrauma. 2012;29(1):66–74.

Cheng L, Gosseries O, Ying L, et al. Assessment of localisation to auditory stimulation in post-comatose states: use the patient's own name. BMC Neurol. 2013;13:27.

Cincotta M, Giovannelli F, Chiaramonti R. No effects of 20 Hz-rTMS of the primary motor cortex in vegetative state: a randomised, sham-controlled study. Cortex. 2015;71:368–76.

Corazzol M, Lio G, Lefevre A, et al. Restoring consciousness with vagus nerve stimulation. Curr Biol. 2017;27(18):R994–6.

Cruse D, Chennu S, et al. Bedside detection of awareness in the vegetative state: a cohort study. Lancet. 2011;378(9809):2088–94.

DeFina PA, Fellus J, Thompson JW. Improving outcomes of severe disorders of consciousness. Restor Neurol Neurosci. 2010;28(6):769–80. https://doi.org/10.3233/RNN-2010-0548.

van Erp WS, Lavrijsen JC, van de Laar FA, Vos PE, Laureys S, Koopmans RT. The vegetative state/unresponsive wakefulness syndrome: a systematic review of prevalence studies. Eur J Neurol. 2014;21(11):1361–8. https://doi.org/10.1111/ene.12483. Epub 2014 Jul 21.

Giacino JT, Ashwal S, Childs N, et al. The minimally conscious state: definition and diagnostic criteria. Neurology. 2002;58(3):349–53.

Giacino JT, Whyte J, Bagiella E, et al. Placebo-controlled trial of amantadine for severe traumatic brain injury. N Engl J Med. 2012;366(9):819–26.

Giacino JT, Katz DI, Schiff ND, Whyte J, Ashman EJ, Ashwal S, Barbano R, Hammond FM, Laureys S, GSF L, Nakase-Richardson R, Seel RT, Yablon S, TSD G, Gronseth GS, Armstrong MJ. Practice guideline update recommendations summary: disorders of consciousness: report of the Guideline Development, Dissemination, and Implementation Subcommittee of the American Academy of Neurology; the American Congress of Rehabilitation Medicine; and the National Institute on Disability, Independent Living, and Rehabilitation Research. Neurology. 2018;91(10):450–60.

Godbolt AK, Stenson S, et al. Disorders of consciousness: preliminary data supports added value of extended behavioural assessment. Brain Inj. 2012;26(2):188–93.

Godbolt AK, Deboussard CN, et al. Disorders of consciousness after severe traumatic brain injury: a Swedish-Icelandic study of incidence, outcomes and implications for optimizing care pathways. J Rehabil Med. 2013;45(8):741–8.

Godbolt AK, Stenberg M, et al. Subacute complications during recovery from severe traumatic brain injury: frequency and associations with outcome. BMJ Open. 2015;5(4):e007208.

Jennett B, Plum F. Persistent vegetative state after brain damage. A syndrome in search of a name. Lancet. 1972;1(7753):734–7.

Jox RJ, Bernat JL, Laureys S, Racine E. Disorders of consciousness: responding to requests for novel diagnostic and therapeutic interventions. Lancet Neurol. 2012;11(8):732–8.

Katz DI, Polyak M, et al. Natural history of recovery from Brain Injury after prolonged disorders of consciousness: outcome of patients admitted to inpatient rehabilitation with 1-4 year follow-up. Prog Brain Res. 2009;177:73–88.

Laureys S, Celesia GG, Cohadon F, Lavrijsen J, León-Carrión J, Sannita WG, Sazbon L, Schmutzhard E, von Wild KR, Zeman A, Dolce G, European Task Force on Disorders of Consciousness. Unresponsive wakefulness syndrome: a new name for the vegetative state or apallic syndrome. BMC Med. 2010;8:68.

Magee WL, O'Kelly J. Music therapy with disorders of consciousness: current evidence and emergent evidence-based practice. Ann N Y Acad Sci. 2015;1337:256–62.

Monti MM, Vanhaudenhuyse A, et al. Willful modulation of brain activity in disorders of consciousness. N Engl J Med. 2010;362(7):579–89.

Padilla R, Domina A. Effectiveness of sensory stimulation to improve arousal and alertness of people in a coma or persistent vegetative state after traumatic brain injury: a systematic review. Am J Occup Ther. 2016;70(3):7003180030p1-8. https://doi.org/10.5014/ajot.2016.021022.

Pape TL, Rosenow JM, Steiner M. Placebo-controlled trial of familiar auditory sensory training for acute severe traumatic brain injury: a preliminary report. Neurorehabil Neural Repair. 2015;29(6):537–47.

Ragazzoni A, Cincotta M, Giovannelli F, Cruse D, Young GB, Miniussi C, Rossi S. Clinical neurophysiology of prolonged disorders of consciousness: from diagnostic stimulation to therapeutic neuromodulation. Clin Neurophysiol. 2017;128(9):1629–46.

Royal College of Physicians. Prolonged disorders of consciousness. National clinical guidelines. 2013. http://www.rcplondon.ac.uk/resources/prolonged-disorders-consciousness-national-clinical-guidelines.

Schiff ND. Recovery of consciousness after brain injury: a mesocircuit hypothesis. Trends Neurosci. 2010;33(1):1–9. https://doi.org/10.1016/j.tins.2009.11.002. Epub 2009 Dec 1.

Schnakers C, Vanhaudenhuyse A, et al. Diagnostic accuracy of the vegetative and minimally conscious state: clinical consensus versus standardized neurobehavioral assessment. BMC Neurol. 2009;9:35.

Seel RT, Sherer M, et al. Assessment scales for disorders of consciousness: evidence-based recommendations for clinical practice and research. Arch Phys Med Rehabil. 2010;91(12):1795–813.

Thonnard M, Gosseries O, Demertzi A, Lugo Z, Vanhaudenhuyse A, Bruno MA, Chatelle C, Thibaut A, Charland-Verville V, Habbal D, Schnakers C, Laureys S. Effect of zolpidem in chronic disorders of consciousness: a prospective open-label study. Funct Neurol. 2013;28(4):259–64. https://doi.org/10.11138/FNeur/2013.28.4.259.

Vanhoecke J, Hariz M. Deep brain stimulation for disorders of consciousness: systematic review of cases and ethics. Brain Stimul. 2017;10(6):1013–23. https://doi.org/10.1016/j.brs.2017.08.006. Epub 2017 Aug 24.

Whyte J, Myers R. Incidence of clinically significant responses to zolpidem among patients with disorders of consciousness: a preliminary placebo controlled trial. Am J Phys Med Rehabil. 2009;88(5):410–8. https://doi.org/10.1097/PHM.0b013e3181a0e3a0.

Whyte J, Nordenbo AM, et al. Medical complications during inpatient rehabilitation among patients with traumatic disorders of consciousness. Arch Phys Med Rehabil. 2013;94(10):1877–83.

83 Specific Paediatric Concerns

Olga Calcagnile, Catherine Aaro Jonsson, and Ingela Kristiansen

Recommendations

Level I

There are insufficient data to support a level I recommendation for this topic.

Level II

There are insufficient data to support a level II recommendation for this topic.

Level III

It is recommended that service providers should consider attention remediation to assist recovery and to involve family members as active treatment providers in the rehabilitation plan.

Tips, Tricks and Pitfalls

- The developing brain is more vulnerable to the effects of traumatic brain injury (TBI), and younger age is not a positive outcome predictor.
- Fine motor skills are more affected than gait after trauma.
- Post-traumatic epilepsy (PTE) is a severe consequence of TBI.
- PTE is less common among young children, and the incidence increases from the age of 15.
- About 50% of children with PTE after severe traumatic brain injury (sTBI) develop an intractable epilepsy.
- Post-traumatic headache has a higher prevalence after mild TBI than more severe TBI.
- In sTBI, chronic headache is mostly reported among younger children.
- Balance hope of recovery and awareness of deficits when giving early information to parents.
- The fastest improvement in recovery happens during the first 1–2 years after injury. Rehabilitation is needed to optimize recovery and the re-entry into everyday life.
- Patients with severe injuries tend to fall behind in long-term cognitive

O. Calcagnile (✉)
Department of Paediatric Medicine, Halland Regional Hospital, Halmstad, Sweden

C. A. Jonsson
Child and Youth Rehabilitation, Östersunds Hospital, Östersund, Sweden
e-mail: catherine.aaro.jonsson@regionjh.se

I. Kristiansen
Department of Women's and Children's Health, Uppsala University and Uppsala University Childrens' Hospital, Uppsala, Sweden
e-mail: ingela.kristiansen@kbh.uu.se

© Springer Nature Switzerland AG 2020
T. Sundstrøm et al. (eds.), *Management of Severe Traumatic Brain Injury*,
https://doi.org/10.1007/978-3-030-39383-0_83

development, but outcome differs considerably between individuals.
- The most typical cognitive deficits are related to attention, processing speed, problem-solving and memory.
- Social deficits are linked to functions such as inhibitory control, mental flexibility, communicative abilities and the understanding of other people's thoughts and feelings.
- Both social and cognitive functioning are promoted in familiar settings with few distractors.
- Family function is a predictor of cognitive and social outcome. Families need help to understand TBI-related deficits and how to cope with them.
- Recovery should be promoted through individualized rehabilitation with family and network integration.
- Promote recovery by assessment of cognitive and social function in the early recovery phase. These assessment results should be utilized in the planning of rehabilitation interventions and also the preparation of the return to home and school.
- There is a clear risk of chronic cognitive and social deficits. Assessment after the recovery phase aids long-term prognostication.
- If lingering deficits are found, functioning in everyday life can still improve with coping strategies. Those include having intellectual knowledge of deficits, being able to recognize when deficits actually disturb function and, finally, being able to plan in advance how to maximize functioning.

83.1 Overview

For many years, there has been the widespread opinion that TBI in the paediatric population would generate fewer long-term sequelae due to the high capacity of brain plasticity in children compared to adults. However, new studies have opened the debate on how instead the developing brain is more vulnerable to TBI. In animal models, for instance, it has been shown that post-injury apoptotic cell death increases in immature brains, that cerebral blood flow and metabolism are age-dependent and finally that biomarkers may be development specific (Giza et al. 2007).

Outcome reports on paediatric population are very limited, and only few recommendations have been identified for paediatric severe TBI (sTBI).

83.2 Sensorimotor Consequences

Strictly sensorimotor outcomes are seldom reported in recent articles. Sensorimotor functions involve both sensory and motor activity and pathways. Motor disabilities are often judged as less incapacitating than cognitive and social impairments; however, enduring sensorimotor deficit can also lead to significant reduction in quality of life. After sTBI, paediatric patients often regain sensorimotor skills and gait, but balance, speed and fine motor tasks are impaired even several years after trauma. Fine motor skills seem to be more affected than gait after trauma, especially considering speed and coordination (Kuhtz-Buschbeck et al. 2003).

Injury localization has been shown in several studies not to be a predictor for long-term outcome. It is important to keep in mind that the brain is a qualitative organ and very limited injuries may have a devastating impact (Lambregts et al. 2018). As for the other aspects of long-term neurological outcome, younger age is not a positive predictor. In relation to sensorimotor functions, pre-school children do not recover faster compared to older children. The duration of loss of consciousness and a higher number of injured brain areas have been identified as negative outcome predictors (Kuhtz-Buschbeck et al. 2003).

Nevertheless, studies have shown that children suffering from TBI have a better general neurological outcome compared to children with non-traumatic brain injuries (nTBI) (e.g. tumours, infections, encephalopathies). An explanation could be that nTBIs often generate more deep and diffuse pathology while TBI is often more focal (Lambregts et al. 2018). However, it is important to keep in mind that also TBI may present a diffuse pathology, especially when dealing with diffuse axonal injuries (DAI).

83.3 Post-traumatic Seizures in Children and Adolescents

Post-traumatic epilepsy (PTE) is a severe consequence of all types of TBI, from mild to severe. Post-traumatic seizures (PTS) occur within 7 days from injury and can be prophylactically treated with anti-epileptic drugs. PTE, on the other hand, may develop even after 15 years from the original trauma, and prophylactic anti-epileptic treatment to avoid debut of PTE has been shown to be ineffective. PTE occurs at all ages, but some aspects are specific for the paediatric population (Keret et al. 2018).

The mechanisms of PTE are so far not fully understood. Particular interest has lately been focused on the neuroinflammation processes that follow the initial injury cascade and how this process is related to epileptogenesis. In children, the brain may be more affected by the inflammatory cascade, thus being more vulnerable to develop seizures; however, findings are still inconclusive (Lucke-Wold et al. 2015).

PTS seems to occur with a higher frequency among children younger than 7 years compared to late adolescents and adults (respectively around 30% of young children with sTBI and 8% of late adolescents). On the other hand, PTE is less common among young children. PTE incidence increases from the age of 15 (8–15% of sTBI) to reach a maximal incidence among the elderly (Evans and Shachter 2018; Christensen et al. 2009; Keret et al. 2018).

There is no agreement between different studies on what may be the key risk factors for developing PTE; however, researchers agree that there is a clear connection between PTE and the severity of TBI. In some studies, PTE was associated even with the length of hospitalization, but that could as well be the consequence of more severe injuries. Some head computed tomography (CT) findings (contusions, oedema and haemorrhages, and the presence of skull fractures) are also considered additional risk factors. Nevertheless, children with PTS do not have a higher risk to develop PTE (Christensen et al. 2009; Keret et al. 2018).

Moreover, around 40–50% of children with PTE after sTBI develop an intractable epilepsy; their quality of life is poorer compared to children that have suffered a similar injury, but have not developed epilepsy. PTE is a clear negative outcome predictor and has even been associated with developmental delay and increased mortality (Keret et al. 2018).

83.4 Post-traumatic Chronic Pain in Children and Adolescents

Chronic pain syndromes are often caused by TBI. Studies in the adult population have shown a high prevalence for chronic headache, shoulder pain, complex regional pain and peripheral nerve impairments. In the paediatric population on the other hand, studies mostly focus on prevalence of chronic headache leaving the other aspects of the chronic pain syndrome mostly unreported (Nampiaparampil 2011).

Contrary to the general belief, post-traumatic headache has a higher prevalence after mild TBI (mTBI) than after more severe injuries. Chronic headache affects mostly teenage girls (around 40–50% of girls 12 months after mTBI compared to 15% of boys) and often has a migraine component. This mirrors the adult population where post-traumatic headache is more prevalent among women that have suffered a mTBI (Blume et al. 2012). A different scenario concerns sTBI. In this case, chronic headache is mostly reported among younger children (more than 30% of children 5–12 years old) with no difference between sexes. These results support the theory that developing brains are more sensitive to TBI than adolescent or adult brains (Blume et al. 2012). There is no correlation between the localization of head trauma and the site where headache will develop, and all forms of headache syndromes are represented (migraine, tension headache, etc.).

The last aspect that should be considered is the major limitation when dealing with paediatric reports. Except for late adolescents, studies are mostly based on parental reports, and data should be handled with caution. Moreover, in the paediatric population, it is difficult to isolate the prevalence of headache that is the result of trauma from any headache syndrome that would have manifested itself over time. Nevertheless, headache prevalence seems to be significantly higher among paediatric TBI patients than among age- and sex-matched controls (Blume et al. 2012).

83.5 Cognitive and Social Long-Term Outcome

Moderate and severe TBIs are often collapsed to a joint group in paediatric. This chapter therefore partly also includes findings from the moderate TBI literature. The knowledge base of cognitive outcome of TBI has been growing during the last decades, while the understanding on social outcome is largely premature and limited. The connections between white matter and grey matter within the frontal and temporal lobes are the most common locations of axonal injuries (Vik et al. 2006). Frontal regions are most frequently involved in focal TBI (Mendelsohn et al. 1992). These injury-prone regions have a prolonged developmental trajectory throughout childhood and adolescence (Gogtay et al. 2004) and are strongly connected to cognitive and social functions (Anderson et al. 2017). Accordingly, both cognitive (Aaro Jonsson et al. 2009; Aaro Jonsson et al. 2014; Anderson et al. 2012; Babikian and Asnarow 2009; Ewing-Cobbs et al. 1997; Halldorsson et al. 2013; Horneman and Emanuelson 2009; Treble-Barna et al. 2017a) and social functions are vulnerable after paediatric TBI (Anderson et al. 2017; Beauchamp and Anderson 2010; Halldorsson et al. 2013; Fyrberg et al. 2007; Horneman et al. 2005; Wilkinson et al. 2017; Renström et al. 2012; Rosema et al. 2012; Ryan et al. 2016a; Ryan et al. 2018). It is recommended that service providers should consider attention remediation to assist recovery (van't Hooft et al. 2005; Butler and Copeland 2002) and that service providers should consider involving family members as active treatment providers in the rehabilitation plan (Braga et al. 2005).

83.6 Cognitive Outcome

A meta-analytic review reports attention, processing speed, problem-solving and memory as the cognitive functions most at risk after sTBI in childhood or adolescence (Babikian and Asnarow 2009). Three years after injury, the patients with sTBI tend to fall behind the development of peers, but the heterogeneity between patients is large, and the result appears to be influenced by a subgroup of children with the most severe deficits (Babikian and Asnarow 2009). Large heterogeneity is one of the most common results in outcome studies of paediatric TBI, even within severity groups (Chapman et al. 2001). Independently from severity of TBI, fatigue and an overwhelming, sustained sense of exhaustion is commonly reported after injury (Crichton et al. 2017; Ponsford et al. 2012); it is connected to cognitive, physical, affective components and impairs social and school functioning (Crichton et al. 2017). Long-term cognitive outcome after TBI in childhood is influenced by several factors as presented in Fig. 83.1.

Post-traumatic amnesia (PTA) is found to be a stronger predictor than Glasgow Coma Scale (GCS) of long-term functioning and participation in daily life for school-aged children and adolescents (Briggs et al. 2015). Susceptibility weighted imaging (SWI) is shown to be more sensitive than CT in detecting traumatic lesions and can be used to predict cognitive outcome after paediatric TBI (Ryan et al. 2016b).

Brain reserve capacity (BRC) refers to variations in previous insults, genetics or exposure to neurotoxic agents at some time prior to receiving a brain injury, giving individuals a different BRC (Dennis et al. 2007). In the event of an accident or illness affecting the brain, individuals with

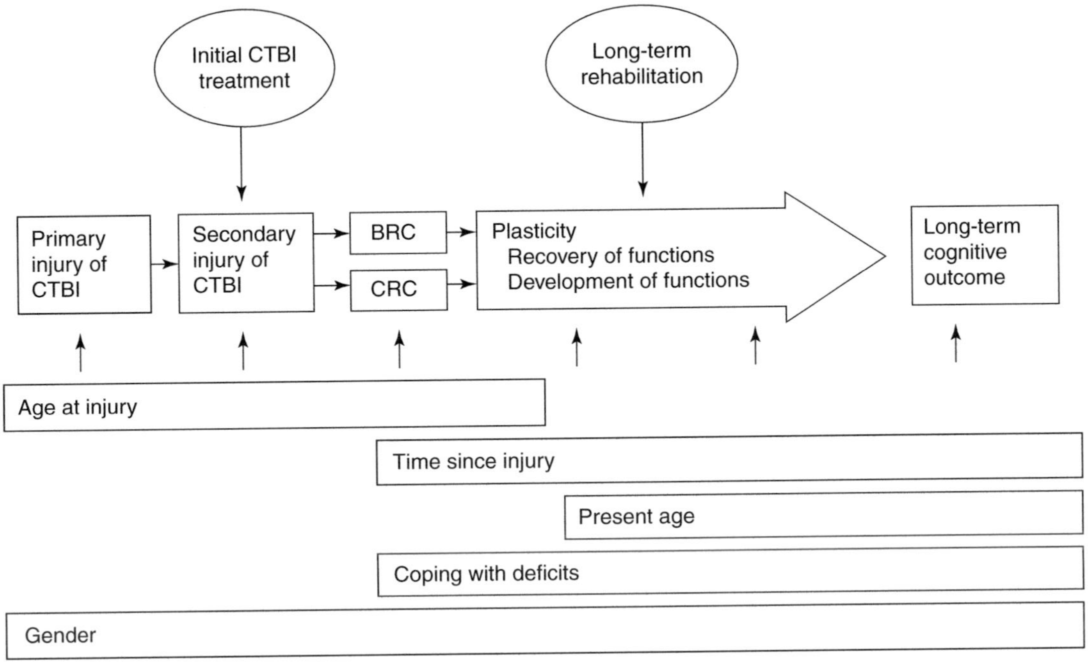

Fig. 83.1 Modifiers of long-term cognitive outcome of childhood TBI (CTBI), from Aaro Jonsson 2013

higher levels of BRC will be deficit-free for longer period of time than individuals with lower levels (Dennis et al. 2007).

The concept of cognitive reserve capacity (CRC) concerns the way in which these networks are used (Stern 2002), and pre-injury behavioural functioning has been reported to be a predictor of post-injury behavioural functioning (Catroppa and Anderson 2008; Fay et al. 2009).

Plasticity is the underlying function of brain recovery. It works through modulation of the neurogenesis, through changes in the strength of synapses and reorganization of neural circuits (Johnston 2009).

Age at Injury. Severe injuries received at a younger age are associated with a poorer outcome (Anderson et al. 2000, 2005). The recovery of older children from sTBI is better than that of younger ones and is more closely aligned to the recovery seen in adults (Anderson et al. 2000). Developing skills are more vulnerable than established skills (Anderson et al. 2000; Slomine et al. 2002; Lehnung et al. 2001; Kaufman et al. 2017), possibly reflecting that injury at the time of myelination can disrupt development of connectivity and constrain organization of networks mediating cognitive skills (Levin 2003). Kaufman et al. (2017) describe rehabilitation with children as working with a moving target. It occurs within the context of an ongoing developmental process, since children may have to relearn the skills they just established, while peers are moving on learning new tasks.

Cognitive outcome differs with the *time since injury*. The most pronounced recovery occurs during the first year after the injury (Chadwick et al. 1981; Ewing-Cobbs et al. 1997; Yeates et al. 2002). Since sTBI often results in impaired cognitive abilities, development is at large risk of being affected by reduced cognitive functions. A neuropsychological assessment in the early stage of recovery provides guidance on how to promote recovery, while an assessment after 1–2 years provides long-term prognostic information of deficits.

The *present age* at assessment, influences the character of the cognitive deficits. Frontal damage acquired early in life may exhibit its most prominent sequelae in later childhood when the executive and self-regulating processes associated with the frontal lobe are critical to psychological development (Taylor and Alden 1997). Outcome can also vary depending on the different expectations that the child or adolescent receives from the environment at various ages.

Coping with Deficits. Family function predicts cognitive long-term outcome (Anderson et al. 2012). In a study of parental burden conducted within the first months of their children's TBI, Stacin et al. (2008) found that a higher age at injury was related to higher levels of parental stress. It may be explained by concerns relating to a return to school and expectations related to academic performance. An alternative reason put forward by the authors is that deficits in cognitive neuropsychological functions may be more apparent in older children, thus contributing to the burden of the parents of the children in this age group. The use of denial as a coping strategy was related to an increase in parental burden and distress (Stacin et al. 2008).

Gender seems to influence outcome after TBI, although very few results of the influence of gender have been reported from the paediatric population. Girls have been shown to have stronger memory function than boys after injury (Donders and Hoffman 2002; Donders and Woodward 2003).

83.7 Social Outcome

Social function refers to the way an individual operates in a social environment by relying on social skills and interacting with others (Beauchamp and Anderson 2010). Younger age at insult (Ryan et al. 2016a), pre-injury function, injury severity, mental health of the parents and the child's self-esteem (Catroppa et al. 2017) are predictors of poorer social outcomes after TBI. A brain insult has an impact on post-injury social functions, but the social support an individual with TBI receives also influences the recovery trajectory (Ryan et al. 2016a). Thus, both injury and non-injury factors should be considered when identifying children at risk for long-term difficulties in social and behavioural domains.

Social competence is intimately linked with cognitive functions as inhibitory control and mental flexibility (Treble-Barna et al. 2017b; Levan et al. 2016), as well as communicative functions, such as expressive and receptive abilities (Fyrberg et al. 2007). Deficits of social function are associated with negative consequences for school performance (Treble-Barna et al. 2017a; Anderson et al. 2017), quality of life and general welfare (Ryan et al. 2016a). In daily life, a person with social dysfunction induced by an sTBI can be slower in the perception of the social interaction and more impulsive. Social functioning can be facilitated in familiar situations with few distractors, while the opposite may increase social problems.

Brain regions identified as contributing to social cognitive skills are represented as a "social network" comprising the prefrontal cortex, temporo-parietal junction, insula and amygdala (Anderson et al. 2017). Due to the vulnerability of these brain regions, it is likely that injuries in these specific areas will disrupt developing social networks in the immature brain (Anderson et al. 2017). Accordingly, right frontal pole thickness has been found to predict social problems (Levan et al. 2016). Children with sTBI have been found to have poorer functions related to the concept of Theory of Mind (ToM) (Ryan et al. 2016b). This implies limitations in the basic ability to understand other people's beliefs, based on knowledge of what others know. It also implies the understanding of how indirect speech, involving irony and empathy, can influence the listener. sTBI patients have been shown to have significantly poorer ToM, which on the other hand has been associated with more frequent behaviour problems and abnormal social brain network morphology (Ryan et al. 2016b). Furthermore, poorer ToM and pragmatic language were predicted by subacute alterations in diffusivity of the dorsal cingulum and middle cerebellar peduncles 2 years after injury (Ryan et al. 2018).

A nationwide Swedish register study investigated long-term medical and social outcomes associated with TBI in childhood (Sariaslan et al. 2016). All individuals born between 1973 and 1985, who had sustained one or more TBIs before the age of 25 years, were investigated. Outcomes were compared with unaffected siblings, thus accounting for the possibility that risks for negative social outcome were apparent in the families. They found that TBI consistently predicted later risk of premature mortality, psychiatric inpatient admission, psychiatric outpatient visits, disability pension, welfare recipiency and low educational attainment. The risks were not found among uninjured siblings. Effects were stronger for those with more severe injuries, repeated TBI and older age at first injury (Sariaslan et al. 2016).

References

Aaro Jonsson C, Smedler A-C, Leis Ljungmark M, Emanuelson I. Long-term cognitive outcomeafter neurosurgically treated childhood traumatic brain injury. Brain Inj. 2009;23:1008–16.

Aaro Jonsson C, Catroppa C, Godfrey C, Smedler AC, Anderson V. Cognitive recovery and development after traumatic brain injury in childhood: a person-oriented, longitudinal study. J Neurotrauma. 2013;30:76–83.

Aaro Jonsson C, Emanuelson IM, Smedler AC. Variability in quality of life 13 years after traumatic brain injury in childhood. Int J Rehabil Res. 2014;37(4):317–22.

Anderson V, Catroppa C, Morse C, Haritou F, Rosenfeld J. Recovery of intellectual ability following traumatic brain injury severity and age at injury. Pediatr Neurosurg. 2000;32:282–90.

Anderson V, Catroppa C, Morse S, Haritou F, Rosenfeld J. Functional plasticity or vulnerability after early brain injury? Pediatrics. 2005;116:1374–82.

Anderson V, Godfrey C, Rosenfeld JV, Catroppa C. Predictors of cognitive function and recovery 10 years after traumatic brain injury in young children. Pediatrics. 2012;129:254–61.

Anderson V, Beauchamp MH, Yeates KO, Crossley L, Ryan N, Hearps S, Catroppa C. Social competence at two years after childhood traumatic brain injury. J Neurotrauma. 2017;34:2261–71.

Babikian T, Asnarow R. Neurocognitive outcomes and recovery after pediatric TBI: meta-analytic review of the literature. Neuropsychology. 2009;23:283–96.

Beauchamp MH, Anderson V. SOCIAL: an integrative framework for the development of social skills. Psychol Bull. 2010;136:39–64.

Blume HK, Vavilala MS, Jaffe KM, Koepsell TD, Wang J, Temkin N, Durbin D, Dorsch A, Rivara FP. Headache after pediatric traumatic brain injury: a cohort study. Pediatrics. 2012;129(1):e31–9.

Braga LW, Da Paz Junior AC, Ylvisaker M. Direct clinician-delivered versus indirect family-supported rehabilitation of children with traumatic brain injury: a randomized controlled trial. Brain Inj. 2005;19:819–31.

Briggs R, Brookes N, Tate R, Lah S. Duration of post-traumatic amnesia as a predictor of functional outcome in school-age children: a systematic review. Dev Med Child Neurol. 2015;57:618–27.

Butler RW, Copeland DR. Attentional processes and their remediation in children treated for cancer: a literature review and the development of a therapeutic approach. J Int Neuropsychol Soc. 2002;8:115–24.

Catroppa C, Anderson V. Outcome and predictors of functional recovery 5 years following pediatric traumatic brain injury (TBI). J Pediatr Psychol. 2008;33:707–18.

Catroppa C, Hearps S, Crossley L, Yeates K, Beauchamp M, Fusella J, Anderson V. Social and behavioral outcomes following childhood traumatic brain injury: what predicts outcome at 12 months post-insult? J Neurotrauma. 2017;34:1439–47.

Chadwick O, Rutter M, Shaffer D, Shrout PE. A prospective study of children with head injuries: IV, specific cognitive deficits. J Clin Neuropsychol. 1981;3:101–20.

Chapman SB, McKinnon L, Levin HS, Song J, Meier MC, Chiu S. Longitudinal outcome of verbal discourse in children with traumatic brain injury: three-year follow-up. J Head Trauma Rehabil. 2001;16:441–55.

Christensen J, Pedersen MG, Pedersen CB, Sidenius P, Olsen J, Vestergaard M. Long-term risk of epilepsy after traumatic brain injury in children and young adults: a population-based cohort study. Lancet. 2009;373(9669):1105–10.

Crichton A, Babl F, Oakley E, Greenham M, Hearps S, Delzoppo C, Hutchison J, Beauchamp M, Anderson V. Prediction of multidimensional fatigue after childhood brain injury. J Head Trauma Rehabil. 2017;32:107–16.

Dennis M, Yeates KO, Taylor HG, Fletcher JM. Brain reserve capacity, cognitive reserve capacity, and age-based functional plasticity after congenital and acquired brain injury in children. In: Stern Y, editor. Cognitive reserve. Theory and applications. New York: Taylor and Frances; 2007. p. 53–83.

Donders J, Hoffman NM. Gender differences in learning and memory after pediatric traumatic brain injury. Neuropsychology. 2002;16(4):491–9.

Donders J, Woodward H. Gender as a moderator of memory after traumatic brain injury in children. J Head Trauma Rehabil. 2003;18:106–15.

Evans RW, Shachter SC. Post-traumatic seizures and epilepsy; 2018. Retrieved from https://www.uptodate.com/contents/post-traumatic-seizures-and-epilepsy

Ewing-Cobbs L, Fletcher JM, Levin HS, Francis DJ, Davidson K, Miner ME. Longitudinal neuropsychological outcome in infants and preschoolers with traumatic brain injury. J Int Neuropsychol Soc. 1997;3:581–91.

Fay TB, Yeates KO, Wade S, Drotar D, Stacin T. Predicting longitudinal patterns of functional deficits in children with traumatic brain injury. Neuropsychology. 2009;23:271–82.

Fyrberg Å, Marchioni M, Emanuelson I. Severe acquired brain injury: rehabilitation of communicative skills in children and adolescents. Int J Rehabil Res. 2007;30:153–7.

Giza CC, Mink RB, Madikians A. Pediatric traumatic brain injury: not just little adults. Curr Opin Crit Care. 2007;13(2):143–52.

Gogtay N, Giedd JN, Lusk L, Hayashi KM, Greenstein D, Vaituzis C, Nugent TF III, Herman DH, Clasen LS, Toga AW, Rapaport JL, Thompson PM. Dynamic mapping of human cortical development during childhood through early childhood. PNAS. 2004;101:8174–9.

Halldorsson JG, Arnkelsson GB, Tomasson K, Flekkoy KM, Magnadottir HB, Arnarson EO. Long-term outcome of medically confirmed and self-reported early traumatic brain injury in two nationwide samples. Brain Inj. 2013;27:1106–18.

Horneman G, Emanuelson I. Cognitive outcome in children and young adults who sustained severe and moderate traumatic brain injury 10 years earlier. Brain Inj. 2009;23:907–14.

Horneman G, Folkesson P, Sintonen H, von Wendt L, Emanuelson I. Health related quality of life of adolescents and young adults 10 years after serious traumatic brain injury. Int J Rehabil Res. 2005;28:245–9.

Johnston MV. Plasticity in the developing brain: implications for rehabilitation. Dev Disabil Res Rev. 2009;15:94–101.

Kaufman JN, Lahey S, Slomine BS. Pediatric rehabilitation psychology: rehabilitating a moving target. Rehabil Psychol. 2017;62:223–6.

Keret A, Shweiki M, Bennett-Back O, Abed-Fteiha F, Matoth I, Shoshan Y, Benifla M. The clinical characteristics of posttraumatic epilepsy following moderate-to-severe traumatic brain injury in children. Seizure. 2018;58:29–34.

Kuhtz-Buschbeck JP, Hoppe B, Gölge M, Dreesmann M, Damm-Stünitz U, Ritz A. Sensorimotor recovery in children after traumatic brain injury: analyses of gait, gross motor, and fine motor skills. Dev Med Child Neurol. 2003;45(12):821–8.

Lambregts SAM, Van Markus-Doornbosch F, Catsman-Berrevoets CE, Berger MAM, De Kloet AJ, Hilberink SR, Roebroeck ME. Neurological outcome in children and youth with acquired brain injury 2-year post-injury. Dev Neurorehabil. 2018;21(7):465–74.

Lehnung M, Leplow B, Herzog A, Benz B, Ritz A, Stolze H, Mehdorn M, Ferstl R. Children's spatial behaviour is differentially affected after traumatic brain injury. Child Neuropsychol. 2001;7:59–71.

Levan A, Black G, Mietchen J, Baxter L, Brock Kirwan C, Gale SD. Right frontal pole cortical thickness and executive functioning in children with traumatic brain injury: the impact on social problems. Brain Imaging Behav. 2016;10:1090–5.

Levin HS. Neuroplasticity following non-penetrating traumatic brain injury. Brain Inj. 2003;17:665–74.

Lucke-Wold BP, Nguyen L, Turner RC, Logsdon AF, Chen YW, Smith KE, Huber JD, Matsumoto R, Rosen CL, Tucker ES, Richter E. Traumatic brain injury and epilepsy: Underlying mechanisms leading to seizure. Seizure. 2015;33:13–23. Devi E

Mendelsohn D, Levin HS, Bruce D, Lilly M, Harward H, Culhane KA, Eisenberg HM. Late MRI after head injury in children: relationship to clinical features and outcome. Childs Nerv Syst. 1992;8:445–52.

Nampiaparampil DE. Chronic headache after pediatric brain injury: a systematic review. J Behav Brain Sci. 2011;1:81–6.

Ponsford J, Ziino C, Parcell D, Shekleton J, Roper M, Redman JR, Phipps-Nelson J, Rajaratnam S. Fatigue and sleep disturbance following traumatic brain injury—their nature, causes, and potential treatments. J Head Trauma Rehabil. 2012;27:224–33.

Renström B, Söderman K, Domellöf E, Emanuelson I. Self-reported health and influence on life situation 5-8 years after paediatric traumatic brain injury. Brain Inj. 2012;26:1405–14.

Rosema S, Crowe L, Anderson V. Social function in children and adolescents after traumatic brain injury: a systematic review 1989–2011. J Neurotrauma. 2012;29:1277–91.

Ryan NP, Catroppa C, Godfrey C, Noble-Haeusslein LJ, Shultz SR, O'Brien TJ, Anderson V, Semple BD. Social dysfunction after pediatric traumatic brain injury: a translational perspective. Neurosci Biobehav Rev. 2016a;64:196–214.

Ryan N, Catroppa C, Beare R, Silk TJ, Crossley L, Beauchamp M, Yeates KO, Anderson V. Theory of mind mediates the prospective relationship between abnormal social brain network morphology and chronic behavior problems after pediatric traumatic brain injury. Soc Cogn Affect Neurosci. 2016b;11:683–92.

Ryan NP, Genc S, Beauchamp MH, Yeates KO, Hearps S, Catroppa C, Anderson VA, Silk TJ. White matter microstructure predicts longitudinal social cognitive outcomes after paediatric traumatic brain injury: a diffusion tensor imaging study. Psychol Med. 2018;48:679–91.

Sariaslan A, Sharp DJ, D'Onofrio BM, Larsson H, Fazel S. Long-Term outcomes associated with traumatic brain injury in childhood and adolescence: a nationwide swedish cohort study of a wide range of medical and social outcomes. PLoS Med. 2016;13:e1002103.

Slomine B, Gerring J, Grados MA, Vasa R, Brady KD, Christensen JR, Denckla MB. Performance on measures of 'executive function' following pediatric traumatic brain injury. Brain Inj. 2002;16:759–72.

Stacin T, Wade S, Walz NC, Yeates KO, Taylor GH. Traumatic brain injuries in early childhood: initial impact on the family. J Dev Beh Pediatr. 2008;29:253–61.

Stern Y. What is cognitive reserve? Theory and research application of the reserve concept. J Int Neuropsychol Soc. 2002;8:448–60.

Taylor G, Alden J. Age-related differences in outcomes following childhood brain insults: an introduction and overview. J Int Neuropsychol Soc. 1997;3:555–67.

Treble-Barna A, Schultz H, Minich N, Taylor HG, Yeates KO, Stancin T, Wade SL. Long-term classroom functioning and its association with neuropsychological and academic performance following traumatic brain injury during early childhood. Neuropsychology. 2017a;31:486–98.

Treble-Barna A, Zang H, Zhang N, Taylor HG, Yeates KO, Wade S. Long-term neuropsychological profiles and their role as mediators of adaptive functioning after traumatic brain injury in early childhood. J Neurotrauma. 2017b;34:353–62.

van't Hooft I, Anderssson K, Bergman B, Sejersen T, von Vendt L, Bartfai A. Beneficial effect from a cognitive training programme on children with acquired brain injuries demonstrated in a controlled study. Brain Inj. 2005;19:511–8.

Vik A, Kvistad KA, Skandsen T, Ingebrigtsen T. Diffuse axonal injury in traumatic brain injury. Tidsskr Nor Laegeforen. 2006;22:2940–4.

Wilkinson A, Dennis M, Simic N, Taylor MJ, Morgan BR, Frndova H, Choong K, Cambells C, Fraser D, Anderson V, Guerguerian A-M, Schachar R, Hutchison J. Brain biomarkers and pre-injury cognition are associated with long-term cognitive outcome in children with traumatic brain injury. BMC Pediatr. 2017;17:173.

Yeates KO, Taylor HG, Wade SL, Drotar D, Stacin T, Minich N. A prospective study of short- and long term neuropsychological outcomes after traumatic brain injury in children. Neuropsychology. 2002;16:514–23.

84 Socioeconomic Consequences

Olli Tenovuo, Marek Majdan, and Nada Andelic

84.1 Overview

All analyses have shown that traumatic brain injury (TBI) is a major public health problem, also from a socioeconomic viewpoint. A recent review estimated that in the US, the annual costs of TBI for mankind are about 400 billion US dollars, representing 0.5% of the total annual global output (Maas et al. 2017). As discussed later in this chapter, calculations of costs do not account for many indirect consequences and may thus be gross underestimates. While milder cases constitute the vast majority of TBIs and therefore have a major socioeconomic impact, at an individual level, the severe cases are much more expensive in all respects. Considering the vast impact of TBIs on public health and economy, the funding for TBI research has severely lagged behind compared to many other, less significant health problems (Zitnay et al. 2008). This situation has started to change first during the last few years, mainly due to investments triggered by the big number of military TBIs in the United States (https://tier7.us/tbi-funding-cdmrp/) and the International Initiative for Traumatic Brain Injury Research (InTBIR) initiative (Tosetti et al. 2013; https://intbir.nih.gov).

O. Tenovuo (✉)
Department of Clinical Medicine, Turku Brain Injury Centre, Turku University Hospital, University of Turku, Turku, Finland

M. Majdan
Department of Public Health, Faculty of Health Sciences and Social Work, Trnava University, Trnava, Slovak Republic
e-mail: mmajdan@truni.sk

N. Andelic
Department of Physical Medicine and Rehabilitation, Oslo University Hospital Ullevål, Oslo, Norway

Research Centre for Habilitation and Rehabilitation Models and Services, Faculty of Medicine, Institute of Health and Society, University of Oslo, Oslo, Norway
e-mail: nada.hadzic-andelic@medisin.uio.no

84.2 Costs for Acute Care of Severe TBIs

Severe TBI is a major medical emergency, requiring in most cases high-level specialized care in trauma centers, treatment at intensive care unit (ICU) often for long periods, as well as long stay in hospital and rehabilitation centers. The costs for acute care of severe TBI consist of emergency care at the accident site; transport; multidisciplinary care at the emergency department (ED), ICU, and wards; surgical measures; consultations; imaging and laboratory costs; medications; and (sub)acute rehabilitation. At an individual level, these costs may of course be highly variable—from those who die at the scene, to those who need ICU care for several weeks, multiple operations, and several months' in-hospital care. In one Finnish study from the year 2009, the mean treat-

© Springer Nature Switzerland AG 2020
T. Sundstrøm et al. (eds.), *Management of Severe Traumatic Brain Injury*,
https://doi.org/10.1007/978-3-030-39383-0_84

ment cost for cases with severe TBI was 16,380 € (Tuominen et al. 2012). This is in line with some other reports, giving direct medical costs of about 18,030 € and 21,500 € during the first post-injury year (Chen et al. 2012; Scholten et al. 2015). A more recent Finnish study reported 39,809 $ average costs for the first post-injury year in severe TBI (Raj et al. 2018). However, for those with very serious TBI, total hospitalization costs in the trauma center and local hospitals are considerably higher during the first year post-injury (about 130,000 €) (Andelic et al. 2014).

There is no reliable data about the percentage of cases with severe TBI among those admitted to hospital. Undoubtedly, all cases with severe TBI who are alive at the ED will be admitted, but the severity of the others admitted may be variable, depending on the local policy and resources, not taking into account the variable definitions of severe TBI. This is reflected, e.g., in the preliminary results of the Collaborative European NeuroTrauma Effectiveness Research in TBI (CENTER-TBI) data (www.center-tbi.eu), showing surprisingly that about one-third of cases (>1600 cases in 20 European countries) with TBI treated at the ICU had "mild" TBI based on the Glasgow Coma Score (GCS) (unpublished data). Using an estimate that about one-third of hospital admissions have severe TBI, this would mean about 700,000 cases in Europe annually (Majdan et al. 2016). Based on these figures, the direct medical costs for severe TBI in Europe are about 14 billion € annually. In addition, a study looking at hospital admissions due to TBI in 25 European countries found high variability in the proportion of TBI treated as day cases (e.g., admitted but discharged the same day), which can reflect different care policies across the countries and make comparisons even harder (Majdan et al. 2016).

84.3 Severe TBI and Late Socioeconomic Sequels

Severe TBI leads to significant costs in terms of long-term rehabilitation and outpatient care. However, limited cost data exists in European countries. In a Norwegian 5-year follow-up study, the average costs per patient for in-hospital rehabilitation were about 70,000 € (SD 60000 €). The cost for the first year following the injury accounted for more than 90% of the total 5-year hospital-based rehabilitation of patients with severe TBI (Andelic et al. 2014). The few reports having tried to estimate the total costs of TBI, have suggested that only about 15% of total costs are caused by direct medical costs (Finkelstein et al. 2006). The indirect socioeconomic consequences of severe TBI are innumerous (Tenovuo et al. 2013), and most of them have been studied very little. Roughly, these can be divided to lost life years, lost productivity (=inability to work), and other indirect consequences, which include socioeconomic sequels for the individual, proxies, working environment, health care, social security, and legal system as well as intangible costs (the quantification of pain, social and psychological limitations, and reduced physical functioning).

84.3.1 Lost Years of Life

Severe TBI causes lost years of life not only as acute mortality but also as increased risk for late mortality and reduced life expectancy. An estimated 82,000 deaths because of TBI occur in Europe each year (Majdan et al. 2016), causing on the average 24.3 years of life lost (YLL), which is considered as the social cost (Majdan et al. 2017). The value of a lost life year has not been agreed upon internationally and may be considered to depend on the GDP of the country in question. Most estimates use values from about 50,000 € to 130,000 € per lost life year (e.g., Yabroff et al. 2008). Using these figures, the socioeconomic value of TBI deaths in Europe would equal from about 100 to 260 billion annually.

By definition, a TBI resulting in death shortly after the injury belongs naturally to the severe TBI category. However, the mortality from TBI is not confined to acute mortality only (Ventura et al. 2010). There are several studies, which show a permanent excess mortality after a TBI compared to normal age- and sex-matched population

(Brooks et al. 2015a, b). The effect size in various studies differs, and a meta-analysis of these was performed within the Global Burden of Disease study, which shows that persons after TBI have a 2.18 times higher risk of death, compared to the general population (Haagsma et al. 2016). The reduced life expectancy from TBI has been estimated to be 6 years (Haagsma et al. 2016) and has been shown to be highly dependent on the severity of the injury (Brooks et al. 2015a, b). Calculations of costs from this increased late mortality and reduced life expectancy have not been published. As increased late mortality and reduced life expectancy are "two sides of the same coin", an estimate of the socioeconomic cost can however be made. With about 700,000 cases of severe TBI annually in Europe, a 6-year reduction in the expected remaining life results in 3.2 million YLLs per year. Using the same value as above, this would mean a cost between 160 and 416 billion €. Thus, when giving an equal value for every YLL, the increased late mortality after a severe TBI causes higher costs than the acute mortality.

84.3.2 Lost Productivity

Lost productivity after a TBI, which is one of the indirect economic costs, results either from inability to return or stay at work or from reduced working capacity. Several studies and meta-analyses have assessed return to work after a TBI (Saltychev et al. 2013; Sigurdardottir et al. 2018). As expected, the risk for inability to work is highest after a severe TBI. This risk, however, depends on social and cultural factors, such as the level of social security, degree of employment in the society, and professional profile of the society. In these respects, the differences within Europe are much smaller than differences, e.g. between European countries and low-income countries in Africa and Asia.

A Finnish study gave a mean cost of 1.4 million € for lost productivity after a severe TBI (Tuominen et al. 2012). As the mean age of patients with TBI has risen, this cost might have diminished during the last 10 years. On the other hand, also salaries and GDP have risen, which probably compensates the age shift in TBI incidence. Using the calculations from the abovementioned study, early retirement from TBI would cause about 150 billion € extra costs annually in Europe. This is in line with estimates done in the United States.

The percentage of patients who return to work after a severe TBI is variable, not least because of inclusion criteria used for this kind of studies. In a Norwegian study, about 50% of preinjury-employed patients with severe TBI returned to work (Sigurdardottir et al. 2018), and similar figures have been published in other studies. On the other hand, a Danish nationwide study showed that only 16% of those with severe TBI achieved a stable position in work-life (Odgaard et al. 2017). Even fewer studies have assessed the working ability and productivity in those who have returned to work. A study done in patients with mild TBI showed that many patients have lowered productivity despite having returned to work (Silverberg et al. 2018). Due to the lack of proper studies, it is not possible to estimate the costs of lowered productivity in those who return and stay at work after a severe TBI.

84.3.3 Other Indirect Costs

Severe TBI is a condition, which greatly affects not only the person her/himself, but also his/her family, relatives, friends, and working community. The socioeconomic costs of the consequences have been scarcely studied. Only the caregiver burden has been assessed, as well as how a severe TBI in a parent affects children or vice versa, but not from an economic viewpoint. However, clinical experience clearly shows that a severe TBI in the family causes distress, mental problems, and loss of productivity in the family members; especially in case of children, these may have lifelong consequences.

Even if persons after TBI do not suffer from physical disabilities, they are often not able to go back to normal life (Humphreys et al. 2013), and the fact that they remain living with their families causes distress in family members even 4 years post-injury (Brooks et al. 1986; Jacobs 1988). This stress tends to be higher in partners than parents and correlates well with the injury severity. Young families have most problems coping with TBI and its consequences (Verhaeghe et al. 2005). A study following up patients for 24 years after TBI showed that tasks, such as financial management or shopping, were causing difficulties in most cases, while only about a third of patients returned to full-time employment (Colantonio et al. 2004).

Several studies and reviews have shown that TBI is not only an event, but also the start of a chronic health condition that predisposes for many medical problems, e.g. increased risk for new TBIs, psychiatric disorders, and neurodegenerative disease. The costs of this increased morbidity are unknown—they are partly covered by the cost estimate from reduced life expectancy, but not fully, with e.g. all direct medical costs from these consequences excluded.

Severe TBI especially at younger age predisposes for alienation with its severe societal and socioeconomic consequences. Patients with severe TBI are often permanently unable to take care of official and economic issues and are thus in need for various social services. In addition, medicolegal problems are common and cause burden for the legal system. A nationwide study from Sweden showed how TBI before adulthood had a significant impact on later psychiatric morbidity, need for welfare benefits, low educational attainment, and premature mortality (Sariaslan et al. 2016). All these aforementioned indirect consequences cause socioeconomic costs, which are poorly known but undoubtedly very significant.

84.4 Conclusions

The socioeconomic costs of severe TBI are known to be remarkable, but as many indirect, yet very costly consequences, have not been covered in the studies done, all existing figures are probably severe underestimates. In Europe alone, epidemiological data and cost analyses suggest that annual costs may exceed 500 billion €, depending, e.g. on how the value of human life is calculated. It should be noted that socioeconomic analyses of TBI have many uncertainties and that there may be significant differences between countries and cultures. In any case, as a more detailed analysis of socioeconomic costs of severe TBI in Europe alone as shown in this chapter gives a similar figure, as has been suggested for global annual costs from all TBIs (Maas et al. 2017), it is possible that the costs of TBI for our society are far more than any estimates have suggested.

References

Andelic N, Ye J, Tornas S, Roe C, Lu J, Bautz-Holter E, et al. Cost-effectiveness analysis of an early-initiated, continuous chain of rehabilitation after severe traumatic brain injury. J Neurotrauma. 2014;31:1313–20.

Brooks N, Campsie L, Symington C, Beattie A, McKinlay W. The five year outcome of severe blunt head injury: a relative's view. J Neurol Neurosurg Psychiatry. 1986;49:764–70.

Brooks JC, Shavelle RM, Strauss DJ, Hammond FM, Harrison-Felix CL. Long-term survival after traumatic brain injury part I: external validity of prognostic models. Arch Phys Med Rehabil. 2015a;96:994–9.

Brooks JC, Shavelle RM, Strauss DJ, Hammond FM, Harrison-Felix CL. Long-term survival after traumatic brain injury part II: life expectancy. Arch Phys Med Rehabil. 2015b;96:1000–5.

Chen A, Bushmeneva K, Zagorksi B, Colantonio A, Parsons D, Wodchis WP. Direct cost associated with acquired brain injury in Ontario. BMC Neurol. 2012;12:76.

Colantonio A, Ratcliff G, Chase S, Kelsey S, Escobar M, Vernich L. Long-term outcomes after moderate to severe traumatic brain injury. Disabil Rehabil. 2004;26:253–61.

Finkelstein EA, Corso PS, Miller TR. The Incidence and Economic Burden of Injuries in the United States. New York, NY: Oxford University Press; 2006.

Haagsma JA, Graetz N, Bolliger I, et al. The global burden of injury: incidence, mortality, disability-adjusted life years and time trends from the Global Burden of Disease study 2013. Inj Prev. 2016;22:3–18.

Humphreys I, Wood RL, Phillips CJ, Macey S. The costs of traumatic brain injury: a literature review. Clinicoecon Outcomes Res. 2013;5:281–7.

Jacobs HE. The Los Angeles head injury survey: procedures and initial findings. Arch Phys Med Rehabil. 1988;69:425–31.

Maas AIR, Menon DK, Adelson PD, et al. Traumatic brain injury – integrated approaches to improve prevention, clinical care, and research. Lancet Neurol. 2017;16:987–1048.

Majdan M, Plancikova D, Brazinova A, Rusnak M, Nieboer D, Feigin V, Maas A. Epidemiology of traumatic brain injuries in Europe: a cross-sectional analysis. Lancet Public Health. 2016;1:e76–83.

Majdan M, Plancikova D, Maas A, et al. Years of life lost due to traumatic brain injury in Europe: a cross-sectional analysis of 16 countries. PLoS Med. 2017;e1002331:14.

Odgaard L, Johnsen SP, Pedersen AR, Nielsen JF. Return to work after severe traumatic brain injury: a nationwide follow-up study. J Head Trauma Rehabil. 2017;32:E57–64.

Raj R, Bendel S, Reinikainen M, Hoppu S, Luoto T, Ala-Kokko T, Tetri S, Laitio R, Koivisto T, Rinne J, Kivisaari R, Siironen J, Higgins A, Skrifvars MB. Temporal trends in healthcare costs and outcome following ICU admission after traumatic brain injury. Crit Care Med. 2018;46:e302–9.

Saltychev M, Eskola M, Tenovuo O, Laimi K. Return to work after traumatic brain injury: a systematic review. Brain Inj. 2013;27:1516–27.

Sariaslan A, Sharp DJ, D'Onofrio BM, Larsson H, Fazel S. Long-term outcomes associated with traumatic brain injury in childhood and adolescence: a nationwide Swedish cohort study of a wide range of medical and social outcomes. PLoS Med. 2016;13:e1002103.

Scholten AC, Haagsma JA, Andriessen TM, Vos PE, Steyerberg EW, van Beeck EF, Polinder S. Health-related quality of life after mild, moderate and severe traumatic brain injury: patterns and predictors of suboptimal functioning during the first year after injury. Injury. 2015;46:616–24.

Sigurdardottir S, Andelic N, Wehling E, Anke A, Skandsen T, Holthe OO, Manskow US, Roe C. Return to work after severe traumatic brain injury: a national study with a one-year follow-up of neurocognitive and behavioural outcomes. Neuropsychol Rehabil. 2018 Apr;18:1–17.

Silverberg ND, Panenka WJ, Iverson GL. work productivity loss after mild traumatic brain injury. Arch Phys Med Rehabil. 2018;99:250–6.

Tenovuo O, Bullock MR, Zafonte RD. International systems of care and research agendas. In: Zasler ND, Katz DI, Zafonte RD, editors. Brain injury medicine – principles and practice. New York, NY: Demos Medical; 2013.

Tosetti P, Hicks RR, Theriault E, Phillips A, Koroshetz W, Draghia-Akli R, Workshop Participants. Toward an international initiative for traumatic brain injury research. J Neurotrauma. 2013;30:1211–22.

Tuominen R, Joelsson P, Tenovuo O. Treatment costs and productivity losses caused by traumatic brain injuries. Brain Inj. 2012;26:1697–701.

Ventura T, Harrison-Felix C, Carlson N, et al. Mortality after discharge from acute care hospitalization with traumatic brain injury: a population-based study. Arch Phys Med Rehabil. 2010;91:20–9.

Verhaeghe S, Defloor T, Grypdonck M. Stress and coping among families of patients with traumatic brain injury: a review of the literature. J Clin Nurs. 2005;14:1004–12.

Yabroff KR, Bradley CJ, Mariotto AB, Brown ML, Feuer EJ. Estimates and projections of value of life lost from cancer deaths in the United States. J Natl Cancer Inst. 2008;100:1755–62.

Zitnay GA, Zitnay KM, Povlishock JT, et al. Traumatic brain injury research priorities: The Conemaugh International Brain Injury Symposium. J Neurotrauma. 2008;25:1135–52.

Subacute MR Imaging: Traumatic Axonal Injury, Brainstem Lesions and Prognostic Factors

85

Toril Skandsen, Kent Gøran Moen, and Anne Vik

Recommendations

Level I

There is insufficient data to support a Level I recommendation for this topic.

Level II

Extensive traumatic axonal injury has been associated with less favourable outcome, and many of these lesions are best depicted on MRI in the early phase. Patients with severe TBI should therefore preferably be examined with magnetic resonance imaging (MRI) within the first few weeks.

Level III

There are no Level III recommendations for this topic.

Tips, Tricks and Pitfalls

Important MRI Findings and Sequences

- Most patients with severe TBI have traumatic axonal injury (TAI), more often in younger than elderly patients.
- Commonly, patients have TAI in concert with other lesions, such as contusions and haematomas.
- Primary brainstem injury is common; most of these are TAI lesions.
- Patients with low acute Glasgow Coma Scale (GCS) scores, not explained by increased intracranial pressure, may have bilateral TAI lesions in brainstem and/or thalamus.

T. Skandsen (✉)
Faculty of Medicine and Health Sciences, Department of Neuromedicine and Movement Science, Norwegian University of Science and Technology (NTNU), Trondheim, Norway

Department of Physical Medicine and Rehabilitation, St. Olav's Hospital, Trondheim University Hospital, Trondheim, Norway
e-mail: toril.skandsen@ntnu.no

K. G. Moen
Faculty of Medicine and Health Sciences, Department of Neuromedicine and Movement Science, Norwegian University of Science and Technology (NTNU), Trondheim, Norway

Department of Radiology, Nord-Trøndelag Hospital Trust, Levanger Hospital, Levanger, Norway
e-mail: kent.g.moen@ntnu.no

A. Vik
Department of Neuromedicine and Movement Science, Norwegian University of Science and Technology (NTNU), Trondheim, Norway

Department of Neurosurgery, St. Olav's Hospital, Trondheim University Hospital, Trondheim, Norway
e-mail: anne.vik@ntnu.no

© Springer Nature Switzerland AG 2020
T. Sundstrøm et al. (eds.), *Management of Severe Traumatic Brain Injury*,
https://doi.org/10.1007/978-3-030-39383-0_85

- Patients with a normal computed tomography (CT) scan may have TAI.
- Patients with a CT scan showing only a few subcortical punctate haemorrhages, or modest peri-mesencephalic subarachnoid or intraventricular haemorrhage, may have widespread TAI.
- Fluid-attenuated inversion recovery (FLAIR): look for high signal in the corpus callosum and dorsal part of the brainstem indicating TAI (Fig. 85.1) and non-haemorrhagic cortical contusions in the frontal and temporal lobes. These lesions attenuate with time.
- Susceptibility-weighted imaging (SWI) or T2∗GRE: look for small dark spots (microbleeds) indicating TAI (Fig. 85.2).

Prognosis: Information to the Family

- Clinical MRI often reveals lesions not previously detected by CT, so emphasize that this was to be expected.
- The most serious finding is that of widespread TAI with bilateral brainstem or thalamic involvement. Statistically, this implies a high risk of severe disability, but notably, also some of these patients eventually have a favourable outcome.

MRI Quality, Timing and Precautions

- MRI examination in the acute or subacute phase needs to be planned, and communication with the neuroradiologist is essential.
- For intensive care unit (ICU) patients that require continuous monitoring or assisted ventilation, the MRI must be planned in cooperation with the staff. Local conditions, such as the number of monitoring ports on the MRI system, MRI compatibility of equipment, distance to the MRI unit and access to anaesthesiology personnel during the examination, can be decisive for timing of the examination.
- The scan protocol takes 30–60 min, and even small patient movements can cause motion artefacts that severely reduce the quality of the scans.
- Many patients will enter a phase with confusion and agitation (post-traumatic amnesia) during recovery. One should therefore consider light sedation during scanning or let a nurse sit close to the patient during scanning in order to repeat the instructions and keep the patient calm.
- To obtain scans of high quality and an assessment by a neuroradiologist experienced with severe TBI, it may be beneficial to perform MRI while the patient is still in the trauma centre.

Contraindications and Precautions

- Early MRI is not decisive for the acute neurosurgical treatment and can first be performed when the patient's condition is stable regarding intracranial pressure and vital body functions.
- Some external orthopaedic fixations are too magnetic to be in the MRI scanner. Internal orthopaedic fixations, as well as material used in craniofacial surgery, are usually compatible with MRI.

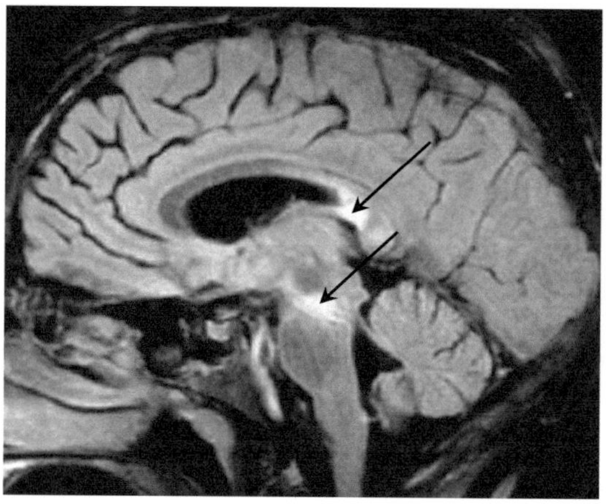

Fig. 85.1 Sagittal FLAIR image. *Arrows* show lesion in the corpus callosum and upper brainstem indicating DAI

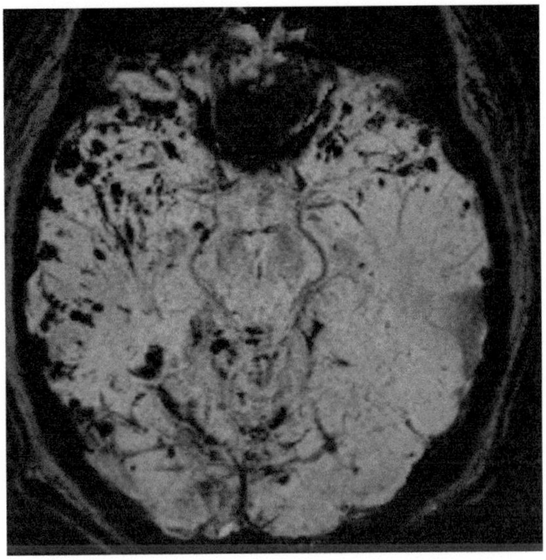

Fig. 85.2 Transversal T2∗-weighted gradient echo image shows micro-haemorrhages in the white matter indicating DAI

85.1 Overview

Computed tomography (CT) is insufficient in the diagnosis of diffuse axonal injury (DAI) and brainstem injury. Such injuries are very common and clinically important in severe traumatic brain injury (TBI), especially in the context of high-energy trauma. Magnetic resonance imaging (MRI) is the superior image modality to gain an overview of the traumatic lesions in the brain parenchyma. The neuroanatomic and prognostic information provided by MRI is important during the subacute phase of clinical management and rehabilitation. Thus, MRI should be considered in all patients with severe TBI.

The lesions in TAI are either haemorrhagic or non-haemorrhagic. The haemorrhagic lesions mostly consist of microbleeds, detected with a T2∗-weighted gradient echo sequence or susceptibility-weighted imaging. The non-haemorrhagic lesions are best visible in T2-weighted imaging, especially fluid-attenuated inversion recovery (FLAIR). Since the non-haemorrhagic lesions attenuate over time, MRI should preferably be performed during the first few weeks post-injury, in order to depict these.

85.2 Background

85.2.1 Clinical MRI in Patients with Severe TBI

MRI is more sensitive than CT in detection of traumatic parenchymal lesions (Gentry et al. 1988; Yuh et al. 2013) and thus better demonstrates the brain damage. MRI has been recommended if the patient's clinical condition is worse than what should be expected based on the CT scan (Parizel et al. 2005; Wintermark et al. 2015). But, regardless of focal lesions that often are revealed in severe TBI, the CT scan may only show the tip of the iceberg of potential lesions present. It should therefore be emphasized that only MRI can reliably depict important traumatic pathoanatomic entities such as traumatic axonal injury (TAI), non-haemorrhagic contusions, brainstem lesions and early trauma-induced ischemia. Thus, it is now recommended that patients with severe TBI should be examined with clinical MRI, preferably during the first 2–4 weeks (Moen et al. 2014; Mutch et al. 2016; Cicuendez et al. 2019).

85.2.2 The MRI Sequences Used in Head Injury

Today, a typical MRI scan protocol in head trauma is performed without contrast at a system with a field strength of 1.5 or 3 T and consists of T1- and T2-weighted imaging, fluid-attenuated inversion recovery (FLAIR) sequence, diffusion-weighted imaging (DWI) and T2∗-weighted gradient echo sequence (GRE) or susceptibility-weighted imaging (SWI) (Haacke et al. 2010; Mutch et al. 2016).

FLAIR is a T2-weighted sequence where the high T2 signal from the cerebral spinal fluid is suppressed, while the signal from traumatic brain oedema or gliosis remains bright, thus increasing the detectability of tissue injury (Fig. 85.1). In the acute and subacute stage, FLAIR sequences are used for the detection of oedema, while in the chronic stage, the hyperintensities represent gliotic scarring secondary to the TBI (Parizel et al. 2005).

T2∗GRE and SWI reveal very small haemorrhages associated with TAI, often referred to as 'microbleeds'. These techniques utilize the paramagnetic properties of the degradation products of haemoglobin which induce a focal signal loss, a 'blooming effect', and the haemorrhages appear dark on the scan (Fig. 85.2). The sensitivity to detect microbleeds is better at higher field strengths (Scheid 2007), and SWI is far more sensitive to blood products than T2∗GRE (Haacke et al. 2009).

Diffusion-weighted imaging is a technique which provides image contrast, resulting from the Brownian movements of water molecules in the brain tissue (Schaefer 2001). DWI can reliably distinguish between vasogenic oedema (increased diffusion) and cytotoxic oedema (restricted diffusion). DWI is most useful in the acute phase and could identify white matter lesions not seen on other conventional sequences during the first 48 h (Huisman et al. 2003). The DWI contains both diffusion and T2 information. These images are compared to the computed apparent diffusion coefficient (ADC) map where the T2 effects have been eliminated while the diffusion effects remain. The areas that appear bright on the DWI scan are dark on the ADC map if they represent restricted diffusion.

85.2.3 Traumatic Axonal Injury

Traumatic axonal injury (TAI), here used synonymously with the alternative term 'diffuse axonal injury', is an important injury type in TBI. TAI has been related to the rotational and deceleration forces associated with high-energy traumas, as traffic accidents, some sports accidents and falls from high heights. However, trauma with lower energy may lead to TAI. It has previously been called 'shearing injury'. The initial mechanical strain and the following cellular events eventually leading to disconnection or recovery of the axons are complex processes and still not fully understood, but primary axotomy is considered to be uncommon (Smith et al. 2013).

In cohort studies, TAI has been found in the majority of patients under the age of 65 with severe TBI who survived the acute phase. TAI was often depicted in concert with other lesions such as contusions and haematomas (Lagares et al. 2009; Skandsen et al. 2010).

The clinical course of TAI is characterized by initial loss of consciousness which is followed by a period of post-traumatic confusion that can last for weeks (Povlishock and Katz 2005). Patients without large contusions or haematomas, who do not wake up or exhibit severe agitation and confusion when sedation is stopped, often have a widespread TAI that cannot be diagnosed with CT.

The patterns of lesions depicted in the white matter with MRI were found to be identical to what had previously been found in the autopsy and animal studies (Gentry et al. 1988; Adams et al. 1989). Thus, in several MRI studies, a modified grading of TAI has been used: TAI stage 1 (lesions confined to the lobar white matter in the hemispheres or cerebellum), TAI stage 2 (lesions in corpus callosum) and TAI stage 3 (lesions in the brainstem). Lesions in the deep nuclei such as basal ganglia and thalami have not been included in this classification. However, most lesions depicted in these locations are increasingly recognized as TAI lesions and are typically found in patients with TAI in other locations (Moe et al. 2018).

Clinical MRI does not show the axonal injury directly; rather TAI is indirectly depicted as oedema (non-haemorrhagic) or small microbleeds surrounding the axons. The microbleeds are depicted with either T2∗GRE or SWI and are typically visible for a long time, months or years (Moen et al. 2012). In contrast, the non-haemorrhagic lesions attenuate during the first weeks and thus may be missed if MRI is performed late (Moen et al. 2012).

85.2.4 Brainstem and Thalamus Injury

Traumatic brainstem injury can be characterized as primary, directly caused by the forces of the trauma, or secondary, resulting from the ischaemia associated with herniation of the brain.

Primary brainstem lesions comprise TAI, which are the most common, contusions, haemorrhages and lacerations (Blumbergs et al. 2008). The pons and mesencephalon are predilection sites, and the lesions may be unilateral or bilateral. TAI in the thalamus is often seen in conjunction with TAI in the brainstem, both of which are lesions seldom depicted on CT (Moe et al. 2018). Contusions in the brainstem are seldom. These are typically superficial with a unilateral distribution and without other signs of widespread TAI. These are hypothesized to be caused by direct impact from the free edge of the tentorium.

With the increasing use of early MRI, it has been shown that brainstem injury is present in almost half of patients with severe TBI surviving the acute phase (Firsching et al. 2001; Skandsen et al. 2011; Hilario et al. 2012). Especially, the unilateral lesions in the brainstem and thalamus are associated with higher GCS score and hence may be seen also in less severe TBI (Moe et al. 2018). In contrast, patients with bilateral TAI lesions in the brainstem or in the thalamus have been found to have especially low level of consciousness in the acute phase (Moe et al. 2018). Other clinical signs in surviving patients with injury in the brainstem and thalamus are prolonged disorder of consciousness, central motor signs with paresis, spasticity or abnormal posturing, dysphagia and ophthalmoplegia. Periods of autonomic dysfunction (paroxysmal sympathetic hyperactivity) with hypertonia, tachycardia, rigidity and profuse sweating can be observed.

85.2.5 Prognosis: Traumatic Axonal Injury, Brainstem Injury and Thalamus Injury

Patients with mild and moderate TBI may also have TAI. Hence, the presence of TAI does not rule out a good outcome. However, recent studies have found that especially the extent of TAI in the splenium of the corpus callosum and in the brainstem as well as in the thalamus is associated with an increased risk of disability (Moen et al. 2014, Cicuendez et al. 2017, Haghbayan et al. 2017, Cicuendez 2019). These studies also showed that the prognostic models including MRI findings had a better discriminatory capacity than models with the established prognostic factors identified in the IMPACT and CRASH models.

In a systematic review and meta-analysis, brainstem injury was strongly associated with increased risk of death and severe disability (Haghbayan et al. 2017). Moreover, some studies using early MRI have found that bilateral involvement of the brainstem was a particularly severe finding (Firsching et al. 1998; Skandsen et al. 2011; Hilario et al. 2012). However, patients with brainstem lesions may have a good outcome, and that is important to bear in mind when counselling the family on individual cases.

Location in the brainstem also matters, and TAI lesions in the substantia nigra and tegmentum (Abu Hamdeh et al. 2017) or within brainstem nuclei of the ascending arousal network (Izzy et al. 2017) correlated more strongly with a poor recovery.

85.2.6 Advanced MR Methods

Several methods require post-processing of MRI data and are therefore less available in clinical diagnostics today. Examples are diffusion tensor imaging (DTI), MR spectroscopy, functional magnetic resonance imaging (fMRI) and different methods for measurement of brain volumes. Since DTI is increasingly used in MRI research and is proposed to be a sensitive biomarker of TAI, this method will be briefly described.

In nerve fibres, diffusivity is greater in the direction of the axon (axial) than perpendicular to the fibres, diffusion anisotropy. DTI is based on sampling of diffusion-weighted images for many directions (Le Bihan et al. 2001) and computation of an index of the diffusion anisotropy, e.g., fractional anisotropy (FA) values (Marquez de la Plata et al. 2011). If the microstructure of the axon is damaged (as in TBI), this can result in decreased axial diffusivity and lower FA values.

Both micro-haemorrhagic and non-haemorrhagic TAI lesions are associated with damage of the underlying white matter microstructure in DTI studies (Moen et al. 2016; Toth et al. 2018). But DTI also depicts axonal damage where the white matter appears to be normal in clinical MRI sequence (Hulkower et al. 2013); it is therefore potentially a more sensitive method for detecting TAI. In a longitudinal DTI study of very severe TBI, it could be demonstrated that normalization of the DTI indices was larger in the patients who recovered function (Sidaros et al. 2008).

DTI is expected to become more useful in the diagnostic work-up of single patients in the clinic with the development of normative databases of, e.g., FA values in different brain areas in healthy humans (Haacke et al. 2010; Douglas et al. 2015). However, recent reviews concluded that DTI is not yet ready for use in individual patients with TBI and that more longitudinal data are needed (Hulkower et al. 2013; Douglas et al. 2015).

85.3 Specific Paediatric Concerns

Children with severe TBI are at risk for long-lasting social and cognitive problems and learning disabilities. It is important for the paediatricians, rehabilitation professionals and neuropsychologists to have a thorough diagnostic of the brain injury, and like for adults, MRI findings can inform about prognosis (Smitherman et al. 2016). We recommend that MRI is performed in all cases of severe paediatric TBI. One should consider performing the examination while the child is still under sedation to avoid additional anaesthesia later.

References

Abu Hamdeh S, Marklund N, Lannsjo M, Howells T, Raininko R, Wikstrom J, Enblad P. Extended anatomical grading in diffuse axonal injury using MRI: hemorrhagic lesions in the substantia nigra and mesencephalic tegmentum indicate poor long-term outcome. J Neurotrauma. 2017;34(2):341–52.

Adams JH, Doyle D, Ford I, Gennarelli TA, Graham DI, McLellan DR. Diffuse axonal injury in head injury: definition, diagnosis and grading. Histopathology. 1989;15(1):49–59.

Blumbergs P, Reilly P, Vink R. Trauma. Greenfield's neuropathology. London: Edward Arnold Ltd.; 2008. p. 733–832.

Cicuendez M, Castano-Leon A, Ramos A, Hilario A, Gomez PA, Lagares A. Prognostic value of corpus callosum injuries in severe head trauma. Acta Neurochir. 2017;159(1):25–32.

Cicuendez M, Castano-Leon A, Ramos A, Hilario A, Gomez PA, Lagares A. The added prognostic value of magnetic resonance imaging in traumatic brain injury: the importance of traumatic axonal injury when performing ordinal logistic regression. J Neuroradiol. 2019;46(5):299–306.

Douglas DB, Iv M, Douglas PK, Anderson A, Vos SB, Bammer R, Zeineh M, Wintermark M. Diffusion tensor imaging of TBI: potentials and challenges. Top Magn Reson Imaging. 2015;24(5):241–51.

Firsching R, Woischneck D, Diedrich M, Klein S, Ruckert A, Wittig H, Dohring W. Early magnetic resonance imaging of brainstem lesions after severe head injury. J Neurosurg. 1998;89(5):707–12.

Firsching R, Woischneck D, Klein S, Reissberg S, Dohring W, Peters B. Classification of severe head injury based on magnetic resonance imaging. Acta Neurochir. 2001;143(3):263–71.

Gentry LR, Godersky JC, Thompson B. MR imaging of head trauma: review of the distribution and radiopathologic features of traumatic lesions. AJNR Am J Neuroradiol. 1988;150:101–10.

Haacke EM, Mittal S, Wu Z, Neelavalli J, Cheng YC. Susceptibility-weighted imaging: technical aspects and clinical applications, part 1. AJNR Am J Neuroradiol. 2009;30(1):19–30.

Haacke EM, Duhaime AC, Gean AD, Riedy G, Wintermark M, Mukherjee P, Brody DL, DeGraba T, Duncan TD, Elovic E, Hurley R, Latour L, Smirniotopoulos JG, Smith DH. Common data elements in radiologic imaging of traumatic brain injury. J Magn Reson Imaging. 2010;32(3):516–43.

Haghbayan H, Boutin A, Laflamme M, Lauzier F, Shemilt M, Moore L, Zarychanski R, Douville V, Fergusson D, Turgeon AF. The prognostic value of MRI in moderate and severe traumatic brain injury: a systematic review and meta-analysis. Crit Care Med. 2017;45(12):e1280–8.

Hilario A, Ramos A, Millan JM, Salvador E, Gomez PA, Cicuendez M, Diez-Lobato R, Lagares A. Severe traumatic head injury: prognostic value of brain stem injuries detected at MRI. AJNR Am J Neuroradiol. 2012;33(10):1925–31.

Hulkower MB, Poliak DB, Rosenbaum SB, Zimmerman ME, Lipton ML. A decade of DTI in traumatic brain injury: 10 years and 100 articles later. AJNR Am J Neuroradiol. 2013;34(11):2064–74.

Huisman TA, Sorensen AG, Hergan K, Gonzalez RG, Schaefer PW. Diffusion-weighted imaging for the evaluation of diffuse axonal injury in closed head injury. J Comput Assist Tomogr. 2003;27(1):5–11.

Izzy S, Mazwi NL, Martinez S, Spencer CA, Klein JP, Parikh G, Glenn MB, Greenberg SM, Greer DM, Wu O, Edlow BL. Revisiting grade 3 diffuse axonal injury: not all brainstem microbleeds are prognostically equal. Neurocrit Care. 2017;27(2):199–207.

Lagares A, Ramos A, Perez-Nunez A, Ballenilla F, Alday R, Gomez PA, Kaen A, Lobato RD. The role of MR imaging in assessing prognosis after severe and moderate head injury. Acta Neurochir. 2009;151(4):341–56.

Le Bihan D, Mangin JF, Poupon C, Clark CA, Pappata S, Molko N, Chabriat H. Diffusion tensor imaging: concepts and applications. J Magn Reson Imaging. 2001;13(4):534–46.

Marquez de la Plata CD, Yang FG, Wang JY, Krishnan K, Bakhadirov K, Paliotta C, Aslan S, Devous MD, Moore C, Harper C, McColl R, Munro Cullum C, Diaz-Arrastia R. Diffusion tensor imaging biomarkers for traumatic axonal injury: analysis of three analytic methods. J Int Neuropsychol Soc. 2011;17(1):24–35.

Moe HK, Moen KG, Skandsen T, Kvistad KA, Laureys S, Haberg A, Vik A. The influence of traumatic axonal injury in thalamus and brainstem on level of consciousness at scene or admission: a clinical magnetic resonance imaging study. J Neurotrauma. 2018; https://doi.org/10.1089/neu.2017.5252.

Moen KG, Skandsen T, Folvik M, Brezova V, Kvistad KA, Rydland J, Manley GT, Vik A. A longitudinal MRI study of traumatic axonal injury in patients with moderate and severe traumatic brain injury. J Neurol Neurosurg Psychiatry. 2012;83(12):7.

Moen KG, Brezova V, Skandsen T, Haberg AK, Folvik M, Vik A. Traumatic axonal injury: the prognostic value of lesion load in corpus callosum, brain stem, and thalamus in different magnetic resonance imaging sequences. J Neurotrauma. 2014;31(17):1486–96.

Moen KG, Vik A, Olsen A, Skandsen T, Haberg AK, Evensen KA, Eikenes L. Traumatic axonal injury: relationships between lesions in the early phase and diffusion tensor imaging parameters in the chronic phase of traumatic brain injury. J Neurosci Res. 2016;94(7):623–35.

Mutch CA, Talbott JF, Gean A. Imaging evaluation of acute traumatic brain injury. Neurosurg Clin N Am. 2016;27(4):409–39.

Parizel PM, Van Goethem JW, Ozsarlak O, Maes M, Phillips CD. New developments in the neuroradiological diagnosis of craniocerebral trauma. Eur Radiol. 2005;15(3):569–81.

Povlishock JT, Katz DI. Update of neuropathology and neurological recovery after traumatic brain injury. J Head Trauma Rehabil. 2005;20(1):76–94.

Schaefer PW. Applications of DWI in clinical neurology. J Neurol Sci. 2001;186(Suppl 1):S25–35.

Scheid R, Ott DV, Roth H, Schroeter ML, von Cramon DY. Comparative magnetic resonance imaging at 1.5 and 3 Tesla for the evaluation of traumatic microbleeds. J Neurotrauma. 2007;24(12):1811–6

Sidaros A, Engberg AW, Sidaros K, Liptrot MG, Herning M, Petersen P, Paulson OB, Jernigan TL, Rostrup E. Diffusion tensor imaging during recovery from severe traumatic brain injury and relation to clinical outcome: a longitudinal study. Brain. 2008;131(2):559–72.

Skandsen T, Kvistad KA, Solheim O, Strand IH, Folvik M, Vik A. Prevalence and impact of diffuse axonal injury in patients with moderate and severe head injury: a cohort study of early magnetic resonance imaging findings and 1-year outcome. J Neurosurg. 2010;113(3):556–63.

Skandsen T, Kvistad KA, Solheim O, Lydersen S, Strand IH, Vik A. Prognostic value of magnetic resonance imaging in moderate and severe head injury: a prospective study of early mri findings and one-year outcome. J Neurotrauma. 2011;28(5):1–9.

Smith DH, Hicks R, Povlishock JT. Therapy development for diffuse axonal injury. J Neurotrauma. 2013;30(5):307–23.

Smitherman E, Hernandez A, Stavinoha PL, Huang R, Kernie SG, Diaz-Arrastia R, Miles DK. Predicting outcome after pediatric traumatic brain injury by early magnetic resonance imaging lesion location and volume. J Neurotrauma. 2016;33(1):35–48.

Toth A, Kornyei B, Kovacs N, Rostas T, Buki A, Doczi T, Bogner P, Schwarcz A. Both hemorrhagic and nonhemorrhagic traumatic MRI lesions are associated with the microstructural damage of the normal appearing white matter. Behav Brain Res. 2018;340:106–16.

Wintermark M, Sanelli PC, Anzai Y, Tsiouris AJ, Whitlow CT, A. C. R. H. I. Institute and A. C. R. H. I. Institute. Imaging evidence and recommendations for traumatic brain injury: conventional neuroimaging techniques. J Am Coll Radiol. 2015;12(2):e1–14.

Yuh EL, Mukherjee P, Lingsma HF, Yue JK, Ferguson AR, Gordon WA, Valadka AB, Schnyer DM, Okonkwo DO, Maas AI, Manley GT, Investigators T-T. Magnetic resonance imaging improves 3-month outcome prediction in mild traumatic brain injury. Ann Neurol. 2013;73(2):224–35.

86 Neurodegeneration and Dementia following Traumatic Brain Injury

Niklas Marklund

Recommendations

Level I

There is Level 1 evidence that severe TBI can lead to lasting, chronic consequences including dementias and other neurodegenerative diseases including Parkinson's disease.

Level II

Numerous studies point to an increased aggregation of tau and amyloid-beta in severe TBI.

Level III

Numerous observational studies suggest a link between TBI and neurodegeneration.

Tips and Tricks

- Amyloid-beta (Aβ) aggregates/plaques, the hallmark of Alzheimer's disease (AD), are found at autopsy or in surgically resected brain tissue within the first post-injury hours-days in approximately 30% of severe TBI patients. Carriers of the APOE ε4 allele may have an increased risk for Aβ aggregation.
- In most large population-based studies, TBI is associated with an increased risk of developing AD.
- Chronic traumatic encephalopathy (CTE) and other tauopathies have been associated with TBI. Predominantly, CTE has been linked to sport-related repeated mild TBI. Increased tau aggregation and phosphorylation has been observed in long-term (not short-term) survivors of severe TBI.
- TBI has been linked to an increased risk for Parkinson's disease in large population-based studies.
- The risk for other neurodegenerative disorders, such as frontotemporal dementia, appears to be increased among TBI patients. At autopsy, numerous proteins linked to neurodegeneration have increased expression and/or accumulate in injured axons. The risk factors contributing to post-TBI degeneration have not been established although axonal injury and neuroinflammation are implicated in this process.

N. Marklund (✉)
Department of Clinical Sciences Lund, Neurosurgery, Lund University, Skåne University Hospital, Lund, Sweden
e-mail: niklas.marklund@med.lu.se

© Springer Nature Switzerland AG 2020
T. Sundstrøm et al. (eds.), *Management of Severe Traumatic Brain Injury*, https://doi.org/10.1007/978-3-030-39383-0_86

- PET imaging, at least for Aβ and tau, is increasingly used and may be useful to follow individuals post-TBI to establish the time course for tau and/or Aβ aggregation as well as to develop novel therapies preventing long-term development of dementia and other neurodegenerative disorders.

86.1 General Aspects

This chapter deals with the risks of developing neurodegenerative disorders, including dementia and Parkinson's disease, following traumatic brain injury (TBI). A large number of studies have found evidence for TBI being a chronic brain disorder with often devastating long-term consequences. For instance, when TBI is sustained in childhood, there may be an increased risk of disability, psychiatric illness, and premature death later in life (McKinlay et al. 2002; Masel and DeWitt 2010; Whiteneck et al. 2016; Wilson et al. 2017). In addition, TBI results in excess mortality, not only in the moderate-severe TBIs, but surprisingly also in those individuals with mild TBI (Wilson et al. 2017). As described elsewhere in this book, disabling and persisting cognitive impairment, personality changes, and decreased quality of life are exceedingly common in survivors of severe TBI. Moreover, in contrast to the common notion of a gradual improvement with time in most TBI survivors, a variety of studies indicate that up to one-half of patients show either no improvement or a slow and gradual decline (Millar et al. 2003; McMillan et al. 2012; Corrigan et al. 2014; Moretti et al. 2012; Himanen et al. 2006). In fact, post-TBI neuroimaging studies have found brain atrophy to the same degree as observed in Alzheimer's disease (AD) (Cole et al. 2018). At autopsy, immunohistochemical studies have provided evidence that TBI is a chronic disease process leading to atrophy of cortical and white matter structures associated with persistent neuroinflammation, white matter degeneration, and progressive cortical atrophy at long term following the initial impact (Johnson et al. 2012) and accumulation of numerous proteins related to neurodegeneration (Kenney et al. 2018). As for the clinical studies, the available evidence is summarized below.

86.2 Alzheimer's Disease

Alzheimer's disease (AD) accounts for 60–80% of all dementias. There are recent large-scale population studies finding a risk increase for AD after TBI. Additionally, TBI patients seem to develop AD at a younger age (Mendez et al. 2015) and have an increased risk for mild cognitive impairment, a common precursor of dementia (Perry et al. 2016). It should be mentioned that a number of studies exist that have failed to document this association [see (Mendez 2017; Huang et al. 2018)], including a nation-wide study evaluating early-onset dementias (Nordstrom et al. 2014). Here, the risk of developing young-onset dementia after TBI was examined in ca 800,000 Swedish military recruits, of whom 45,000 sustained a TBI over a three-decade period. In this cohort, the risk for AD was not markedly increased by TBI after multivariate adjustments. However, most reports and meta-analyses conclude that a single moderate to severe TBI is a risk factor for AD. For instance, in a prospective study of US World War II veterans, 548 veterans with a single moderate or severe TBI were compared to 1228 without, an increased risk of both AD and non-AD dementias after TBI was observed (Plassman et al. 2000). A statewide study in California evaluated the association between TBI and dementia in 164,661 patients and found that moderate to severe TBI increased the risk of dementia in patients >55 years old with a hazard ratio (HR) of ≥1.3 (Gardner et al. 2014). In a nation-wide Swedish study (Nordstrom and Nordstrom 2018), all individuals aged ≥50 years ($n \geq$ three million) with a diagnoses of dementia and TBI were tracked, and by using three different cohorts, an increased dementia risk after TBI was found with an adjusted odds ratio of 1.8. This association was strongest in the first post-injury year. It should be noted that all TBI severities were included, but the risk was higher for patients with more severe TBI or multiple TBIs. In a recent Danish study (Fann et al. 2018), 132 093 individuals (4.7%) had at least one TBI during 1977–2013, and 126 734 (4.5%) had incident dementia during 1999–2013. The fully adjusted risk of all-cause dementia in people with a history of TBI was higher (HR 1.24) than in those without a history of TBI, as was the specific risk of AD (HR 1.16). The risk of dementia was highest in the first 6 months after TBI. The younger a person was when sustaining a TBI, the higher the HRs for dementia were when the risk was stratified by the time since TBI. Importantly, TBI victims had an increased risk of dementia also when compared to individuals with non-TBI trauma. Overall, many reports find a relative 2–14-fold risk increase of dementias following TBI, and plausibly the largest meta-analysis to date found an overall odds ratio of 1.4 for AD in TBI victims (Perry et al. 2016) without apparent gender differences. Carriers of the apolipoprotein E (APOE) ε4 alleles have an increased risk for AD. When one APOE ε4 is present, there is a threefold increase that AD will occur at a younger age, one possible reason being impaired proteolytic breakdown and clearance of Aβ. Thus, there may also be a link between this allele and worse outcome in TBI.

86.3 Other Dementias and Neurodegenerative Disorders

An increasing number of selected athletes all having sustained several sport-related concussions/mild TBIs during their career have been observed to develop a dementia-like clinical picture. At autopsy, these athletes were commonly found to show increased irregular deposition of phosphorylated ***tau*** in neurons as well as in glia at the depth of cortical sulci (Mez et al. 2017). Long-term survivors of single, severe TBI also show increased presence of neurofibrillary tangles of tau (Johnson et al. 2012). Using microdialysis, tau levels were markedly higher in patients with severe TBI when the probes were placed in the vicinity of cortical contusions. Furthermore, tau levels correlated with markers for axonal injury indicating an association with white matter pathology and release of tau (Magnoni et al. 2012). Although microdialysis studies are often limited by the lack of adequate controls, this technique is suitable for the acute evaluation of tau, and Aβ, release in severe TBI (Tsitsopoulos and Marklund 2013; Marklund et al. 2009). As for in vivo detection, the rapid development of tau tracers may make positron-emission tomography (PET) imaging a useful tool to study the importance of tau in severe TBI.

A meta-analysis of 22 case studies revealed that TBI increased the risk of *Parkinson's disease (PD)* by 57% with a pooled odds ratio of 1.6 (Jafari et al. 2013). A large retrospective cohort study of 165,799 TBI patients aged ≥55 years implies a 44% risk increase for PD after TBI (Gardner et al. 2014) and adds to other reports finding an association between TBI and PD (Perry et al. 2016; Gardner et al. 2018). Since the study by Gardner and colleagues (Gardner et al. 2014) also found an increased risk for AD, there may be either common denominators or several disease processes leading to a variety of neurodegenerative diseases post-TBI.

Pooled clinical and neuropathologic data from three prospective cohort studies indicate that TBI with a loss of consciousness leads to an increased risk for AD, Lewy body accumulation, progression of parkinsonism, as well as PD (Crane et al. 2016). The risk is higher in those with a more severe injury. Importantly, even in those injured prior to the age of 25, there was an increased risk suggesting markedly prolonged duration of the pathological processes leading to neurodegeneration.

In addition to the previously reported studies on AD and PD, TBI can also increase the risk of non-AD dementias with a focus on *frontotemporal dementias (FTD)* (Huang et al. 2018). A retrospective case-control study of 80 FTD patients and 124 controls demonstrated that TBI increases the risk of developing FTD with an odds ratio of 3.3 (Rosso et al. 2003). A larger retrospective case-control study of 845 veterans found an association between TBI and FTD with an odds ratio of 4.4 (Kalkonde et al. 2012). A large population study from Taiwan evaluating >140,000 patients found a >4 times increased risk of FTD during the coming 4 years following TBI, and this risk increase was particularly pronounced in those aged <65 years (Wang et al. 2015).

86.4 Pathophysiology

Most neurodegenerative disorders have hallmark histological findings. These include abnormal aggregation, misfolding and/or accumulation of proteins such as Aβ aggregates/plaques, neurofibrillary tangles (NFTs) of p-tau, α-synuclein accumulation in PD, and transactive response DNA-binding protein of 43 kDa (TDP-43) in FTD. Why TBI appears to increase these pathological processes is unclear, and whether TBI initiates or merely accelerates this pathophysiology remains unknown. Importantly, although tau and Aβ have received most research attention, multiple proteinopathies may coexist in TBI victims (Kenney et al. 2018).

The hallmark findings of AD, increased deposition of Aβ aggregates/plaques and NFTs of phosphorylated tau, are observed in increased frequency in long-term TBI survivors. The Aβ aggregates have been observed as early as a few hours post-injury in ca 30% of severe TBI patients and have been associated with the formation of potentially neurotoxic Aβ protofibrils and oligomers (Abu Hamdeh et al. 2018). These findings were more pronounced in the carriers of the known AD-associated APOE ε4 genotype. Also in individuals surviving many years following a single severe TBI, there is increased Aβ aggregation (Johnson et al. 2012). In contrast, the other hallmark finding of AD, NFTs have not been observed early post-injury, although this pathology is found at the time of death in higher density and in wider distribution in brains of long-term survivors of single severe TBI. The reasons for the increased tau and Aβ aggregations have not been established, although they have been linked to axonal and white matter pathology and a persistent inflammatory response. To date, most information of TBI-related pathology comes from histological analyses from surgically resected brain tissue or from autopsy material. Rather recently, ever improving PET techniques using tracers for tau or Aβ have shown promise in following TBI-related pathology in vivo and over time. To date, there are no therapies counteracting the disease drivers for neurodegeneration post-TBI, and these novel techniques are likely instrumental in developing novel treatment options. Tissue analysis of Aβ aggregates/plaques post-TBI has been performed both at autopsy (Roberts et al. 1994; Smith and Weingart 2012) and in surgically resected tissue (Abu Hamdeh et al. 2018; Ikonomovic et al. 2004; Furst and Bigler 2016). In these studies, ca 30% of TBI patients had plaques/aggregates of Aβ, occurring across all age groups and as early as a few hours post-injury. In the postmortem study of patients with a single moderate-severe TBI surviving 1–47 years, Aβ was also found in approximately 30% of the cases (Johnson et al. 2012; Johnson et al. 2009). Aβ aggregation has been linked to axonal injury, since accumulation of Aβ is observed in injured axons after TBI (Smith et al. 2003; Chen et al. 2009). Amyloid precursor protein (APP), the hallmark immunohistochemical marker of axonal injury, also accumulates in damaged axons and co-localizes with β-secretase (BACE1) and the presenilin subunit (PS1) of γ-secretase, providing the means for cleavage of APP into Aβ (Chen et al. 2009). The Aβ species accumulating in the axonal bulbs of brains from TBI patients is Aβ42, the peptide most prone to aggregate into plaques (Uryu et al. 2007). In the presence of the APOE ε4 allele, the Aβ clearance is impaired, and this may increase the formation of neurotoxic Aβ protofibrils and oligomers, leading to increased Aβ aggregation (Abu Hamdeh et al. 2018). It should be mentioned that the plaques observed acutely in TBI are not identical to those observed in AD. Those found in TBI are more diffuse in nature than those found in advanced AD (Ikonomovic et al. 2004).

Tau, a microtubule-associated protein found in axons, forms the hyperphosphorylated aggregates (NFTs) found in the brains of AD patients and of individuals suffering from the neurodegenearive disorders named tauopathies. Chronic traumatic encephalopathy (CTE) is considered one of these tauopathies. In experimental TBI, there is an increased expression, as well as phosphorylation, of ***tau*** (Tsitsopoulos and Marklund 2013). This early tau phosphorylation is observed in injured axons and white matter, although not in the neuronal cell body or dendrites (Ojo et al. 2016). A small subset of patients have been found to display p-tau immunoreactivity in acute postmortem TBI brains (Smith et al. 2003; Uryu et al. 2007). Tau-positive glia cells have also been found in the brains of up to 20% of severe TBI patients (Smith et al. 2003; Uryu et al. 2007). Long-term survivors of a single severe TBI have shown increased presence of NFTs at autopsy. This increase was noted only in those patients surviving longer than 4–5 months post-injury (Johnson et al. 2012). NFTs have been most prominently found in the superficial cortical layers, with clustering in the depths of the sulci. This accumulation pattern has not been observed in controls in whom most tau pathology situates in the transentorhinal cortex and hippocampus (Johnson et al. 2012). In TBI patients younger than 60 years of age, 34% had tau pathology, whereas tau was only observed in 9% of controls (Johnson et al. 2012). There are some crucial differences between the tau pathology observed in TBI and that in AD. For instance, there is much more astrocytic tau in CTE compared to AD. Additionally, NFTs are preferentially deposited in layers II and III of the post-TBI cortex in contrast to the preferential deposition of tau in layers V and VI in AD.

Obviously, tissue histopathology is merely for postmortem diagnostics and research purposes, not for therapeutics or patient follow-up. Novel tools to follow Aβ and tau aggregation in vivo are rapidly being developed. The use of molecular imaging such as PET to detect and to monitor amyloid and tau deposition and neuroinflammation is rapidly improving. These tools have allowed researchers to visualize the pre-mortem deposition of Aβ using, e.g., Pittsburgh compound B (PiB) or flutemetamol. Tau tracers are also rapidly being improved and used for the detection of tauopathies and AD pathology. Research in TBI using these novel tools is still scarce, but an increasing number of studies are ongoing. These studies may lead to an increased understanding of the post-TBI disease process and to the development of, e.g., antibody-based treatment (Lee et al. 2018; Scott et al. 2016; Gatson et al. 2016; Ramlackhansingh et al. 2011).

86.5 Conclusions

Most, but not all, population-based studies indicate that TBI leads to increased risk of developing various neurodegenerative disorders such as FTD, AD, CTE, and PD.

Tissue analysis of TBI victims, either from surgically resected tissue or at autopsy, indicates that TBI results in a number of proteinopathies (e.g., accumulation of amyloid-beta, tau, and TDP-43), persisting or exacerbating for many years post-injury. Thus, TBI appears to elicit a polypathology, which may be related to axonal injury. In the near future, this neurodegenerative process can be followed in vivo with the aid of recently developed PET tracers, possibly enabling the development of novel treatment options.

References

Abu Hamdeh S, Waara ER, Moller C, Soderberg L, Basun H, Alafuzoff I, et al. Rapid amyloid-beta oligomer and protofibril accumulation in traumatic brain injury. Brain Pathol. 2018;28(4):451–62.

Chen XH, Johnson VE, Uryu K, Trojanowski JQ, Smith DH. A lack of amyloid beta plaques despite persistent accumulation of amyloid beta in axons of long-term survivors of traumatic brain injury. Brain Pathol. 2009;19(2):214–23.

Cole JH, Jolly A, de Simoni S, Bourke N, Patel MC, Scott G, et al. Spatial patterns of progressive brain volume loss after moderate-severe traumatic brain injury. Brain. 2018;141(3):822–36.

Corrigan JD, Cuthbert JP, Harrison-Felix C, Whiteneck GG, Bell JM, Miller AC, et al. US population estimates of health and social outcomes 5 years after rehabilitation for traumatic brain injury. J Head Trauma Rehabil. 2014;29(6):E1–9.

Crane PK, Gibbons LE, Dams-O'Connor K, Trittschuh E, Leverenz JB, Keene CD, et al. Association of traumatic brain injury with late-life neurodegenerative conditions and neuropathologic findings. JAMA Neurol. 2016;73(9):1062–9.

Fann JR, Ribe AR, Pedersen HS, Fenger-Gron M, Christensen J, Benros ME, et al. Long-term risk of dementia among people with traumatic brain injury in Denmark: a population-based observational cohort study. Lancet Psychiatry. 2018;5(5):424–31.

Furst AJ, Bigler ED. Amyloid plaques in TBI: incidental finding or precursor for what is to come? Neurology. 2016;86(9):798–9.

Gardner RC, Burke JF, Nettiksimmons J, Kaup A, Barnes DE, Yaffe K. Dementia risk after traumatic brain injury vs nonbrain trauma: the role of age and severity. JAMA Neurol. 2014;71(12):1490–7.

Gardner RC, Byers AL, Barnes DE, Li Y, Boscardin J, Yaffe K. Mild TBI and risk of Parkinson disease: a chronic effects of neurotrauma consortium study. Neurology. 2018;90(20):e1771–e9.

Gatson JW, Stebbins C, Mathews D, Harris TS, Madden C, Batjer H, et al. Evidence of increased brain amyloid in severe TBI survivors at 1, 12, and 24 months after injury: report of 2 cases. J Neurosurg. 2016;124(6):1646–53.

Himanen L, Portin R, Isoniemi H, Helenius H, Kurki T, Tenovuo O. Longitudinal cognitive changes in traumatic brain injury: a 30-year follow-up study. Neurology. 2006;66(2):187–92.

Huang CH, Lin CW, Lee YC, Huang CY, Huang RY, Tai YC, et al. Is traumatic brain injury a risk factor for neurodegeneration? A meta-analysis of population-based studies. BMC Neurol. 2018;18(1):184.

Ikonomovic MD, Uryu K, Abrahamson EE, Ciallella JR, Trojanowski JQ, Lee VM, et al. Alzheimer's pathology in human temporal cortex surgically excised after severe brain injury. Exp Neurol. 2004;190(1):192–203.

Jafari S, Etminan M, Aminzadeh F, Samii A. Head injury and risk of Parkinson disease: a systematic review and meta-analysis. Mov Disord. 2013;28(9):1222–9.

Johnson VE, Stewart W, Graham DI, Stewart JE, Praestgaard AH, Smith DH. A neprilysin polymorphism and amyloid-beta plaques after traumatic brain injury. J Neurotrauma. 2009;26(8):1197–202.

Johnson VE, Stewart W, Smith DH. Widespread tau and amyloid-beta pathology many years after a single traumatic brain injury in humans. Brain Pathol. 2012;22(2):142–9.

Kalkonde YV, Jawaid A, Qureshi SU, Shirani P, Wheaton M, Pinto-Patarroyo GP, et al. Medical and environmental risk factors associated with frontotemporal dementia: a case-control study in a veteran population. Alzheimers Dement. 2012;8(3):204–10.

Kenney K, Iacono D, Edlow BL, Katz DI, Diaz-Arrastia R, Dams-O'Connor K, et al. Dementia after moderate-severe traumatic brain injury: coexistence of multiple proteinopathies. J Neuropathol Exp Neurol. 2018;77(1):50–63.

Lee BG, Leavitt MJ, Bernick CB, Leger GC, Rabinovici G, Banks SJ. A systematic review of positron emission tomography of tau, amyloid beta, and neuroinflammation in chronic traumatic encephalopathy: the evidence to date. J Neurotrauma. 2018;35(17):2015–24.

Magnoni S, Esparza TJ, Conte V, Carbonara M, Carrabba G, Holtzman DM, et al. Tau elevations in the brain extracellular space correlate with reduced amyloid-beta levels and predict adverse clinical outcomes after severe traumatic brain injury. Brain. 2012;135(Pt 4):1268–80.

Marklund N, Blennow K, Zetterberg H, Ronne-Engstrom E, Enblad P, Hillered L. Monitoring of brain interstitial total tau and beta amyloid proteins by microdialysis in patients with traumatic brain injury. J Neurosurg. 2009;110(6):1227–37.

Masel BE, DeWitt DS. Traumatic brain injury: a disease process, not an event. J Neurotrauma. 2010;27(8):1529–40.

McKinlay A, Dalrymple-Alford JC, Horwood LJ, Fergusson DM. Long term psychosocial outcomes after mild head injury in early childhood. J Neurol Neurosurg Psychiatry. 2002;73(3):281–8.

McMillan TM, Teasdale GM, Stewart E. Disability in young people and adults after head injury: 12-14 year follow-up of a prospective cohort. J Neurol Neurosurg Psychiatry. 2012;83(11):1086–91.

Mendez MF. What is the relationship of traumatic brain injury to dementia? J Alzheimers Dis. 2017;57(3):667–81.

Mendez MF, Paholpak P, Lin A, Zhang JY, Teng E. Prevalence of traumatic brain injury in early versus late-onset Alzheimer's disease. J Alzheimers Dis. 2015;47(4):985–93.

Mez J, Daneshvar DH, Kiernan PT, Abdolmohammadi B, Alvarez VE, Huber BR, et al. Clinicopathological evaluation of chronic traumatic encephalopathy in players of american football. JAMA. 2017;318(4):360–70.

Millar K, Nicoll JA, Thornhill S, Murray GD, Teasdale GM. Long term neuropsychological outcome after head injury: relation to APOE genotype. J Neurol Neurosurg Psychiatry. 2003;74(8):1047–52.

Moretti L, Cristofori I, Weaver SM, Chau A, Portelli JN, Grafman J. Cognitive decline in older adults with a history of traumatic brain injury. Lancet Neurol. 2012;11(12):1103–12.

Nordstrom A, Nordstrom P. Traumatic brain injury and the risk of dementia diagnosis: A nationwide cohort study. PLoS Med. 2018;15(1):e1002496.

Nordstrom P, Michaelsson K, Gustafson Y, Nordstrom A. Traumatic brain injury and young onset dementia: a nationwide cohort study. Ann Neurol. 2014;75(3):374–81.

Ojo JO, Mouzon BC, Crawford F. Repetitive head trauma, chronic traumatic encephalopathy and tau: Challenges in translating from mice to men. Exp Neurol. 2016;275(Pt 3):389–404.

Perry DC, Sturm VE, Peterson MJ, Pieper CF, Bullock T, Boeve BF, et al. Association of traumatic brain injury with subsequent neurological and psychiatric disease: a meta-analysis. J Neurosurg. 2016;124(2):511–26.

Plassman BL, Havlik RJ, Steffens DC, Helms MJ, Newman TN, Drosdick D, et al. Documented head injury in early adulthood and risk of Alzheimer's disease and other dementias. Neurology. 2000;55(8):1158–66.

Ramlackhansingh AF, Brooks DJ, Greenwood RJ, Bose SK, Turkheimer FE, Kinnunen KM, et al. Inflammation after trauma: microglial activation and traumatic brain injury. Ann Neurol. 2011;70(3):374–83.

Roberts GW, Gentleman SM, Lynch A, Murray L, Landon M, Graham DI. Beta amyloid protein deposition in the brain after severe head injury: implications for the pathogenesis of Alzheimer's disease. J Neurol Neurosurg Psychiatry. 1994;57(4):419–25.

Rosso SM, Landweer EJ, Houterman M, Donker Kaat L, van Duijn CM, van Swieten JC. Medical and environmental risk factors for sporadic frontotemporal dementia: a retrospective case-control study. J Neurol Neurosurg Psychiatry. 2003;74(11):1574–6.

Scott G, Ramlackhansingh AF, Edison P, Hellyer P, Cole J, Veronese M, et al. Amyloid pathology and axonal injury after brain trauma. Neurology. 2016;86(9):821–8.

Smith WS, Weingart S. Emergency neurological life support (ENLS): what to do in the first hour of a neurological emergency. Neurocrit Care. 2012;17(Suppl 1):S1–3.

Smith DH, Chen XH, Iwata A, Graham DI. Amyloid beta accumulation in axons after traumatic brain injury in humans. J Neurosurg. 2003;98(5):1072–7.

Tsitsopoulos PP, Marklund N. Amyloid-beta peptides and tau protein as biomarkers in cerebrospinal and interstitial fluid following traumatic brain injury: a review of experimental and clinical studies. Front Neurol. 2013;4:79.

Uryu K, Chen XH, Martinez D, Browne KD, Johnson VE, Graham DI, et al. Multiple proteins implicated in neurodegenerative diseases accumulate in axons after brain trauma in humans. Exp Neurol. 2007;208(2):185–92.

Wang HK, Lee YC, Huang CY, Liliang PC, Lu K, Chen HJ, et al. Traumatic brain injury causes frontotemporal dementia and TDP-43 proteolysis. Neuroscience. 2015;300:94–103.

Whiteneck GG, Cuthbert JP, Corrigan JD, Bogner JA. Risk of negative outcomes after traumatic brain injury: a statewide population-based survey. J Head Trauma Rehabil. 2016;31(1):E43–54.

Wilson L, Stewart W, Dams-O'Connor K, Diaz-Arrastia R, Horton L, Menon DK, et al. The chronic and evolving neurological consequences of traumatic brain injury. Lancet Neurol. 2017;16(10):813–25.

Part XI

Research in Severe TBI

Niklas Marklund

Neurointensive Care Unit as a Platform for Advanced Clinical Research

87

Per Enblad, Tim Howells, and Lars Hillered

Recommendations

It is not possible to recommend how the optimal neurointensive care (NIC) platform for advanced clinical research should be organized and equipped according to evidence-based medicine principles. Instead, the following advices are given according to the experience from our own and other centers. We believe it is fundamental that the NIC unit is organized in a way that research and development are integrated with routine care. It is also of outmost importance that controlled and standardized conditions are created for the management of the patients. Finally, we believe that information technology systems set up for acquisition and analysis of the large amounts of monitoring data generated will provide unique possibilities for explorative clinical research and that this approach will be beneficial for clinical research and for management and outcome of the patients (Elf et al. 2002).

87.1 Overview

The neurointensive care (NIC) unit provides an excellent environment for clinical explorative research. Continuous multimodality monitoring of physiological parameters (e.g., arterial blood pressure and temperature) and intracranial parameters (e.g., intracranial pressure, cerebral perfusion pressure, brain tissue oxygenation, neurochemistry, and neurophysiology) and computerized collection of high-resolution data, make it possible to obtain a direct insight into human brain injury processes. The use of modern imaging techniques, such as magnetic resonance imaging (MRI) and positron emission tomography (PET), is enhancing our understanding of the mechanisms underlying these processes. New monitoring techniques can be validated and critical thresholds defined. The NIC unit also plays an important role in translational research bridging the gap between the laboratory and the patients and in the development of new treatment and management strategies. The Uppsala NIC unit is an important platform in our Centre of Excellence Neurotrauma (www.neurotrauma.se) and played a central role in recent network activities: the BrainIT Group (www.brainit.org) and Uppsala Berzelii Technology Centre for Neurodiagnostics (http://www.ufold.uu.se/Partners/Uppsala_Berzelii_Technology_Centre_for_Neurodiagnostics/).

The aims of this chapter are first to describe the cornerstones of the NIC research platform and second to give a few examples of research in which important knowledge was gained by taking advantage of this platform.

P. Enblad (✉) · T. Howells · L. Hillered
Department of Neuroscience, Neurosurgery, Uppsala University, Uppsala, Sweden
e-mail: per.enblad@neuro.uu.se

© Springer Nature Switzerland AG 2020
T. Sundstrøm et al. (eds.), *Management of Severe Traumatic Brain Injury*,
https://doi.org/10.1007/978-3-030-39383-0_87

Tips, Tricks, and Pitfalls

- Establish a research group including various different competences, e.g., neurosurgeons, neurointensivists, research nurses, engineers, programmers, and statisticians.
- Involve all members of the staff in the research projects and give them regular feedback.
- Try to make all graduated members of the research group responsible for their own parts of the overall research program to avoid conflicts.
- Try to establish interdisciplinary network activities to enable translation of knowledge between basic science, technological science, and the NIC setting.

87.2 Background

87.2.1 Organization of the Neurointensive Care Unit

It is important to create a culture for all members of the NIC staff where research and development is integrated with clinical routine. The goal should be to create a controlled and standardized management environment for the patients resembling the conditions in the laboratory in terms of maintaining clear and consistent standards for patient care. This can be achieved by implementation of standardized management protocol systems similar to the Good Laboratory Practice (GLP) standards. It is also of outmost importance to establish a multidisciplinary research group comprising, e.g., neurosurgeons, neurointensivists, neurophysiologists, neurochemists, research nurses, engineers, programmers, and statisticians.

87.2.2 Multimodality Monitoring and Computerized Data Acquisition and Analysis Systems

Multimodality monitoring generates enormous amounts of valuable data. It is crucial to set up a computer-based system for collection and acquisition of data. One example is the Odin Monitoring System software (formerly the Edinburgh Browser), which has been developed over several years by the computer scientist Tim Howells in collaboration with clinicians, initially in Edinburgh and during the last decades in Uppsala. This system can be networked to all beds in the NIC unit for collection, analysis and visualization of demographic data, physiological minute-by-minute monitoring data, and treatment data. The software has been extended to include functions for high-resolution waveform data analysis, which can be used in autoregulation and compliance studies. Another computer system specially designed for NIC is the ICM+ software developed at the University of Cambridge by Peter Smielewski and Marek Czosnyka. This software is focused on signal acquisition and processing and has been used extensively in autoregulation and compliance studies and also in the management of hydrocephalus patients. The Sensometrics software developed at the National Hospital in Oslo has also been used extensively in brain injury research, based on the analysis of intracranial and systemic pressure signals. A fourth example is the ICUpilot system developed by the former CMA Microdialysis AB, currently manufactured by M Dialysis AB in Sweden (www.mdialysis.com) for integration and analysis of microdialysis and other monitoring data. Other software systems are also available on the market.

87.3 Illustrative NIC Research Projects

87.3.1 High-Resolution Waveform Data Analysis for Monitoring of Autoregulation and Compliance

Earlier, the dominant school of intensive care management of patients with traumatic brain injury (TBI) held that the most critical factor was maintaining cerebral perfusion pressure (CPP) (Rosner et al. 1995). Other neurosurgical centers have taken a more cautious approach to elevating CPP (CPP-oriented therapy) and have focused primarily on lowering intracranial pressure (ICP) (ICP-oriented therapy) (Elf et al. 2002; Eker et al. 1998). A study of CPP and ICP management strategies involving our own center found evidence that some patients responded better to CPP oriented management and others did better when given ICP-oriented treatment (Howells et al. 2005). We also found that pressure autoregulation status was the key to determining the optimal strategy. The Brain Trauma Foundation guidelines have moved in this direction, recommending that CPP management be carefully targeted based in part on pressure autoregulation status (Bratton et al. 2007). Most measures of autoregulation used are based on the response of ICP to changes in systemic blood pressure. The best available measure for continuous assessment of autoregulation status is the Pressure Reactivity Index (PRx) from the Cambridge group, calculated as a moving correlation coefficient between 40 consecutive samples of values for ICP and mean arterial blood pressure averaged for a period of 5 s (Czosnyka et al. 1997; Guendling et al. 2006). PRx is well validated as a measure of pressure autoregulation, but the best way of using PRx in routine clinical decision-making remains to be established. It is therefore important to refine our understanding of existing measures of autoregulation and to develop new measures, with the goal of clinical application clearly in mind. Modern NIC software systems including functions for high-resolution waveform data analysis provide an excellent tool for such studies.

The monitoring of intracranial compliance in NIC may provide valuable information about intracranial compensatory volume reserve and risk of developing high ICP. Various approaches have been used to estimate intracranial compliance (Marmarou et al. 1975; Robertson et al. 1989; Yau et al. 2002; Czosnyka et al. 2001). There is currently no compliance monitoring method that is widely used in practical clinical care. The most widely studied measures of intracranial compliance are computed from the ICP waveform. One such ICP waveform-based measure of compliance is the RAP index, which has been validated in a number of clinical studies (Castellani et al. 2009; Czosnyka et al. 2007; Kim et al. 2009; Timofeev et al. 2008a, b). The RAP index is calculated as the moving correlation between mean ICP and the ICP pulse amplitude over a time window of about 4 min. The ICP pulse amplitude itself has also been studied and validated as a measure of compliance (Czosnyka et al. 2001; Bentsen et al. 2008; Eide and Sorteberg 2007, 2011). A third metric that has been proposed is the ascending slope of the ICP pulse waveform (Contant et al. 1995). Compliance-based management of subarachnoid hemorrhage according to the ICP pulse amplitude has been the subject of a randomized clinical trial (RCT), showing promising results (Eide et al. 2011). Future NIC studies within this field may foster the development of compliance monitoring into a valuable clinical management tool.

87.3.2 Development of Neurochemical Monitoring Methods from Bench to Bed

Based on cerebral microdialysis (MD) studies in our animal models of stroke and traumatic brain injury (TBI) in the 1980s in collaboration with Ungerstedt et al. (Hillered et al. 1989; Nilsson et al. 1990), we set out to explore the usefulness of MD monitoring in the NIC setting in patients with TBI and subarachnoid hemorrhage (SAH). Our seminal observations strongly supported a potentially important role for MD as a neurochemical monitoring tool (Persson and Hillered 1992). The MD method has eventually become a widespread tool for neurochemical monitoring and research in neurosurgery and NIC with over 1400 publications on PubMed to date. MD is a unique tool for harvesting of neurochemical signals in the human brain and has together with neuroimaging methods (CT, PET, MRI) provided important new insights into the neurochemistry of acute human brain injury. MD is currently used in the NIC setting mainly for energy metabolic monitoring, monitoring of cellular distress biomarkers, and protein biomarker sampling and as an emerging tool in neuropharmacology (Hutchinson et al. 2015).

87.3.2.1 Energy Metabolic Monitoring

Low-molecular-weight cutoff MD in the NIC setting has been chiefly used for monitoring of energy metabolic perturbation (glucose, lactate, pyruvate, lactate/pyruvate ratio (LPR)), excitotoxicity (glutamate), membrane phospholipid degradation/oxidative stress (glycerol), and urea metabolism, driven by the availability of dedicated point-of-care analytical tools (M Dialysis AB, Solna, Sweden). There are numerous reviews on the application of MD in clinical neurosurgery, with a few of the most recent referred to here (Hutchinson et al. 2015; Zeiler et al. 2017a, b; Helbok and Beer 2017). The following discussion will focus on TBI.

Ischemic Energy Metabolic Crisis Following TBI

Based on pioneering work of Graham and colleagues in the 1970s, ischemia was identified as an important component of severe TBI. This concept was based on autopsy data from patients succumbing to severe TBI (Graham et al. 1978). In the NIC setting, much effort is directed towards minimizing secondary ischemia owing to intracranial hypertension and low perfusion pressure, to prevent progression of the primary brain damage. Studies have been done to validate MD biomarkers of cerebral ischemia using, e.g., PET. In particular, the LPR has been suggested to be a sensitive and specific marker of ischemia (Enblad et al. 1996, 2001; Hutchinson et al. 2002). Another advantage of the LPR (unlike individual MD biomarkers) is that it is a quantitative measure, independent of the extraction efficiency of the MD catheter (Persson and Hillered 1996). A number of validation studies collectively suggest a typical MD-biomarker pattern of ischemia as shown in Table 87.1.

Nonischemic Energy Metabolic Crisis Following TBI

In recent years, due to the refinement of modern NIC as well as preventive measures in the society with e.g. safer cars and a variety of protective gears, the most severe injuries are fewer, and the problem of overt secondary ischemia has diminished. Instead the complexity of energy metabolic alterations following TBI has been increasingly acknowledged. With the combined use of multimodal monitoring and neuroimaging methods, a new concept of nonischemic energy metabolic crisis has emerged (see Hillered and

Table 87.1 Typical MD-marker pattern of overt cerebral ischemia

	Glucose	Lactate	Pyruvate	LPR
Ischemia	↓↓	↑↑	↓↓	↑↑

↓↓ marked decrease, ↑↑ marked increase, *LPR* lactate/pyruvate ratio (For references, see Hillered et al. (2005) and Hutchinson et al. (2015))

Enblad 2008). Using MD-LPR as a surrogate end point marker, studies by the Houston and UCLA groups revealed that the occurrence of high LPR levels (LPR >30–40) without hypoxia/ischemia measured by brain tissue oximetry and PET, respectively, was surprisingly frequent after TBI (Hlatky et al. 2004; Vespa et al. 2005). Apparently, such LPR elevations were often characterized by a pyruvate close to or only slightly below the critical level (Table 87.2), but without a dramatic lactate and LPR increment (or critically low brain pO_2). This phenomenon was tentatively named Type 2 LPR elevation (Hillered et al. 2006) to be distinguished from the classical Type 1 LPR elevation seen in ischemia, with more pronounced pyruvate reductions (and critically low brain pO_2) in combination with a markedly increased lactate and LPR (Table 87.1). The Type 2 LPR phenomenon may reflect several possible energy metabolic changes following TBI, including a relative shortage of brain glucose (in spite of normal or high blood glucose), dysfunction of the glycolytic pathway, shunting of glucose to competing pathways such as the pentose phosphate pathway (Dusick et al. 2007), and perturbed mitochondrial function (Nielsen et al. 2013). Thus, the emerging picture is that the post-traumatic brain may frequently suffer from a complex nonischemic energy metabolic crisis unrelated to classical hypoxia/ischemia. The potential importance of nonischemic energy crisis as a secondary injury mechanism following clinical TBI was suggested by data showing an association between low brain glucose during NIC and poor 6-month clinical outcome (Vespa et al. 2003). In a study by Timofeev et al. (2011) on 223 TBI patients, multivariate logistic regression analysis showed that high levels of MD-glucose and LPR (together with PRx and age) were independent predictors of mortality whereas high MD-pyruvate was associated with reduced mortality. Apparently, in addition to MD-glucose and LPR, MD-pyruvate is a biomarker of energy metabolic crisis that deserves increased attention in NIC.

Spreading Depolarization (SD) Following Acute Brain Injury

SD is a depolarization wave spreading across the cerebral cortical surface observed in the 1940s following brain injury in experimental animals as a cortical spreading depression (Leao 1947). SD in the form of peri-infarct depolarization is thought to be an important mechanism for the recruitment of penumbral tissue to infarction in experimental stroke (Gill et al. 1992). Because of the difficulty involved in measuring SD, it was not until 2002 that SD was reported to occur in the human brain following acute injury using subdural strip electrodes (Strong et al. 2002). It has now become clear that SD is a common feature of human TBI and neurovascular brain injury. In patients who have undergone craniotomy, SD occurs in 50–60% of TBI and in 70% of SAH patients (Feuerstein et al. 2010). SD is thought to be an important secondary injury mechanism by challenging the energy metabolic capacity of the brain tissue to restore ion homeostasis. By the use of rapid sampling MD in combination with subdural strip electrodes, SDs have been shown to lead to marked, transient reductions of MD-glucose and concomitant increases of MD-lactate, posing a risk of brain glucose depletion when occurring repeatedly, despite an adequate blood supply (Hashemi et al. 2009; Feuerstein et al. 2010). Thus, the SD phenomenon may be an additional important mechanism leading to nonischemic energy metabolic crisis following TBI.

Table 87.2 Tentative critical MD levels in secondary cerebral energy crisis

	Glucose	Lactate	Pyruvate	LPR
Critical level	<1.0 mmol/L	>3.0 mmol/L	<120 μmol/L	>30

Conservatively chosen based on Reinstrup et al. (2000), Schulz et al. (2000), Oddo et al. (2008), Meierhans et al. (2010), and Hutchinson et al. (2015)

Brain Glucose and Insulin Management in the NIC Setting

Experimental studies decades ago suggested that hyperglycemia at the onset of cerebral ischemia aggravates brain damage by producing more pronounced lactic acidosis leading to increased oxidative stress (Siesjo 1981; Li et al. 1999). There is evidence that hyperglycemia in the acute phase of TBI is associated with poor outcome irrespective of injury severity (Liu-DeRyke et al. 2009). Correcting hyperglycemia >10 mmol/L was shown to reduce mortality after severe TBI (Jeremitsky et al. 2005), and many neurosurgical centers avoid blood glucose values >10 mmol/L as a routine precaution. A new direction was taken by van den Berghe and colleagues, presenting evidence that keeping blood glucose between 4.4 and 6.1 mmol/L reduced morbidity and mortality in surgical and medical intensive care patients (Van den Berghe et al. 2001, 2006). This data created widespread attention even though follow-up studies failed to confirm the positive effects of tight glycemic control in surgical and medical critical care patients (Arabi et al. 2008; Brunkhorst et al. 2008). In the NIC setting, tight glycemic control (5.0–6.7 mmol/L) produced signs of metabolic distress (reduced MD-glucose and increased MD-LPR and MD-glutamate) without any improvement in 6-month outcome in severe TBI patients (Vespa et al. 2006). Along the same line, Oddo and colleagues showed that tight glycemic control (4.4–6.7 mmol/L) in NIC patients with severe traumatic and neurovascular brain injury was associated with an increased prevalence of energy metabolic crisis (brain MD-glucose <0.7 mmol/L + MD-LPR >40), associated with a higher mortality rate at discharge (Oddo et al. 2008). Data from Meierhans and colleagues studying brain energy metabolic alterations with MD at different blood glucose levels in 20 patients with severe TBI support the notion that MD-glucose levels below 1 mmol/L should be avoided and suggest that the optimal blood glucose range may be 6–9 mmol/L in the NIC setting (Meierhans et al. 2010).

In summary, both hyper- and hypoglycemia are important adverse factors in the NIC setting. It has become increasingly clear that low brain glucose is a common phenomenon during NIC, putting the acutely injured brain at risk for secondary energy metabolic crisis and aggravated brain damage related to the phenomena discussed above. Conversely, blood glucose levels >10 mmol/L should be avoided (Jeremitsky et al. 2005). The need for controlling brain glucose, particularly to avoid critically low levels frequently observed despite a normal or high blood glucose, has in our view strengthened the indication for brain glucose monitoring with MD in the NIC setting, although a specific treatment algorithm remains to be assessed.

87.3.2.2 Monitoring of Cellular Distress Biomarkers

MD-glutamate and MD-glycerol are widely used biomarkers of cellular distress caused by excitotoxicity and membrane phospholipid degradation/oxidative stress, respectively, in the NIC setting. These biomarkers can be readily analyzed at the bedside with the dedicated MD analyzers available in many neurosurgical centers worldwide. MD-glutamate was recommended as a useful biomarker in NIC monitoring at the Stockholm Consensus Meeting on MD monitoring (Bellander et al. 2004). The importance of MD-glutamate as a biomarker in TBI patients was emphasized by the Houston group demonstrating a relationship between MD-glutamate and mortality as well as 6-month functional outcome in a prospective study on 165 severe TBI patients (Chamoun et al. 2010). In the Cambridge study, averaged MD-glutamate levels were significantly higher in TBI patients who died (Timofeev et al. 2011). In the consensus statement from the 2014 International Microdialysis Forum in Cambridge, monitoring of MD-glutamate is an option and may be useful for estimating prognosis in TBI (Hutchinson et al. 2015). Although widely used, there is still concern as to the precise interpretation of the biomarker signals. For example, glutamate accumulation in the interstitial fluid (ISF) following brain injury may be derived from several different sources and by different mechanisms, making the interpretation problematic (see Hillered et al. 2005). Also, glycerol accumulation in the ISF following brain injury may reflect different phenomena, including increased membrane phospholipid degradation, oxidative stress, and de novo synthesis from glucose. Recent data using ^{13}C-labeled glucose and MD suggest that de novo synthesis from glucose following experimental TBI only accounts for a few percent of the MD-glycerol signal (Clausen et al. 2011), leaving membrane phospholipid degradation and oxidative stress as the dominating sources of the MD-glycerol signal. Oxidative stress following TBI is thought to be closely associated with excitotoxicity, i.e., glutamate-mediated intracellular accumulation of Ca^{2+} leading to, e.g., phospholipase activation, membrane phospholipid degradation, and formation of arachidonic acid (see Hillered et al. 2005). Another end product of this phospholipid degradation process is glycerol (Marklund et al. 1997), which has also been implicated as a biomarker of oxidative stress (Lewen and Hillered 1998; Merenda et al. 2008). In an attempt to validate glycerol as a biomarker of oxidative stress, we performed a study on MD-8-iso-$PGF_{2\alpha}$, a widely used biomarker of oxidative stress, in six patients with severe TBI (Clausen et al. 2012). We found a significant, strong correlation between MD-8-iso-$PGF_{2\alpha}$ and MD-glycerol and between MD-8-iso-$PGF_{2\alpha}$ and MD-glutamate, supporting the close association between oxidative stress and excitotoxicity also in the human brain following TBI, and that the MD-glycerol signal is reflecting oxidative stress to a large degree. In the 2014 Consensus statement, monitoring of MD-glycerol is an option in TBI as a biomarker of cerebral injury (Hutchinson et al. 2015).

In summary, MD-glutamate and MD-glycerol provide important neurochemical information on excitotoxic and oxidative stress-related secondary injury following acute brain injury in the NIC setting. These biomarkers may become increasingly useful for proof-of-principle testing before moving to large-scale clinical trials and as surrogate end point markers in neuroprotective drug development.

87.3.2.3 Protein Biomarker Sampling

Biomarkers are currently predicted to play an increasingly important role in future NIC. The introduction of high-molecular-weight cutoff (100 kDa or more) MD catheters, potentially allowing for studies on the proteomics of acute brain injury, has lately been met with considerable enthusiasm. The basic assumption is that sampling of protein biomarkers directly in the injured human brain by MD delivers neurochemical signals with an improved temporal and spatial resolution compared to conventional protein biomarker sampling from vCSF or blood. MD thus offers a unique opportunity for biomarker sampling in the brain, potentially avoiding both dilution and chemical degradation of the protein biomarkers. A number of feasibility studies have been published reporting the potential of monitoring various proteins in the NIC setting, including cytokines (Hillman et al. 2005; Helmy et al. 2009, 2010; Zeiler et al. 2017b), amyloid-β and Tau protein (Brody et al. 2008; Marklund et al. 2009), VEGF and FGF2 (Mellergard et al. 2010), and other proteins (for references, see Dahlin et al. 2010; Maurer 2010). However, several methodological issues have emerged, such as potential perfusion fluid loss, low and unstable protein recovery, and biofouling, questioning the robustness of high-molecular-weight cutoff MD methodology (Dahlin et al. 2010). Apparently, protein trafficking across such MD membranes is a highly complex process involving a number of aspects potentially affecting the in vivo protein and fluid recovery, such as various physical properties of proteins, membrane biofouling, and encapsulation (Helmy et al. 2009; Dahlin et al. 2010). When a foreign material is inserted into a living organism, a tissue response will occur, starting with protein adsorption to the material surface followed by the interaction with host cells leading to a phenomenon called biofouling (Anderson et al. 2008). Biofouling has severe implications for MD, as it may lead to decreased protein recovery and inflammatory responses and limit the duration of accurate in vivo sampling (Wisniewski et al. 2001). Biofouling of MD catheters following 42-h in vivo dialysis in human brain has been documented by electron microscopy (Helmy et al. 2009). Because of the methodological issues involved with in vivo MD protein sampling, we started a multidisciplinary collaborative effort within the Uppsala Berzelii Technology Centre for Neurodiagnostics (http://www.ufold.uu.se/Partners/Uppsala_Berzelii_Technology_Centre_for_Neurodiagnostics/) to improve our understanding of the mechanisms involved with protein trafficking across high-molecular-weight cutoff MD membranes. The main results from this project were that addition of Dextran 500 (kDa) to the crystalloid MD perfusate stabilized the microfluidity over the MD membrane, resulting in a more stable fluid recovery close to the targeted 100% level for stable diffusion across the MD membrane (Dahlin et al. 2010). Furthermore, by modification of the high MWCO MD membrane surface with Pluronic F-127 (Poloxamer 407), we could demonstrate a dramatic reduction of protein adsorption to the MD membrane (Dahlin et al. 2012). This modified MD methodology was validated in a porcine model of acute brain injury (Purins et al. 2011), showing that the fluid recovery was stable and close to 100% during the stepwise ICP intervention. This effect was accompanied by a more robust protein biomarker sampling performance (Dahlin et al. 2014). The same MD method was recently used in a diffuse TBI model in rats to monitor 27 protein biomarkers of inflammation during the first 6 hours after injury that were difficult to study in patients (Clausen et al. 2019). We are striving to translate the use of this MD methodology into the NIC setting, pending further research on the safety of the surface modification in the human brain. Meanwhile, we have developed a new MD perfusate with a Dextran 500 additive in collaboration with M Dialysis AB, an industrial partner in the Uppsala Berzelii Centre. This perfusate was recently CE certified for human use and available as a clinical tool for MD biomarker sampling (M Dialysis AB, Stockholm, Sweden).

Finally, we started to use a novel powerful analytical technology within the Uppsala Berzelii Centre project for multiplexed protein biomarker analyses in very small MD samples. The methodology called Proximity Extension Assay (PEA) utilizes assays with dual oligonucleotide-conjugated antibodies for each antigen. Antigen binding is followed by an enzymatic ligation of the oligonucleotides and quantitative real-time polymerase chain reaction (qPCR) amplification, with a very high sensitivity and specificity (Assarsson et al. 2014). PEA allows for simultaneous analysis of up to 92 biomarkers in 1 μL samples. Our working hypothesis is that the combination of MD and PEA technology will provide a powerful tool for temporal mapping of biomarkers for complex secondary injury mechanisms, such as neuroinflammation, directly in the human brain (Hillered et al. 2014). Thus far, we have used several PEA panels to screen for ~500 potential biomarkers in MD samples every 3 h over the first 5 days upon arrival of the TBI patients to our NIC unit. Secondly, we have used a dedicated PEA panel for temporal mapping of 92 biomarkers of inflammation in a similar manner. This study provides a unique data set with individual temporal trends for 69 potential inflammatory biomarkers in patients with TBI, supporting our hypothesis that the combination of MD and PEA is a powerful tool to map the complex inflammatory cascade in the injured human brain (Dyhrfort et al. 2019). The technique offers new possibilities of protein profiling of complex secondary brain injury pathways.

Additionally, in collaboration with Olink Proteomics AB, industrial partner in the Uppsala Berzelii Centre, we have developed a prototype of a dedicated PEA panel of 21 promising biomarkers of TBI aimed for bedside use in the NIC unit. This panel is currently being validated in MD samples from TBI patients in another parallel study in progress.

87.3.2.4 Neuropharmacology

Cerebral microdialysis is considered to have a great potential for monitoring of free target drug concentrations and as a tool in clinical drug development in the NIC setting (Helmy et al. 2007). This concept was put forth by Alves et al. (2003) in a study with the glutamate release inhibitor Topiramate®, showing that the initial dose given systemically had to be raised markedly to achieve adequate free drug concentration in NIC patients with severe TBI. The study also showed that MD may be used as a surrogate end point tool in the NIC setting to obtain proof of concept, in this case lowering of interstitial glutamate levels

(Alves et al. 2003). Another example is a study by Ederoth et al. (2004) measuring free morphine concentrations in TBI patients. Finally, a recent clinical study using an IL1 receptor antagonist (Anakinra®, clinically approved for rheumatoid arthritis) as an anti-inflammatory treatment in severe TBI patients showed that the endogenous MD levels of IL1ra in the brain could be markedly elevated by the drug administration (Helmy et al. 2014). The authors also nicely demonstrated that the treatment altered the MD pattern of inflammatory biomarkers in the brain as a surrogate end point effect, strongly supporting the potential for MD in drug development.

References

Alves OL, Doyle AJ, Clausen T, Gilman C, Bullock R. Evaluation of topiramate neuroprotective effect in severe TBI using microdialysis. Ann N Y Acad Sci. 2003;993:25–34.

Anderson JM, Rodriguez A, Chang DT. Foreign body reaction to biomaterials. Semin Immunol. 2008;20:86–100.

Arabi YM, Dabbagh OC, Tamim HM, Al-Shimemeri AA, Memish ZA, Haddad SH, Syed SJ, Giridhar HR, Rishu AH, Al-Daker MO, Kahoul SH, Britts RJ, Sakkijha MH. Intensive versus conventional insulin therapy: a randomized controlled trial in medical and surgical critically ill patients. Crit Care Med. 2008;36:3190–7.

Assarsson E, Lundberg M, Holmquist G, Björkesten J, Thorsen SB, Ekman D, Eriksson A, Rennel Dickens E, Ohlsson S, Edfeldt G, Andersson AC, Lindstedt P, Stenvang J, Gullberg M, Fredriksson S. Homogenous 96-plex PEA immunoassay exhibiting high sensitivity, specificity, and excellent scalability. PLoS One. 2014;9(4):e95192.

Bellander BM, Cantais E, Enblad P, Hutchinson P, Nordström CH, Robertson C, Sahuquillo J, Smith M, Stocchetti N, Ungerstedt U, Unterberg A, Olsen NV. Consensus meeting on microdialysis in neurointensive care. Intensive Care Med. 2004;30:2166–9.

Bentsen G, Stubhaug A, Eide PK. Differential effects of osmotherapy on static and pulsatile intracranial pressure. Crit Care Med. 2008;36:2414–9.

Bratton SL, Chestnut RM, Ghajar J, McConnell Hammond FF, Harris OA, Hartl R, Manley GT, Nemecek A, Newell DW, Rosenthal G, Schouten J, Shutter L, Timmons SD, Ullman JS, Videtta W, Wilberger JE, Wright DW. Guidelines for the management of severe traumatic brain injury. IX. Cerebral perfusion thresholds. J Neurotrauma. 2007;24(Suppl. 1):S59–64.

Brody DL, Magnoni S, Schwetye KE, Spinner ML, Esparza TJ, Stocchetti N, Zipfel GJ, Holtzman DM. Amyloid-beta dynamics correlate with neurological status in the injured human brain. Science. 2008;321:1221–4.

Brunkhorst FM, Engel C, Bloos F, Meier-Hellmann A, Ragaller M, Weiler N, Moerer O, Gruendling M, Oppert M, Grond S, Olthoff D, Jaschinski U, John S, Rossaint R, Welte T, Schaefer M, Kern P, Kuhnt E, Kiehntopf M, Hartog C, Natanson C, Loeffler M, Reinhart K. Intensive insulin therapy and pentastarch resuscitation in severe sepsis. N Engl J Med. 2008;358:125–39.

Castellani G, Zweifel C, Kim DJ, Carrera E, Radolovich DK, Smielewski P, Hutchinson PJ, Pickard JD, Czosnyka M. Plateau waves in head injured patients requiring neurocritical care. Neurocrit Care. 2009;11:143–50.

Chamoun R, Suki D, Gopinath SP, Goodman JC, Robertson C. Role of extracellular glutamate measured by cerebral microdialysis in severe traumatic brain injury. J Neurosurg. 2010;113:564–70.

Clausen F, Hillered L, Gustafsson J. Cerebral glucose metabolism after traumatic brain injury in the rat studied by (13)C-glucose and microdialysis. Acta Neurochir. 2011;153(3):653–8.

Clausen F, Marklund N, Lewen A, Enblad P, Basu S, Hillered L. Interstitial F2-isoprostane 8-iso-PGF$_{2\alpha}$ as a biomarker of oxidative stress following severe human traumatic brain injury. J Neurotrauma. 2012;29(5):766–75.

Clausen F, Marklund N, Hillered L. Acute inflammatory biomarker responses to diffuse traumatic brain injury in the rat monitored by a novel microdialysis technique. J Neurotrauma. 2019;36(2):201–11. https://doi.org/10.1089/neu.2018.5636. [Epub ahead of print].

Contant CF, Robertson CS, Crouch J, Gopinath SP, Narayan RK, Grossman RG. Intracranial pressure waveform indices in transient and refractory intracranial hypertension. J Neurosci Methods. 1995;57:15–25.

Czosnyka M, Smielewski P, Kirkpatrick P, Laing RJ, Menon D, Pickard JD. Continuous assessment of the cerebral vasomotor reactivity in head injury. Neurosurgery. 1997;41:11–9.

Czosnyka M, Czosnykja ZH, Whitfield PC, Donovan T, Pickard JD. Age dependence of cerebrospinal pressure-volume compensation in patients with hydrocephalus. J Neurosurg. 2001;94:482–6.

Czosnyka M, Smielewski P, Timofeev I, Lavinio A, Guazzo E, Hutchinson P, Pickard JD. Intracranial pressure: more than a number. Neurosurg Focus. 2007;22(5):E10.

Dahlin AP, Wetterhall M, Caldwell KD, Larsson A, Bergquist J, Hillered L, Hjort K. Methodological aspects on microdialysis protein sampling and quantification in biological fluids: an in vitro study on human ventricular CSF. Anal Chem. 2010;82:4376–85.

Dahlin AP, Hjort K, Hillered L, Sjödin MO, Bergquist J, Wetterhall M. Multiplexed quantification of proteins adsorbed to surface-modified and non-modified microdialysis membranes. Anal Bioanal Chem. 2012;402(6):2057–67.

Dahlin AP, Purins K, Clausen F, Chu J, Sedigh A, Lorant T, Enblad P, Lewén A, Hillered L. Refined microdialysis method for protein biomarker sampling in acute brain injury in the neurointensive care setting. Anal Chem. 2014;86(17):8671–9.

Dusick JR, Glenn TC, Lee WN, Vespa PM, Kelly DF, Lee SM, Hovda DA, Martin NA. Increased pentose phosphate pathway flux after clinical traumatic brain injury: a [1,2-(13)C(2)]glucose labelling study in humans. J Cereb Blood Flow Metab. 2007;27:1593–602.

Dyhrfort P, Shen Q, Clausen F, Thulin M, Enblad P, Kamali-Moghaddam M, Lewén A, Hillered L. Monitoring of protein biomarkers of inflammation in human traumatic brain injury using microdialysis and proximity extension assay technology in neurointensive care. J Neurotrauma. 2019;36:2872–85.

Ederoth P, Tunblad K, Bouw R, Lundberg CJ, Ungerstedt U, Nordstrom CH, Hammarlund-Udenaes M. Blood-brain barrier transport of morphine in patients with severe brain trauma. Br J Clin Pharmacol. 2004;57(4):427–35.

Eide PK, Sorteberg W. Association among intracranial compliance, intracranial pulse pressure amplitude and intracranial pressure in patients with intracranial bleeds. Neurol Res. 2007;29:798–802.

Eide PK, Bentsen G, Sorteberg A, Martinsen PB, Stubhaug A, Sorteberg W. Effect of intracranial pressure (ICP) versus ICP wave amplitude guided intensive care management on acute clinical state and 12 months outcome in patients with aneurysmal subarachnoid hemorrhage, a randomized and blinded single-center trial. Neurosurg Focus. 2011;30(2):A1.

Eker C, Asgeirsson B, Grande PO, Schalen W, Nordstrom CH. Improved outcome after severe head injury with a new therapy based on principles for brain volume regulation and preserved microcirculation. Crit Care Med. 1998;26:1881–6.

Elf K, Nilsson P, Enblad P. Treatment results of patients with traumatic brain injury improved by refined neurointensvie care. The Uppsala experience of an organised secondary insult programme. Crit Care Med. 2002;30:2129–34.

Enblad P, Valtysson J, Andersson J, Lilja A, Valind S, Antoni G, Långström B, Hillered L, Persson L. Simultaneous intracerebral microdialysis and positron emission tomography performed in the detection of ischemia in patients with subarachnoid hemorrhage. J Cereb Blood Flow Metab. 1996;16:637–44.

Enblad P, Frykholm P, Valtysson J, Silander HC, Andersson J, Fasth KJ, Watanabe Y, Långström B, Hillered L, Persson L. Middle cerebral artery occlusion and reperfusion in primates monitored by microdialysis and sequential positron emission tomography. Stroke. 2001;32:1574–80.

Feuerstein D, Manning A, Hashemi P, Bhatia R, Fabricius M, Tolias C, Pahl C, Ervine M, Strong AJ, Boutelle MG. Dynamic metabolic response to multiple spreading depolarizations in patients with acute brain injury: an online microdialysis study. J Cereb Blood Flow Metab. 2010;30:1343–55.

Gill R, Andine P, Hillered L, Persson L, Hagberg H. The effect of MK-801 on cortical spreading depression in the penumbral zone following focal ischaemia in the rat. J Cereb Blood Flow Metab. 1992;12:371–9.

Graham DI, Adams JH, Doyle D. Ischaemic brain damage in fatal non-missile head injuries. J Neurol Sci. 1978;39:213–34.

Guendling K, Smielewski P, Czosnyka M, Lewis P, Nortje J, Timofeev I, Hutchinson PJ, Pickard JD. Use of ICM+ software for on-line analysis of intracranial and arterial pressures in head-injured patients. Acta Neurochir Suppl. 2006;96:108–13.

Hashemi P, Bhatia R, Nakamura H, Dreier JP, Graf R, Strong AJ, Boutelle MG. Persisting depletion of brain glucose following cortical spreading depression, despite apparent hyperaemia: evidence for risk of an advers effect of Leao's spreading depression. J Cereb Blood Flow Metab. 2009;29:166–75.

Helbok R, Beer R. Cerebrospinal fluid and brain extracellular fluid in severe brain trauma. Handb Clin Neurol. 2017;146:237–58.

Helmy A, Carpenter KL, Hutchinson PJ. Microdialysis in the human brain and its potential role in the development and clinical assessment of drugs. Curr Med Chem. 2007;14:1525–37.

Helmy A, Carpenter KL, Skepp er JN, Kirkpatrick PJ, Pickard JD, Hutchinson PJ. Microdialysis of cytokines: methodological considerations, scanning electron microscopy, and determination of relative recovery. J Neurotrauma. 2009;26:549–61.

Helmy A, Carpenter KL, Menon DK, Pickard JD, Hutchinson PJ. The cytokine response to human traumatic brain injury: temporal profiles and evidence for cerebral parenchymal production. J Cereb Blood Flow Metab. 2010;31:658–70.

Helmy A, Guilfoyle MR, Carpenter KL, Pickard JD, Menon DK, Hutchinson PJ. Recombinant human interleukin-1 receptor antagonist in severe traumatic brain injury: a phase II randomized control trial. J Cereb Blood Flow Metab. 2014;34(5):845–51.

Hillered L, Enblad P. Nonischemic energy metabolic crisis in acute brain injury. Crit Care Med. 2008;36:2952–3.

Hillered L, Hallström Å, Segersvärd S, Persson L, Ungerstedt U. Dynamics of extracellular metabolites in the striatum after middle cerebral artery occlusion in the rat monitored by intracerebral microdialysis. J Cereb Blood Flow Metab. 1989;9:607–16.

Hillered L, Vespa PM, Hovda DA. Translational neurochemical research in acute human brain injury: the current status and potential future for cerebral microdialysis. J Neurotrauma. 2005;22:3–41.

Hillered L, Dahlin AP, Clausen F, Chu J, Bergquist J, Hjort K, Enblad P, Lewén A. Cerebral microdialysis for protein biomarker monitoring in the neurointensive care setting—a technical approach. Front Neurol. 2014;5:245.

Hillered L, Persson L, Nilsson P, Ronne-Engstrom E, Enblad P. Continuous monitoring of cerebral metabolism in traumatic brain injury: a focus on cerebral microdialysis. Current Opinion in Critical Care. 2006;12(2):112–8.

Hillman J, Aneman O, Anderson C, Sjogren F, Saberg C, Mellergard P. A microdialysis technique for routine measurement of macromolecules in the injured human brain. Neurosurgery. 2005;56:1264–8.

Hlatky R, Valadka AB, Goodman JC, Contant CF, Robertson CS. Patterns of energy substrates during ischemia measured in the brain by microdialysis. J Neurotrauma. 2004;21:894–906.

Howells T, Elf K, Jones P, Ronne-Engström E, Piper I, Nilsson P, Andrews P, Enblad P. Pressure reactivity as a guide in the treatment of cerebral perfusion pressure in patients with brain trauma. J Neurosurg. 2005;102:311–7.

Hutchinson PJ, Gupta AK, Fryer TF, Al-Rawi PG, Chatfield DA, Coles JP, O'Connell MT, Kett-White R, Minhas PS, Aigbirhio FI, Clark JC, Kirkpatrick PJ, Menon DK, Pickard JD. Correlation between cerebral blood flow, substrate delivery, and metabolism in head injury: a combined microdialysis and triple oxygen positron emission tomography study. J Cereb Blood Flow Metab. 2002;22:735–45.

Hutchinson PJ, Jalloh I, Helmy A, Carpenter KL, Rostami E, Bellander BM, Boutelle MG, Chen JW, Claassen J, Dahyot-Fizelier C, Enblad P, Gallagher CN, Helbok R, Hillered L, Le Roux PD, Magnoni S, Mangat HS, Menon DK, Nordström CH, O'Phelan KH, Oddo M, Perez Barcena J, Robertson C, Ronne-Engström E, Sahuquillo J, Smith M, Stocchetti N, Belli A, Carpenter TA, Coles JP, Czosnyka M, Dizdar N, Goodman JC, Gupta AK, Nielsen TH, Marklund N, Montcriol A, O'Connell MT, Poca MA, Sarrafzadeh A, Shannon RJ, Skjøth-Rasmussen J, Smielewski P, Stover JF, Timofeev I, Vespa P, Zavala E, Ungerstedt U. Consensus statement from the 2014 international microdialysis forum. Intensive Care Med. 2015;41(9):1517–28.

Jeremitsky E, Omert LA, Dunham CM, Wilberger J, Rodriguez A. The impact of hyperglycemia on patients with severe brain injury. J Trauma. 2005;58:47–50.

Kim DJM, Czosnyka Z, Keong N, Radolovich D, Smielewski P, Sutcliffe M, Pickard JD, Czosnyka M. Index of cerebrospinal compensatory reserve in hydrocephalus. Neurosurgery. 2009;64:494–502.

Leao AA. Further observations on the spreading depression of activity in the cerebral cortex. J Neurophysiol. 1947;10:409–14.

Lewen A, Hillered L. Involvement of reactive oxygen species in membrane phospholipid breakdown and energy perturbation after traumatic brain injury in the rat. J Neurotrauma. 1998;15:521–30.

Li PA, Liu GJ, He QP, Floyd RA, Siesjo BK. Production of hydroxyl free radical by brain tissues in hyperglycemic rats subjected to transient forebrain ischemia. Free Radic Biol Med. 1999;27:1033–40.

Liu-DeRyke X, Collingridge DS, Orme J, Roller D, Zurasky J, Rhoney DH. Clinical impact of early hyperglycemia during acute phase of traumatic brain injury. Neurocrit Care. 2009;11:151–7.

Marklund S, Salci K, Lewén A, Hillered L. Glycerol as a marker for post-traumatic membrane phospholipid degradation in rat brain. Neuroreport. 1997;8:1457–61.

Marklund N, Blennow K, Zetterberg H, Ronne-Engstrom E, Enblad P, Hillered L. Monitoring of brain interstitial total tau and beta amyloid proteins by microdialysis in patients with traumatic brain injury. J Neurosurg. 2009;110:1227–37.

Marmarou A, Shulman K, La Morgese J. Compartmental analysis of compliance and outflow resistance of the CSF system. J Neurosurg. 1975;43:523–34.

Maurer MH. Proteomics of brain extracellular fluid (ECF) and cerebrospinal fluid (CSF). Mass Spectrom Rev. 2010;29:17–28.

Meierhans R, Bechir M, Ludwig S, Sommerfeld J, Brandi G, Haberthür C, Stocker R, Stover JF. Brain metabolism is significantly impaired at blood glucose below 6 mM and brain glucose below 1 mM in patients with severe traumatic brain injury. Crit Care. 2010;14:R13.

Mellergard P, Sjogren F, Hillman J. Release of VEGF and FGF in the extracellular space following severe subarachnoidal haemorrhage or traumatic head injury in humans. Br J Neurosurg. 2010;24:261–7.

Merenda A, Gugliotta M, Holloway R, Levasseur JE, Alessandri B, Sun D, Bullock MR. Validation of brain extracellular glycerol as an indicator of cellular membrane damage due to free radical activity after traumatic brain injury. J Neurotrauma. 2008;25:527–37.

Nielsen TH, Olsen NV, Toft P, Nordström CH. Cerebral energy metabolism during mitochondrial dysfunction induced by cyanide in piglets. Acta Anaesthesiol Scand. 2013;57(6):793–801.

Nilsson P, Hillered L, Ponten U, Ungerstedt U. Changes in cortical extracellular levels of energy related metabolites and amino acids following concussive brain injury in rats. J Cereb Blood Flow Metab. 1990;10:631–7.

Oddo M, Schmidt JM, Carrera E, Badjatia N, Connolly ES, Presciutti M, Ostapkovich ND, Levine JM, Le Roux P, Mayer SA. Impact of tight glycemic control on cerebral glucose metabolism after severe brain in jury: a microdialysis study. Crit Care Med. 2008;36:3233–8.

Persson L, Hillered L. Chemical monitoring of neurosurgical intensive care patients using intracerebral microdialysis. J Neurosurg. 1992;76:72–80.

Persson L, Hillered L. Intracerebral microdialysis. J Neurosurg. 1996;85:984–5.

Purins K, Sedigh A, Molnar C, Jansson L, Korsgren O, Lorant T, Tufveson G, Wennberg L, Wiklund L, Lewén A, Enblad P. Standardized experimental brain death model for studies of intracranial dynamics, organ preservation, and organ transplantation in the pig. Crit Care Med. 2011;39:512–7.

Reinstrup P, Stahl N, Mellergard P, Uski T, Ungerstedt U, Nordstrom CH. Intracerebral microdialysis in clinical practice: baseline values for chemical markers during wakefulness, anesthesia, and neurosurgery. Neurosurgery. 2000;47:701–9.

Robertson CS, Narayan RK, Contant CF, Grossman RG, Gokaslan ZL, Pahwa R, Caram P, Bray RS, Sherwood A. Clinical experience with a continuous monitor of intracranial compliance. J Neurosurg. 1989;71:673–80.

Rosner MJ, Rosner SD, Johnson AH. Cerebral perfusion pressure: management protocol and clinical results. J Neurosurg. 1995;83:949–62.

Schulz MK, Wang LP, Tange M, Bjerre P. Cerebral microdialysis monitoring: determination of normal and ischemic cerebral metabolisms in patients with aneurysmal subarachnoid hemorrhage. J Neurosurg. 2000;93:808–14.

Siesjo BK. Cell damage in the brain: a speculative synthesis. J Cereb Blood Flow Metab. 1981;1:155–85.

Strong AJ, Fabricius M, Boutelle MG, Hibbins SJ, Hopwood SE, Jones R, Parkin MC, Lauritzen M. Spreading and synchronous depressions of cortical activity in acutely injured human brain. Stroke. 2002;33:2738–43.

Timofeev I, Czosnyka M, Nortje J, Smielewski P, Kirkpatrick P, Gupta A, Hutchinson P. Effect of decompressive craniectomy on intracranial pressure and cerebrospinal compensation following traumatic brain injury. J Neurosurg. 2008a;108:66–73.

Timofeev I, Dahyot-Fizelier C, Keong N, Nortje J, Al-Rawi PG, Czosnyka M, Menon DK, Kirkpatrick PJ, Gupta AK, Hutchinson PJ. Ventriculostomy for control of raised ICP in acute traumatic brain injury. Acta Neurochir Suppl. 2008b;102:99–104.

Timofeev I, Carpenter KL, Nortje J, Al-Rawi PG, O'Connell MT, Czosnyka M, Smielewski P, Pickard JD, Menon DK, Kirkpatrick PJ, Gupta AK, Hutchinson PJ. Cerebral extracellular chemistry and outcome following traumatic brain injury: a microdialysis study of 223 patients. Brain. 2011;134(Pt 2):484–94.

Van den Berghe G, Wouters P, Weekers F, Verwaest C, Bruyninckx F, Schetz M, Vlasselaers D, Ferdinande P, Lauwers P, Bouillon R. Intensive insulin therapy in the critically ill patients. N Engl J Med. 2001;345:1359–67.

Van den Berghe G, Wilmer A, Hermans G, Meersseman W, Wouters PJ, Milants I, Van Wijngaerden E, Bobbaers H, Bouillon R. Intensive insulin therapy in the medical ICU. N Engl J Med. 2006;354:449–61.

Vespa PM, McArthur D, Q'Phelan K, Glenn T, Etchepare M, Kelly D, Bergsneider M, Martin NA, Hovda DA. Persistently low extracellular glucose correlates with poor outcome 6 months after human traumatic brain injury despite a lack of increased lactate: a microdialysis study. J Cereb Blood Flow Metab. 2003;23:865–77.

Vespa P, Bergsneider M, Hattori N, Wu HM, Huang SC, Martin NA, Glenn TC, McArthur DL, Hovda DA. Metabolic crisis without brain ischemia is common after traumatic brain in jury: a combined microdialysis and positron emission tomography study. J Cereb Blood Flow Metab. 2005;25:763–74.

Vespa P, Boonyaputthikul R, McArthur DL, Miller C, Etchepare M, Bergsneider M, Glenn T, Martin N, Hovda D. Intensive insulin therapy reduces microdialysis glucose values without altering glucose utilization or improving the lactate/pyruvate ratio after traumatic brain injury. Crit Care Med. 2006;34:850–6.

Wisniewski N, Klitzman B, Miller B, Reichert WM. Decreased analyte transport through implanted membranes: differentiation of biofouling from tissue effects. J Biomed Mater Res. 2001;57:513–21.

Yau Y, Piper I, Contant C, Citerio G, Kiening K, Enblad P, Nilsson P, Ng S, Wasserberg J, Kiefer M, Poon W, Dunn L, Whittle L. Multi-centre assessment of the Spiegelberg compliance monitor: interim results. Acta Neurochir Suppl. 2002;81:167–70.

Zeiler FA, Thelin EP, Helmy A, Czosnyka M, Hutchinson PJA, Menon DK. A systematic review of cerebral microdialysis and outcomes in TBI: relationships to patient functional outcome, neurophysiologic measures, and tissue outcome. Acta Neurochir. 2017a;159(12):2245–73.

Zeiler FA, Thelin EP, Czosnyka M, Hutchinson PJ, Menon DK, Helmy A. Cerebrospinal fluid and microdialysis cytokines in severe traumatic brain injury: a scoping systematic review. Front Neurol. 2017b;8:331.

Current State of the Art in Neurotrauma Research

88

Andrew I. R. Maas, David K. Menon, and Niklas Marklund

Recommendations

Level I

There are numerous studies at an evidence Level I evaluating neuroprotective therapies with promising *preclinical* documentation. None of these have found improved outcome over control treatments in severe traumatic brain injury (TBI).

Level II

There are numerous studies at an evidence Level II evaluating therapies with promising *preclinical* documentation. Although promising results of an experimental therapy were obtained in a few of these reports, none could be confirmed at an evidence Level I.

Level III

There are numerous high-quality experimental studies both in rodents and in higher-order species finding treatments that modulate key pathogenic mechanisms and improve histological and/or behavioral outcome.

There are examples of single-center or non-randomized trials finding clinical benefit of an experimental therapy, results that await confirmation in larger trials or that later failed at the multicenter, randomized controlled trial stage.

88.1 Introduction

Traumatic brain injury (TBI) has been described as "the most complex disease of the most complex organ in the human body." Neurotrauma research poses formidable challenges, and these have to be addressed and overcome in order to advance clinical care. This is much needed as the currently available evidence underpinning guideline recommendations for treatment of patients with TBI is not strong. Of the 27 recommendations in the fourth edition of the Guidelines for the Management of Severe TBI, only eight are based on evidence of high or moderate quality, and of these, only one is graded as a Level I recommendation, the highest level (Carney et al. 2017). Despite ostensibly convincing evidence for efficacy of many putative neuroprotective

A. I. R. Maas (✉)
Department of Neurosurgery, Antwerp University Hospital and University of Antwerp, Edegem, Belgium
e-mail: andrew.maas@uza.be

D. K. Menon
Division of Anaesthesia, University of Cambridge, Cambridge, UK

Neurosciences Critical Care Unit, Addenbrooke's Hospital, Cambridge, UK

N. Marklund
Department of Clinical Sciences Lund, Neurosurgery, Lund University, Skåne University Hospital, Lund, Sweden

© Springer Nature Switzerland AG 2020
T. Sundstrøm et al. (eds.), *Management of Severe Traumatic Brain Injury*,
https://doi.org/10.1007/978-3-030-39383-0_88

agents in experimental studies, translation to the clinic has failed, and there are as yet no neuroprotective agents available with proven clinical benefit. Why is this? Is that perhaps because benefits of targeting one isolated mechanism get lost amidst the complexity of TBI in the clinical situation with many confounding features? Does it then make sense to target only a single mechanism, in the hope of finding a "silver bullet"? Have clinical trials been well conducted with sufficiently large sample sizes and appropriate end points? Are currently accepted end points sufficiently sensitive to detect benefits in all severities of TBI? Does it make sense to expect to find benefit 6 months after injury following a specific treatment that was used only in the first few days?

Research in neurotrauma should be a "closed loop," in which experimental research informs clinical management and treatment through translational research and feedback from the clinical setting informs design and targets for experimental research—in other words, "from bench to bedside and back." In the clinical setting, we now much better appreciate the heterogeneity of TBI as a disease and have come to recognize that the concept of "one size fits all" does not apply to TBI. Current research has a strong focus on developing precision medicine approaches, aimed to better characterize TBI in (subgroups of) patients and to permit appropriate targeting of therapy. It is here that experimental research has yielded huge progress in better understanding the pathophysiologic processes and their detection in TBI.

In this chapter, we aim to present the current state of the art in neurotrauma research with a specific focus on experimental, translational, and clinical research.

88.2 Experimental Neurotrauma Research

Animal models of TBI have long been used to explore pathogenic mechanisms and to evaluate novel therapies in TBI. Without doubt, key discoveries of relevance for human TBI have emerged from such animal experiments. In view of the TBI complexity and heterogeneity, a variety of animal models are needed to mimic the different facets of human TBI. Across numerous reports using these models, hundreds of pharmacological compounds have been found efficacious on histological and/or behavioral outcome. However, when evaluated in clinical randomized controlled trials (RCTs), none of these promising compounds were able to achieve an improved outcome in the complex clinical situation (see below). Although there are numerous reasons for the failure of the RCTs, thoroughly discussed in this chapter, concerns have been raised on the validity of the experimental TBI models and whether they at all can be used to develop successful human therapies. The key question is thus: can the complexity of severe human TBI be mimicked by preclinical models? In the following paragraphs, we address this question by describing key animal models and their limitations, species used, and experimental trial design. Later in this chapter, translational approaches to explore key experimental findings in the human setting are described.

88.2.1 Common Animal Models, Their Strengths, and Limitations

The heterogeneity of human TBI (Saatman et al. 2008) calls for the use of different TBI models (Marklund 2016). The most common ones are listed in Table 88.1.

To mimic a focal TBI/contusions, the controlled cortical impact (CCI) is the most widely used. Here, a craniotomy is performed, and a piston delivers an impact to the exposed dura. The depth of the impact is adjusted according to the hypothesis of the study, and the CCI is fast, reproducible, and easy to use. It can be used in any species, and even if it is considered a predominately focal TBI model, it has aspects of widespread neurodegeneration (Marklund 2016; Hall et al. 2005). It has advantages in the study of contusion development as well as cell death mechanisms. Commonly, the injury

Table 88.1 Examples of animal models, and the human TBI subtype they aim to mimic

TBI subtype	Animal model	Strengths	Limitations
Contusion/ focal TBI	CCI	Easy and fast to perform, adjustable injury level	Craniotomy, too large lesion, white matter injuries
	Weight drop (Feeney)	Adjustable injury level	Imprecise impact mechanism
Diffuse	I/A	Widespread axonal injury	Not, e.g., for mice or pigs
	cFPI	Widespread axonal injury, brain stem pathology	Mortality, technically challenging
	Nonimpact acceleration	Mimics diffuse axonal injury, produces unconsciousness	In NHP and pigs/piglets only, costs and ethics
Mixed	lFPI	Adjustable, mimics human pathophysiology	Mortality, technically challenging
	Weight drop (Shohami)	Easy, fast, no craniotomy needed	Used only in mice

CCI controlled cortical impact, *FPI* Fluid percussion injury, *c* central, *l* lateral, *I/A* impact acceleration (Marmarou model), *NHP* nonhuman primate

involves a large part of the hemisphere and may in many studies have been too extensive to be clinically relevant.

To mimic a diffuse TBI, the most common rodent models are the impact/acceleration model (Marmarou) in rats and the central (midline) fluid percussion injury (cFPI) model. They both produce widespread axonal injury, although they may not replicate all features of diffuse axonal injury as observed in humans. One advantage of the cFPI model is its use in both rats and mice as well as in the pig, although it is technically challenging. At impact, an apnea and post-traumatic seizures are observed, and there is some immediate mortality. For the study of axonal pathology post-TBI, both models provide relevant information that has to some extent been replicated in the human setting (Flygt et al. 2013; Thomas et al. 2018; Ma et al. 2019).

To mimic a "mixed" TBI, e.g., a model with features of both focal/contusional and diffuse TBI, the lateral FPI model (Thompson et al. 2005) and the weight drop model as developed by Shohami and co-workers (Liraz-Zaltsman et al. 2018) are useful. There is here a more substantial component of axonal injury, but a less extensive contusion when compared to the CCI model. The injury mechanisms (impact and brain displacement) and the resulting behavioral impairment and histological characteristics appear clinically relevant (Thompson et al. 2005).

Important strengths of animal models include the possibility for strict control of physical parameters, injury mechanisms, baseline characteristics such as genetics, age and gender, and the use of histological end points (Risling et al. 2019). The vast majority of experimental TBI research is performed in the rodent species. Although the differences to the human anatomy and structure pose key limitations, it should be noted that important features observed in human TBI, such as the development of post-traumatic seizures, oligodendrocyte death, axonal injury, as well as post-traumatic white and grey matter atrophy are also observed in the rodent (Flygt et al. 2016; Bolkvadze and Pitkanen 2012; Bramlett and Dietrich 2002; Pischiutta et al. 2018). Perhaps the most important limitation of the rodent model is that none mimics a severe TBI. Only in the pig/piglet and in particular the nonhuman primate is prolonged unconsciousness observed when the nonimpact acceleration models are used (Sorby-Adams et al. 2018). Thus, it is incorrect to state that a rodent TBI is "severe", at least in comparison with the definition used in humans. Instead, injury severity in rodents can be assessed using a combination of the peak pressure (in the fluid percussion model), post-traumatic apnea and/or righting reflex time, weight loss and intracranial pressure increases, lesion volume, and behavioral outcomes such as the neurological severity scores.

88.2.2 Species Used

Due to their availability, low costs, reproducibility, and large amount of available normative data, rodents will continue to be extensively used in experimental TBI research. Rodent studies enable detailed dissection of numerous injury mechanism using modern molecular biology techniques that include genetic manipulations. However, there are limited similarities between the rodent and human brains. Rodents have large olfactory bulbs, small cerebral cortices, arranged differently than the human cortex, and a small white matter proportion compared with higher species. In addition, the cortex of higher-order species contains numerous high-velocity neurons due to their enhanced processing capacity (Marklund and Hillered 2011; Cai and Wang 2016). In contrast to rodents, large animal species have well-developed meninges, and rodents do not develop herniation due to mass lesion to the extent humans do. In view of the importance of axonal injury in humans, the different thresholds to injury in gray and white matter tissue are an additional limitation to the translatory value of rodents in TBI research in view of their smaller white matter tracts (Cai and Wang 2016). Furthermore, in their comprehensive review of the different TBI-induced changes in cerebral glucose metabolism, inflammatory processes, axonal integrity, and water homeostasis, Agoston and colleagues (Agoston et al. 2019) showed that there are huge interspecies differences in the time course of the trajectories of these pathogenic events. For instance, the immediate post-injury increase in glucose uptake lasts 3–6 h in animals and 7–10 days in humans, and the TBI-induced neuroinflammatory response may be 4–30 times faster in rats than in humans (Agoston et al. 2019). Thus, a "rat day" may be markedly different than a "human day." How to evaluate long-term consequences of TBI in species with such vast differences in life expectancies also remains controversial. Perhaps most importantly, rodent brains are lissencephalic, whereas the brains of humans and other higher-order species are gyrencephalic (Marklund and Hillered 2011). These important differences have somewhat shifted the focus to using large animal models in TBI research (Sorby-Adams et al. 2018). A variety of species including canine, feline, ovine, porcine, and nonhuman primate (NHP) models have been used. To date, the majority of large-animal studies use pigs and sheep. FPI, CCI, and penetrating TBI models have been used in sheep in occasional reports, although pigs, long considered to mimic human physiology (Finnie 2012), dominate TBI research to date. Although the cFPI model was previously common, the CCI model is currently the most widely used in the pig (Sorby-Adams et al. 2018). In addition, the nonimpact acceleration models were successfully used in adult miniature pig and later modified for use in piglets. With these models, increased ICP, reduced CPP, and brain oxygenation have been observed (Friess et al. 2011). In contrast to rodent models, porcine models have also successfully been used to study brain edema, resuscitation and polytrauma, and hemorrhagic TBI. It was suggested (Sorby-Adams et al. 2018) that preclinical guidelines established in experimental stroke could be used also for TBI. Here, large animal models should be the last preclinical step before commencement of clinical trials. However, as we argue in the coming sections of this chapter, this may not be enough for successful translation of therapies into the clinical setting.

88.2.3 Study Design and Outcome Measures

The causes for the repeated failures of RCTs in TBI are multifactorial. Contributing factors may be, e.g., profound inter-center variability in clinical care, wrong dose and time window of the administered drug, and patient heterogeneity, among many others. However, the preclinical studies preceding the clinical development should also be critically assessed. Obvious concerns are whether the TBI models used to evaluate the drug reflect the clinical conditions and whether patient heterogeneity is adequately addressed in the experimental stage. For instance, the vast majority of rodent TBI research is conducted on young male animals, which does not reflect current clinical epidemiology. Furthermore, the time window for initiation of treatment is commonly much shorter in the experimental setting than what later is used in the RCT. Importantly, prolonged time windows should be explored, as should the brain penetration of the evaluated compound. Furthermore, the outcome measures used in experimental TBI may not sufficiently compare with the human situation (Hanell and Marklund 2014). Factors such as communication difficulties, personality disorders, psychological issues, and quality of life factors are all crucial to human outcome, but difficult to assess in animals. However, more complex outcome measures are possible and recommended also in experimental TBI research. It could also be considered that standard animal housing is too sensory deprived to allow clinically relevant research and that an environmental enrichment design should be used more often. There are thus numerous methods to improve the translational value of experimental TBI research, and additional strategies are provided in the coming section of this chapter.

The answer to the question if the complexity of clinical TBI is mimicked by preclinical models, may well be "not really" or at best "only in part." This is particularly true for severe TBI, and at most a moderate level of TBI severity is achieved in most studies. It is recommended that the researcher aim to refine the animal model for maximum clinical applicability and whenever possible, try to establish key findings also in the human setting (tissue, neuroimaging, biomarkers). Another strategy is to explore promising pharmacological approaches in a preclinical multicenter setting. The Operation Brain Trauma Therapy (OBTT) consortium in the USA (Kochanek et al. 2018) is one example of such strategy, and a similar European initiative is ongoing across several centers. While rodents will continue to have a dominating role in TBI research, especially in studies exploring injury mechanisms and in initial evaluation of potential therapies, the use of large animal models will likely become increasingly important in the near future.

88.3 Translational Research in Neurotrauma

Translational research in TBI is complex and challenging. As reviewed in the previous paragraphs, experimental models do not fully replicate the mix of heterogeneous pathologies seen in human TBI, and disease biology may differ between animal models and the human brain. Standardization can be achieved in the experimental setting, but in the more "dirty" clinical setting, extracranial injuries and second insults contribute to the disease process. Uncertainty exists on how pharmacokinetics of novel drugs can be translated from animal models to the clinical situation and how experimental studies may inform timing and duration of drug administration. More detailed understanding of the type, impact, and temporal profile of pathophysiological processes in human TBI is necessary to inform choice, timing, and duration of drug therapy.

88.3.1 Current Approaches: Problems, Pitfalls, and Opportunities

The traditional approach to translational research is to first perform early phase I clinical trials to test human toxicology in healthy volunteers; then proceed to phase II studies for safety testing, dose finding studies, and proof of concept in patients with the disease; and finally conduct phase III efficacy oriented studies (Fig. 88.1). This conventional translational drug development pipeline is based on drugs that emerge from preclinical models and are sequentially tested in phase I clinical trials for human toxicology and then phase II and III clinical trials to evaluate efficacy (Fig. 88.1). It is now increasingly recognized that many older preclinical studies may have been poorly designed to facilitate clinical translation, since either the disease model or the way in which the drug was used bore inadequate relevance to human disease (Janowitz and Menon 2010). More recent efforts have focused on better preclinical studies, with a procedural rigor that replicates human clinical trials in terms of

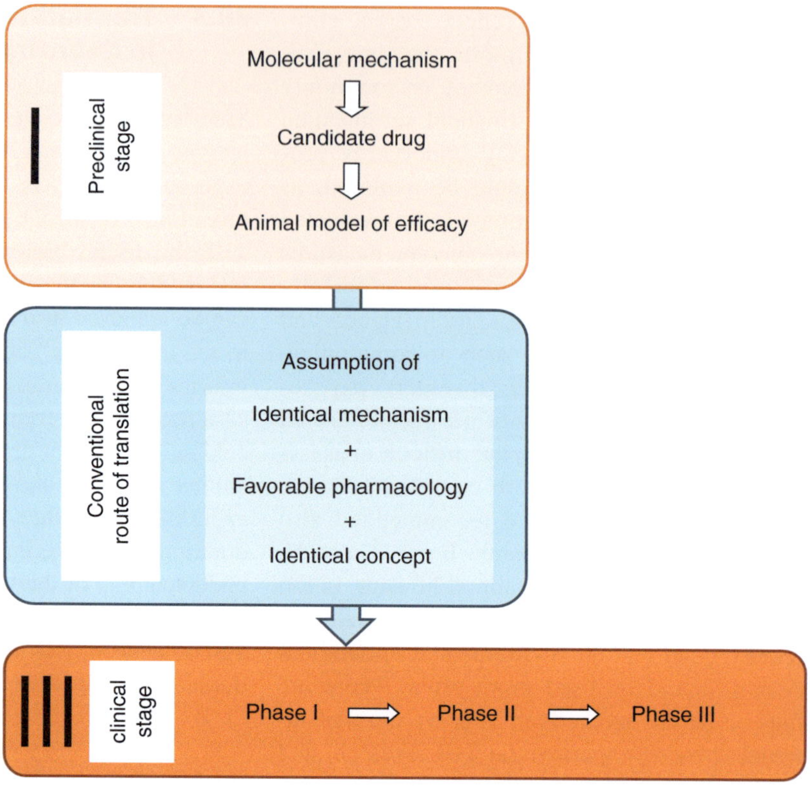

Fig. 88.1 Conventional approach to translational research

predefined hypotheses, strict protocols, blinded assessment of outcome, and stringent assessment of replicability of results (Kochanek et al. 2016). These efforts merit strong endorsement and will undoubtedly improve the state in which new investigational therapies are delivered by preclinical scientists to the clinical translational pipeline. However, even where such preclinical studies are optimally designed, this conventional translational pathway makes assumptions that are unsafe and may well be wrong. These include expectations that:

- The molecular mechanisms demonstrated in animal models have the same temporal profile and outcome impact in human TBI.
- Regional pharmacokinetics and biodistribution of new drugs are identical in animal models and human disease.
- Pharmacodynamic models that have been developed in the laboratory (e.g., receptor kinetics) can be directly replicated in human TBI.

These expectations have led to the assumption that efficacy demonstrated in experimental models targeted primarily to contusional brain injury or diffuse injury will hold across the broad and heterogeneous spectrum of clinical TBI. Evidence shows that these assumptions were wrong for a large proportion of neuroprotective compounds evaluated in clinical TBI in the past (Janowitz and Menon 2010) and that these errors persist in more recent trials of investigational drugs in TBI (Stein 2015). We need a better translational model for drug development.

One suggested option (Sorby-Adams et al. 2018) has been to test novel drugs that initially have shown efficacy in rodent models in larger gyrencephalic species (cats, dogs, primates) before moving into clinical studies. This approach has some merit, particularly in demonstrating drug safety in a second species. It may also demonstrate efficacy against physiological targets (such as intracranial hypertension), which are less prominent in rodent models. However, we would argue that testing the drug higher up the evolutionary ladder still does not provide a faithful representation of its efficacy in man. Once preclinical safety testing is complete, and TBI models demonstrate efficacy of a molecule, we believe that the evaluation of such a candidate molecule would be best served by a translational pipeline which:

- Rapidly and effectively determines whether the molecular mechanism that has been effectively targeted in experimental models exists in human TBI, how much it contributes to human disease, when it is initiated, and how long it remains active. It would also be critical to identify and validate molecular or imaging biomarkers of this mechanism.
- Determines whether the agent, when administered by the intended route, in a dose that is demonstrated to be safe by preclinical testing, reaches its putative site of action in the brain in concentrations that are adequate to modulate the molecular process it is targeted at.
- Establishes that the agent, at the brain concentrations achieved in human TBI, modulates the target mechanism in a way that modifies levels of biomarkers that quantify it.

These requirements are best met by a translational pipeline that incorporates strong elements of experimental medicine. This approach to developing new pharmacological therapies is made more practicable by the tools that have been used to improve clinical TBI outcomes through non-pharmacological approaches. These improvements in clinical outcome have been largely based on our ability to monitor and treat physiological targets (e.g., intracranial pressure (ICP), brain hypoxia, and changes in brain chemistry), coupled with the use of neuroimaging for diagnosis and prognostication. The monitoring and diagnostic modalities developed in this context can be used to create more rational paradigms of neuroprotective drug development. These tools provide opportunities to investigate disease biology, proof of mechanism (PoM), pharmacokinetic validation, and proof of concept (PoC) in small, carefully selected cohorts of patients at an early stage of drug development. They include the following.

88.3.2 Access to Tissue Biofluids and Tissue

Access to cerebrospinal fluid (CSF) is commonly available in more severe patients with TBI, either through ventriculostomies inserted for intracranial pressure (ICP) monitoring or CSF drainage for raised ICP, or at the time of placement of a ventriculoperitoneal shunt at the subacute stage in the small proportion of patients who have persistent post-traumatic hydrocephalus. This last subset of patients also provides a cohort in whom CSF can be relatively easily accessed at chronic stages after TBI. Access to CSF enables detection of molecular biomarkers of disease processes and neural injury, which allows us to establish the presence and magnitude of a pathophysiological process (e.g., cytokines to characterize neuroinflammation), document its point of initiation and subsequent time course in clinical TBI (thus determining windows for the initiation and duration of therapy), and quantify the effect of interventions against the target.

Cerebral microdialysis (CMD) now forms part of routine clinical monitoring in several centers worldwide (Hutchinson et al. 2015). The primary aim of CMD, in terms of clinical practice, is to monitor cerebral energy metabolism (through measurement of glucose, lactate, and pyruvate levels), glutamate release, and glycerol generation (as a marker of membrane phospholipid breakdown in ongoing tissue injury). However, particularly with the advent of CMD catheters with 100-kDa cutoffs (Hutchinson et al. 2005), there is the increasing opportunity to access the brain extracellular fluid to measure levels of biomolecules (Oddo and Hutchinson 2018) and also determine if novel drugs can achieve therapeutically relevant concentrations in the brain following human TBI (Helmy et al. 2016). Such assessment of regional pharmacokinetics (PK) of new agents can form part of a phase II study. However, modern microdosing approaches to studying drug biodistribution (see below), coupled with ultrasensitive assays, may allow us to examine blood–brain barrier penetration with small (and pharmacodynamically ineffective—and hence safe) doses of novel agents at a relatively early stage of drug development. Finally, CMD can be used to demonstrate that novel agents result in changes in levels of downstream mediators as expected from their biology—as proof of concept (Helmy et al. 2016). Increasingly, CMD is being used to interrogate metabolic pathways in the brain (Gallagher et al. 2009; Carpenter et al. 2014), and analysis of these results may suggest the use of novel energy substrates, whose efficacy can be tested in preliminary studies using CMD (Stovell et al. 2018).

TBI is one of the few acute neurological diseases in which routine clinical management provides access to brain tissue at the time of the acute insult. Resection of space occupying contusions, undertaken as part of a management strategy to control ICP, provides (in the form of the margins of the resected contusion tissue) a targeted sampling of the traumatic penumbra, where pathophysiology is most active and where many agents might be expected to have their prime site of action. These tissue samples can be used to document pathophysiology and measure drug levels.

While the discussion above has (appropriately) focused on access to tissue and biofluids in the brain, it is important to recognize that the expanding role for blood biomarkers in the routine clinical management of TBI (Mondello et al. 2011) offers opportunities for translational research. First, biomarker measurement in humans may provide a bridge to emerging rigorous preclinical research that uses biomarkers as an intermediate outcome (Mondello et al. 2016). Second, biomarker measurement may allow more secure diagnosis of TBI, especially in milder injury or CT-negative patients with severe injury (who may have diffuse axonal injury), and stratify patients prognostically (Turgeon et al. 2013). Further, changes in biomarker level relate to disease evolution, and modulation of such evolution by drugs can provide evidence of their effect - either good or bad (Scott et al. 2018). Finally, while some biomarkers, such as microRNAs (Mateen et al. 2017) are being pursued for their diagnostic and prognostic potential, they may also offer options for therapy.

88.3.3 Neuroimaging of Pathophysiology, Disease Evolution, and Drug Distribution

Neuroimaging in TBI conventionally employs X-ray computed tomography, which is primarily used for detecting surgical lesions and providing prognostic information. However, serial CT imaging also provides a marker of disease evolution in TBI, since it quantifies lesion progression, and the change in imaging from baseline at presentation thus represents an intermediate end point of drug efficacy. An example is the use of novel (possibly genetically targeted) interventions acting on the ABCC8/TRPM4 locus to reduce edema after TBI (Jha et al. 2019). More recently, magnetic resonance imaging (MRI) has shown enormous promise in TBI and can aid in characterizing acute pathophysiology—examples include differentiating cytotoxic from vasogenic edema and detecting traumatic axonal injury. Serial imaging can also be used to demonstrate disease progression in the acute (Newcombe et al. 2013) and chronic (Newcombe et al. 2016) phases. MRI can also show evidence of benefit from acute interventions—such as the reversal of pericontusional cytotoxic edema by acute normobaric hyperoxia (Veenith et al. 2017). The ability to measure change from baseline, and to examine the effect of interventions to modulate such disease progression, may increase sensitivity to detect drug benefit in early stage studies and identify patient subgroups most likely to benefit.

In terms of molecular imaging, the modality with the best track record is positron emission tomography (PET) (Sorby-Adams et al. 2018). Oxygen PET is increasingly being used as a research tool in clinical TBI to characterize acute physiology of energy failure, providing information not just on classical ischemia, but also novel mechanisms such as diffusion hypoxia

(Menon et al. 2004; Veenith et al. 2016) and mitochondrial dysfunction (Vespa et al. 2005). Critically, these same approaches can be used to show whether interventions can improve (Nortje et al. 2008) or worsen (Coles et al. 2007) energy metabolism in TBI. More recently, PET ligands for the Translocator Protein (TSPO) have been used to label activated microglia and image neuroinflammation in the acute (Donat et al. 2017) and chronic (Ramlackhansingh et al. 2011) phase after TBI. Such imaging of neuroinflammation can also be used as a proximate end point to examine the efficacy of drugs that modulate neuroinflammation (Scott et al. 2018)—and integrating the measurement of blood biomarkers into these studies can help dissect mechanistic efficacy from possible benefit. There is also enormous current interest in using a range of PET ligands to image amyloid (Hong et al. 2014) and tau (Mohamed et al. 2019) deposition after TBI. Given the increasing recognition that TBI can be a chronic disease in a subgroup of patients, such imaging is critical to identify patient subsets that show such pathology. Given that interventions aimed at these neurodegenerative processes may take years to decades to show clinical benefit, serial imaging with such ligands, underpinned by serial MRI to examine changes in evolving tissue fate, provides a key realistic means of early demonstration of efficacy of interventions that target accumulation of such molecules. Finally, although not yet applied to TBI, microdosing with PET, the administration of subtherapeutic concentrations of a radiolabeled version of target molecules, coupled with the high sensitivity of PET imaging, allows characterization of regional pharmacokinetics and calibration of drug–target interactions (Burt et al. 2017). The technique can quantify receptor occupancy and assess competing candidate molecules, or different doses of a single candidate drug, in humans in the clinical setting in which the drug might be deployed. This allows choices to be made between competing candidate compounds at an early stage and provides a rational approach to drug development, shortening critical time lines and possibly increasing success rate for drug development from current levels.

88.3.4 Intermediate and Late Imaging End Points

In TBI, functional outcome is most commonly assessed at 6–12 months post-injury, which poses a logistic challenge and results in large proportions of missing outcomes (Richter et al. 2019). Consequently, physiological markers, such as ICP, have been suggested as a surrogate outcome. However, although severe intracranial hypertension may be a marker of mechanistic efficacy and is known to be a predictor of mortality, it has a less robust (or no) relationship to the more relevant end point of functional outcome (Balestreri et al. 2006). Brain imaging may provide a more relevant surrogate outcome by identifying the impact of an intervention on tissue fate. Although conventional MRI outperforms CT for assessing tissue survival (Amyot et al. 2015), it is an insensitive measure of selective neuronal loss and covert axonal injury (Newcombe et al. 2011). Newer imaging techniques provide the opportunity to study the effects of drugs on more subtle markers of injury, such as tissue injury and neuronal survival. While late MRI can provide useful intermediate outcome measures, based on volume loss on conventional sequences (Marcoux et al. 2008), diffusion tensor imaging can detect occult microstructural injury (Newcombe et al. 2011). Some injury mechanisms in TBI may result in selective neuronal loss (SNL) rather than pan-necrosis; SNL can be detected with ^{1}H-MR spectroscopy (Marcoux et al. 2008) and PET with the benzodiazepine ligand, [11C]-flumazenil (Kawai et al. 2010).

88.3.5 Reverse Translation: The Role of Genomics

Thus far, we have focused on how a range of tools applicable to clinical TBI may be used to transport drugs that have emerged from preclinical research through the translational pipeline. However, the imminent availability of results from genome-wide association studies may offer additional opportunities. Conventionally, genomics has been promoted for improved stratification of patients in trials and perhaps the selection of patients more likely to respond to a given intervention. However, genomic medicine may also provide opportunities for a paradigm altering approach, by identifying therapeutic targets that emerge from a data-driven, unbiased analysis of the genetic variations that drive TBI outcome. Emerging examples, thus far based on candidate gene analysis, support this paradigm and may hold most promise in the repurposing of established drugs with known safety profiles in other indications for use to improve outcomes in TBI. This framework has led to the preclinical (and phase II) evaluation of glibenclamide (Jha et al. 2018a, b) as a treatment for cerebral edema post-TBI (through its action on SUR1/ABCC8, which is now known to drive edema development in TBI and stroke) and maraviroc (an anti-HIV agent) as a treatment in TBI models (Joy et al. 2019).

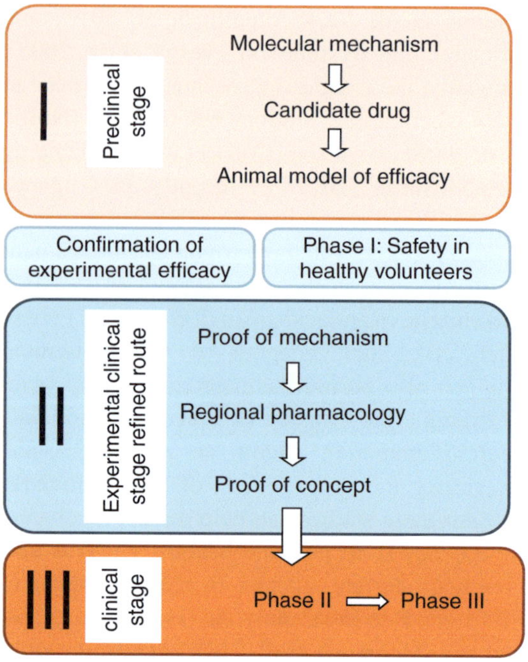

Fig. 88.2 Alternative approach to translational research

88.3.6 Translational Outlook

Thus, many clinical monitoring techniques in TBI can be used in translational research, and these opportunities could be utilized systematically to overcome some of the obstacles and pitfalls during translational research in TBI. The comprehensive failure of attempts at translating neuroprotection in TBI may be partly due to an incomplete understanding of human disease biology and partly to missed opportunities for optimization of drug design and dosage during early translation. Emerging experience over the last few years suggests that the tools used for clinical monitoring in TBI could address these issues. The impact of such research on pharmacology and disease biology could be large because the multitude of potentially useful treatments far surpasses not just the financial investment and time available for drug development, but also (and perhaps more critically) access to patient populations for trials.

We propose the systematic introduction of an additional stage in drug development for TBI (Fig. 88.2) that incorporates experimental medicine. The recent substantial refinement in clinical research tools, coupled with the previous failure of conventional approaches, makes TBI a prime target for such a strategy. However, such a refinement of translational research should also benefit drug development in other diseases and organ systems.

88.4 Clinical Research

Clinical research in neurotrauma is a dynamic and challenging field. Over the years, epidemiology in high-income countries is changing, approaches to management have evolved, and new technologies have been introduced to monitor the more severely injured patients. Most research originates from high-income countries, but over 90% of neurotrauma occurs in low- and middle-income countries (LMICs). Initiatives have been taken to address this discordance. The Lancet Commission on Global Surgery called attention for the lack of neurosurgical services in many LMICs and strongly advocated universal access to safe, affordable surgical and anesthesia care when needed saves lives, prevents disability, and promotes economic growth. This is particularly relevant to neurotrauma and its research. The WFNS-WHO Liaison Committee (Meara et al. 2015) actively seeks to advance the care for neurotrauma in LMICs, and the NIHR Global Health Research Group on Neurotrauma was established and is coordinated by Cambridge University (http://neurotrauma.world/). They initiated the Global Neurotrauma Outcomes Study (GNOS: https://globalneurotrauma.com), which is currently enrolling across the world. GNOS aims to provide a global picture of the management and outcomes of patients undergoing emergency surgery for TBI. In addition, this will establish a platform and clinical network to facilitate future research in global neurotrauma and neurosurgery.

Research in TBI has had a strong focus on patients with moderate to severe TBI. The greatest burden of TBI is, however, caused by mild TBI. The CENTER-TBI registry that enrolled patients across all severities showed that 81% of all patients were classified as having a mild TBI. Of patients seen in the Emergency Room and discharged or admitted to the hospital ward, approximately 95% had a mild TBI. Importantly, 28% of these had not attained a full recovery at 6 months after injury. These data highlight a need for increased research efforts in mild TBI.

RCTs are considered the gold standard for generating evidence in medical research to support treatment recommendations. In TBI, challenges are posed by the heterogeneity of the population—in terms of type of injury, clinical severity, and variations in treatment. Approaches commonly used to reduce heterogeneity have employed strict enrollment criteria, typically focusing on prognostic variables and pre-injury morbidity. Such approach is statistically inefficient (Roozenbeek et al. 2009, 2012) and reduces generalizability of findings. Importantly, elderly patients (≥65 years of age) are consequently disenfranchised from research to improve their outcome, and these constitute 28% of the TBI population in a recent study (Maas et al. 2015). Recognition of the relevance of large-scale observational studies to generate high-quality evidence is increasing. Comparative effectiveness research (CER) can exploit the heterogeneity of TBI in terms of type of injury, management, and outcome and would permit assessment of therapeutic approaches in real-world situations. This is, however, methodologically challenging because of a high risk of "confounding by indication": Patients receiving a specific intervention are not selected at random, but decisions on treatment approaches are influenced by patient characteristics, disease course, physician preferences, and other uncontrolled factors. As a consequence, finding an association between an intervention and outcome may not be causal. An illustrative example would be finding an association between ICP monitoring (generally performed in the sickest patients) and poorer outcome. In all TBI research, it is important to recognize the continuum of care along the chain of trauma care (Fig. 88.3), which may substantially influence the chance of finding benefits in the acute hospital phase.

If severe second insults occur in the prehospital phase, the battle may already be lost no matter how good and effective hospital care may be. Likewise, if benefits may occur from a novel intervention in the acute hospital setting, it may be impossible to demonstrate efficacy at 6 months if such benefits are not consolidated by good post-acute care. This may have occurred in the BEST TRIP trial on ICP (Chesnut et al. 2012) conducted in two LMICs, where post-acute care was completely lacking.

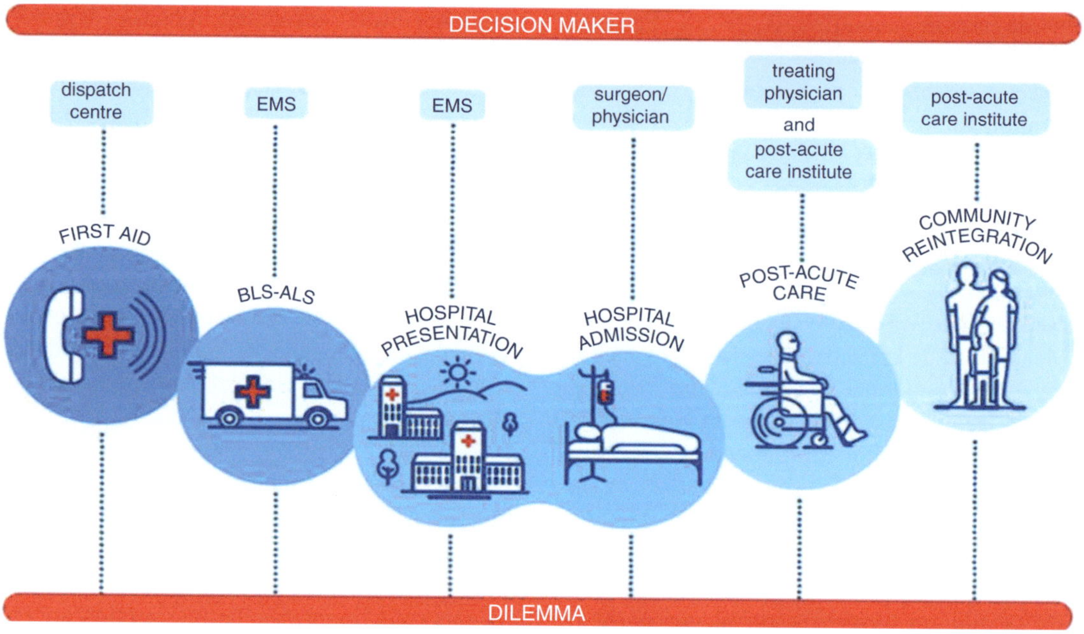

Fig. 88.3 The chain of trauma care

88.5 Clinical Trials in TBI

Most RCTs have been conducted in patients with moderate to severe TBI. Many of these trials have been underpowered, and only few showed statistically significant results. In a systematic review of 191 completed RCTs (Phase 2 and Phase 3), Bragge et al. (Bragge et al. 2016) found that only 26 could be considered robust (high quality with sufficient numbers), of which six showed a statistically significant effect (three positive and three negative). Table 88.2 presents an overview of large Phase 3 trials (published and unpublished), conducted in moderate to severe TBI.

Of the 32 RCTs listed in this table, four concerned surgical management, six concerned medical management, and 22 aimed to demonstrate efficacy of putative neuroprotective agents. Since 2000, an increase can be noted in investigator-driven RCTs on medical or surgical management. Of the 16 RCTs that started recruitment in 2000 or later, seven (44%) investigated medical or surgical management, compared to only 3/16 (19%) in older RCTs. Overall, the results have been disappointing: Only four RCTs showed lower mortality or better outcome in the intervention group, six showed higher mortality or poorer outcome, and 22 found no significant effect between intervention groups.

88.5.1 RCTs on Neuroprotective Agents

Of the 22 RCTs on neuroprotective agents, three reported higher mortality (CRASH, SNX-111, and Magnesium (Roberts et al. 2004; Temkin et al. 2007)). One RCT on a neuroprotective agent (HIT III: Nimodipine) showed benefit (Harders et al. 1996). The most convincing evidence came from the CRASH trial: This was a mega trial that enrolled 10,008 patients and reported increased mortality and poorer long-term outcome in the intervention group (methylprednisolone). This trial forms the evidence base for the Level I Guideline recommendation not to use steroids for the treatment of TBI. The beneficial effects of nimodipine in patients with traumatic subarachnoid hemorrhage, reported in HIT III, should be interpreted with caution. First,

Table 88.2 Overview of large phase III trials in moderate to severe TBI (published and unpublished)

Study + agent	Mechanism targeted/treatment approach	Study population	N pat	Start of treatment	Year of study	Status	Published/ reference	Result
POLAR hypothermia	Various intracerebral processes	GCS ≤ 8	511	≤3 h	2010–2017	Completed	Cooper et al. (2018)	No significant difference
RESCUEicp	Decompressive craniectomy vs standard care for raised ICP	Abnormal CT and raised ICP	408	Within 6 h of randomization	2004–2014	Completed	Hutchinson et al. (2016)	Decreased mortality, but higher number of patients with disability
STITCH	Early surgery vs standard care for contusions	Early surgery within 12 h vs initial conservative management	170	≤48 h	2009–2012	Halted by funding agency	Gregson et al. (2015)	Mortality significantly lower in early surgery group
Eurotherm	Various intracerebral processes	ICU admission for TBI and ICP monitoring within 10 days of injury	387	ICP > 20 mmHg for at least 5 min	2009–2014	Stopped for safety reasons	Andrews et al. (2018)	Outcome significantly poorer in hypothermia group
EPO-TBI	Multiple targets	GCS 3–12	606	≤24 h	2010–2014	Completed	Nichol et al. (2015)	No effect on 6-month GOSE, possibly lower mortality in patients without a mass lesion
EPO	Multiple targets	GCS motor score ≤ 6	200	≤6 h	2006–2012	Completed	Robertson et al. (2014)	No significant effect
Hydrocortisone + fludrocortisone vs placebo	Prevention of hospital acquired pneumonia	GCS ≤ 8	336	≤24 h	2010–2012	Completed	Asehnoune et al. (2014)	No significant effect, but trend to efficacy in subgroup with adrenal insufficiency
SYNAPSE/progesterone studies	Multiple targets	GCS ≤ 8	1179	≤8 h	2010–2013	Completed	Skolnick et al. (2014)	No significant effect

(continued)

Table 88.2 (continued)

Study + agent	Mechanism targeted/treatment approach	Study population	No. pat.	Start of treatment	Year of study	Status	Published/ reference	Result
PROTECT III/progesterone studies	Multiple targets	GCS 4–12	882	≤4 h	2010–2013	Terminated for reasons of futility	Wright et al. (2014)	No significant effect
BEST TRIP	ICP guided management vs clinical imaging guided management	GCS ≤ 8	324	≤48 h	2008–2011	Completed	Chesnut et al. (2012)	No significant difference
CRASH-2 IBS tranexamic acid	Fibrinolysis	GCS ≤ 14	270	≤8 h	2008–2010	Completed	Perel et al. (2012)	No significant effect on 28-day mortality
DECRA	Early decompressive craniectomy vs standard care	GCS ≤ 8 and ICP monitoring ICP > 20 for 15 min within a 1-h period	155	≤48 h	2002–2010	Completed	Cooper et al. (2011)	Poorer outcome on the GOSE
The Brain Trial	Bradykinin (β2 receptor) antagonist	GCS ≤ 12	228	≤8 h	2007	Terminated	Shakur et al. (2009)	No significant effect
SAFE study Subgroup analysis of patients with TBI	Saline vs albumin	GCS ≤ 13	460	No time limit specified; used as resuscitation fluid up to 28 days after ICU admission	2001–2003	Completed; subgroup analysis	SAFE Study Investigators; Australian and New Zealand Intensive Care Society Clinical Trials Group; Australian Red Cross Blood Service; George Institute for International Health and Myburgh (2007)	Significantly higher mortality in patients treated with albumin

Pharmos/dexanabinol (Maas 2006)	Glutamate excitotoxicity, lipid peroxidation, inflammatory response	Motor score 2–5 + CT abnormalities	861	≤ 6 h	2000–2004	Completed	Maas et al. (2006)	No significant effect
CRASH/steroid trial (Roberts 2004)	Inflammatory response/edema	GCS < 15	10,008	≤8 h	2000–2004	Completed	2005 (CRASH trial) collaborators (Roberts et al. 2004)	Higher mortality
Magnesium	Various intracerebral processes	GCS 3–12 and/or intracranial surgery	499	≤8 h	1998–2004	Completed	Roberts et al. (2004), Temkin et al. (2007)	Poorer outcome at low dose Higher mortality at high dose
Large versus limited decompressive craniectomy	Standard large craniectomy vs limited craniectomy	GCS 4–8 Unilateral contusion or swelling with mass effect	486	Not specified	1998–2001	Completed	Jiang et al. (2005)	Significantly better outcome in patients with large decompressive craniectomy
Pfizer/CP-101606	Glutamate excitotoxicity	GCS 4–8	404	≤8 h	1997–2000	Completed	Yurkewicz et al. (2005)	*Non*-significant effect
Parke Davis/SNX-111	Calcium channel blocker	GCS 4–8	237	≤12 h	1997–1998	Terminated by DSMB for safety reasons	No	Higher mortality
NABIS/hypothermia	Various intracerebral processes	GCS 3–8 Motor score 1–5	392	≤6 h	1994–1998	Halted	Clifton et al. (2001)	No effects on outcome Reduced incidence of ICP, 30 mmHg

(continued)

Table 88.2 (continued)

Study + agent	Mechanism targeted/treatment approach	Study population	No. pat.	Start of treatment	Year of study	Status	Published/ reference	Result
CBF targeted management	Cerebral ischemia	Motor score ≤5	189	≤12 h	1994–1997	Completed	Robertson et al. (1999)	No significant effects on outcome Decreased incidence of desaturation episodes Increased incidence of ARDS
Saphir/D-CPP-ene	Glutamate excitotoxicity	Not obeying commands, 1 reactive pupil	924	≤12 h	1995–1997	Completed	No	No significant effect reported
Cerestat/aptiganel	Glutamate excitotoxicity	GCS 4–8 GCS 3 if pupils are reactive	532	≤8 h	1996–1997	Terminated	No	No significant effect
Selfotel	Glutamate excitotoxicity	GCS 4–8	693	≤8 h and within 4 h of admission	1994–1996	Terminated	Morris et al. (1999)	No significant effect
Eliprodil study	Glutamate excitotoxicity	GCS 4–8	452	≤12 h	1993–1995	Completed	No	No significant effect reported
Tirilazad domestic trial	Lipid peroxidation	GCS ≤ 8: 85% GCS 9–12: 15%	1155	≤4 h	1991–1994	Terminated	No	No significant effect reported
Tirilazad international trial	Lipid peroxidation	GCS ≤ 8: 85% GCS 9–12: 15%	1120	≤4 h	1992–1994	Completed	Marshall et al. (1998)	No significant effect
Bradycor/CP-0127	Bradykinin (β2 receptor) antagonist	GCS 3–8	139	≤8 h	1996	Completed	(Marmarou et al. (1999)	12% improvement in fav. outcome ($P = 0.26$)
PEG-SOD	Free radical damage	GCS ≤ 8	1562	Within 8	1993–1995	Completed	Young et al. (1996)	No significant difference
HIT IV Nimodipine	Calcium mediated damage	GCS < 15 + traumatic subarachnoid hemorrhage	592	≤12 h	1997–1999	Completed	No	No significant effect

HIT III Nimodipine	Calcium mediated damage	TSAH	123	≤12 h	1994	Completed	Harders et al. (1996)	Significant reduction in unfavorable outcome
HIT II Nimodipine	Calcium mediated damage	Not obeying commands	852	12 h of not obeying commands within 24 h of injury	1989–1991	Completed	A multicenter trial of the efficacy of nimodipine on outcome after severe head injury (1994)	No significant effect on overall population
HIT I Nimodipine	Calcium mediated damage	Not obeying commands	351	24 h	1987–1989	Completed	Bailey et al. (1991)	No significant effect
Dexamethasone-mega dose trial	Various intracerebral processes	GCS ≤ 13	300	≤3 h	1986–1989	Completed	Gaab et al. (1994)	No significant effect
Triamcinolone steroid trial	Various intracerebral processes	Severe head injury, not further defined	396	≤4 h	1985–1990	Completed	Grumme et al. (1995)	No significant effect

In red are the surgical trials, in green medical management trials, and with no color the medication/neuroprotection trials the trial was relatively small ($n = 123$), it was not considered as robust in the systematic review by Bragge et al. (Bragge et al. 2016), and larger trials in the broader population of severe TBI failed to show benefit of nimodipine.

88.5.2 RCTs on Medical Management

Of the six RCTs on medical management, two showed poorer outcome in the intervention group (SAFE study and Eurotherm). The SAFE study was a large-scale RCT investigating the benefits of 4% albumin over saline as resuscitation fluid in 6997 patients admitted to the ICU (Finfer et al. 2004). While in the overall population no differences were found in outcome between intervention groups, in a subgroup analysis of 460 patients with moderate to severe TBI, mortality was significantly higher in patients treated with albumin (SAFE Study Investigators; Australian and New Zealand Intensive Care Society Clinical Trials Group; Australian Red Cross Blood Service; George Institute for International Health and Myburgh 2007). As a consequence, albumin is no longer recommended in the treatment of TBI.

Eurotherm was designed as a pivotal RCT to demonstrate benefit of hypothermia in the treatment of patients with severe TBI (Andrews et al. 2015). Originally designed to recruit 1800–2000 patients, the protocol was later amended to a sample size of 600 patients. The trial was stopped for safety reasons after recruitment of 387 patients in 47 centers from 18 countries. Outcome as assessed by the GOSE at 6 months after injury was significantly poorer in the hypothermia group and mortality significantly higher. While Eurotherm allowed recruitment of patients up to 10 days after injury, the POLAR study (Cooper et al. 2018), which was in part conducted in parallel, aimed to initiate hypothermia as soon as possible, preferably already in the prehospital phase. This study recruited 511 patients and found no significant effect of hypothermia. The poorer outcome with hypothermia in Eurotherm and the absence of beneficial effects of hypothermia in POLAR have been considered reasons for abandoning the use of hypothermia in TBI by some. However, patients recruited to POLAR had relatively mild injury—few required therapy for refractory intracranial hypertension. While POLAR is a key study in informing us about the failure of *prophylactic hypothermia as a universal primary neuroprotective intervention* in TBI, it tells us little about whether it could provide benefit in the context of *refractory intracranial hypertension as a rescue therapy*. In this situation, the benefits of ICP control may outweigh the known hazards associated with the intervention. We need a study that specifically addresses the use of *therapeutic* (not prophylactic) hypothermia in this context—which is where it is most commonly employed by centers that continue to use it. The contextual contrast here is similar to that between DECRA and RESCUEicp (see below). Like RESCUEicp, the population for such a study would be less than 20% of the ICU TBI population—the study would not be easy to recruit to and complete, but is essential if we are to have high-quality evidence to adopt or discard the use of hypothermia in this setting.

88.5.3 RCTs on Surgical Management

Four large-scale RCTs have been conducted on the surgical management of TBI with a focus on decompressive craniectomy and the surgical treatment of contusions—all showing a significant effect. Jiang et al. in a study on 486 patients with severe TBI who required a decompressive craniectomy convincingly demonstrated that a large craniectomy resulted in better outcome compared to a more limited decompression (Jiang et al. 2005). The DECRA trial, however, showed that the early use of Decompressive Craniectomy (DC) for modest increases of ICP in patients with diffuse injuries was associated with poorer outcome (Cooper et al. 2011). In contrast, RESCUEicp (Randomized Evaluation of Surgery with Craniectomy for Uncontrollable Elevation of Intracranial Pressure) targeted refractory severe intracranial hypertension (Hutchinson et al. 2016). This trial showed a significant reduction in mortality in patients treated with DC, but this came at the cost of a 9% increase in survival with severe dependence at 6 months. However, at 12 months, there were 13% more survivors who were independent at home.

The different results obtained in DECRA versus RESCUEicp may be related to the different populations studied (in DECRA, only patients with diffuse injuries), to indications/timing (early DC in DECRA vs refractory raised ICP in RESCUEicp), or to complications of DC performed in these different settings. RESCUEicp has highlighted that long-term outcome evaluation is advisable, and the ethical concerns of possibly increasing severe dependence by performing a DC should motivate taking individual wishes of patients and their relatives into consideration when considering to perform a DC. It should be noted that neither study addresses primary decompression in patients operated for a mass lesion. This is currently ongoing in RESCUE-ASDH. The STITCH trial (Surgical Trial in Traumatic Intracerebral Haemorrhage) investigated benefits of early surgery versus an initial conservative approach in patients with contusion (Gregson et al. 2015). Unfortunately, the trial was stopped after inclusion of 170 patients due to an administrative decision of the funding agency. This is regrettable as on analysis mortality in patients undergoing early surgery was significantly reduced, but no statistically significant effect on the primary end point of functional outcome (GOSE at 6 months) could be demonstrated due to the relatively low sample size. The results of and issues raised by RCTs on the surgical management of TBI strongly motivate future research to identify subgroups of patients who are most likely to benefit and also those who are not likely to benefit.

88.5.4 Observational Studies and the Potential of Individual Patient Data Analyses Across Studies

Much of our understanding of and care for TBI have come from observational studies.

Previous observational studies include the Traumatic Coma Data Bank (TCDB) in the USA, the Core Data Survey of the European Brain Injury Consortium (Eisenberg et al. 1990; Murray et al. 1999), and studies by the Trauma Audit and Research Network (TARN) in the UK (http://www.tarn.ac.uk). The TCDB unequivocally demonstrated adverse consequences of secondary insults (hypoxia and hypotension), and the TARN (Patel et al. 2005) showed a 2.15-fold increase in the odds of death adjusted for case mix for patients with severe TBI treated in non-neurosurgical center compared to those treated at a neurosurgical center. This forms a strong argument for transferring and treating all patients with severe head injury in a setting with 24-h neurosurgical facilities. In contrast to common belief, participation in an observational study may by itself promote quality of care for the individual patient. Sir Graham Teasdale, one of the world leaders in the field of TBI, when asked if he would ever personally consent to participation in a clinical trial on TBI once answered that he certainly would, but would wish to be allocated to the placebo group. This reflects the understanding that patients allocated to a placebo group within a trial may benefit from closer scrutiny of their clinical course and better adherence to guidelines while not being exposed to any additional risk of an investigational treatment. Similar benefits apply to observational studies.

The potential of meta-analyses across studies was clearly demonstrated by the International Mission on Prognosis and Analysis of randomized Controlled Trials in TBI (IMPACT) studies (Maas et al. 2007). The IMPACT studies aimed to improve the design and analyses of clinical trials by analyzing individual patient data across eight RCTs and three observational studies. These studies laid the basis for standardization of data collection in TBI (Common Data Elements: https://www.commondataelements.ninds.nih.gov), developed prognostic models for moderate and severe TBI, and proposed recommendations for increasing statistical power in RCTs (Maas et al. 2013). These recommendations included targeting of a broad population, applying covariate adjustment, and using an ordinal analysis rather than the traditional dichotomization of outcome. The IMPACT prognostic models remain current and are the most widely used and best validated models for predicting outcome. Substantial differences in outcome were demonstrated: On analyses of data from 9578 patients recruited in 265 centers, the risk of unfavorable outcome was 3.3 times higher between centers at the lower end of the outcome range compared to those at the higher end (97.5th versus 2.5th percentile) (Lingsma et al. 2011). In a similar analysis of 9987 patients from the CRASH trial that also enrolled subjects from LMICs, a 6.6-fold difference was found. These differences in outcome highlight the potential for comparative effectiveness research in large-scale observational studies. Observational studies, however, have suffered from a relative lack of funding as reviewers for grant applications often demand hypothesis-driven research. Recognition of the relevance of observational studies has substantially increased over the past 5 years and is embodied by the formal establishment of InTBIR (International Initiative for Traumatic Brain Injury Research: http://intbir.nih.gov) as collaboration of funding agencies. Over 11 large-scale studies are currently being conducted under the umbrella of InTBIR. The largest are CENTER-TBI (Collaborative European NeuroTrauma Effectiveness Research in TBI: www.Center-tbi.eu) and CREACTIVE (Collaborative Research on Acute Traumatic brain Injury in intensive care medicine) in Europe and TRACK-TBI (Transforming Research and Clinical Knowledge in Traumatic Brain Injury) and ADAPT (Approaches and Decisions in Acute Pediatric TBI Trial) in the USA. Overall, the InTBIR studies will likely include over 40,000 patients with TBI of all severities, many of whom will provide data on genomics, biomarkers, and imaging to facilitate precision medicine approaches for TBI. The concept of large-scale observational studies combined with CER has attracted global interest, and projects are evolving in Australia, China, and India.

88.6 The Future of Clinical Research in TBI

While RCTs will remain a major pillar for demonstrating effectiveness of specific interventions and management strategies for TBI, we anticipate an increased focus on high-quality prospective observational studies, which have a large potential for developing precision medicine approaches and, when subjected to CER, identification of best practices. An increased focus of research should be targeted to patients with milder forms of TBI, and studies across all severities need to include elderly patients, a subgroup in which the incidence of TBI is increasing rapidly but is currently seldom included in clinical studies. Research on TBI should be stimulated in LMICs to address specific aspects of management in these settings.

TBI is a global disease that requires global efforts to prevent its occurrence in the general population and to improve outcome for patients. TBI has a rich history of academic collaborations, and existing networks should be strengthened and new networks developed. This will require commitment from governmental and nongovernmental funding agencies, which currently only have few mechanisms to support TBI research on a global basis.

88.7 Summary

This chapter aimed to summarize past, present, and future research in TBI. It is clear that there have never been better tools available to study the complexity of TBI than those existing today. With rapidly developing methodology for neuroimaging, monitoring, pharmacology, and big data analysis, the use of large observational studies will expand our knowledge of the pathobiology of TBI. To enable the translation of therapies to clinical benefit, refined animal models are needed. The rodent models should be used to dissect pathogenic mechanisms and to screen for novel therapeutic options. It is likely that higher-order species, particularly the pig/piglet models, should be used more extensively prior to embarking on large-scale clinical studies. In addition, improved translational efforts are being evaluated where experimental medicine will play an important role. Here, small but extensively characterized cohorts of patients will be studied using detailed monitoring that will include tissue, biomarker, and imaging analysis. Although RCTs are considered the gold standard, challenges are posed by the heterogeneity of the TBI population in terms of type of injury, clinical severity, and variations in treatment. As such, TBI research may specifically benefit from large-scale observational studies in the setting of comparative effectiveness research. More focus should be on research in LMICs since TBI is truly a global disease with increasing incidence worldwide. To explore novel therapies, existing networks should be strengthened and new networks developed. These factors will presumably all need to be improved in order to develop precision medicine approaches to the individual TBI patient.

References

A multicenter trial of the efficacy of nimodipine on outcome after severe head injury. The European Study Group on Nimodipine in severe head injury. J Neurosurg. 1994;80(5):797–804.

Agoston DV, Vink R, Helmy A, Risling M, Nelson D, Prins M. How to translate time: the temporal aspects of rodent and human pathobiological processes in traumatic brain injury. J Neurotrauma. 2019;36(11):1724–37.

Amyot F, Arciniegas DB, Brazaitis MP, Curley KC, Diaz-Arrastia R, Gandjbakhche A, et al. A review of the effectiveness of neuroimaging modalities for the detection of traumatic brain injury. J Neurotrauma. 2015;32(22):1693–721.

Andrews PJ, Sinclair HL, Rodriguez A, Harris BA, Battison CG, Rhodes JK, et al. Hypothermia for intracranial hypertension after traumatic brain injury. N Engl J Med. 2015;373(25):2403–12.

Andrews PJ, Sinclair HL, Rodriguez A, Harris B, Rhodes J, Watson H, et al. Therapeutic hypothermia to reduce intracranial pressure after traumatic brain injury: the Eurotherm3235 RCT. Health Technol Assess. 2018;22(45):1–134.

Asehnoune K, Seguin P, Allary J, Feuillet F, Lasocki S, Cook F, et al. Hydrocortisone and fludrocortisone for prevention of hospital-acquired pneumonia in patients with severe traumatic brain injury (Corti-TC): a double-blind, multicentre phase 3, randomised placebo-controlled trial. Lancet Respir Med. 2014;2(9):706–16.

Bailey I, Bell A, Gray J, Gullan R, Heiskanan O, Marks PV, et al. A trial of the effect of nimodipine on outcome after head injury. Acta Neurochir. 1991;110(3–4):97–105.

Balestreri M, Czosnyka M, Hutchinson P, Steiner LA, Hiler M, Smielewski P, et al. Impact of intracranial pressure and cerebral perfusion pressure on severe disability and mortality after head injury. Neurocrit Care. 2006;4(1):8–13.

Bolkvadze T, Pitkanen A. Development of post-traumatic epilepsy after controlled cortical impact and lateral fluid-percussion-induced brain injury in the mouse. J Neurotrauma. 2012;29(5):789–812.

Bragge P, Synnot A, Maas AI, Menon DK, Cooper DJ, Rosenfeld JV, et al. A state-of-the-science overview of randomized controlled trials evaluating acute management of moderate-to-severe traumatic brain injury. J Neurotrauma. 2016;33(16):1461–78.

Bramlett HM, Dietrich WD. Quantitative structural changes in white and gray matter 1 year following traumatic brain injury in rats. Acta Neuropathol. 2002;103(6):607–14.

Burt T, John CS, Ruckle JL, Vuong LT. Phase-0/microdosing studies using PET, AMS, and LC-MS/MS: a range of study methodologies and conduct considerations. Accelerating development of novel pharmaceuticals through safe testing in humans—a practical guide. Expert Opin Drug Deliv. 2017;14(5):657–72.

Cai B, Wang N. Large animal stroke models vs. rodent stroke models, pros and cons, and combination? Acta Neurochir Suppl. 2016;121:77–81.

Carney N, Totten AM, O'Reilly C, Ullman JS, Hawryluk GW, Bell MJ, et al. Guidelines for the management of severe traumatic brain injury, fourth edition. Neurosurgery. 2017;80(1):6–15.

Carpenter KL, Jalloh I, Gallagher CN, Grice P, Howe DJ, Mason A, et al. (13)C-labelled microdialysis studies of cerebral metabolism in TBI patients. Eur J Pharm Sci. 2014;57:87–97.

Chesnut RM, Temkin N, Carney N, Dikmen S, Rondina C, Videtta W, et al. A trial of intracranial-pressure monitoring in traumatic brain injury. N Engl J Med. 2012;367(26):2471–81.

Clifton GL, Miller ER, Choi SC, Levin HS, McCauley S, Smith KR Jr, et al. Lack of effect of induction of hypothermia after acute brain injury. N Engl J Med. 2001;344(8):556–63.

Coles JP, Fryer TD, Coleman MR, Smielewski P, Gupta AK, Minhas PS, et al. Hyperventilation following head injury: effect on ischemic burden and cerebral oxidative metabolism. Crit Care Med. 2007;35(2):568–78.

Cooper DJ, Rosenfeld JV, Murray L, Arabi YM, Davies AR, D'Urso P, et al. Decompressive craniectomy in diffuse traumatic brain injury. N Engl J Med. 2011;364(16):1493–502.

Cooper DJ, Nichol AD, Bailey M, Bernard S, Cameron PA, Pili-Floury S, et al. Effect of early sustained prophylactic hypothermia on neurologic outcomes among patients with severe traumatic brain injury: the POLAR randomized clinical trial. JAMA. 2018;320(21):2211–20.

Donat CK, Scott G, Gentleman SM, Sastre M. Microglial activation in traumatic brain injury. Front Aging Neurosci. 2017;9:208.

Eisenberg HM, Gary HE Jr, Aldrich EF, Saydjari C, Turner B, Foulkes MA, et al. Initial CT findings in 753 patients with severe head injury. A report from the NIH Traumatic Coma Data Bank. J Neurosurg. 1990;73(5):688–98.

Finfer S, Bellomo R, Boyce N, French J, Myburgh J, Norton R, et al. A comparison of albumin and saline for fluid resuscitation in the intensive care unit. N Engl J Med. 2004;350(22):2247–56.

Finnie JW. Comparative approach to understanding traumatic injury in the immature, postnatal brain of domestic animals. Aust Vet J. 2012;90(8):301–7.

Flygt J, Djupsjo A, Lenne F, Marklund N. Myelin loss and oligodendrocyte pathology in white matter tracts following traumatic brain injury in the rat. Eur J Neurosci. 2013;38(1):2153–65.

Flygt J, Gumucio A, Ingelsson M, Skoglund K, Holm J, Alafuzoff I, et al. Human traumatic brain injury results in oligodendrocyte death and increases the number of oligodendrocyte progenitor cells. J Neuropathol Exp Neurol. 2016;75(6):503–15.

Friess SH, Ralston J, Eucker SA, Helfaer MA, Smith C, Margulies SS. Neurocritical care monitoring correlates with neuropathology in a swine model of pediatric traumatic brain injury. Neurosurgery. 2011;69(5):1139–47; discussion 47.

Gaab MR, Trost HA, Alcantara A, Karimi-Nejad A, Moskopp D, Schultheiss R, et al. "Ultrahigh" dexamethasone in acute brain injury. Results from a prospective randomized double-blind multicenter trial (GUDHIS). German Ultrahigh Dexamethasone Head Injury Study Group. Zentralbl Neurochir. 1994;55(3):135–43.

Gallagher CN, Carpenter KL, Grice P, Howe DJ, Mason A, Timofeev I, et al. The human brain utilizes lactate via the tricarboxylic acid cycle: a 13C-labelled microdialysis and high-resolution nuclear magnetic resonance study. Brain. 2009;132(Pt 10):2839–49.

Gregson BA, Rowan EN, Francis R, McNamee P, Boyers D, Mitchell P, et al. Surgical Trial in Traumatic IntraCerebral Haemorrhage (STITCH): a randomised controlled trial of early surgery compared with initial conservative treatment. Health Technol Assess. 2015;19(70):1–138.

Grumme T, Baethmann A, Kolodziejczyk D, Krimmer J, Fischer M, von Eisenhart Rothe B, et al. Treatment of patients with severe head injury by triamcinolone: a prospective, controlled multicenter clinical trial of 396 cases. Res Exp Med (Berl). 1995;195(4):217–29.

Hall ED, Sullivan PG, Gibson TR, Pavel KM, Thompson BM, Scheff SW. Spatial and temporal characteristics of neurodegeneration after controlled cortical impact in mice: more than a focal brain injury. J Neurotrauma. 2005;22(2):252–65.

Hanell A, Marklund N. Structured evaluation of rodent behavioral tests used in drug discovery research. Front Behav Neurosci. 2014;8:252.

Harders A, Kakarieka A, Braakman R. Traumatic subarachnoid hemorrhage and its treatment with nimodipine. German tSAH Study Group. J Neurosurg. 1996;85(1):82–9.

Helmy A, Guilfoyle MR, Carpenter KLH, Pickard JD, Menon DK, Hutchinson PJ. Recombinant human interleukin-1 receptor antagonist promotes M1 microglia biased cytokines and chemokines following human traumatic brain injury. J Cereb Blood Flow Metab. 2016;36(8):1434–48.

Hong YT, Veenith T, Dewar D, Outtrim JG, Mani V, Williams C, et al. Amyloid imaging with carbon 11-labeled Pittsburgh compound B for traumatic brain injury. JAMA Neurol. 2014;71(1):23–31.

Hutchinson PJ, O'Connell MT, Nortje J, Smith P, Al-Rawi PG, Gupta AK, et al. Cerebral microdialysis methodology—evaluation of 20 kDa and 100 kDa catheters. Physiol Meas. 2005;26(4):423–8.

Hutchinson PJ, Jalloh I, Helmy A, Carpenter KL, Rostami E, Bellander BM, et al. Consensus statement from the 2014 international microdialysis forum. Intensive Care Med. 2015;41(9):1517–28.

Hutchinson PJ, Kolias AG, Timofeev IS, Corteen EA, Czosnyka M, Timothy J, et al. Trial of decompressive craniectomy for traumatic intracranial hypertension. N Engl J Med. 2016;375(12):1119–30.

Janowitz T, Menon DK. Exploring new routes for neuroprotective drug development in traumatic brain injury. Sci Transl Med. 2010;2(27):27rv1.

Jha RM, Molyneaux BJ, Jackson TC, Wallisch JS, Park SY, Poloyac S, et al. Glibenclamide produces region-dependent effects on cerebral edema in a combined injury model of traumatic brain injury and hemorrhagic shock in mice. J Neurotrauma. 2018a;35(17):2125–35.

Jha RM, Elmer J, Zusman BE, Desai S, Puccio AM, Okonkwo DO, et al. Intracranial pressure trajectories: a novel approach to informing severe traumatic brain injury phenotypes. Crit Care Med. 2018b;46(11):1792–802.

Jha RM, Desai SM, Zusman BE, Koleck TA, Puccio AM, Okonkwo DO, et al. Downstream TRPM4 polymorphisms are associated with intracranial hypertension and statistically interact with ABCC8 polymorphisms in a prospective cohort of severe traumatic brain injury. J Neurotrauma. 2019;36(11):1804–17.

Jiang JY, Xu W, Li WP, Xu WH, Zhang J, Bao YH, et al. Efficacy of standard trauma craniectomy for refractory intracranial hypertension with severe traumatic brain injury: a multicenter, prospective, randomized controlled study. J Neurotrauma. 2005;22(6):623–8.

Joy MT, Ben Assayag E, Shabashov-Stone D, Liraz-Zaltsman S, Mazzitelli J, Arenas M, et al. CCR5 is a therapeutic target for recovery after stroke and traumatic brain injury. Cell. 2019;176(5):1143–57.e13.

Kawai N, Maeda Y, Kudomi N, Yamamoto Y, Nishiyama Y, Tamiya T. Focal neuronal damage in patients with neuropsychological impairment after diffuse traumatic brain injury: evaluation using (1)(1)C-flumazenil positron emission tomography with statistical image analysis. J Neurotrauma. 2010;27(12):2131–8.

Kochanek PM, Bramlett HM, Shear DA, Dixon CE, Mondello S, Dietrich WD, et al. Synthesis of findings, current investigations, and future directions: operation brain trauma therapy. J Neurotrauma. 2016;33(6):606–14.

Kochanek PM, Dixon CE, Mondello S, Wang KKK, Lafrenaye A, Bramlett HM, et al. Multi-center preclinical consortia to enhance translation of therapies and biomarkers for traumatic brain injury: operation brain trauma therapy and beyond. Front Neurol. 2018;9:640.

Lingsma HF, Roozenbeek B, Li B, Lu J, Weir J, Butcher I, et al. Large between-center differences in outcome after moderate and severe traumatic brain injury in the international mission on prognosis and clinical trial design in traumatic brain injury (IMPACT) study. Neurosurgery. 2011;68(3):601–7; discussion 7–8.

Liraz-Zaltsman S, Slusher B, Atrakchi-Baranes D, Rosenblatt K, Friedman Levi Y, Kesner E, et al. Enhancement of brain d-serine mediates recovery of cognitive function after traumatic brain injury. J Neurotrauma. 2018;35(14):1667–80.

Ma X, Aravind A, Pfister BJ, Chandra N, Haorah J. Animal models of traumatic brain injury and assessment of injury severity. Mol Neurobiol. 2019;56:5332.

Maas AI, Murray G, Henney H 3rd, Kassem N, Legrand V, Mangelus M, et al. Efficacy and safety of dexanabinol in severe traumatic brain injury: results of a phase III randomised, placebo-controlled, clinical trial. Lancet Neurol. 2006;5(1):38–45.

Maas AI, Marmarou A, Murray GD, Teasdale SG, Steyerberg EW. Prognosis and clinical trial design in traumatic brain injury: the IMPACT study. J Neurotrauma. 2007;24(2):232–8.

Maas AI, Murray GD, Roozenbeek B, Lingsma HF, Butcher I, McHugh GS, et al. Advancing care for traumatic brain injury: findings from the IMPACT studies and perspectives on future research. Lancet Neurol. 2013;12(12):1200–10.

Maas AI, Menon DK, Steyerberg EW, Citerio G, Lecky F, Manley GT, et al. Collaborative European NeuroTrauma effectiveness research in traumatic brain injury (CENTER-TBI): a prospective longitudinal observational study. Neurosurgery. 2015;76(1):67–80.

Marcoux J, McArthur DA, Miller C, Glenn TC, Villablanca P, Martin NA, et al. Persistent metabolic crisis as measured by elevated cerebral microdialysis lactate-pyruvate ratio predicts chronic frontal lobe brain atrophy after traumatic brain injury. Crit Care Med. 2008;36(10):2871–7.

Marklund N. Rodent models of traumatic brain injury: methods and challenges. Methods Mol Biol. 2016;1462:29–46.

Marklund N, Hillered L. Animal modelling of traumatic brain injury in preclinical drug development: where do we go from here? Br J Pharmacol. 2011;164(4):1207–29.

Marmarou A, Nichols J, Burgess J, Newell D, Troha J, Burnham D, et al. Effects of the bradykinin antagonist Bradycor (deltibant, CP-1027) in severe traumatic brain injury: results of a multi-center, randomized, placebo-controlled trial. American Brain Injury Consortium Study Group. J Neurotrauma. 1999;16(6):431–44.

Marshall LF, Maas AI, Marshall SB, Bricolo A, Fearnside M, Iannotti F, et al. A multicenter trial on the efficacy of using tirilazad mesylate in cases of head injury. J Neurosurg. 1998;89(4):519–25.

Mateen BA, Hill CS, Biddie SC, Menon DK. DNA methylation: basic biology and application to traumatic brain injury. J Neurotrauma. 2017;34(16):2379–88.

Meara JG, Leather AJ, Hagander L, Alkire BC, Alonso N, Ameh EA, et al. Global surgery 2030: evidence and solutions for achieving health, welfare, and economic development. Lancet. 2015;386(9993):569–624.

Menon DK, Coles JP, Gupta AK, Fryer TD, Smielewski P, Chatfield DA, et al. Diffusion limited oxygen delivery following head injury. Crit Care Med. 2004;32(6):1384–90.

Mohamed AZ, Cumming P, Gotz J, Nasrallah F, Department of Defense Alzheimer's Disease Neuroimaging Initiative. Tauopathy in veterans with long-term posttraumatic stress disorder and traumatic brain injury. Eur J Nucl Med Mol Imaging. 2019;46(5):1139–51.

Mondello S, Papa L, Buki A, Bullock MR, Czeiter E, Tortella FC, et al. Neuronal and glial markers are differently associated with computed tomography findings and outcome in patients with severe traumatic brain injury: a case control study. Crit Care. 2011;15(3):R156.

Mondello S, Shear DA, Bramlett HM, Dixon CE, Schmid KE, Dietrich WD, et al. Insight into pre-clinical models of traumatic brain injury using circulating brain damage biomarkers: operation brain trauma therapy. J Neurotrauma. 2016;33(6):595–605.

Morris GF, Bullock R, Marshall SB, Marmarou A, Maas A, Marshall LF. Failure of the competitive N-methyl-D-aspartate antagonist Selfotel (CGS 19755) in the treatment of severe head injury: results of two phase III clinical trials. The Selfotel Investigators. J Neurosurg. 1999;91(5):737–43.

Murray GD, Teasdale GM, Braakman R, Cohadon F, Dearden M, Iannotti F, et al. The European brain injury consortium survey of head injuries. Acta Neurochir. 1999;141(3):223–36.

Newcombe VF, Outtrim JG, Chatfield DA, Manktelow A, Hutchinson PJ, Coles JP, et al. Parcellating the neuroanatomical basis of impaired decision-making in traumatic brain injury. Brain. 2011;134(Pt 3):759–68.

Newcombe VF, Williams GB, Outtrim JG, Chatfield D, Gulia Abate M, Geeraerts T, et al. Microstructural basis of contusion expansion in traumatic brain injury: insights from diffusion tensor imaging. J Cereb Blood Flow Metab. 2013;33(6):855–62.

Newcombe VF, Correia MM, Ledig C, Abate MG, Outtrim JG, Chatfield D, et al. Dynamic changes in white matter abnormalities correlate with late improvement and deterioration following TBI: a diffusion tensor imaging study. Neurorehabil Neural Repair. 2016;30(1):49–62.

Nichol A, French C, Little L, Haddad S, Presneill J, Arabi Y, et al. Erythropoietin in traumatic brain injury (EPO-TBI): a double-blind randomised controlled trial. Lancet. 2015;386(10012):2499–506.

Nortje J, Coles JP, Timofeev I, Fryer TD, Aigbirhio FI, Smielewski P, et al. Effect of hyperoxia on regional oxygenation and metabolism after severe traumatic brain injury: preliminary findings. Crit Care Med. 2008;36(1):273–81.

Oddo M, Hutchinson PJ. Understanding and monitoring brain injury: the role of cerebral microdialysis. Intensive Care Med. 2018;44(11):1945–8.

Patel HC, Bouamra O, Woodford M, King AT, Yates DW, Lecky FE, et al. Trends in head injury outcome from 1989 to 2003 and the effect of neurosurgical care: an observational study. Lancet. 2005;366(9496):1538–44.

Perel P, Al-Shahi Salman R, Kawahara T, Morris Z, Prieto-Merino D, Roberts I, et al. CRASH-2 (Clinical Randomisation of an Antifibrinolytic in Significant Haemorrhage) intracranial bleeding study: the effect of tranexamic acid in traumatic brain injury—a nested randomised, placebo-controlled trial. Health Technol Assess. 2012;16(13):iii–xii, 1–54.

Pischiutta F, Micotti E, Hay JR, Marongiu I, Sammali E, Tolomeo D, et al. Single severe traumatic brain injury produces progressive pathology with ongoing contralateral white matter damage one year after injury. Exp Neurol. 2018;300:167–78.

Ramlackhansingh AF, Brooks DJ, Greenwood RJ, Bose SK, Turkheimer FE, Kinnunen KM, et al. Inflammation after trauma: microglial activation and traumatic brain injury. Ann Neurol. 2011;70(3):374–83.

Richter S, Stevenson S, Newman T, Wilson L, Menon DK, Maas AIR, et al. Handling of missing outcome data in traumatic brain injury research: a systematic review. J Neurotrauma. 2019;36:2743.

Risling M, Smith D, Stein TD, Thelin EP, Zanier ER, Ankarcrona M, et al. Modelling human pathology of traumatic brain injury in animal models. J Intern Med. 2019;285(6):594–607.

Roberts I, Yates D, Sandercock P, Farrell B, Wasserberg J, Lomas G, et al. Effect of intravenous corticosteroids on death within 14 days in 10008 adults with clinically significant head injury (MRC CRASH trial): randomised placebo-controlled trial. Lancet. 2004;364(9442):1321–8.

Robertson CS, Valadka AB, Hannay HJ, Contant CF, Gopinath SP, Cormio M, et al. Prevention of secondary ischemic insults after severe head injury. Crit Care Med. 1999;27(10):2086–95.

Robertson CS, Hannay HJ, Yamal JM, Gopinath S, Goodman JC, Tilley BC, et al. Effect of erythropoietin and transfusion threshold on neurological recovery after traumatic brain injury: a randomized clinical trial. JAMA. 2014;312(1):36–47.

Roozenbeek B, Maas AI, Lingsma HF, Butcher I, Lu J, Marmarou A, et al. Baseline characteristics and statistical power in randomized controlled trials: selection, prognostic targeting, or covariate adjustment? Crit Care Med. 2009;37(10):2683–90.

Roozenbeek B, Lingsma HF, Maas AI. New considerations in the design of clinical trials for traumatic brain injury. Clin Investig (Lond). 2012;2(2):153–62.

Saatman KE, Duhaime AC, Bullock R, Maas AI, Valadka A, Manley GT, et al. Classification of traumatic brain injury for targeted therapies. J Neurotrauma. 2008;25(7):719–38.

SAFE Study Investigators; Australian and New Zealand Intensive Care Society Clinical Trials Group; Australian Red Cross Blood Service; George Institute for International Health, Myburgh J, et al. Saline or albumin for fluid resuscitation in patients with traumatic brain injury. N Engl J Med. 2007;357(9):874–84.

Scott G, Zetterberg H, Jolly A, Cole JH, De Simoni S, Jenkins PO, et al. Minocycline reduces chronic microglial activation after brain trauma but increases neurodegeneration. Brain. 2018;141(2):459–71.

Shakur H, Andrews P, Asser T, Balica L, Boeriu C, Quintero JD, et al. The BRAIN TRIAL: a randomised, placebo controlled trial of a bradykinin B2 receptor antagonist (Anatibant) in patients with traumatic brain injury. Trials. 2009;10:109.

Skolnick BE, Maas AI, Narayan RK, van der Hoop RG, MacAllister T, Ward JD, et al. A clinical trial of progesterone for severe traumatic brain injury. N Engl J Med. 2014;371(26):2467–76.

Sorby-Adams AJ, Vink R, Turner RJ. Large animal models of stroke and traumatic brain injury as translational tools. Am J Physiol Regul Integr Comp Physiol. 2018;315(2):R165–R90.

Stein DG. Embracing failure: what the phase III progesterone studies can teach about TBI clinical trials. Brain Inj. 2015;29(11):1259–72.

Stovell MG, Mada MO, Helmy A, Carpenter TA, Thelin EP, Yan JL, et al. The effect of succinate on brain NADH/NAD(+) redox state and high energy phosphate metabolism in acute traumatic brain injury. Sci Rep. 2018;8(1):11140.

Temkin NR, Anderson GD, Winn HR, Ellenbogen RG, Britz GW, Schuster J, et al. Magnesium sulfate for neuroprotection after traumatic brain injury: a randomised controlled trial. Lancet Neurol. 2007;6(1):29–38.

Thomas TC, Ogle SB, Rumney BM, May HG, Adelson PD, Lifshitz J. Does time heal all wounds? Experimental diffuse traumatic brain injury results in persisting histopathology in the thalamus. Behav Brain Res. 2018;340:137–46.

Thompson HJ, Lifshitz J, Marklund N, Grady MS, Graham DI, Hovda DA, et al. Lateral fluid percussion brain injury: a 15-year review and evaluation. J Neurotrauma. 2005;22(1):42–75.

Turgeon AF, Lauzier F, Burns KE, Meade MO, Scales DC, Zarychanski R, et al. Determination of neurologic prognosis and clinical decision making in adult patients with severe traumatic brain injury: a survey of Canadian intensivists, neurosurgeons, and neurologists. Crit Care Med. 2013;41(4):1086–93.

Veenith TV, Carter EL, Geeraerts T, Grossac J, Newcombe VF, Outtrim J, et al. Pathophysiologic mechanisms of cerebral ischemia and diffusion hypoxia in traumatic brain injury. JAMA Neurol. 2016;73(5):542–50.

Veenith TV, Carter EL, Grossac J, Newcombe VFJ, Outtrim JG, Nallapareddy S, et al. Normobaric hyperoxia does not improve derangements in diffusion tensor imaging found distant from visible contusions following acute traumatic brain injury. Sci Rep. 2017;7(1):12419.

Vespa P, Bergsneider M, Hattori N, Wu HM, Huang SC, Martin NA, et al. Metabolic crisis without brain ischemia is common after traumatic brain injury: a combined microdialysis and positron emission tomography study. J Cereb Blood Flow Metab. 2005;25(6):763–74.

Wright DW, Yeatts SD, Silbergleit R, Palesch YY, Hertzberg VS, Frankel M, et al. Very early administration of progesterone for acute traumatic brain injury. N Engl J Med. 2014;371(26):2457–66.

Young B, Runge JW, Waxman KS, Harrington T, Wilberger J, Muizelaar JP, et al. Effects of pegorgotein on neurologic outcome of patients with severe head injury. A multicenter, randomized controlled trial. JAMA. 1996;276(7):538–43.

Yurkewicz L, Weaver J, Bullock MR, Marshall LF. The effect of the selective NMDA receptor antagonist traxoprodil in the treatment of traumatic brain injury. J Neurotrauma. 2005;22(12):1428–43.

Index

© Springer Nature Switzerland AG 2020
T. Sundstrøm et al. (eds.), *Management of Severe Traumatic Brain Injury*,
https://doi.org/10.1007/978-3-030-39383-0

MIX
Papier aus verantwortungsvollen Quellen
Paper from responsible sources
FSC® C105338

FSC
www.fsc.org

If you have any concerns about our products,
you can contact us on
ProductSafety@springernature.com

In case Publisher is established outside the EU,
the EU authorized representative is:
Springer Nature Customer Service Center GmbH
Europaplatz 3, 69115 Heidelberg, Germany

Printed by Libri Plureos GmbH
in Hamburg, Germany